FELINE MEDICINE AND THERAPEUTICS

KV-039-476

FELINE MEDICINE AND THERAPEUTICS

EDITED FOR THE BRITISH SMALL ANIMAL
VETERINARY ASSOCIATION BY

E. A. CHANDLER
BVetMed, FRCVS

C. J. GASKELL
BVSc, PhD, DVR, MRCVS

AND

R. M. GASKELL
BVSc, PhD, MRCVS

SECOND EDITION

**Blackwell
Science**

© 1985, 1994 by
Blackwell Science Ltd
Editorial Offices:
Osney Mead, Oxford OX2 0EL
25 John Street, London WC1N 2BL
23 Ainslie Place, Edinburgh EH3 6AJ
238 Main Street, Cambridge
    Massachusetts 02142, USA
54 University Street, Carlton
    Victoria 3053, Australia

Other Editorial Offices:
Arnette Blackwell SA
    224, Boulevard Saint Germain
    75007 Paris, France

Blackwell Wissenschafts-Verlag GmbH
    Kurfürstendamm 57
    10707 Berlin, Germany

    Zehetnergasse 6
    A-1140 Wien
    Austria

All rights reserved. No part of this publication
may be reproduced, stored in a retrieval system,
or transmitted, in any form or by any means,
electronic, mechanical, photocopying,
recording or otherwise, except as permitted by
the UK Copyright, Designs and Patents Act
1988, without prior permission of the publisher.

First published in 1985
Reprinted 1987
Japanese translation 1989
Spanish translation 1990
Second edition 1994
Reprinted 1995
Reissued in paperback 1996

Set by Excel Typesetters Company, Hong Kong
Printed in Great Britain
at the Alden Press Limited,
Oxford and Northampton
Bound by Hartnolls Ltd, Bodmin, Cornwall

The Blackwell Science logo is a trade mark of
Blackwell Science Ltd, registered at the United
Kingdom Trade Marks Registry

DISTRIBUTORS

Marston Book Services Ltd
PO Box 269
Abingdon
Oxon OX14 4YN
(*Orders*: Tel: 01235 465500
        Fax: 01235 465555)

USA
Blackwell Science, Inc.
238 Main Street
Cambridge, MA 02142
(*Orders*: Tel: 800 215-1000
        617 876-7000
        Fax: 617 492-5263)

Canada
Copp Clark, Ltd
2775 Matheson Blvd East
Mississauga, Ontario
Canada, L4W 4P7
(*Orders*: Tel: 800 263-4374
        905 238-6074)

Australia
Blackwell Science Pty Ltd
54 University Street
Carlton, Victoria 3053
(*Orders*: Tel: 03 9347-0300
        Fax: 03 9349-3016)

A catalogue record for this title
is available from the British Library

ISBN 0-632-04133-1

Library of Congress
Cataloging-in-Publication Data

Feline medicine and therapeutics
    edited for the British Small Animal
    Veterinary Association
    by E.A. Chandler, C.J. Gaskell, R.M. Gaskell.
    – 2nd ed.
            p.   cm.
    Includes bibliographical references
    and index.
    ISBN 0-632-04133-1
  1. Cats – Diseases.   I. Chandler, E.A.
  II. Gaskell, C.J.   III. Gaskell, Rosaline M.
  IV. British Small Animal Veterinary Association.
  SF985.F45   1994
  636.8′0896 – dc20

Contents

Contents

List of Colour Plates

List of Colour Plates

Contributors

R. S. ANDERSON BVMS, PhD, MRCVS, *University of Liverpool, Department of Veterinary Clinical Science and Animal Husbandry, Veterinary Field Station, 'Leahurst', Neston, Wirral, Merseyside L64 7TE*

D. BENNETT BSc, BVetMed, PhD, DSAO, MRCVS, *University of Liverpool, Department of Veterinary Clinical Science and Animal Husbandry, Small Animal Hospital, Crown Street, Liverpool, Merseyside L7 7EX*

M. BENNETT BVSc, PhD, MRCVS, *University of Liverpool, Department of Veterinary Clinical Science and Animal Husbandry, Veterinary Field Station, 'Leahurst', Neston, Wirral, Merseyside L64 7TE*

A. C. BLAXTER BVMS, BA, PhD, MRCVS, *People's Dispensary for Sick Animals, 556 Bath Road, Brislington, Bristol, Avon BS4 3J2*

B. BROCHIER DVM, PhD, *Department of Virology-Immunology, Faculty of Veterinary Medicine, University of Liège, B-43, Sart Tilman, 4000 Liège, Belgium*

I. H. BURGER BSc, PhD, *Waltham Centre for Pet Nutrition, Waltham-on-the-Wolds, Melton Mowbray, Leicestershire LE14 4RT*

S. DAWSON BVMS, PhD, MRCVS, *University of Liverpool, Department of Veterinary Pathology, Veterinary Field Station, 'Leahurst', Neston, Wirral, Merseyside L64 7TE*

R. J. EVANS MA, PhD, VetMB, MRCVS, *University of Cambridge, Department of Clinical Veterinary Medicine, Madingley Road, Cambridge CB3 0ES*

P. A. FLECKNELL MA, VetMB, PhD, DLAS MRCVS, *University of Newcastle upon Tyne, Comparative Biology Centre, The Medical School, Framlington Place, Newcastle upon Tyne NE2 4HH*

C. J. GASKELL BVSc, PhD, DVR, MRCVS, *University of Liverpool, Department of Veterinary Clinical Science and Animal Husbandry, Small Animal Hospital, Crown Street, Liverpool, Merseyside L7 7EX*

R. M. GASKELL BVSc, PhD, MRCVS, *University of Liverpool, Department of Veterinary Pathology, Veterinary Field Station, 'Leahurst', Neston, Wirral, Merseyside L64 7TE*

T. J. GRUFFYDD-JONES BVetMed, PhD, MRCVS, *University of Bristol, Department of Clinical Veterinary Science, Langford House, Langford, Bristol, Avon BS18 7DU*

D. A. HARBOUR BSc, PhD, *University of Bristol, Department of Clinical Veterinary Science, Langford House, Langford, Bristol, Avon BS18 7DU*

C. D. HOPPER BVSc, BSc, PhD, MRCVS, *University of Bristol, Department of Clinical Veterinary Science, Langford House, Langford, Bristol BS18 7DU*

O. JARRETT BVMS, PhD, MRCVS, FRSE, *University of Glasgow, Department of Veterinary Pathology, Veterinary School, Bearsden Road, Bearsden, Glasgow G61 1QH*

J. G. LANE BVetMed, FRCVS, *University of Bristol, Department of Clinical Veterinary Science, Langford House, Langford, Bristol, Avon BS18 7DU*

R. A. MUGFORD BSc, PhD, *PO Box 23, Chertsey, Surrey KT16 0PU*

P.-P. PASTORET DVM, PhD, *Department of Virology-Immunology, Faculty of Veterinary Medicine, University of Liège, B-43, Sart Tilman, 4000 Liège, Belgium*

H. C. RUTGERS DVM, MSc, DIP ACVIM, MRCVS, *University of London, Royal Veterinary College, Department of Small Animal Medicine and Surgery, Hawkshead Lane, North Mymms, Hatfield, Hertfordshire AL9 7TA*

J. SANSOM BVSc, DVOphthal, MRCVS, *The Animal Health Trust, Unit of Comparative Ophthalmology, Lanwades Park, Kennett, Newmarket, Suffolk CB8 7PN*

A. H. SPARKES BVetMed, MRCVS, *The Feline Centre, University of Bristol, Department of Clinical Veterinary Science, Langford House, Langford, Bristol, Avon BS18 7DU*

M. E. STODDART BVetMed, BSc, PhD, DVR, MRCVS, *Tableland, Burton Row, Brent Knoll, Somerset TA9 4BW*

K. L. THODAY BVetMed, PhD, DVD, MRCVS, *The University of Edinburgh, Department of Veterinary Clinical Studies, Royal (Dick) School of Veterinary Studies, Summerhall, Edinburgh EH9 1QH*

A. H. M. VAN DEN BROEK BVSc, DVR, FRCVS, *The University of Edinburgh, Department of Veterinary Clinical Studies, Royal (Dick) School of Veterinary Studies, Summerhall, Edinburgh EH9 1QH*

K. WILLOUGHBY BVMS, MRCVS, *University of Liverpool, Department of Veterinary Clinical Science and Animal Husbandry, Veterinary Field Station, 'Leahurst', Neston, Wirral, Merseyside L64 7TE*

J. M. WILLS BVetMed, PhD, MRCVS, *Waltham Centre for Pet Nutrition, Waltham-on-the-Wolds, Melton Mowbray, Leicestershire LE14 4RT*

P. R. WOTTON BVSc, PhD, MRCVS, *University of Bristol, Department of Clinical Veterinary Science, Langford House, Langford, Bristol, Avon BS18 7DU*

A. I. WRIGHT BVSc, MRCVS, *University of Bristol, Department of Clinical Veterinary Science, Langford House, Langford, Bristol, Avon BS18 7DU*

Preface to the Second Edition

It is now 11 years since the first edition of *Feline Medicine and Therapeutics* was published, and while knowledge of the cat has advanced rapidly the primary object of this book has remained the same – to help veterinary surgeons and students to practise the art and science of feline medicine. As such, many of the comments in the preface to the first edition remain true, although the old-fashioned perception of the cat as just a small dog has receded rapidly as understanding has grown.

Cats continue to increase in popularity as companion animals and in many parts of the world they number more than dogs as household pets. As one might expect, owners and breeders are becoming increasingly knowledgeable on feline ailments and health requirements. *Feline Medicine and Therapeutics* aims to satisfy the demand for up to date scientific information for veterinary surgeon and owner alike and will bring further improvements in the care of the feline species.

As befits the increase in veterinary knowledge, this second edition is significantly larger than the first with perhaps the most notable addition being a chapter on the feline immunodeficiency virus. It now seems remarkable that such an important infection of the cat was not appreciated such a short time ago. Other chapters have increased in size to accomodate new information and in a number the expertise of new authors or coauthors is welcomed.

As before the editors and authors are pleased to recognize the contributions of others to the information within this book. There are now many experts working in the field of feline medicine and their role in adding to the now very considerable amount of available information is acknowledged with sincere gratitude.

E. A. CHANDLER
C. J. GASKELL
R. M. GASKELL

Preface to the First Edition

Feline Medicine and Therapeutics has been produced primarily for the practising veterinary surgeon and students. The subject of feline medicine is one that until relatively recently was not well covered in the undergraduate veterinary course. In the past few years, however, the number of pet cats, and the interest in them, has risen appreciably and with it the need for information on feline disease. As this knowledge grew, the view of the cat as a small dog rapidly became outdated as the range of metabolic idiosyncrasies and specific disease problems became obvious. In recognizing this difference, the BSAVAs textbook *Feline Medicine and Therapeutics* has been produced as a companion to *Canine Medicine and Therapeutics* and has attempted to draw together as contributors those with direct experience in feline medicine.

The Editors recognize the problem that, unlike its sister volume on the dog, there are some deficiencies in certain sections on the organ systems. This represents an absolute lack of information in the species and the authors have been unwilling, quite correctly, to extrapolate information from other species where more data are available. In some cases, lack of material on disease conditions in the cat represents lack of research due to economic restraints within academic institutes, or within the cat fancy, but in others the cat demonstrates a generally healthier situation than, for instance, in the dog.

As the title suggests this book is primarily on medicine and therapeutics, but authors have occasionally described surgical techniques when this is relevant to the treatment of a medical condition.

The Editors and authors would like to acknowledge the role of many colleagues, organizations and grant-awarding bodies for their contribution to this rapid increase in knowledge of feline matters. In particular, the Feline Advisory Bureau in Britain has played a major role in the support of feline studies through its Clinical Research Scholarships. Inevitably much of the work referred to in this volume is that of others and it is gratefully acknowledged.

E. A. CHANDLER
C. J. GASKELL

PART 1
MAJOR SYSTEMS

Chapter 1 / The Skin

A. H. M. VAN DEN BROEK
AND K. L. THODAY

INTRODUCTION

Until the beginning of the last decade, it was a commonly held belief that little was known about skin diseases of cats. However, Scott (1980) ably showed that this was not the case by listing and discussing more than 1000 references on the subject in his excellent monograph *Feline Dermatology 1900–1978*. The 1980s provided an explosion of knowledge about feline dermatology with Scott providing comprehensive reviews of the material published between 1979 and 1982 (Scott, 1984), between 1983 and 1985 (Scott, 1987a), and between 1986 and 1988 (Scott, 1990).

SKIN BIOLOGY

The skin constitutes the major interface between an animal and its environment. In this role it has several highly specialized and diverse functions which combine to promote the survival and propagation of the animal. In relation to the external environment it provides protection (a barrier to the penetration of physical and chemical agents, microbiological organisms and radiation, plus camouflage markings and danger signals), information (sensory perception) and also, through pheromone secretion, contributes to successful reproduction of the species. In respect of the internal environment, it plays a crucial part in homeostasis by providing a barrier which prevents the loss of water, electrolytes and macromolecules and through its contribution to thermoregulation. In addition, it is important in vitamin D synthesis, plays a role in vitamin, mineral and fat storage, and makes a limited contribution to the excretion of waste products. Function is related to structure, and this is dealt with in the following sections.

Embryology

In the fetus, a single layer of ectodermal cells gives rise to the epidermis. Subsequently, cells from the basal layer of the epidermis differentiate into epithelial germs. These develop into the hair follicle and the sebaceous, epitrichial (apocrine) and atrichial (eccrine) glands. At the same time, neural crest cells (derived from ectoderm) and bone marrow cells (derived from mesoderm) migrate to and infiltrate the basal cell layer of the epidermis giving rise to melanocytes and Langerhans' cells respectively. Beneath the fetal ectodermal cells is the dermis, derived from mesoderm and composed of mesenchymal cells dispersed in a matrix of ground substance. The mesenchymal cells differentiate into fibroblasts and lipocytes. Subsequently, collagen fibres produced by fibroblasts, and later elastic fibres are deposited in the ground substance matrix.

Gross and microscopic anatomy

Feline skin is very thin, ranging in thickness from 0.37 mm (lateral aspect of the distal limbs) to 1.9 mm (dorsum), compared to that of dogs (0.5 mm to 5 mm respectively). It is also more pliable, elastic and extensible than that of dogs.

The skin is composed of two distinct layers, the epidermis (outer layer) and the dermis (inner layer) and is supported by the hypodermis (subcutis).

The epidermis

The epidermis varies in thickness from 12 to 45 μm (mean 25 μm). Consequently, lesions such as vesicles, bullae and pustules are transient, rupturing readily.

It comprises four or five layers of cells: an inner, basal cell layer, the stratum basale, which multiplies and differentiates sequentially into the stratum spinosum, granulosum, lucidum (where present) and finally the outer layer of cells, the stratum corneum. The stratum granulosum is discontinuous and best developed in the epidermis of the footpads, while the stratum lucidum is usually only distinguished in the footpads and planum nasale. The stratum corneum is thicker in lightly haired or glabrous (non-hairy) skin than in hairy skin and is thickest in the footpads and planum nasale. Scattered among the basal cells there may be melanocytes, Langerhans' (dendritic) cells and Merkel's cells. Melanocytes are found mainly in the epidermis of the lip, footpads, planum nasale, prepuce, scrotum, dorsal tail, pinnae, circumanal area, umbilical skin of the fetus and in hair bulbs. Melanocytes are responsible for the synthesis of melanin, which is found in varying concentrations in the different cell strata of the epidermis. Langerhans' cells are antigen-presenting cells and are involved in immune responses; Merkel's cells are specialized, slow-adapting, tactile cells located in dome-shaped projections of the skin (tylotrich pads).

The stratum corneum is coated and permeated by a continuously renewed protective emulsion, which is composed of lipids (free fatty acids, mono- and triglycerides, cholesterol, mono- and diester waxes and squalene), proteins (including immunoglobulins), pheromones and salts. This protective film, formed principally by the secretion of sebaceous and epitrichial glands, plays a vital role in protection against microorganisms and excessive water loss.

The dermis

The dermis constitutes a connective tissue support for the epidermis. In the superficial dermis, immediately below the basal cell layer in a matrix of hyaluronic acid and chondroitin sulphate, are fine collagen fibres running parallel to the epidermis and an interlacing network of elastic fibres. Below these are thicker, more densely but irregularly arranged collagen fibres and a denser network of elastic fibres. Located in interstitial spaces are fibroblasts, histiocytes (scavengers of degenerate cells) and mast cells. Other cells (lymphocytes, plasma cells, neutrophils and eosinophils) are transient visitors except in certain diseases.

The hypodermis

Located below the dermis, the hypodermis is a further layer of connective tissue containing adipose tissue deposited in a network of thick bands of collagen fibres and numerous elastic fibres. It provides additional support and enhances the shock-absorbing capacity of skin.

Epidermal appendages

The epidermal appendages comprise the sebaceous glands, epitrichial (apocrine) sweat glands, atrichial (eccrine) sweat glands, anal sacs, hair follicles and nails.

SEBACEOUS GLANDS

These are exocrine alveolar glands discharging lipids into hair follicles, with which they are usually associated. They occur rarely in glabrous skin, where they discharge directly onto the surface of the skin.

Sebaceous glands vary in number and size, being largest and most numerous on the lips and upper eyelids (tarsal glands), dorsal aspect of the tail, prepuce, scrotum, circumanal glands and anal glands.

Sebaceous glands do not appear to be innervated. Although their activity in man and laboratory animals is influenced by hormones, non-endocrine factors may also be involved (Thody & Shuster, 1989).

SWEAT GLANDS

These are saccular or coiled exocrine glands comprising inner secretory cells surrounded by myoepithelial cells, and an outer sheath of fibrocytes. Epitrichial sweat glands discharge a proteinaceous secretion into the hair follicles with which they are associated. Atrichial sweat glands occur rarely in glabrous skin but are present in the footpads. In both these locations they discharge directly onto the surface of the skin.

Sweat glands are largest in the mucocutaneous areas and on the lips, face and dorsal aspect of the pads.

Sweat gland activity is probably controlled by a combination of neural (sympathetic and cholinergic) and non-neural factors (Jenkinson & McEwan, 1990).

ANAL SACS

These are located between the internal and external anal sphincters and are lined by large, specialized sebaceous and epitrichial glands.

HAIR

Cats' hair has been subdivided into three types: primary (guard) hair; awn hair (thinner hairs and possessing a subapical swelling); and secondary (down, undercoat) hair. The ratio of primary to secondary hairs is 1:10 (Baker, 1974). All hairs have the same basic structure consisting of a central core, the medulla, surrounded by cortical cells (which contain pigment giving the hair its particular colour), and an outer layer, the cuticle.

Large primary hair follicles have two to five satellite clusters of hairs made up of three smaller primary hairs surrounded by six to 12 secondary hair follicles. The central primary hair possesses its own pilosebaceous unit while the satellite clusters share a common follicle opening and pilosebaceous unit. Associated with the pilosebaceous unit is the arrector pili muscle. This is composed of smooth muscle, has cholinergic innervation and is about a quarter to a half of the diameter of the central primary hair follicle. It originates in the superficial epidermis and inserts on a bulge on the hair follicle.

The activity of hair follicles is cyclic and divided into three phases. *Anagen* is a period of activity producing new hair (0.25 to 0.3 mm per day) which grows up the follicle displacing telogen hairs. This is followed by *catagen*, a brief transitional phase when hair growth ceases and the hair bulb begins to degenerate. *Telogen* is a resting phase during which the hair is retained dead in the follicle and subsequently lost. Follicular activity in cats follows a mosaic pattern and is dominated by photoperiod (Baker, 1974), with the greatest activity occurring in summer and least in winter. Ambient temperature, various hormones and diseases also influence follicular activity.

Sinus hairs and tylotrich hairs have a specialized tactile function. Sinus hairs are found on the muzzle, above the eyes and the palmar aspect of the carpus and constitute an element of a complex, slow-adapting mechanoreceptor while tylotrich hairs, located on the tylotrich pads, are part of what are thought to be rapid-adapting mechanoreceptors.

NAILS (CLAWS)

These specialized structures are direct continuations of the dermis and epidermis. They have prehensile, locomotor and protective functions.

Blood vessels

The blood supply to the skin is organized with three intercommunicating plexuses of arteries and veins. The superficial plexus lies immediately below the epidermis; the middle plexus at the level of the sebaceous glands; and the deep plexus at the interface of the dermis and hypodermis.

Nerves

The skin is abundantly supplied with afferent and efferent nerve fibres. Afferent fibres run from a variety of mechanoreceptors (Merkel's cells, Ruffini endings, sinus hair, tylotrich hair, Pacinian corpuscles, Meissner's corpuscles, Krause corpuscles), nociceptors and thermoreceptors and mediate the sensations of touch, pain, itch, heat and cold.

Efferent fibres supply blood vessels, sweat glands and arrector pili muscles.

THE APPROACH TO THE SKIN CASE

To reach a definitive diagnosis in feline dermatological cases, a systematic approach is essential. As in investigating diseases of any system, a detailed history, physical examination and confirmatory tests, where indicated, should always precede management.

The depth of the approach will vary from case to case. In some, the appearance of the condition may be immediately suggestive of its aetiology and a simple investigation will be all that is required. In many cases, however, the cause of the condition is not immediately apparent and a comprehensive approach will be required. This should be carried out when the patient is first presented and before therapy has modified the presenting signs.

The approach to the skin case may be summarized as a 10-point plan (Table 1.1).

Table 1.1 The approach to the skin case – a 10-point plan.

1 Owner's complaint
2 Identify the patient:
    Breed
    Sex
    Age
3 Preliminary examination
4 General medical history
5 Specific dermatological history
6 Lifestyle:
    Diet
    Environment
7 Contagion:
    Other animals
    Human contacts
8 Physical examination:
    General
    Skin
9 Laboratory and other diagnostic tests
10 Analyse data for diagnosis

1 Owner's complaint

This is the reason for the presentation of the cat to the veterinary surgeon. The commonest owners' complaints in feline dermatology are pruritus and alopecia but others include excoriation, swelling and papulocrustous (miliary) dermatitis.

2 Identify the patient

Information about the breed, sex and age of the animal is the first link in the chain between the owner's complaint and diagnosis. Some breeds may be prone to certain diseases, e.g. the Persian to the Chediak–Higashi syndrome. There are sex predispositions to certain dermatoses, e.g. tail gland hyperplasia in the entire male, hyperadrenocorticism in the female. Some diseases are more common at certain ages, e.g. dermatophytosis in young animals, neoplasia in the old.

3 Preliminary examination

Before taking a full history, it is helpful to make a preliminary examination of the animal. Without prejudging the case, it allows emphasis to be placed on certain aspects, e.g. contact dermatitis occurs mainly on ventral surfaces. A generalized dermatosis is, therefore, unlikely to be related to a contact agent unless the animal has been bathed in it.

4 General medical history

History-taking is one of the arts of veterinary science and a good pet-side manner is a valuable asset to the clinician. Owners often purposely or unconsciously withhold relevant information. Remarks between owners or from children may be very pertinent. It is easy to lead clients unintentionally and questions should be phrased in a way which minimizes this risk.

Skin changes are common in systemic disease and a general medical history is therefore essential in investigating skin cases. Relevant topics which should be included, together with examples of diseases which may result in skin lesions, are given below and discussed later in the text.

• Vaccination status: herpesvirus and calcivirus have been recovered from feline skin lesions.

• Worming status: endoparasite hypersensitivity is purported to occur rarely in cats.

• Previous illnesses: many systemic diseases result in skin changes.

• Current medications: virtually any type of skin lesion may be precipitated by drug administration in any particular individual.

• Appetite: is often decreased in systemic illness but may be increased in hyperadrenocorticism, diabetes mellitus or hyperthyroidism.

• Thirst: polyuria/polydipsia may result from nephropathy, hepatopathy, hyperadrenocorticism, diabetes mellitus or hyperthyroidism.

• Digestive tract: maldigestion or malabsorption may present to the dermatologist because of skin and coat changes, resulting from fat, vitamin or other micronutrient deficiencies. Vomiting or diarrhoea occasionally accompany food hypersensitivity.

• Urinary tract: some owners may notice polyuria but not polydipsia.

• Respiratory tract: respiratory signs may be present in lung metastases from a skin tumour.

• Exercise tolerance: may change in many systemic diseases.

Having assembled a comprehensive body of information about the patient's general health, the clinician should then proceed to specific questioning about the skin disorder.

5 Specific dermatological history

Routine questioning should aim to establish:
• The duration of the problem.
• The initial distribution. Many diseases have specific early predilection sites, a knowledge of which is very helpful in suggesting possible diagnoses. By the time of initial presentation, the lesions may have become too generalized for the initial distribution to be obvious.
• The morphology of the original lesions and any changes during progression to the appearance at presentation.

• Whether pruritus is present. The presence or absence of pruritus is the single most important sign at the outset of a dermatological investigation but is notoriously difficult to establish in cats. Cats essentially only scratch at their heads and, when pruritic, lick clsewhere. Such excessive grooming may be carried out secretly, unseen by the owners.

• If pruritus is present, did it occur from the outset of the dermatosis or develop subsequently?

• Is the condition painful rather than pruritic? This differentiation may be extremely difficult for the owner to make.

• Whether the problem has a seasonal occurrence.

• Whether ectoparasites have been seen by the owner and whether the animal is regularly treated with a topical parasiticide.

• Whether the patient has received any treatment, either by the owner with pet shop remedies, or by another veterinary surgeon. Previous treatments may completely alter the clinical appearance of a dermatosis.

6 Lifestyle

Diet

It is possible to produce a myriad of skin lesions by feeding diets deficient in various substances but these rarely occur naturally. Food hypersensitivity is occasionally seen and the dietary constituents should be listed, not forgetting titbits.

Environment

Contact dermatitis is seen occasionally in cats. Information about the environment should include whether the cat is allowed in the house and whether it is allowed in every room. The fabrics and chemicals with which it comes into contact should be noted.

7 Contagion

Other animals

It is important to determine if the client has other pets and if so, whether they have skin disease.

Human contacts

The skin health of the family should be assessed, bearing in mind the zoonotic potential of, particularly, fleas, *Cheyletiella* and *Notoedres* mites and the dermatophytes. The appearance of such conditions in the unfortunate owner is often suggestive of the cause of the animal's dermatosis and, where possible, it is helpful to examine human lesions (Thoday, 1979).

While the history required before carrying out a physical examination may, at first sight, seem extensive, it takes little time to obtain in a first opinion situation by an experienced clinician who is then in an informed position to proceed.

8 Physical examination

General

A general physical examination of the cat should be carried out before examining the skin. Specific details are beyond the scope of this chapter.

Skin

The skin is exceptional as a system in that its gross pathology can be directly observed. Good lighting is therefore of paramount importance. A combination light and magnifying lens may be found to be useful.

Initially, a general impression of the cat should be gained, determining whether it is alert or lethargic, obese or thin. The distribution of the lesions (localized or generalized, symmetrical or asymmetrical) should be assessed. Symmetrical lesions may result from internal causes whereas external causes often produce a characteristically irregular distribution. Close inspection of the skin should then follow, the examiner moving systematically from head to tail and from dorsum to ventrum, finally turning the cat over to examine the undersurfaces. The hair and skin should be palpated, noting their quality and texture. An impression should be gained of the skin's thickness, elasticity and temperature. The degree of pruritus should be assessed by light digital stimulation in affected and non-affected areas. Areas of alopecia should be examined and the ease of epilation of the remaining hair noted. Where

necessary, the hair should be clipped to reveal the extent, severity and nature of the lesions. Trichograms (microscopic examination of the distal ends of at least 20 hairs from affected areas) may be useful if spontaneous or self-epilation of hair is difficult to establish (discussed further under 'Feline symmetric alopecia', see p. 68).

The skin pathology should be classified according to accepted terminology. Quite commonly, the morphology of skin lesions may be the only guide to diagnosis. Primary lesions are the direct result of the disease process and are diagnostically valuable. Secondary lesions result from modification of primary lesions due to such things as scratching and secondary bacterial infection. They are of little value in diagnosis, merely complicating the clinical picture.

The information obtained from the examination is best recorded on a line diagram (Fig. 1.1). These can be reproduced very cheaply or inked stamps are available commercially for stamping case cards. They have a number of advantages over a purely written description, as they provide a quick and potentially accurate method of assembling large amounts of information. They can be used to record gross changes in the disease process and they enable the clinician speedily to refresh his/her memory of a case on subsequent visits.

9 Laboratory and other diagnostic tests

General techniques

TOTAL EOSINOPHIL COUNT

The eosinophil fulfils a large number of roles. They are effector cells in hypersensitivity responses, participate in the reduction of inflammation, are involved in host defence mechanisms against extracellular parasites and are phagocytic. Thus, blood eosinophilia may occur in a number of diseases of cats, and in the absence of other definable causes it may still be a useful indicator of various types of skin diseases.

As eosinophilia frequently occurs in flea-bite hypersensitivity (Scott *et al.*, 1986) it supports this

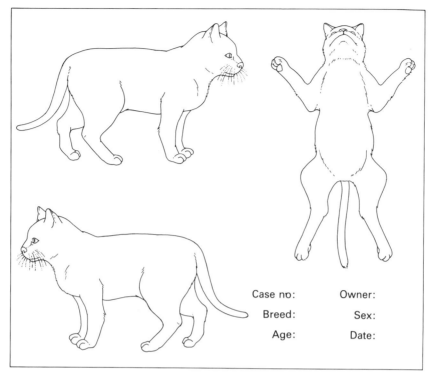

Fig. 1.1 Sheet of line diagrams used by the authors for case recording.

diagnosis when clinical signs are suggestive but fleas or their faeces cannot be recorded (Thoday, 1990a). It may occur in atopic disease (Scott *et al.*, 1986), food hypersensitivity (White & Sequoia, 1989) and is usual in eosinophilic plaque and may be seen in eosinophilic granuloma, particularly when oral lesions are present (Muller *et al.*, 1989). Blood eosinophilia is helpful in distinguishing idiopathic from definitively diagnosable causes of feline symmetric alopecia (Thoday, 1990a). Other possible cutaneous causes of blood eosinophilia include the hypereosinophilic syndrome (Scott *et al.*, 1985) and mast cell tumours (Thoday, 1990a).

BIOCHEMICAL TESTS

Routine biochemical tests are commonly used in the diagnosis of systemic diseases with skin manifestations (see later) and are therefore of direct value in dermatological practice. The de-

tailed discussion of such tests is beyond the scope of this chapter.

SKIN BIOPSY

In the last decade, veterinary dermatohisto-pathology has come of age as a discipline in its own right. A number of pathologists with specific training and expertise in dermatohistopathology are available in the USA and are beginning to emerge in the UK. In order to obtain the most information from skin biopsy, clinicians must select the appropriate areas of skin, excise them and preserve them carefully and separately, and send a detailed history to the histopathologist.

In cats, biopsies may occasionally be obtained under local anaesthesia in amenable individuals but a combination of local anaesthesia and heavy sedation or general anaesthesia alone is usually required. Although many pathologists still prefer material taken by the elliptical excision technique (as this provides a larger sample) (Thoday, 1981a) most clinicians now use a disposable 6–8 mm biopsy punch for ease and speed. However, fragile lesions (e.g. vesicles or bullae) or deep lesions, involving the subcutis, together with most skin tumours, should be biopsied by elliptical excision.

Care should be taken to select representative, non-excoriated lesions. As a guide, a minimum of three biopsies should be taken from each case. Early lesions provide most information but middle and late lesions are sometimes helpful. Intact vesicles or bullae are required in the bullous autoimmune diseases. The biopsy should include the transition zone from diseased to apparently normal skin. The hair should be carefully clipped (never shaved), but the skin should not be cleaned. Where local anaesthesia is used, the agent of choice is 1% lignocaine without adrenaline administered subcutaneously. This agent minimizes the risk of artefactual changes which may occur when adrenaline is included (Henfrey *et al.*, 1991). Whichever technique is used, a full-thickness incision is made, the skin grasped gently by the subcutaneous fat and subsequently dissected free of it. The wound is closed with simple interrupted, non-absorbable sutures.

The specimen should be gently blotted free of blood with a swab and placed subcutis down on a piece of card to prevent curling. The line of demarcation between affected and non-affected tissue should be marked on the card in pencil before placing in 10% buffered formol saline (most inks are discoloured by this preservative). The stage of the lesion should clearly be marked on the container. For direct immunofluorescence testing, biopsies must be snap frozen in liquid nitrogen and subsequently held at −70°C (impractical for many practitioners) or preserved and transported in Michel's fixative. Ideally, separate lesions should be taken for histopathological examination and immunofluorescence testing but, where this is not possible, two halves of the biopsy may be satisfactory. In such cases, it will be found simpler to make the central incision prior to excision of the biopsy.

A succinct but comprehensive history should accompany the submitted specimens.

Ectoparasitic infestations
A number of techniques may be employed in the diagnosis of ectoparasitic infestations.

DIRECT OBSERVATION
The larger ectoparasites such as ticks, fleas and lice are easily found macroscopically, aided, if necessary, by a magnifying lens and light. Small species such as *Cheyletiella*, *Otodectes* and *Trombicula* mites may be similarly observed with care and can be removed for microscopic examination using a moistened cotton bud or dissecting needle.

COAT BRUSHINGS OR COMBINGS
Coat brushings are a useful aid to diagnosis in flea and *Cheyletiella* infestation. Spraying with a parasiticide followed by combing or brushing onto a light-coloured surface frequently reveals the presence of fleas or flea faeces when even a diligent search of the coat has failed. Flea faeces are comma-shaped, brown or black, and can be distinguished from pieces of grit as, when they are placed on moist cotton wool or filter paper, a reddish brown band forms around them due to their blood content. *Cheyletiella* mites may be revealed by brushing the coat onto a dark surface and observing the slow-moving, minute, white specks ('walking dandruff'). Microscopic examination of the brushings is necessary to confirm the diagnosis.

ADHESIVE TAPE COLLECTION
Suitable material for the diagnosis of *Cheyletiella* infestation may be obtained by repeatedly pressing a piece of clear adhesive tape onto an affected area that has been carefully clipped free of hair. The tape is then stuck onto a glass slide and examined microscopically.

THE SKIN SCRAPING
The examination of skin scrapings is one of the most valuable procedures in dermatology but

remains grossly underused in feline skin disease. It will confirm a diagnosis of *Cheyletiella* infestation, feline scabies and demodicosis.

It is vital to select the area for scraping with care, always using a predilection site for the suspected disease even when lesions are widespread. Excoriated lesions should be avoided as the parasites may have been shed from them with the rubbed-off cellular debris. The hair overlying the lesions should be thoroughly but carefully removed using sharp electric clippers. This is time-consuming, particularly with uncooperative patients, but it prevents contaminating the sample with hair and reduces subsequent difficulties with microscopy. The area should be moistened with 5% potassium hydroxide to facilitate adherence of the material to the scalpel blade. A blunt blade should be used and the depth of the scraping varied depending on the suspected disease, e.g. shallow for *Cheyletiella* spp. and deep, producing slight capillary ooze, for *Notoedres cati* and *Demodex* spp. Deep scrapings should always be collected where the possible causal parasite is unknown. After removing the sample, the area is then swabbed with cotton wool moistened with water.

Ideally, the accumulated material is examined immediately but this may not be possible in a practice situation. The material may be suitably stored by pressing another microscope slide on top of it and retained in an envelope. It should be prepared for examination by mixing with a few drops of 5–20% potassium hydroxide and divided into small aliquots. Each is then gently warmed (to increase the rate of clearing) or left for one hour after covering with a cover slip. The slide is then scanned systematically. Large amounts of material may likewise be divided into aliquots or may be gently warmed in a test tube with potassium hydroxide, the fluid centrifuged and the supernatant discarded prior to examining the deposit microscopically.

INVESTIGATION OF THE HABITAT

Where confirmation of a diagnosis of infestation with facultative parasites such as fleas is difficult, material for examination may be collected by vacuum-cleaning the environment or by shaking articles such as the animal's bedding over a sheet of plastic.

Bacterial infections

The skin of healthy cats has a resident microbial population currently thought to include *Micrococcus* spp., α-haemolytic streptococci, *Acinetobacter* spp. (Krogh & Kristensen, 1976) and *Staphylococcus simulans* (Devriese *et al.*, 1984). In addition, various other coagulasenegative staphylococci (*S. capitis, S. cohrii, S. epidermidis, S. haemolyticus, S. hominis, S. saprophyticus, S. sciuni, S. warneri* and *S. xylosus*) (Mardh *et al.*, 1978; Biberstein *et al.*, 1984; Devriese *et al.*, 1984; Cox & Hoskins, 1985) have been isolated from healthy cat skin depending on their environments. Transient organisms (β-haemolytic streptococci, *Escherichia coli, Proteus mirabilis, Pseudomonas* spp., *Alcaligenes* spp., coagulase-positive staphylococci (*S. aureus, S. hyicus* and *S. intermedius*) and some of the coagulase-negative staphylococci above) may be routinely cultured from the skin, do not multiply there and are of no significance unless they become involved in a pathological process as secondary invaders (Muller *et al.*, 1989). Thus, the recovery of untyped bacteria gives little information to the clinician.

Open lesions are frequently contaminated and, where possible, taking samples from such sites should be avoided. Ideally, intact pustules should be opened with a 25 gauge needle and contained pus absorbed onto a swab, or material expressed to the surface and treated likewise, or swabs introduced into discharging sinuses. Impression smears may be made on a microscope slide and stained with Gram's stain or a rapid stain such as Diff-Quik. For bacterial culture, transport medium should be used to prevent the dessication and death of sensitive bacteria in transit.

Biopsies of pyoderma lesions are useful in recurrent superficial or deep pyodermas and, in the latter, may aid in the diagnosis of mycobacterial infections or underlying mycoses.

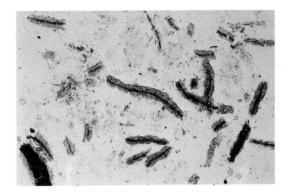

Fig. 1.2 *Microsporum canis* infection. Arthrospores obliterate the anatomical features of affected hairs (magnification × 45).

Dermatophyte infections

Whilst laboratory examinations for dermatophytes are technically simple, they require considerable experience in their interpretation, if false positive results are to be avoided.

EXAMINATION UNDER ULTRAVIOLET (WOOD'S) LIGHT

Microsporum canis is the most important cause of dermatophytosis in cats and the vast majority of strains fluoresce at some stage of infection when exposed to ultraviolet (Wood's) light (Pepin & Oxenham, 1987). A positive result is an apple-green fluorescence of the hair (Plate 1.1) which must be carefully distinguished from the bluish appearance of dust, the irridescence of some topically applied preparations and the true fluorescence of, for example, tetracyclines. Fluorescence is not shown by affected skin or laboratory fungal cultures. Where present, fluorescent hairs should always be selected for further investigations.

DIRECT MICROSCOPY

Prior to collection of material for microscopic examination and culture, the area should be soaked with 70% alcohol to reduce bacterial contamination. Normal hairs are unlikely to be infected. With lesions that fluoresce, affected hairs should be chosen; otherwise, damaged hairs with broken or thickened roots should be selected. They should be plucked with epilation forceps, not cut, and scales and crusts removed by scraping with a blunt scalpel blade. The most active infection occurs at the periphery of the lesion but severely affected hairs may be found elsewhere, and should not be overlooked.

An alternative method is to brush the coat with a toothbrush or scalp brush sterilized in 0.1% chlorhexidine solution for 30 minutes (the Mackenzie brush technique) (Mackenzie, 1961) transferring accumulated material for direct microscopy by shaking onto a slide and for culture by shaking or by gently pushing the bristles or teeth into the medium. The method is particularly useful for rapid screening of large numbers of animals in cat colonies.

The material should be cleared in 5–20% potassium hydroxide and then examined microscopically in subdued light. Material may also be stained using lactophenol cotton blue or blue-black ink. Fungal arthrospores are seen as small, spherical, refractile structures in chains or as a mosaic sheath around the hair. Hyphae may be seen as filaments, sometimes fragmenting into arthrospores. *Microsporum* spp. infected hairs have a collar of arthrospores, often obliterating the anatomical features of the hair (Fig. 1.2). Although a similar arrangement may be seen in severe infections with *Trichophyton* spp., a chain arrangement together with hyphae is usually observed.

FUNGAL CULTURE

Definitive diagnosis of fungal infection is made by identification of the organism after culture. Sabouraud's dextrose agar is still the most satisfactory culture medium for practitioner use. Its slight acidity and added antibacterial agents inhibit bacterial growth and cyclohexamide reduces the growth of contaminating, saprophytic fungi. Dermatophyte test medium (DTM) is readily available to practitioners. Used correctly and with an understanding of possible reactions occurring in it, it can be a useful adjunct to diagnosis in practice. DTM is based on Sabouraud's dextrose agar with added phenol red as indicator. Initially

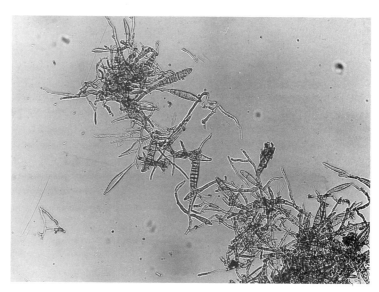

Fig. 1.3 *Microsporum canis.* Typical spindle-shaped macroconidia. Sabouraud's dextrose agar (magnification × 270).

amber, it turns red as a result of alkaline metabolites produced after utilization of its protein during dermatophyte growth (usually within 3 to 7, but occasionally up to 14 days after inoculation). When the protein is exhausted, dermatophytes then utilize carbohydrate and the medium returns to its original amber colour. Saprophytic fungi initially utilize carbohydrate, producing neutral or acid metabolites without a colour change. When the carbohydrate is exhausted (usually after 14 days) they will also utilize protein, producing a red coloration. Thus, cultures on DTM should never be more than 14 days old when read. The typical colony pigmentation, which is a useful diagnostic feature, is masked by the colour change in DTM and ideally, the medium should only be used in conjunction with plain Sabouraud's agar.

A small quantity of the material to be cultured is gently but firmly pressed onto the surface of the medium and the container lid loosely replaced as aerobic conditions are necessary for growth. Large inocula should be avoided as they produce overgrowth of contaminants. Incubation is carried out for 1 to 2 weeks at room temperature in an enclosed area containing a water-filled vessel to prevent dessication. Most common dermatophytes produce growth in this time but the culture should be retained for 1 month before concluding that it is negative. The organism is identified by the morphology of the colony, the colour changes produced during growth and the microscopic appearance of the macroconidia in wet preparations (Fig. 1.3).

BIOPSY
Skin biopsy stained appropriately is a rapid and essentially accurate method of diagnosing dermatophytosis and is occasionally diagnostic when other tests are negative.

Endocrine diseases
Many non-specific and specific, often dynamic-function, tests are employed in the diagnosis of endocrine diseases with dermatological manifestations. These are described later in the text as each disease is discussed and in Chapter 12 on the endocrine system.

Hypersensitivities
The methods used in the investigation of hypersensitivity dermatoses depend on the nature of the suspected allergen(s).

ECTOPARASITE HYPERSENSITIVITY

These tests are discussed under the relevant sections.

FOOD HYPERSENSITIVITY

The most commonly used and reliable test for the diagnosis of food hypersensitivity in cats is the elimination (restriction, 'hypoallergenic') diet or 'test-meal'. Although guidelines for the formulation of elimination diets may be made, the diet chosen in any individual case is decided on after a careful consideration of the animal's usual feeding regimen.

Ideally, the new diet should be formulated from foods never or rarely previously fed. Agents should be free of colourings, flavourings or preservatives. Where the cat eats as the owner, a single, fresh protein source should be selected according to low frequency of feeding. A carbohydrate source is not required during the diagnostic stage of the investigation. The authors usually use rabbit, turkey, chicken or fish (obtained from shops supplying the foods for human consumption) or, where owners are unwilling to prepare fresh food, commercially available restriction diets or tinned lamb-based baby food, (approximately in order of preference). Pet shops should not be used as sources of foods for elimination diets as it is possible that such foodstuffs may contain more than one protein source. Similarly, simply changing from one proprietary foodstuff to another is unsatisfactory in the investigation of food hypersensitivity.

Occasionally, short-term oral antibacterial agents and/or oral glucocorticoids may be necessary to reduce inflammation and pruritus, thus breaking the itch-scratch cycle, in the first few days only of dietary testing.

The diet should be cooked in the same way and without additives during the time of dietary testing and fed to the exclusion of all other foodstuffs (including milk). In addition, all palatable medications (including vitamin/mineral supplements) must be discontinued. Cats should be confined to the house to prevent feeding elsewhere.

The diet should be fed for at least 3 weeks and the animal reinspected by the veterinary surgeon to ascertain possible changes in the symptoms and signs (particularly a reduction in pruritus). On the uncommon occasions on which initial concurrent drug therapy is used to break the itch-scratch cycle, the test period should be extended to at least 4 weeks. As many dermatoses wax and wane to some degree independently of management practices, it is essential that should any improvement be borderline, the diet is continued for a further 4 weeks and the animal reinspected. Occasionally, animals may be hypersensitive to the agents chosen for the elimination diet (e.g. if it forms part of the tinned food normally fed). In such cases, the animal may or may not show an exacerbation of its signs on dietary restriction. Thus, if there has been little or no improvement at reinspection, a second diet formulated from an unrelated protein source should be fed for a further 3 weeks and the animal reassessed. Where improvement is partial, the possibilities of other concurrent hypersensitivities (e.g. flea-bite hypersensitivity or atopic disease) may need to be investigated.

Once improvement in the condition, as a result of elimination dietary testing, is confirmed, one pure foodstuff at a time should be added to the diet and fed for 7–10-day periods. Initially, foods added should be those making up a significant proportion of the previous diet and those which were fed fairly frequently. Dietary hypersensitivities are usually restricted to one or a very small number of substances. Where the allergen is an animal protein, identification is relatively simple. However, vegetable proteins and colourings, flavourings and preservatives in proprietary diets may all be responsible for the signs and identification of such allergens may be extremely difficult.

As cats are particularly fastidious with respect to the foods they will eat, owners should be strongly encouraged to determine the offending allergen. Where this is impossible, the authors use a feline prescription diet (Feline Selected Protein Diet). Where this leads to a recurrence of clinical signs, a balanced diet is compiled from 'safe' foods, where necessary adding daily a taurine supplement and eggs for additional protein. Clam juice has usually been recommended as a good source of taurine. However, Pion *et al.* (1989) reported that maintenance and therapeutic requirements of cats for taurine would require the consumption of 0.25 l and 1 l respectively of clam juice daily! Taurine tablets are available from UK health food shops, and Pion *et al.* (1989) recommended supplementation if the plasma taurine concentration falls to less than 40 nmol/l.

Where the specific allergen is identified, elimination from the diet results in long-term remission of signs. Should they recur, the feeding of the allergen in 'hidden' form (e.g. milk in chocolate) or additional hypersensitivities should be investigated.

Most veterinary dermatologists believe that intradermal testing for food hypersensitivity is unreliable and such tests are not in widespread use. Radioallergosorbent testing (RAST) to determine specific IgE against food allergens correlates with the history and dietary testing in approximate 50% of affected humans but such data are unavailable for cats. Leucocytotoxicity testing against foods is diagnostically valueless in man and probably also in cats.

ATOPIC DISEASE
Atopic disease is diagnosed from the history, physical examination and intradermal testing.

A positive result in intradermal testing depends on the reaction of the test allergen with specific IgE antibody on the surface of mast cells. There is general agreement that aqueous allergens should be used. The usual concentration is 1000 protein nitrogen units (PNU) per ml with the exception of housedust and housedust mite which may be irritant above 250 PNU.

If glucocorticoids have been administered, the test must be delayed until at least 3 weeks after the cessation of the duration of activity of the glucocorticoid used. Other forms of therapy, such as antihistamines and sedatives, should be stopped at least 10 days before testing. In cats, the procedure should be carried out under ketamine restraint at a dose of 5–10 mg/kg administered intramuscularly. A portion of the thorax is clipped with electric clippers, the injection sites marked with an indelible felt pen and an intradermal injection of 0.05 ml of each individual allergen is made together with histamine (positive) and diluent (negative) control. Mixes of allergens are not recommended since the concentration of each individual allergen in the mix may be too low to elicit a positive response. Pollens employed are based on their prevalence in the geographical area.

Positive reactions in cats tend to be smaller, flatter, less well-circumscribed and less erythematous than in dogs, with the reaction peaking between 5 and 15 minutes after injection. In cats, they are more easily visualized by sideways illumination in a darkened room. They are graded either on the mean diameter in two directions (in mm) or from 0 (the size of the negative control reaction) to + + + + (the size of the histamine control). By convention, using the former method, positive reactions are defined as either having a diameter at least 5 mm greater than the negative control or being equal to or larger than the mean of the negative and positive controls or, using the latter method, as a + + or greater reaction. Positive reactions indicate only the presence of skin-sensitizing IgE antibodies. Test reactions must, therefore, be closely correlated with the history.

There are numerous possible causes of false positive and false negative reactions. False positive reactions may result from extracts which are too concentrated or are contaminated. False negative reactions are most commonly due to the prior use of glucocorticoids or antihistamines but may also result from faulty technique, out-of-date extracts or using allergen mixes. As the shelf-life of concentrated extracts is much shorter when they have been diluted, stock allergens should ideally be maintained in concentrations of 20 000 PNU and diluted to testing strength every 2 months.

CONTACT HYPERSENSITIVITY
The investigation of contact hypersensitivity in small animal dermatology is a time-consuming and tedious procedure for both owner and veterinary surgeon. Environmental restriction is dif-

ficult for owners and, indeed, may be impossible in all but the most motivated of clients in a house which is open-plan or where small children forget to close doors. Patch testing is a technically difficult procedure in patients whose efforts are directed solely at the removal of the test substances. Luckily, contact hypersensitivity appears to be very rare in cats as this species manifests a very poor Type IV response. The following regimen for the investigation of contact hypersensitivity is a modification of that routinely used by the authors for dogs. On only very rare occasions will practitioners find it necessary to employ it in cats.

Although cases of allergic contact dermatitis usually improve when hospitalized, the complete change of environment removes other potential allergens (foods, inhalants) and thus merely confirms an environmental agent as causal. Similar comments apply to house cats which are kennelled or restricted in a garage or garden shed. However, where restriction in the home environment is impossible, improvement on hospitalization, transfer of the patient to a friend's home, or kennelling or housing out of the home, with negative results on elimination diet and intradermal testing, gives circumstantial evidence for a diagnosis of contact dermatitis.

In long-standing cases, it may be necessary to reduce the inflammatory response and secondary skin changes with glucocorticoids or antibacterial agents for a few days prior to initiating environmental restriction. Where seasonal allergens (e.g. grass pollens) are suspected, the cat should be kept away from grass. Where an allergen in the home is suspected, the cat is confined to one room while its routine and diet remain unchanged. Kitchens are often the best location for confining the cat as many have relatively inert floors which are rarely allergenic and they frequently communicate with the garden so the cat can easily be excluded from the rest of the house. The owner is requested to remove any blankets and rugs and the kitchen floor is washed with clean water with no added soap or detergent. Most owners accept this inconvenient regimen once they understand the rationale.

Whether the suspected allergen is out-of-doors or in the house, animals with chronic skin changes should dramatically improve after only 14 days without exposure to the allergen and re-examination should show a marked reduction in the severity of the lesions and the degree of pruritus. If grass pollen hypersensitivity is suspected, when the animal is free of symptoms and signs, the animal should be allowed contact with the grass to demonstrate recurrence of signs. Where the allergen is in the home, the cat should be allowed into one additional room at a time for 10 days at a time. If the signs recur during this time, the room containing the possible allergen has been located. By careful removal and reintroduction of articles in the room, it is possible to confirm which article is the cause of the response.

Where the suspicion of contact dermatitis remains after investigation of the immediate environment, the clinician's attention should be directed to places the cat visits regularly. Contact hypersensitivity has also been recorded to drugs (e.g. neomycin).

Confirmation of the allergen can be made by patch testing although there appears to be only one such positive test report in the literature (Thoday, 1985). Alternatively, patch testing may be carried out without previous environmental restriction tests. Glucocorticoids must be stopped for a minimum of 3 weeks from the maximum duration of the drug's activity before patch testing. There are no standard patch testing kits available for veterinary use in the UK. However, kits are available for human use, or sympathetic hospitals may be prepared to make up agents in petrolatum at suitable dilutions for use in animals. Walton (1977a) has suggested concentrations and vehicles for patch testing in the dog and until further information is available, these should be used for cats. However, many allergens (e.g. components of carpets) are not in liquid/suspension form. Such agents may be used in solid form or, rarely, attempts may be made to extract constituents in various solvents.

There are two types of procedure, open testing and closed testing. For each, hair should be clipped over the lateral thorax 1 or 2 days before the test and an Elizabethan collar and bandaging of the ipsilateral hindfoot may be necessary to prevent interference with the test sites.

Open patch tests may be used for liquids or suspensions of suspected allergens. A drop of the test solution is applied to the skin (over the clipped lateral thorax) and the solvent allowed to evaporate. The site is checked at 24, 48, 72, 96 and 120 hours, a positive reaction being shown by an erythematous response at the test site. Open testing is considerably less satisfactory than the closed technique.

Although there are a number of ways of carrying out closed patch testing, the simplest and most accurate is by employing Finn Chambers (Plate 1.2). These testing aids are aluminium discs firmly attached to adhesive tape. Solid agents may be placed in the chamber or liquids/suspensions may be absorbed onto the filter paper supplied. The discs have a raised edge which, on removal, should show an indentation in the skin indicating close contact between the allergen and the skin. Where such an indentation is not visible, the particular allergen should be retested.

The filled chambers are stuck over the clipped lateral thorax, supported by a conforming bandage and covered with a light wrap, or, in animals determined to remove the allergens, adhesive tape. After 48 hours, the patches are removed, the test sites marked and inspected daily for a further 3 days (i.e. inspected at 48, 72, 96 and 120 hours). Positive reactions are shown by erythema, oedema, papules, vesicles or pustules or bullae. Erosions or ulcerations may be noted but such responses are suggestive of irritant rather than hypersensitivity responses. They may be graded as:

    0 = No response
    + = Erythema only
   ++ = Erythema, oedema and papules
  +++ = Erythema, oedema, many papules
        and vesicles
 ++++ = Large confluent blisters

False positive responses may result from irritant reactions, pressure and friction effects, severe adhesive tape reaction and patch contamination. False negative responses may result from interference with patches, inadequate leaching out of the allergen from solids, inadequate concentration of the allergen and, possibly, variations in local sensitivity.

Hypersensitivity responses may be distinguished from irritant reactions by repeating the positive reactors on a control animal (a positive response indicating an irritant reaction) or by using lower concentrations of the positive test substances (continued positive responses suggesting hypersensitivity). Removal of the offending agent from the environment should produce resolution of the signs and reintroduction, relapse within 1–3 days.

Autoimmune dermatoses

The definitive diagnosis of conditions such as the pemphigus complex and systemic and discoid lupus erythematosus requires carefully conducted histological techniques and immunofluorescence tests which are beginning to become commercially available in the UK.

HISTOLOGY

The selection, excision and preservation of material for histological examination has been dealt with previously (p. 9).

The classical histological lesions seen in many of these diseases are very suggestive of the particular condition, but in practice these changes may be extremely difficult to demonstrate. Success depends on a number of factors. The correct lesion must be carefully selected, avoiding those that are old, infected or self-traumatized. The examination of multiple sections of repeated biopsies is essential if the classical pathology is to be regularly recognized.

DIRECT IMMUNOFLUORESCENCE TESTING

This technique is used to identify deposits of immunoglobulin and/or complement (C3) in involved tissue by means of the fluorescent antibody technique. In cats, it relies on the principle that anti-feline immunoglobulin and anti-feline C3 prepared in another species will fix to feline immunoglobulin or C3 present in tissue sections. If the anti-feline antisera are conjugated with fluorescein isothiocyanate, this fixation may be visualized by means of fluorescence microscopy. The position of the fluorescence and therefore of the deposited immunoglobulin or C3 is significant. Standard controls are essential for correct diagnosis.

As previously discussed, formol saline destroys the antigenicity of the deposited immunoglobulin and material must be preserved and transported either by freezing in liquid nitrogen or by immersion in Michel's fixative (Michel *et al.*, 1972).

INDIRECT IMMUNOFLUORESCENCE TESTING
This technique demonstrates the presence of circulating autoantibodies which may occur in some autoimmune skin diseases. These antibodies will bind to sections of relevant tissues and can be visualized by fluorescence microscopy using anti-feline antisera conjugated with fluorescein isothiocyanate, as described under the direct test. Standard controls are again essential.

In the pemphigus complex sections of fresh oral or oesophageal mucosa are used, skin generally being less satisfactory. However, the technique is rarely used in cats as it often gives false negative results. Antinuclear antibody (ANA) may be demonstrated by the technique in pemphigus erythematosus and in systemic lupus erythematosus. Rat liver is the usual preferred tissue substrate.

10 Analyse data for diagnosis

At the conclusion of the investigation the clinician should analyse the information obtained to determine the likely diagnosis.

CONGENITAL AND HEREDITARY DISORDERS

Alopecias
   Alopecia universalis
   Hereditary hypotrichosis
   Pili torti
Pigmentation defects
   Chediak–Higashi syndrome
Abnormalities of structural integrity
   Aplasia cutis
   Cutaneous asthenia

Miscellaneous conditions
   Hair shaft abnormality in Abyssinian cats

Summary

A number of hereditary and/or congenital skin disorders have been described in cats. Congenital conditions are present at birth and may be hereditary or due to some influence occurring during gestation. Tardive conditions are not present at birth but develop subsequently, usually in the first year of life. The heritability of some conditions is poorly documented.

Congenital/hereditary disorders are usually not amenable to more than symptomatic therapy. In most conditions the affected animals should not be used for breeding.

These conditions may be classified conveniently as those presenting primarily with alopecia, pigmentation defects or abnormalities of structural integrity, together with miscellaneous conditions.

Alopecias

Alopecia universalis (Sphinx cat, Canadian hairless cat)
Alopecia universalis is a rare, hereditary disease resulting in generalized alopecia due to complete absence of primary hairs and limited numbers of abnormal secondary hairs. Regrettably it has been bred for selectively to produce this so-called 'breed'. The breed standard for Sphinx cats requires a covering of fine hair on the face, paws, scrotum, tip of the tail and the back.

Trauma incurred by the rasping action of the tongue results in reluctance to groom and consequently the accumulation of desquamated keratin and sebaceous and epitrichial (apocrine) gland secretions on the skin and in the nail folds. These give the skin an oily feel and rancid smell. Histologically there is a complete absence of primary hair follicles and a reduced number of secondary hair follicles.

Antiseborrhoeic shampoos (e.g. 1% selenium sulphide) are used as necessary to control the greasiness and odour. Material accumulating in the nail folds is best removed manually.

Hereditary hypotrichosis

Hereditary hypotrichosis (less than the normal amount of hair), has been reported in the Siamese (autosomal recessive trait) (Letard, 1938), Devon Rex (Thoday, 1981b) and in a Mexican breed of cat (modes of inheritance not determined). The condition may be generalized or regional. The Devon Rex was seen as an adult and had bilaterally symmetric trunk hypotrichosis (Plate 1.3). When mated with an unrelated Devon Rex, five kittens born to it were similarly affected but when crossed with a Burmese, all progeny had normal coats. The Siamese cats were born with a downy covering of secondary hairs. These were rapidly lost and affected areas were effectively alopecic by 2 weeks of age. Subsequently, there was some hair regrowth but this was again lost when the kittens were 6 months old. Histopathological examination of biopsies demonstrated small, poorly developed, primary hair follicles devoid of hairs and a reduced number of secondary hair follicles.

There is no treatment and affected animals should not be bred.

Pili torti

Pili torti is an inherited, autosomal dominant trait characterized in man by a 90–360° rotation of the hair shaft about its long axis. It has been diagnosed tentatively in a litter of kittens resulting from a sibling mating (Geary & Baker, 1986).

Apparently normal at birth, the kittens rapidly lost hair and at 18 days were presented with a sparse covering of readily epilated hair, a mild periocular dermatitis, pedal dermatitis and paronychia. Subsequently, all kittens developed systemic signs (undiagnosed cause) and either died or were euthanased.

Examination of epilated hair with light microscopy and scanning electron microscopy revealed flattening and clockwise rotation of the hair shaft through 360°.

Pigmentation defects

Chediak–Higashi syndrome (oculocutaneous albinism)

The Chediak–Higashi syndrome is an hereditary, autosomal recessive condition of blue-smoke, light-green, light-yellow or light-yellow-green-eyed Persian cats affecting membrane-bound organelles of various cell types.

It is characterized by partial oculocutaneous hypopigmentation, associated with an increase in size but a decrease in number of melanin granules in hair and skin and abnormal granulation of leucocytes. There is decreased fundic pigmentation, photophobia, red rather than yellow-green fundic reflectivity, bilateral nuclear cataracts (in most affected animals, developing from 3 months of age) and a bleeding tendency (Kramer *et al.*, 1977; Prieur *et al.*, 1979). In man it has also been associated with increased susceptibility to infection and the development of lymphoma but this has not been described in cats.

Diagnosis is supported by detection of abnormally large, eosinophilic, sudanophilic, peroxidase-containing granules in neutrophils or enlarged but reduced numbers of melanin granules in hair shafts, follicles and skin.

There is currently no treatment for this condition.

Abnormalities of structural integrity

Aplasia cutis (epitheliogenesis imperfecta)

Aplasia cutis is an hereditary, congenital discontinuity of the squamous epithelium. It is rare in cats (Scott, 1980), and the mode of inheritance in this species is unknown.

Clinically it is distinguished by well-demarcated areas of absence of epithelium resulting in ulceration of skin and/or mucosa, accompanied by secondary infection and possibly septicaemia. Histologically it is characterized by the absence of epidermis and adnexa in affected areas of skin.

Treatment is not usually successful. If limited areas are involved skin grafting may be of benefit, although the wisdom of such treatment is debatable. Large defects are not treatable.

Cutaneous asthenia (Ehlers–Danlos-like syndrome, dermatosparaxis)

The term 'cutaneous asthenia' embraces a number of hereditary, congenital connective tissue disorders which result in increased skin fragility, hyperextensibility and laxity. Both dominant and recessive traits have been identified in cats.

Classically, the skin of affected cats is soft, loosely attached to subcutaneous tissue and may hang in folds, particularly around the head and limbs (Plate 1.4). Irregular, thin, white scars provide evidence of skin fragility. Minor trauma (venepuncture, clipping, restraint) may result in gaping (fish-mouth) tears. Although sub-cutaneous haematomas occasionally develop in traumatized areas there is, characteristically, minimal bleeding when the skin tears. Recessive cutaneous asthenia only rarely shows the hyper-extensibility and laxity of joints commonly seen in affected humans.

Diagnosis is based on the clinical findings, skin extensibility index and histopathological and ultrastructural changes. The extensibility index is calculated by lifting a fold of skin on the dorsal lumbar surface to its maximum height without causing pain and is calculated as:

$$\text{Extensibility index (\%)} = \frac{\text{Vertical height of skin fold}}{\text{Body length (occipital crest to tail base)}} \times 100$$

Affected cats have a skin extensibility index of more than 19% (Patterson & Minor, 1977; Freeman *et al.*, 1987).

Light microscopic examination may reveal dis-orientation, fragmentation and shortening of collagen fibres, haphazard packing of fibres into bundles and disorganized interweaving of fibre bundles, or may be normal. Electron microscopy may demonstrate abnormalities in collagen fibril morphology (wide variation in diameter and ir-regular contours of fibrils) and disorganized packing of fibrils into fibres. Biochemical studies are necessary to confirm abnormalities of collagen metabolism. In the recessive form, there is a deficiency of procollagen peptidase and accumu-lation of procollagen.

There is no treatment. Environmental restric-tion and surgical declawing may be necessary to minimize trauma of the skin. Any wounds should be promptly sutured using horizontal mattress sutures.

Miscellaneous conditions

Hair shaft abnormality in Abyssinian cats
An abnormal expansion of the medulla at the top of the whiskers and guard hairs has recently been reported in three Abyssinian cats (Wilkinson & Kristensen, 1989).

An onion-shaped swelling was observed at the top of the whiskers (all cases) and guard hairs (two cases). Occasionally a second swelling was detected along the hair shaft. Involvement of the guard hairs imparted a rough, brittle and lustreless appearance to the coat.

Microscopic examination of the hairs indicated that the swelling was due to expansion of the medulla. The epidermis, dermis, hair follicles and adnexae appeared normal.

ENDOCRINE AND METABOLIC DISEASES

Acromegaly
Hyperadrenocorticism
  Spontaneous
  Iatrogenic
Hyperthyroidism
Hypothyroidism
  Congenital or juvenile onset
  Iatrogenic
Diabetes mellitus
Xanthomatosis
Mucopolysaccharidosis
Renal and hepatic disease
Maldigestion and malabsorption

Summary
With the exception of congenital and juvenile-onset hypothyroidism and mucopolysaccharidosis these conditions are usually seen in middle-aged to old cats. Only mucopolysaccharidosis has a breed predilection (Siamese cats); hyperadreno-corticism is seen most frequently in female cats, and acromegaly shows a preponderance in male cats.

In these conditions, cutaneous lesions, though of varied importance, are relatively minor manifestations of systemic diseases. Endocrine disturbances may be accompanied by symmetric alopecia, and seborrhoea but not usually pruritus. Seborrhoea sicca and variable, though usually low-grade pruritus may be present in renal disease, hepatic disease, maldigestion and malabsorption. Cutaneous nodules occur in xanthomatosis and may be present in mucopolysaccharidosis.

Acromegaly

Acromegaly has recently been documented in cats (Peterson, 1988; Peterson *et al.*, 1990). It is usually caused by a growth hormone-secreting pituitary tumour resulting in overgrowth of connective tissue, bone and viscera and the development of insulin-resistant diabetes mellitus.

Cutaneous changes (thickening of the skin and development of excessive skin folds particularly in the region of the head and neck) may accompany the major signs of polyuria and polydipsia which are associated with insulin-resistant diabetes mellitus. There may be cardiomegaly (with or without a systolic murmur, gallop rhythm and congestive cardiac failure), hepatomegaly, nephromegaly (with or without renal failure), enlarged endocrine organs, large head, mandible, tongue and abdomen and weight gain.

The diagnosis is supported by laboratory findings of hyperglycaemia, glycosuria, hypercholesterolaemia and azotaemia and confirmed by detection of raised plasma growth hormone concentrations.

As treatment with somatostatin analogues has proved unsuccessful (Peterson, 1988) pituitary ^{60}Co teletherapy may be of value in treating feline acromegaly.

Hyperadrenocorticism (hyperadrenocorticalism, hyperadrenocorticoidism, Cushing's-like disease, Cushing's-like syndrome)

Both spontaneous and iatrogenic hyperadrenocorticism (HAC), though uncommon, are now well recognized in cats. Spontaneous HAC usually results from excessive adrenocorticotrophic hormone production by pituitary tumours or less commonly hypertrophy; functional adrenal gland tumours are rare. Despite the glucocorticoid resistance of cats, iatrogenic HAC may result from excessive glucocorticoid (Thoday, 1985) and megestrol acetate therapy. Cats with spontaneous or iatrogenic HAC are predisposed to develop diabetes mellitus.

Cutaneous lesions include bilaterally symmetrical alopecia, seborrhoea and a thin, inelastic, hyperpigmented, easily torn and bruised skin. In the authors' experience, cutaneous lesions are uncommon in iatrogenic HAC. The major clinical signs are polyuria, polydipsia, polyphagia and abdominal enlargement. Muscle wasting, obesity or weight loss and hepatomegaly have also been noted (Nelson *et al.*, 1988; Peterson, 1988).

Tentative diagnosis is made on the basis of history and clinical signs, supported by laboratory findings, i.e. hyperglycaemia, glucosuria (which reflect the susceptibility of these cats to diabetes mellitus), hypercholesterolaemia, eosinopenia, lymphopenia and leucocytosis. The diagnosis is confirmed by an excessive increase in plasma cortisol concentration following stimulation with adrenocorticotrophic hormone (ACTH) (see Chapter 12). At present low- and high-dose dexamethasone suppression tests have not been adequately standardized for routine use in cats though it appears that the latter may be of diagnostic value (Peterson, 1988).

Unilateral or bilateral adrenalectomy currently appears to be the most successful means of treating adrenal tumours and hyperplasia, respectively. Traditionally, the use of *o,p'*-DDD (mitotane) has been discouraged in cats because of the susceptibility of the species to chlorinated hydrocarbons. However, the drug appears to be well tolerated in 75% of cats (Zerbe *et al.*, 1987) but does not appear to be particularly effective in controlling HAC (Nelson *et al.*, 1988; Zerbe, 1989). Treatment with metyrapone has had varied success while ketoconazole appears to be ineffective in producing adrenocortical suppression and may be hepatotoxic (Willard *et al.*, 1986). ^{60}Co teletherapy may be of value in treating HAC due to pituitary tumours (Nelson *et al.*, 1988).

Hyperthyroidism (thyrotoxicosis)

Hyperthyroidism is a common, multisystemic disorder of cats. Cutaneous signs include excessive shedding of hair, patchy or symmetrical alopecia (Plate 1.5), dry or greasy seborrhoea, a matted hair coat (Plate 1.6), excessive nail growth and thin pliable skin (Thoday & Moonay, 1992a) which are probably associated with behavioural changes resulting in decreased or increased grooming together with direct effects on the skin of excessive concentrations of thyroid hormones (Peterson *et al.*, 1983; Thoday, 1986a, 1988). The major clinical signs are weight loss despite polyphagia, tachycardia and other cardiac abnormalities, polyuria/polydipsia, hyperactivity, diarrhoea and vomiting.

Diagnosis is based on the history, physical examination including the presence of goitre, and is confirmed by elevated resting concentrations of serum triiodothyronine (T_3) and/or thyroxine (T_4).

Surgical thyroidectomy is the preferred treatment in a practice situation for younger or otherwise healthy individuals. Alternatives are the use of radioactive iodine (^{131}I) or chronic administration of antithyroid drugs (carbimazole (UK) or methimazole (USA)) (Thoday & Moonay, 1992b).

Hypothyroidism

Naturally occurring hypothyroidism occurs rarely in cats. Congenital and juvenile onset hypothyroidism have been documented (Arnold *et al.*, 1984; Peterson, 1988) but despite putative evidence (clinical signs and low serum plasma T_4 concentrations) naturally occurring adult-onset hypothyroidism has yet to be definitely diagnosed. Iatrogenic hypothyroidism (Peterson & Turrel, 1986), resulting from the treatment of hyperthyroidism, is the most common cause for the development of feline hypothyroidism. Experimental hypothyroidism has also been reported (Thoday, 1986b, 1989, 1990b).

Clinically, congenital hypothyroidism is characterized by a decreased number of primary hairs and predominance of undercoat, disproportion-

ate dwarfism, lethargy and bradycardia (Arnold *et al.*, 1984). Iatrogenic and experimental hypothyroidism are associated with non-pruritic seborrhoea sicca, matted hair coat due to failure to groom, alopecia of the lateral and medial distal halves of both pinnae and broadening of the muzzle due to myxoedema. With the exception of the pinnae, bilaterally symmetrical alopecia does not develop and hair removed by clipping regrows (Thoday, 1986b, 1989, 1990b). Experimentally, weight gain is not noted although bradycardia and subnormal rectal temperature occur (Thoday, 1990b).

Diagnosis is based on history and clinical signs, suggested by subnormal serum thyroxine (T_4) and triiodothyronine (T_3) concentrations and confirmed by the failure of serum T_4 concentrations to rise adequately 6 hours after the intravenous injection of 0.5 IU/kg bovine TSH (Thoday, 1990b).

Treatment for congenital or iatrogenic hypothyroidism comprises daily oral T_4 supplementation at a dose of 10 μg/kg twice daily, subsequently adjusted depending on the clinical response and, where necessary, serum T_4 and T_3 concentrations 4 to 6 and 12 hours after administration on a twice-daily dosing regimen.

Diabetes mellitus

Diabetes mellitus may be associated with a variety of cutaneous changes including a dry hair coat, generalized seborrhoea sicca with or without pruritus, thinning of the skin, symmetrical pinnal and ventral abdominal alopecia, pyoderma, demodicosis and xanthomatosis. These resolve with successful treatment of the diabetes. Additional clinical signs may occur if the diabetes is associated with acromegaly or hyperadrenocorticism (see above).

Xanthomatosis

Xanthomatosis is a disorder of lipid metabolism resulting in the intracellular accumulation of abnormal quantities of sudanophilic material and is associated with hyperlipidaemia, hypertriglyceridaemia and hypercholesterolaemia. In cats, this condition has been associated with naturally occurring and megestrol acetate-induced diabetes mellitus (Kwochka & Short, 1984; Jones *et al.*, 1985) and presumed idiopathic familial hyperlipoprotcinaemia (Jones *et al.*, 1983), but may also occur without evidence of abnormal fat metabolism (Fawcett *et al.*, 1977).

The skin lesions comprise cutaneous papules and plaques which may become ulcerated, and soft, well-circumscribed, single or multiple subcutaneous nodules of variable size. These are usually located over the head, trunk and proximal extremities.

The diagnosis is confirmed by detection of histiocytes packed with sudanophilic material on histopathological examination of biopsies of the lesions.

Xanthomas regress spontaneously if the underlying condition is controlled.

Mucopolysaccharidosis

Mucopolysaccharidosis (MPS), a lysosomal storage disease, is associated with arylsulphatase B deficiency (Maroteaux–Lamy syndrome or MPS VI) and has been described in Siamese cats (Jezyk *et al.*, 1977; Haskins *et al.*, 1979). Cutaneous nodules located on the head, swollen eyelids and thickened skin may occur. In addition, affected cats have a broad flat face, small ears, diffuse corneal clouding, retinal atrophy and skeletal and neurological abnormalities and fail to grow.

Diagnosis is confirmed by the demonstration of excessive amounts of urinary glycosaminoglycans. The condition is progressive and although successful treatment by bone marrow transplantation has been reported (Gasper *et al.*, 1984) it is inadvisable to breed from cats with this hereditary disease.

Renal and hepatic disease

Seborrhoea sicca and diffuse thinning of the hair may be seen in end-stage renal disease and hepatic disease (Plate 1.7). Low-grade pruritus is a less frequent cutaneous manifestation of these diseases.

Maldigestion and malabsorption

These are uncommon syndromes in cats but may be accompanied by a dry or greasy seborrhoea, with or without pruritus, in association with the development of essential fatty acid and fat-soluble vitamin deficiencies.

BACTERIAL INFECTIONS

Cellulitis and abscess
Impetigo and ecthyma
Folliculitis and furunculosis
Actinomycosis and nocardiosis
Corynebacterial infection
Plague
Mycobacterial infections
   Cutaneous tuberculosis
   Feline leprosy
   Opportunistic mycobacterial granulomas
Bacterial pseudomycetoma
Dermatophilosis
Bacterial paronychia and pyonychia

Summary

With the exception of abscesses and cellulitis, bacterial infections are rare in cats. Impetigo and ecthyma occur in kittens, and feline leprosy is seen most frequently in cats aged between 1 and 3 years, but no other age, breed or sex predispositions appear to have been recorded. Cutaneous manifestations of bacterial infections are varied and include pustular dermatitis, folliculitis, plaques, ulcers, furunculosis, cellulitis, abscesses, pyogranulomatous nodules and sinuses discharging pus which may contain granules. Drainage lymph nodes may be enlarged and systemic signs (pyrexia, anorexia and depression) may occur.

In all persistent or recurrent infections it is essential to identify the causal organisms (impression smear, biopsy, culture), carry out antibacterial sensitivity testing and investigate the possibility of accompanying immunosuppressive diseases (e.g. feline leukaemia (FeLV) and immunodeficiency (FIV) infections, diabetes mellitus and neoplasia).

Cellulitis and subcutaneous abscess

These conditions are common, particularly in the entire male, usually result from cat bites and scratches and consequently often involve the head, tail base and limbs. The causal bacteria introduced by these injuries are part of the normal oral flora and comprise mixed populations of aerobes (*Pasteurella multocida*, β-haemolytic streptococci) and anaerobes (*Bacteroides* spp., *Fusobacterium* spp., *Peptostreptococcus* spp.) (Love *et al.*, 1978; Scott, 1980).

Early clinical signs are pain, lameness, swelling and small crusts, which cover puncture wounds, local lymphadenopathy, malaise and pyrexia. Subsequently, cellulitis may develop in locations with little subcutaneous tissue (limbs and tail) but elsewhere abscesses may occur. If these are untreated, possible sequelae include periostitis, septic arthritis, osteomyelitis, otitis media, sinusitis, rhinitis and pyothorax (Joshua, 1971, 1972).

Prophylactic oral or parenteral penicillin is always indicated when puncture wounds are present. Cellulitis should be treated with systemic penicillins and hot fomentations. Abscesses should be encouraged to develop by hot fomentations alone and, subsequently, should be drained following a generous ventral incision and flushed with diluted 20 volumes hydrogen peroxide or 2% chlorhexidine solution. Flushing should be repeated daily until the wound heals.

Normally, healing following appropriate therapy is rapid. Failure to heal or recurrence of infection at the same site may be associated with involvement of other tissues, the presence of anaerobic bacteria (including *Actinomyces* spp. or *Nocardia* spp.), fungi, mycoplasmas, immunosuppression (e.g. FeLV or FIV infections, diabetes mellitus or neoplasia) or the presence of a foreign body (e.g. a fragment of tooth).

In most entire male cats, castration is helpful in reducing the incidence of cat bite infections.

Impetigo and ecthyma

These are rare conditions of young kittens attributed to 'over-zealous mouthing' by the mother. A pustular dermatitis, associated with *Pasteurella multocida* and β-haemolytic streptococci, occurs principally on the neck, withers and back but may become more extensive. The occurrence of systemic signs, depression, anorexia and pyrexia, is variable. Treatment comprises systemic antibacterial agents (penicillin, ampicillin, amoxycillin) and topical cleansing with chlorhexidine or aluminium acetate (Scott, 1980).

Folliculitis and furunculosis

These are rare conditions attributed to infection with β-haemolytic streptococci and coagulase-positive staphylococci and *Pasteurella multocida* (Scott, 1980). They may affect the chin, where they may complicate feline acne, and occasionally involve the face and trunk.

Clinical signs of folliculitis include papules, pustules (from which hairs emerge), crusts (erupted pustules), erosions, ulcers and hair loss. Furunculosis, (resulting from rupture of infected hair follicles) may be associated with draining tracts and cellulitis. Pruritus, pain and local lymphadenopathy are variable.

Bacterial culture and sensitivity testing should be undertaken before instituting treatment with systemic antibacterial agents and daily cleansing with ethyl alcohol (acne), chlorhexidine solution or 2.5% benzoyl peroxide.

Actinomycosis and nocardiosis

Actinomycosis and nocardiosis occur rarely in cats. *Actinomyces* spp. (*A. bovis* and *A. viscosus*) are normal residents of the cat's mouth and gastrointestinal tract, and cutaneous infection may result from bites, scratches, penetrating foreign bodies and wound contamination. *Nocardia* spp. (*N. asteroides*, *N. brasiliensis* and *N. caviae*) are soil saprophytes and infection may occur by inhalation and ingestion in addition to contamination of skin wounds. Immunosuppressive diseases may predispose to infection with *N. asteroides*.

Cutaneous lesions, manifested as pyogranulomatous nodules and abscesses with multiple discharging tracts, occur most frequently on the limbs but may be located elsewhere. In nocardiosis the discharge may be tomato soup-like in colour and consistency and may contain 'sulphur' granules, while in actinomycosis it invariably contains 'sulphur' granules but may be yellow, grey or reddish-brown in colour. The presence of these granules (dense aggregates of bacterial colonies) in pyogranulomatous lesions characterizes the formation of actinomycotic mycetoma. A primary respiratory form (pleural effusion and empyema), or abdominal form (ascites, organ abscesses), vertebral osteomyelitis, central nervous system (CNS) lesions and disseminated infection, may also occur, particularly in nocardiosis.

Diagnosis and differentiation between actinomycosis and nocardiosis rely on identification of the causal bacteria in smears of exudate (Ziehl–Neelsen stain), after crushing the mycelial clumps (Gram's, Hanks' acid-fast, Ziehl–Neelsen stains), by culture or by histological examination of biopsy specimens (Brown and Bren's, Gomori's methenamine silver stains).

Prior to treatment, the patient should be examined for foreign bodies (actinomycosis) and immunodeficiency or immunosuppressive diseases (nocardiosis) and appropriate treatment carried out where indicated. Therapy should combine prolonged and high-concentration antibacterial therapy. Although a large number of antibacterial agents (e.g. penicillins, sulphonamides, trimethoprim-potentiated sulphonamides) have been recommended to treat actinomycosis and nocardiosis, our current treatment of choice for nocardiosis is with oral clindamycin together with lavage of the tracts using diluted 20 volume hydrogen peroxide twice daily. Oral sodium or potassium iodide (30–100 mg daily in dilute solution) has effective proteolytic actions, thinning discharges, increasing drainage and removing foci of infection. Concentrated solutions may result in gastric irritation and vomiting and should not be used. Parmaceutical preparations of potassium iodide are not currently available in the UK and potassium iodate may be used in its place.

Treatment should be continued for at least 4 weeks after complete clinical remission has been obtained (see Chapter 23).

Corynebacterial infections

Apparent infection with *Corynebacterium* spp. has been associated with plaque-like lesions and multiple discharging sinuses over the inguinal fat pads of obese cats (Wilkinson, 1981), while *Rhodococcus* (*Corynebacterium*) *equi* has been cultured from a cutaneous abscess in a cat (Higgins & Paradise, 1980) and from a case of bilateral forelimb cellulitis with sinuses discharging a cream to green or bloody pus (Elliot *et al.*, 1986) (Plate 1.8).

Treatment with a prolonged, high dosage of an appropriate antibacterial agent determined by bacterial culture and sensitivity testing is required.

Plague

Yersinia pestis, the cause of bubonic plague, may be transmitted to cats by rodent bites or fleas. Though cosmopolitan, it is of importance only in Asia, Africa and some regions of the USA. It produces cutaneous abscesses and draining sinuses often located on the head and limbs, local lymphadenopathy, high fever, septicaemia, depression and anorexia. Because of the public health risk all suspected cases should be treated with great care.

Diagnosis is by identification of the organism by culture or immunofluorescence of impression smears or by demonstration of a fourfold increase in antibody titres from the acute to convalescent stages.

Treatment is by drainage of abscesses, flushing with 1% povidone iodine and antibacterial therapy (streptomycin (the therapy of choice), tetracycline or chloramphenicol). Flea control, to prevent further spread of the infection, is essential.

Mycobacterial infections

Tuberculosis

Tuberculosis, caused by *Mycobacterium bovis* or, less frequently, *M. tuberculosis*, is now a rare condition manifested cutaneously by solitary or multiple plaques, nodules and ulcers and abscesses which may discharge a thick yellow-green pus. Lesions usually occur on the head, neck or limbs. Drainage lymph nodes may be enlarged and infected and occasionally develop discharging sinuses. Systemic signs (anorexia, depression, pyrexia and weight loss) may be present.

Diagnosis is suggested by the demonstration of the Gram-positive, acid-fast bacilli in smears or biopsy material and confirmed by culture or guinea pig inoculation.

After positive diagnosis, the public health authorities should be notified and the cat euthanased (see Chapter 23).

Feline leprosy
Feline leprosy is a rare, cosmopolitan, pyogranulomatous condition occurring most frequently in young cats and caused by unidentified acid-fast bacteria (now not thought to be *Mycobacterium lepraemurium*, the rat leprosy bacillus). The cutaneous lesions, usually located on the head, limbs and ventrum, are similar in nature to those seen in tuberculosis (single or multiple plaques, nodules, ulcers, abscesses and tracts discharging a serosanguinous fluid). The lesions do not spread but enlarge slowly. Local lymphadenopathy may occur but systemic signs are infrequent.

Diagnosis requires demonstration of acid-fast bacteria (Ziehl–Nielsen stain) in impression smears or biopsies and ruling out a diagnosis of tuberculosis by guinea pig inoculation.

The preferred treatment is by surgical excision where possible, possibly in combination with administration of tetracycline, dapsone at a dosage of 1 mg/kg twice daily (Wilkinson, 1988) or clofazimine at a dosage of 8 mg/kg/day orally (Mundell, 1990). Neither dapsone nor clofazimine is licensed for use in cats. Dapsone may cause haemolytic anaemia and neurotoxicity and should be used with caution.

Opportunistic mycobacterial granulomas (atypical mycobacterial granulomas)
Opportunistic mycobacterial granulomas may result from cutaneous penetration or wound contamination by any of several mycobacteria that

are soil saprophytes, including *M. xenopi*, *M. fortuitum*, *M. chelonei*, *M. phlei* and *M. smegmatis*.

Lesions are similar in location and nature to those seen in feline leprosy. Diagnosis is made by demonstration of acid-fast organisms in impression smears or biopsy material and their identification on the basis of cultural and biochemical characteristics.

Some cases regress spontaneously. Where possible, wide surgical excision without suturing, allowing the wound to heal by granulation, is the treatment of choice. This should be combined with antibacterial therapy (kanamycin or gentamycin). Response to treatment is variable and, if poor, euthanasia may be appropriate.

Bacterial pseudomycetoma (cutaneous bacterial granuloma botryomycosis)

Bacterial pseudomycetoma describes a pyogranulomatous lesion often with discharging sinuses, caused by non-branching bacteria and characterized by the presence of compact bacterial colonies or grains. Infection is introduced by bites, trauma or contamination of wounds and the subsequent development of a granulomatous reaction may result from the host's inability to eliminate the organism, or a hypersensitivity response to it.

Diagnosis is based on histopathological examination of lesions and demonstration of bacteria (Gram's or Brown and Bren's stains).

Treatment is by radical surgical excision and antibacterial therapy, based on bacterial sensitivity testing. Antibacterial therapy alone is not effective as the tissue response prevents adequate drug penetration. Walton *et al.* (1983) described the development, following multiple bite wounds, of a pyogranulomatous panniculitis with sinuses in an ovariohysterectomized female cat. A coagulase-positive staphylococcus and *Streptococcus canis* were isolated from the lesions. Resolution occurred following surgical excision of affected tissue combined with amoxycillin therapy.

Dermatophilosis
(cutaneous streptothrichosis)

Dermatophilus congolensis, thought to be transmitted from carrier farm animals, is a very rare, opportunistic cause of cutaneous pyogranulomatous disease in cats. Cutaneous inflammation, trauma, parasites and moisture predispose to infection.

The lesions described include sinuses draining subcutaneous masses involving the popliteal lymph node (Jones, 1976) or located in the popliteal area (Miller *et al.*, 1983; Carakostas *et al.*, 1984) and from a paw (Carakostas *et al.*, 1984). Pyogranulomatous lesions have also been found on the base of the tongue and in the bladder (O'Hara & Cordes, 1963).

Diagnosis relies on demonstration of the characteristic 'railroad track' alignment of organisms in purulent exudate or crushed crusts using Gram's, Giemsa's or Wright's stains. Organisms may also be identified in biopsy material and by culture.

Treatment comprises removal of crusts, systemic antibacterial therapy with ampicillin or amoxycillin and, if indicated, surgical excision of granulation tissue. Elimination of any precipitating factors (e.g. moisture, trauma, parasitic infestations) may lead to spontaneous resolution.

Bacterial paronychia and pyonychia

Bacterial paronychia and pyonychia are uncommon disorders in cats and are almost invariably secondary to another disease, notably trauma, fungal infections, parasitic infestations, contact dermatitis, autoimmune diseases, immunosuppression (e.g. feline leukaemia and immunodeficiency virus infections, diabetes mellitus and glucocorticoid therapy). Of these predisposing diseases FeLV infection and pemphigus foliaceus are probably the most common.

Although bacterial culture and antibacterial sensitivity tests followed by appropriate antibacterial therapy are indicated, investigation must be directed at identifying the underlying cause of the condition.

VIRAL DISEASES

Feline leukaemia virus infection
Feline immunodeficiency virus infection
Feline calicivirus and feline herpesvirus infection
Feline sarcoma virus infection
Pseudorabies virus infection
Cow pox infection

Feline leukaemia virus

Cutaneous conditions associated with feline leukaemia virus (FeLV)-positive cats include bacterial infections (recurrent abscesses, cellulitis, paronychia/pyonychia (Plate 1.9), fungal infections, neoplasia (lymphosarcoma, fibrosarcoma, liposarcoma, multiple cutaneous horns), generalized seborrhoea, eosinophilic plaque, severe pruritus and poor wound healing (Cotter *et al.*, 1975; Center *et al.*, 1982). It is therefore prudent to investigate the FeLV status of cats presenting with these signs, particularly those cats with recurrent or poorly responsive cutaneous infections. Increased susceptibility to infections and neoplasia and poor wound healing may be attributed to the immunosuppressive activity of FeLV. However, the causal association between FeLV and eosinophilic plaque, pruritus and seborrhoea is not clear. Despite the association of immunosuppression and recurrent bacterial infection, it appears that control achieved in these cases by combining antibacterial agents and glucocorticoids is superior to that achieved by antibacterial agents alone (Scott, 1987b).

Diagnosis is made by detection of viral antigens or by virus isolation (see Chapter 15).

Feline immunodeficiency virus

Cutaneous conditions associated with feline immunodeficiency virus (FIV)-positive cats include chronic otitis externa (Pedersen *et al.*, 1987), pustular dermatitis, gingivitis, stomatitis and squamous cell carcinoma of the digits (Hosie *et al.*, 1989). Diagnosis is confirmed by antibody detection (see Chapter 16).

Feline calicivirus and feline herpesvirus infection

Feline calicivirus has been isolated from vesicles, erosions and ulcers located on the feet as well as the oral cavity of a young cat (Cooper & Sabine, 1972) (see Chapter 14). The lesions cleared with symptomatic therapy. Viral particles morphologically consistent with feline calicivirus have also been observed in samples obtained from eosinophilic ulcers and granuloma (Neufield *et al.*, 1980) though their significance is unknown.

Feline herpesvirus has been isolated from cutaneous ulcers located on the thorax, abdomen and limbs of cats (Johnson & Sabine, 1971; Flecknell *et al.*, 1979). Oral ulceration also occurred in all of these cases. Two of the cases reported (Flecknell *et al.*, 1979) were treated with two doses of feline rhinotracheitis and calicivirus vaccine, ampicillin and, topically, with a 1% solution of 5-iodo-2'-deoxyuridine (an antiviral agent). Both responded well but when treatment was discontinued one cat relapsed.

Erosive changes at the medial canthi (Plate 1.10) and around the nares have been seen in cats subsequent to administration of combined intranasal feline calcivirus/herpes virus vaccines.

Feline sarcoma virus

The feline sarcoma virus, facilitated by FeLV (Carpenter *et al.*, 1987) induces multiple cutaneous fibrosarcomas in cats less than 3 years old (Hardy, 1981) (see section below, 'Cutaneous Neoplasms').

Cowpox virus (Orthopoxvirus)

A considerable number of cases of cowpox virus infection in cats have now been reported from the UK and elsewhere in Europe (Thomsett *et al.*, 1978; Gaskell *et al.*, 1983; Martland *et al.*, 1983).

The cutaneous lesions may be pruritic and are variable in character, including erythematous macules, papules and plaques, crusts overlying purulent ulcers and ulcerated nodules. Initial lesions are usually solitary and often located on the head, neck or forelimb but become generalized (Plate 1.11). Buccal ulceration and systemic signs such as pyrexia, anorexia, dyspnoea, coryza and diarrhoea may also occur.

Antibody titres in paired blood samples are helpful in diagnosis, which is confirmed by demonstration of characteristic intracytoplasmic inclusion bodies in epithelial cells or identification of the virus in crusts by electron microscopy (reviewed by Bennett, 1989).

Most cats recover spontaneously though broad-spectrum antibacterial cover is indicated to control secondary bacterial infections. Those animals developing pneumonia or pleural effusion should be investigated for immunosuppression (e.g. concurrent FeLV or FIV infection) and may die or require euthanasia. Glucocorticoids are always contraindicated as they exacerbate the condition.

Cats may transmit cowpox virus infection to man (Bennett, 1989) (see Chapter 18).

Pseudorabies (Aujeszky's disease, mad itch)

Pseudorabies, caused by herpesvirus suis, has been documented in cats (Horvarth & Papp, 1967).

Pruritus is a less consistent clinical feature in cats than dogs and in one series of naturally occurring cases was recorded in only 58.7% of animals (Horvath & Papp, 1967). It appears to be manifested most frequently as rubbing of one side of the head. Intense pruritus and self-mutilation are uncommon.

Diagnosis depends on a history of contact with pigs or ingestion of pigmeat, clinical signs of encephalitis (muscular tremors, salivation, opisthotonus, paralysis and convulsions) and virus isolation (clotted blood or tonsillar tissue) and identification using fluorescent antibody techniques.

The disease progresses rapidly and affected cats usually die 24 hours after onset of clinical signs (Howard, 1986) though some cases may survive for 7 days. No reliable treatment has yet been reported (see Chapter 20).

PROTOZOAL DISEASES

Toxoplasmosis

Toxoplasmosis is a multisystemic disease which may rarely causes nodular cutaneous lesions in cats (Frenkel *et al.*, 1987).

Leishmaniasis

Leishmaniasis, a disease endemic in the Mediterranean, Middle and Far East, areas of Central America and Central Africa, occurs rarely in cats and may be seen in the UK in quarantined animals.

Infection usually occurs as a result of the bites of blood-sucking sandflies but may also be introduced through wounds by direct contact. Reported skin lesions include ulcers covered by a crust and located on the lips, nose, eyelids and pinnae.

Diagnosis requires the demonstration of the organism (Giemsa's stain) in biopsies of affected skin. Successful treatment of feline leishmaniasis has not been reported.

FUNGAL DISEASES

Superficial mycoses
  Dermatophytoses
  Dermatomycoses
    Candidiasis
    Malassezia infection
    Trichosporonosis
Subcutaneous mycoses
  Sporotrichosis
  Phaeohyphomycosis
  Eumycotic mycetoma and fungal pseudo-mycetoma
Systemic mycoses
  Cryptococcosis
  Coccidioidomycosis
  Blastomycosis
  Histoplasmosis
  Paecilomycosis

Summary

Superficial mycoses are caused by fungi that may be primary animal or human pathogens, part of the cat's normal flora or found in soil. Dermatophytes constitute the most common fungal infections of cats, the other infections in this group being rare. Subcutaneous and systemic mycoses are caused by fungi occurring naturally in soil, decaying organic material and on plants. All are uncommon opportunistic pathogens of cats. They have been reported in the USA but are very rare in the UK and elsewhere in Europe.

The cutaneous lesions of dermatophytosis are superficial, varied and not usually accompanied by systemic signs. Lesions associated with dermatomycoses tend to be localized to the mouth and mucocutaneous areas (candidiasis) or ears (*Malassezia* infection) and may rarely be associated with systemic signs (candidiasis). Trichosporonosis, subcutaneous mycoses and systemic mycoses are associated with nodular granulomatous lesions, which may ulcerate and develop draining tracts, discharging pus onto the skin. The presence of granules composed of dense aggregates of fungal filaments in the pus distinguishes mycetomas from other subcutaneous mycoses. Although subcutaneous mycoses rarely become disseminated systemically they may be accompanied by systemic signs of illness. In contrast, systemic mycoses are rarely confined to the skin and clinical signs due to involvement of the respiratory, skeletal and central nervous systems and ocular lesions may be evident.

Superficial mycoses

Superficial mycoses are fungal infections of keratinized tissues: the stratum corneum, hair and nails. Dermatophytoses are infections of these tissues by species belonging to the genera *Microsporum*, *Trichophyton* and *Epidermophyton*. Dermatomycoses are infections of these tissues with non-dermatophytes.

Dermatophytosis (ringworm)

Dermatophytes are variably contagious, infecting animals and man by direct and indirect contact, and are extremely robust, surviving in the environment for 12 to 52 months. All cats are susceptible to dermatophytosis but certain factors may predispose to infection (Table 1.2).

Dermatophytes are particularly efficient parasites, frequently causing minimal reaction on the skin of their usual host, but a more severe response in species to which they are not adapted. All species of dermatophyte probably originated in the soil. They may be classified according to the following.

1 Host preference
  (a) Anthropophilic (primary pathogens of man, rarely transmitted to animals and incapable of surviving in soil)
  (b) Zoophilic (primary pathogens of animals, commonly transmitted to man and only rarely isolated from soil)
  (c) Geophilic (normally inhabit soil, occasionally infect animals)
2 Position of fungal spores on or in the hair
  (a) Ectothrix – almost all zoophilic species
  (b) Endothrix – some common anthropophilic species
3 Culture characteristics
4 In human medicine, the position on the body
  M. canis, a zoophilic fungus, is isolated from 94% of feline cases in the UK (Wright, 1989) and

Table 1.2 Factors predisposing to dermatophyte infections.

Age – young animals predisposed (low skin fatty acid concentrations, lack of acquired immunity)
Lack of acquired resistance
Defective cell-mediated immunity
Skin defects – abraded or microabraded skin probably required for establishment of initial infection
Nutritional deficiencies – in particular protein and vitamin A
Existing systemic disease
Climate – high temperature, high humidity

From Thoday (1981b) with kind permission.

is the principal cause of dermatophytosis in the USA (Kaplan & Ajello, 1959). The cat is probably its natural host and asymptomatic carrier states in this species are frequent. Although *T. mentagrophytes*, which has zoophilic and anthropophilic forms, commonly affects rodents, which constitute a potential source of infection for cats, it is only occasionally isolated from cases of feline dermatophytosis. *M. gypseum*, a geophilic fungus, is isolated infrequently from cats in the USA, and very rarely from cats in the UK.

Dermatophytes invade hair in the anagen phase and fungal hyphae advance downwards along the hair keratin to Adamson's fringe, the upper limit of mitotic activity in the hair root.

Clinically, the classical lesion of 'ringworm' is a rapidly growing circular area of alopecia involving the head and limbs (Plate 1.12a). However, it is essential to appreciate that cutaneous signs of dermatophytosis are extremely variable and include single or multiple, localized or generalized, circular or irregular lesions of alopecia, broken hair, scale, crusts, areas of increased dermal pigmentation, generalized seborrhoea sicca, secondary bacterial infection which occasionally may cause folliculitis and furunculosis, and onychomycosis. Pruritus and self-inflicted lesions may also occur, particularly in association with *T. mentagrophytes* infection (Plate 1.13), which may also cause granulomatous lesions.

Infections with *M. canis* are occasionally manifested as miliary, papulocrustous eruptions and rarely mycetomas. Kerion formation, the development of localized, inflamed, oedematous plaques with secondary bacterial infection and draining tracts, occurs occasionally following folliculitis or furunculosis and may constitute a hypersensitivity reaction. The fine, long-haired breeds such as the Persian may be almost symptomless carriers of *M. canis*. Such cases are potentially very important in the spread of the disease in catteries and the home.

Tentative diagnosis is suggested by the history, particularly involvement of in-contact animals or owners (Plate 1.12b) and by physical examination. Confirmation depends on demonstration of fungal infection. This may be achieved by UV light and direct microscopical examinations, by culture or skin biopsy (see above).

Dermatophytosis may be a self-limiting disease; spontaneous remission commonly occurs within 1–6 months and mild cases may not require drug therapy. A total body clip, with reclipping as necessary, to expose hidden lesions and facilitate topical treatment is advised in all cases. This seemingly time-consuming and costly procedure is, in fact, time-saving and economical because it reduces the duration of treatment and is well-tolerated by cats and clients (with prior warning) alike. Hair clippings should be disposed of carefully by burning.

Localized topical treatment of dermatophytosis is usually of less value in animals than in man because the coat makes application difficult, the usually widespread nature of the infection makes localized topical therapy impractical, and the lack of patient co-operation causes difficulties during and after application. It is not usually recommended by the authors. Total body dips, containing 2% lime sulphur, which is allowed to dry on, has been reported to be effective by Scott (1980), but, to the authors' knowledge, is not readily available in Britain. Povidine iodine has been found to be of value by the authors but may irritate and stain cats. A 0.2% solution of enilconazole applied as a total body rinse twice weekly for 4 weeks has been reported from France to be very effective in the management of feline dermatophytosis but it is not licensed for use in cats in the UK.

All severe or chronic cases, except pregnant queens, should be treated with the fungistatic antibiotic griseofulvin. The daily dose, of micro-size formulation usually recommended for cats is 15–20 mg/kg. However, these figures were based on metabolism studies carried out in man. Scott (1980) considers this may be ineffective in many feline cases and daily doses of 25–132 mg/kg have been used. Absorption of griseofulvin is enhanced and risk of vomiting reduced if it is administered with a fatty meal (2.5–5.0 ml corn oil). In all cases treatment should be continued for at least 2 weeks after clinical resolution has occurred and cultures are negative. If onychomycosis has

occurred, longterm (6–12 months) griseofulvin therapy may be required and if involvement of nails is extensive surgical amputation of nails may prove the most effective form of treatment. Griseofulvin is teratogenic and its use is contraindicated in pregnancy. It may also provoke idiosyncratic, dose-unrelated drug reactions presenting clinically as depression, anorexia, vomiting, diarrhoea, ataxia, jaundice, anaemia, neutropenia, ataxia and angioedema (Helton *et al.*, 1986; Kunkle & Meyer, 1987).

In addition to treating clinically affected cats, all in-contact animals should be screened for infection. All dermatophyte-positive animals should be treated as indicated above while dermatophyte-negative in-contact animals should receive the therapeutic dose of griseofulvin for 14 days. As dermatophytes survive in the environment for up to 52 months (Muller *et al.*, 1989), contaminated disposable items should be destroyed, and the environment vacuum-cleaned weekly with the bag and its contents being disposed of by burning. Where possible, fomites and the environment should be disinfected using iodine, formalin (10% solution), sodium hypochlorite (5% solution), chlorhexidine or steam. A procedure for elimination of fungal infection from catteries (Dawson & Noddle, 1968) is summarized in Table 1.3. Success depends on its vigorous and persistent application.

Treatment with ketoconazole (10–20 mg/kg/day given orally in divided doses) is effective (Woodard, 1983). But, unfortunately, adverse side effects are common and include anorexia, vomiting, diarrhoea, fever, depression and neurological abnormalities. It may also be tetragenic owing to the higher incidence of adverse effects and the occurence of ketoconazole resistant strains of *M. canis*, griseofulvin remains the drug of choice for the systemic treatment of feline dermatophytosis. Ketoconazole is not licensed for use in cats in the UK. The management of local lesions with radiofrequency current hypothermia (Lueker & Kainer, 1981) and treatment by vaccination (Mosher *et al.*, 1977) require further evaluation.

Table 1.3 Elimination of dermatophytosis from cat colonies.

1 Assess existing infection (physical examination, Wood's lamp, Mackenzie brush technique and culture)
2 Isolate and treat positive or carrier cases. Dose negative group prophylactically with griseofulvin for 2 weeks to prevent spread of infection
3 Use routine hygienic precautions when feeding and cleaning the two groups
4 Clean cattery with suitable disinfectants at weekly intervals
5 Reassess negative group after 2 weeks
6 Isolate and assess new cats (physical examination, Wood's lamp, Mackenzie brush technique and culture) prior to admission to the colony
7 Reject or treat positive cases

Dermatomycoses

CANDIDIASIS (MONILIASIS)

Candida albicans, a dimorphic fungus, is, in the yeast phase, a normal resident of the mucosae of the mouth, alimentary, genital and upper respiratory tracts. It may result in disease, usually in association with immunosuppression (e.g. FeLV or FIV infections, diabetes mellitus, glucocorticoid therapy), chronic debilitation or prolonged antibacterial therapy.

Lesions are characteristically whitish-grey plaques overlying non-healing erosions and may be found in the mouth, at mucocutaneous junctions and on nail folds.

Diagnosis depends on identification of the organism in scrapings and biopsy samples or following its culture.

Topical treatment with gentian violet (1 : 10 000 in 10% alcohol), nystatin, amphotericin B or miconazole is often adequate, though the latter may cause irritant reactions. Ketoconazole given orally (5–10 mg/kg twice daily) is effective. Amphotericin B may be used systemically in severe, unresponsive cases but is potentially severely nephrotoxic. Regimens for amphotericin B administration vary. Foil (1986) advised

0.25–0.5 mg/kg administered intravenously, over 5 to 10 minutes, in 50 ml dextrose (5% solution). To reduce renal toxicity this should be preceded and followed by intravenous administration of a 0.9% sodium chloride solution (5 ml/kg). Treatment is repeated three times weekly to a total dose of 4 mg/kg.

MALASSEZIA (PITYROSPORUM) INFECTION

Malassezia pachydermatis (*Pityrosporum canis*), a yeast, has been isolated from the normal external ear canal of cats and may occasionally be involved in the genesis of otitis externa (see 'Diseases of Specialized Cutaneous Areas', p. 74). Topical treatment with miconazole or nystatin is advised.

TRICHOSPORONOSIS

Infection with these saprophytic yeasts, which are found in soil, has been reported to cause cutaneous and nasal granulomata in cats after bites and is enhanced by immunosuppressive drugs or diseases (Doster *et al.*, 1987). There is currently no known treatment.

Subcutaneous mycoses

Subcutaneous mycoses are fungal infections which have penetrated, usually by trauma, to viable tissues beyond the keratinized layers of the skin. Systemic dissemination is rare. All the causal fungi occur naturally in soil or on plants, all are uncommon opportunistic pathogens of cats in the USA but are very rare in Europe.

Clinically, lesions are subcutaneous nodules and granulomata which may ulcerate and develop tracts discharging pus. The presence of granules in the pus distinguishes eumycotic mycetomas from other subcutaneous mycoses.

Sporotrichosis

Sporotrichosis is caused by *Sporothrix* (*Sporotrichium*) *schenckii*. Although the fungus shows universal distribution, it requires high humidity and temperature and clinical cases are unlikely to be encountered in the UK.

A spherical nodule, sometimes becoming

alopecic, ulcerated and discharging creamy pus, or crusty circular lesions and areas of necrosis, develop at the site(s) of entry (*cutaneous form*); infection may subsequently spread along lymphatics (*cutaneous-lymphatic form*) and may rarely become disseminated.

Diagnosis depends on isolation of the organism by culture of pus or biopsy material.

Successful treatment of the cutaneous form with 0.1 ml/kg sodium iodide administered orally as a 20% solution twice daily in milk or food has been reported (Scott, 1980). Two months' treatment with ketoconazole (5 mg/kg twice daily) alone resulted in only partial resolution of the cutaneous-lymphatic form (Burke *et al.*, 1983) but the subsequent combined administration of ketoconazole and sodium iodide achieved complete resolution. Amphotericin B has also been used successfully (Attelburger, 1988).

Phaeohyphomycosis

Phaeohyphomycosis results from infection with members of the Dematiaceae (brown or black pigmented fungi), notably *Phialophora verrucosa*, *Exophiala jeanselmei*, *Drechslera spicifera*, *Cladosporium* spp., *Stemphylium* spp. and *Moniliella suaveolens*. These produce single or multiple subcutaneous nodules, which may become ulcerated, develop tracts and discharge pus the colour of which reflects the pigmentation of the causal fungi. Systemic dissemination may occur but is rare.

Diagnosis is supported by histopathological demonstration of hyaline or dark-walled septate hyphae in affected tissue and confirmed by culture of the causal fungi from samples of discharge or biopsy material.

Possible treatments include surgical excision of nodules, oral ketoconazole (Sousa *et al.*, 1984), amphotericin B alone or combined with 5-fluorocytosine (McKeever *et al.*, 1983) or a combination of these. Local recurrence may occur.

Eumycotic mycetomas and fungal pseudomycetoma

Mycetomas are localized chronic granulomatous reactions characterized by the presence of granules (grains) composed of dense aggregates of fungal or bacterial filaments and provoked by mycotic or actinomycotic infections of skin, subcutaneous tissue or bone. Sinuses frequently develop and discharge granules and pus onto the skin. Haematogenous dissemination of infection is rare. Mycetomas resulting from actinomycotic infections have been discussed previously.

Eumycetomas are produced by the eumycotic fungi *Curvularia geniculata*, *Pseudoallescheria boydii*, *Aspergillus* spp., *Madurella* spp. and *Cephalosporium* spp. (Emmons *et al.*, 1977). These are normally present in soil, on plants or in decaying organic material and are introduced into subcutaneous tissue by penetrating wounds. In cats eumycetoma due to *Cephalosporium potronii* (van den Akker, 1952), *Madurella grisea* (Holzworth, 1987a) and a member of the genus *Torula* (van den Broek & Thoday, 1987) (Plate 1.14) have been reported.

Pseudomycetoma is a rare, subcutaneous infection caused by dermatophytes or nonactinomycete bacteria. *M. canis* and *Trichophyton* spp. have been reported to cause pseudomycetoma, over the flanks of cats, characterized by firm nodules and ulcers with variable discharge (Bourdin *et al.*, 1975; Tuttle & Chandler, 1983; Miller & Goldschmidt, 1986; Yager *et al.*, 1986).

Treatment for mycetomas and fungal pseudomycetomas comprises radical surgical excision accompanied by amphotericin B (mycetomas) or griseofulvin (fungal pseudomycetomas) and an antibacterial agent if appropriate.

Systemic mycoses

Systemic mycoses are fungal infections of internal organs. Cutaneous involvement results from secondary haematogenous dissemination or direct skin infection by trauma, inoculation or contamination of wounds. The organisms are contracted from the soil or decaying organic material (see Chapter 23).

Cryptococcosis (torulosis, European blastomycosis)

Cryptococcus neoformans is a saprophytic, yeast-like organism found in soil, particularly in association with pigeon droppings, which provide it with creatinine as a source of nitrogen. It has a worldwide distribution. Infection with *C. neoformans* principally involves the upper respiratory tract, central nervous system, eyes and skin.

Multiple cutaneous or subcutaneous granulomas or abscesses are frequently located on the head and may ulcerate and exude a gelatinous or mucosanguinous fluid. The drainage lymph nodes may be enlarged. Immunosuppression, particularly impaired cell-mediated immunity, may increase susceptibility to infection and thus the FeLV and FIV status of affected cats should be investigated.

Successful treatment with amphotericin B combined with 5-fluorocytosine has been reported (Prevost *et al.*, 1982).

Coccidioidomycosis

Coccidioides immitis is a soil organism limited to the south-western USA, Mexico and South America.

Cutaneous lesions (chronic draining abscesses or discharging sinuses) result from contamination of wounds or dissemination from pulmonary infections. Clinical signs related to respiratory, skeletal and ocular lesions may also be evident.

Blastomycosis (North American blastomycosis)

Blastomyces dermatitidis is a dimorphic fungus, entering the yeast phase in animal tissues. Its habitat (probably soil) is yet to be determined but is geographically limited to Canada, the USA, Central and South America, and Africa. Skin infection follows dissemination from the lungs or introduction into the skin by trauma or inoculation and produces granulomatous, draining cutaneous lesions. The major clinical signs are associated with respiratory tract lesions though CNS and ocular lesions also occur.

Histoplasmosis

Histoplasma capsulatum is a dimorphic fungus found in soil, especially that enriched by faeces from birds and bats. It has a wide geographical distribution in temperate and tropical climates.

It becomes a yeast in animal tissues and may cause granulomatous, ulcerated or draining cutaneous lesions. However, upper and lower respiratory tract signs are most common. Ocular, skeletal and rarely CNS involvement also occur.

Paecilomycosis

Digital granuloma and nasal infection caused by *Paecilomyces fumosoroseus* has been reported in a cat (Elliot *et al.*, 1984). Treatment with oral ketoconazole and surgery was unsuccessful.

ALGAL DISEASES

Protothecosis

Prototheca spp. are saprophytic, colourless algae, with a worldwide distribution. Mammalian infection rarely occurs but may be predisposed to by immunosuppression. In cats, large, solitary, granulomatous, subcutaneous masses located on the head (Finnie & Chloe, 1981) or a limb (Kaplan *et al.*, 1976; Chloe & Allinson, 1982) have been reported. *Prototheca wickerhamii* was isolated from the lesions involving limbs.

Diagnosis is made by identification of the organism in biopsy material.

Treatment is by radical surgical excision. Amphotericin B alone (Mayhall *et al.*, 1976) or combined with tetracycline (Venezio *et al.*, 1982) has been used successfully to treat human protothecosis but data on such treatment regimens for cats are not available.

PARASITIC DISEASES

Helminth parasites
  Anatrichosomiasis
  Dracunculosis
Arthropod parasites
  Arachnida

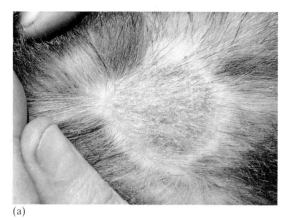

(a)

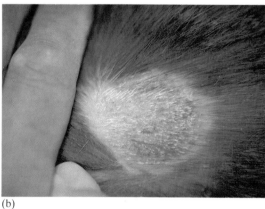

(b)

Plate 1.1 The textbook 'ringworm' lesion. The appearance of *Microsporum canis* infection (a) before and (b) during illumination by ultraviolet (Wood's) lamp. (Reproduced with permission from Thoday, 1979, 1981b.)

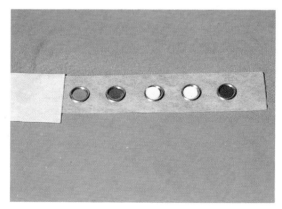

Plate 1.2 Finn Chambers. Adhesive tape attached aluminium discs into which test allergens may be placed direct or absorbed onto the papers supplied.

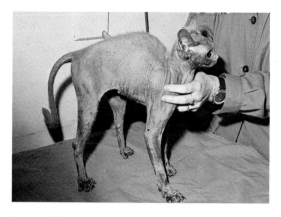

Plate 1.3 Hereditary hypotrichosis in a female Devon Rex cat.

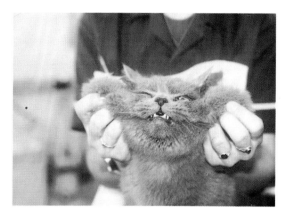

Plate 1.4 Skin hyperextensibility in a cat with cutaneous asthenia. (Courtesy of D.I. Grant.)

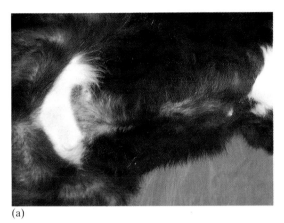

(a)

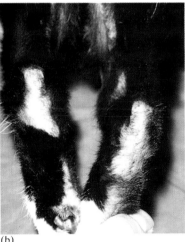

(b)

Plate 1.5 Hyperthyroid, 16-year-old, neutered female domestic short-haired cat. (a) Diffuse thinning of hair over the ventral thorax, abdomen and medial thighs. (b) Patchy alopecia over the caudal hocks. (Reproduced with permission from Thoday, 1988.)

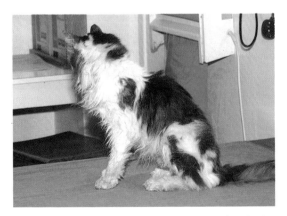

Plate 1.6 Hyperthyroid, 15-year-old, neutered male domestic long-haired cat. The coat condition is poor with numerous mats. (Reproduced with permission from Thoday, 1988.)

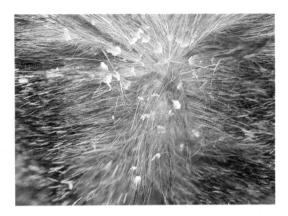

Plate 1.7 Seborrhoea sicca in a cat with chronic hepatic disease. (Reproduced with permission from Thoday, 1981b.)

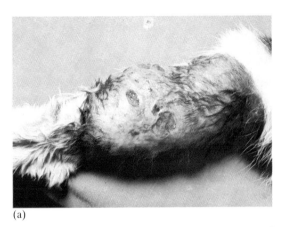

(a)

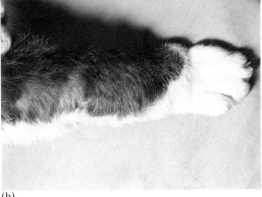

(b)

Plate 1.8 *Rhodococcus (Corynebacterium) equi* cellulitis. (a) Before and (b) 9 weeks after beginning antibacterial therapy.

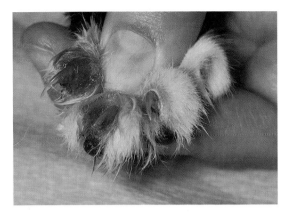

Plate 1.9 Paronychia associated with feline leukaemia virus infection in a 4-year-old, neutered female domestic long-haired cat.

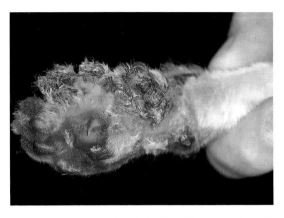

Plate 1.11 Orthopoxvirus infection. (Courtesy of G.H. Sture.)

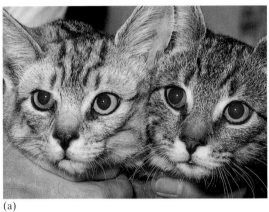

(a)

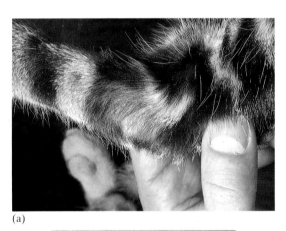

(a)

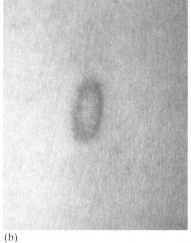

(b)

(b)

Plate 1.10 (a) Alopecia and erosions at the nasal canthi of two 16-week-old kittens subsequent to intranasal administration of a combined herpesvirus/calicivirus vaccine. These lesions were not secondary to clinical conjunctivitis and ocular discharges. (b) A close-up view of one of the cats. (Courtesy of B.M. Corcoran.)

Plate 1.12 Dermatophytosis: *Microsporum canis* infection on the (a) elbow of a kitten and (b) the thorax of its owner.

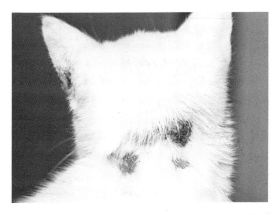

Plate 1.13 Dermatophytosis: *Trichophyton mentagrophytes* infection.

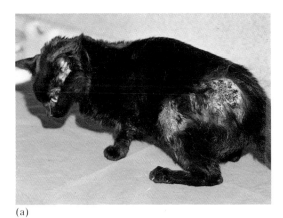

(a)

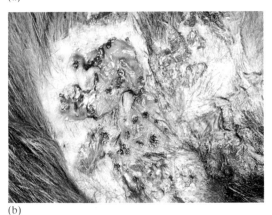

(b)

Plate 1.14 Subcutaneous mycosis: (a), (b) infection with a fungus of the form genus *Torula*. The black granules are aggregations of fungal hyphae.

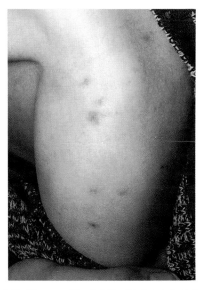

Plate 1.15 Human *Cheyletiella blakei* infestation: the maculopapular lesions are often in groups of three.

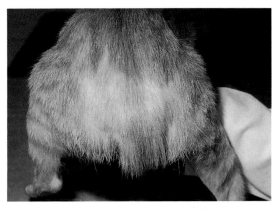

Plate 1.16 Flea infestation: alopecia and broken hairs over the dorsal lumbosacral area.

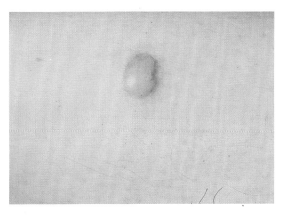

Plate 1.17 Bullous eruption due to *Ctenocephalides felis* bite: human leg.

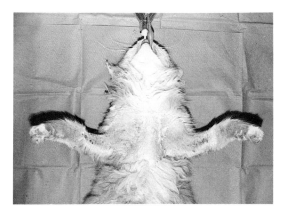

Plate 1.18 Chemical irritant dermatitis: turpentine substitute was used to remove paint from the coat. (Reproduced with permission from Thoday, 1981b.)

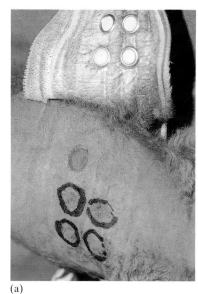

(a)

(b)

Plate 1.19 Patch testing as an aid to distinguish chemical irritant dermatitis from contact hypersensitivity. (a) (b) The test substance (wax furniture polish) has produced a bulla when tested undiluted but minimal response in graded dilutions. The irritant nature of the reaction was confirmed by evoking similar responses on another of the owner's cats which had no evidence of skin disease.

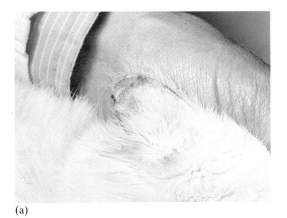

(a)

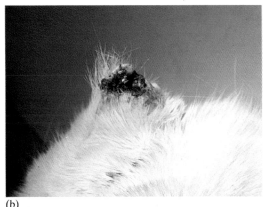

(b)

Plate 1.20 Feline solar dermatitis. (a) Early lesion of the left ear showing alopecia and curling of the cartilage. (b) The right ear of the same cat: squamous cell carcinoma formation.

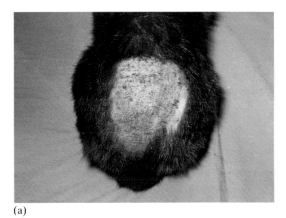

(a)

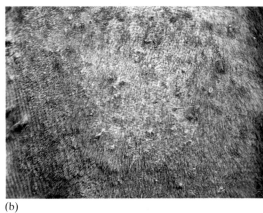

(b)

Plate 1.21 (a) Papulocrustous (miliary) eruption due to flea bite hypersensitivity. The hair has been clipped from the cat's dorsal lumbosacral area to demonstrate the lesions. (b) Close-up of the lesions. (Reproduced with permission from Thoday, 1981b.)

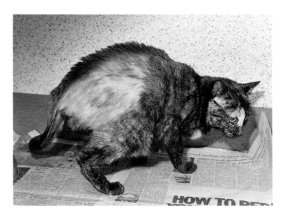

Plate 1.22 Food hypersensitivity: pruritus with resultant self-inflicted injury caused fracture of hairs and alopecia over a large but solitary area. (Reproduced with permission from Thoday, 1981b.)

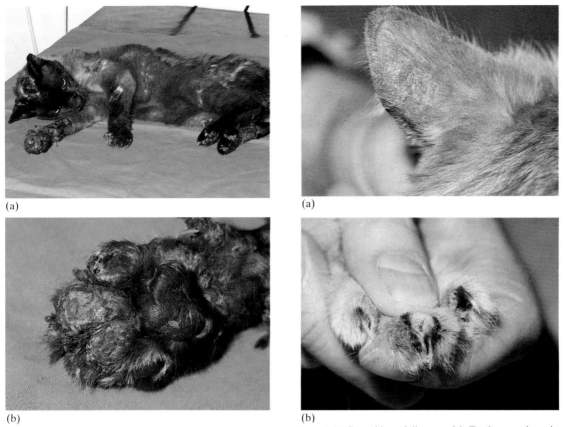

(a)

(b)

Plate 1.23 Pemphigus foliaceus: (a) Widespread distribution in this 14-year-old neutered female Tonkinese cat. (b) Hyperkeratosis of pads of the right forefoot.

(a)

(b)

Plate 1.24 Pemphigus foliaceus: (a) Erythema, alopecia and crusts on the pinna. (b) Paronychia and pyonychia.

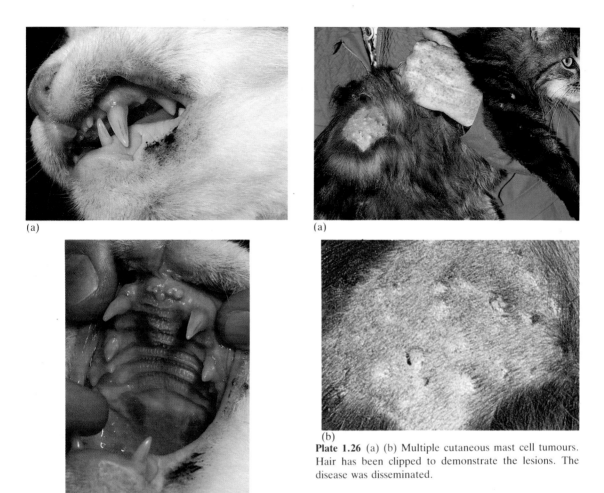

(a)

(a)

(b)

(b)
Plate 1.26 (a) (b) Multiple cutaneous mast cell tumours. Hair has been clipped to demonstrate the lesions. The disease was disseminated.

Plate 1.25 Systemic lupus erythematosus: (a) Labial erosions and crusts. (b) Erosions and ulcers on the hard and soft palates. (Courtesy of Julie I. Henfrey.)

Tick infestation
Otodectes infestation
Feline scabies
Sarcoptes scabiei infestation
Lynxacarus radovskyi infestation
Cheyletiella infestation
Demodicosis
Trombicula infestation
Dermanyssus gallinae infestation
Insecta
  Flea infestation
  Pediculosis
  Myiasis
  Cuterebriasis

Summary

Flea infestation and *Otodectes* infestation occur frequently, tick, *Trombicula* and *Cheyletiella* infestation are seen less commonly and the remaining conditions are uncommon in cats. Anatrichosomiasis, dracunculosis, cuterebriasis and cat fur mite infestation have not been reported in the UK.

No age, breed or sex incidence for parasitic infestations have been observed in cats except in *Otodectes* infestation, which is particularly common in kittens. A seasonal incidence occurs in *Trombicula* and tick infestations, myiasis, cuterebriasis and, less commonly now that central heating of houses has become commonplace, flea infestation. Immunosuppressive diseases predispose to demodicosis.

Some conditions may be associated with particular signs such as discharging cutaneous nodules/cysts (anatrichosomiasis and cuterebriasis), ulcerated footpads (dracunculosis), otitis externa (*Otodectes* infestation), salt and pepper appearance of the coat (pediculosis, cheyletiellosis, *Lynxacarus radovskyi* infestation) and ulceration and undermining of the skin (myiasis). In other conditions, cutaneous signs are diverse but often include a variable degree of pruritus, alopecia, seborrhoea and papulocrustous (miliary) eruptions. With some of the infestations, in-contact owners and/or animals may also have cutaneous lesions.

Helminth parasites

Anatrichosomiasis

Anatrichosomiasis, resulting from infestation with migrating larvae of the nematode *Anatrichosoma cutaneum*, has been reported in a South African cat presented with lameness, necrosis, sloughing and ulceration of the footpads of all four feet (Lange *et al.*, 1980).

Diagnosis was based on demonstration of adult worms (females 42 mm long) and bioperculate eggs within the epidermis.

Dracunculosis

Dracunculosis, resulting from infestation with *Dracunculus medinensis*, has been reported in cats in the USA (Scott, 1980). Infection is acquired by drinking water containing the parasite's intermediate crustacean host. Adult worms produced pruritic nodules, located on the limbs or trunk, which discharged a milky-white exudate.

Diagnosis is based on identification of larvae in the exudate and treatment is by surgical excision of nodules or administration of thiabendazole.

Arthropod parasites

Tick infestation

Ticks are not host-specific and although several species may affect the cat, infestation is uncommon (Scott, 1980). In the UK, infestations with *Ixodes hexogonus* and *I. ricinus* occur most frequently.

They are usually located on the head, ears, neck or limbs. Although, potentially, tick bites may provoke irritation or pruritus they generally appear to cause little discomfort and affected cats are presented because the owner has noticed a 'cyst' or 'growth'.

Numerous different methods for removing ticks have been proposed (Scott, 1980) but gentle manual extraction, using mosquito forceps to grasp the capitulum as close as possible to the skin, is very effective. If the mouthparts are not completely extracted, they may provoke a granulomatous, foreign body reaction. Such a reaction sometimes occurs in the absence of mouthpart retention, suggesting a chronic immunological response (perhaps due to arthropod antigens bound to dermal collagen), which may sometimes be aborted by intralesional glucocorticoids. Otherwise, reactions should be removed surgically. If several ticks are present, manual removal should be combined with the use of a parasiticidal powder or spray to eliminate undetected parasites.

Otodectes cynotis infestation

Otodectes cynotis is an obligate, relatively large, non-burrowing mite and the commonest cause of otitis externa in cats, especially kittens. Occasionally it causes cutaneous lesions elsewhere, notably on the head, interscapular area, base of the tail and paws.

In the external ear canal it provokes irritant and hypersensitivity reactions resulting in the production of a thick, granular, reddish-black discharge and predisposing to secondary bacterial infections. The degree of pruritus varies and if severe may be accompanied by excoriations of the pinnae, head shaking and formation of aural haematomata. Cutaneous lesions include localized alopecia, erythema, scale and crust formation. These are associated with a variable degree of pruritus.

Diagnosis is by visualizing the white mite by direct auroscopic inspection or by microscopic identification of the mite in exudate taken from the ear or in scrapings from cutaneous lesions. Occasionally the mites may cause lesions on in-contact humans.

Treatment of uncomplicated otodectic otitis by instillation of parasiticidal ear drops into the external ear canal twice weekly is usually effective and should be continued 2 weeks beyond clinical cure (usually 4 weeks). A 0.5% solution of amitraz in 50% propylene glycol instilled into the ear canal (Bussiéras & Chermette, 1986) and ivermectin (1 mg in cats less than 5 kg; 1.5 mg in cats more than 5 kg) injected subcutaneously (Schneck, 1988) have also been reported to be effective but are not licensed for use in cats in the UK. As the mite is highly contagious, all in-contact animals should be treated at the same time. In cases with severe pruritus or secondary bacterial infection,

use of a preparation combining anti-inflammatory, antibacterial, antimycotic and parasiticidal therapy may be indicated. If cutaneous lesions are also present, if the condition persists or rapidly recurs or in multi-animal households, the whole body should be treated with a suitable parasiticide (e.g. dichlorvos/fenitrothion or pyrethrins/ pyrethroids). In persistent or recurrent infestations it may also be necessary to introduce measures, similar to those used for flea control, to eliminate the mite from the environment.

Feline scabies

Feline scabies is an intensely irritating, highly contagious, scaling dermatosis caused by infestation with the burrowing mite *Notoedres cati*. The mite is an obligatory parasite, the female laying eggs in intraepidermal burrows and surviving for only a few days off the host. Its life cycle is completed in 17 days. The disease is very rare in the UK.

Clinically, feline scabies is characterized by intensely pruritic cutaneous lesions comprising erythema, scale, crusts and lichenification. These are accompanied by excoriations, alopecia and secondary bacterial infection. Lesions are usually concentrated on the ears, head and neck but may spread to the elbows, feet and genitalia. Regional lymphadenopathy may occur. Affected cats may have a mouse-like odour. In a single case the only clinical sign of infestation was a mild dorsal scale (Thoday, 1985).

The diagnosis is suggested by the clinical signs, and supported by involvement of other animals in the household and, possibly, of the owners (pruritic papulocrustous lesions classically on the arms and trunk). Microscopic identification of the mite (which has a similar appearance to *Sarcoptes scabiei* var. *canis* but is smaller with a dorsal anus and concentric striations) in skin scrapings confirms the diagnosis.

Treatment with parasiticidal shampoos (1% selenium sulphide) once weekly until 2 weeks after clinical remission is usually effective. If indicated, this should initially be combined with glucocorticoids and antibacterial agents to reduce pruritus and manage secondary bacterial infection. In-contact cats, dogs and rabbits should be similarly treated. Amitraz as 0.025% washes (Bussiéras & Chermette, 1986) and ivermectin (1 mg/kg) given by subcutaneous injection (Muller *et al.*, 1989) have also been used successfully but are not licensed for use in cats in the UK.

Sarcoptes scabiei infestation

A number of confirmed cases of infestation with the canine scabies mite (terminal anus and transverse striations) have been described in cats (Bussiéras, 1984; Hawkins *et al.*, 1987; Kershaw, 1989).

The lesions consisted of erythematous papules, yellow-grey crusts and scales, and involved the tail, scrotum, perineum, medial and caudal aspects of the hindlegs and feet. Pruritus was absent to intense.

In one case, (Kershaw, 1989), weekly treatment with 1% sulphur baths for 6 weeks and a bromocyclen spray for a further 3 weeks was successful.

It has been suggested that immunodeficiency may predispose to the establishment of these infestations.

Lynxacarus radovskyi (cat fur mite) infestation

Infestation of cats with *Lynxacarus radovskyi*, a rare parasite of cats, has been reported in Australia, USA, Puerto Rico and Fiji (reviewed by Scott, 1984) but not, as yet, Europe. The mites do not appear to be highly contagious.

Clinically the infestation imparts a 'salt and pepper' appearance to the coat due to the mite attaching to the distal part of the hair shaft. Affected cats may also develop a patchy alopecia, seborrhoea sicca and generalized papulocrustous eruptions. Pruritus is absent or minimal.

Diagnosis is made by identification of mites on hair samples, skin scrapings or adhesive tape impression.

Treatment with parasiticidal baths once a week for 3 weeks is usually effective.

Cheyletiella infestation

Infestation with *Cheyletiella* spp. is uncommon in cats. *C. blakei* is the species usually found in cats, while *C. yasguri* and *C. parasitovorax* may be present if in-contact dogs or rabbits are infested. *Cheyletiella* spp. are surface-living, obligate parasites just visible to the naked eye, the life cycle of which is completed in 34 days. Adult females may survive up to 10 days off the host while larvae, nymphs and adult males die within 2 days.

Infestations occur principally along the dorsum and in some cats are asymptomatic while in others a variety of clinical signs occur, including seborrhoea sicca, papulocrustous eruptions and a variable degree of pruritus. Occasionally pruritus may occur in the absence of cutaneous lesions.

Diagnosis is suggested by the clinical signs, the observation of 'walking dandruff' (with or without a magnifying lens) and of the occurrence, on the owner, of grouped (often in threes), pruritic, maculopapulovesicular eruptions (Plate 1.15). Microscopic identification of the mites or their eggs in coat brushings or superficial skin scrapings or material collected by adhesive tape confirms the diagnosis. The mites are characterized by prominent palpi (accessory mouthparts) and setae (combs) located terminally on their legs, while their eggs are oval and attached to hairs by only one pole. In cases with minimal or no cutaneous lesions, faecal flotation may facilitate recovery of the mites. The species of mite involved may be determined by the shape of the sensory organ on genu 1: cone-shaped, *C. blakei*; globoid, *C. parasitovorax*; heart-shaped, *C. yasguri*.

Treatment with 1% selenium sulphide washes once weekly for 4 weeks, is usually successful in eliminating the parasite. In-contact animals should be similarly treated and the environment treated with an insecticidal spray. Powders and sprays may not be effective in eradicating infestations on animals as mites are shielded by epidermal debris.

Demodicosis

Demodicosis has been reported rarely in cats and has been associated with concurrent potentially immunosuppressive diseases such as FeLV and FIV infections, upper respiratory tract infections, toxoplasmosis, diabetes mellitus, hyperadreno-corticism, glucocorticoid administration and systemic lupus erythematosus (reviewed by Chesney, 1989). Infestations may be due to *Demodex cati*, which is located in hair follicles and is not contagious; some, though, are caused by a currently unnamed species which infests the stratum corneum (Conroy *et al.*, 1982). This newly described species is relatively short and has a broad, blunted abdomen.

Cutaneous lesions may be focal, multifocal or, very rarely, generalized and are usually located on the head (nose, eyelids and periocular area), pinnae, and body. Typically alopecia, with or without erythema, seborrhoea and hyperpigmentation are present. Follicular papules, secondary pyoderma and a moderate to severe degree of pruritus may also occur. In some cases the only clinical feature is ceruminous otitis externa.

Diagnosis relies on identification of the mite in deep skin scrapings, pus samples or, in cats with ceruminous otitis, smears from ear swabs. In all cases, the possibility of underlying immunosuppressive diseases should be investigated.

Though localized areas of demodicosis may heal spontaneously, treatment of all cases is advised. Presumably because of the often superficial location of feline demodicosis, successful therapy has been reported with such simple regimens as weekly pyrethrin-carbamate shampoos and weekly malathion or 2% lime-sulphur dips. Treatment with amitraz, fenchlorphos and phosmet has also been reported to be effective (Medleau *et al.*, 1988). However, in cats, total body applications of amitraz have been associated with anorexia, depression and malodorous faeces and neither it, nor fenchlorphos or phosmet are licensed for use in cats in the UK. In addition to controlling the parasite, any underlying immunosuppressive disease should be corrected if possible.

Trombicula (Neotrombicula) autumnalis (harvest mite, berry bug, chigger) infestation
Only the larvae of *Trombicula autumnalis*, a free-living mite, are parasitic. Infestation, obtained from grassland or wooded areas, occurs seasonally during late summer and autumn.

Larvae are usually located on the head (particularly the ears) and feet. Less commonly they may be found elsewhere. Infestation may be asymptomatic or provoke a papulocrustous reaction accompanied by a variable degree of pruritus and self-inflicted damage.

Tentative diagnosis is made on the basis of season and distribution of lesions. It is confirmed by macro- or microscopic identification of the 0.2 mm, orange to red, six-legged larvae.

Treatment with one application of a reliable parasiticide (dichlorvos/fenitrothion spray, pyrethrin/pyrethroid powder or spray, selenium sulphide, sulphur or monosulfiram washes) is adequate as breeding does not occur on the host, but may need to be repeated if reinfestation occurs. Rarely, short-term glucocorticoids may be required to control severe pruritus.

Dermanyssus gallinae infestation
Dermanyssus gallinae, the red mite of poultry, may also parasitize wild and cage birds and rarely mammals. Normally it hides during the day in nests or in crevices and cracks in poultry houses or cages and emerges at night to feed. Its life cycle can be completed in 7 days but may extend to 5 months depending on opportunities to feed, it being able to survive without feeding for many months.

Infestation of cats is associated with papulocrustous lesions and pruritus commonly affecting the face, dorsum and limbs.

Diagnosis may be suggested by the history (access to a poultry house) and is confirmed by macro- or microscopic identification of the 0.7 mm long mites. These are yellow-white in colour when fasting and red after feeding.

Treatment of affected cats with selenium sulphide washes is effective but parasiticidal sprays must be used in the environment to prevent reinfestation.

Insecta

Flea infestation

Flea allergy dermatitis (FAD) is the most important single cause of skin disease in cats in the UK. The species most commonly identified on cats are *Ctenocephalides felis* (94%), *Spilopsyllus cuniculi* (the rabbit flea; 4%) and *Archeopsyllus erinacei* (the hedgehog flea; 1%) (W.P. Beresford Jones & M.R. Geary, personal communication).

Fleas are facultative parasites. Eggs may be laid in the environment or on the host. In optimal conditions adults normally live for a year but separated from the host may survive for only 3 to 4 months. In favourable environmental conditions (moderate ambient temperature and high humidity) the life cycle may be completed in 14 days but may be arrested in adverse conditions.

Although irritant responses to flea bites may produce clinical signs, hypersensitivity reactions (Types I and IV) together with cutaneous basophil hypersensitivity are probably most important. The typical signs are pruritus and papulocrustous (miliary) eruptions distributed along the dorsum (particularly the lumbosacral area) (Plate 1.16), the posteromedial aspect of the hindlimbs, the ventral abdomen, the head and the neck. These may be accompanied by excoriations, alopecia due to fractured hair shafts, acute moist dermatitis, seborrhoea sicca and secondary pyoderma. Eosinophilic granuloma or plaques and symmetrical alopecia may also occur with or without miliary eruptions.

A tentative diagnosis is made on the basis of clinical signs, and is supported by the detection of flea faeces and/or fleas on the cat. However, cats are fastidious washers and fleas may be transient visitors to the cat's skin so neither may be identified. Eosinophilia may be helpful in differentiating flea-allergic dermatitis from idiopathic feline symmetrical alopecia (Thoday, 1986b, 1990a). The occurrence of skin lesions on other animals in the home and on the owners (papular urticaria and bullae; Plate 1.17), and response to treatment support the diagnosis positive reactions to the intradermal injection of flea antigen.

Successful treatment depends on the institution of an intense, persistent programme of flea eradication directed at both the affected animals and their environment. Affected and in-contact animals should be sprayed or dusted with an effective parasiticide possessing residual action, e.g. dichlorvos/fenitrothion or pyrethrins/pyrethroids (the latter being the only safe parasiticides for use on kittens).

The environment should be vacuum-cleaned thoroughly, especially in sites where the animal sleeps, and then sprayed ideally with an insect growth regulator such as methoprene alone or in combination with a parasiticide or a parasiticidal spray (e.g. iodophenophos/dichlorvos). The contents of the dustbag should be burned. This programme should be repeated regularly until control is achieved. Methoprene spraying may be used continually in the environment of severely affected animals. Flea collars are of little value in controlling flea infestation and may cause contact irritation or hypersensitivity. Hyposensitization has been used to attempt to modulate the immune response to flea saliva antigen in cats, but reports of its value are not encouraging.

Pediculosis

Pediculosis is infestation by lice. These parasites are obligatory, host-specific insects capable of surviving in the environment for only a few days. Pediculosis is uncommon in cats and is sometimes associated with debility or neglect. It is usually due to the biting louse *Felicola subrostratus*, although *Trichodectes canis*, the biting louse of dogs, has been found on kittens and aged cats (Wilkinson, 1966).

The clinical signs vary and include papulocrustous eruptions, seborrhoea sicca, dorsal and symmetrical alopecia and variable pruritus. These may be accompanied by a variable degree of pruritus. Some cats may be asymptomatic carriers.

Diagnosis is made by identification of the parasite or its eggs, which are cemented to the hair shaft along one side in contrast to those of *Cheyletiella*, which are attached to the hair shaft at only one pole of the egg. Thorough treatment with a suitable parasiticide usually results in rapid clearing of the condition. Parasiticidal treatment should be repeated once a week for 4 weeks. Short-term glucocorticoids may be used if the pruritus is severe.

Myiasis (fly strike)
Cutaneous myiasis is a rare, seasonal (summer) condition of cats, in individuals predisposed by debility, injury and neglected wounds. Blowflies (calliphorids) and flesh flies (sarcophagids) deposit their eggs in the coat in areas often contaminated with urine, faeces and other discharges. The usual areas involved are those round the anus, genitalia, eyes, nose and any discharging wounds. The resultant larvae produce proteolytic enzymes that cause cutaneous ulceration, which may become extensive.

Treatment requires clipping away hair to expose the full extent of the lesions, and manual removal of all larvae, followed by gentle cleaning of affected tissue and topical application of a suitable antibacterial agent. In addition, the coat (but not the lesions) should be treated with a suitable parasiticide and the predisposing cause of the condition determined and treated.

Cuterebriasis
Cuterebriasis is a rare seasonal (summer/autumn) condition caused by larvae of *Cuterebria* spp. flies. Adult flies deposit their eggs on stones or on plants near rabbit and rodent burrows and these may be transferred to the coat of cats passing through these areas. After hatching, larvae may parasitize cats, penetrating the skin in the submandibular or neck area, or being ingested when the cat grooms. They subsequently undergo an aberrant migration or develop in a 1-cm subcutaneous swelling which discharges a sanguinous fluid through a fistula (Kazacos *et al.*, 1980).

Treatment is by manual extraction of the larva and drainage of the swelling. Crushing of the larva should be avoided as irritant or allergic reactions may be produced against retained material. Healing, following drainage, is usually slow.

DISEASES DUE TO HYMENOPTERA

Bee and wasp stings
Cats are occasionally stung by bees and wasps during the summer months, particularly in the early or late parts of the season when these insects are torpid. Young, inquisitive animals are most commonly affected, usually on the face or feet. Pain followed by local inflammation (hyperaemia and oedema) develops and, in some animals, anaphylaxis may occur.

Treatment is by extraction of the sting, where present, and the application, if feasible, of cold compresses. Glucocorticoids may be required in severe cases and, because of the risk of airway obstruction due to oedema, should always be given if the lesion is in the oral cavity. Antihistamines are of limited value.

ENVIRONMENTAL DISEASES

Trauma
    Contusions, abrasions and lacerations
    Foreign bodies
Contact irritants/and chemical burns
    Physical irritant dermatitis
    Chemical irritant dermatitis
    Chemical burns
Poisons
    Thallium
    Chlorinated naphthalene
Ultraviolet radiation
    Actinic keratoses
    Feline solar dermatitis
Temperature
    Temperature-dependent coat colour
    Thermal burns
    Frostbite

Traumatic diseases

Contusions, abrasions and lacerations
A variety of traumatic events may produce contusions, abrasions and lacerations. In most instances, contusions do not require treatment. Abrasions should be clipped free of hair, gently

cleaned and dressed with an emollient ointment such as zinc and castor oil. Lacerations should be thoroughly cleaned using chlorhexidine solution (0.05%), which has broad-spectrum antibacterial activity, debrided if necessary and then closed, obliterating dead space and inserting drains if appropriate. Systemic antibacterial therapy may be required.

Foreign bodies

Foreign bodies (grass awns, splinters of wood, gravel, glass etc.) may occasionally result in skin lesions in cats. If affecting the feet and legs they may be associated with lameness. Often there is a discharging sinus which may respond temporarily to antibacterial agents. Aural foreign bodies provoke sudden-onset, violent head-shaking and scratching of the affected ear.

Management is by surgical removal of the foreign body.

Contact irritants and chemical burns

Physical irritant dermatitis

Physical irritants such as sand and gravel rarely cause contact dermatitis in cats. Clinically the lesions are usually limited to interdigital erythema.

Diagnosis is based on history and clinical signs and confirmed by confirmation of remission of lesions on avoidance, and recurrence following provocative exposure.

Chemical irritant dermatitis

Chemical irritant contact dermatitis is uncommon in cats. It may be caused by a variety of chemicals (Table 1.4), referred to as primary irritants which, on direct contact with the skin, provoke an inflammatory response which is not mediated by hypersensitivity reactions.

The distribution of the lesions is determined by the area(s) exposed to the irritant and degree of protection afforded by the hair covering in these areas. The relatively glabrous ventral surfaces are the sites most usually affected. Particularly susceptible areas are the chin, axillae (Plate 1.18), inner aspects of the pinnae, the ventral thorax

Table 1.4 Agents reported to have caused chemical irritant dermatitis in cats.

Flea collars	Various oils and greases
Insecticides	Wax polish
Kerosene	Highly chlorinated water
Turpentine	Iodine compounds
Paint	Quaternary ammonium compounds
Tars	Naphthols
Phenols	Fertilizers
Cresols	Acids
Various soaps	Salt
Various topical medicaments	Benzoyl peroxide

Adapted from Scott (1980).

and abdomen, the medial aspects of the hindlimbs, the perineum and feet. If the irritant is a liquid, any part of the body may be involved.

Lesions vary from mild erythema and papules with or without pruritus to crusts, excoriations and pyotraumatic dermatitis. In severe cases, ulceration and necrosis, which usually result in pain, may occur. Secondary infection commonly results.

Diagnosis is made on the basis of the history, physical examination, avoidance, provocative exposure and patch testing. Reactions to concentrated but not diluted agents under test (Plate 1.19) suggest irritant rather than hypersensitivity responses. The irritant nature of the reaction may be confirmed by evoking similar responses on a control animal. Histopathological examination of skin biopsies is not diagnostic.

Treatment comprises topical dressings to clean or neutralize the irritant (Swarfega is a 'universal' solvent). Tar may be removed by soaking with vegetable oil. Subsequently, emollient creams (e.g. zinc and castor oil) or topical and systemic glucocorticoids and antibacterial agents may be required. Prevention depends on elimination or avoidance of the irritant.

Flea collars impregnated with dichlorvos or occasionally carbamates have been reported to result in chemical irritant contact dermatitis in cats, although it has been suggested that a small number of cases may result from contact hyper-sensitivity (Muller, 1970). Though initially local-ized to the immediate area of contact the clinical signs are said, on occasions, to become more generalized. The lesions reported range from ery-thema, alopecia and scaling to oedema, erosions and ulceration with secondary bacterial infection. Pruritus, pain and lethargy may also occur.

Diagnosis is based on the history and clinical signs. Treatment includes removal of the collar, clipping and cleaning of the area, and appli-cation of emollient or glucocorticoid/antibacterial creams to the affected area and systemic gluco-corticoids and antibacterial agents if necessary.

The authors believe that flea collar dermatitis is a very rare problem in cats. They have recognized it on only two occasions.

Chemical burns
These may be caused by acids or alkalis. They present similarly to thermal burns although with alkalis, the skin may change to a white and brown colour and may feel soft and gelatinous.

Immediate treatment is by dilution of the agent with water. Long-term management is as for thermal burns (see below).

Poisons

Thallium poisoning (thallotoxicosis)
The use of thallium, a rodenticide, is illegal in the UK. Cutaneous signs of thallium toxicosis are essentially of historic interest. They were seen in chronic thallium poisoning and comprised alopecia, erythema, crust formation and skin necrosis. These initially involved the pinnae, lips and eyelids but later became generalized.

Chlorinated naphthalene poisoning
Chlorinated naphthalene poisoning associated with exposure to wood preservatives has been described in cats (Wagener & Krüger, 1953). Lesions consisted of bilateral alopecia and hyper-keratosis of the eyelids and nose.

Ultraviolet radiation-related diseases

Actinic keratoses
These result from excessive exposure to UV light of skin lacking pigment or an adequate covering of hair, and they may be precursors of squamous cell carcinomas.

Actinic keratoses are solitary or multiple areas of erythema, hyperkeratosis, crusting and some-times plaque formation. Histopathological exam-ination reveals premalignant epidermal changes of atypia and dysplasia. Management is by sur-gical excision or cryotherapy. In human medicine, 5-fluorouracil has been used but information on this therapy in cats is not available.

Feline solar dermatitis
Feline solar dermatitis is a phototoxic reaction to UV light. It occurs in exposed areas of the skin lacking pigment and inadequately protected by hair, such as the pinnae and less frequently the eyelids, nose and lips of white cats or cats which are white over these areas. Blue-eyed white cats, living in sunny climates, are predisposed.

Solar dermatitis is manifested initially as ery-thema and hair loss at the borders of the pinnae. Subsequently, scale and crust formation, pain and then self-inflicted damage occur, resulting in further hair loss and in exposure of more skin to UV light. Lesions may initially heal during the winter months but become progressive and over successive years may result in curling of the pinnae due to deformation of the cartilage (Plate 1.20a) and may culminate in the development of ul-cerating squamous cell carcinoma (Plate 1.20b).

Diagnosis is based on the history and physical appearance. Biopsy of lesions is of value in deter-mining whether or not neoplasia has developed.

Treatment in the early stages is by keeping cats out of the sun during the sunniest part of the day (10.00 to 16.00 hours) and protection by use of topical sunscreen preparations containing para-aminobenzoic acid. In practice, amputation of the poorly protected pinnal tips is the most re-liable form of treatment, and, where possible, should be carried out before the development of neoplasia. If neoplasia has ensued, radical surgical excision of the pinnae is indicated. Cosmetically, the result is satisfactory and the prognosis is good as metastases are rare.

Although in one study, no relationship could be demonstrated between the condition and erythropoietic protoporphyria, an oral combination of beta-carotene and canthaxanthin (10–15 mg daily dose of active carotenoids reducing to 4–5 mg daily) was effective in treating the early stages of the condition and preventing recurrence on re-exposure to sunlight (Irving *et al.*, 1982).

Temperature-related conditions

Temperature-dependent coat colour
In certain breeds (the Siamese, Himalayan, Balinese and Burmese), hair colour is determined by the temperature-dependent activity of an enzyme involved in the synthesis of melanin. Low temperatures increase enzyme activity and high temperatures reduce its activity. This phenomenon gives rise to the points (nose, ears, feet and tail tip) seen in these breeds. It is also responsible for the regrowth of lighter hair over a previous site of inflammation (where the temperature has been higher) and darker hair over a shaved area (where the temperature was reduced because of loss of insulation), and for the changes in coat colour associated with Horner's syndrome (the Aguirre syndrome) in these breeds. These colour changes are not permanent and the hair reverts to its normal colour in the next growth phase provided the source of the temperature change has been reversed.

Thermal burns
Thermal burns are uncommon in cats. They may result from a number of causes, e.g. spillage of boiling water or hot oil, biting of electric wires or walking on the hotplate of a cooker, and may result in partial-thickness (incomplete) or full-thickness (complete) destruction of the skin, which is often followed by secondary infection, particularly with *Pseudomonas aeruginosa*.

Partial-thickness burns are manifested as erythematous, oedematous, moist and painful areas with a persistent capillary blood flow and possibly vesicle formation and the matting of hair by exudate. Full-thickness burns result in an area of avascular, insensitive, inelastic, necrotic skin covered by matted hair. Gentle removal or sloughing of this reveals ulcerated, suppurating tissue.

Burns, depending on their depth and extent, have two major sequelae: hypovolaemic shock and sepsis. Immediate treatment in all cases involves cooling the affected areas with cold water or ice. Cats with extensive burns will require intensive care, comprising fluid therapy, pain management and wound care to minimize infection and reduce the risk of sepsis. In all cases, clipping, removal of all dead tissue and debris and gentle cleaning of the affected area with saline or a mild detergent soap are essential. Subsequently the affected area should be cleaned three times daily, topical antibacterial agents (e.g. silver sulphadiazine) applied and the area protected by petrolatum gauze or an occlusive hydrocolloid dressing securely taped or bandaged in place. Systemic antibacterial agents are ineffective. Should the eschar become infected, semi-synthetic penicillins, which diffuse well in tissue, should be injected below the eschar (Goodwin, 1984). If sepsis occurs, antibacterial therapy should be based on blood culture and sensitivity testing and given intravenously. The burn should be monitored until the full extent and depth of the area affected is evident (usually 10 days). It is then possible to debride the necrotic skin and close the wound by direct apposition of healthy skin. If the area involved is too great, skin grafts may be required.

Frostbite
Frostbite occurs in regions with sub-zero temperatures. It is rare in the UK. It principally affects the poorly insulated ear tips but occasionally the tail tip, the scrotum and the feet may be involved. These are cool, pale and lack sensation but become erythematous and painful as they thaw. In severe cases tissue becomes necrotic and sloughs and the local haircoat may turn white.

Frozen tissue requires gentle handling. The affected tissue should be rapidly thawed by application of lukewarm water. When thawed, the areas may be hyperaemic and painful and self-trauma must be prevented. Provided the structure has not been completely devitalized, healing occurs quickly. Necrotic tissue should be removed surgically but this should be delayed for a few days as more tissue may be viable than initially estimated.

NUTRITIONAL DISORDERS

Obesity
Malnutrition
Fat-responsive dermatosis
Vitamin E deficiency
Vitamin A deficiency
Biotin deficiency
Riboflavin deficiency
Niacin deficiency
Pyridoxine deficiency
Zinc deficiency
Iodine deficiency

Summary

Obesity occurs occasionally but the other conditions are rarely seen. The cutaneous lesions of most dietary deficiencies include varying degrees of dry or greasy seborrhoea and alopecia, little or no pruritus and may be accompanied by involvement of other body systems. The exceptions are vitamin E deficiency (painful subcutaneous swellings) and experimental niacin deficiency (oral ulceration). Dietary deficiencies are unlikely to occur in cats fed proprietary diets (see Chapter 24).

Obesity

This is far less common in cats than dogs. It may occur due to overfeeding or lack of exercise or be associated with disease (acromegaly, iatrogenic hypothyroidism or hyperadrenocorticism) or drug therapy (megestrol acetate or glucocorticoids).

The main cutaneous lesions are bilaterally symmetrical, erythematous, moist areas of inflammation involving intertriginous areas of the axillae, groin and intermammary areas. These are sometimes accompanied by secondary bacterial infection.

The primary therapeutic aim is to reduce the cat's weight by dieting, increasing chances for exercise, stopping drug therapy or investigating underlying disease processes. Topical zinc and castor oil or antibacterial/glucocorticoid creams and, if necessary, systemic antibacterial agents and glucocorticoids may provide adequate short-term therapy. Glucocorticoids should not be employed in cases resulting from naturally occurring or iatrogenic hyperadrenocorticism.

Malnutrition

This may occasionally be encountered in neglected animals. The skin may be dry, seborrhoeic and susceptible to secondary bacterial infection.

Fat-responsive dermatosis

In most animals, essential fatty acids (EFA) are derived from dietary *cis*-linoleic acid and alpha-linolenic acid by carbon chain elongation and desaturation. In the cat, minimal activity of desaturase enzymes results in reduced utilization of these particular fatty acids and consequently a dependence on dietary EFA, supplied by a high meat diet, to meet most of its EFA requirement.

Experimental EFA deficiency results in a greasy seborrhoeic hair coat, slow wound healing, reduced growth rate, loss of weight, anoestrus and testicular hypoplasia (Rivers & Frankel, 1980; MacDonald *et al.*, 1984). The natural occurrence of EFA deficiency is suggested by cutaneous lesions such as a dry or greasy seborrhoeic skin and hair coat responsive to dietary fat supplementation (Scott, 1980). However, as some of the cases reported were fed balanced diets and had no evidence of impaired fat absorption (maldigestion, malabsorption) or utilization (hepatic disease) the term fat-responsive dermatosis is preferred to EFA deficiency.

Diagnosis is based on the clinical signs and response to dietary fat supplementation with equal volumes (2.5–5.0 ml/day) of vegetable oil and lard, or evening primrose oil. Dietary supplementation may be required indefinitely.

Vitamin E deficiency (pansteatitis, yellow fat disease)

Common in the 1960s, pansteatitis now occurs only sporadically. Though associated with diets high in polyunsaturated fish oils, particularly tuna fish, it has also been reported in cats fed excessive cod-liver oil, various tinned foods and rarely liver (O'Donnell & Hayes, 1987). Vitamin E may be inactivated by oxidation in the presence of high concentrations of unsaturated fatty acids, rancidity and food processing. Deficiency of vitamin E allows lipid peroxidation resulting in the formation of ceroid, a yellow pigment, and its deposition in adipose tissue provoking inflammation.

Clinically, pansteatitis is manifested by pyrexia, anorexia, reluctance to move and resentment of handling. Firm and lumpy subcutaneous and abdominal fat may be detected by palpation, where this is tolerated.

Diagnosis is suggested by the dietary history and clinical signs, supported by the presence of leucocytosis (neutrophilia and sometimes eosinophilia) and confirmed by macroscopic, UV light and histopathological examination of fat biopsies. Affected fat varies in colour from deep yellow to orange-brown and glows yellow-orange under UV light when fixed in formalin. Histologically, it is characterized by infiltration of neutrophils, lymphocytes, plasma cells and macrophages and the presence of ceroid (possibly an intermediate peroxidation/polymerization product of lipid metabolism) in fat cells, macrophages and foreign body giant cells.

Treatment comprises dietary change, oral α-tocopherol acetate supplementation (25–75 IU twice daily) and glucocorticoids to reduce inflammation. If necessary, diazepam (2.5–5 mg/cat/day) may be useful in stimulating appetite. Intravenous injection of diazepam is preferred as its appetite-stimulating ability appears to be reduced following intramuscular or oral administration.

Vitamin A deficiency

Experimental vitamin A deficiency has been recorded in cats (Gerschoff *et al.*, 1957).

Clinically, the cutaneous lesions include poor hair coat, patchy alopecia, seborrhoea and comedone formation. Ocular lesions (conjunctivitis, keratitis sicca and retinal degeneration), reproductive abnormalities (testicular atrophy, aspermatogenesis, anoestrus and foetal loss), bronchopneumonia, anorexia, weight loss and muscle wasting may also occur.

Diagnosis should be confirmed by demonstration of a low plasma vitamin A concentration: less than 1.4 µmol/l suggests deficiency, and less than 0.52 µmol/l confirms deficiency (O'Donnell & Hayes, 1987).

As cats cannot convert vitamin A precursors (carotenoids) to the active form (retinol), vitamin A supplementation is required. Oral vitamin A supplementation (400 IU/kg/day) for 10 days or a single parenteral injection of aqueous vitamin A (6000 IU/kg) are usually an adequate treatment for any deficiency. As cats are susceptible to vitamin A toxicity, treatment must be carefully regulated.

Biotin deficiency

Clinically, experimental biotin deficiency results in the accumulation of dried discharges around the mouth, nose and eyes followed by alopecia of the extremities and then the body with generalized leucotrichia and seborrhoea. In addition there may be anorexia, weight loss and diarrhoea (Carey & Morris, 1977).

Although papulocrustous (miliary) dermatitis has been attributed to biotin deficiency (Joshua, 1959) it is unlikely that such deficiency occurs naturally.

Riboflavin deficiency

An experimentally induced, marginal riboflavin deficiency resulted in periauricular and periorbital alopecia, epidermal atrophy, cataract formation and testicular hypoplasia (Gerschoff *et al.*, 1959).

Niacin (nicotinic acid) deficiency

Clinical signs of niacin deficiency include ulceration of the tongue and palate accompanied by profuse salivation, anorexia, diarrhoea and weight loss (Heath *et al.*, 1940).

Pyridoxine deficiency

Experimental pyridoxine deficiency results in seborrhoea accompanied in some cases by alopecia of the face (temporal, periauricular, nasal and perioral areas) and extremities (Norton, 1987).

Zinc deficiency

Experimental dietary zinc deficiency in kittens resulted in reduced appetite and weight gain and the development of variable cutaneous lesions consisting of scaly or crusty, ulcerative lesions at the mucocutaneous junction of the lips and nasal philtrum, thinning of the hair coat, retarded hair growth and seborrhoea (Kane *et al.*, 1981).

Naturally occurring zinc deficiency has not been reported in cats.

Iodine deficiency

Experimentally induced in kittens and adult cats, prolonged dietary iodine deficiency may cause hypothyroidism (see above).

IMMUNOLOGICAL DISEASES

Immunological diseases affecting the skin of cats may be classified as hypersensitivities, autoimmune disorders, immune-mediated disorders, diseases of probable immune-mediation and immunodeficiencies.

Hypersensitivities
  Urticaria and angioedema
  Drug eruption
  Ectoparasite hypersensitivities
    Fleas
    Ticks

  Otodectes cynotis
  Notoedres cati
  Trombicula autumnalis
  Endoparasite hypersensitivities
    Roundworm
    Tapeworm
    Hookworm
  Food hypersensitivity
  Atopic disease
  Contact hypersensitivity
  Bacterial and fungal hypersensitivity

Hypersensitivities

Summary
Repeated or prolonged encounters with the same or cross-reacting antigens provoke an immune response which normally facilitates elimination of the antigen from the body. However, in some individuals, modulation of the immune response is impaired and the antigen-antibody or antigen-immune competent cell interaction results in tissue damage. These injurious interactions are termed hypersensitivity (allergic) reactions.

Four types of hypersensitivity reactions are recognized (Coombs & Gell, 1975); all have been implicated in the conditions being considered and all entail the release of various mediators including histamine, leukotrienes and proteases, which cause inflammation and pruritus.

Type I reactions are characterized by the interaction of antigen with IgE antibody bound to mast cells or basophils. Although IgE has not yet been characterized in cats there is considerate evidence for its occurrence. Type I hypersensitivity is thought to be involved in urticaria and angioedema, drug, ecto- and endoparasite hypersensitivity, food hypersensitivity, atopic disease and drug eruption.

Type II reactions are mediated by the interaction of antibody (IgG or IgM), with or without complement, or immunocompetent cells with self antigen(s) on body tissues and result in cytotoxicity or cytolysis. This reaction characterizes autoimmunity but has also been incriminated in drug eruptions.

Type III reactions are distinguished by the combination of antigen with circulating antibody to form microcomplexes which become deposited in the walls of blood vessels. They have been implicated in drug hypersensitivity.

Type IV reactions are mediated by T-effector cells which secrete numerous lymphokines when confronted with the sensitizing antigen. This reaction is responsible for contact hypersensitivity and may be involved in food hypersensitivity, flea allergic dermatitis, *Otodectes* infestation and drug eruption.

Estimates of the incidence of each condition vary. However, flea allergic dermatitis is probably the most important single cause of skin disease in cats; food hypersensitivity and atopic disease are considerably less common but are being diagnosed with increasing frequency; the other conditions listed are rare. No breed or sex predisposition has been reported. Age of onset is usually 3–5 years in flea allergic dermatitis and thought to be 6 months to 2 years in atopy (Scott, 1987b). Food and contact hypersensitivity commonly require 2 years' exposure to the offending allergen before clinical signs are manifest (Walton, 1977a,b).

Pruritus is the cardinal sign of cutaneous hypersensitivity. This may be localized or generalized and is often accompanied by excoriations and broken hair due to self-inflicted trauma. Hair loss, secondary seborrhoea and rarely pyoderma may also be present. Miliary dermatitis, eosinophilic plaque, symmetrical alopecia and urticaria-angioedema may be associated with hypersensitivity reactions.

Urticaria and angioedema (hives)

Urticaria (wheals) and angioedema (large oedematous swellings) are rare in cats. They have been associated with the use of antisera and vaccines (FeLV antisera, feline panleucopenia vaccine), transfusions, drugs (penicillin and tetracycline), foods, insect stings and bites, plants and intestinal parasites (Muller *et al.*, 1989) and may be mediated by immune (Types I and III hypersensitivity reactions) and non-immune mechanisms which cause increased capillary permeability.

Reactions may be localized or generalized, are usually transient but may be recurrent. Either reaction may be accompanied by pruritus, leakage of serum or haemorrhage.

Diagnosis is based on the history, physical examination and thorough investigation to eliminate possible causes, which may be difficult to identify, particularly in chronic cases.

Management rests on elimination and/or avoidance of any identified trigger. If indicated, symptomatic treatment with adrenaline (1:1000 solution, 0.1–0.2 ml injected subcutaneously, intramuscularly or intravenously) or prednisolone (1 mg/kg twice daily administered intramuscularly, intravenously or orally) may be given. Antihistamines, although of no value in the treatment of existing reactions, may be used to prevent anticipated reactions and in the management of chronic cases.

Ectoparasite hypersensitivities

Hypersensitivity reactions may be important in the response of cats to infestation with a number of ectoparasites. Details of the clinical aspects of these conditions are presented in the section above on parasitic diseases.

FLEA BITE HYPERSENSITIVITY DERMATITIS (FLEA ALLERGY DERMATITIS)

Although many authors feel that flea bites are capable of inducing significant clinical reactions without hypersensitivity being involved, Halliwell (1985) has suggested that such reactions always involve hypersensitivity (Plate 1.21). As in dogs, it is probable that Types I and IV hypersensitivity reactions and cutaneous basophil hypersensitivity are of prime importance in the genesis of this problem in cats.

TICKS

Tick bites provoke cutaneous basophil hypersensitivity reactions in guinea pigs (Allen, 1973) and cattle (Allen *et al.*, 1977) and may be involved in the genesis of tick-bite granulomata. After excluding foreign-body reactions to retained mouthparts, these persistent lesions can often be aborted by intralesional glucocorticoids.

OTODECTES CYNOTIS

Weisbroth *et al.* (1974) have presented evidence for the involvement of Type I and III hypersensitivity responses in current (and presumed previous) infestations with *O. cynotis*.

NOTOEDRES CATI

In addition to mechanical irritation, Type I and IV hypersensitivity reactions have been implicated in the genesis of pruritus in human scabies (Falk & Bolle, 1980). It is probable that *Notoedres cati* provokes similar reactions.

TROMBICULA AUTUMNALIS

The variable intensity of reactions to *Trombicula* infestations between animals suggests the occurrence of hypersensitivity reactions in some cats.

Endoparasite hypersensitivity

Hypersensitivity reactions (possibly Type I) to roundworms, tapeworms and hookworms have been reported (Scott, 1980) but appear to be rare. The clinical signs observed are pruritus, papulocrustous dermatitis and seborrhoea sicca. Diagnosis is supported by the observation of eggs or tapeworm segments on faecal examination and response to treatment.

Food hypersensitivity

Virtually any food has the potential to provoke a hypersensitivity reaction. However, in each case usually only one dietary item is involved and this has often been fed for several years prior to the development of a reaction. Rarely, two or more related foods (e.g. beef and milk) may be incriminated. Clinically, food hypersensitivity, which may involve Types I, III and IV reactions to dietary allergens, is indistinguishable from food intolerance and idiosyncrasy, neither of which involve immune mechanisms.

The clinical signs are varied and may be focal, multifocal or generalized. Pruritus and alopecia may be localized (Plate 1.22), particularly to the head and neck, or generalized and may be accompanied by erythema, excoriations, recurrent urticaria-angioedema, recurrent chemosis with or without epiphora, papulocrustous erup-

tions, eosinophilic plaques or ulcers, symmetrical alopecia, seborrhoea and otitis externa. Gastrointestinal signs (vomiting, diarrhoea and colic, lymphocytic-plasmocytic colitis), respiratory distress, malaise and peripheral lymphadenopathy have been reported infrequently (White & Sequoia, 1989). Multisystem involvement is rare. Clinical signs may be intermittent if the offending dietary item is not fed continuously.

Diagnosis relies on dietary restriction (discussed previously) as intradermal skin testing and radioallergosorbent tests are unreliable. Management involves excluding the offending foodstuff from the diet. Where owners are unwilling or unable to comply, glucocorticoids may be used to produce some measure of control but food hypersensitivity frequently is poorly responsive to drug therapy.

Atopic disease

Atopic disease is a Type I hypersensitivity reaction. The observation of clinical signs typical of atopy, the occurrence of positive intradermal tests and subsequently a good response to hyposensitization and the demonstration of passive cutaneous anaphylaxis have provided putative evidence for the existence of atopy in cats and recent studies have provided immunological evidence for the occurence of IgE in cats (De Boer *et al.*, 1993), although a genetic predisposition to atopy has not been demonstrated.

The clinical signs, often first manifested when the cat is 6 months to 2 years old (Scott, 1987b), may be seasonal or non-seasonal and include pruritus, in particular of the face, neck and paws, accompanied by excoriations, secondary infections and seborrhoea. Lesions of the eosinophilic granuloma complex, papulocrustous eruptions and symmetrical alopecia may also occur. In one study (Gross *et al.*, 1986), 9% of cats with miliary dermatitis were diagnosed as atopic. Cats with cutaneous signs of atopy may also exhibit signs of feline asthma (Halliwell & Gorman, 1989). Diagnosis relies on the use of intradermal tests (discussed above).

Feline atopic disease may be managed in a number of ways. These include avoidance of relevant allergens, antihistamines (H_1 receptor blocking drugs), essential fatty acid supplementation, glucocorticoids and hyposensitization. Avoidance of relevant allergens is not possible in most cases. The antihistamine chlorpheniramine (2 mg/cat orally twice daily) is often effective. Essential fatty acid supplementation (evening primrose oil with or without fish oil) has been used to modify the inflammatory reaction caused by atopic disease in humans and dogs but its value in the control of feline atopy has not yet been reported. Glucocorticoids are highly effective but may produce serious adverse effects in the long term. To minimize these risks, short-acting glucocorticoids such as prednisolone or prednisone are essential if long-term use is required. They should be given orally at a dosage of 1–2 mg/kg twice daily until pruritus is controlled. Thereafter, double the daily dose is given on alternate evenings, tapering this gradually to that which just fails to control the signs, thus ensuring that the lowest possible amount is being used.

Hyposensitization involves the repeated injection of initially increasing doses of causal allergen(s) in an attempt to modify the immune response so that signs subside or disappear. Reedy (1982) reported a 75% improvement in 10 of 15 cats hyposensitized. In view of its potential side-effects, the use of megestrol acetate should be avoided.

Drug eruption

On clinical grounds, hypersensitivity reactions are thought to be the most common cause of drug eruptions in man but the situation is not clear in cats. Any drug has the potential to provoke one or more of the four types of hypersensitivity reaction. Drugs incriminated in adverse cutaneous reactions (including drug eruption) in cats are listed in Table 1.5.

Clinical signs associated with drug hypersensitivity can mimic virtually any dermatosis but commonly include pruritus, erythema, urticaria-angioedema, papulocrustous eruptions and alopecia. Toxic epidermal necrolysis and erythema multiforme may also be associated with drug hypersensitivity reactions.

Investigation of drug hypersensitivity necessitates the withdrawal of all drugs (unless the risks of so doing outweigh the benefits of diagnosis) and substitution, if essential, of chemically unrelated drugs. Remission of clinical signs, sometimes several weeks after drug withdrawal, supports a tentative diagnosis of drug eruption. Theoretically, provocative exposure could confirm the diagnosis but this may involve unacceptable risks (Wilcke, 1986).

Contact hypersensitivity

In humans, contact hypersensitivity is mediated by Type IV and less commonly Type I (contact urticaria) responses. It has been produced experimentally in the cat (Schultz & McGuire, 1982). However, although occasional reports of clinical cases have occurred, only one (neomycin hypersensitivity) appears to have been confirmed by patch testing (Thoday, 1985).

Clinical signs include pruritus, erythema, papulovesicular eruptions and increased pigmentation. These usually occur on contact sites in areas where the hair is thin (the ventrum, medial aspect of the hindlimbs and ventral aspects of the paws and neck) but may be generalized if the allergen is present in a liquid or aerosol, or focal (e.g. otitis externa) if the allergen is a drug. Similar clinical signs occur with contact irritants. However, reaction to these is immediate, not requiring a prolonged period of sensitization, and is likely to involve more than one cat in a multi-cat household.

Investigation relies on avoidance of the suspected contact allergen for a 3-week period; this has been discussed above. Treatment is by avoidance of the allergen if possible. If this is impossible, topical or systemic glucocorticoids may provide limited control.

Bacterial and fungal hypersensitivity

Bacterial and fungal hypersensitivity have been suspected in cats. MacDonald *et al.* (1972) reported successful treatment of a chronic bacterin dermatosis using an autogenous bacterium. Fungal hypersensitivity has been postulated in association with lesions of miliary dermatitis in

Table 1.5 Adverse cutaneous reactions to drugs in cats: incriminated drugs and resultant lesions.

Drug	Lesion
Antibacterial agents	
Sulphasoxizole	Papulocrustous dermatitis, alopecia
Penicillin	Papulocrustous dermatitis, urticaria-angioedema
Hetacillin	Multifocal alopecia, pruritus, toxic epidermal necrolysis
Ampicillin	Multifocal alopecia, pruritus, toxic epidermal necrolysis, pemphigus foliaceus-like disease
Cephaloridine	Papulocrustous dermatitis, toxic epidermal necrolysis
Cephalexin	Papulocrustous dermatitis
Tetracycline	Urticaria-angioedema
Gentamycin	Erythema, alopecia, pruritus
Neomycin	Contact dermatitis
Antifungal agents	
Griseofulvin	Papulocrustous dermatitis
Miconazole	Contact dermatitis
Parasiticides	
Dichlorvos	Contact dermatitis
Carbamates	Contact dermatitis
Dichlorophen	Crusts, caseous paronychia
Antithyroid agents	
Propylthiouracil	Facial swelling, pruritus
Methimazole	Pruritus, excoriations
Glucocorticoids	
Various (particularly depot preparations) when administered subcutaneously	Alopecia, atrophy
Prednisolone	Atrophy, fragility
Antihistamines	
Cimetidine	Pemphigus foliaceus-like disease
Anticonvulsants	
Phenytoin	Atrophy, fragility
Vaccines and antisera	
Panleucopenia vaccine	Angioedema
Leukaemia virus vaccine	Erythema, alopecia, angioedema
Combined intranasal herpesvirus/calicivirus vaccine	Alopecia, erosions
Parenteral water in oil emulsion	Lipophagic granuloma
Leukaemia virus antiserum	Toxic epidermal necrolysis
Anaesthetic agents and bases	
Polyoxyethylated castor oil	Erythema, angioedema
Benzocaine skin cream	Methaemoglobinaemia
Miscellaneous	
Aurothioglucose	Erythema multiforme

cats due to *M. canis*, and in kerion formation, a highly inflamed, nodular lesion associated with fungal and bacterial infection.

Autoimmune diseases

Pemphigus complex
   Pemphigus vulgaris
   Pemphigus foliaceus
   Pemphigus erythematosus
Systemic lupus erythematosus
Discoid lupus erythematosus
Cold agglutinin disease

Summary

These autoimmune disorders result from Type II and III hypersensitivity reactions. In Type II reactions antibody (IgG or IgM), with or without complement or immunocompetent cells, interacts with self antigens present on body tissues. Examples include the pemphigus complex and cold agglutinin disease. In Type III hypersensitivity reactions, immune complexes are deposited on basement membranes in vascular endothelium or in tissues. Examples include systemic lupus erythematosus (SLE) and discoid lupus erythematosus (DLE).

The autoimmune dermatoses are uncommon to rare conditions. Pemphigus foliaceus has the highest incidence in cats in the USA (Scott *et al.*, 1987) and in the UK. No breed, sex or age predisposition have been reported.

The pemphigus complex and SLE and DLE are usually bilaterally symmetrical, erosive to ulcerative, crusting, scaling dermatoses involving the face, ears and paws. Systemic signs such as anorexia, pyrexia and depression may also occur.

The pemphigus complex

In these conditions, autoantibody directed against the glycocalyx of keratinocytes or the intercellular cement results in the formation of intraepidermal vesicles and bullae. These are transient and rupture (cat epidermis is thin and rubbing is common) to give rise to erosions and, less commonly, ulcers surrounded by epidermal collarettes and erythema and subsequently crusting, scaling lesions with secondary bacterial infection with

hair loss. Gentle rubbing of the border of vesicles or erosions may cause peeling of the superficial layer of skin (Nikolsky's sign), which is indicative of impaired intercellular binding. The degree of pruritus and pain accompanying the lesions is variable. Depending on their severity, these conditions may be accompanied by local lymphadenopathy and systemic signs, anorexia, pyrexia and depression. Cyclic phases of spontaneous remission and exacerbation may occur.

Pemphigus vulgaris is a severe and potentially life-threatening disease. It involves the oral mucous membranes and hard palate, where bullae may occasionally be detected, and the mucocutaneous junction of the lips, eyelids and nares. Occasionally the ears and paws are also affected.

Pemphigus foliaceus usually involves the planum nasale, periorbital area and ears initially but may become more generalized, affecting the trunk and abdomen, pads (hyperkeratosis) and in most cases the nail folds (paronychia and pyonychia) (Plates 1.23 & 1.24). In some cases, only the foot pads are affected. Onychomadesis may be seen. Mucocutaneous and oral cavity involvement is unusual.

Pemphigus erythematosus, a relatively benign disease, appears to be limited to the face, particularly the bridge of the nose and ears. It may result in reduced skin pigment (leucoderma) predisposing to photodermatitis. Oral lesions have not been documented.

Diagnosis is supported by detection of acantholytic keratinocytes and neutrophils in impression smears of lesions (Tzanck test) and is confirmed by characteristic histopathology and positive direct immunofluorescence testing of early lesional and perilesional biopsies. Histopathologically, pemphigus vulgaris is characterized by acantholysis and suprabasilar cleft formation which leaves the basal cells adhering to the basement membrane like a 'row of tombstones'. Pemphigus foliaceus and erythematosus display acantholysis and subcorneal clefting. Immunofluorescence gives a 'chicken mesh' appearance throughout the epidermis with all three forms. In pemphigus erythematosus there may also be linear basement membrane zone fluorescence and a positive antinuclear antibody (ANA) titre suggesting that the disease may be a cross-over syndrome between pemphigus and lupus erythematosus.

Treatment requires vigorous immunosuppressive therapy with systemic glucocorticoids, prednisolone (1–3 mg/kg initially twice daily) being the drug of choice. When substantial improvement occurs, the total daily dose may be given once daily. Once remission is achieved, alternate-day therapy with the minimum dose required to control the condition should be instituted. Chrysotherapy (gold salt therapy) using aurothioglucose or sodium aurothiomalate, has also been used successfully in cats as an adjunctive or alternative form of therapy. Using aurothioglucose, intramuscular test doses of 1 mg and 2 mg are given 1 week apart to detect idiosyncratic reactions to gold and, in their absence, followed by 1 mg/ kg weekly until a clinical improvement occurs, usually after 6–12 weeks. Subsequently, a monthly maintenance dose of 1 mg/kg is administered. Gold salts are mildly immunosuppressive, anti-inflammatory and have anti-complement activity. They require careful laboratory monitoring to detect possible side-effects (anaemia, nephrotoxicity and hepatotoxicity). Cats are very susceptible to azathioprine toxicity. It should be used very cautiously if at all in the initial treatment of the pemphigus complex (Beale, 1988) and may not be appropriate for long-term maintenance in cats as, in one study (Caciola, 1984), leucopenia occurred in 50% of cats treated with eight doses. Minimizing exposure to direct sunlight and the application of sunscreens may also benefit cases with pemphigus erythematosus.

Whatever treatment is used, some cats may go into temporary or permanent remission (particularly with pemphigus foliaceus and erythematosus) and need only intermittent or no further treatment.

Systemic lupus erythematosus

The precise aetiology of systemic lupus erythematosus (SLE) is unknown but it is thought that genetic predisposition, impaired T-suppressor cell function (possibly a result of lymphocytotoxic antibody activity), viral infection, hormonal influences, UV light and interaction of drugs with nuclear material may all be involved. These result in clones of B-cells producing antibodies against self antigens on various body tissues. Cutaneous signs are thought to result principally from the deposition of autoantibody-antigen complexes (Type III hypersensitivity reaction) at the epidermal basement membrane.

The cutaneous manifestations of SLE include erythema, erosions, ulcers, crusts, scales, hypopigmentation and hair loss involving the face, nasal and periorbital areas and the ears and peripheral lymphadenopathy. Pruritus, seborrhoea, paronychia and ulcers of the lip, palate (Plate 1.25) and nose, and proliferative gingivitis may also occur. SLE is a multisystemic disease and cutaneous signs may be accompanied by depression, anorexia, pyrexia, weight loss, anaemia, leucopenia, glomerulonephritis and inflammatory polyarthritis.

Histopathological examination of skin biopsies reveals hydropic or lichenoid changes in the basal cell layer of the epidermis, which may be accompanied by evidence of thickening of the basement membrane zone, a perifollicular, mononuclear cell infiltrate, myxoedema and subepidermal vacuolation. Direct immunofluorescence testing demonstrates a 'lupus band' of immunoglobulin and/or complement at the basement membrane zone.

Different schemes, proposed as a basis for diagnosing SLE in dogs, may also provide the basis for its diagnosis in cats (Bennett, 1987; Halliwell & Gorman, 1989). Bennett (1987) suggests the fulfilment of three criteria: detection of antinuclear antibody in the blood; clinical evidence for the involvement of two or more body systems, i.e. dermatitis, autoimmune haemolytic anaemia, immune-mediated thrombocytopenia, polyarthritis, glomerulonephritis; and demonstration of immunopathological features consistent with involvement of these systems. If only one or two of the criteria are satisfied only a tentative diagnosis can be made. Halliwell and Gorman (1989) propose positive serology (positive antinuclear factor titre or lupus erythematosus cell preparation) together with two major clinical signs (non-infective polyarthritis, dermatosis with histopathology and immunofluorescence compatible with SLE, Coombs' positive anaemia, glomerulonephritis with significant proteinuria, thrombocytopenia or neutropenia of unknown aetiology, polymyositis) or one major and two minor (pyrexia of unknown origin, CNS signs, pleuritis) clinical signs.

Treatment is initiated with a high dose of oral prednisolone (2–3 mg/kg twice daily) which is reduced to the minimum alternate-day maintenance dose once remission is achieved. If the disease is non-responsive or becomes refractory to prednisolone, concurrent use of cyclophosphamide, or aurothioglucose, should be considered. Exposure to sunlight should be minimized as UV light may exacerbate skin lesions. If other body systems are involved additional therapeutic measures should be instituted if indicated (see Chapter 3).

Discoid lupus erythematosus
Discoid lupus erythematosus (DLE) has recently been described in cats (Willemse & Koeman, 1989). DLE is similar in aetiology to SLE and produces cutaneous lesions which mimic those of SLE and include vesicles, ulcers, papules and pustules on the pinnae, scale and crust formation on the pinnae, footpads, body and around the eyes, and hypopigmentation of the footpads. However, unlike SLE, lesions of DLE are limited to the skin. Diagnosis was based on the history, clinical signs, histopathology of skin biopsies which was similar to that of SLE but included the presence of Civatte (colloid) bodies, demonstration of a lupus band of immunoglobulin at the basement membrane zone with direct immunofluorescence and the failure to demonstrate autoimmune involvement of other body systems. Treatment with glucocorticoids was effective.

Cold agglutinin disease
This condition results from ischaemia following the obstruction of peripheral blood vessels with red blood cells agglutinated by autoantibody

(IgM) which is reactive at low temperatures. It has been associated with upper respiratory tract infection in cats. The extremities of the body are particularly susceptible and clinically the condition is characterized by erythema, cyanosis then necrosis, and sloughing and ulceration of the borders of the pinnae, the nose, the tip of the tail and the paws. Diagnosis is confirmed by demonstration of autoagglutination of blood mixed with an anticoagulant at 4°C. The reaction is reversed on warming to 37°C. A positive Coombs' test at 4°C is of questionable value.

Management should involve correction of precipitating factors, where possible, avoidance of cold and immunosuppressive drug therapy.

Immune-mediated disorders
Vasculitis
Vasculitis is thought to be mediated by Type III hypersensitivity reactions although Type I hypersensitivity responses may be important in triggering immune complex deposition in blood vessel walls. In humans, development of this condition may be associated with concurrent infections, neoplasia and SLE, may be precipitated by drugs or vaccinations or may be idiopathic.

Typically, cutaneous vasculitis results in focal ulceration of the extremities (paws, pinnae and tail), lips and oral mucosa or vaccination sites (Schmeitzel, 1986). It has been diagnosed tentatively (Scott, 1987b) in a cat presented with recurrent ulceration of the footpads, pinnae and lips. Histopathological examination of the lesions, revealing destruction of neutrophil nuclei, was compatible with the diagnosis.

Treatment includes correction of any underlying conditions and administration of systemic glucocorticoids or possibly dapsone.

Disorders of probable immune-mediation
Relapsing polychondritis
In humans, similarities between relapsing polychondritis rheumatoid arthritis and SLE have supported the suggestion that this condition results from interaction of autoantibodies and mucopolysaccharides.

A tentative diagnosis of relapsing polychondritis was made in a cat which was presented clinically with painful, swollen, curled, erythematous pinnae (Scott, 1987a). The diagnosis was supported by histopathological examination, which demonstrated lymphoplasmacytic infiltration, loss of cartilage basophilia and cartilage necrosis. The cat was lost to follow-up. In man the condition responds well to systemic glucocorticoids or dapsone.

Sterile granuloma syndrome
Sterile granuloma syndrome has been reported in cats (Conroy, 1983), which were presented clinically with multiple, occasionally solitary, erythematous nodules and plaques usually involving the head and extremities.

Cultures for microorganisms are sterile. Response to systemic glucocorticoids is good and has led to the suggestion of an immune basis for this condition. However, recurrence of the lesions is common.

Alopecia areata
Genetic, endocrine, psychological and, more recently, immune-mediated factors have been implicated in the pathogenesis of alopecia areata in humans.

Clinically, this condition is distinguished by a non-inflammatory, focal or multifocal, well-circumscribed alopecia and has been observed occasionally in cats (Conroy, 1979). Diagnosis is based on histopathology and requires the observation of characteristic 'swarm of bees' accumulations of mononuclear cells around the inferior segment of anagen hair follicles. The lesions have been reported to respond to sublesional injections of triamcinolone but there is no definitive evidence that they are beneficial.

Immunodeficiency disorders
Cutaneous manifestations arising from immunosuppression in feline leukaemia virus infection and feline immunodeficiency virus infection are discussed in the relevant sections under 'Viral Diseases' above.

CUTANEOUS NEOPLASMS

Summary
The skin is the second most common site for the development of neoplasia in cats and gives rise to a diverse range of primary neoplasms. Surveys of these tumours (McVean *et al.*, 1978; Thoday, 1981b; Bostock, 1986; Carpenter *et al.*, 1987) indicate that the majority are malignant and that, excluding tumours of the ear canal, four types of tumour (basal cell tumours, fibrosarcomas, mast cell tumours and squamous cell carcinomas) account for approximately 60% of all feline skin tumours. Most skin tumours occur in middle-aged to old cats but no sex predisposition has been noted. Siamese cats are reported to have a lower incidence of skin tumours than other breeds (Dorn *et al.*, 1968) but may have a higher incidence of basal cell and mast cell tumours (Carpenter *et al.*, 1987).

As the majority of feline skin tumours are malignant, the rate of tumour growth, the degree of local invasiveness and the nature of the drainage lymph nodes should be evaluated in every case. If indicated, radiographic examination of the thorax and abdomen should be undertaken for evidence of metastases.

Impression smears are of value in diagnosing mast cell tumours (Plate 1.26) but it is strongly advised that in each case, tentative diagnosis is confirmed by histopathological examination. Where indicated, this will facilitate institution of the appropriate postoperative therapy. As tumour handling may precipitate an intravascular and intralymphatic tumour cell shower, disseminating tumour cells, wide excision biopsies (1 cm minimum) with minimal tumour handling are preferred to incisional biopsies. If multiple tumours are present, at least two should be submitted for histopathological examination before concluding that they represent the same type of neoplasm.

Where possible, wide surgical excision accompanied, if indicated, by amputation, local drainage lymph node removal and postoperative chemotherapy, is the treatment of choice. In some instances this is impractical or impossible and other forms of therapy may be required. For example, radiotherapy combined with hyperthermia may be necessary to treat squamous cell carcinomas successfully, while chemotherapy may be indicated in the treatment of cutaneous lymphoma and multiple mast cell tumours. In view of the potential toxic and immunosuppressive effects of chemotherapy, complete blood counts, renal and hepatic function tests and FeLV and FIV status should be evaluated before deciding to institute treatment.

Table 1.6 lists the important cutaneous neoplasms of cats. Table 1.7 lists the important non-neoplastic tumours. Details of the incidence, clinical features and management of these neoplasms and non-neoplastic tumours are given in Tables 1.8 and 1.9.

Table 1.6 Important cutaneous neoplasms.

Epithelial neoplasms
  Papilloma
  Intracutaneous cornifying epithelioma
  Squamous cell carcinoma
  Basal cell tumour
  Hair follicle tumours
    Trichoepithelioma
    Dilated pore of Winer
    Pilomatrixoma
  Sebaceous gland tumours
    Nodular sebaceous hyperplasia
    Sebaceous adenoma
    Sebaceous epithelioma
    Sebaceous adenocarcinoma
  Sweat gland tumours
    Epitrichial (apocrine) cyst
    Epitrichial (apocrine) adenoma
    Epitrichial (apocrine) adenocarcinoma
    Atrichial (eccrine) adenoma
    Atrichial (eccrine) adenocarcinoma
  Epithelioid sarcoma
Mesenchymal neoplasms
  Fibroma
  Fibrosarcoma
  Myxoma and myxosarcoma

Table 1.6 *Continued*

  Undifferentiated sarcoma
  Nodular fasciitis
  Leiomyoma and leiomyosarcoma
  Schwannoma
  Lipoma
  Liposarcoma
  Tumours of vascular origin
    Haemangioma
    Haemangiosarcoma
    Haemangiopericytoma
    Lymphangioma and lymphangiosarcoma
  Mast cell tumour

Lymphohistiocytic neoplasms
  Histiocytoma
  Fibrous histiocytoma
  Malignant fibrous histiocytoma (extraskeletal giant cell tumour)
  Cutaneous lymphoma
    Primary lymphoma
      Non-epitheliotropic forms (B-cell origin)
      Epitheliotropic forms (T-cell origin)
        Mycosis fungoides-like disease
    Secondary lymphoma
  Alopecia mucinosa
  Cutaneous plasmacytoma
    Primary cutaneous plasmacytoma
    Secondary cutaneous plasmacytoma

Melanocytic neoplasms
  Melanoma

Secondary skin neoplasms

Table 1.7 Non-neoplastic tumours.

Cutaneous cysts
  Epidermoid cysts
  Follicular cysts
Keratoses
  Actinic keratoses
  Cutaneous horn
Naevi
  Organoid
  Melanocytic
Inflammatory polyp

Table 1.8 Incidence, clinical features and management of feline skin tumours.

Tumour	Incidence	Patient predisposition	Site predisposition	Gross appearance	Behaviour	Treatment	Comments
EPITHELIAL TUMOURS							
Papilloma	Rare	Middle-aged to old	Head, eyelids, feet	Usually solitary. Small, well-circumscribed. May be pedunculated or cauliflower-like. Alopecic, occasionally ulcerated and bleeding	Benign	None or surgical excision, cryotherapy, or electrotherapy	
Intracutaneous cornifying epithelioma (keratoacanthoma)	Very rare				Benign	Surgical excision	One questionable report
Squamous cell carcinoma	Common	Blue-eyed, white-haired, middle-aged to old	Hypopigmented, sparsely or non-haired skin (particularly pinnae, lips, nose, eyelids)	Usually solitary, sometimes multiple. Firm, poorly circumscribed and ulcerated. Occasionally proliferative	Malignant. Highly locally invasive but slow to metastasize (local lymph nodes and lungs)	Wide surgical excision or amputation (digits). Also cryotherapy, electrosurgery, hyperthermia, radiotherapy, chemotherapy	Exposure to ultraviolet light correlates with development
Basal cell tumour	Common	Siamese, middle-aged to old	Head, neck, thorax	Usually solitary, occasionally multiple. Variable size, often oval-round, firm, raised, well-circumscribed nodules. May be pedunculated. Often pigmented. May be alopecic, ulcerated and bleeding	Usually benign and slow-growing. Rarely malignant; may metastasize to local lymph nodes	Wide surgical excision or cryotherapy	Most common melanotic skin neoplasm
Hair-follicle tumours Trichoepithelioma	Rare	Middle-aged	Possibly head	Usually solitary, occasionally multiple. Small, round, firm, raised, well-circumscribed. May be alopecic and ulcerated	Benign	None, wide surgical excision, cryotherapy, electrotherapy	
Dilated pore of Winer	Rare	Old, male	Face and neck	Solitary. Round, firm, raised, well-circumscribed with wide-mouthed, keratin-filled, central pore	Benign	None or surgical excision	
Pilomatrixoma	Very rare			Solitary. Round, soft to firm, raised, well-circumscribed. May be alopecic and ulcerated	Benign	None, surgical excision, cryotherapy	

	Frequency	Age	Location	Clinical features	Behaviour	Treatment	Comments
Sebaceous gland tumours							
Nodular sebaceous hyperplasia Adenoma	Uncommon	Middle-aged		Usually solitary, may be multiple. Usually small, firm, raised, well-circumscribed. May be lobulated (nodular hyperplasia, epithelioma), pedunculated (external ear canal); may be alopecic and ulcerated	Benign	None, surgical excision, cryotherapy, electrosurgery	
Epithelioma	Very rare	Middle-aged to old					
	Very rare	Middle-aged to old	Head, external ear canal				
Adenocarcinoma	Very rare	Middle-aged to old		Solitary. Variable size, firm, raised, poorly-circumscribed. May be alopecic and ulcerated	Malignant, locally invasive, rarely metastasizes	Wide surgical excision, cryotherapy, electrosurgery	
Sweat gland tumours Epitrichial (apocrine and ceruminous) glands							
Cysts	Rare (apocrine) Frequent (ceruminous)	Middle-aged	Head (apocrine) Ear canal (ceruminous)	Solitary, often multiple. Small, oval-round, fluctuant, raised, well-circumscribed, blue-black occasionally pinkish colour (ceruminous gland). May be alopecic	Benign	None, wide surgical excision (lateral wall resection or external ear canal ablation if affecting the ear), cryotherapy, electrosurgery	Ceruminous gland lesions are often accompanied by otitis externa
Adenoma	Frequent	Middle-aged to old	Head and neck (apocrine) Ear canal (ceruminous)	Usually small, firm, raised, fluctuant, well-circumscribed, white/red/ blue-black colour. Rarely ulcerated	Benign	Benign	
Adenocarcinoma	Frequent	Middle-aged to old	Ear canal (ceruminous)	Variable size, firm, poorly circumscribed. May be inflamed, ulcerated and bleeding	Malignant, highly locally invasive. May metastasize (local lymph nodes and lungs)	Wide surgical excision (lateral wall resection or external ear canal ablation if affecting the ear)	

continued on p. 58

Table 1.8 *Continued*

Tumour	Incidence	Patient predisposition	Site predisposition	Gross appearance	Behaviour	Treatment	Comments
Atrichial (eccrine)							
Adenoma	Very rare		Confined to footpads	Solitary. Firm, well to poorly-circumscribed May be ulcerated	Benign	Wide surgical excision	
Adenocarcinoma	Very rare				Malignant, locally invasive		
Epithelioid sarcoma	Rare	Middle-aged	Proximal limbs	Solitary. Firm, poorly circumscribed nodules. May be ulcerated	Malignant. May metastasize (local lymph nodes and lungs)	Wide surgical excision	
MESENCHYMAL TUMOURS							
Fibroma	Uncommon	Middle-aged to old	External ear canal, limbs and body	Solitary. Small, soft to firm, well-circumscribed. May be pedunculated, alopecic and ulcerated	Benign	None, wide surgical excision, cryotherapy, electrosurgery	
Fibrosarcoma	Common	Wide age range	Head, proximal limbs	Solitary, may be multiple. Variable size, firm, poorly circumscribed. May be alopecic and ulcerated	Malignant, locally invasive, occasionally metastasize (lungs)	Wide surgical excision, amputation, chemotherapy. Local recurrence common	Feline sarcoma virus (facilitated by FeLV) induces multiple fibrosarcomas in cats less than 3 years old
Myxoma and myxosarcoma (fibrosarcoma with abundant myxomatous substance)	Rare	Old		Solitary, poorly circumscribed, wide variation in shape	Myxoma – benign; myxosarcoma – malignant. Locally infiltrative. Rarely metastasizes (lungs)	Wide surgical excision. Local recurrence is common	
Undifferentiated sarcoma	Rare	Old	Footpads	Pads soft, ulcerated and painful	Malignant, locally invasive, slow to metastasize	Wide surgical excision	

	Incidence	Age	Site	Gross appearance	Behaviour	Treatment	Comments
Nodular fasciitis (aggressive fibromatosis)	Rare		Face	Solitary or multiple. Variable size, firm, poorly circumscribed	Benign	Wide surgical excision. Glucocorticoids. Local recurrence may occur	May represent an aggressive inflammatory process suggestive of locally invasive neoplasia
Leiomyoma and leiomyosarcoma	Very rare			Solitary. Firm, well-circumscribed	Leiomyoma – benign; leiomyosarcoma – malignant	Wide surgical excision	
Schwannoma	Uncommon	Middle-aged	Head, neck and forelimbs	Variable size, firm, well- to poorly circumscribed. White to pinkish-grey in colour. May ulcerate	Often malignant, rarely metastasizes	Wide surgical excision, amputation. Local recurrence	
Lipoma	Uncommon	Middle-aged to old	Thorax, abdomen, proximal limbs	Solitary or multiple. Variable size, soft to firm (fibrolipoma) usually well-circumscribed. May be infiltrative (lipomatosis). Occasionally pedunculated	Benign	Surgical excision	
Liposarcoma	Very rare	Old		Usually solitary, occasionally multiple, poorly circumscribed, may ulcerate.	Malignant. Locally invasive but rarely metastasizes (local lymph nodes and lungs)	Wide surgical excision	Has been induced experimentally by injection of FeLV

continued on p. 60

Table 1.8 *Continued*

Tumour	Incidence	Patient predisposition	Site predisposition	Gross appearance	Behaviour	Treatment	Comments
Tumours of vascular origin							
Haemangioma	Rare	Middle-aged to old	Limbs, flank head and neck	Usually solitary, but may be multiple. Small, firm to fluctuant, well-circumscribed. Red to bluish-black colour. Alopecic. May ulcerate and bleed	Benign	None, wide surgical excision, cryotherapy, electrosurgery	C-type viral particles isolated from one subcutaneous haemangioma
Haemangiosarcoma	Uncommon	Middle-aged to old	Head, axillae, inguinal area, limbs	Usually solitary. Variable size, soft and friable, poorly circumscribed. Red-black colour. Often ulcerate and bleed	Malignant. May be quiescent then grow rapidly. Highly locally invasive. Occasionally metastasize (lungs)	Wide surgical excision. Local recurrence	Poor prognosis
Haemangiopericytoma	Very rare			Solitary. Friable to firm, multinodular	Rarely metastasize	Surgical excision	
Lymphangioma	Very rare	Wide age range	Ventrum limbs	Variable size, cystic fluctuant swelling possibly discharging a pale-yellow fluid	Benign	Wide surgical excision.	
Lymphangiosarcoma	Rare				Locally invasive, rarely metastasize (lungs)	Local recurrence common	Poor prognosis
Mast cell tumour	Common	Siamese, older males	Head, neck	Solitary or multiple, variable size, soft to firm, raised nodules/plaques. Poorly to well-circumscribed. May be erythematous, ulcerated and pruritic	Usually benign, may be malignant. May metastasize (local lymph nodes and lungs). May be accompanied by splenomegaly and hepatomegaly	Wide surgical excision for solitary tumours, chemotherapy for disseminated tumours (glucocorticoids alone or in combination with other agents; no evidence combination therapy is superior to glucocorticoids alone). Radiotherapy. Local recurrence or dissemination common	

LYMPHOHISTIOCYTIC TUMOURS

Tumour	Incidence	Age	Location	Clinical features	Behaviour	Treatment	Comments
Histiocytoma	Very rare		Possibly head	Solitary. Small, firm, dome to button-shaped, well-circumscribed	Benign	None, surgical excision, cryotherapy, electrosurgery	
Fibrous histiocytoma	Rare		Face, limbs	Multiple. Firm, poorly circumscribed, may be alopecic	Benign but locally invasive. Does not metastasize	Surgical excision, glucocorticoids	
Malignant fibrous histiocytoma (extraskeletal giant cell tumour)	Rare	Middle-aged to old	Limbs and neck	Solitary. Variable size and shape, poorly circumscribed	Malignant, locally invasive, does not metastasize	Radical surgical excision or amputation	Poor prognosis
Cutaneous lymphoma — Primary lymphoma Non-epitheliotropic (B-cell origin) Epitheliotropic (T-cell origin) Mycosis fungoides	Rare	Middle-aged to old	Generalized or multifocal, rarely solitary	Nodules/plaques or ulcers. May be accompanied by inflammation, exfoliative dermatitis and pruritus	May be accompanied by lymphomegaly, hepatomegaly and splenomegaly in later stages	Chemotherapy (glucocorticoids, cyclophosphamide, vincristine)	
Secondary lymphoma	Rare	Middle-aged to old		Plaques or nodules. May ulcerate. Commonly pruritic	Accompanied by signs of other system involvement (alimentary, thymic, multicentric)	As for other lymphomas	Results from dissemination from other sites. Poor prognosis
Alopecia mucinosa	Rare		Head, ears, neck	Areas of alopecia and scaling			Precursor of mycosis fungoides
Plasmacytoma	Very rare			Raised, firm, well-circumscribed. May be ulcerated	May be confined to the skin (primary) or associated with myelomatosis (multiple myeloma) (secondary)	Surgical excision if primary	May be accompanied by monoclonal gammopathy if associated with myelomatosis

continued on p. 62

Table 1.8 *Continued*

Tumour	Incidence	Patient predisposition	Site predisposition	Gross appearance	Behaviour	Treatment	Comments
MELANOCYTIC TUMOURS Melanoma	Rare	Middle-aged to old	Head, ears eyelids	Solitary. Variable size. Macules/nodules/plaques. Brown to black to light colour. May be pedunculated, alopecic and ulcerated (malignant)	Usually malignant, rapid growth, commonly metastasize (local lymph nodes and lungs)	Radical surgical excision, radiotherapy. Poor prognosis	Have been produced experimentally by injection of feline sarcoma virus
SECONDARY SKIN NEOPLASIA (Metastasis to skin from other organs)	Rare						
Examples: Bronchogenic carcinoma			Digits	Ulcerative lesions			
Pancreatic and jejunal adenocarcinoma			Umbilical area	Cutaneous nodules			
Mammary gland adenocarcinoma			Head	Subcutaneous nodules			

Table 1.9 Incidence, clinical features and management of feline non-neoplastic tumours.

Tumour	Incidence	Patient predisposition	Site predisposition	Gross appearance	Behaviour	Treatment	Comments
Cutaneous cysts							
Epidermoid cysts	Uncommon		Head, neck, proximal limbs	Usually solitary, occasionally multiple. Well-circumscribed, round, fluctuant to firm. May discharge a grey/yellow/white cheesy material		Surgical excision	Should never be manually evacuated (increased chance of expression into dermis/subcutis with foreign body reaction and infection)
Follicular cysts (milia)	Common			Small, white to yellow, resembling pustules		None or surgical excision	Develop from retention of follicular or glandular products
Keratoses							
Actinic keratoses		*See* squamous cell carcinoma	*See* squamous cell carcinoma	Solitary or multiple. Erythema, scale, crust and occasionally nodule/plaque formation	Premalignant state, capable of progression to squamous cell carcinoma	Surgical excision, cryotherapy, possibly topical 5-fluorouracil	Result from excessive exposure to ultraviolet light
Cutaneous horn	Uncommon		Footpads (in association with feline leukaemia virus infection), neck, axillae	Multiple (footpads) or solitary, firm horn-like projections		Surgical excision. No satisfactory treatment for leukaemia virus-associated cutaneous horns	May be idiopathic, associated with feline leukaemia virus infection, or arise from papillomas, basal cell tumours or keratoacanthomas

continued on p. 64

Table 1.9 *Continued*

Tumour	Incidence	Patient predisposition	Site predisposition	Gross appearance	Behaviour	Treatment	Comments
Naevi (circumscribed developmental defects)							
Organoid (hair follicle and epitrichial sweat glands) / Melanocytic	Rare		Head, (proximal limbs (organoid), trunk (melanocytic)	Single or multiple. Soft to firm nodules (organoid); brown to black macules or papules (melanocytic). Well-circumscribed, may be pedunculated		None, surgical excision or cryotherapy	
Inflammatory polyp	Common		External ear canal, nasal cavity, nasopharynx, middle ear	Pedunculated mass. May be associated with otitis externa		Gentle traction (lateral vertical canal resection, slit soft palate if necessary)	

numbers of lymphocytes and neutrophils. Histopathological examination of lesions is characterized by infiltration with plasma cells often containing prominent Russell's bodies.

Many cases are asymptomatic and therapy may not be warranted. Some cases undergo spontaneous remission. Treatment, if indicated, is with immunosuppressive doses of prednisolone (e.g. 2.2 mg/kg twice daily) and/or chrysotherapy. Once satisfactory remission is achieved, doses of prednisolone and aurothioglucose are reduced to maintenance levels or discontinued.

Erythema multiforme

Erythema multiforme is an uncommon, acute, inflammatory condition affecting the skin and/or mucous membranes. It is currently considered to be a hypersensitivity reaction and has been associated in man and dogs with drug therapy, infections, neoplasia and connective tissue disorders or may be idiopathic. In cats it has been described in association with administration of penicillin and aurothioglucose (Scott *et al.*, 1987). The lesions are variable and may consist of symmetrical erythematous maculopapular eruptions, involving the body and proximal extremities and healing centrally while continuing to spread peripherally to produce annular (target) or arciform lesions, urticarial plaques or vesicles and bullae. Maculopapular eruptions commonly produce no systemic signs (erythema multiforme minor) but when extensive, vesiculobullous or ulcerative lesions occur and animals may be systemically ill (erythema multiforme major, Stevens–Johnson syndrome).

Histopathological changes accompanying erythema multiforme vary with the nature of the lesion but typically comprise hydropic degeneration of the epidermal basal cells, single cell necrosis of keratinocytes, perivascular infiltration of lymphocytes and macrophages or full-thickness coagulation necrosis of epithelium.

Erythema multiforme may be a mild, self-limiting disease, with spontaneous remission occurring within several weeks. However, in all cases, potentially triggering causes should be investigated and treated where possible. The use and efficacy of systemic glucocorticoids in the management of erythema multiforme is both controversial and doubtful.

Toxic epidermal necrolysis (Lyell's syndrome)

Toxic epidermal necrolysis (TEN) is a vesicobullous and ulcerative disorder currently thought to be mediated by immune mechanisms. In humans and dogs it may be associated with drug administration, systemic disease (e.g. infections, neoplasia, toxins) or may be idiopathic. In cats, it has only been recorded in association with drug administration (cephaloridine, hetacillin, ampicillin and feline leukaemia virus antiserum) (Scott *et al.*, 1987).

It is characterized clinically by mucocutaneous vesicles and bullae, which are succeeded by ulceration, epidermal collarette formation and a positive Nikolsky's sign (apparently normal skin which wrinkles on rubbing). These are accompanied by a variable degree of cutaneous pain, anorexia, pyrexia and depression.

The histopathology of lesional biopsies is characteristic irrespective of cause. There is full-thickness coagulation necrosis of the epidermis with dermo-epidermal cleft formation and minimal dermal inflammation.

Treatment depends on identification and elimination, where possible, of the precipitating cause. This must be combined with supportive and symptomatic therapy (fluids, antibacterial agents, topical agents). The use of systemic glucocorticoids is controversial, most workers believing they are not helpful and possibly contraindicated.

In humans, there is a close overlap between erythema multiforme major and TEN, and differentiation may be confusing. Erythema multiforme major may precede TEN and the patient may show both types of lesion (Champion, 1986; Pye, 1986). In addition, Lyell (1990) himself has recently written that the term 'toxic epidermal necrolysis (TEN) has come to the end of its useful life because what I thought was a single entity of scalded skin has turned out to be three separate diseases', these being staphylococcal scalded skin syndrome, generalized bullous fixed drug eruption and a group for which he proposes the name exanthematic necrolysis to cover the conditions in the remainder of the TEN group together with erythema multiforme major. The value of this contribution in reclassifying TEN and erythema multiforme in other species has not yet been evaluated.

Hypereosinophilic syndrome

This condition is rare and is characterized by a persistent circulating eosinophilia and eosinophilic infiltration of various organs (gastrointestinal tract, liver, spleen, bone marrow, lymph nodes) and sometimes the skin. The cutaneous signs include pruritus, maculopapular erythema and severe excoriations. Cutaneous histopathological examination reveals a perivascular dermatitis with eosinophilic infiltration (Scott *et al.*, 1985). The condition responds poorly to systemic glucocorticoids.

Lichenoid dermatoses

Lichenoid dermatoses are rare skin disorders possibly resulting from T-lymphocyte-mediated cytotoxicity directed against keratinocytes (Scott, 1989). Only one case of feline lichenoid dermatitis appears to have been reported (Buerger & Scott, 1988).

The lesions observed were bilaterally symmetrical and comprised characteristically grouped, angular, erythematous, flat-topped papules with a hyperkeratotic, scaly surface. In some areas, these coalesced forming hyperkeratotic, alopecic plaques. No systemic illness was reported.

Diagnosis was based on the history, physical examination and histopathological examination of skin biopsies. Lichenoid dermatoses are characterized histopathologically by interface dermatitis with hydropic degeneration of basal cells, necrotic apoptotic keratinocytes (Civatte bodies) and band-like infiltration of mononuclear cells at the dermo-epidermal junction.

Lichenoid dermatoses undergo spontaneous regression over a variable period of time (7 months in the case above). In other species, treatment by surgical excision is effective but medical therapy appears to be of little or no benefit.

Disorders associated with alopecia

Excessive moulting

Hair shedding in cats is governed principally by photoperiod and to a lesser degree by environmental temperature. In outdoor cats living in colder environments excessive physiological shedding in spring and autumn may result in transient coat thinning.

Pre-auricular alopecia

Sparseness of hair in the temporal area, extending from the eye to the ear, may be observed, particularly in short-haired cats. It is a physiological rather than a pathological condition and requires no treatment.

Feline symmetric alopecia

Feline symmetric alopecia (FSA) is a relatively new name for a condition previously termed feline endocrine alopecia, which itself has numerous hormonal synonyms. FSA is an advance in nomenclature for a syndrome which is clearly multifactorial and for which no endocrine aetiology had been proven. However, where the aetiology is determined, the term 'feline symmetric alopecia' should be used only descriptively, with the term *idiopathic feline symmetric alopecia (IFSA)* being reserved for cases of unknown cause.

Known causes of FSA include dermatophytosis, demodicosis (Scott, 1980, 1984), flea infestation (possibly associated with flea bite hypersensitivity), pediculosis, telogen defluxion, psychogenic alopecia (Thoday, 1986b, 1990a), food hypersensitivity and atopic disease (Kunkle, 1989), and hyperthyroidism (Thoday, 1990c). However, 53% of the cases in one study were idiopathic (Thoday, 1990a).

Whatever the cause of the syndrome, the possible sites affected are similar although the combination may vary between cases. In IFSA, the sites affected, in decreasing order, are: the ventral abdomen; medial, lateral and caudal hindlegs; forelegs (elbow to carpus); anogenital region; lateral abdomen; ventral and lateral thorax and the axillae. Generally, there is diffuse thinning of hair over affected sites rather than total alopecia and with or without a well-demarcated division between affected and non-affected areas (Plate 1.29a). Where animals are removing the hair themselves, the remaining hairs are well-anchored but may be fractured. Where the hair is being lost spontaneously, it is easily epilated. Whatever the cause, there are commonly no skin changes. Papules, crusts and erythema suggest parasitic infestations or hypersensitivity responses.

Diagnostically, the most important factor to establish is whether or not the hair is being removed by the cat. This is notoriously difficult as many owners will genuinely believe the cat to be non-pruritic as cats are commonly secret groomers. Therefore, trichograms should be carried out in all affected cats. The distal ends of at least 20 epilated hairs are examined microscopically. Evidence of fracture of the distal hair shaft suggests that the cat is removing the hair. Regrettably, many cats epilate rather than fracture the hair and in these, fractured hair shafts are not seen.

Definitive diagnosis of the cause of FSA is made from the history, physical examination and macro- and microscopic examinations for ectoparasites and for dermatophytes by UV light examination, microscopically or on culture, T_4 and T_3 determinations, dietary restriction and provocative testing for food hypersensitivity and intradermal testing for atopic disease. If fleas or flea faeces are not identified, intensive flea-control measures should be undertaken early in the investigation as fleas may still be causal. Where a specific aetiology is determined, it is treated accordingly. Eosinophilia may result from a number of causal diseases. A raised eosinophil count ($>1.5 \times 10^9$/l) had a 91% predictive value in ruling out IFSA in one study (Thoday, 1990a). Evidence of hair regrowth during the wearing of an Elizabethan collar for a 6-week period confirms that the cat is responsible for its hair loss and this procedure should always precede treatment for IFSA. A study in a small number of IFSA cats suggested that some animals may have low thyroid reserve (Thoday, 1990a).

The symptoms of IFSA are primarily aesthetic and thus the clinician must always question whether treatment is actually justified. However, many clients require attempts at management of IFSA. Although there is no proof that affected animals are hypothyroid, in one study 73% of cats responded totally and 15% partially to treatment with liothyronine sodium (T_3) at an initial dose of 40 µg/day, increasing by 20 µg every third day to a maximum of 100 µg/day, the total daily dose being divided into two (Thoday, 1990a) (Plate 1.29b). Twelve weeks after beginning therapy, cats should be sampled 3 hours after half the daily dosage of liothyronine sodium for both plasma T_4 and T_3 concentrations, which should be low or undetectable and within the reference range respectively. Where serum T_3 concentrations exceed the reference range, the T_3 dosage should be reduced. Continuous lower dose therapy (commonly 40 µg twice daily) is usually needed to maintain the coat. Other drugs used for the treatment of IFSA include megestrol acetate and oral or depot-injectable testosterone but side-effects are significantly more common and serious than with T_3.

Psychogenic alopecia and dermatitis
The term 'psychogenic alopecia' describes hair loss resulting from excessive localized licking and chewing, which is provoked by a disturbed behaviour pattern. Although rarely diagnosed in the UK, until relatively recently the condition was regularly reported from the USA. However, currently it is felt that many affected animals have physical disease entities, particularly hypersensitivity responses, and the incidence of diagnosis of psychogenic alopecia and dermatitis has fallen dramatically (K.W. Kwochka, personal communication).

True psychogenic alopecia and dermatitis may be a manifestation of anxiety or stress induced by moving to a new home, acquisition of a new cat or arrival of a new baby, but may also be a habit precipitated by local skin irritation. The condition occurs in cats of any age, sex and breed but is seen most frequently in Siamese, Burmese, Himalayan and Abyssinian cats ('highly-strung' breeds).

Clinically, focal or multifocal areas of alopecia, with broken and/or self-epilated hair, may be present (Plate 1.30). These are frequently located on the dorsum, medial thigh and ventral abdomen but may occur on the limbs and perianal or genital areas and are sometimes accompanied by variable degrees of inflammation, erosion and secondary infection. In Siamese and Himalayan cats whose coat colour is temperature-dependent, hair may regrow a darker colour in previously affected sites.

Diagnosis is based on the history, physical signs, confirmation of self-induced alopecia and dermatitis (see FSA), and elimination of physical causes for the lesions.

Before instituting treatment, it is important to investigate and, if possible, remove the underlying cause of the behavioural disturbance. Tranquillizers such as diazepam (1–2 mg/cat twice daily), sedatives such as phenobarbitone (2.2–6.6 mg/kg twice daily) and mood modifiers (progestogens such as megestrol acetate – see 'Eosinophilic ulcer' – and medroxyprogesterone acetate, 75–100 mg/cat every 2–3 months) may be used therapeutically and reduced to minimum dosage where the precipitating cause cannot be identified or removed.

Telogen defluxion (telogen effluvium, telogen defluvium)
Telogen defluxion may be precipitated by physiological stress such as gestation or lactation, disease states and certain drugs (e.g. ampicillin and sulphonamides). These result in curtailment of the anagen phase of the hair cycle and the consequent synchronous entry of large numbers of hairs into the telogen phase. Abnormal quantities of hair are therefore readily lost by grooming or friction and a localized or generalized, often symmetrical alopecia may result (Plate 1.31).

No specific treatment is required. The haircoat will return to normal following resolution of the underlying condition.

Anagen defluxion
This is a rare condition characterized by symmetrical truncal alopecia, which follows a temporary interruption in hair growth due to stress (infections, surgery, drugs) and is caused by fracture of hair shafts. Arrested hair growth is associated with defective keratinization of the hair shaft predisposing to fracture of hairs at that point, when normal hair growth resumes (Miller, 1990).

Pinnal alopecia
Periodic pinnal alopecia occurs in some Siamese cats. The cause is unknown and the hair regrows spontaneously after several months. No treatment is required.

Collar frictional alopecia
Alopecia resulting from simple friction between coat and collar is common in cats. When the collar is removed, there is a well-demarcated area of frequently total alopecia often completely circling the neck and the skin is smooth, shiny and shows no inflammatory response, thus simply differentiating the condition from flea collar dermatitis.

The lesion associated with collar frictional alopecia is pathognomonic for the condition. Removing the collar results in resolution.

Disorders of pigmentation
Periocular leucotrichia
Periocular leucotrichia (reduction of pigment in hairs of the mask resulting in a 'halo-like' or 'goggles' appearance round the eyes) has been described in Siamese cats (Scott, 1984). It occurs more frequently in females than males and appears to be associated with stress factors such as oestrus, pregnancy, systemic disease and dietary deficiency.

The condition is transient, resolving spontaneously as new hair grows in.

Unilateral periocular depigmentation (Aguirre syndrome)
This syndrome involving unilateral failure of hair pigmentation occurs in Siamese cats and may be associated with Horner's syndrome or corneal necrosis with uveitis and upper respiratory tract infections (Simon, 1985).

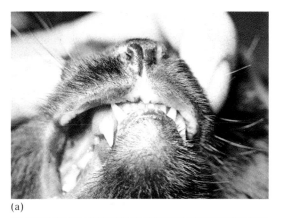

(a)

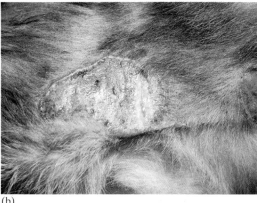

(b)

Plate 1.27 Indolent ulcer. (a) Lip ulcer. Surgical excision was curative. (Reproduced with permission from Thoday, 1981b.) (b) Trunk ulcer.

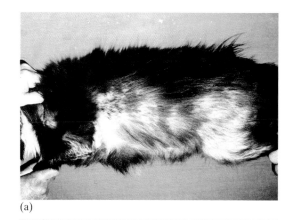

(a)

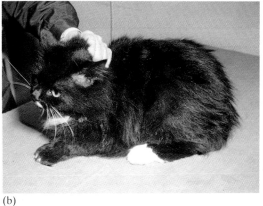

(b)

Plate 1.29 Idiopathic feline symmetric alopecia. (a) A 10-year-old, neutered female domestic short-haired cat with widespread alopecia. (b) The same cat 18 weeks after beginning treatment with liothyronine sodium.

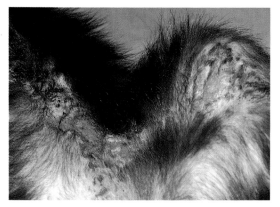

Plate 1.28 Eosinophilic plaque secondary to flea bite hypersensitivity on the abdomen and medial stifle.

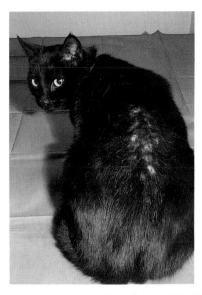

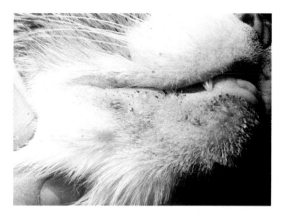

Plate 1.32 Acne: the area has been clipped to demonstrate the lesions. (Reproduced with permission from Thoday, 1981b.)

Plate 1.30 Psychogenic alopecia and dermatitis. The precipitating cause could not be identified but the problem was managed satisfactorily with diazepam.

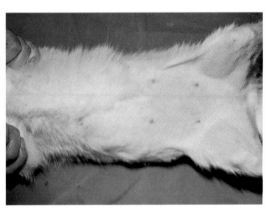

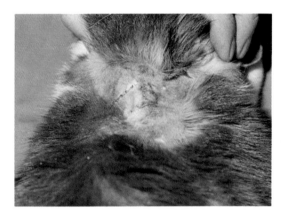

Plate 1.33 Cutaneous atrophy over the neck region due to subcutaneous injection of a depot glucocorticoid preparation. Continued pruritus due to flea infestation (the original cause of the glucocorticoid administration) has resulted in additional self-inflicted erosions.

Plate 1.31 Telogen defluxion: 12 weeks post-partum. The cat was pregnant again.

Lentigo simplex

This condition is of unknown aetiology. It has been described in orange cats usually beginning when they are less than 1 year old and characterized by a macular melanosis restricted to the lips, gums, eyelids and nose. Initially small foci of intense melanosis, the lesions enlarge and may coalesce. No additional clinical signs occur (Scott, 1987c). Recently, a case of generalized lentigine formation was described in a silver, domestic short-haired cat (Nash & Paulsen, 1990). Although the cat had developed lentigines on the head before 6 months of age, they began to increase in number and to affect the trunk when it was 3 years of age.

Histopathological examination reveals hypermelanosis of the basal cell layer and adjacent keratinocytes.

No treatment is known or necessary. Lentigo simplex does not predispose to melanoma.

Disorders affecting cutaneous and subcutaneous fat

Panniculitis

Panniculitis (inflammation of subcutaneous fat) is a condition of multiple aetiology including, in cats, infections, immune disorders, nutritional deficiency and, most frequently, idiopathy (Scott & Anderson, 1988). It has no age, breed or sex predispositions.

Feline panniculitis is manifested by the development of single or occasionally multiple, initially deep-seated nodules usually on the ventrum or ventrolateral thorax. These become fluid-filled and rupture, resulting in ulcers and sinuses which discharge thick, sometimes bloody, often oily material. The lesions may or may not be painful and heal slowly leaving depressed scars. The development of lesions may be preceded by systemic signs, such as pyrexia and depression, appropriate to the underlying cause.

Diagnosis is based on the history, physical examination, aspiration cytology ('foamy' lipid-containing macrophages) and is confirmed by the histological examination of excision biopsies. These demonstrate fat necrosis, foamy lipid-containing macrophages and foreign body giant cells. Determination of the specific cause of panniculitis necessitates examination of biopsy material using special stains and the culture of biopsy material to eliminate the possibility of microbiological organisms and investigations to rule out immune disorders and nutritional deficiencies. Accompanying clinical signs may indicate the probable cause in some cases (e.g. multisystem involvement if associated with SLE).

Treatment comprises identification and correction of the underlying cause. Excision of solitary lesions may be curative. Oral vitamin E supplementation with dietary change is effective for pansteatitis. Idiopathic (sterile) panniculitis should be treated with 2 mg/kg oral prednisolone twice daily until healing occurs and then tapered. Some cases may require intermittent or alternate-day prednisolone therapy.

Subcutaneous fat sclerosis

This condition, manifested clinically as a painless, extensive subcutaneous plaque, has been described in a 1-year-old, male, neutered, short-haired domestic cat (Buerger & Walton, 1987).

Histopathological examination revealed subcutaneous fibrosis with minimal fat necrosis and inflammation. The condition did not respond to glucocorticoids and euthanasia was carried out.

Seborrhoeic disorders

Acne

Acne is a dermatosis characterized by comedo (blackhead) formation. Feline 'acne' describes the plugging of hair follicles located on the chin and, less commonly, those on the lip with keratin and sebum (Plate 1.32). Except for a mild, diffuse symmetrical alopecia there are often no further clinical signs but sometimes there is accompanying infection with *Pasteurella multocida*, β-haemolytic streptococci and coagulase-positive staphylococci and the development of papules and pustules. Occasionally, this progresses to follicular rupture (furunculosis) and sinus formation. In these cases submandibular lymphadenopathy, pyrexia and depression may occur.

The aetiology of the condition is uncertain, it has no breed, sex or age predisposition, and has been ascribed to a predilection to seborrhoea, a failure to wash the area adequately, especially after eating, and inability of telogen hairs to push accumulations of keratin and sebum out of the hair follicle infundibulum.

In many cases of feline acne, no treatment is required although comedones may be expressed manually. In more severe cases, the area may be treated with 50–100% ethyl alcohol as a lipid solvent or with cleansing and antibacterial agents such as chlorhexidine or 2.5% benzoyl peroxide. The latter is also a follicular flushing agent. If secondary bacterial infection has become established these measures should be combined with systemic antibacterial therapy (trimethoprim/ sulphonamide combination, ampicillin, amoxycillin, tetracycline or erythromycin). Topical therapy may have to be continued indefinitely (3–4 times weekly) in order to keep the animal asymptomatic.

The authors have successfully used 13-*cis*-retinoic acid (isotretinoin) administration (5 mg once daily for 12 weeks and then 5 mg every second day) to treat one severe case and the feeding of raw liver (for its vitamin A content) (2 oz per week) to treat another. Isotretinoin is not licensed for use in cats in the UK.

Tail-gland hyperplasia (stud tail)
Although termed 'stud' tail, this condition also occurs in females and neutered males. It describes the accumulation of waxy secretions on the dorsal aspect of the tail, an area rich in epitrichial (apocrine) and modified sebaceous glands. Clinically, these accumulations are usually associated with yellowish-grey, oily material which may result in matting or thinning of the hair, and hyperpigmentation. Occasionally, secondary bacterial infection may result in folliculitis and furunculosis.

Treatment is by clipping out the affected area and gentle cleaning (see 'Feline acne'). Although the aetiology of the condition is unknown, it may be associated with the failure of some confined cats to clean this area. Remission of the condition may therefore be avoided by allowing the cat as much freedom as possible. Castration has no effect on the condition and though progestogens

may be beneficial, their use should be avoided if possible.

Feline seborrhoea
Seborrhoea is uncommon in cats and invariably secondary to an underlying disorder. Seborrhoea sicca (white-grey scale with dry skin and hair coat) may be associated with ecto- and endoparasitic infestations, fungal infections, nutritional deficiencies and metabolic disorders. Seborrhoea oleosa (greasy skin and hair coat) has been associated with FeLV infection, SLE, chronic liver disease and drug eruptions (Scott, 1987a).

Treatment should be directed at the underlying cause and may be combined with 1% selenium sulphide shampoos and dietary supplementation with essential fatty acids.

Miscellaneous disorders
Papulocrustous dermatitis (miliary dermatitis)
Multiple papulocrustous eruptions are a common reaction of feline skin to cutaneous insults and occur in many conditions. These may be broadly grouped as: ectoparasitic infestations (flea infestation, pediculosis, *Otodectes cynotis*, *Notoedres cati*, *Cheyletiella* spp., *Trombicula* spp., *Demodex* spp., *Lynxacarus radovskyi* infestations), some of which are undoubtedly associated with hypersensitivity responses; other hypersensitivity disorders (drugs, foods, atopic disease, contactants, endoparasites); infections (bacteria, fungi); and a group of miscellaneous disorders (dietary deficiency, contact dermatitis). Despite this extensive list, flea-bite hypersensitivity causes the vast majority of cases of papulocrustous dermatitis in cats in the UK (Thoday, 1985) and hypersensitivity responses in general are the commonest cause of papulocrustous eruptions in cats (Gross *et al.*, 1986).

Clinically the miliary lesions are accompanied by a variable degree of pruritus, self-inflicted lesions and lymphadenopathy. Occasionally, temperament changes, restlessness and aggression may occur.

In all cases it is essential to eliminate the known possible causes of miliary dermatitis before classifying a case as idiopathic. To accomplish this it is advised that the investigation is planned with the owner and then adhered to strictly. Although the investigation of any case should be tailored appropriately to the individual pet and owner, it may conveniently be staged as follows:

Stage 1: Take a complete history. Ensure a balanced diet. If indicated eliminate possible involvement of drugs by withdrawal of non-essential medications or substitution of chemically unrelated drug(s) for 3 weeks.

Stage 2: (a) Eliminate possible involvement of ectoparasites (physical examination, coat brushings and skin scrapings). As fleas are the most important single cause of papulocrustous dermatitis it is advised that even when there is no evidence of their involvement, a month's programme of intensive flea control is instituted (see section above on ectoparasites).

(b) At the same time, eliminate possible involvement of dermatophyte infection by collecting hair and scale for direct microscopal examination and culture.

(c) Rule out possible endoparasite involvement by faecal examination.

Stage 3: Eliminate possible involvement of food hypersensitivity by dietary restriction.

Stage 4: Eliminate atopic disease by intradermal testing.

Stage 5: Biopsy.

Stage 6: Eliminate possible involvement of bacterial infection by instituting a 3–6 week course of a systemic antibacterial agent (e.g. trimethoprim and sulphadiazine).

Stage 7: Re-evaluate possible involvement of an environmental agent (atopic disease, very rarely a contact agent) by hospitalization.

If, on completion of the investigation, no specific cause is identified, the case may be considered idiopathic and treated with glucocorticoids or, in the absence of response, progestogens (see 'Eosinophilic granuloma "complex"'). However, because of associated side-effects, progestogens should be avoided wherever possible.

Skin fragility/atrophy

Acquired excessive skin fragility, manifested by easy tearing of the skin, has been documented in

association with drug administration (phenytoin: Barthold *et al.*, 1980; prednisolone: Scott *et al.*, 1982) and systemic disease (dysautonomia: Sharp, 1987; cholangiosarcoma: Regnier & Pieraggi, 1989).

Although dermal atrophy was also documented in the cat receiving phenytoin (5–8 mg/kg/day for 3 weeks) electron microscopic examination revealed depletion but no structural abnormality of the collagen. Discontinuation of the drug resulted in resolution of the condition. Atrophy of dermal collagen has been reported in iatrogenic hyperadrenocorticism (Scott *et al.*, 1982). Localized alopecia, and thinning of the skin with epidermal and dermal atrophy may result from subcutaneous administration of glucocorticoids (particularly depot preparations) (Plate 1.33). Abnormally thin skin but no hyperextensibility was noted in the cat with cholangiosarcoma. In this case histopathological examination revealed dermal atrophy and electron microscopic examination demonstrated disorganization of collagen fibrils and fibres and abnormal diameters and cross-sectional shape of collagen fibrils.

Skin necrosis associated with urethral rupture

Extensive skin necrosis associated with subcutaneous infiltration by urine as a consequence of traumatic urethral rupture (in one case a bite and in the other iatrogenically as a result of catheterization) has been described in two cats (Holt, 1989). Both cases were managed successfully by skin grafting.

Ear margin necrosis

Bilateral necrosis and sloughing of the ear may be associated with frostbite, solar dermatitis, cold agglutinin disease and vasculitis and has been reported in cats with serious febrile systemic disease, haematological disorders (Holzworth, 1987b) and decomposed scallop poisoning (Scott, 1987b).

Arteriovenous fistula

An arteriovenous fistula is a direct communication between an artery and vein bypassing the capillary bed and is rare in cats. Although arteriovenous fistulae may be congenital, the cases of peripheral arteriovenous fistulae reported in cats appear to be acquired as a result of trauma (Slocum *et al.*, 1973; Furneau *et al.*, 1974), although recurrent arteriovenous fistula has been reported in a cat with hyperthyroidism (Harari *et al.*, 1984).

Lesions may be associated with oedema, hair loss, pain, secondary infection and haemorrhage and are characterized by pulsating vessels, a continuous machinery murmur and sometimes palpable thrills.

Diagnosis is confirmed by arteriography and treatment requires surgical excision of the lesion or amputation of the affected digit/limb.

DISEASES OF
SPECIALIZED CUTANEOUS AREAS

Diseases of the external ear
  Otitis externa
  Aural haematoma
  Aural neoplasia
Diseases of the eyelids
  Entropion and ectropion
  Blepharitis
  Neoplasia
Diseases of the anal sacs
  Impaction
Diseases of the nails
  Paronychia and pyonychia
  Abnormal nail growth

Diseases of the external ear

Otitis externa

Otitis externa is an acute or chronic inflammation of the epithelial lining of the external auditory meatus and may extend to involve the pinna. Any one or a combination of several different factors may be involved in its genesis. The most important single cause, especially in kittens, is the parasitic mite *Otodectes cynotis*. Other parasites (*Demodex* spp., *Notoedres cati*, *Trombicula autumnalis*), foreign bodies, polyps and neoplasia (particularly ceruminous gland adenomas and adenocarcinomas) may also cause otitis externa.

Bacteria (*Staphylococcus intermedius* and β-haemolytic streptococci and, less frequently, *Pasteurella multocida*, *Pseudomonas aeruginosa*, *Proteus* spp. and *Escherichia coli*), with yeasts such as *Malassezia pachydermatis* (*Pityrosporum canis*) may be cultured, and occasionally fungi (*Microsporum canis* and *Trichophyton mentagrophytes*) may also be involved. However, the role of these infectious agents in initiating otitis is debatable. In most cases, it is probable that they are secondary invaders taking advantage of favourable changes in the microclimate of the ear canal to multiply and establish themselves. Once this is accomplished, they exacerbate and perpetuate any inflammatory process.

The degree of irritation produced by otitis externa varies markedly between individuals and is not related to the apparent severity of the lesions. Common clinical manifestations of otitis externa are twitching and scratching the affected ear(s) and shaking the head. Occasionally aural haematomata develop.

Diagnosis is made on the basis of physical signs and auroscopic examination. However, thorough investigation is necessary to ascertain the specific cause in each case. *Otodectes cynotis*, which is white and retreats from the light source, and foreign bodies and neoplasms may be detected by auroscopic examination. Ceruminous discharges are associated with seborrhoeic conditions, *Demodex cati* infestation and *M. pachydermatis*; reddish brown to black waxy discharges with *Otodectes cynotis* infestation; purulent discharges with bacterial infections; and dry crusty lesions may be associated with fungal infection.

In many cases, auroscopic examination may reveal only non-specific evidence of otitis externa: an accumulation of a variable amount of discharge, accompanied by inflammation, swelling, occasionally ulceration and, in chronic otitis, hyperplasia or verrucose proliferations of the epithelium. Swabs of the discharge should be examined microscopically for mites (*Demodex cati* and *Otodectes cynotis*) and cultured, if indicated, for bacteria, yeasts and fungi. Initial examination should be followed, if necessary, by gentle but thorough cleaning of the ear canal

(0.5% hexetidine solution) or, if the discharge is waxy, a ceruminolytic agent such as squalene. Re-examination should subsequently be carried out to establish the patency of the tympanic membrane. Hypersensitivity reactions (drugs, foods, atopic disease) may also be causal.

Successful treatment necessitates correction of the underlying cause and elimination of secondary infections. Topical therapy is adequate to control most infections providing a generous quantity of the therapeutic agent is instilled into the ear canal to ensure adequate penetration. In severe cases, systemic treatment may be required. A large number of topical preparations are available for the treatment of otitis externa. There is no universal panacea and specific therapy should be selected for each case, avoiding complex formulations where these are unnecessary. Anti-yeast agents are commonly included as constituents of proprietary ear dressings. Where *M. pachydermatis* is the apparent cause or the result of ceruminous otitis, it may be controlled by acidifying the ear canal using 13% aluminium acetate solution (Burow's solution). Powders tend to form aggregates and usually fail to reach the tympanic membrane and should therefore be avoided.

In cases failing to respond promptly or recurring frequently, treatment should be discontinued and all possible predisposing systemic and local factors should be investigated carefully. To facilitate aural examination, the cat should be sedated or anaesthetized, the ear canals examined thoroughly, the patency of the tympanic membrane checked, and aural swabs sent for culture and antibacterial sensitivity testing. Appropriate therapy or further investigations should then be instituted. Where cases respond to therapy with subsequent exacerbation on continued or repeated treatment, a contact hypersensitivity to a constituent of the otic preparation should be suspected.

If no predisposing factor can be identified and the condition continues to recur, continued therapy or vertical canal resection or ablation should be considered.

Aural haematoma

Haematoma of the pinnae usually occurs in association with otitis externa as a result of traumatization of blood vessels running between the skin and concave aspect of the pinnal cartilage.

Treatment includes investigation and correction of the underlying cause and surgical incision and drainage of the haematoma and subsequent obliteration of dead space to prevent its reformation. Recently, Kuwahara (1986) has suggested that aspiration and flushing of the haematoma followed by dexamethasone instilled directly into the haematoma cavity or, alternatively and less satisfactorily, given daily intravenously, produced results superior to those obtained surgically. These observations remain to be confirmed by other workers.

Aural neoplasia

Benign polyps and apocrine (ceruminous) gland adenoma, adenocarcinomas and squamous cell carcinoma are the most important tumours of the ear canal (see 'Cutaneous neoplasms' above).

Diseases of the eyelids

Entropion and ectropion

These are uncommon in cats. Entropion (inversion of the eyelids) occurs more frequently in Persian cats than other breeds. It may result in blepharospasm, excessive lachrimation and ulcerative keratitis. Ectropion (eversion of the eyelids) usually results from chronic conjunctivitis or cicatricial healing of a wound.

Both conditions are treated by surgical correction.

Blepharitis

Blepharitis (inflammation of the skin of the eyelid) may be caused by bacterial (*Staphylococcus intermedius*) or fungal (*Microsporum canis*) infections or infestations with ectoparasites (*Notoedres cati*, *Demodex* spp.). Inflammation, alopecia, and crust and scale formation may be evident. Diagnosis of the cause depends on the history, physical examination, examination of skin scrapings for evidence of parasitic infestations or fungal infections, and bacterial and fungal cultures.

Treatment must be appropriate to the specific cause.

Neoplasia

Squamous cell carcinoma is the most common eyelid tumour of cats (see 'Environmental diseases' and 'Cutaneous neoplasms' above).

Diseases of the anal sacs

Impaction

Anal sac impaction is seen occasionally in cats. Signs include licking and rubbing the anal area, pain on defaecation, scooting, tail chasing, perianal inflammation and tailhead alopecia (Miller, 1990). These are relieved by manual expression of the sacs.

Disease of the nails

Nails and nailbeds are susceptible to trauma and a variety of disease processes including bacterial and fungal infections and autoimmune disorders.

Paronychia and pyonychia

Paronychia is inflammation of the soft tissue surrounding the nail, while pyonychia is a purulent infection in this area. They are commonly seen together and result most frequently from bacterial and occasionally yeast (candidal paronychia) and fungal (onychomycosis) infections. Bacterial infections are usually secondary to immunosuppression (e.g. FeLV and FIV infections, diabetes mellitus) autoimmune diseases (pemphigus foliaceus, SLE) and, occasionally, contact dermatitis. Primary bacterial infections are rare.

Diagnosis includes examination and culture for bacteria, yeasts and fungi, submission of biopsy material for histopathological examination and direct immunofluorescence testing and investigation of possible causal immunosuppressive disease.

Treatment must be directed at correcting the underlying cause and elimination of any second-ary infection. Exposure and drainage of infection may require removal of the nail-plate.

Abnormal nail growth

Geriatric cats which have abnormal nail growth and which fail to wear down their nails, and hyperthyroid cats with abnormally rapid nail growth may periodically require nail trimming.

APPENDIX

Drugs and materials mentioned in the text may be obtained as shown:

Adrenaline 1–1000: (Bimeda UK).

Aluminium acetate: Aluminium acetate solution BPC (Burow's solution).

Amitraz: Aludex Mange Mite Wash (Hoechst).

Amphotericin B: Fungizone (E.R. Squibb & Sons).

Aurothioglucose: Solganol (Schering (USA)).

Azathioprine: Imuran (Wellcome).

Benzoyl peroxide: Oxydex (C-Vet); Paxcutol (Virbac).

Betacarotene: Carotin (Prosana (Australia)); Salatene (Roche (Australia, USA)).

Biopsy punch: (Stiefel Laboratories)

Blue-black ink: Quink (Parker Pen Company).

Carbimazole: Neo-Mercazole (Nicholas Laboratories).

Cetrimide: Cetavlon Solution 40% (Imperial Chemical Industries Pharmaceuticals).

Chlorhexidine: Hibitane (Imperial Chemical Industries Pharmaceuticals).

Chlorpheniraine: Piriton (Allen & Hanburys).

Clofazimine: Lamprene (Geigy Pharmaceuticals).

Cyclophosphamide: Endoxana (Boehringer Ingelheim).

Dapsone: Dapsone tablets B.P.

Dermatophyte Test Medium: Fungassay (C-Vet).

Diazepam: Valium (Roche).

Dichlorvos/fenitrothion: Nuvan Top (Ciba-Geigy Agrochemicals).

Diff-Quik: (Merz & Dade, AG (Switzerland)).

Enilconazole: Imaverol (Janssen).

Essential fatty acid supplements (evening primrose oil and fish oil):

Efavet 330, Efavet Regular (Efamol Vet).

Ethyl alcohol: Alcohol (95%) B.P. Dilute with water to required concentration.

Feline Selected Protein Diet; Waltham.

Finn Chambers: (Associated Hospital Supplies, PO Box 4, Pershore, Worcestershire).

5-Fluorocytosine (flucytosine): Alcobon (Roche). Available to hospitals only.

Gentian violet: (BDH).

Griseofulvin: Grisovin (Coopers Pitman-Moore).

Hydrogen peroxide: Hydrogen peroxide solution B.P.

Intradermal allergen solutions: (ARTU Biologicals, Postbus 612, AP Lelystad, Holland; HAL Allergenen Laboratorium BV, Postbus 1007, 2001 Haarlem, Holland).

5-Iodo, 2'-deoxyuridine: Virudox (Bioglan Laboratories); Herpid (Boehringer Ingelheim).

Iodofenphos/dichlorvos: Nuvan Staykil (Ciba-Geigy Agrochemicals).

Isotretinoin: Roaccutane (Roche). Available to hospitals only.

Ivermectin: Ivomec (MSD Agvet).

Ketoconazole: Nizoral (Janssen).

Lactophenol Cotton Blue: (BDH).

Levamisole: Levacide (Norbrook Laboratories); Nilverm (Coopers Pitman-Moore).

Lignocaine: Xylocaine (Astra Pharmaceuticals).

Liothyronine sodium: Tertroxin (Coopers Pitman-Moore).

Malathion: Derbac M Liquid, Suleo-M Lotion (International Laboratories); Prioderm Cream Shampoo, Prioderm Lotion (Napp Laboratories).

Medroxyprogesterone acetate: Perlutex (Leo Laboratories).

Megestrol acetate: Ovarid (Coopers Pitman-Moore).

Methimazole: Tapazole (Eli Lilly (USA)).

Methoprene: Acclaim (Sanofi Animal Health).

Methoprene/permethrin: Acclaim Plus (Sanofi Animal Health).

Metyrapone: Metopirone (Ciba Laboratories).

Michel's fixative: Proprietary preparation not available. Composition see Muller *et al.* (1989) p. 442.

Monosulfiram: Tetmosol (Imperial Chemical Industries Pharmaceuticals).

Nystatin: Nystan (E.R. Squibb & Son).

o,p'-DDD: Lysodren tablets (Bristol Laboratories); capsules (Assistance Publique (France)).

Patch testing kit: (Associated Hospital Supplies, PO Box 4, Pershore, Worcestershire).

Phenobarbitone: Phenobarbitone tablets (APS Ltd).

Potassium iodate: Potassium iodate tablets (Cambridge Selfcare Diagnostics).

Povidone iodine: Pevidine (BK Veterinary Products).

Prednisolone: Prednisolone tablets (Veterinary Drug Co).

Prednisone: Prednisone B.P.

Pyrethrins/Pyrethroids: Head-To-Tail Powder, Head-To-Tail Spray (Coopers Pitman-Moore); Pybuthrin Powder (Veterinary Drug Co).

Selenium sulphide: Seleen (Sanofi Animal Health).

Silver sulphadiazine: Flamazine (Smith & Nephew Pharmaceuticals).

Sodium aurothiomalate: Myocrisin (May & Baker).

Sodium iodide: Sodium iodide injection B.P.C.

Squalene: Sebumol eardrops (Willow Francis).

Swarfega: (Deb Chemical Proprietaries).

Taurine: L-Taurine (Cantassium Vitamins).

Testosterone: Orandrone (tablets); Androject, Durateston (injectable) (Intervet UK).

Thiabendazole: Mintezol (Merck, Sharp & Dohme).

Thyroxine: Soloxine (Daniels pharmaceuticals).

Vincristine: Oncovin (Eli Lilly).

Vitamin A: Vitamin A water miscible Type 100 (Roche).

Vitamin E: Tocovite (Arnolds Veterinary Products); Vita E (Bioglan); Ephynal (Roche).

Zinc and castor oil cream: Zinc and Castor Oil cream/ointment B.P.

REFERENCES AND FURTHER READING

General

Muller G.H., Kirk R.W. & Scott D.W. (1989) *Small*

Animal Dermatology, 4th edn. W.B. Saunders, Philadelphia. The standard text on small animal skin diseases.

Scott D.W. (1980) Feline dermatology 1900–1978: A monograph. *J. Am. Anim. Hosp. Ass.* **16**, 303–459.

Scott D.W. (1984) Feline dermatology 1979–1982: Introspective retrospections. *J. Am. Anim. Hosp. Ass.* **20**, 537–64.

Scott D.W. (1987a) Feline dermatology 1983–1985: 'The secret sits'. *J. Am. Anim. Hosp. Ass.* **23**, 255–74.

Scott D.W. (1990) Feline dermatology 1986–1988: Looking to the 1990s through the eyes of many counsellors. *J. Am. Anim. Hosp. Ass.* **26**, 515–37.

The authors are pleased to acknowledge the value of these four excellent literature reviews by D.W. Scott in the preparation of this chapter.

Others

Allen J.R. (1973) Tick resistance: basophils in skin reactions of resistant guinea pigs. *Int. J. Parasitol.* **3**, 195–200.

Allen J.R., Doube B.M. & Kemp D.H. (1977) Histopathology of bovine stain reactions to Ixodes holocyclus. *Can. J. Comp. Med.* **41**, 27–35.

Arnold U., Opitz M., Grosser I., Bader R. & Eigenmann J.E. (1984) Goitrous hypothyroidism and dwarfism in a kitten. *J. Am. Anim. Hosp. Ass.* **20**, 753–8.

Attelberger M.H. (1988) Subcutaneous mycoses. In Barlough J.E. (ed) *Manual of Small Animal Infectious Diseases.* Churchill Livingstone, New York, pp. 277–90.

Baker K.P. (1974) Hair growth and replacement in the cat. *Br. Vet. J.* **130**, 327–35.

Barthold S.W., Kaplan B.J. & Schwartz A. (1980) Reversible dermal atrophy in a cat treated with phenytoin. *Vet. Pathol.* **17**, 469–76.

Beale K.M. (1988) Azathioprine for treatment of immune-mediated diseases of dogs and cats. *J. Am. Vet. Med. Ass.* **192**, 1316–8.

Bennett D. (1987) Canine systemic lupus erythematosus. In Grunsell C.S.G., Hill F.W.G. & Raw M.-E. (eds) *Veterinary Annual*, 27th Issue. Scientechnica, Bristol, pp. 350–6.

Bennett M. (1989) Cowpox in cats. *In Practice* **11**, 244–7.

Biberstein E.C., Jang S.S. & Hirsh D.C. (1984) Species distribution of coagulase-positive staphylococci in animals. *J. Clin. Microbiol.* **19**, 610–5.

Bostock D.E. (1986) Neoplasms of the skin and subcutaneous tissues in dogs and cats. *Brit. Vet. J.* **142**, 1–19.

Bourdin M., Destombes P., Parodi A.L., Drouhet E. & Segretain G. (1975) Première observation d'un mycétoma à *Microsporum canis* chez un chat. *Recueil de Médecine Vétérinaire* **151**, 475–80.

Buerger R.G. & Scott D.W. (1988) Lichenoid dermatitis in a cat: A case report. *J. Am. Anim. Hosp. Ass.* **24**, 55–9.

Buerger R.G. & Walton D.K. (1987) Subcutaneous fat sclerosis in a cat. *Compen. Cont. Educ. Pract. Vet.* **9**, 1198–201.

Burke M.J., Grauer G.F. & Macy D.W. (1983) Successful treatment of cutaneolymphatic sporotrichosis in a cat with ketoconazole and sodium iodide. *J. Am. Anim. Hosp. Ass.* **19**, 542–7.

Bussiéras J. (1984) A rare case of sarcoptic mange in a cat. *Practique Medicale et Chirugicale de l'Animal de Compaigne* **19**, 375–7.

Bussiéras J. & Chermette R. (1986) Amitraz and canine demodicosis. *J. Am. Anim. Hosp. Ass.* **22**, 779–82.

Caciolo P.L., Nesbitt G.H. & Hurvitz A.I. (1984) Pemphigus foliaceus in eight cats and results of induction therapy using azathioprine. *J. Am. Anim. Hosp. Ass.* **20**, 571–7.

Carakostas M.C., Miller R.I. & Woodward M.G. (1984) Subcutaneous dermatophilosis in a cat. *J. Am. Vet. Med. Ass.* **185**, 675–6.

Carey C.J. & Morris J.G. (1977) Biotin deficiency in the cat and the effect on hepatic proprionyl CoA carboxylase. *J. Nutr.* **107**, 330–4.

Carpenter J.L., Andrews L.K. & Holzworth J. (1987) Tumors and tumor-like lesions. In Holzworth J. (ed) *Diseases of the Cat: Medicine and Surgery*, vol. 1. W.B. Saunders, Philadelphia, pp. 406–596.

Center S.A., Scott D.W. & Scott F.W. (1982) Multiple cutaneous horns on the foot pads of a cat. *Feline Practice* **12**(4), 26–30.

Champion R.H. (1986) Disorders affecting small blood vessels: Erythema and telangiectasia. In Rook A., Wilkinson D.S., Ebling F.S.G., Champion R.H. & Buxton J.L. (eds) *Textbook of Dermatology*, 4th edn, vol. 2. Blackwell Scientific Publications, Oxford, pp. 1081–97.

Chesney C.J. (1989) Demodicosis in the cat. *J. Small Anim. Pract.* **30**, 689–95.

Chloe P.J. & Allinson J.F. (1982) Prototheocosis in a cat. *J. Am. Vet. Med. Ass.* **180**, 78–9.

Conroy J.D. (1979) Immune-mediated diseases of skin and mucous membranes. In Ettinger S.J. (ed) *Textbook of Veterinary Internal Medicine*, vol. 2. W.B. Saunders, Philadelphia, pp. 2140–58.

Conroy J.D. (1983) An overview of immune-mediated mucocutaneous diseases of the dog and cat. II. Other diseases based on immunologic mechanisms. *Am. J. Dermatopathol.* **5**, 593–9.

Conroy J.D., Healey M.C. & Bane A.G. (1982) New *Demodex* sp. infesting a cat: A case report. *J. Am. Anim. Hosp. Ass.* **18**, 405–7.

Coombs R.R.A. & Gell P.G.H. (1975) Classification of

allergic reactions responsible for clinical hypersensitivity and disease. In Gell P.G.H. & Coombs R.R.A. (eds) *Clinical Aspects of Immunology*. Blackwell Scientific Publications, Oxford, p. 761.

Cooper L.M. & Sabine M. (1972) Paw and mouth disease in a cat. *Austral. Vet. J.* **48**, 644.

Cotter S.M., Hardy W.D.H. & Essex M. (1975) Association of feline leukaemia virus with lymphosarcoma and other disorders in the cat. *J. Am. Vet. Med. Ass.* **166**, 449–54.

Cox H.U. & Hoskins J.D. (1985) Distribution of staphylococcal species on clinically healthy cats. *Am. J. Vet. Res.* **46**, 1824–8.

Dawson C.O. & Noddle B.M. (1968) Treatment of *Microsporum canis* ringworm in a cat colony. *J. Small Anim. Pract.* **9**, 613–20.

De Boer D.J., Saban R., Schultz K.T. & Bjorling D.E. (1993) Feline IgE. Preliminary Evidence of its existence and crossreactivity with Canine IgE. In Ihrke P.J., Mason I.S. & White S.D. (eds) *Advances in Veterinary Dermatology*. vol. 2. Pergamon Press, Oxford. pp. 51–62.

Devriese L.A., Nzuambe D. & Godard C. (1984) Identification and characterisation of staphylococci isolated from cats. *Vet. Microbiol.* **9**, 279–85.

Dorn C.R., Taylor D.O.N., Schneider R., Hibbard H.H. & Klauber M.R. (1968) Survey of animal neoplasms in Alameda and Contra Costa counties, California. II. Cancer morbidity in dogs and cats from Alameda county. *J. Natl Cancer Inst.* **40**, 307–18.

Doster A.R., Erickson E.D. & Chandler F.W. (1987) Trichosporonosis in two cats. *J. Am. Vet. Med. Ass.* **190**, 1184–6.

Elliot G.S., Whitney M.S., Reed W.M. & Tuite J.F. (1984) Antemortem diagnosis of paecilomycosis in a cat. *J. Am. Vet. Med. Ass.* **184**, 93–4.

Elliot G., Lawson G.H.K. & Mackenzie C.P. (1986) *Rhodococcus equi* in cats. *Vet. Rec.* **118**, 693–4.

Emmons C.W., Binford C.H., Utz J.P. & Kwon-Chung K.J. (1977) *Medical Mycology*, 3rd edn. Lea & Febiger, Philadelphia.

Falk E.S. & Bolle R. (1980) In vitro demonstration of specific immunologic hypersensitivity to scabies mite. *Br. J. Dermatol.* **103**, 367–73.

Fawcett J., Demaray S.Y. & Altman N. (1977) Multiple xanthomatosis in a cat. *Feline Practice* **7**(3), 31–3.

Finnie J.W. & Chloe P.J. (1981) Cutaneous protothecosis in a cat. *Austral. Vet. J.* **57**, 307–8.

Flecknell P.A., Orr C.M., Wright A.I., Gaskell R.M. & Kelly D.F. (1979) Skin ulceration associated with herpesvirus infection in cats. *Vet. Rec.* **104**, 313–5.

Foil, C.S. (1986) Antifungal agents in dermatology. In Kirk R.W. (ed) *Current Veterinary Therapy IX: Small Animal Practice*. W.B. Saunders, Philadelphia, pp. 560–5.

Freeman L.J., Hegreberg G.A. & Robinette J.D. (1987) Ehlers–Danlos syndrome in dogs and cats. *Seminars Vet. Med. Surg. (Small Animal)* **11**, 221–7.

Frenkel J.K., Kier A.B., Wagner J.E. & Holzworth J. (1987) Protozoan diseases. In Holzworth J. (ed) *Diseases of the Cat: Medicine and Surgery*, vol. 1. W.B. Saunders, Philadelphia, pp. 359–405.

Furneau R.W., Pharr J.W. & McManus J.L. (1974) Arteriovenous fistula following dew-claw removal in a cat. *J. Am. Anim. Hosp. Ass.* **10**, 569–73.

Gaskell R.M., Gaskell C.J., Evans R.J., Dennis P.E., Bennett A.M., Udall M.C., Voyle C. & Hill T.J. (1983) Natural and experimental pox virus infection in the domestic cat. *Vet. Rec.* **112**, 164–70.

Gasper P.W., Thrall M.A., Wenger D.A., Macy D.W., Gilette E.L., Kesel M.L. & Hoover F.A. (1984) Installment of arylsulphatase B activity in a mucopolysaccharidosis VI Siamese cat by bone marrow transplantation. *Vet. Clin. Pathol.* **13**(1), 29.

Geary M.R. & Baker K.P. (1986) The occurrence of pili torti in a litter of kittens in England. *J. Small Anim. Pract.* **27**, 85–8.

Gerschoff S.N., Andrus S.B., Hegsted D.M. & Lentini E.A. (1957) Vitamin A deficiency in cats. *Lab. Invest.* **6**, 227–40.

Gerschoff S.N., Andrus S.B. & Hegsted D.M. (1959) The effect of the carbohydrate and fat content of the diet upon the riboflavin requirement of the cat. *J. Nutr.* **68**, 75–88.

Goodwin C.W. (1984) Current burn treatment. *Adv. Surg.* **18**, 145–76.

Gross T.L., Kwochka K.W. & Kunkle G.A. (1986) Correlation of histologic and immunologic findings in cats with miliary dermatitis. *J. Am. Vet. Med. Ass.* **189**, 1322–5.

Halliwell R.E.W. (1985) Cited by Kwochka K.W. & Bevier D.E. (1987) Flea dermatitis. In Nesbitt G.H. (ed) *Dermatology*. Churchill Livingstone, New York, pp. 21–55.

Halliwell R.E.W. & Gorman N.T. (eds) (1989) Atopic Disease *Veterinary Clinical Immunology*. W.B. Saunders, Philadelphia, pp. 232–52.

Harari J., MacCoy D.M., Johnson A.L. & Tranquilli W.J. (1984) Recurrent peripheral arteriovenous fistula and hyperthyroidism in a cat. *J. Am. Anim. Hosp. Ass.* **20**, 759–64.

Hardy W.D. (1981) The feline sarcoma viruses. *J. Am. Anim. Hosp. Ass.* **17**, 981–97.

Haskins M.E., Jezyk P.F. & Patterson D.F. (1979) Mucopolysaccharide storage disease in three families of cats with arylsulphatase B deficiency. Leucocyte studies and carrier identification. *Pediatric Res.* **13**, 1203–10.

Hawkins J.A., McDonald R.K. & Woody B.J. (1987) *Sarcoptes scabiei* infestation in a cat. *J. Am. Vet. Med.*

Ass. **190**, 1572–3.

Heath M.K., McQueen J.W. & Spies T.D. (1940) Feline pellegra. *Science* **92**, 514.

Helton K.A., Nesbitt G.H. & Caciolo P.C. (1986) Griseofulvin toxicity in cats: Literature review and report of seven cases. *J. Am. Anim. Hosp. Ass.* **22**, 453–8.

Henfrey J.I., Thoday K.L. & Head K.W. (1991) Comparison of three local anaesthetic techniques for skin biopsy in dogs. *Vet. Derm.* **2**, 21–7.

Higgins R. & Paradis M. (1980) Abscess caused by *Corynebacterium equi* in a cat. *Can. Vet. J.* **21**, 63–4.

Holt P.E. (1989) Hindlimb skin loss associated with urethral rupture in two cats. *J. Small Anim. Pract.* **30**, 406–9.

Holzworth J. (1987a) Mycotic diseases. In Holzworth J. (ed) *Diseases of the Cat: Medicine and Surgery*, vol. 1. W.B. Saunders, Philadelphia, pp. 320–58.

Holzworth J. (1987b) The ear. In Holzworth J. (ed) Diseases of the Cat: Medicine and Surgery, vol. 1. W.B. Saunders, Philadelphia, pp. 725–38.

Horvath Z. & Papp L. (1967) Clinical manifestations of Aujeszky's disease in the cat. *Acta Veterinaria Hungarica* **17**, 49–54.

Hosie M., Sparkes A. & Hopper C. (1989) Feline immunodeficiency virus. *In Practice* **11**, 87–95.

Howard D.R. (1986) Pseudorabies in dogs and cats. In Kirk R.W. (ed) *Current Veterinary Therapy IX: Small Animal Practice*. W.B. Saunders, Philadelphia, pp. 1071–2.

Irving R.A., Day R.S. & Eales L. (1982) Porphyrin values and treatment of feline solar dermatitis. *Am. J. Vet. Res.* **43**, 2067–9.

Jezyk P.F., Haskins M.E., Patterson D.F., Mellman W.J. & Greenstein M. (1977) Mucopolysaccharidosis in a cat with arylsulphatase B deficiency: A model of Maroteaux Lamoy syndrome. *Science* **198**, 834–6.

Johnson R.P. & Sabine M. (1971) The isolation of herpesvirus from skin ulcers in domestic cats. *Vet. Rec.* **89**, 360–3.

Jones B.R., Wallace A., Harding D.R.K., Hancock W.S. & Campbell C.H. (1983) Occurrence of idiopathic, familial hyperchylomicronaemia in a cat. *Vet. Rec.* **112**, 543–7.

Jones B.R., Wallace A., Hancock W., Harding D.R.K. & Johnstone A.C. (1985) Cutaneous xanthomata associated with diabetes mellitus in a cat. *J. Small Anim. Pract.* **26**, 33–41.

Jones R.T. (1976) Subcutaneous infection with *Dermatophilus congolensis* in a cat. *J. Comp. Pathol.* **86**, 415–21.

Joshua J.O. (1959) The use of biotin in certain skin diseases of the cat. *Vet. Rec.* **71**, 102.

Joshua J.O. (1971) Abscesses and their sequelae in cats. Part 1. *Feline Practice* **1**(2), 9–12.

Joshua J.O. (1972) Abscesses and their sequelae in cats. Part 2. *Feline Practice* **2**(1), 22–3.

Kane E., Morris J.G., Rogers Q.R., Ihrke P.J. & Cupps P.T. (1981) Zinc deficiency in the cat. *J. Nutr.* **111**, 488–95.

Kaplan W. & Ajello L. (1959) Oral treatment of spontaneous ringworm in cats with griseofulvin. *J. Am. Vet. Med. Ass.* **135**, 253–61.

Kaplan W., Chandler F.W., Holzinger E.A., Plue R.E. & Dickinson R.O. (1976) Prototothecosis in a cat: First recorded case. *Sabouraudia* **14**, 281–6.

Kazocos K.R., Bright R., Johnson K.E., Anderson K.L. & Cantwell H.D. (1980) *Cuterebra* sp. as a cause of pharyngeal myiasis in cats. *J. Am. Anim. Hosp. Ass.* **16**, 773–6.

Kershaw A. (1989) *Sarcoptes scabiei* infestation in a cat. *Vet. Rec.* **124**, 537–8.

Kramer J.W., Davis W.C. & Prieur D.J. (1977) The Chediak–Higashi syndrome of cats. *Lab. Invest.* **36**, 554–62.

Krogh H.V. & Kristensen S. (1976) A study of skin diseases in dogs and cats. II. Microflora of the normal skin of dogs and cats. *Nor. Vet. Med.* **28**, 459–63.

Kunkle G.A. (1989) Miliary dermatitis, eosinophilic granuloma complex and symmetric hypotrichosis as manifestations of feline allergy. In Kirk R.W. (ed) *Current Veterinary Therapy X: Small Animal Practice*. W.B. Saunders, Philadelphia, pp. 583–6.

Kunkle G.A. & Meyer D.J. (1987) Toxicity of high doses of griseofulvin in cats. *J. Am. Vet. Med. Ass.* **191**, 322–3.

Kuwahara J. (1986) Canine and feline aural haematomas: Results of treatment with corticosteroids. *J. Am. Anim. Hosp. Ass.* **22**, 641–7.

Kwochka K.W. & Short B.G. (1984) Cutaneous xanthomatosis and diabetes mellitus following long-term therapy with megestrol acetate in a cat. *Comp. Cont. Ed. Prac. Vet.* **6**, 185–92.

Lange A.L., Verster A., Amstel S.R.van & Ley R. de la (1980) *Anatrichiosoma* sp. infestation in the footpads of a cat. *J. S. Afr. Vet. Ass.* **51**, 227–9.

Letard E. (1938) Hairless Siamese cats. *J. Hered.* **29**, 173–5.

Love D.N., Jones R.F., Bailey M. & Johnson R.F. (1978) Isolation and characterisation of bacteria from abscesses in the subcutis of cats. *J. Med. Microbiol.* **12**, 207–12.

Lueker D.C. & Kainer R.A. (1981) Hyperthermia for the treatment of dermatomycosis in dogs and cats. *Vet. Med. Small Anim. Clinician* **76**, 658–9.

Lyell A. (1990) Requiem for toxic epidermal necrolysis. *Br. J. Dermatol.* **122**, 837–46.

MacDonald K.R., Greenfield J. & McCausland H.D. (1972) Remission of staphylococcal dermatitis by autogenous bacterin therapy. *Can. Vet. J.* **13**, 45–8.

MacDonald M.L., Anderson B.C., Rogers Q.R., Buffington C.A. & Morris J.G. (1984) Essential fatty acid requirements of cats: pathology of essential fatty acid deficiency. *Am. J. Vet. Res.* **45**, 1310–7.

MacEwen E.G. & Hess P.W. (1987) Evaluation of the effect of immunomodulation on the feline eosinophilic granuloma complex. *J. Am. Anim. Hosp. Ass.* **23**, 519–26.

McKeever P.J., Caywood D.D. & Perman V. (1983) Chromomycosis in a cat: Successful medical treatment. *J. Am. Anim. Hosp. Ass.* **19**, 533–6.

MacKenzie D.W. (1961) The extra-human occurrence of *Trichophyton tonsurans* var-*sulfureum* in a residential school. *Sabouraudia* **1**, 58–64.

McEwan Jenkinson D. (1990) Sweat and sebaceous glands and their function in domestic animals. In von Tscharner C. & Halliwell R.E.W. (eds) *Veterinary Dermatology*, vol. 1. Ballière Tindall, London, pp. 429–51.

McVean D.W., Monlux A.W., Anderson P.S., Silberg S.L. & Roszel J.F. (1978) Frequency of canine and feline tumours in a defined population. *Vet. Pathol.* **15**, 700–15.

Mardh P.A., Hovelius K. & Nilsonn P.O. (1978) Coagulase-negative, novobiocin-resistant staphylococci on the skin of animals and man, on meat and in milk. *Acta. Vet. Scand.* **19**, 243–53.

Martland M.F., Fowler S., Poulton G.J. & Baxby D. (1983) Pox virus infection in a domestic cat. *Vet. Rec.* **112**, 171–2.

Mayhall C.G., Miller C.W., Eisen A.Z., Kobayashi G.S. & Medoff G. (1976) Cutaneous prototothecosis. Successful treatment with amphotericin B. *Arch. Dermatol.* **112**, 1749–52.

Medleau L., Brown C.A., Brown S.A. & Jones C.S. (1988) Demodicosis in cats. *J. Am. Anim. Hosp. Ass.* **24**, 85–91.

Michel B., Milner Y. & David K. (1972) Preservation of tissue-fixed immunoglobulins in skin biopsies of patients with lupus erythematosus and bullous diseases – preliminary report. *J. Invest. Dermatol.* **59**, 449–52.

Miller R.I., Ladds P.W., Hayes D.P. & Trueman K.F. (1983) Probable dermatophilosis in two cats. *Austral. Vet. J.* **60**, 155–6.

Miller W.H. (1990) Symmetrical truncal hair loss in cats. *Compen. Cont. Educ. Pract. Vet.* **12**, 461–70.

Miller W.H. & Goldschmidt M. (1986) Mycetomas in the cat caused by a dermatophyte. *J. Am. Anim. Hosp. Ass.* **22**, 255–60.

Mosher C.L., Langendoen K. & Stoddard P. (1977) Treatment of ringworm (*Microsporum canis*) with an inactivated vaccine. *Vet. Med. Small Anim. Clinician* **72**, 1343–5.

Muller G.H. (1970) Flea collar dermatitis in animals. *J. Am. Vet. Med. Ass.* **157**, 1616–26.

Mundell A.C. (1990) The use of clofazamine in the treatment of three cases of feline leprosy. In von Tschamer C. & Halliwell R.F.W. (eds) *Advances in Veterinary Dermatology* vol. 1. Balliere Tindall, London. p. 451.

Nash S. & Paulsen D. (1990) Generalised lentigines in a silver cat. *J. Am. Vet. Med. Ass.* **196**, 1500–1.

Nelson R.W., Feldman E.C. & Smith M.C. (1988) Hyperadrenocorticism in cats: Seven cases (1978–1987). *J. Am. Vet. Med. Ass.* **193**, 245–50.

Neufield J.L., Burton L. & Jeffrey K.R. (1980) Eosinophilic granuloma in a cat. Recovery of virus particles. *Vet. Pathol.* **17**, 97–9.

Norton A. (1987) Cited by Scott D.W. (1990) Feline dermatology 1986–1988: Looking to the 1990s through the eyes of many counsellors. *J. Am. Anim. Hosp. Ass.* **26**, 515–37.

O'Donnell J.A. & Hayes K.C. (1987) Nutrition and nutritional disorders. In Holzworth J. (ed) *Diseases of the Cat: Medicine and Surgery*, vol. 1. W.B. Saunders, Philadelphia, pp. 15–42.

O'Hara P.J. & Cordes D.O. (1963) Granulomata caused by *Dermatophilus* in two cats. *N.Z. Vet. J.* **11**, 151–4.

Patterson D.F. & Minor R.W. (1977) Hereditary fragility and hyperextensibility of the skin of cats. *Lab. Invest.* **37**, 170–9.

Pedersen N.C., Ho E.W., Brown M.L. & Yamamoto J.K. (1987) Isolation of a T-lymphotropic virus from domestic cats with an immunodeficiency-like syndrome. *Science* **235**, 790–3.

Pepin G.A. & Oxenham M. (1987) Feline dermatophytosis. The diagnosis of subclinical infection and its relevance to control. *Proc. Br. Vet. Dermatol. Study Group. Vet. Dermatol. Newsletter* **11**, 21–3.

Peterson M.E. (1988) Endocrine disorders in cats: Four emerging diseases. *Compend. Cont. Educ. Pract. Vet.* **10**, 1353–62.

Peterson M.E. & Turrel J.M. (1986) Feline hyperthyroidism. In Kirk R.W. (ed) *Current Veterinary Therapy IX: Small Animal Practice.* W.B. Saunders, Philadelphia, pp. 1026–33.

Peterson M.E., Kintzer P.P., Cavanagh P.G., Fox P.R., Ferguson D.C., Johnson G.F. & Becker D.V. (1983) Feline hyperthyroidism: Pretreatment clinical and laboratory evaluation of 131 cases. *J. Am. Vet. Med. Ass.* **183**, 103–10.

Peterson M.E., Taylor R.S., Greco D.S., Nelson R.W., Randolph J.F., Foodman M.S., Moroff S.D., Morrison S.W. & Lothrop C.D. (1990) Acromegaly in 14 cats. *J. Vet. Int. Med.* **4**, 192–201.

Pion P., Power H.T., Rogers Q.R. & Kittleson M. (1989) Taurine for cats. *J. Am. Vet. Med. Ass.* **194**, 1005–6.

Prevost E., McKee J.M. & Crawford P. (1982) Successful medical management of severe feline cryptococcosis. *J. Am. Anim. Hosp. Ass.* **18**, 111–9.

Prieur D.J., Collier L.L., Bryan G.M. & Meyers K.M.

(1979) The diagnosis of feline Chediak–Higashi syndrome. *Feline Practice* **9**(5), 26–32.

Pye R.H. (1986) Bullous eruptions. In Rook A., Wilkinson D.S., Ebling F.J.G., Champion R.H. & Buxton J.L. (eds) *Textbook of Dermatology*, 4th edn., vol. 2. Blackwell Scientific Publications, Oxford, pp. 1619–63.

Reedy, L.M. (1982) Results of allergy testing and hyposensitisation in selected feline skin diseases. *J. Am. Anim. Hosp. Ass.* **18**, 618–23.

Regnier A. & Pieraggi M.T. (1989) Abnormal skin fragility in a cat with cholangiosarcoma. *J. Small Anim. Pract.* **30**, 419–23.

Rivers J.D. & Frakel T.L. (1980) Fat in the diet of cats and dogs. In Anderson R.S. (ed) *Nutrition of the Dog and Cat.* Pergamon, Oxford, pp. 67–9.

Schmeitzel L.P. (1986) Cited by Mutter G.H., Kirk R.W. & Scott D.W. (1989) Immunological diseases. In *Small Animal Dermatology*. W.B. Saunders, Philadelphia, pp. 427–574.

Schneck G. (1988) Use of ivermectin against ear mites in cats. *Vet. Rec.* **123**, 599.

Schultz K.T. & McGuire H.C. (1982) Chemically-induced delayed hypersensitivity in the cat. *Vet. Immunol. Immunopathol.* **3**, 585–90.

Scott D.W. (1987b) The skin. In Holzworth J. (ed) *Diseases of the Cat: Medicine and Surgery*, vol. 1. W.B. Saunders, Philadelphia, pp. 619–75.

Scott D.W. (1987c) Lentigo simplex in orange cats. *Companion Anim. Pract.* **1**, 23–5.

Scott D.W. (1989) Lichenoid dermatoses in dogs and cats. In Kirk R.W. (ed) *Current Veterinary Therapy X: Small Animal Practce.* W.B. Saunders, Philadelphia, pp. 614–5.

Scott D.W. & Anderson W.I. (1988) Panniculitis in dogs and cats: a retrospective analysis of 78 cases. *J. Am. Anim. Hosp. Ass.* **24**, 551–9.

Scott D.W., Manning T.O. & Reimers (1982) Iatrogenic Cushing's syndrome in the cat. *Feline Practice* **12**(2), 30–6.

Scott D.W., Randolph J.F. & Walsh K.M. (1985) Hypereosinophilic syndrome in a cat. *Feline Practice* **15**(1), 22–30.

Scott D.W., Walton D.K. & Slater M.R. (1986) Miliary dermatitis: A feline cutaneous reaction pattern. *Proc. Second Annual Kal Kan Symp.* **2**, 11–8.

Scott D.W., Walton D.K., Slater M.R., Smith C.A. & Lewis R.M. (1987) Immune-mediated dermatoses in domestic animals: ten years after. II. *Compend. Cont. Educ. Pract. Vet.* **9**, 539–53.

Sharp N.J.H. (1987) Factors relating to the aetiology and pathogenesis of feline and equine dysautonomias. *J. Small Anim. Pract.* **28**, 397–400.

Simon M. (1985) Observation clinique. Dépigmentation périoculaire chez deux chats siamois. *Pratique Medicale & Chirurgicale de l'Animal de Compagnie* **20**, 49–50.

Slocum B., Colgrove D.J. & Carrig C.B. (1973) Acquired arteriovenous fistula in two cats. *J. Am. Vet. Med. Ass.* **162**, 271–5.

Sousa C.A., Ihrke P.J. & Culbertson R. (1984) Subcutaneous phaeohyphomycosis (*Stemphilium* sp. and *Cladosporium* sp. infections) in a cat. *J. Am. Vet. Med. Ass.* **185**, 673–5.

Thoday K.L. (1979) Skin diseases of dogs and cats transmissible to man. *In Practice* **1**(1), 5–15.

Thoday K.L. (1981a) Investigative techniques in small animal clinical dermatology. *Br. Vet. J.* **137**, 133–54.

Thoday K.L. (1981b) Skin diseases of the cat. *In Practice* **3**(6), 22–35.

Thoday K.L. (1985) The skin. In Chandler E.A., Gaskell C.J. & Hilbery A.D.R. (eds) *Feline Medicine and Therapeutics*, 1st edn. Blackwell Scientific Publications, Oxford, pp. 3–37.

Thoday K.L. (1986a) Clinical, biochemical and immunological studies of feline thyroid function. PhD Thesis, University of Edinburgh.

Thoday K.L. (1986b) Differential diagnosis of symmetric alopecia in the cat. In Kirk R.W. (ed) *Current Veterinary Therapy IX: Small Animal Practice.* W.B. Saunders, Philadelphia, pp. 545–53.

Thoday K.L. (1988) Feline hyperthyroidism – A review of the literature. In Chandler E.A. (ed) *Advances in Small Animal Practice 1.* Blackwell Scientific Publications, Oxford, pp. 120–58.

Thoday K.L. (1989) Feline hypothyroidism: An experimental study. *Proc. Br. Vet. Dermatol. Study Group. Vet. Dermatol. Newsletter* **12**, 5–8.

Thoday K.L. (1990a) Aspects of feline symmetric alopecia. In von Tscharner C. & Halliwell R.E.W. (eds) *Advances in Veterinary Dermatology Volume 1.* Ballière Tindall, London, pp. 47–69.

Thoday K.L. (1990b) Clinical features of experimentally-induced hypothyroidism in cats. In von Tscharner C. & Halliwell R.E.W. (eds) *Advances in Veterinary Dermatology Volume 1.* Ballière Tindall, London, pp. 482–3.

Thoday K.L. (1990c) The thyroid gland. In Hutchison M. (ed) *Manual of Small Animal Endocrinology.* British Small Animal Veterinary Association, Cheltenham, pp. 25–57.

Thoday K.L. & Mooney C.T. (1992a) Historical, clinical and laboratory features of 126 hyperthyroid cats. *Vet. Rec.* **131**, 257–264.

Thoday K.L. & Mooney C.T. (1992b) Medical Management of Feline Hyperthyroidism. In Kirk's Current Veterinary Therapy XI: Small Animal Practise. W.B. Saunders, Philadelphia.

Thody A.J. & Shuster S. (1989) Control and function of sebaceous glands. *Physiol. Rev.* **69**, 383–416.

Thomsett L.R., Baxby D. & Denham E.M.H. (1978)

Cowpox in the domestic cat. *Vet. Rec.* **103**, 567.

Tuttle P.A. & Chandler F.W. (1983) Deep dermatophytosis in a cat. *J. Am. Vet. Med. Ass.* **183**, 1106–8.

Van den Akker S. (1952) Een Schimmelinfectie (*Cephalosporium potronii*) in de mandholte van een kat. *Tijdschrieft voor Diergeneeskunde* **77**, 515–6.

Van den Broek A.H.M. & Thoday K.L. (1987) Eumycetoma in a British cat. *J. Small Anim. Pract.* **28**, 827–31.

Venezio F.R., Lavoo E., Williams J.E., Zeiss C.R., Caro W.A., Mangkorkanok-Mark M. & Phair J.P. (1982) Progressive cutaneous prototSthecosis. *Am. J. Clin. Pathol.* **77**, 485–93.

Wagener K. & Krüger A. (1953) Experimentelle Hyperkeratose ('X-disease') bei Katzen and Hunden. *Deutsche Tieraztliche Wochenschnift* **60**, 312–5.

Walton D.K., Scott D.W. & Manning T.O. (1983) Cutaneous bacterial granuloma (botryomycosis) in a dog and cat. *J. Am. Anim. Hosp. Ass.* **19**, 537–41.

Walton G.S. (1977a) Allergic contact dermatitis. In Kirk R.W. (ed) *Current Veterinary Therapy VI: Small Animal Practice.* W.B. Saunders, Philadelphia, pp. 571–5.

Walton G.S. (1977b) Allergic responses to ingested allergens. In Kirk R.W. (ed) *Current Veterinary Therapy VI: Small Animal Practice.* W.B. Saunders, Philadelphia, pp. 575–9.

Weisbroth S.H., Powell M.B., Roth L. & Scher S. (1974) Immunopathology of naturally occurring otodectic otoacariasis in the domestic cat. *J. Am. Vet. Med. Ass.* **165**, 1088–93.

White S.D. & Sequoia D. (1989) Food hypersensitivity in cats: 14 cases (1982–1987). *J. Am. Vet. Med. Ass.* **194**, 692–5.

Wilcke J.R. (1986) Allergic drug reactions. In Kirk R.W.

(ed) *Current Veterinary Therapy IX: Small Animal Practice.* W.B. Saunders, Philadelphia, pp. 444–8.

Wilkinson G.T. (1966) Diseases of the skin. In *Diseases of the Cat.* Pergamon Press, Oxford, pp. 183–99.

Wilkinson G.T. (1981) An overview of feline skin disease in Australia. In: *Proceedings of the Post-Graduate Committee in Veterinary Science*, No. 57, pp. 277–84. Refresher course on dermatology, University of Sydney.

Wilkinson G.T. (1988) Mycobacterial infections. In Barlough J.E. (ed) *Manual of Small Animal Infectious Diseases.* Churchill Livingstone, New York, pp. 213–24.

Wilkinson G.T. & Kristensen T.S. (1989) A hair abnormality in Abyssinian cats. *J. Small Anim. Pract.* **30**, 27–8.

Willard M.D., Nachreiner R.F., Howard V.C. (1986) Effect of long-term administration of ketoconazole in cats. *Am. J. Vet. Res.* **47**, 2510–3.

Willemse T. & Koeman J.P. (1989) Discoid lupus erythematosus in cats. Vet. *Dermatol.* **1**, 19–24.

Woodard D.C. (1983) Ketoconazole therapy for *Microsporum* spp. dermatophytes in cats. *Feline Practice* **13**(5), 28–9.

Wright A.I. (1989) Ringworm in dogs and cats. *J. Small Anim. Pract.* **30**, 242–9.

Yager J.A., Wilcock B.P., Lynch J.A. & Thompson A.R. (1986) Mycetoma-like granuloma in a cat caused by *Microsporum canis*. *J. Comp. Pathol.* **96**, 171–6.

Zerbe C.A. (1989) Feline Hyperadrenocorticism. In Kirk R.W. (ed) Current Veterinary Therapy X: Small Animal Practise. W.B. Saunders, Philadelphia.

Zerbe C.A., Nachreiner R.F., Dunstan R.W. & Dalley J.B. (1987) Hyperadrenocorticism in a cat. *J. Am. Vet. Med. Ass.* **190**, 559–63.

Chapter 2 / The Nervous System

R. J. EVANS

INTRODUCTION

Neurology is an inexorably logical subject. There is a strong correlation between structure and function in the nervous system and for both there are marked segmental and hierarchical relationships. Ablation of a structure by a pathological process leads to loss or modification of its function. This change of function may be detected by systematic neurological examination and the cause of the deficit presumed by extrapolation. Many, but not all, nervous system lesions are anatomically localized and damage specific structures. It is thus important to have a thorough appreciation of the anatomy and physiology of the nervous system to make sound neurological diagnoses.

Although nervous system function is ordered, the nervous system is also highly interactive and integrative. The systems within it which perform individual functions are extensively interconnected to achieve the total coordination of bodily function necessary to survival. Thus many of the functional systems have, or connect with, pathways projecting throughout the nervous system, both centrally and peripherally. A lesion may involve only one functional system, for example the vestibular position sensors of the ear, but, because of this interactive nature of nervous information processing and signalling, it may produce widespread effects including changes in equilibrium, gait and eye movement.

For the same reasons signs resulting from damage to different structures may overlap. Viewed in isolation a single clinical sign may therefore be referable to more than one system. Nystagmus may be physiological or may arise from lesions of the vestibular system, cerebellum, visual system or brainstem tracts. It is thus a synthesis and appreciation of the overall pattern of signs which enables one to deduce the site or sites which have been damaged (and sometimes the type of lesion). For example, if a cat has damage to the trigeminal nerve and also to the ipsilateral seventh and eighth cranial nerves, the lesion must be at a point where these structures lie close together, i.e. in the cerebellopontine angle. If, on the other hand, a lesion damages the ophthalmic division of the trigeminal nerve together with the third, fourth and sixth cranial nerves, the problem must lie around the orbit. Signs which aid determination of the site of a lesion may loosely be called localizing signs. An important correlate of this which will be stressed repeatedly throughout this chapter is the need for thoroughness in neurological examination; shortcuts are to be avoided since they may lead to critical information being overlooked. Conversely, diagnostic aids are relatively less helpful for neurological diseases than they are for those of other systems and are no substitute for thorough history-taking and examination.

Neurological diagnosis in the cat is made more challenging by the large number of generalized diseases which affect the feline nervous system, often resulting in lesions at a number of sites within the nervous system (Table 2.1). Thus it is more common to see multifocal signs in nervous diseases of cats than in other species. These disseminated conditions include genetic disorders,

Table 2.1 Diseases associated with multifocal signs.

Generalized metabolic disorders
  Hyperammonaemia (hepatic encephalopathy)
  Hypocalcaemia
  Hypoglycaemia
  Hypokalaemia
  Uraemia*

Hereditary degenerations* (see Table 2.6)

Infective/inflammatory processes
  Actinomycosis
  Angiostrongylosis
  Aspergillosis
  Blastomycosis
  Coccidioidomycosis
  Cryptococcosis
  Cutebriasis
  Dirofilariasis
  Feline immunodeficiency virus (FIV)
  Feline infectious peritonitis (FIP)*
  Feline spongiform encephalopathy (FSE)
  Histoplasmosis
  Meningitides/generalized infections
  Nocardiosis
  Protothecosis
  Pseudorabies
  Rabies
  Toxocariasis
  Toxoplasmosis

Neoplasms (particularly lymphosarcomas)*

Asterisks indicate common conditions.

infective, degenerative and neoplastic conditions. The diagnosis of these conditions will frequently rest more heavily on diagnostic aids than is the case for those diseases with localized lesions.

In writing this chapter the intention has been to emphasize and to provide literature references for those conditions which are specific to the cat, in which the incidence in the cat is unusually high, whose pathology or clinical signs in the cat are unusual or which have been recently or insufficiently recognized. In particular it seemed important to underline the growing awareness of the diversity of neurological disorders in the cat. Thus well-recognized conditions for which the diagnosis and treatment are both established and

well documented may appear relatively under-represented. Sources of information dealing with these well-documented aspects of feline neurology will be found amongst those listed under 'Further Reading'. Feline dysautonomia appeared just before the first edition of this textbook was prepared and only preliminary results were available at that time. Although feline dysautonomia has decreased significantly in incidence since that time and the signs in recent cases have been less severe, the aetiology remains unknown and the possibility must exist that it will again become common and clinically important. For these reasons it has been given a relatively extended treatment.

THE DIAGNOSTIC APPROACH TO THE NEUROLOGICAL PATIENT

Disease of other systems may affect the nervous system secondarily, or may mimic nervous disorders. The clinician should not therefore assume that nervous disease is present in a patient presented with an appropriate owner complaint. The initial aim should be to establish the nature of the complaint. A full medical history, including previous illness, is taken. A full general examination is mandatory.

The information from the history, the results of the general examination and, if necessary, laboratory examinations for metabolic and haematological abnormalities (see pages 87–88 and Chapter 4), will enable the clinician to assess whether this is a putative neurological complaint. If so, there are three diagnostic questions to be answered.

1 What component(s) of the nervous system is(are) injured? (see above)
2 What is the nature of the lesion?
3 What is the inciting cause?

To this end, a full neurological examination is required. An incomplete neurological examination is of little value and may be positively misleading. Adequate time must be allowed for full assessment of the neurological patient; neurology is not a discipline that can be rushed. Many specific details of neurological examination are referred to in those sections of this chapter which deal with particular components of the nervous system. The material has been arranged on this basis because it seems more coherent to consider the physiology, examination and diseases of particular subsystems in unified discussions. There are, however, certain general aspects of neurological examination which are discussed here because of their relevance to the examination of any patient with a suspected nervous disorder.

In carrying out neurological examinations, the order in which tests are performed is not *per se* particularly important but it is vital to have a fixed procedure so that no part of the examination is inadvertently overlooked. Meticulous written recording of the results, stage by stage during the examination, including noting those features that are normal, is also a very helpful discipline not only for the immediate assessment of the patient, but more so for comparison at subsequent examinations when it can be of major diagnostic or prognostic significance to establish whether progression or recovery has occurred. Accurate neurological diagnosis and prognosis is often critically dependent on such sequential assessments of the patient and this is particularly so in the cat because of the high incidence of generalized, neoplastic and degenerative diseases, which are progressive in nature and which affect the nervous system.

First, it is important to inspect the patient from some distance without interfering. At this stage, general appearance should be assessed, including the degree of alertness of the patient, general bodily condition and whether there are any asymmetries or deformities which might indicate muscle wasting. The aspect and symmetry of the face deserves particular attention. Abnormalities can be a useful cue to finding cranial nerve deficits. Time spent playing with the animal both at long range, in the time-honoured fashion of getting it to chase balls or pieces of string, as well as directly is well rewarded since the examiner cannot exercise a cat in the disciplined way in which he might a horse or dog. Play allows a thorough inspection of the gait at slow and fast pace as well as during straight progression and turning. Play also permits the fatigability of the patient and any weakness to be assessed. This phase of the examination should be carried out on a surface that provides reasonable friction. It is difficult for the patient and misleading for the examiner if the floor is smooth and slippery. Since cats are often resentful of the more detailed aspects of neurological examination, the more information gained at this stage the better. After this general assessment the author usually moves on to assess the cranial nerves (see pp. 101–106). The eyes and ears should also be examined at this time.

Assessment of the postural and proprioceptive reactions in the cat is difficult because of the recalcitrant nature of many patients; the author has found that it is generally impossible to carry out the wheelbarrow, hemiwalking and hemistanding manoeuvres with cats. A simplified system must therefore be used. It is possible to perform the knuckling test with each paw in turn for assessment of proprioception, the normal response being for the patient to return its paw to the usual resting position. This can be complemented by placing a piece of paper under each foot in turn and slowly sliding it away from the body. The normal animal will promptly move the limb back under the body. Placing responses are also of value. The tactile placing response is performed with the eyes of the patient covered. The animal is brought up to a tabletop so that the anterior aspect of the forelimbs touches the edge. The patient then puts its paws onto the tabletop if normal. The visual placing response is performed in the same fashion but with the eyes uncovered. The placing reflexes involve the higher centres. The tactile placing reflex depends on intact sensory and motor areas of cortex as well as ascending and descending spinal pathways. The visual placing reflex involves a relatively restricted area of the visual cortex as well as motor cortex and descending pathways. The extensor thrust response of the hindlimbs when the animal is lowered onto a surface is also of value. This is a spinal reflex involving the L4 and L5 segments.

Of the tendon reflexes involving spinal reflex

arcs, the patellar, triceps and Achilles tendon reflexes can be readily elicited in the cat, but the author has found the biceps response impossible to test reliably and omits this. The assessment of muscle tone is unreliable because of the propensity of the patient to resist all interferences.

In testing for pain perception, it is important to remember first that the cat is capable of inflicting unpleasant injury to the examiner with much more speed and efficiency than most dogs: the patient should be well restrained. Second, it must be remembered that many cats are far more stoical than the average dog. To test pain a claw on each foot should be compressed near its base using artery forceps. The withdrawal of a limb in response to pain represents a positive (spinal level reflex) withdrawal response; it does not indicate conscious (cortical) pain perception, which is only assured if the animal turns to inspect the site of insult or there is some facial, vocal or concerted response. It must be remembered that sensory nerve distribution areas are less discrete in the cat than in the dog (Hekmatpanah, 1961).

Having made a diagnosis, it is important to both cat and owner to assess the prognosis and whether the condition is treatable. This will depend not only on the inciting cause and localization of the lesion, but also on its severity. The assessment of severity is discussed, where appropriate, in relation to individual conditions.

Ancillary aids

There are specific circumstances in which radiology, electrophysiology and clinical pathology have a part to play in the investigation of nervous disorders, but the value of ancillary aids in neurology is often overestimated. In particular, there is relatively little that can be achieved using electrophysiological aids that cannot also be realized by astute clinical observation.

Clinical pathology

Haematological and biochemical investigations have two distinct roles in the investigation of patients with putative neurological disorders.

There are many systemic disorders which may present with nervous signs due to functional CNS disturbance; for example, metabolic disturbances (see below) and the involvement of the CNS in pyogranulomatous feline infectious peritonitis. Others may present with signs which mimic those of nervous disease, for example weakness and collapse associated with hypokalaemia or coma associated with hypo- or hyperglycaemia. Thus a major role for clinical pathology is in the identification of such systemic disturbances, and in these cases haematological and biochemical examination of peripheral blood is useful. Examination of peripheral blood is of more restricted value with diseases which primarily involve nervous tissue although it may be of assistance when inflammatory or systemic disease is suspected. Urine analysis may occasionally be helpful, for example if diabetes mellitus is suspected to underlie neurological signs, but faecal analysis has little value since parasitic infections involving the CNS are rarely if ever patent at the time that neurological signs are detected. Examination of the cerebrospinal fluid (CSF) can be of considerable value but even this is not of general utility. Since there is significant risk attached to CSF collection in the cat it is wise to weigh the results of the general clinical examination, neurological examination and peripheral blood examinations to assess the likely nature of the disease process. Cerebrospinal fluid may reflect changes in the meninges, choroid or CNS parenchyma. In the latter case only lesions close to the surface significantly affect CSF. The most florid changes are found in conditions affecting the meninges and in inflammatory disease. CSF changes can be minimal or absent in spinal cord compression and degenerations.

Systemic metabolic disturbances which may present with clinical signs

Systemic conditions encountered in the cat which may give rise to neurological disturbance or to signs which resemble those of nervous disease include the following (see also Table 2.1):

Hypoxia. This may give rise to ataxia, weakness, collapse, seizures or coma. There are many

causes but those amenable to detection by haematological examination include haemorrhage,
severe anaemia, methaemoglobinaemia and
other toxic haemoglobinopathies, hyperviscosity associated with myeloma or polycythaemia and thromboembolism.

Hypoglycaemia. This results in dullness and depression, neuromuscular weakness, seizures
and coma and may result from insulin overdose, starvation, and glycogen storage disease
Type I. Although rare, functional pancreatic
islet cell tumours with associated hypoglycaemia and neurological signs do occur in
the cat (McMillan *et al.*, 1985).

Hyperglycaemia. In uncontrolled diabetes mellitus this may present as depression, neuromuscular weakness or coma.

Hypokalaemia. This is discussed on p. 121.

Hypercalcaemia. This may result from functional
parathyroid tumours, as a result of calcium
mobilization from bone in lymphosarcoma or
multiple myeloma, or from dietary calcium:
phosphorus imbalance or excessive administration of vitamin D. It may give rise to depression and neuromuscular weakness.

Hypocalcaemia. This results in ataxia, depression, muscular tremors and/or, at its most
severe, marked tetany. It may be encountered
during lactation (see Chapter 7), occasionally in
pregnancy and in ethylene glycol intoxication.

Uraemia. In acute or decompensated chronic
renal failure uraemia may present as depression, muscle weakness, tremors, seizures or
tetany.

Hyperammonaemia. This is associated with portosystemic shunts, or hepatic failure, and is
discussed on page 97–98.

Clinical chemistry

It will be apparent that measurements of plasma
glucose, ketone bodies, cholesterol, plasma proteins, potassium, calcium, urea, creatinine and
ammonia have value in distinguishing the most
common of the generalized abnormalities from
genuine neurological disorders. In the case of
hyperammonaemia measurement of plasma bile
acids may also be of value. Blood lead deter-

minations are of value if lead poisoning is suspected. For further details of clinical chemical
investigations see Evans (1989a).

Haematology

Haematological changes are generally an inconstant and unreliable feature in feline neurological
disorders. Leucocytosis may be absent or of varying intensity in encephalitis, myelitis and abscessation, but is often florid in meningitis. Changes
in blood leucocyte counts are rare in fungal or
protozoal infections of the CNS but when they do
occur may predominantly involve the mononuclear cells. In toxoplasmosis leucopenia may precede leucocytosis. In feline infectious peritonitis
there is usually a mild neutrophilia with a slight
left shift, moderate non-regenerative anaemia and
hypergammaglobulinaemia. Polycythaemia vera
and plasma cell myeloma are primary haematological conditions which increase blood viscosity
and give rise to a variety of variable episodic
neurological signs including weakness, disorientation, collapse and convulsions. Their diagnosis
rests upon appropriate haematological investigation (see Chapter 4 and Evans, 1989a).

Serology

Serology is of limited value but should be performed when toxoplasmosis (see Chapter 25) or
cryptococcosis (see Chapter 23) are suspected.
Feline infectious peritonitis (FIP) titres may also
be of some value but their interpretation remains
controversial (see Chapter 17).

Cerebrospinal fluid collection and analysis

Cerebrospinal puncture is usually performed between the occipital bone and the first cervical
vertebra, so as to enter the cisterna magna. It
may also be performed in the lumbar region
(using the technique described for myelography).
Cerebrospinal fluid collection is contraindicated
if intracranial pressure is likely to be significantly
raised or there is a space-occupying lesion within
the cranial cavity. Cisternal CSF collection should
not be undertaken if there are cranial fractures or
cervical vertebral instability.

Cisternal puncture is performed in the anaesthetized intubated animal and thus anaesthetic risk is also a contraindication. The region is shaved. Surgical asepsis is required. The neck is firmly flexed and propped in a horizontal position. The landmarks are the occipital protuberance and the wings of the atlas. The spinal needle is inserted in the midline midway between the occipital protuberance and a line joining the wings of the atlas. The needle is slowly advanced directing it towards the nose. The procedure is more difficult than in the dog: there is less tissue to penetrate and the changes in resistance as the needle passes through fascial planes and as it enters the cistern are difficult to discern. The needle should be advanced with great caution and the stylet should be removed from time to time to ascertain whether the cistern has been entered. Once CSF flows from the needle, a three-way tap and manometer should be attached and CSF pressure measured. The normal range is 50–125 mmH$_2$O depending upon the depth of anaesthesia. A maximum of 2 ml of CSF should then be withdrawn slowly and split between EDTA and heparin tubes, and a sterile bijou.

Colour and turbidity should be assessed. The cells should be counted, differentiated and examined for evidence of inflammatory or neoplastic cells. Protein and glucose should be measured. Gram's stain should be performed on smears and the fluid cultured. In neoplastic involvement, tumour cells may be found in smears from a centrifuged pellet, otherwise the CSF is, in general, normal, although its pressure may be markedly increased. CSF changes in infections are discussed on p. 126. In trauma, xanthochromia or fresh blood are common findings.

For more detailed discussion of the role of CSF analysis in neurological diagnosis the reader is referred to Evans (1989a).

Radiology and other imaging techniques

Radiological evaluation is of limited value in intracranial disease. It is of much greater value in spinal cord dysfunction. Neuroradiographic techniques, particularly the critical question of patient positioning to obtain unambiguous views, and neuroradiological interpretation are thoroughly discussed by Luttgen *et al.* (1988) and Davies (1989).

Skull radiography and radiology are beyond the scope of this chapter. Radiography may be helpful in diagnosis of otitis media, of hydrocephalus and of bony lesions of the skull or vertebral column of neurological significance. Contrast techniques have rarely been applied to intracranial disease in the cat although they are potentially of value.

Plain radiographs are an essential component of the assessment of spinal cord dysfunction. When space-occupying lesions are suspected, myelography is also of substantial value. Lumbar injection used to be the preferred route for the administration of contrast media for myelography in the cat. However, with the availability of newer non-ionic water-soluble compounds such as metrizamide, iopamidol or iohexol, cisternal administration can now be performed with confidence, although the anatomical constraints noted in the discussion of CSF collection are relevant. For a detailed account of myelography in the cat the reader is referred to Wheeler *et al.* (1985).

Where they are available, more advanced methods such as computed tomography and magnetic resonance imaging can be of considerable value for identifying and localizing lesions within the parenchyma of the CNS (LeCouteur *et al.*, 1983).

Electrophysiology

Electromyography and measurement of nerve conduction velocities are becoming more widely used in feline neurology although experience is still limited compared with that in dogs. Electromyography can reveal reduced nerve conduction velocity, for example in the neuropathies associated with diabetes mellitus and with FIV infection. The reader is referred to Duncan (1989) for details of these techniques. Evoked potential measurements are of value in the assessment of hearing in the cat as they are in the dog (Wilkes, personal communication).

Electroencephalography

Electroencephalography has some value in cerebral hemisphere disease as a confirmatory investigation, but there are many complications in obtaining diagnostically useful recordings and considerable expertise is required for interpretation. It is most valuable where there is a focal lesion which can be localized by this means and in distinguishing acquired from idiopathic epilepsy. The reader is referred to Barker (1989) for detailed discussion.

DISEASES OF THE CEREBRAL HEMISPHERES AND ASSOCIATED STRUCTURES

The cranial cavity anterior to the tentorium cerebelli houses five structures that are closely integrated and may be considered together for the purposes of clinical neurology. They are the midbrain, the cerebral hemispheres, the thalamus, the hypothalamus and the pituitary gland. In the cat, a number of disease processes may affect these structures: tumours, trauma and intoxication are common, encephalitides and ischaemic and vascular conditions are not.

Disease processes in this area produce local effects. Tumours (whether of brain substance, the meninges or extradural space), inflammatory processes and interference with vascular perfusion may all produce local tissue necrosis. While the centre of the lesion is thus effectively ablated and function is lost, the periphery may act as an excitatory focus. The site of the lesion is more important than its size. Small lesions in the thalamus may produce very much more severe signs than large lesions in some areas of cortex.

More disseminated effects may also arise. Any of the insults under consideration may produce brain swelling due to oedema. Secondary hydrocephalus may occur with tumours and infections, due to compressive or inflammatory occlusion of CSF circulation respectively. Space-occupying lesions (tumours, haemorrhage, oedema or hydrocephalus) can cause raised intracranial pressure. This in turn may produce herniation of the cerebral hemispheres under the tentorium cerebelli. This results in compression of the brainstem. Compressive changes may decrease vascular perfusion and give rise to ischaemic necrosis. Slight tentorial herniation induces vertical nystagmus, moderate herniation and tetraparesis; when herniation becomes severe the grave features noted in the discussion of cerebral trauma develop. Raised intracranial pressure may also give rise to papilloedema (p. 101), which is a very significant sign.

The major signs of disease of the cerebral hemisphere may be very generalized or there may be localizing signs. There may be changes of temperament including depression, failure to respond to the owner, unusual viciousness or docility. There may also be loss of feeding, defecation or urination habits. Circling, which is wide and which may be intermittent, is seen in about 40% of cases. The direction of the circling is to the side of the lesion in about 70% of these (Nafe, 1979). In the remainder the sidedness is variable or consistently away from the lesion. Epileptiform fits (see p. 93) are a less frequent sign of cerebral hemisphere involvement and may develop after other signs.

Localizing signs have been less closely studied in cats than in dogs. Motor cortex involvement may cause contralateral hemiparesis or ataxia. In sensory cortex involvement, the postural reactions in the contralateral limbs may be markedly depressed or absent. Prefrontal lobe lesions may produce dummy-like behaviour. The localizing value of optic and olfactory nerve signs is discussed below.

Congenital conditions

These are discussed on p. 127.

Acquired conditions

Trauma

Cranial trauma in cats is relatively common, most often arising from road traffic accidents but also from falls from high buildings and pellet or bullet injuries. It is generally severe, readily evident and often rapidly fatal, particularly since there is a tendency for the cranial sutures to separate. Impact injury to the head may, however, result in brain lesions in the presence or absence of skull fractures. The brain may suffer contusion, laceration, concussion or haemorrhage. Diagnosis may be straightforward if there is a clear history or external evidence of trauma. These can, however, sometimes be misleading. In the absence of definite evidence, other conditions producing cerebral dysfunction will need to be considered (see Tables 2.1–2.5 and 2.7).

Mildly affected animals may be obtunded and show disorientation. There may be mild ataxia with normal reflexes of the cranial nerves. Transient anisocoria may be noted, but the pupils will still be reactive to light. Consciousness is retained throughout. Close observation for 24–48 hours is, however, essential in case the delayed development of haemorrhage, brain oedema or infection leads to deterioration in condition and a need for more intensive treatment.

In moderate trauma there may be coma, dullness and altered consciousness, or temporary loss of consciousness (2–5 minutes). Consideration should be given to other conditions which may impair consciousness (see below and Table 2.4). Coma may occur terminally in many conditions in the cat, as well as in shock. Many intoxications may also produce coma (see Chapter 28). Metaldehyde, alphachloralose and ethylene glycol poisoning have all occurred in cats. Seizures may also be present. Other common signs encountered in cases of cerebral trauma include contralateral or bilateral visual defects, and upper motor neuron paresis of one or more limbs. Less often there may be impairment of conscious proprioception or of postural reflexes.

In cases of moderate trauma, the development of brain oedema may lead to tentorial herniation and worsening of the condition due to brainstem compression. The signs of brainstem compression are the development of unilateral and then bilateral pupillary dilatation together with a progressive transition from consciousness to coma. Muscle tone may progress from mild weakness to rigidity and then flaccidity. Tentorial herniation may develop after hours or days. The development of these signs indicates the need for urgent medical measures to reduce brain oedema or the need for surgical decompression.

Severe injury will be revealed by presentation with sudden onset of florid and diffuse signs. There is generally coma and there may be seizures. Coma may arise because of severe brainstem injury or because of generalized cerebral hemisphere dysfunction. In severe trauma both are usually present. Other signs include upper motor neuron tetraparesis, decerebrate rigidity, crossed extensor reflexes and occasionally the perineal mass response. The pupils are usually fixed and bilaterally miotic. Complete pupillary dilatation may develop preterminally. Respiration is shallow and irregular. Cranial nerve defects in the presence of a severe brainstem lesion indicate a poor prognosis. Assessment of the oculovestibular reflexes (p. 103) is valuable in comatose animals. Absence of these indicates a grave prognosis.

MANAGEMENT

The management of cerebral trauma cases is primarily medical although surgical intervention may sometimes be indicated to elevate fractures or to decompress the cranial cavity. The immediate steps in management should be instituted before neurological assessment is attempted. A patent airway should be established, haemorrhage should be controlled and the treatment of shock commenced. In conscious animals in severe pain, narcotic analgesics may be indicated. It should be noted, however, that their administration prejudices further neurological monitoring and may worsen respiratory depression of central origin (see Chapter 27).

The primary aim of medical management is the reduction of brain oedema and prevention of its progression. The latter may be achieved by administration of a soluble preparation of a glucocorticoid, for example dexamethasone free alcohol or methylprednisolone sodium succinate, preferably intravenously with the initial dose within 1 hour of injury. In animals with mild signs, 0.1 mg/kg of dexamethasone should be given twice daily for 2 or 3 days. In cases of intermediate severity dexamethasone should be given three times daily at a dose of 1 mg/kg on the first day, 0.3 mg/kg on the second day and at 0.1 mg/kg for two further days. Severely affected animals should receive 2 mg/kg dexamethasone 8-hourly on the first day, 1 mg/kg three times a day on the second day, and 0.5 mg/kg three times on the third day. Therapy with 0.1 mg/kg twice daily can then be continued for as long as necessary. In severe cases methylprednisolone sodium succinate may be administered at a dose of 30 mg/kg.

In severe cases further measures may be indicated to reduce existing brain oedema, provided that there is no fracture or other evidence for intracranial haemorrhage. Mannitol in 20% solution, 2 g/kg, should be administered by intravenous infusion on three occasions separated by an interval of 4–6 hours. Frusemide at 1 mg/kg may be given 6-hourly. There should be careful attention to monitoring hydration status, urine output, and fluid and electrolyte balance. Animals in the milder groups, in which deterioration occurs, should receive similarly vigorous therapy, particularly if there is evidence of subtentorial herniation. Antibiotics should be administered as necessary.

PROGNOSIS
In all degrees of severity of injury recovery may be remarkably good with no or minor residual deficits. Clearly, however, the probability of successful treatment is inversely related to the gravity of the injury.

Inflammatory disease
Inflammatory central nervous system disease of the cat is usually due to infection and is frequently multifocal (see p. 124), although toxoplasmosis and feline infectious peritonitis (FIP) may produce focal cerebral signs, as may also feline spongiform encephalopathy and feline immunodeficiency virus infection.

Neoplasia and other space-occupying lesions
Space-occupying lesions should perhaps more accurately be called expanding lesions. They may be tumours, abscesses or parasitic cysts. Because

the cranial cavity is inexpansible, growth of these lesions not only results in local destruction, but also in raised intracranial pressure and therefore in consequential changes remote from the site of the prime lesion.

The major signs of anterior fossa lesions have already been discussed. With space-occupying lesions additional signs are often present. Visual abnormalities are discussed on p. 102. There is often weakness on the contralateral side, manifested as a tendency to fall to that side. Unilateral cortical lesions may produce contralateral sensory loss. Incoordination and ataxia may also occur with variable degrees of severity. The identification of localizing signs is an important component in establishing the presence of a space-occupying lesion.

Tumours are the only common space-occupying lesions in the cat. Tumours developing within the brain may be primary or they may be metastases from primary lesions elsewhere. Metastatic involvement of the central nervous system in the cat appears to be extremely rare, arising mainly with osteosarcomas and squamous cell carcinomas. Aesthesioneuroblastomas arising in the nasal cavity may invade the cranium (Smith *et al.*, 1989).

Meningiomas are the most common primary brain tumours in the cat, and the tela choroidea of the third ventricle appears to be a site of predilection (Luginbuhl, 1961). Lymphosarcomas are also common. Reports differ as to the frequency of occurrence of astrocytomas, but they are also relatively common. Pituitary chromophobe adenomas and pituicytomas appear, from the findings of Zaki and Hurvitz (1976), to be more common than has generally been suggested. Ependymomas, oligodendrogliomas and lymphosarcomas may be multiple.

Treatment
Symptomatic treatment with glucocorticoids and anticonvulsants may produce an abatement of signs for a period ranging from days to months. Surgical removal of tumours cannot be considered routinely practicable although it has been achieved for neoplasms accurately located by

computed tomography (LeCouteur *et al.*, 1983) Angiographic localization or electroencephalography may be helpful in localizing lesions in some cases. Only meningiomas are unlikely to recur after excision. Radiotherapy is also a possibility if lesions can be accurately localized (LeCouteur *et al.*, 1983). In the majority of cases, however, radical treatment is impractical and the long-term prognosis remains hopeless.

ABSCESSES
Cerebral abscesses are very rare in the cat, but may arise from spread of nasal or frontal sinus infections.

PARASITIC LESIONS
These are uncommon but coenurus cysts of *Taenia* spp. occur and show signs typical of space-occupying lesions. Aberrant dirofilariasis (Fakushima *et al.*, 1984) and at least four cases of cuterebriasis have been reported (Hatziolos, 1966; McKenzie *et al.*, 1978).

DEGENERATIONS
Inherited degenerative conditions most commonly present as progressive ataxia in kittens and are discussed under that heading (see below).

Extensive laminar necrosis of cerebral cortex may follow the anoxia of cardiac arrest (usually during general anaesthesia). Cortical necrosis occurs when the anoxia is prolonged beyond about 4 minutes, and increases in severity with increased duration of arrest. The clinical signs are prolonged unconsciousness, seizures, cortical blindness and cranial nerve palsies. Cerebral oedema also develops and after shorter periods of anoxia may be the only change.

Treatment
The aim of treatment is the control of brain oedema. Glucocorticoids and if necessary mannitol should be administered, employing the regime described for severe cranial injury.

Ischaemic encephalopathy
There are a number of reports of a spontaneously occurring ischaemic encephalopathy affecting mature cats of both sexes. The onset is acute. Severe depression and mild to moderate ataxia develop, together with predominantly unilateral cerebral signs. There may also be pyrexia and occasionally dilated pupils. CSF examination often reveals mild elevations of protein concentration and mononuclear cell number. Partial resolution occurs, but there are often residual behavioural changes, with increased aggressiveness being common, or long-term visual defects of cortical type, although some cats may recover completely.

At post-mortem examination, degenerative changes of variable severity are found (Kornegay, 1981). These range from mild unilateral laminar cortical necrosis to severe infarction of both grey and white matter of the cerebral hemisphere and frank cavitation. In severe cases the thalamus may also be involved and occasionally lesions may be present in the brainstem and produce signs related to that area. The cause is unknown, and in many cases no reason for ischaemia is evident. It has been suggested that the condition is a consequence of focal granulomatous meningoencephalitis (Zaki & Nafe, 1980). In other cases vasculitis has been recorded and there is a record of thrombosis of the middle cerebral artery. It is possible that this is an end-stage condition that may arise from a number of aetiologies.

There is no specific treatment, but it has been suggested that glucocorticoids may be helpful early in the course.

SEIZURES

Seizures are not a common clinical sign in the cat. Seizures, also known as fits or convulsions, are the manifestation of spontaneous paroxysmal discharge of a group of nerve cells, which may spread to involve large areas of the cerebrum. Fits usually occur as discrete episodes and are often recurrent. In feline practice, generalized, grand-mal seizures are the most commonly recognized. There is widespread intermittent contraction and relaxation of skeletal muscles. Occasionally, however, partial fits due to a non-spreading epileptogenic focus may be recognized.

In these cases there may be a variety of behavioural abnormalities.

Despite being uncommon, fits are an important clinical sign: they are alarming to the owner; they may be life-threatening and their differential diagnosis may present considerable difficulty.

The causes of convulsions are numerous (Table 2.2). It is commonly stated that idiopathic epilepsy is a rare cause of fits in the cat and that seizures are more usually a sign of organic disease (Kay, 1975). This is not the author's experience; none the less, it is very important that a thorough diagnostic protocol is employed in seizure cases, since organic causes are not negligible. The causes of convulsions may be divided into those that are extracranial and those that arise within the cranial cavity. The extracranial causes act primarily by metabolic effects on the brain. They include renal disease, acute or chronic acquired liver disease, portosystemic shunting, hypoxia, hypoglycaemia and hypocalcaemia associated with lactation. With the exception of renal disease, they are all relatively uncommon causes. Cats are very susceptible to a wide range of intoxicants which induce seizures. Fits may arise as a result of direct neurotoxic effects or secondarily to hepatotoxicity or nephrotoxicity. Chlorinated hydrocarbons, organophosphorus compounds, ethylene glycol, phenols, lead and inorganic or organic mercury are possible causes in the cat. These intoxications are discussed in Chapter 28 and by Evans (1988).

Intracranial causes of fits are more diverse and are more commonly encountered (Table 2.2). Brain injury may cause convulsions immediately or they may be a delayed consequence due to glial scarring. Any cerebral inflammatory disease may cause seizures. Feline infectious peritonitis in its dry (pyogranulomatous) form, toxoplasmosis and meningoencephalitis are possible causes. Fits may occur in rabies. Any of the space-occupying lesions discussed previously may precipitate convulsions. In thiamine deficiency convulsions are a prominent feature late in the course of the disease. They are common in anoxic cerebral degeneration and may also be a feature of lysosomal storage diseases.

Table 2.2 Conditions associated with seizures.

Idiopathic epilepsy*

Degenerations
  Cerebral ischaemia
  Storage diseases and other heritable degenerations (see Table 2.6)
  Thiamine deficiency

Generalized metabolic derangements
  Hyperammonaemia (hepatic encephalopathy)
  Hypocalcaemia
  Hypoglycaemia
  Uraemia*

Intoxications
  Alphachloralose
  Benzoic acid
  Ethylene glycol*
  Lead
  Organochlorine pesticides*
  Organophosphorus pesticides
  Phenolics
  Strychnine

Inflammatory disease
  Blastomycosis
  Cryptococcosis
  Feline infectious peritonitis (FIP)*
  Granulomatous meningoencephalitis
  Meningitis
  Pseudorabies (Aujeszky's disease)
  Rabies
  Toxoplasmosis
  Other encephalitides

Space-occupying lesions
  Abscesses
  Coenurus cysts
  Filariae
  Hydrocephalus
  Neoplasms*
  Oestrid larvae

Trauma*

Asterisks indicate common conditions.

Animals with organic intracranial disease will usually have detectable neurological deficits in the periods between fits and may have other clinical signs. If organic intracranial disease can be ruled out and there is no clinical or clinical pathological evidence of the extracranial causes, a diagnosis of idiopathic epilepsy may be made. These animals must, however, be regularly monitored for the development of focal signs or progressive changes indicating that organic disease has been overlooked.

Clinical features

GENERALIZED SEIZURES

Grand-mal and Jacksonian-type generalized seizures are encountered in cats. Grand-mal seizures are most common and have no localizing features. As a general rule a fit (or ictus) occurs as a component of a characteristic series of changes. Initially, there is a premonitory period of behavioural abnormality before convulsions are seen. In this stage of prodrome or aura the cat may appear vacant or frightened, seek attention or hide, sit in unusual postures, cry out or become aggressive. Fits often begin when the animal is dozing or asleep. The prodrome is followed by the convulsive episode, which usually lasts 1–3 minutes. The animal falls to the ground with limbs extended and there is then bilaterally symmetrical muscular activity, which characteristically includes paddling and running movements and jaw-champing. Pupillary dilatation and salivation are also present and involuntary urination and defecation are not uncommon. Consciousness is temporarily lost. After subsidence of motor activity and recovery of consciousness the animal may rise but there is then a period of post-ictal depression.

Jacksonian seizures are the consequence of initial irritation of a focus, which spreads to give generalized cerebral activity after a short period. In consequence, there are initial focal signs related to the location of the lesion, for example movements of a single limb or isolated chewing movements, before the full generalized pattern develops.

PARTIAL SEIZURES

Partial seizures are the consequence of a localized epileptogenic focus from which activity does not spread. Signs relate to the site of the focus and may therefore be much more difficult to detect. There may be localized motor activity if the motor cortex is involved, but a focus in other areas may produce vague behavioural signs such as transient confusion, apparent blindness, fear-behaviour or apparent attention to non-existent objects.

Diagnosis

DIFFERENTIATING FEATURES

The above features tend to be characteristic of idiopathic epilepsy. There may be difference of detail in fits of other causes which suggest this to be the case; unfortunately these features are not sufficiently constant to be relied upon for diagnosis. Seizures due to hypoglycaemia tend to follow strenuous activity and are preceded by a period of muscle flaccidity or by trembling. Those due to intoxicants and to thiamine deficiency may in some cases be precipitated by handling or stimulation. Convulsions due to intoxicants may be prolonged or more regularly recurrent and may progress to coma. The prodrome may not be detectable in fits due to organic disease. Convulsions associated with space-occupying lesions tend to become progressively more frequent and severe, but other seizures may also show this pattern.

True seizures must be distinguished from the tetanic limb extension of tetanus and of strychnine poisoning. Classically in these situations stimulation readily induces rigid limb extension, opisthotonos and apnoea. There are no repetitive movements and consciousness is not lost. However, such discrimination is not always easy.

HISTORY

In history-taking several features should be noted. Age of onset is important. Idiopathic epilepsy is often, although not invariably, a disease of young cats; tumours are generally problems of aged cats. Organic disease is suggested if other signs develop prior to or simultaneously with the onset of seizures. The owner should be questioned carefully about diet and about the possibility of exposure to toxins. The context in which fits occur and their natural history should also be established.

EXAMINATION

A thorough routine examination is essential before proceeding to neurological examination. Detectable neurological abnormalities between fits suggest organic brain disease. In the absence of such signs, there may be quiescent or extremely local intracranial disease or the cause may be extracranial.

ANCILLARY AIDS

Ancillary examinations are of substantial value. Haematological examination may confirm suspicions of inflammatory disease or reveal evidence of lead poisoning. Where extracranial disease is suspected, the appropriate biochemical parameters should be investigated. To rule out some common metabolic causes of seizures blood urea, alanine aminotransferase (ALT), alkaline phosphatase (AlkP), fasting blood glucose and serum calcium should be measured. CSF examination is valuable only if organic brain disease is suspected. Radiography is primarily useful in trauma or hydrocephalus.

Electroencephalography can be useful as a confirmatory investigation and may assist in localization and characterization of a lesion, but in the majority of cases a diagnosis may be reached without it. It is not a substitute for a good history and examination.

STATUS EPILEPTICUS

A proportion of affected animals may have fits of increasing severity and frequency which eventually merge, or they may have one prolonged fit. The animal then passes into the condition of prolonged loss of consciousness with intermittent or continuous seizure activity referred to as status epilepticus. Status epilepticus may lead to hyperthermia and irreversible brain changes and death. It is a neurological emergency and must be controlled as soon as possible.

Prophylaxis and therapy of epilepsy

Therapy for epilepsy falls into two categories: prevention of convulsions and treatment of status epilepticus.

PROPHYLACTIC MEASURES

These have two components. If the seizures are due to organic disease, then appropriate treatment of the underlying cause should be instituted where possible. Where convulsions are due to idiopathic epilepsy, or in cases of organic disease where primary therapy is not possible or fails, anti-epileptic drugs may be used in prophylactic control of fits.

Prophylactic drug therapy presents some problems in the cat, and is not indicated following a single fit or if the frequency of fits is low, since all the available drugs have undesirable side-effects (see also Chapter 27). The prophylactic agents of choice are phenobarbitone and diazepam.

The important pharmacological feature of the anticonvulsant drugs is that they act by lowering the general excitability of the brain and thus reducing the probability of initiation of seizure activity. Thus steady blood and brain concentrations of the drug must be maintained regardless of whether fits occur. This requires continuous and regular administration. Sudden cessation can result in rebound with severe convulsions; they must be tailed off gradually. Stabilization of therapy is therefore a long-term matter of trial and systematic adjustment of dose. Any chosen dose level must be tried for at least 2 weeks and then the balance of effect on seizure frequency and degree of sedation assessed before it is accepted as satisfactory or alteration made. Once stabilization is achieved, prophylaxis may be needed indefinitely, but if no fits occur over 12 months it is sensible to test withdrawal of therapy. If fits increase in frequency during prophylactic treatment it may be necessary to increase dose levels. If prophylaxis is to be successful it is essential that both owner and veterinary surgeon thoroughly appreciate the effects of and the importance of adherence to the regime.

The usual dosage requirement of phenobarbitone is in the range 7–30 mg b.i.d. or t.i.d. and this may be adjusted in 3–6 mg steps. For diazepam, doses in the range 1–5 mg b.i.d. or t.i.d. are usually effective and adjustments may be made in 0.5–2 mg steps.

TREATMENT OF STATUS EPILEPTICUS

Status epilepticus is a medical emergency. The animal should be briefly assessed and an airway established if necessary. Oxygen may be required if there is hypoxia. The animal should be protected from self-inflicted injury. The drug of choice for control of the seizures is diazepam. Initially 5–10 mg is administered intravenously. If after 10 minutes convulsions continue, this is increased to effect or up to a maximum total dose of 20 mg. If the latter is ineffective, phenobarbitone is given intravenously up to a maximum dose of 60 mg, or general anaesthesia may be induced with pentobarbitone. Over-medication should be avoided. Fluid therapy may be needed. Careful medical and neurological monitoring is essential. Oral anticonvulsant therapy should be initiated as soon as possible.

Prolonged or recurrent seizures due to intoxication may be managed in the same way as status epilepticus.

Prognosis

Clearly where organic disease underlies fits, this determines the prognosis. Animals with idiopathic epilepsy may be kept seizure-free for months or even indefinitely with carefully regulated medication. More animals than one might wish lapse into fatal status epilepticus; this number could almost certainly be reduced by more skilled management.

Thiamine deficiency
(see also Chapter 24)

A number of CNS signs are possible, including fits. The condition is a degenerative encephalopathy which arises in some cats fed a diet consisting substantially or entirely of fish, and is due to high levels of thiaminase (Jubb *et al.*, 1956). Very rarely it may be seen with unsupplemented diets of cooked meat, since thiamine is heat labile. The condition is uncommon. It resembles Chastek paralysis of mink and fox.

Signs

Animals show progressive inappetence. There is ataxia and dysmetria: the gait is peculiar with high, weaving leg movements and the head is ventroflexed so that the chin is tucked in. The pupils are dilated and slow to respond to light and there may be papilloedema and peripapillary neovascularization. Vestibular reflexes are absent. Spasticity may occur and the animals may walk stiffly on their toes; tone is heightened by handling. The tail is held erect. Convulsions are common. Advanced cases become semicomatose, cry continuously and show opisthotonos and maintained extensor tone.

Diagnosis

In life diagnosis is based on clinical signs and dietary history. At post-mortem examination there are bilaterally symmetrical lesions in the inferior colliculi, medial vestibular, lateral geniculate and oculomotor nuclei and other nuclei of the brainstem. Haemorrhagic necrosis is the prominent feature of the lesions. Occasionally diffuse cerebrocortical degeneration is also present.

Treatment

The diet should be changed. Early in the disease clinical signs may be reversible by low doses of thiamine (1–5 mg IM). Later, when coma has set in, 50–100 mg (IV or IM) should be given daily until a response is obtained, but prognosis is poor in advanced cases. Residual ataxia may remain for 2 or 3 weeks.

Hepatic encephalopathy

Hepatic encephalopathy is generally detected during the first 6 months of life, when it is usually associated with the presence of portosystemic shunts (Vulgamott *et al.*, 1980). Rarely it is a consequence of hepatic failure in the older animal. The initial sign is frequently ptyalism, but encephalopathic signs soon develop (Blaxter *et al.*, 1988). The neurological signs associated with hepatic encephalopathy include behavioural changes, ataxia, visual disturbances, mydriasis, depression and/or excitement. Seizures may be a prominent feature. The neurological signs occur episodically and are exacerbated after feeding. A small proportion of affected cats are stunted. The neurological signs are associated with functional CNS derangement secondary to one or more metabolic alterations. There is failure adequately to clear from the blood ammonia generated by the gut flora and from amino acid metabolism. Resting blood ammonia levels are increased and there is a reduced tolerance to an oral challenge with ammonium salts. CNS ammonia levels may be extremely high. Accumulation of mercaptans, produced by gut bacteria, short-chain fatty acids, indole metabolites and middle-molecules together with alterations in the ratio of aromatic to branched-chain aliphatic amino acids in the plasma have also been implicated. Mercaptans are neurotoxic. Altered ammonia levels, the imbalance in amino acids and alterations in GABA metabolism may have secondary CNS effects to decrease excitatory amino acid transmitter levels, perturb 5-HT and noradrenaline concentrations, and to induce synthesis of monoamine false transmitters. Disturbances in CNS energy metabolism and sodium-potassium ATPase may also contribute to the neurological dysfunction. For an account of the diagnosis of the condition, which rests mainly on investigation of liver blood supply and function, and for its treatment, see Chapter 8.

Intoxications

For detailed discussion of intoxications the reader is referred to Chapter 28 and to Evans (1988). Lead, organophosphorus and organochlorine compounds are important causes of seizures and are discussed briefly in this context.

Lead

Lead poisoning is rarely diagnosed in cats, but may be more common than is generally suspected. The predominant neurological signs are lethargy, or hyperexcitability and seizures, depending upon the individual. Inappetence, constipation and vomiting may also be noted. The blood lead levels associated with toxicity in the cat have not been adequately defined. See Chapter 28 for further details.

Organochlorine insecticides

Poisoning with organochlorine compounds is encountered quite frequently (Gruffydd-Jones *et al.*, 1981; Evans, 1988). Marked hyperexcitability is the predominant feature. There are muscle tremors, generally progressing to intermittent or continuous seizures. Ataxia, depression, wasting, alopecia and ptyalism may also be noted. Treatment is by non-specific control of seizures, using phenobarbitone or diazepam, calcium infusions and supportive therapy.

Organophosphorus and carbamate insecticides

These compounds are inhibitors of acetylcholinesterase and result in the accumulation of acetylcholine both peripherally and centrally. Cats are often exposed to multiple sources due to the use of flea collars, insecticidal aerosols for flea control on the animal and in the environment and of vaporizing strips, and toxicity due to cumulative effects is therefore relatively common. The clinical signs are due to neuromuscular and autonomic overactivity. Respiratory distress which progresses to apnoea is life-threatening. Seizures, coma, vomiting, diarrhoea, excessive salivation and lacrimation are also prominent signs. Treatment consists of giving the muscarinic antagonist atropine intravenously (0.2 mg/kg or to effect) together with an intramuscular dose of 0.2 mg/kg. The intravenous dose should be repeated as necessary. If it is available and can be administered within 4 hours, pralidoxime (20–40 mg/kg) is of value for the treatment of organophosphorus intoxication but is contraindicated in carbamate intoxication.

BEHAVIOURAL ABNORMALITIES

Inappropriate behavioural traits in cats may arise in diverse ways (Table 2.3). Frequently they are psychogenic in origin or reflect normal patterns of behaviour which are unacceptable to the owner or with which the owner is unacquainted. For further discussion of these the reader is referred to Chapter 26. Behavioural abnormalities may, however, reflect neurological disease or disorders of other body systems, particularly where there

Table 2.3 Conditions associated with behavioural changes or behaviour unacceptable to the owner.

Normal behaviour
   Oestrus behaviour*
   Fighting/territorial behaviour*
   Hunting
   Spraying*
   Territorial scratching*

Disease of other systems
   Hyperthyroidism*
   Pain
   Diarrhoea
   Cystitis
   Urinary incontinence
   Cardio-respiratory distress

Functional brain disorders
   CNS-active drugs
   Hepatic encephalopathy
   Psychomotor seizures
   Uraemic encephalopathy*

Organic brain disorders
   Diabetes insipidus
   FIP*
   Hereditary degenerative disorders (see Table 2.6)
   Ischaemic encephalopathy
   Lead poisoning
   Mercury poisoning
   Neoplasms*   ⎫ Hypothalamic lesions
   Other space-occupying lesions ⎭ frequently responsible
   Pseudorabies
   Rabies (common in some countries)
   Thiamine deficiency
   Toxoplasmosis

Psychogenic
   Spraying*
   Aberrant defecation and/or urination*
   Exaggeration of normal aggressiveness*
   Excessive grooming*
   Tail chasing*

Asterisks indicate common problems.

has been a change in behaviour patterns. It is important to consider such possibilities. In most cases cats with behavioural changes consequent upon neurological disorders or disease of other body systems will generally have other signs. These conditions are therefore discussed else- where in this chapter or in the appropriate chapters of this text. It should be noted, however, that behavioural abnormalities may occur alone in psychomotor seizures and may be the first signs to appear in rabies, pseudorabies and spongiform encephalopathy.

LETHARGY, ALTERED AWARENESS OR CONSCIOUSNESS, AND COMA

Lethargy, altered awareness or consciousness, and coma can be the result of disease of the cerebrum, brainstem or meninges, disseminated CNS pathology, or systemic diseases with secondary effects on the brain (Table 2.4). The differential diagnosis is therefore very wide and many of the conditions involved may also cause behavioural changes or seizures. The relevant neurological conditions are discussed elsewhere in this chapter. The diagnosis of the systemic conditions is discussed briefly in the section of this chapter on diagnostic aids but other chapters should be consulted as appropriate.

BRAINSTEM LESIONS

Brainstem lesions which show localized signs do so because they involve the central or peripheral components of the third to twelfth cranial nerves and are discussed in the following section.

Minor non-localizable lesions may produce unilateral or bilateral upper motor neuron paresis and loss of proprioception from the limbs. As the severity of the lesion increases, sensory deficits become more severe. Severe lesions produce coma or severe obtundation. Such lesions are often associated with trauma and usually involve cerebral damage too. The consequences and assessment of severe brainstem damage are dis- cussed in the section dealing with cerebral trauma. Non-localizable brainstem signs may be produced by feline infectious peritonitis, toxoplasmosis or cryptococcosis.

CRANIAL NERVE DEFICITS

Cranial nerve deficits are of considerable im- portance not only because of their deleterious

Table 2.4 Conditions associated with altered consciousness, lethargy and coma.

Generalized conditions
  Shock*
  Hypoglycaemia
  Hyperglycaemia
  Anaemia*
  Hyperviscosity
    Polycythaemia
    Myeloma
  Hypoadrenocorticism
  Hypokalaemia
  Hypoxia*
  Weakness/muscle wasting/cachexia*
  Pyrexia/septicaemia/viraemia*
  Uraemia*
  Hyperammonaemia (hepatic encephalopathy)

Central nervous system causes
  Encephalitides
    Blastomycosis
    Cryptococcosis
    FIP*
    Pseudorabies (Aujeszky's disease)
    Rabies
    Toxoplasmosis
  Hereditary degenerations (see Table 2.6)
  Hydrocephalus
  Intoxications
    Alphachloralose*
    Barbiturates
    Carbamates
    Ethylene glycol*
    Lead
    Metaldehyde*
    Narcotics
    Phenolics
    Salicylates
  Meningitides
    Bacterial
    Blastomycosis
    Cryptococcosis
  Narcolepsy
  Subdural empyema†
  Space-occupying lesions
    Abscesses
    Coenurus cysts
    Filariae
    Hydrocephalus
    Neoplasms*
    Oestrid larvae
  Hypoxia*
  Thiamine deficiency
  Trauma*

† Dow *et al.*, 1988.
Asterisks indicate common conditions.

effects, but also because they provide information for the localization of both intracranial and extracranial lesions. Cranial nerves may be involved in lesions either singly or in groups and at any point along their course. Thus, from the single or associated palsies, it may be possible to establish which part is affected by the lesion – whether the nuclei, the pathway within the brain substance, the point of exit, the intraosseous part or the extracranial part of the nerve.

Cranial nerves II, III, IV and VI and the cervical sympathetic trunk: neuro-ophthalmology

Neuro-ophthalmological examination is an important and revealing aspect of the neurological examination. In the context of this chapter only a superficial discussion is possible and for further information the reader is referred to Petersen-Jones (1989).

Cranial nerve II

The second cranial nerve (optic nerve) conveys the fibres of the visual pathway from the retina to the optic chiasma, where the fibres enter the optic tract after partial decussation. The optic tracts pass to the lateral geniculate bodies on their respective sides where they synapse. Between these points, fibres diverge to pass to the pretectal region and mediate visual reflexes. From each lateral geniculate body an optic radiation passes to the ipsilateral occipital (visual) cortex.

Cranial nerve III

The third cranial (oculomotor) nerve originates from the oculomotor nucleus and conveys motor fibres to the ventral, dorsal and medial rectus muscles and inferior oblique muscles of the orbit, and also to the levator palpebrae superioris muscle. It emerges from the brainstem close to the crus cerebri and passes to the orbit through the cavernous sinus. The oculomotor nerve also conveys parasympathetic fibres from the Edinger–Westphal nuclei, which receive fibres from the pretectal region, thus completing the pupillary light response reflex arc. The partial decussation of the optic chiasma and connections between the pretectal nuclei convey the consensual light reflex.

Cranial nerve IV

The fourth cranial (trochlear) nerve arises from its nucleus in the mesencephalon and decussates before emerging from the brainstem dorsally and cranial to the cerebellar peduncles. It courses downwards and forwards and leaves the skull through the orbital fissure to innervate the superior oblique (trochlear) muscle.

Cranial nerve VI

The sixth cranial (abducens) nerve arises from its nucleus at the level of the posterior cerebellar peduncle, the fibres leaving the brainstem ventromedial to the fifth, seventh and eighth nerves. From here it passes forwards on the base of the skull and through the orbital fissure into the orbit where it innervates the lateral rectus and retractor bulbi muscles. The third, fourth and sixth nerves together control ocular position and movement.

Cervical sympathetic trunk

The cervical sympathetic trunk is not a cranial nerve. However, it provides substantial innervation to elements within the eye, orbital structures and the upper eyelid (Fig. 2.1). Interference with this pathway produces a diagnostically valuable composite of neuro-ophthalmological signs (Horner's syndrome). It is therefore appropriate

to discuss its anatomy at this point. The pathway of sympathetic innervation originates in the hypothalamus and passes through the midbrain to synapse on sympathetic preganglionic neurons in the thoracolumbar spinal cord. Axons from these cells leave the cord and enter the sympathetic trunk and pass cranially, synapsing with the postganglionic neurons in the superior cervical ganglion. From here, axons enter the skull and pass through the middle ear joining the ophthalmic nerve (branch of V) by way of whose branches they are distributed, entering the orbit through the orbital fissure.

Neuro-ophthalmological signs

All neuro-ophthalmological examinations should include a comprehensive ophthalmological examination to eliminate intraocular causes of visual and pupillary abnormalities. In testing the menace reflex a transparent screen should be placed between the hand and the patient so that draughts do not induce false-positive results.

Ophthalmological examination may reveal optic atrophy if there is involvement of the optic nerves. The disc appears shrunken and pale with atrophic or absent vessels. Papilloedema is an important sign of raised intracranial pressure: the disc appears raised and oedematous with a blurred outline. The veins are engorged and may be seen to dip over the raised edge of the disc. Uveitis is a significant finding. It is not uncommonly present in cases of feline infectious peritonitis (FIP) involving the central nervous system or in toxoplasmosis.

BLINDNESS

Lesions of the optic nerve, chiasma and tract produce blindness, but of differing character depending upon the site of the lesion. The pupillary reflexes are also differently affected by lesions at different sites (Figs. 2.2 and 2.3).

A complete optic nerve lesion produces unilateral blindness in that eye with a slightly dilated pupil and obliteration of the direct pupillary reflex, and the consensual reflex on illumination of that eye. Illumination of the other eye produces normal direct and consensual responses.

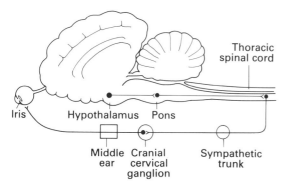

Fig. 2.1 Sympathetic innervation of the iris.

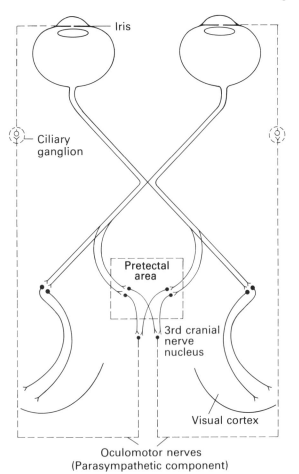

Fig. 2.2 The pathway of the light reflex.

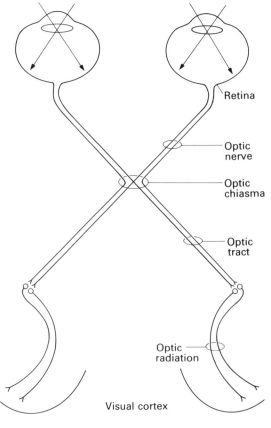

Fig. 2.3 The visual pathway.

This is a rare combination in the cat, but may be produced by intraorbital tumours, in which case the eye will be proptosed and may be fixed because of third, fourth and sixth nerve involvement.

Tumours in the pituitary fossa compress or ablate the optic chiasma. Small tumours may cause visual field defects; larger ones result in total blindness with complete absence of pupillary responses (see above).

Lesions of the optic tract produce blindness in the contralateral visual field with responsive pupils, as do lesions in the lateral geniculate nucleus, optic radiation or optic cortex. This is

known as cortical blindness, and is total with bilateral lesions.

Hereditary blindness due to progressive retinal atrophy is seen in Abyssinian cats (Narfstrom, 1985). Affected animals may be presented at any age from a few months onwards and have dilated pupils and very sluggish or absent pupillary light reflexes. On ophthalmoscopic examination there is a characteristic tapetal hyper-reflectivity together with atrophy of the retinal blood vessels. Familial degeneration of photoreceptors has been recorded (West-Hyde & Buyukmihci, 1982) as has bilateral optic nerve aplasia (Barnett & Grimes, 1974). Retinal degeneration is also a feature of some storage diseases (see below) and of taurine deficiency (see Chapter 24). FIP, toxoplasmosis, cryptococcosis and lymphosarcoma can all give rise to blindness, which may be due to central or to retinal involvement.

NYSTAGMUS

Nystagmus may be defined as a disturbance of ocular posture characterized by more or less rhythmic oscillations of the eyes. Nystagmus may be a normal or a pathological phenomenon. It is a common feature of vestibular disease, because of the vestibulo-ocular connections contained in the medial longitudinal fasciculus, but it may also occur in a variety of other circumstances.

Detailed observation of the features of nystagmus are required to define it. It is necessary to note the following: whether it is spontaneous, induced by head movement or induced by fixation of the eyes; whether it is differentiated into fast and slow phases and if so in which direction is the quick phase; how fast it is; the extent of the excursion and the variability. Fine or well-compensated nystagmus may only be visible with the ophthalmoscope. The various forms of nystagmus are discussed briefly below.
1 Normal (physiological) nystagmus. Optokinetic nystagmus when following a series of objects moving across the visual field is quite normal.
2 Pathological nystagmus. Spontaneous nystagmus arises from vestibular lesions. In peripheral disease it is horizontal and the rapid phase is towards the normal side. In central disease, vertical nystagmus may also be seen. Vestibular nystagmus rapidly becomes reduced in extent due to compensation.
3 Positional nystagmus. Positional nystagmus occurs when the head is moved relative to the body (the vestibular-ocular reflexes). In peripheral disease it is unchanging. In central vestibular disease it alters in character as the head position is varied.
4 Fixating nystagmus. Fixating nystagmus is a characteristic nystagmus which is a form of intention tremor: when attempting to fixate an object the eyes gradually drift to the rest position and are then flicked back to fix on the object. It is claimed that the fast phase is more marked

towards the side of the lesion, but the author is unable to confirm this.
5 Nystagmus of blindness is very variable.
6 Cats will rarely tolerate attempts to induce caloric nystagmus.

Nystagmus of Siamese cats
A congenital nystagmus is found in the Siamese breed. The condition is characterized by episodic occurrence of bursts of rapid and fine horizontal eye movements. It is benign and is a physiological adaptation to abnormal central projections.

STRABISMUS

If strabismus, or squint, is suspected the head should be systematically moved vertically and horizontally: in squints, conjugate eye movements are maintained. In lesions of the vestibular system or the medial longitudinal fasciculus, conjugate gaze is normal in some positions and abnormal in others. In all third, fourth and sixth nerve palsies vision is normal unless the optic nerve is also damaged. Lesions within the orbit may give rise to complex deficits in which Horner's syndrome (see below) is also present.

Cranial nerve III palsies
Deficits of the third cranial nerve may arise from compression, contusion or ablation of the oculomotor nucleus or the nerve. They produce ventrolateral strabismus, pupillary dilatation and ptosis (due to paralysis of levator palpebrae superioris). Isolated deficits of the third nerve are almost invariably a sign of tentorial herniation. Early in herniation the deficit is unilateral and there is ipsilateral pupillary dilatation. As herniation progresses, dilatation becomes bilateral.

Cranial nerve IV palsies
Damage to the trochlear nerve causes rotation of the eyeball some 45° clockwise about its horizontal axis. Fourth nerve palsies are rare. They most commonly occur in conjunction with a third nerve palsy because of the close proximity of their nuclei, or with third and sixth nerve deficits because of lesions in the brainstem, the basilar region (when other cranial nerves may be

affected), the orbital fissure or orbit (in which case the ophthalmic division of the trigeminal nerve is also involved).

Cranial nerve VI palsies
Sixth nerve palsies may occur alone from lesions of the brainstem. Most commonly they occur with deficits of the third and fourth nerves because of lesions in the regions cited in the previous paragraph. The eye is deviated medially.

Positional strabismus
In vestibular disease the disturbance of ocular posture may also result in a positional strabismus in which the eye on the affected side is deviated towards the ground. In peripheral disease this is constant; in central disease it may disappear in some positions of the head.

Congenital strabismus of Siamese cats
A congenital convergent strabismus is encountered in Siamese cats. It is a response to an abnormal projection pattern of the optic nerve fibres. As with the congenital nystagmus of Siamese cats, it is benign and is not amenable to correction. In some cases the dominant white gene may mask the characteristic Himalayan albinism pattern of hair coloration in Siamese cats. Such 'crypto-Siamese' cats may also show the strabismus.

HORNER'S SYNDROME
Horner's syndrome is a complex of abnormalities produced by interruption of the sympathetic supply to the eye, orbit and periorbital smooth muscle. It is usually unilateral. There is enophthalmos, slight ptosis, protrusion of the nictitating membrane and pupillary constriction. The pupil remains reactive. Horner's syndrome may be caused by injury to the neural pathway anywhere along its course.

The site of the lesion may be identified by the associated neurological signs. Traumatic injuries and other spinal cord abnormalities (see below) may affect the pathway in the upper cervical region, in which case there is associated hemiplegia or tetraplegia, or in the cervico-

thoracic region, in which case there is usually an upper motor neuron deficit of the hindlimbs and a lower motor neuron deficit of the forelimbs. Brachial plexus injury may also interrupt the pathway at the level of the thoracic ventral roots.

The sympathetic trunk may be affected by trauma, by lymphosarcoma or by neurofibromas; Horner's syndrome occurs alone in this eventuality. Otitis media may involve the fibres as they cross the middle ear cavity; there are associated vestibular and sometimes facial nerve signs. Retrobulbar lesions may produce Horner's syndrome associated with ophthalmic nerve and second, third, fourth and sixth nerve deficits.

Other cranial nerves

Cranial nerve I
The function of the first cranial (olfactory) nerve is difficult to test and some neurologists doubt the value of the evaluation. Examination of the response to a non-irritant aromatic substance such as oil of cloves (obtainable from retail pharmacists) on cotton wool and comparison with a control pledget has some value.

The first cranial nerve is very short, consisting of bundles of fibres passing through the cribriform plate to the olfactory bulb. Lesions in the region of the cribriform plate may involve the nerve either unilaterally or bilaterally. Bilateral involvement produces anosmia. There is often an associated nasal discharge. If the lesion extends intracranially, the optic nerves or chiasma are likely to be involved, as is the frontal lobe. Blindness, absence of pupillary reflexes and mental changes are therefore commonly associated with first nerve involvement.

Cranial nerve V
The fifth cranial (trigeminal) nerve takes origin from three nuclei. The motor nucleus is located in the pons. The sensory fibres pass to two separate nuclei which extend caudally from the pons. The sensory and motor fibres emerge from the pons just ventral to the cerebellum, often as separate bundles which then fuse. This point of emergence is close to that of the seventh and

eighth nerves. The nerve enters the trigeminal canal in the petrous temporal bone where the trigeminal ganglion is situated. From here three branches emerge: the ophthalmic, which is the principal sensory nerve to the orbit; the maxillary nerve sensory to the skin of the cheek, the side of the face and the soft and hard palates and upper jaw. The mandibular nerve is the motor nerve to muscles of mastication and provides sensory innervation to the remainder of the face and to the lower jaw and tongue (but not supplying taste buds).

Damage to the motor division of the trigeminal nerve by the jamming of objects across the back of the mouth is much less common than in dogs, but can occur. There is flaccid paralysis of the muscles of mastication. If this is unilateral the jaw may hang asymmetrically, pulled to the unaffected side. If it is bilateral the jaw hangs flaccidly and chewing is impossible. Subsequently there may be muscular fibrosis and contracture which may result in a very limited capacity to open the mouth. The prognosis is poor.

Deficits of the ophthalmic division have already been discussed above in the section dealing with neuro-ophthalmology.

Complex abnormalities involving the trigeminal nerve arise in the cerebellopontine angle syndrome, which is dealt with below in the discussion of vestibular disease.

Cranial nerve VII

The seventh cranial (facial) nerve originates from a nucleus in the medulla. Its fibres pass around the sixth nerve nucleus close to the floor of the fourth ventricle before emerging close to the eighth nerve, passing through the petrous temporal bone and crossing round the posterior border of the mandible before being distributed to the muscles of the face.

Facial nerve palsies are common because of the numerous sites at which the nerve is vulnerable. The clinical signs are a flaccid paralysis of the facial muscles so that the cheek hangs in a loose, drooping fashion and may fill with food. The eye cannot be closed, the ear is immobile and the nostril on the affected side cannot be dilated.

The eyelid paralysis may lead to corneal drying and ulceration. In chronic lesions there may be marked contracture of the affected side.

Facial nerve paralysis without accompanying deficits may follow trauma such as superficial damage from blows to the face. The facial nerve is also susceptible to involvement in otitis media and interna. Lesions in the region of the sixth nerve nucleus may affect this nerve and also involve the facial nerve fibres as they pass round it producing a combined deficit. The facial nerve is also involved in the cerebellopontine angle syndrome (see page 109) and neoplasms are a common cause of lesions.

Cranial nerve VIII

The eighth cranial (vestibulocochlear) nerve has two divisions: the cochlear division concerned with hearing and the vestibular division concerned with equilibrium sense. The two divisions emerge from the medulla and cross to enter the petrous temporal bone where they are distributed to their respective end organs. Vestibular diseases, otitis media and interna and the cerebellopontine angle syndrome are discussed in connection with ataxia on page 109.

DEAFNESS

Deafness is difficult to assess subjectively in the cat. Often the owner's long-term impressions may be the most useful indication. Until recently there has been no convenient instrumental method of assessing hearing loss, but the application of auditory evoked potentials now offers this possibility. An otoscopic examination is an integral part of any neurological examination.

CONGENITAL DEAFNESS

There are several gene systems determining varying degrees of coat whiteness in the cat. Of these the dominant white gene is associated with deafness. Heterozygous or homozygous possession of this gene produces a pure white coat with full penetrance. The gene also has effects on eye colour, although the effects on the eye and ear are due to pleiotropy and are not fully penetrant. Up to 80%, but not all, of such cats may be deaf. Ear involvement may be unilateral or bilateral. They may have two blue eyes, two yellow eyes, or may be odd-eyed. The deafness is the result of degeneration of the organ of Corti and there is no treatment (Elverland & Mair, 1980). Affected cats are able to live a normal life, but are at increased risk of being involved in road traffic accidents. True albino cats (see also Chapter 1), with white coats and pink eyes, have normal hearing.

ACQUIRED DEAFNESS

Damage to the external ear, the middle ear, the sensory apparatus, the eighth nerve or its cochlear nuclei may all produce acquired deafness, as in theory may involvement of tracts and the auditory cortex. The causes are numerous, but acquired deafness is rarely diagnosed.

The petrous temporal bone and its contents may occasionally be damaged in skull trauma (see p. 90) when there may be bleeding from the external auditory meatus and the tympanic membrane may also be ruptured. Vestibular signs will usually be present and often there will be associated internal haemorrhage producing severe brainstem compromise. Treatment is as described for cerebral trauma.

Degenerative deafness may occur with increasing age, as cochlear sensitivity is reduced. It is difficult to detect. Deafness due to intoxication is not uncommon. The cat is very sensitive to the ototoxic effects of aminoglycoside antibiotics such as streptomycin (see Chapter 27), but deafness may also occur in other intoxications. Deafness due to aminoglycoside antibiotics is usually irreversible.

Tumours may also cause deafness. Very rarely neurofibromas of the eighth nerve may cause slowly progressive cochlear and vestibular signs. The eighth nerve is involved in the cerebellopontine angle syndrome (see p. 109) and may be affected by bony tumours of the petrous temporal bone.

Otitis media and interna are common in the cat and may produce unilateral and bilateral deafness. Vestibular signs are more prominent and auditory deficits seem to be surprisingly rare.

Ninth, tenth and eleventh cranial nerves

The ninth (glossopharyngeal), tenth (vagus) and eleventh (accessory) nerves have many closely related functions and are difficult to test neurologically, although the gag reflex is a means of assessing the ninth and tenth nerves. The tenth and eleventh nerves may also be assessed by the oculocardiac reflex if the trigeminal nerve is known to be intact. The accessory nerve's spinal component innervates muscles stabilizing the scapula (trapezius, sternocephalicus and brachiocephalicus) and lesions may sometimes produce elevation of the dorsum of the scapula. Detectable involvement of these nerves is rare in the cat, but the author has encountered it in one animal with caudal extension of a cerebellopontine angle lesion.

Twelfth cranial nerve

The twelfth cranial (hypoglossal) nerve arises from the ventrolateral surface of the medulla oblongata close to the foramen magnum. It leaves the skull through the hypoglossal foramen and passes in a wide loop to innervate the intrinsic muscles of the tongue and muscles associated with the hyoid apparatus.

Abnormalities of tongue shape, position and movement are the most obvious signs of lesions. Early on, there may be flaccidity and if the lesion is unilateral the tongue is drawn to the opposite side. Bilateral lesions produce inability to withdraw the tongue into the mouth. Later there is atrophy and fibrosis with a contracted corrugated tongue, which may be drawn to the affected side if the lesion is unilateral.

The involvement of the twelfth nerve is not uncommon in animals with cerebellopontine angle lesions, presumably due to compression of the brainstem or slight herniation through the foramen magnum. Trauma may sometimes injure the nerve in its extracranial course.

ATAXIA

Ataxia is the term applied to incoordination of gait. It is by far the most common neurological presenting sign in the cat. Its differentiation is of major diagnostic significance. Unfortunately this can present real difficulty because of the very wide range of causes. Often it may require great care to distinguish it from weakness or localized paralysis, particularly in uncooperative patients. In any case it is often associated with these signs. Table 2.5 lists the causes of incoordination of gait in the cat.

Many peripheral and central nervous structures are involved in coordinating equilibrium. The peripheral detectors of conscious and unconscious proprioception and their spinal long tracts and central relays, the vestibular system and to a lesser extent the visual system all acquire and process relevant sensory data and there is also cerebral cortical involvement. The motor cortex, descending upper motor neuron long tracts, lower motor neuron and spinal reflexes are all involved in motor control. The cerebellum is a servo-like comparator: sensory data relating to position and movement are related to motor control output and the latter is adjusted to remove any discrepancy between the predetermined and achieved results. Many routine or repetitive movements are heavily dependent on cerebellar function.

Ataxia can arise from lesions affecting any of the above structures. The ataxia may have characteristic features which allow one to localize the lesion, as for example with vestibular or cerebellar lesions. Often, however, one must rely on associated signs for precise localization. It must be remembered that disease may be multifocal.

Cerebellum

Cerebellar dysfunction produces a characteristic pattern of abnormalities. There is generalized hypotonia and there may be hyper-reflexia. Incoordination involves all four limbs and the head. To compensate for this, the animal adopts a wide-based stance. The animal is unable to correct movements, hence often they overshoot the intended range (dysmetria). Dysmetria is most often manifested as hypermetria, with a high-stepping gait. There is an intention tremor and

Table 2.5 Conditions associated with ataxia.

Non-neural causes of incoordination
Arthritides*
Cardiopulmonary dysfunction
Fractures*
Hyperviscosity syndrome
Hypoxia
Metabolic derangements
 Hypercalcaemia
 Hypocalcaemia
 Hypoglycaemia (including glycogenosis)
 Hypokalaemia
 Hypoxia
Myopathies
Severe anaemia*
Shock*
Sedative drugs

Ataxia of cerebral origin: deficient postural reactions with mild gait abnormality
Degenerations
 Ischaemic encephalopathy*
 Thiamine deficiency
Space-occupying lesions
 Abscesses
 Coenurus cysts
 Filariae
 Hydrocephalus
 Neoplasms*
 Oestrid larvae
Trauma

Ataxia of vestibular origin: circling, head-tilt, loss of balance and vestibular nystagmus
Congenital vestibular disease
Acquired peripheral vestibular disease
 Neoplasms
  Lymphosarcomas
  Neurofibromas
 Idiopathic feline vestibular syndrome
 Ototoxicity
  Aminoglycoside antibiotics
  Arsenical and mercurial compounds
  Chlorhexidine
  Iodine compounds
  Quaternary ammonium compounds
Acquired central vestibular disease
Degenerations
 Hereditary degenerations (see Table 2.6)
 Thiamine deficiency

continued on p. 108

Table 2.5 *Continued*

Inflammatory diseases
   Cryptococcosis
   FIP
   Micro-abscessation of the brainstem
   Nocardiosis
   Other meningitides/encephalitides
   Toxoplasmosis
Intoxications
   Lead
   Mercury
Space-occupying lesions
   Abscesses
   Hydrocephalus
   Neoplasms
      Glioma
      Meningioma
      Lymphosarcomas
      Neurofibromas (extensions from VIIIth nerve)
Trauma

Ataxia of cerebellar origin: dysmetria/hypermetria,
intention tremor, wide-based gait and fixating nystagmus
Congenital
   Cerebellar hypoplasia due to:
      Non-inflammatory cerebellar hypoplasia
      Panleucopenia
Acquired
   Degenerations
      Hereditary degenerations (see Table 2.6)
      Thiamine deficiency
   Inflammatory disease
      Cryptococcosis
      FIP
      Toxoplasmosis
      Other meningitides/encephalitides
   Space-occupying lesions
      Neoplasms
         Astrocytoma
         Osteosarcomas involving the cranial vault or
            temporal bone
      Abscesses
      Coenurus cysts
   Trauma

Ataxia due to lesions of the spinal cord
Degenerative
   Cervical intervertebral disc disease

Degenerative (*continued*)
   Fibrocartilaginous embolism and degenerative
      myelopathy
   Hereditary degenerations (see Table 2.6)
   Syringomyelia
Inflammatory
   Abscessation
   Aberrant parasite migration
   Cryptococcosis
   Discospondylitis
   FIP
   Meningitis/encephalitis/myelitis
   Polio (encephalo) myelitis
   Toxoplasmosis
   Vertebral osteomyelitis/abscess
Intoxications
   Chronic organophosphorus intoxication
   Mercurial poisoning
   Organochlorine compounds
Space-occupying lesions
   Abscesses
   Discospondylitis
   Epidural/subdural haemorrhage
   Exostoses due to hypervitaminosis A
   Haematomas
   Intervertebral disc disease
   Multiple cartilaginous exostoses
   Neoplasms
      Glioma
      Lymphosarcoma
      Meningioma
      Metastases
      Neurofibroma/schwannoma
      Osteosarcoma/chondrosarcoma
   Vertebral osteomyelitis/abscess
Trauma
   Fractures
   Haematomyelia
   Intervertebral disc disease
   Progressive myelomalacia
   Subluxations

Disorders of peripheral nerve
Exostoses due to hypervitaminosis
Ischaemic neuromyopathy

continued on p. 109

Table 2.5 *Continued*

Intoxications
  Lead
  Mercury
  Arsenic
Multiple cartilaginous exostoses
Neoplasms*
Polyneuropathies
  Chronic relapsing polyradiculoneuritis
  Diabetes mellitus
  Hyperchylomicronaemia
  Hypertrophic polyneuropathy
  Niemann – Pick disease
  Non-inflammatory polyneuropathy
Trauma*

Asterisks indicate common problems.

fixating nystagmus, probably as a consequence of cortical compensatory adjustment.

Fine head tremor is commonly noted. Loss of equilibrium may be total with a staggering gait and a pronounced tendency to fall sideways or backwards. Cerebellar involvement is usually bilateral with symmetrical signs. Rarely, unilateral involvement is encountered and signs are then usually, but not invariably, ipsilateral.

Congenital cerebellar disease: cerebellar hypoplasia due to feline panleucopenia virus
Significant cerebellar development occurs at around the time of birth and for some days afterwards. Infection with feline panleucopenia virus *in utero* or immediately after birth seriously damages the external germinal layer and also Purkinje cells (Kilham *et al.*, 1971). The resulting cerebellar hypoplasia produces a characteristic syndrome. The degree of hypoplasia and severity of associated signs are rather variable.

The signs are apparent as soon as the kittens attempt to walk, at around 4 weeks, and may become more apparent as activity increases. Nystagmus is usually absent. The lesion is non-progressive and compensatory changes may lead to some improvement, although signs persist throughout life. This serves to distinguish cerebellar hypoplasia from the conditions causing progressive incoordination in kittens and young cats, in which the signs become worse with time (see below). Fortunately the frequency of this disease has fallen as uptake of panleucopenia vaccination has increased and it is now quite rare. It should be noted that pregnant queens should not be vaccinated with live panleucopenia vaccines since this may cause cerebellar hypoplasia in the offspring.

Occasionally non-inflammatory cerebellar hypoplasia is encountered in kittens. Its cause is unknown.

Acquired cerebellar disease
Trauma may sometimes cause acute-onset, non-progressive cerebellar signs, from which there may be some recovery. It is rare for these to occur alone; usually there will be accompanying cerebral or brainstem involvement.

Inflammatory disease may cause acquired cerebellar disease. Diffuse meningitis is uncommon, but may involve the cerebellum. Feline infectious peritonitis, toxoplasmosis, spongiform encephalopathy, and very rarely cryptococcosis may involve the cerebellum. Usually other brain areas are also involved. The pyogranulomatous meningoencephalitis of feline infectious peritonitis does from time to time produce pure cerebellar signs. Haematological and CSF examinations are often helpful in establishing the inflammatory nature of the lesion and in differentiating the causes.

Space-occupying lesions may affect the cerebellum. There are reports of coenurus cysts occurring here. More commonly encountered are tumours and abscesses. Meningiomas may compress the cerebellum, as may osteosarcomas. Astrocytomas are also encountered. Cerebellomedullary and cerebellopontine abscesses occur secondary to otitis media and involve the cerebellum ipsilaterally. Again haematological and CSF examinations are helpful.

Vestibular disease and the cerebellopontine angle syndrome

Vestibular disease is common. Most often this is

due to otitis media and otitis interna, but other possible causes cannot be ignored.

The peripheral vestibular apparatus is located in the petrous temporal bone. The vestibular division of the eighth cranial nerve, together with the cochlear division, passes through the internal auditory meatus and enters the brainstem at the junction of the pons and medulla. The vestibular fibres then make connections in the vestibular nuclei or pass to the cerebellum via the posterior cerebellar peduncle.

From the vestibular nuclei there are widespread connections which influence cortical and spinal control of movement and equilibrium. Diagnostically, a particularly important set of connections is to the oculomotor, trochlear and abducens nerve nuclei via the medial longitudinal fasciculus. This pathway is involved in the control of eye position and movement, and the generation of normal vestibular nystagmus. Lesions which may produce abnormalities of eye co-ordination are discussed on p. 103.

The signs produced by a lesion involving the vestibular system differ depending upon whether the damage involves the peripheral components (sense organ and nerve) or the central components (the vestibular nuclei or vestibular projections).

Both peripheral and central lesions are characterized by a head tilt. This is always to the side of the lesion when it is peripheral, and is usually so when it is central. The head is turned to the same side. If the defect is bilateral, head tilt is often not present and only symmetrical ataxia is observed. A head tilt alone is not diagnostic of vestibular disease: it may be behavioural, anatomical or muscular in origin.

Tight circling, again usually to the side of the lesion, is characteristic of both central and peripheral disease. The animal is usually reluctant to turn to the opposite side. The animal has decreased tone in the forelimb on the affected side, to which it may also fall. Animals with peripheral lesions may lean to the affected side. The trunk may be curved to the side of the lesion. There may be vomiting.

The righting response is abolished. Marked rolling towards the side of the lesion may be encountered with both peripheral and central involvement. This is often transient.

With otitis media there will usually be fetid otorrhoea and pain on palpation, and there may also be intermittent head shaking.

Accompanying signs due to involvement of adjacent neurological structures are important in differentiating central and peripheral lesions. Peripheral lesions may involve the facial nerve and the cervical sympathetic fibres producing facial paralysis and Horner's syndrome. Central lesions do not involve the sympathetic fibres and Horner's syndrome is not seen. However, the roots of the fifth, sixth and seventh cranial nerves may be involved producing a combined deficit. Hearing is lost in the affected ear. Involvement of the brainstem and of the cerebellum may produce ipsilateral hemiparesis and hypermetria, deficiencies of conscious proprioception and head-bobbing. Space-occupying lesions of the cerebellopontine and cerebellomedullary angles are common and produce a progressively developing involvement of these central structures. This is known as the cerebellopontine angle syndrome. The cerebellar signs are often eclipsed by the vestibular involvement. Late in the course of such lesions hypoglossal nerve involvement may also be seen. Meningiomas and lymphosarcomas are not uncommon at this site and abscessation due to spread of otitis commonly occurs. Such spread may also cause brainstem micro-abscessation. Otitis media/interna should be vigorously treated by middle-ear irrigation followed by systemic antibiotics or by bulla osteotomy if advanced.

In the case of lesions in the middle ear, radiography is often helpful. Radiographs may reveal increased density of the tympanic bulla, which may be accompanied by thickening of its wall. Haematological examination is not helpful in differentiating the cause of the lesion.

Congenital vestibular disease
Congenital vestibular disease may be seen in kittens of a number of breeds. Siamese kittens from affected litters develop signs at 3–4 weeks of age. There is marked head tilt with mild ataxia and no

nystagmus. Normal vestibular nystagmus may be absent. Deafness has been recorded in one case. The signs disappear by 3–4 months of age, although occasionally there may be recurrences. No abnormality has been found on pathological examination. The condition may have a hereditary basis.

Burmese kittens may present with severe rolling at or soon after birth or later, with a head tilt and severe asymmetrical ataxia. The signs are non-progressive. No lesions have been identified and again a hereditary basis is suspected.

Congenital vestibular syndromes have been identified in other breeds, including Birmans and British Creams. These appear to defy classification at present. In some cases presentations resembling those described in Siamese and Burmese have been seen in the same litter. Many animals recover; these are more often those that show later head tilts rather than those rolling at birth.

In investigating apparently congenital cases of vestibular disease it must be realised that otitis can occur very early in life, and this must be excluded.

Acquired vestibular disease

PERIPHERAL
Otitis media and interna have already been discussed (see pp. 109–110).

Trauma may fracture the petrosal bone causing deafness and vestibular signs. There may be bleeding from the external ear and the tympanic membrane may be ruptured. Often intracranial haemorrhage or contusion may cause severe brainstem damage.

Ototoxicity
The cat is very susceptible to the toxic action of the aminoglycoside antibiotics upon the vestibular system (Hawkins & Lurie, 1952; Hawkins *et al.*, 1953) and this is discussed further in Chapter 27. Vestibular disease can also be induced by salicylates and by heavy metals, notably organic mercurials and arsenicals. Other intoxications, amongst which methyl mercury is notable, may also produce vestibular damage. Lane (1985) has

emphasized the sensitivity of the feline vestibular apparatus to iodine compounds, quaternary ammonium compounds and chlorhexidine. These are all compounds which have been used for irrigation of the ear and which can induce vestibular disease.

Neoplasms
Tumours of the vestibular nerve occur occasionally. These are most commonly neurofibromas and result in slowly progressive, unilateral vestibular signs and deafness. Central signs appear when the lesion begins to compress the brainstem.

Lymphosarcomas involving the tympanic bulla or the petrous temporal bone also produce vestibular signs but they are an uncommon occurrence in this site.

Idiopathic feline vestibular syndrome
An acquired vestibular syndrome of unknown cause develops acutely in cats of all ages and either sex (Burke *et al.*, 1985). The condition appears to occur most commonly in the late summer and early autumn. There is severe unilateral ataxia with a head tilt. The animal falls or rolls to that side. The animal may cower and cry out persistently. There is a spontaneous horizontal nystagmus, directed to the side opposite to that to which the head tilts, which abates over a few days. It is claimed that head oscillations may parallel the nystagmus. Positional nystagmus is present and may persist for some time after the spontaneous nystagmus has been lost. The signs slowly disappear although sometimes there is slight residual head tilt or asymmetrical ataxia. Treatment has no effect on the outcome and is not required.

CENTRAL
Severe trauma may cause central vestibular involvement; the consequent deficit is often permanent. The effects of central space-occupying lesions have been discussed on pp. 92–93. The bacterial, viral, fungal or protozoal infections of the brain or meninges may all produce vestibular signs, but there are usually other neurological abnormalities. The haemorrhagic necrosis of

thiamine deficiency involves the vestibular nuclei. Ataxia is a feature of the condition and vestibular signs may be the only ones early in its course.

PROGRESSIVE NERVOUS SYSTEM DEGENERATION IN KITTENS

There exists a large group of inherited abnormalities that cause progressive central nervous system degenerative changes. These may be divided into two groups: the storage diseases and a small miscellaneous group (Table 2.6).

It is often difficult to account for the clinical signs on a neuroanatomical basis, but these diseases have some characteristic features which

Table 2.6 Hereditary nervous degenerative diseases.

Disease	Breed
Storage diseases	
Ceroid lipofuscinosis	Siamese
Globoid cell leucodystrophy, Krabbe's disease	DSH
Glycogen storage disease type I	DSH
GM1	DSH
GM1 gangliosidosis type II	Siamese
GM2 gangliosidosis Tay–Sachs' disease	DSH
Mannosidosis	Persian
Metachromatic leucodystrophy	DSH
Mucopolysaccharidosis I Hurler's syndrome	DSH
Mucopolysaccharidosis VI (Maroteaux–Lamy syndrome)	Siamese
Sphingomyelinosis (Niemann–Pick disease)	Siamese
Inadequately defined	Abyssinian
Other heritable degenerations	
Familial spongiform degeneration	Egyptian Mau
Motor neuron disease	DSH
Neuroaxonal dystrophy	DSH
Progressive retinal atrophy	Abyssinian

References: Blakemore (1975), Haskins *et al.* (1979a,b,c, 1981), Kelly & Gaskell (1976), Narfstrom (1985), Norby & Thuline (1970), Van den Bergh *et al.* (1977), Vandevelde *et al.* (1982), Woodward *et al.* (1974).

enable one to identify them as falling into this category. Accurate diagnosis of the exact condition then requires highly specialized laboratory investigations. But these are, however, well worth while since characterization allows for selective breeding to avoid recurrences. The conditions are recessive and heterozygotes can usually be identified as such.

The following generalizations can be made about these conditions. They are rare and, as inheritance is generally as an autosomal recessive trait, only single members of a litter are likely to be affected. Specific diseases are present in particular breeds and often there is a history of inbreeding. Affected animals are usually normal at birth but fail to grow as rapidly as their normal littermates. The majority of these conditions present as neurological disorders in young animals. The clinical signs vary somewhat, but usually there is marked ataxia, or ascending paralysis or a combination of these. The disease is invariably slowly progressive and eventually fatal.

Storage diseases

Storage diseases are inborn errors of metabolism. In many of the conditions lysosomal degradative enzymes are deficient. Lysosomes are membrane-bound intracellular structures containing a population of degradative enzymes, each enzyme having a specific substrate. In a lysosomal storage disease the genetically determined lack of one of these enzymes results in the accumulation of its substrate in lysosomes. The accumulation cannot readily be disposed of and eventually affects cell function; disease then results. All cells are affected and a variety of signs may be seen, but neurons, being non-dividing cells, are particularly susceptible, hence the prominence of nervous disease. In the case of deficiency of enzymes of glycogen metabolism glycogen accumulates in the cytoplasm.

A number of these conditions are well recognized in the cat (Table 2.6). Indeed, they appear to be more common in the cat than in other species. Others are probably present in the population. Animals fulfilling the criteria noted above deserve further investigation. The activity of appropriate enzymes is measured, often using leucocytes as the source. Otherwise histological, histochemical or electron-microscopic evidence of storage may be sought in biopsy specimens. The appropriate organ or tissue for biopsy depends upon which condition is most probable. A laboratory should be consulted concerning appropriate biopsy sites. For detailed discussion of these conditions the reader is referred to Blakemore (1975) and to Evans (1989b).

Miscellaneous group

The other inherited conditions showing progressive degenerative CNS changes include spongiform degeneration in the Egyptian Mau; hereditary neuroaxonal dystrophy in domestic short hairs, and lower motor neuron paralysis due to neurofilament accumulation in domestic short hairs.

PARESIS AND PARALYSIS

Paresis and paralysis are often confused. Paralysis is the complete loss of voluntary muscle control to the affected region. In contrast paresis refers to muscular weakness of neural origin; it may be regarded as a state of partial paralysis. Paraplegia refers to paralysis of both hindlimbs; hemiplegia to the paralysis of both the hind- and forelimbs on one side of the body; tetraplegia (or quadriplegia) to paralysis of all four limbs.

Both paresis and paralysis may result from lesions at any level of the descending motor pathway. They are, however, most commonly associated with diseases of the brainstem, spinal cord or of peripheral nerves. As with intracranial disease, full assessment of signs is the key to identification of the site of the lesion. Paralysis due to damage of upper motor neurons has different characteristics from that due to lower motor neurons. This is of some help in identifying the level of lesion.

Spinal cord

The localization of lesions within the spinal cord depends upon the craniocaudal segmental organ-ization of its function and of the spinal nerves. The importance of the distinction between upper and lower motor neuron lesions has already been mentioned. The motor neurons of the ventral horn of the spinal cord, whose axons pass to the skeletal muscles, are known as the lower motor neurons. The neurons of the descending motor pathway from the cerebral cortex to the lower motor neurons are known as the upper motor neurons.

Lower motor neuron injury effectively removes the spinal outflow from the muscles supplied. Thus, there is loss of voluntary motor activity and of segmental reflexes. The muscle becomes flaccid and no longer resists passive movement. It also rapidly undergoes atrophy and later fibrosis and contracture unless reinnervated. Fibrillations precede flaccidity. If the lesion is irritative, gross fasciculation may precede it. Lower motor neuron injury is thus associated with flaccid paralysis and absent or reduced reflexes.

Upper motor neuron injury denervates the lower motor neurons and produces some disinhibition of the lower cell. After a brief period of flaccidity, tone increases over a period of 1–5 days. It may also be possible by passive stretch to elicit rhythmical contractions known as clonus. The segmental reflexes remain intact and fairly rapidly become hyperactive. Abnormal reflexes also appear, of which the most significant is the crossed extensor reflex. This paralysis with hyperreflexia, hypertonia and clonus is characteristic of upper motor neuron injury.

Clearly, an injury at any level will damage not only the lower motor neurons of that segment, producing local flaccid paralysis, but also the upper motor neurons, so that spastic paralysis is produced caudal to the lesion (Fig. 2.4). Since flaccid and spastic paralysis are easily differentiated only in the limbs and tail, this is not a subtle means of localization. None the less, the pattern will indicate whether the lesion is above the level of the brachial plexus outflow, at that level, between the brachial and lumbosacral outflows, at the level of the latter outflow, or behind it. Lesions involving one or few cord segments are termed transverse myelopathies. Multifocal

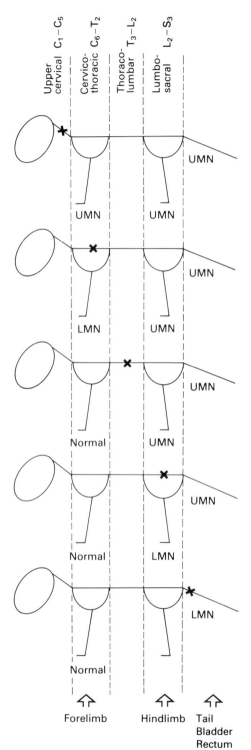

Forelimb   Hindlimb   Tail
Bladder
Rectum

lesions or those involving many segments are described as disseminated myelopathies. Accurate definition of this segmental involvement requires assessment of sensory function, particularly at the level at which the panniculus reflex ceases and anaesthesia appears, since these can be assessed on a segmental basis.

Paralysis of the anus and bladder may be of upper motor neuron type (lesions cranial to S1), in which case the anal reflex is present and reflex bladder emptying occurs. Lesions in the region S1–S3 or of the peripheral outflow cause lower motor neuron loss of bladder and anal control, so that there is urinary retention and overflow coupled with faecal incontinence. Lesions cranial to C5 may cause diaphragmatic paralysis since the phrenic nerve outflow is at C4 and those in the region C1–T5 may cause Horner's syndrome.

The cauda equina also lies within the spinal canal and lesions here produce dysfunction of these nerves. The resulting syndrome comprises lower motor neuron paralysis of the bladder and rectum; a flaccid anaesthetic tail; perineal anaesthesia; and weakness and incoordination or paralysis of the hindlimbs. Injuries to the tail base may avulse the more caudal nerve roots producing tail and bladder paralysis and anaesthesia of the perineum and tail.

Since they are largely within the spinal canal and may be separately affected, the spinal nerve roots merit mention at this point. A lesion of a dorsal root and its ganglion produces sensory dysfunction of one dermatome. Ventral root lesions produce a lower motor neuron deficit in the muscles receiving innervation from that root.

Assessment of a spinal cord lesion depends upon a number of factors. First, it is of significance whether the lesion is unilateral or bilateral. Second, the severity of signs should be considered. It is important to determine which functional modalities are lost. Mild lesions abolish only conscious proprioception. With increasing severity, voluntary motor function, superficial

Fig. 2.4 Distribution of signs with lesions at different sites along the spinal cord.

pain sensation and finally deep pain sensation are lost sequentially. Third, the speed of development of the lesion must be considered. Slowly developing lesions allow physiological compensations to take place and produce considerably milder signs than do acute lesions of the same extent and severity. From this it may be concluded that in traumatic injury the prognosis is closely related to the severity of loss of spinal cord function. In other conditions, the prognosis is likely to be much more closely related to the nature of the inciting cause.

In spinal cord disease, plain radiography and myelography are of substantial value not only in confirming the craniocaudal localization of lesions, but also in assessing the nature of the abnormality and giving some idea of its size.

Spinal cord disease

CONGENITAL

Congenital spinal cord and spinal column malformations are a hereditary feature of the Manx breed. Similar malformations occur sporadically in other breeds and are discussed on p. 127.

ACQUIRED

Trauma

Impact is a common cause of spinal cord dysfunction. It may cause contusion, laceration or severance with associated oedema. In addition, there may be haemorrhage, which may be subdural or extramedullary producing cord compression. Following very mild injury there may be oedema only. Vertebral injuries will often be present as well. There may be complete or partial fracture with or without complete or partial dislocation (Griffiths, 1978; McKee, 1990). Compression fractures may also occur.

Traumatic injuries may involve any region of the spinal column. Those in the sacral and tail areas are most common. The cord extends to L6 in the cat so that bony injuries down to this level may affect the substance of the cord. The paralysis and ataxia caused by spinal cord trauma are non-progressive from about 24 hours after the injury.

MANAGEMENT

The medical management of spinal cord injury aims primarily to reduce oedema and is essentially as described for cerebral trauma (see pp. 91–92). Doses of glucocorticoids, as recommended above for treatment of cranial trauma (see pp. 91–92) may be employed. Methylprednisolone sodium succinate appears to be more effective than dexamethasone in reducing the consequences of cord trauma (Hoerlein *et al.*, 1985). Cage rest is essential. The cat should be confined in the minimum possible space. In mild cases medical management may be all that is required. Initially, muscle spasms may protect the site against displacement. Movement is, however, a problem once recovery is under way, since it may produce or aggravate displacement and produce further spinal cord damage. Internal fixation is certainly practicable in cats and may be combined with hemilaminectomy. Hemilaminectomy decompresses the cord and relieves the effects of oedema and haematomyelia but is less effective than methylprednisolone in acute spinal damage (Hoerlein *et al.*, 1985). Surgery is only of value if carried out promptly. It is not a substitute for the medical management of oedema, and is rarely undertaken. The reader is referred to textbooks of surgery for details of surgical technique.

Cats tolerate external casts poorly although they have been employed as a means of immobilizing spinal fracture sites. Long-term (2–4 weeks) sedation of these patients with diazepam or phenobarbitone may be a preferable alternative. In the early stages, use of narcotic analgesics may also produce useful sedation as well as pain relief (see Chapter 27).

Interference with micturition is a significant problem. With upper motor neuron lesions of bladder and total loss of bladder control there may be excessive sphincter tone. In this circumstance manual emptying is difficult and may rupture the bladder. Phenoxybenzamine or acepromazine are of value for relieving functional sphincter tone, and bethanecol may be used to increase bladder wall tone. Intermittent catheterization or, better, an indwelling catheter is indicated. Fluid therapy and intravenous alimentation may be needed early in the course of therapy of severe cases. Diligent nursing is essential to prevent the formation of decubitus ulcers and to keep the animal free of secretions and excreta. Antibiotic therapy may be needed if catheterization results in cystitis.

Intervertebral disc disease

Intervertebral disc degeneration is common in cats, although clinical disease arising from it is very rare (Heavner, 1971). Disc degeneration occurs progressively with increasing age, and protrusion and prolapse are common in the cervical and lumbar regions. Disc calcification does not generally occur in the cat. Other causes must be eliminated before considering disc degeneration to be the cause of paresis and ataxia. Rarely cervical disc rupture can result in focal myelomalacia and posterior paralysis. In a case in which deep pain sense was spared, hemilaminectomy and durotomy resulted in a successful outcome (Salisbury & Cook, 1985).

Inflammatory disease

NON-INFECTIOUS
Spinal meningitis may follow myelography.

INFECTIOUS
Feline infectious peritonitis may produce diffuse leptomeningitis of the spinal cord (Legendre & Whitenack, 1975) as well as pyogranulomatous myelitis. The disease is chronic and progressive. The severity and distribution of signs are very variable. Cryptococcosis may cause a very similar clinical picture.

Suppurative meningitis may arise by spread from tail-bite abscesses, vertebral osteomyelitis or discospondylitis. Severe pain is present. These lesions are irritative and local hyperaesthesia is not uncommon. There is often, but not invariably, fever. Haematological examination and radiography are helpful in diagnosis. Osteomyelitis or abscessation may cause the cauda equina syndrome.

Toxoplasma gondii may produce a multifocal myelitis with diffuse signs. Cerebrospinal fluid examination is helpful in confirming these conditions and in differentiating between them.

Degenerations

Lysosomal storage diseases may present with an early ascending paresis and spinal ataxia. This is a relatively prominent feature with the lipidoses. Degenerative myelopathy of acute onset due to fibrocartilaginous emboli has been recorded (Zaki *et al.*, 1976). The onset is sudden, there is no pain, and the signs are non-progressive. It is rare. A slowly progressive degenerative myelopathy (Mesfin *et al.*, 1980) of unknown cause also occurs rarely.

Space-occupying lesions

Space-occupying lesions are an important cause of slowly progressive ataxia. Tumours account for nearly half the cases of spinal cord disease encountered in the cat (Wheeler, 1989), but vertebral abscesses and discospondylitic lesions may occasionally have the same effect, as may haemorrhage.

TUMOURS
Tumours affecting the spinal cord may lie in three locations. They may be extradural; they may lie in the subdural and subarachnoid space; or they may be intramedullary.

Extradural tumours are most frequently lymphosarcomas (Northington & Juliana, 1978). Others encountered rarely include meningiomas, schwannomas and neurofibromas originating from spinal nerve roots, osteosarcomas and chondrosarcomas (Shell *et al.*, 1987), lipomas and metastatic masses.

Tumours in the space between the dura and the cord are commonly meningiomas. Lymphomas, and very rarely metastases, may also be encountered. Intramedullary tumours are usually of neuroectodermal origin.

Tumours in all these sites produce progressive spinal cord dysfunction, which usually develops very slowly. Pain may be present early in the course, but generally disappears later. Occasionally irritative features may be present. Treatment with glucocorticoids may produce temporary remission of signs. Extradural tumours may be accessible to surgery, but this is rarely warranted.

Vertebral osteomyelitis and discospondylitis

Vertebral osteomyelitis and discospondylitis are both relatively common. Haematological and radiographic examinations will usually establish the diagnosis. A marked neutrophilia and left-shift are usually present (Norsworthy, 1979). Long-term therapy (up to 6 weeks) with an anti-microbial agent is indicated (Kornegay, 1983). Wherever possible the organism should be identified by culture and its sensitivity determined. If that is not possible the antibiotics of choice are the cephalosporins, ampicillin, amoxycillin or clavulanate-potentiated amoxycillin.

Cage rest is essential, and sedation with pheno-barbitone tablets (0.5–2 mg/kg), to limit mobility, and analgesia with codeine tablets (0.25–1.0 mg/kg) are also of value.

Multiple cartilaginous exostoses

This condition has most commonly been recorded in Siamese and in domestic short hairs. Many partially calcified exostoses develop from the cortex of bone. They commonly arise from the vertebral bodies and the vertebral spinous processes, particularly of the cervical and lumbar regions. The animals are generally presented as young adults. Cervical cord compression may give rise to tetraparesis whilst lumbar involvement leads to paraparesis. A proportion of these animals survive and develop little in the way of neurological signs but the worst affected cases will require euthanasia.

Intoxications

Progressive spinal ataxia and paresis may follow 10–14 days after acute organophosphorus insecticide or tri-O-cresyl phosphate intoxication (Abou-Donia *et al.*, 1983). Methylmercury poisoning may also produce progressive spinal cord dysfunction. Generalized weakness and trembling, associated with widespread status spongiosus of CNS white matter has been reported following exposure to hexachlorophane (Thompson *et al.*, 1987). Mild paresis and spinal ataxia have been the only signs in some cases of poisoning with organochlorine compounds.

Spinal pain, hyperaesthesia and hypersensitivity

It is not uncommon to encounter cats with spinal pain or hyperaesthesia. The conditions affecting the spinal cord and column should be considered in the differential diagnosis as should panosteitis and myositis. Often no organic cause can be found for the signs, although a proportion of these cases are positive for feline leukaemia virus.

Localized hypersensitivity elsewhere may arise from irritative lesions; for example, cats with lesions impinging on the trigeminal nerve may be hyperaesthetic about the face on the affected side and may mutilate it. Other forms of mutilation, such as that in which Siamese cats may pluck large areas bald, appear to be behavioural (see Chapter 26).

In generalized hyperexcitability, the following should be considered: tetanus; rabies; Aujeszky's disease (pseudorabies); toxoplasmosis; FIP; cryptococcosis; thiamine deficiency; hypoglycaemia; hypocalcaemia; and intoxication by strychnine, alphachloralose, organophosphorus or organochlorine compounds. The differentiation of the tetany of tetanus and strychnine poisoning from seizures is discussed on p. 126. Strychnine and alphachloralose intoxications are discussed in Chapter 28.

Peripheral nervous system

The peripheral nervous system comprises the cranial nerves, the spinal segmental nerves and the peripheral autonomic nervous system. The cranial nerves are discussed above. The anatomy and physiology of the peripheral nervous system should need no repetition.

Diseases of the peripheral nervous system (PNS)

Trauma is the most common cause of peripheral nerve deficits. The cauda equina syndrome has been discussed (see p. 114). Radial paralysis, brachial plexus injury, and sciatic paralysis are also commonly seen. Peripheral nerve palsies are usually unilateral. Very severe trauma is required to produce bilateral PNS deficits, and other causes, particularly cord lesions, should always be considered when these are seen. Injury may sever, lacerate, stretch or contuse the nerve. Surgical injury to peripheral nerves is more common than one might wish.

TRAUMA

Cauda equina
Spinal column lesions caudal to Co6 will involve the cauda equina (see above) rather than the spinal cord.

Radial nerve paralysis
Selective radial nerve paralysis is much less common than brachial plexus injury. It may be differentiated into high and low paralysis depending on whether the whole limb is affected or the deficit is confined below the elbow joint.

High radial paralysis renders extension of the elbow and carpus impossible. At rest, the paw knuckles over on the ground. In motion, the limb is carried with the elbow flexed or the limb drops at the paw and knuckles at the paw with each step. There is anaesthesia of the dorsolateral forearm. Low radial paralysis causes only knuckling of the paw and anaesthesia of the same skin innervation field. Many animals manage to compensate by flicking the paw as they walk.

Treatment and prognosis. The prognosis is guarded and recovery can be slow. If there is other evidence, such as a penetrating wound or fracture, to suggest that the nerve is severed, surgical repair may be attempted. Otherwise, glucocorticoid therapy for 7–10 days may be helpful, as may physiotherapy. If there is no recovery and the dorsum of the paw becomes ulcerated through scraping the ground, carpal fusion or amputation is indicated.

Brachial plexus injury
Injury of the brachial plexus is usually the result of road traffic accidents or falls from high buildings. The nerve roots of the plexus may be crushed, torn or severed from the spinal cord. Most commonly the C8 and T1 roots are involved, but the fifth, sixth and seventh roots may also be injured. Horner's syndrome occurs if the thoracic ventral roots are severed. Damage to the cervical outflow abolishes the ipsilateral panniculus reflex. In the most severe variant of the condition, there is analgesia of the lateral surface of the arm and of the entire limb distal to the elbow. There is total flaccid motor paralysis with dropping of the elbow, knuckling of the carpus and paralysis of the shoulder flexors. The limb cannot support weight. However, injury to the plexus is often not total and complex variations in the pattern of sensory and motor dysfunction are found. The prognosis is extremely poor if there is any more than mild paresis.

Brachial plexus neoplasms
Neoplasms involving the brachial plexus appear to be rare in the cat, but lymphosarcomas, reticulosis and chondrosarcomas have been recorded (Shell *et al.*, 1987; Sharp, 1989a). Horner's syndrome may be associated with tumours at this site in the cat.

Sciatic nerve paralysis
Sciatic nerve injury often accompanies pelvic or high femoral fractures, but it may also be the consequence of surgical injury, particularly that associated with pinning of fractures of the femur, or inadvertent injection. Usually both components of the nerve are injured, but occasionally one branch is spared.

Typically the animal can bear weight on the limb and the leg is not carried. The hock is dropped and the paw is knuckled. The cranial, lateral and caudal aspects of the leg are anaesthetic distal to the stifle, as are the dorsal, lateral and plantar surfaces of the paw. Fractures in the sacrococcygeal region may also result in urinary incontinence, anal dysfunction and tail paralysis.

The prognosis is rather variable depending upon the degree of injury, and recovery may take up to 16 weeks. Surgical intervention appears to have little effect on the outcome (Jacobson & Schrader, 1987). Conservative treatment is as described for radial nerve paralysis. Self-mutilation can be a problem and amputation may be required.

HYPERVITAMINOSIS A

Hypervitaminosis A is discussed in more detail in Chapters 2 and 24. Vertebral exostoses arising from the dietary imbalance may produce chronic compression of peripheral nerves or of their spinal roots. In consequence, peripheral nerve deficits may contribute to the abnormalities of gait and behaviour seen in this condition. The neurological signs most commonly affect the forelimbs. There is paresis of variable severity and there may be muscle wasting. Areas of skin anaesthesia or hyperaesthesia are often noted. Altered sensory perception may also involve the shoulder and neck. Involvement may be unilateral or bilateral.

Withdrawal of liver from the diet leads to considerable recovery in mild or moderately affected animals. In severe cases, the deficits may persist.

INFLAMMATION

Inflammatory peripheral nerve lesions are rare. Chronic relapsing polyradiculoneuritis has been reported. The signs are episodic with periods of remission and recurrence over several months. High-stepping gait, ataxia, muscle twitching and loss of sensory perception were noted in one report (Flecknell & Lucke, 1978). A polyneuritis with destruction of axons and myelin and lymphoid perivascular cuffing was associated with acute-onset paralysis, fever, jaundice and anaemia (Lane & deLahunta, 1984). Brachial plexus neuropathy can occur following rabies vaccination.

DEGENERATIONS

Ischaemic neuromyopathy

Ischaemic neuromyopathy contributes to the signs of aortic embolism which is in turn a consequence of cardiomyopathy (see Chapter 11). The formation of thrombi in the heart leads to embolism and thus to occlusion of the terminal aorta or of peripheral arteries. Most often there is occlusion of both iliac arteries and this syndrome is the commonest cause of apparent bilateral peripheral nerve paralysis of the hindlimbs. Much less frequently a brachial artery may be occluded with unilateral forelimb paralysis. The release of 5-hydroxytryptamine (5-HT, serotonin) from blood platelets and consequent vasoconstriction may contribute to the development and maintenance of ischaemia (Butler, 1971). The nature of the lesion depends upon the degree of ischaemia; in the worst affected cases muscle necrosis and nerve degeneration occur but milder lesions may result in demyelination which may also be present in the proximal zone of severe lesions.

The clinical signs are dramatic with acute-onset paresis or flaccid paralysis, pain and a weak or absent pulse (Griffiths & Duncan, 1979). Affected limbs may be dragged; sensation and reflexes are generally lost. The limb is cold, particularly distally, and the pads and nail beds are usually cyanotic but may show pallor. The muscles of affected limbs are initially soft and yield to pressure but subsequently come to feel hardened. Biochemical examination may reveal greatly elevated creatine kinase (CK) and alanine aminotransferase (ALT) activities but this is not invariably the case. The prognosis is poor and there is no particularly effective therapy. Many affected animals die acutely, although in those that survive nerve regeneration can occur over a period of weeks to months if the blood supply is reestablished. In such cases motor function begins to return in 1–4 weeks; complete recovery is possible but residual neurological deficits may persist (Griffiths & Duncan, 1979). The prognosis remains guarded because of the persistence of the initiating cardiomyopathy and the likelihood of further embolic episodes.

Surgical intervention for embolectomy has been advocated (Robins *et al.*, 1982), but must be performed with great rapidity to be of any value. Medical management is generally preferable. Analgesia should be instituted. Therapy with aspirin to reduce platelet responsiveness and to minimize the risk of further thromboembolism together with treatment of the cardiomyopathy should be initiated immediately and continued for the remainder of the animal's life. Aspirin should be given at a dose rate of 5–25 mg/kg p.o. every second or third day. See Chapter 27 for further discussion of the use of aspirin in cats. The 5-HT antagonist cyproheptadine may have some value in treatment, as may low-dose heparin, but both appear to be of limited effectiveness.

Diabetes mellitus
Peripheral neuropathy is a feature of human diabetes mellitus and has also been reported in the cat (Kramek *et al.*, 1984). There is weakness, generally of the hindlimbs, muscle atrophy and blunting of reflexes, and quite commonly a plantigrade gait. Nerve conduction velocity is decreased. The condition is a distal axonopathy with secondary demyelination. Careful attention to control of blood glucose concentrations can result in neurological improvement, particularly in recently diagnosed cases.

Niemann–Pick disease
The hereditary neurolipidoses have been discussed previously; however, Niemann–Pick disease is worthy of particular mention in the context of peripheral neuropathies since Cuddon *et al.* (1989) have reported findings on the neuropathy in this condition. The three affected animals were presented at between 1 and 7 months of age. The signs included progressive paraparesis or tetraparesis, hyporeflexia, reduced muscle tone and muscle atrophy. In one case a high-stepping gait described as resembling stringhalt was noted. Diagnosis was based on assay of liver biopsy specimens or cultured skin fibroblasts for the deficient enzyme sphingomyelinase. Foamy mononuclear cells may also be noted in peripheral blood and bone marrow. The peripheral nerve roots are hypomyelinated and there is myelin loss in the peripheral nerves.

Hereditary hyperchylomicronaemia
Hereditary hyperchylomicronaemia appears to be inherited as an autosomal recessive trait (Jones *et al.*, 1986). It is characterized by basal hyperlipaemia, increased triglyceride and cholesterol, which are present predominantly as chylomicrons, and reduced levels of heparin-activated lipoprotein lipase. Neuropathy is noted in about half of the cases, characterized by axonal degeneration due to nerve compression by lipid granulomas. A wide variety of nerves including cranial nerves and the cervical sympathetic trunk may be affected and signs may consequently be extremely varied. Spinal foramina appear to be a predilection site for the formation of lipid granulomas. Lipaemia retinalis is also a common feature. Dietary restriction of fat intake is beneficial in reducing plasma lipid levels and some neurological improvement may follow.

Hypertrophic polyneuropathy
A hypertrophic polyneuropathy resembling hereditary sensorimotor neuropathy in man has been reported in cats (Dahme *et al.*, 1987). Affected individuals showed intention tremor, mild sensory and postural deficits and sluggish tendon reflexes. The pathology of the disease is characterized by atrophy and aberrant regeneration of peripheral myelin.

Non-inflammatory polyneuropathy
Progressive onset of tetraparesis associated with a non-inflammatory polyneuropathy characterized by demyelination and axonal degeneration has been recorded (Shores *et al.*, 1987).

Feline immuno-deficiency virus (FIV)
Peripheral neuropathy associated with FIV has been reported and is discussed in Chapter 16.

NEOPLASIA
Schwannomas and neurofibromas are the only primary tumours of the peripheral nervous system. They may occur at any point on the course of a nerve. Other tumours may invade or compress peripheral nerves and if near their spinal origin may involve more than one nerve. Peripheral nerve tumours produce a slowly developing peripheral nerve palsy which may be preceded by signs of nerve irritation.

INTOXICATION
Lead, thallium or mercury intoxication may produce a peripheral polyneuropathy. Heavy metal intoxications are discussed in Chapter 28.

Muscle and neuromuscular junction

DISEASE OF THE NEUROMUSCULAR JUNCTION

Myasthenia gravis

There are now several reports of the occurrence of myasthenia gravis in the cat (Mason, 1976; Indrieri *et al.*, 1983; Joseph *et al.*, 1988; Cuddon, 1989). Both the acquired (adult) and the congenital forms of the disease have been reported (Indrieri *et al.*, 1983; Joseph *et al.*, 1988; Cuddon, 1989). The disease is due to depressed sensitivity of muscle end-plates to acetylcholine released from motor nerve terminals. In the case of the acquired disease, the condition is immune-mediated and the reduced end-plate sensitivity is due to complexing of acetylcholine receptors by circulating anti-receptor antibody. In the case of congenital disease, there is no antibody involvement and the actual concentration of acetylcholine receptor sites appears to be abnormally low. The signs of the disease are generalized muscular weakness potentiated by exercise, altered phonation, respiratory distress and difficulty in eating. Megoesophagus has been reported but appears to be a less constant finding than in canine myasthenia gravis. It should be possible to confirm the diagnosis by administering 0.2 mg edrophonium bromide under atropine cover (the 'Tensilon test'). This should produce dramatic but temporary relief of the signs and allow the animal to exercise for some minutes without tiring. Therapy is with pyridostigmine bromide orally once daily or neostigmine methyl sulphate intramuscularly twice daily. The dose of the drug must be adjusted for the individual animal, but is likely to be of the order of 0.25 mg for neostigmine methyl sulphate and of the order of 10–30 mg for the pyridostigmine salt. Overdosing produces a cholinergic crisis. Underdosing leads to recurrence of signs. In view of the immune-mediated nature of the acquired condition, therapy with glucocorticoids may be of some value although there is no evidence that they have any dramatic palliative effect.

BOTULISM

Botulism occurs occasionally in cats following the ingestion of material containing the toxins of *Clostridium botulinum*. The major effect of these toxins is to inhibit the release of acetylcholine at the neuromuscular junction nerve ending. Generalized weakness or flaccid paralysis are seen in the absence of other signs. Diagnosis is based on the history, the clinical features and demonstration of the toxin. Electromyography reveals the absence of end-plate potentials. The prognosis is poor but supportive therapy is occasionally successful.

HYPOKALAEMIA

Hypokalaemia occurs in Conn's syndrome (Eger *et al.*, 1983; see also Chapter 12) as a consequence of renal dysfunction (Dow *et al.*, 1987; Fettman, 1989) and as an episodic familial condition in some Burmese cats. It may present as neuromuscular weakness, depression, disorientation or paralysis. Affected animals show a characteristic ventroflexion of the neck. The condition reported by Mason (1988) as a thiamine-responsive hereditary episodic weakness in Burmese cats may actually be this condition.

MYOPATHY

Nutritional myopathies are discussed in Chapter 3.

Autonomic nervous system

FELINE DYSAUTONOMIA: KEY–GASKELL SYNDROME

Feline dysautonomia (also known as feline autonomic polyganglionopathy, dilated pupil syndrome, Key–Gaskell syndrome) was first recognized in the autumn of 1981 and was described the following February by Key and Gaskell (1982). The disease rose to a high incidence by the late summer and autumn of 1982, then abated somewhat before rising to a second highpoint at the same time the following year. Since that time the disease has waned in incidence and become clinically milder. Cases are now recognized only sporadically. The disease has clinical signs which reflect widespread dysfunction of the autonomic nervous system consequent upon pathological changes in autonomic neurons. The condition bears many clinical and pathological similarities to grass-sickness in the horse. The reader who wishes for more detailed information is referred to the Waltham Symposium on the disease (Edney *et al.*, 1987) and to Blaxter and Gruffydd-Jones (1987) and Sharp (1989b).

History
Affected cats have usually been in good health immediately before the development of the disease although a small proportion have exhibited recent gastrointestinal disturbances or upper respiratory tract signs.

Clinical signs
Clinical signs appear over a period varying from 1 to about 7 days. Some or all of the following may be noted:

 1 Pupillary dilation accompanied by absent or reduced pupillary light responses, reduced tear production and protruded membrana nictitans.
 2 A dry crusted nose.
 3 Bradycardia.
 4 Decreased tear production.
 5 Megoesophagus with retching, regurgitation or vomiting.
 6 Prolapse of the nictitating membrane.
 7 Depression.
 8 Dysphagia, anorexia and marked weight loss.
 9 Constipation, sometimes with anal flaccidity and faecal incontinence.
10 Bladder atony with urinary retention and overflow, or urinary incontinence. Secondary bacterial cystitis may develop.
11 A dry mouth, sometimes with secondary infection and diphtheresis.
12 Dehydration, which may be severe.
13 Transient collapse (associated with hypotension).
None of these clinical signs is a constant finding but the first five are the most frequent and the most specific. Most signs have decreased in inci-

dence and severity with time since the disease was recognized in 1981. A small proportion of animals also show abdominal pain. In some cases a mild proprioceptive loss may be present and there may be hindleg or generalized weakness. In a small number of cases skin laxity is encountered and the skin may detach from the underlying tissue.

Diagnosis
Diagnosis in life is based primarily on the constellation of clinical signs. As these have become less marked this has become more difficult and Sharp (1989b) has suggested that an objective means of diagnosis is needed. He has proposed a grading and scoring system to this end.

Radiological investigations may be of some value. Megoesophagus may be detected on plain films, or by barium swallow, in the majority of cases. Pharyngeal dysfunction, delayed gastric emptying and generalized ileus may be present; also the bladder may be distended.

The utility of pharmacological studies of autonomic function for diagnosis has been reported (Canton *et al.*, 1988; Guilford *et al.*, 1988). They assessed ocular responses to application of 0.1% pilocarpine to the cornea. This induces miosis within 10–15 minutes in affected but not in normal animals. Similarly in affected cats a 1:10 000 solution of adrenaline will induce contraction of the nictitating membrane.

Treatment
Affected animals should be rehydrated and ideally should be kept in a darkened room in view of the absence of photomotor responses. Vomiting and regurgitation are major problems and metoclopramide has some value in reducing vomiting. Feeding is best accomplished by nasogastric tube since cats tolerate pharyngostomy extremely poorly. Constipation is a major problem in this condition and the use of liquid paraffin, petroleum jelly or ispaghula husk can be helpful. In severe cases regular enemas may be necessary. Regular bladder emptying by manual expression is re-

quired. Bethanecol hydrochloride* has been used to induce bladder emptying but has not proved particularly successful. Physostigmine, demecarium or pilocarpine ophthalmic drops may be useful to stimulate pupillary constriction, tear production and salivation but must be used with caution since affected animals show enhanced responsiveness to them. Regular instillation of hypromellose eyedrops ('false tears') may be helpful in preventing the development of secondary keratoconjunctivitis sicca.

Regurgitation may give rise to aspiration pneumonia. Urinary retention may lead to secondary bacterial cystitis. The mucous membrane of the mouth may also become secondarily infected. In such cases, appropriate antibacterial therapy should be instituted. Glucocorticoids have been employed in a number of centres, ostensibly to stimulate appetite, but there is little rationale for their use and they appear to be of little value. In view of the anorexia and weight loss in these animals, anabolics are indicated.

Outcome
In the early months after the condition appeared the prognosis was poor, survival being variously estimated as 0 to 30%. As the severity of clinical signs has abated the prognosis has improved and around half of affected cats have survived latterly, although clinical signs may not completely resolve. The likelihood of survival is inversely related to the severity of the clinical signs. Some animals that survive need to eat several times their pre-illness daily food intake to maintain their weight and may be less resistant to stress. Faecal or urinary incontinence can be troublesome and may develop after apparent recovery.

Aetiology and epidemiology
The aetiology of the condition is unknown. For this reason, there has been considerable interest

*Myotonine; Glenwood Laboratories Ltd., Canterbury, Kent, UK.

in its epidemiology in the hope that this may shed some light on the cause.

The condition first appeared in the British Isles and now also occurs in Belgium, Denmark, France, Germany, Holland, Norway, Sweden and Switzerland as well as New Zealand (Edney & Gaskell, 1988). After the appearance of the condition in the autumn of 1981, its incidence increased rapidly. Subsequently, the condition appears to have exhibited a seasonal incidence with a peak in the late summer and early autumn. The affected animals are drawn from both rural and urban environments. There appears to be no predilection for either sex or for intact as opposed to neutered animals. The condition has been encountered in animals of all ages, but there does appear to be a fairly strong disposition for the disease to affect animals under 3 years of age. There is no agreement as to whether there is no breed predisposition, or whether there is a higher relative risk in purebred cats or in those of mixed breeding.

The condition does not appear to be readily transmissible and is sporadic in occurrence. Only a small number of clusters of cases in multi-cat households have been reported. When clusters have occurred in multi-cat households, there have been examples both of related and of non-related animals being affected. Management systems do not appear to have a profound influence on the incidence.

Pathology
The disease is essentially a neurological disorder and no consistent changes are found outside the central and peripheral nervous systems. The major changes in the periphery involve both the sympathetic and parasympathetic divisions of the autonomic nervous system. In long-standing cases there is a marked decrease in the number of neurons in the autonomic ganglia, together with fibrosis and increased numbers of supporting cells. In earlier cases neurons show eosinophilia, loss of Nissl substance and nuclear crenation and pyknosis. The nucleus is displaced to a peripheral position in the perikaryon and the cytoplasm is

frequently vacuolated. Prominent neuronophagic nodules may be present. There is marked loss of neurons and fibres in the myenteric plexus of the gut with severe depletion of neuropeptide transmitters.

Changes are not restricted to the autonomic nervous system. Dorsal root ganglia may also be involved. The small dark neurons are particularly affected, showing similar changes to those found in the autonomic neurons. Within the CNS such changes are encountered in the third, fifth, seventh and twelfth cranial nerve nuclei, the dorsal motor nucleus of the vagus, the nucleus ambiguus of the brainstem and in the intermediolateral and ventral horn grey matter of the spinal cord. Both in the CNS and PNS Wallerian degeneration is present.

Electron microscopical examination of the autonomic ganglia reveals marked neuronal changes in the absence of changes in the satellite cells. The neurons contain cisternae, which would appear to be derived from the endoplasmic reticulum and possibly the Golgi apparatus, and are filled with floccular proteinaceous material (Griffiths *et al.*, 1985). Ribosomal numbers are markedly decreased. Complex membrane whorls and stacks are also present and no normal endoplasmic reticulum or Golgi zone can be identified. Affected axons may also show marked dystrophic ultrastructural changes. These are seen both in myelinated and unmyelinated fibres. There is accumulation of neurotubules, neurofilaments, vesiculotubular membrane profiles and mitochondria.

BLADDER AND VISCERAL DYSFUNCTION

Bladder dysfunction and faecal retention and/or incontinence are seen in a number of circumstances:
- Feline dysautonomia
- Sacral spinal cord lesions
- Avulsion or neurapraxia of sacral spinal nerves
- Injury to the cauda equina
- Vertebral and spinal malformations

Avulsion of the sacral nerve roots and neurapraxia of the pudendal nerve are quite common in the cat as a result of road traffic accidents, attempts to catch or pull cats by their tail, and malicious attempts to swing them by their tail. There is usually urinary retention and overflow, constipation or faecal incontinence and tail flaccidity with complete sensation loss. There may also be weakness, ataxia, sensory loss or paralysis in the hindlimbs. Neurapraxia of the pudendal nerve is the more common of the two occurrences and most cases recover fully with conservative management. Cases of avulsion carry a poor prognosis but in occasional cases autonomous bladder contraction develops sufficiently, although there is no control over when or where urination occurs. In either case manual emptying of the bladder, or an indwelling catheter is required in the interim. Phenoxybenzamine or acepromazine are of value to reduce functional sphincter tone, and bethanecol may be of value to increase detrusor muscle contraction. In about half of a series of cases with sacrococcygeal fractures there was urinary incontinence; the prognosis was good if there was an intact anal reflex and those animals recovered control of micturition within about a month (Smeak & Olmstead, 1985). For a detailed discussion of bladder dysfunction the reader is referred to Sharp (1989b).

MULTIFOCAL SIGNS

Widespread neurological signs suggest a disseminated or multifocal disease process. Such pathology is usually of inflammatory or toxic origin. Feline infectious peritonitis, feline leukaemia virus (which may be associated on rare occasions with bizarre neurological disorders), toxoplasmosis, cryptococcosis and spongiform encephalopathy should be considered, as should organophosphorus, organochlorine, and heavy metal intoxication. Thiamin deficiency and, in young cats, lysosomal storage diseases are also possible causes, as are the inherited system degenerations.

INFECTIONS WITH PROMINENT NEUROLOGICAL SIGNS

Viral infections

Rabies

Rabies should always, however briefly, be considered in the differential diagnosis in any case with neurological signs. It is an acute, contagious, almost invariably fatal disease. Its virology, epidemiology and laboratory diagnosis are considered in Chapter 19. Both furious and dumb rabies occur in the cat. The signs are essentially those of encephalitis and hence are rather variable.

Prodromal phase

In the prodromal phase, there are behavioural changes. The cat may hide, call plaintively, show pica and, commonly, demonstrate increasing irritability. This phase lasts 1–2 days.

Excitement phase

In furious rabies the cat then makes sudden attacks, biting and scratching furiously and often taking persistent hold with its teeth. There may be focal, behavioural, cerebellar, vestibular or cranial nerve signs. If confined, the cat may attack the bars of its cage and any introduced object. The voice characteristically becomes hoarse or strained.

Paralytic phase

Ataxia develops and progresses to ascending paralysis. The episodes of rage disappear as the animal lapses into terminal coma. Death supervenes 3–8 days after signs appear.

Neither drooling nor masseter paralysis is commonly seen in the cat. In dumb rabies there is no stage of marked irritation, but ataxia develops and is followed by paralysis, coma and death.

Aujeszky's disease (pseudorabies)

(see also Chapter 20)
Pseudorabies is rare in the cat (Dow & McFerran, 1963). It is a rapidly progressive condition and cats die within 24–36 hours of the onset of signs. Initially, there is lethargy and anorexia. The cat may hide and may call plaintively. Marked evidence of pruritus develops. The cat licks, gnaws, scratches and rubs a localized area of skin and may severely mutilate it. Twitching of the lips or face may be noted and the animal drools saliva. Terminally, there may be convulsions or coma (Horvath & Papp, 1967).

Feline infectious peritonitis (see Chapter 17)

Feline infectious peritonitis has been referred to repeatedly throughout this chapter. It may produce a severe pyogranulomatous meningitis and encephalomyelitis, which may involve any area of the nervous system and is often multifocal (Kornegay, 1978). The eye is also commonly involved and uveitis or even panophthalmitis may be present. This may be unilateral or bilateral. The disease is chronic and associated with persistent fever. The CSF shows florid abnormality: the protein may reach 0.5 g/dl, much of this being globulin, and the white cell count may exceed 1000 cells/mm^3. The cell population may be monocytic or a large proportion of neutrophils may also be present.

Feline spongiform encephalopathy

Recently a novel spongiform encephalopathy, which resembles scrapie, has been reported in the cat (Wyatt *et al.*, 1990). On clinical and pathological grounds, the condition clearly belongs to the group of transmissible spongiform encephalopathies which includes not only scrapie but also Creutzfeld-Jakob disease in man, bovine spongiform encephalopathy (BSE), mink transmissible encephalopathy and comparable diseases in a number of other species. This relationship is reinforced by the finding of prion protein (PrP) in brains of affected cats. PrP is an altered protein derived from the genome of the host which is present in scrapie and BSE. The etiological agents responsible for these transmissible encephalopathies still await identification, but they clearly have unusual properties, for example their great resistance to inactivation, and are currently thought likely to be atypical viruses. Feline spongiform encephalopathy (FSE) presents with progressive ataxia, particularly involv-

ing the hindlimbs, abnormalities of agonistic behavioural and hyperaesthesia also appear to be
consistent clinical signs. The progressive nature
of the disease is such that euthanasia of affected
animals has generally been carried out 2–3
months after the onset. Additional, less consistent, clinical features have been noted in a
proportion of affected animals. These include
hypersalivation, altered grooming behaviour,
altered head posture, with associated nodding,
muscle fasciculation, polydipsia, polyphagia, difficulty in defecation and urination (Wyatt *et al.*,
1990, 1991). These findings set this condition
apart clinically from other forms of progressive
fcline ataxia.

The epidemiology of the condition is not yet
established but current evidence supports the view
that FSE is a newly emerged disease and it is
suspected that, as for BSE, there may have been
some common vehicle of infection. On histopathological examination lesions are essentially
confined to the central nervous system and occur
throughout the neuraxis. Vacuolation of varying
degree is found in the neuropil and neuronal
perikarya of the grey matter; less marked vacuolation is also found in white matter. In the neuropil many small empty vacuoles are noted and this
change is most marked in the medial geniculate
body, the thalamus, corpus striatum, the deeper
layers of the cerebral cortex and in the cerebellar
cortex. The vacuoles in neuronal perikarya may
be single or multiple and are generally large
and discrete. Perikaryal vacuolation is seen most
markedly in the raphe nuclei, the vesicular nuclei
of the medulla oblongata, the nucleus tractus
solitarius and the nucleus ruber. Vacuolation of
the white matter, together with axonal degeneration, are less marked features but occur particularly in the medulla, especially affecting the
pyramidal tracts.

Other viral infections

Non-suppurative meningoencephalomyelitis and
polioencephalomyelitis, with mononuclear perivascular infiltration and of presumed viral origin,
have been repeatedly reported in the cat (Borland
& McDonald, 1965; Kronevi *et al.*, 1974;

Vandevelde & Braund, 1979; Hoff & Vandevelde,
1981; Strom *et al.*, 1992) and may comprise more
than one condition. The signs are generally slowly
progressive. Fever, posterior ataxia and paresis,
apathy, seizures, nystagmus and head tilt are the
major clinical signs. Hyperaesthesia and seizures
may also occur in some affected animals. No
causal organism has been identified.

Bacterial infections

Bacterial encephalitis is very rare and meningitis,
which may be regionally localized, is only a little
more common. CSF examination is valuable:
organisms may be seen or cultured. Neutrophil
leucocytes are present in abundance and/or the
protein is elevated. Although many antibiotics
penetrate the blood–brain barrier in the presence
of inflammation, and despite the fact that it is
usually contraindicated in the cat (see Chapter
27), chloramphenicol is the antibiotic of choice
for these conditions and for intracranial abscesses.

Tetanus (see also Chapter 23)

Tetanus is uncommon in the cat. It usually follows an accidental wound or castration. Limb
stiffness may be the only feature and this may
involve only one limb. Inability to rise, tetanic
spasms, protrusion of the nictitating membrane
and drawing forward of the tail over the back
are commonly seen (Killingsworth *et al.*, 1977).
Opisthotonos, trismus and risus sardonicus are
rare.

The major differential diagnosis is strychnine
intoxication, in which the spasms are more severe,
but there are periods of intermittent relaxation.
Strychnine poisoning rarely involves the nictitating membrane. Diagnosis is based on the history and signs. Laboratory investigations are of
little importance.

Treatment is directed to neutralization of the
toxin, elimination of the organism and relief of
muscle spasm. Five thousand units of tetanus
antitoxin should be given following a small test
dose. The wound should be debrided and flushed
with hydrogen peroxide. Procaine penicillin G
should be given at a dose of 60 000 IU/kg IM

daily for a minimum of 5 days. Diazepam (2.5 mg IM) or phenobarbitone (2.5 mg IM) four times daily may be used to induce muscle relaxation. The animal should be kept in a quiet, dark environment and attention should be paid to fluid therapy, alimentation and prevention of decubitus ulcers.

Fungal infections (see also Chapter 23)

Cryptococcus neoformans infection has been reported in cats in Britain, although it is rare. None the less the disease is widely distributed; worldwide, *C. neoformans* is the most common fungal infection of the feline CNS (Wilkinson, 1979). Both this organism and *Aspergillus fumigatus* may spread from the nose or sinuses to produce meningitis. Affected cats may present with one or more signs including dullness and depression, ataxia, head pressing, head-tilt, circling, nystagmus and seizures. There may also be optic neuritis, retinitis or uveitis and some affected animals become blind. CSF pressure is very high (up to 400 mmH$_2$O). The organism may be seen in CSF smears and may be isolated. There is a moderate leucocytosis and protein increase in the CSF. Amphotericin B (0.01 mg/kg every other day for 8 weeks) and flucytosine (0.1 mg/kg daily) singly or in combination are the agents of choice for treatment (Prevost *et al.*, 1983) but therapy is rarely successful when there is CNS involvement. The combination has a synergistic effect whilst reducing toxicity. Ketoconazole may also be used and has the advantage of being of low toxicity and being amenable to oral dosing; it may, however, be less effective.

Protozoal infections (see Chapter 23)

Toxoplasma gondii produces diffuse or multifocal nervous system disease. CNS involvement is common in affected cats and the resulting neurological signs include abnormal behaviour, lethargy, anisocoria, blindness, tremor, circling, ataxia, paralysis, opisthotonos and convulsions (Petrak & Carpenter, 1965; Hirth & Nielsen, 1969). There is often an associated uveitis and

prominent muscle, liver or lung involvement. CSF reveals no identifiable organisms, but variable pleiocytosis often dominated by mononuclear cells and increased protein levels. Faecal examination is not helpful in the diagnosis of CNS disease, but serology may be of some value. Often the diagnosis is only made at post-mortem. Treatment is with sulphadiazine and pyrimethamine but is often unsuccessful when there is neurological involvement. Clindamycin 10 mg/kg b.i.d. orally or parenterally has also been employed.

CONGENITAL MALFORMATIONS OF THE NERVOUS SYSTEM

Hydrocephalus

Primary (juvenile) hydrocephalus is not common in the cat. Affected kittens have an open fontanelle and a domed skull. Signs are extremely variable, but are present from birth. There is commonly a visual deficit and ataxia. Dullness, compulsive circling, convulsions and coma may also be seen. The majority of affected kittens die fairly early in life.

Secondary or acquired hydrocephalus may occur as a consequence of trauma, inflammation, including FIP (Krum *et al.*, 1975), or space-occupying lesions interfering with CSF drainage. Intracranial pressure rises progressively and death ensues. Treatment is not a practical proposition.

Hereditary meningoencephalocele

Hereditary meningoencephalocele associated with craniofacial skeletal abnormalities and apparently inherited as an autosomal recessive trait with variable penetrance has been recorded in Burmese cats (Sponenberg & Graf-Webster, 1986).

Spinal dysgenesis

A spectrum of spinal cord and vertebral defects related to abnormalities of neural tube closure during early prenatal development is encountered in Manx cats (Michael *et al.*, 1969). The condition is hereditary and is determined by a semi-lethal autosomal dominant gene. All affected animals are heterozygotes; homozygosity causes intra-uterine death.

Even Manx cats considered to be normal show a variety of manifestations of the condition. They may be described as: normal tailed; stumpy — these individuals have several coccygeal vertebrae and the tail may be severely kinked; rumpy-riser — these animals have from one to seven fused coccygeal vertebrae in an upright position; and rumpy — these individuals have no coccygeal vertebrae (see also Chapter 3).

Many rumpies are clinically abnormal having megacolon, paresis of the hindlimbs and urinary incontinence. 'Abnormal' Manx cats may be much more severely affected. They may have occult spina bifida (unfused vertebral laminae overlain by skin) often representing healed congenital meningocele; meningocele in which the meninges protrude through the defect in the vertebral laminae or myelomeningocele in which spinal cord also protrudes. The skin may or may not be fused over the site of the meningocele or myelomeningocele. Open lesions with CSF leakage occur (Hall *et al.*, 1988). The terminal spinal cord is also abnormal. These animals have faecal incontinence, often with faecolith accumulation; decreased perineal sensation; plantigrade posture; and walk with a rapid, hopping motion. Bladder dysfunction may lead to cystitis and there may be megacolon.

Exencephaly (an imperfect cranium with the brain lying partially outside the skull) and kyphoscoliosis (dorsal and lateral curvature of the spinal column) have also been encountered in Manx cats. Congenitally split neuraxis (neuroschisis) has been encountered in a Burmese cross, open spina bifida in Siamese and Siamese crosses, and occult spina bifida in a Maltese. It is not clear whether these sporadic occurrences have a hereditary origin or are due to teratogens.

REFERENCES

Abou-Donia M.B., Jensen D.N. & Lapadula D.M. (1983) Neurologic manifestations of tri-O-cresyl delayed neuro-toxicity in cats. *Neurobehav. Toxicol. Teratol.* **5**, 431–42.

Barker J. (1989) Electroencephalography. In Wheeler S.J. (ed) *British Small Animal Veterinary Association Manual of Small Animal Neurology.* BSAVA, Cheltenham, pp. 67–76.

Barnett K.C. & Grimes T.D. (1974) Bilateral aplasia of the optic nerve in a cat. *Brit. J. Ophthalmol.* **58**, 663–7.

Blakemore W.F. (1975) Lysosomal storage diseases. *Vet. Ann.* **15**, 242–5.

Blaxter A. & Gruffydd-Jones T.J. (1987) Feline dysautonomia. *In Practice* **9**, 58–61.

Blaxter A.C., Holt P.E., Pearson E.R., Gibbs C. & Gruffydd-Jones T.J. (1988) Congenital portosystemic shunt in the cat: a report of 9 cases. *J. Small Anim. Pract.* **29**, 631–45.

Borland R. & McDonald N. (1965) Feline encephalomyelitis. *Brit. Vet. J.* **121**, 479–82.

Burke E.E., Moise S., DeLahunta A. & Erb N.H. (1985) Review of idiopathic feline vestibular syndrome. *J. Am. Vet. Med. Assoc.* **187**, 941–3.

Butler H.C. (1971) An investigation into the relationship of an aortic embolus to posterior paralysis in the cat. *J. Small Anim. Pract.* **12**, 141–58.

Canton D.D., Sharp N.J.H. & Aguirre G.D. (1988) Dysautonomia in a cat. *J. Amer. Vet. Med. Assoc.* **192**, 1293–6.

Cuddon P.A. (1989) Acquired immune-mediated myasthenia gravis in a cat. *J. Small Anim. Pract.* **30**, 511–6.

Cuddon P.A., Higgins R.J., Duncan I.D., Miller S., Parent J. & Moser A. (1988) Feline Niemann–Pick disease associated polyneuropathy. *Brain* **112**, 1429–43.

Dahme E., Kraft W. & Scabell J. (1987) Hypertrophische Polyneuropathie bei der Katze. *J. Vet. Med. A.* **34**, 271–88.

Davies J.V. (1989) Neuroradiology. In Wheeler S.J. (ed) *British Small Animal Veterinary Association Manual of Small Animal Neurology.* BSAVA, Cheltenham, pp. 85–106.

Dow C. & McFerran J.B. (1963) Aujeszky's disease in the dog and cat. *Vet. Rec.* **75**, 1099–102.

Dow S.W., LeCouteur R.A., Fettman M.J. & Spurgeon T.L (1987) Potassium depletion in cats: hypokalemic polymyopathy. *J. Amer. Vet. Med. Assoc.* **191**, 1563–8.

Dow S.W., LeCouteur R.A., Henik R.A., Jones R.L. & Poss M.L. (1988) Central nervous system infection associated with anaerobic bacteria in two dogs and two cats. *J. Vet. Intern. Med.* **2**, 171–6.

Duncan I.D. (1989) Electromyography and nerve conduction studies. In Wheeler S.J. (ed) *British Small Animal Veterinary Association Manual of Small Animal Neurology.* BSAVA, Cheltenham, pp. 63–6.

Edney A.T.B. & Gaskell C.J. (1988) Feline dysautonomia around the world. *Vet. Rec.* **123**, 451–2.

Edney A.T.B., Gaskell C.J. & Sharp N.J.H. (eds) (1987) Waltham Symposium No. 6. Feline dysautonomia — an emerging disease. *J. Small Anim. Pract.* **28**, 333–416.

Eger C.E., Robinson W.F. & Huxtable C.R.R. (1983) Primary hyperaldosteronism (Conn's syndrome) in a cat: a case report and review of comparative aspects. *J. Small Anim. Pract.* **24**, 293–307.

Elverland H.H. & Mair I.W.S. (1980) Hereditary deafness in the cat. An electron microscopic study of the spiral ganglion. *Acta Otolaryngol.* **90**, 360–7.

Evans R.J. (1988) Poisoning in cats. *Vet. Ann.* **28**, 251–60.

Evans R.J. (1989a) Haematology, biochemistry, cerebrospinal fluid analysis and other clinicopathological investigations. In Wheeler S.J. (ed) *British Small Animal Veterinary Association Manual of Small Animal Neurology.* BSAVA, Cheltenham, pp. 49–62.

Evans R.J. (1989b) Lysosomal storage diseases in dogs and cats. *J. Small Anim. Pract.* **30**, 144–50.

Fakushima E., Hutsell D. & Patton S. (1984) Aberrant dirofilariasis in a cat. *J. Am. Vet. Med. Assoc.* **184**, 199–201.

Fettman M.J. (1989) Feline kaliopenic polymyopathy/nephropathy syndrome. *Vet. Clin. N. Amer. (Small Anim. Pract.)* **19**, 415–32.

Flecknell P.A. & Lucke V.M. (1978) Chronic relapsing polyradiculoneuritis in a cat. *Acta Neuropathol.* **41**, 81–4.

Griffiths I.R. (1978) Spinal cord injuries: a pathological study of naturally occurring lesions in the dog and cat. *J. Comp. Pathol.* **88**, 303–15.

Griffiths I.R. & Duncan I.D. (1979) Ischaemic neuromyopathy in cats. *Vet. Rec.* **104**, 518–22.

Griffiths I.R., Sharp N.J.H. & McCulloch M.C. (1985) Feline dysautonomia (the Key–Gaskell syndrome): an ultrastructural study of autonomic ganglia and nerves. *Neuropathol. Appl. Neurobiol.* **11**, 17–29.

Gruffydd-Jones T.J., Evans R.J., Brown P. & Sullivan K. (1981) Dieldrin poisoning in cats following woodworm treatment. *Vet. Rec.* **108**, 540.

Guilford W.G., O'Brien D.P., Allert A. & Ermeling H.M. (1988) Diagnosis of dysautonomia in a cat by autonomic nervous system function testing. *J. Am. Vet. Med. Assoc.* **193**, 823–8.

Hall J.A., Fettman M.J. & Ingram J.T. (1988) Sodium chloride depletion in a cat with fistulated meningomyelocele. *J. Am. Vet. Med. Assoc.* **192**, 1445–8.

Haskins M.E., Jezyk P.F., Desnick R.J., McDonough S.K. & Patterson D.F. (1979a) Mucopolysaccharidosis in a domestic short-haired cat: a disease distinct from that seen in the Siamese cat. *J. Amer. Vet. Med. Assoc.* **175**, 384–7.

Haskins M.E., Jezyk P.F., Desnick R.J., McDonough S.K. & Patterson D.F. (1979b) Alpha-1-iduronidase deficiency in a cat: a model of mucopolysaccharidosis I. *Paed. Res.* **13**, 1294–7.

Haskins M.E., Jezyk P.F. & Patterson D.F. (1979c) Mucopolysaccharide storage disease in three families of cats with arylsulfatase B deficiency; leukocyte studies and carrier identification. *Paed. Res.* **13**, 1203–10.

Haskins M.E., Jezyk P.F., Desnick R.J. & Patterson D.F. (1981) Animal model of human disease: Mucopolysaccharidosis VI; Maroteaux–Lamy syndrome. Arylsulfatase B-deficient mucopolysaccharidosis in the Siamese cat. *Amer. J. Pathol.* **105**, 191–3.

Hatziolos B.C. (1966) Cutebra larva in the brain of a cat. *J. Amer. Vet. Med. Assoc.* **148**, 787–93.

Hawkins J.E. & Lurie M.H. (1952) The ototoxicity of streptomycin. *Ann. Otol. Rhinol. Laryngol.* **61**, 789–806.

Hawkins J.E., Rahway N.J. & Lurie M.H. (1953) The ototoxicity of dihydrostreptomycin and neomycin in the cat. *Ann. Otol. Rhinol. Laryngol.* **62**, 1128–37.

Heavner J.E. (1971) Intervertebral disk syndrome in the cat. *J. Amer. Vet. Med. Assoc.* **159**, 425–7.

Hirth R.S. & Nielsen S.W. (1969) Pathology of feline toxoplasmosis. *J. Small Anim. Pract.* **10**, 213–21.

Hoerlein B.F., Redding R.W., Hoff E.J. & McGuire J.A. (1985) Evaluation of naloxone, crocetin, thyrotropin releasing hormone, methylprednisolone, partial myelotomy and hemilaminectomy in the treatment of acute spinal cord trauma. *J. Am. Anim. Hosp. Assoc.* **21**, 67–77.

Hoff E.J. & Vandevelde M. (1981) Non-suppurative encephalomyelitis in cats suggestive of a viral origin. *Vet. Pathol.* **18**, 170–80.

Horvath Z. & Papp L. (1967) Clinical manifestations of Aujeszky's disease in the cat. *Acta. Vet. Acad. Sci. Hung.* **17**, 49–54.

Indrieri R.J., Creighton S.R. & Lambert E.H. (1983) Myasthenia gravis in two cats. *J. Am. Vet. Med. Assoc.* **182**, 57–60.

Jacobson A. & Schrader S.C. (1987) Peripheral nerve injury associated with fracture or fracture dislocation of the pelvis in dogs and cats: 34 cases (1978–82). *J. Am. Vet. Med. Ass.* **190**, 569–72.

Jones B.R., Johnstone A.C., Cahill J.I. & Hancock W.S. (1986) Peripheral neuropathy in cats with inherited primary hyperchylomicronaemia. *Vet. Rec.* **119**, 268–72.

Joseph R.J., Carrillo J.M. & Lennon V.A. (1988) Myasthenia gravis in the cat. *J. Vet. Intern. Med.* **2**, 75–9.

Jubb K.V.F., Saunders L.Z. & Coates H.V. (1956) Thiamine deficiency encephalopathy in cats. *J. Comp. Pathol.* **66**, 217–27.

Kay W.J. (1975) Epilepsy in cats. *J. Am. Anim. Hosp. Assoc.* **11**, 77–82.

Kelly D.F. & Gaskell C.J. (1976) Spongy degeneration of the central nervous system in kittens. *Acta Neuropathol.* **35**, 151–8.

Key T. & Gaskell C.J. (1982) A puzzling syndrome in cats associated with pupillary dilatation. *Vet. Rec.* **110**, 160.

Kilham L., Margolis G. & Colby E.D. (1971) Cerebellar ataxia and its transmission in cats by feline panleukopenia virus. *J. Am. Vet. Med. Assoc.* **158**, 888–906.

Killingsworth C., Chiapella A., Veralli P. & deLahunta A. (1977) Feline tetanus. *J. Am. Anim. Hosp. Assoc.* **13**, 209–15.

Kornegay J.N. (1978) Feline infectious peritonitis: the central nervous system form. *J. Am. Anim. Hosp. Assoc.* **14**, 580–4.

Kornegay J.N. (1981) Feline neurology. *Compend. Cont. Educ. Pract. Vet.* **3**, 203–14.

Kramek B.A., Moise N.S., Cooper B. & Raffe R. (1984) Neuropathy associated with diabetes mellitus in the cat. *J. Am. Vet. Med. Assoc.* **184**, 42–5.

Kronevi T., Nordstrom M., Moreno W. & Nilsson P.O. (1974) Feline ataxia due to a non-suppurative meningo-encephalomyelitis of unknown aetiology. *Nord. Vet. Med.* **26**, 720–5.

Krum S., Johnson K. & Wilson J. (1975) Hydrocephalus associated with the noneffusive form of feline infectious peritonitis. *J. Am. Vet. Med. Assoc.* **167**, 746–8.

Lane J.G. (1985) Ototoxicity in the dog and cat. *Vet. Rec.* **117**, 94.

Lane J.R. & DeLahunta A. (1984) Polyneuritis in a cat. *J. Am. Anim. Hosp. Assoc.* **20**, 1006–8.

LeCouteur R.A., Fike J.R., Cann C.E., Turrel J.M., Thompson J.E. & Biggart J.F. (1983) X-ray computed tomography of brain tumors in cats. *J. Am. Vet. Med. Assoc.* **183**, 301–5.

Legendre A.M. & Whitenack D.L. (1975) Feline infectious peritonitis with spinal cord involvement in two cats. *J. Am. Vet. Med. Assoc.* **167**, 931–2.

Luginbuhl H. (1961) Studies on meningiomas in cats. *Am. J. Vet. Res.* **22**, 1030–40.

Luttgen P.J., Braund K.G., Brawner W.R. & Vandevelde M. (1980) A retrospective study of 29 spinal tumours in the dog and cat. *J. Small Anim. Pract.* **21**, 213–26.

Luttgen P.J., Pechman R.D. & Hartsfield S.M. (1988) Neuroradiology. *Vet. Clin. N. Amer. (Small Anim. Pract.)* **18**, 501–28.

McKee W.M. (1990) Spinal trauma in dogs and cats: a review of 51 cases. Vet. Rec. **126**, 285–9.

McKenzie B.E., Lyles D.I. & Clinkscales J.A. (1978) Intracerebral migration of Cutebra larva in a kitten. *J. Am. Vet. Med. Assoc.* **172**, 173–5.

McMillan F.D., Barr B. & Feldman E.C. (1985) Functional pancreatic islet cell tumor in a cat. *J. Am. Anim. Hosp. Assoc.* **21**, 741–6.

Mason K.V. (1976) A case of myasthenia gravis in a cat. *J. Small Anim. Pract.* **17**, 467–72.

Mason K. (1988) A hereditary disease in Burmese cats manifested as an episodic weakness with head nodding and neck ventroflexion. *J. Am. Anim. Hosp. Assoc.* **24**, 147–51.

Michael C.C., Lassman L.P. & Tomlinson B.E. (1969) Congenital anomalies of the lower spine and spinal cord in Manx cats. *J. Pathol.* **97**, 269–76.

Nafe L.A. (1979) Meningiomas in cats: a retrospective clinical study of 36 cases. *J. Am. Vet. Med. Assoc.* **174**, 1224–7.

Narfstrom K. (1985) Progressive retinal atrophy in Abyssinian cats. *Svensk. Vet.* **37**, 821–2.

Norby D.E. & Thuline H.C. (1970) Inherited tremor in domestic cats. *Felis catus* L. *Nature* **227**, 1262–3.

Norsworthy G.D. (1979) Discospondylitis as a cause of posterior paresis. *Feline Pract.* **9**, 39–40.

Northington J.W. & Juliana M.M. (1978) Extradural lymphosarcoma in six cats. *J. Small Anim. Pract.* **19**, 409–16.

Petersen-Jones S.M. (1989) Abnormalities of eyes and vision. In Wheeler S.J. (ed) *British Small Animal Veterinary Association Manual of Small Animal Neurology.* BSAVA, Cheltenham, pp. 141–61.

Petrak M. & Carpenter J. (1965) Feline toxoplasmosis. *J. Am. Vet. Med. Assoc.* **146**, 728–34.

Prevost E., McKee J.M. & Crawford P. (1983) Successful medical management of severe feline cryptococcosis. *J. Am. Anim. Hosp. Assoc.* **18**, 111–4.

Robins G.M., Wilkinson G.T., Menrath V.H., Atwell R.B., & Riesz G. (1982) Long term survival following embolectomy in two cats with aortic embolism. *J. Small Anim. Pract.* **23**, 165–74.

Salisbury S.K. & Cook J.R. (1988) Recovery of neurological function following focal myelomalacia in a cat. *J. Am. Anim. Hosp. Assoc.* **24**, 227–30.

Sharp N.J.H. (1989a) Neurological deficits in one limb. In Wheeler S.J. (ed) *British Small Animal Veterinary Association Manual of Small Animal Neurology.* BSAVA, Cheltenham, pp. 179–206.

Sharp N.J.H. (1989b) Visceral and bladder function: dysautonomia. In Wheeler S.J. (ed) *British Small Animal Veterinary Association Manual of Small Animal Neurology.* BSAVA, Cheltenham, pp. 207–22.

Shell L., Dallman M. & Sponenberg P. (1987) Chondrosarcoma in a cat presenting with forelimb monoparesis. *Compend. Contin. Educ. Pract. Vet.* **9**, 391–8.

Shores A., Braund K.G. & McDonald R.K. (1987) Chronic relapsing polyneuropathy in the cat. *J. Am. Anim. Hosp. Assoc.* **23**, 569–73.

Smeak D.D. & Olmstead M.L. (1985) Fracture/luxations of the sacrococcygeal area in the cat. A retrospective study of 51 cases. *Vet. Surg.* **14**, 319–24.

Smith M.O., Turrel J.M., Bailey C.S. & Cain G.R. (1989) Neurological abnormalities as the predominant signs of neoplasia of the nasal cavity in dogs and cats: seven cases. *J. Am. Vet. Med. Assoc.* **195**, 242–5.

Sponenberg D.P. & Graf-Webster E. (1986) Hereditary meningoencephalocele in Burmese cats. *J. Hered.* **77**, 60.

Thompson J.P., Senior D.F., Pinson D.M. & Moriello

K.A. (1987) Neurotoxicosis associated with the use of hexachloraphene in a cat. *J. Am. Vet. Med. Assoc.* **190**, 1311–2.

Van den Bergh P., Baker M.K. & Lange A.L. (1977) A suspected lysosomal storage disease in Abyssinian cats. Part I: genetic, clinical and clinical pathological aspects. *J. S. Afr. Vet. Assoc.* **48**, 195–9.

Vandevelde M. & Braund K.G. (1979) Polioencephalomyelitis in cats. *Vet. Pathol.* **16**, 420–7.

Vandevelde M., Fankhauser R., Bichsel P., Wiesmann U. & Herschkowitz N. (1982) Hereditary neurovisceral mannosidosis associated with alpha-mannosidase deficiency in a family of Persian cats. *Acta Neuropathol.* **58**, 64–8.

Vulgamott J.C., Turnwald J.C., King G.K., Herring D.S., Hansen J.F. & Boothe H.W. (1980) Congenital portocaval anomalies of the cat: two case reports. *J. Am. Anim. Hosp. Assoc.* **16**, 915–9.

West-Hyde L. & Buyukmihci (1982) Photoreceptor degeneration in a family of cats. *J. Am. Vet. Med. Assoc.* **181**, 243–7.

Wheeler S.J. (1989) Spinal tumours in cats. *Vet. Ann.* **29**, 270–7.

Wheeler S.J., Clayton-Jones D.G. & Wright J.A. (1985) Myelography in the cat. *J. Small Anim. Pract.* **26**, 143–52.

Wilkinson G.T. (1979) Feline cryptococcosis: a review and seven case reports. J. Small Anim. Pract. **20**, 749–68.

Woodward J.C., Collins G.H. & Hessler J.R. (1974) Feline hereditary neuroaxonal dystrophy. *Am. J. Pathol.* **74**, 551–66.

Zaki F.A. & Hurvitz A.I. (1976) Spontaneous neoplasms of the central nervous system of the cat. *J. Small Anim. Pract.* **17**, 773–82.

Zaki F.A. & Nafe L.A. (1980) Ischaemic encephalopathy and focal granulomatous meningoencephalitis in the cat. *J. Small Anim. Pract.* **21**, 429–38.

Zaki F.A., Prata R.G. & Werner L.L. (1976) Necrotizing myelopathy in a cat. *J. Am. Vet. Med. Assoc.* **169**, 228–9.

FURTHER READING

Amann J.F. (1987) Congenital and acquired neuromuscular diseases of young dogs and cats. *Vet. Clin. N. Amer. (Small Anim. Pract.)* **17**, 617–39.

Averill D.R. (1973) Feline neurology. *J. Am. Anim Hosp. Assoc.* **40**, 195–9.

Broeck A.H.M. van den (1987) Horner's syndrome in dogs and cats: a review. *J. Small Anim. Pract.* **28**, 929–40.

Chrisman C. (1982) *Problems in Small Animal Neurology.* Lea & Febiger, Philadelphia.

DeLahunta A. (1977) Feline neurology. *Vet. Clin. N. Am. (Small Anim. Pract.)* **6**, 433–52.

DeLahunta A. (1983) *Veterinary Neuroanatomy and Clinical Neurology*, 2nd edn. W.B. Saunders, Philadelphia.

Evans R.J. (1985) Special neurology of the cat. In Wheeler S.J. (ed) *British Small Animal Veterinary Association Manual of Small Animal Neurology.* BSAVA, Cheltenham, pp. 255–71.

Flanders A. (1986) Feline aortic thromboembolism. *Compend. Cont. Educ. Pract. Vet.* **8**, 473–80.

Frey H.H. (1986) Use of anticonvulsants in small animals. *Vet. Rec.* **118**, 484–6.

Haskins M.E. (1987) Inherited metabolic disorders. In Holzworth J. (ed) *Diseases of the Dog and Cat: Medicine and Surgery*, vol. 1. W.B. Saunders, Philadelphia, pp. 808–19.

Holiday T.A. (1971) Clinical aspects of some encephalopathies of domestic cats. *Vet. Clin. N. Am. (Small Anim. Pract.)* **1**, 367.

Kern T.J. & Erb H.N. (1987) Facial neuropathy in dogs and cats: 95 cases. *J. Am. Vet. Med. Assoc.* **191**, 1604–9.

Nafe L.A. (1984) Topics in feline neurology. *Vet. Clin. N. Am. (Small Anim. Pract.)* **14**, 1289.

Oliver J.E. (1972) Neurologic emergencies in small animals. *Vet Clin. N. Am. (Small Anim. Pract.)* **2**, 341.

Oliver J.E. & Lorenz M.D. (1983) *Handbook of Veterinary Neurologic Diagnosis.* W.B. Saunders, Philadelphia.

Palmer A.C. (1976) *Introduction to Animal Neurology.* Blackwell Scientific Publications, Oxford.

Parker A.J., O'Brien D.P. & Sawchuk S.A. (1983) The nervous system. In Pratt P.W. (ed) *Feline Medicine.* American Veterinary Publications, Santa Barbara.

Selcer R.R. (1980) Trauma to the nervous system. *Vet. Clin. N. Amer. (Small Anim. Pract.)* **10**, 619.

Shell L. (1982) Cranial nerve disorders in dogs and cats. *Compend. Cont. Educ. Pract. Vet.* **4**, 458–67.

Wheeler S.J. (ed) (1989) *British Small Animal Veterinary Association Manual of Small Animal Neurology.* BSAVA, Cheltenham.

Chapter 3 / The Musculoskeletal System

D. BENNETT

INTRODUCTION

The feline patient can cope very well with all manner of musculoskeletal problems and perhaps because of this, the subject of locomotory disease is often neglected in this species. None the less, a lame animal is of concern to an owner and any locomotory disease can certainly interfere with the quality of the animal's life, especially in a species which is expected to be agile and athletic. Many recent advances have been made in the study of musculoskeletal diseases of the cat and several diseases can now be recognized and treated and a prognosis given. There are several possible ways of classifying diseases and the accuracy of any classification depends upon the available information. The classification used here (Table 3.1) is simple and probably most relevant to the clinician.

TRAUMATIC DISEASE

Fractures

Bone fractures are not uncommon in cats. The exact traumatic episode is generally unknown; cats either arrive home or are found in an injured state. Road traffic accidents or falls from a height are the most likely cause. Various surveys have been reported and indicate that the femur, tibia, mandible and pelvis are the most commonly fractured bones (Carter, 1964; Hill, 1977; Knecht, 1978). In a survey of feline pelvic fractures (Bennett, 1975) the average age of cats sustaining pelvic injury was 1.3 years; it is suggested that

young animals learn to cope with their environmental hazards through experience, but the very young cat is more likely to remain close to the home environment and is thus more protected.

The repair of fractures is beyond the scope of this chapter. Various surgical techniques can be used, although conservative treatment is often gratifying as, for example, with pelvic fractures. Recent studies have shown that the external fixator is well tolerated by the cat and can be used to treat a number of fracture problems in this species. The size of the cat is often helpful to the surgeon and, in general, cats are very co-operative orthopaedic patients.

A recent study by May et al. (1991) showed that the routine castration of male kittens resulted in delayed closure of the growth plates. This is probably due to interference with the important physiological role played by androgens in normal growth and physeal maturation. Such an effect may be of orthopaedic portent in cats since an open growth plate is more susceptible to trauma than a closed one.

Luxations/subluxations

Traumatic luxations of joints are seen in cats usually following a suspected road accident or fall from a height. The hip is probably the most commonly dislocated joint of the cat (Fig. 3.1) (Bennett, 1975). This is usually treated successfully by external reduction under general anaesthesia. Strapping of the leg is not advisable in cats, since in most cases they will not tolerate the sling. Recurrent hip luxations may be treated by

Table 3.1 A classification of diseases of the feline musculoskeletal system.

Traumatic disease
Fractures
Luxations/subluxations
Tendons

Bone infections
Bacterial
Mycotic

Metabolic bone diseases
Nutritional secondary hyperparathyroidism
Osteodystrophy of mature cats
Rickets (osteomalacia)
Hypervitaminosis A
Hypovitaminosis A
Renal secondary hyperparathyroidism
Primary hyperparathyroidism
Primary hypoparathyroidism

Arthritis
Traumatic arthritis
Osteoarthritis
Infective arthritis
Immune-based arthritis

Neoplastic and neoplastic-like lesions
Osteocartilaginous exostoses
Extraskeletal osteosarcoma
Extraskeletal osteoma
Parosteal osteoma
Chondrosarcoma
Osteoma
Osteoid osteoma
Multilobular chondromas
Osteoclastoma
Giant cell sarcoma
Spindle cell sarcoma
Fibrosarcoma
Synovioma
Synovial sarcoma
Aneurysmal bone cyst
Fibrous dysplasia
Metastatic neoplasms of bones and joints
Direct extension of neoplasms to bone
Synovial cyst
Synovial osteochondrometaplasia

Inherited, congenital and developmental disorders
Osteogenesis imperfecta
Manx cat
Kinked tail
Polydactylia
Ectrodactylia
Syndactylia
Amelia and hemimelia
Arrested development of long bones of forelimbs
Mandible ramus aplasia
Congenital duplication
Arthrogryposis
Chondrodysplasia
Achondroplasia
Congenital hypothyroidism
Maxillofacial compression
Craniofacial malformation in Burmese
Pectus excavatum
Other skeletal abnormalities
Mucopolysaccharidosis
Patellar luxation
Hip dysplasia
Osteochondrosis
Other congenital abnormalities

Muscle disease
Myositis
Localized myositis ossificans
Generalized myositis ossificans
Aortic thromboembolism
Myasthenia gravis
Hypokalaemic polymyopathy
Burmese sporadic myopathy
Tetanus
Fibrotic myopathy
Dystrophy-like myopathies
Other myopathies
Contracture of the gastrocnemius muscle/tendon

Diseases of the vertebral column
Intervertebral disc protrusions
Spondylosis deformans and ankylosing hyperostosis
Bacterial discospondylitis
Atlantoaxial subluxation

Miscellaneous diseases
Hypertrophic pulmonary osteoarthropathy
Disuse osteopenia
Osteopetrosis
Myelofibrosis osteosclerosis syndrome
Feline hyperaesthesia syndrome
Plasma cell pododermatitis
Feline metaphyseal osteopathy

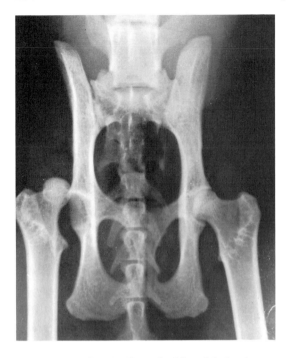

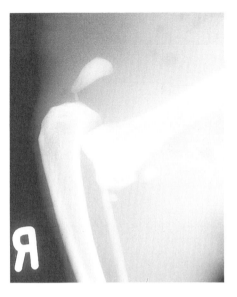

Fig. 3.2 Lateral radiograph of the stifle joint of a cat, showing luxation of the femorotibial joint.

Fig. 3.1 Ventrodorsal radiograph of the pelvis showing an anterodorsal hip luxation.

transarticular pinning (Bennett & Duff, 1980) or by femoral head excision, although cats can often manage well with a permanently luxated hip (Bennett, 1975).

Total luxation or subluxation of the femorotibial joint may occasionally be seen following road traffic injuries (Fig. 3.2). Such luxations are associated with cruciate and collateral ligament rupture. Careful reconstruction of the damaged ligaments is recommended in these cases, although stabilization of the joint with crosspins has been described (Fig. 3.3); the pins are removed after 3 weeks. The same technique has been used by the author to treat antebrachiocarpal luxation in the cat. The femoropatellar joint may also luxate secondary to trauma and usually responds to capsular tightening. The patella may also luxate in association with a dislocated hip joint. The tarsocrural joint is commonly luxated or subluxated, often associated with fractures of the medial and/or lateral malleoli of the hock (Fig. 3.4). Treatment is by fixation of

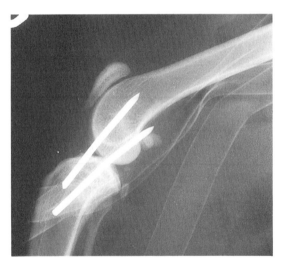

Fig. 3.3 Lateral radiograph of the stifle joint of a cat, showing a cross-pinning technique to stabilize a luxated stifle.

the fractured malleoli, usually by a tension band wiring technique or by reconstructing the collateral ligaments of the hock. Although most ligament tears in cats are associated with major trauma, there is a report suggesting that there

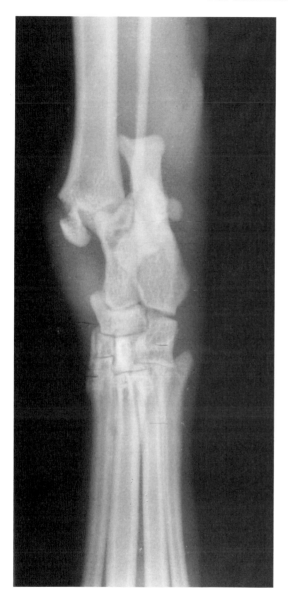

Fig. 3.4 Craniocaudal radiograph of the hock joint showing a bilateral malleolar fracture. There is subluxation of the tibiotarsal joint.

may be a gradual failure of the cranial cruciate rupture akin to that seen in dogs (Janssens *et al.*, 1991; Schrauwers & Appeldoorn, 1991). Furthermore, a tentative association between cruciate failure and cardiomyopathy in the cat has been suggested (Janssens *et al.*, 1991).

Falls may sometimes dislocate the temporomandibular joint, either unilaterally or bilaterally. Occasionally, there is also a fracture of the mandibular symphysis or horizontal/vertical rami. Reduction of the dislocation under anaesthesia is not difficult, using a small rod as a fulcrum inserted into the angles of the jaw. Other joints are less commonly luxated in the cat.

Temporomandibular ankylosis has been reported in the cat (Bennett & Campbell, 1976; Sullivan, 1989). These cats present with difficulty in opening their mouths resulting in difficulty in eating and grooming. There is obvious mechanical impediment to jaw opening and any attempt to force open the jaws produces pain. Radiography may show loss of the temporomandibular joint space and proliferation of bone around the joints which is often most evident within the zygomatic space on the ventrodorsal view. Although there may be no history of trauma, it is thought that this is the most likely explanation. The trauma may occur several months before the onset of clinical signs and in some cases may be severe enough to cause an intra-articular fracture. Surgical resection of part of the zygoma, mandibular condyle and vertical ramus may be necessary to free the ankylosis.

Tendons

Severance of tendons is not uncommon, associated with penetrating foreign bodies, most often glass. Suturing of a severed tendon is always recommended and is imperative for some of the larger tendons, such as that of the gastrocnemius muscle. Many surgeons do not attempt to suture the small digital tendons and although the animal can adjust, a permanent postural defect may remain which would not be acceptable for a show animal. Infection of tendons and tendon sheaths may follow penetrating wounds, particularly bites. Rupture of the Achilles tendon can be seen, particularly in overweight middle-aged cats, as a spontaneous gradual entity. In these cases an obvious severance of the tendon may not be apparent. Surgery of the Achilles tendon must be accompanied by postoperative immobilization of the hock joint in extension, preferably by use of an external fixator. Tendon surgery is again outside the scope of this chapter.

BONE INFECTIONS

Bacterial infective (suppurative) osteomyelitis

Aetiology and pathogenesis
Osteomyelitis is most often caused by a bacterial infection of bone. Bacteria may reach bone by the haematogenous route, by extension from adjacent soft tissues, for example nail bed infections, or by direct contact, for example bite wounds, compound fractures or surgical fixation of fractures. Once bacteria are present, bone mounts an inflammatory response similar to that seen in other tissues.

The severity of the osteomyelitis depends on many factors; for example, the initial site of infection within the bone, the exact organism, the contribution of other disease to bone abnormality, the presence of vascular ischaemia and the animal's age and general health. In some cases, the animal's responses will contain the infection; in others the infection will disseminate within the bone.

Infection may spread subperiosteally or within the Haversian system of cortical bone, or within the medullary cavity. As infection spreads, vascular thrombosis occurs, resulting in localized areas of cortical bone ischaemia, and there may be complete bony death or increased bone production around the area of infection. Complete bone death may result in sequestrum formation where a piece of dead bone sits within a granulation-filled bony depression or involucrum. Alternatively, dead bone may be resorbed and replaced by new bone.

Acute osteomyelitis refers to the early stages described above and where treatment is initiated promptly. Chronic osteomyelitis occurs when the process continues for an extended period of time and may result in disseminated infection within the bone. The most frequent organism is *Staphylococcus* although many other organisms including *Streptococcus* spp. and *Pseudomonas* spp. can be involved; mixed infections are not uncommon. Pure anaerobic or mixed aerobic and anaerobic infections of bone can also occur (Berg *et al.*, 1979; Walker *et al.*, 1983). Anaerobic infections can be difficult to diagnose since special culture conditions are necessary and samples need to be processed within a very short time. Many cases of 'sterile' osteomyelitis are probably due to anaerobic organisms that have failed to grow in the laboratory.

Clinical signs
There is usually an obvious lameness associated with localized bone pain and swelling. Other signs may be related to fracture of the bone, penetrating wound or infected soft tissue; fever and systemic illness may or may not be present. Weight loss may occur, especially in chronic osteomyelitis cases. With chronicity, discharging sinus tracts may be obvious. Local lymph nodes are often enlarged.

Radiography
Osteomyelitis may show bony lysis and/or increased bone density (Fig. 3.5). Periosteal new bone, which may extend a considerable distance along the length of the affected bone, may be present. Sequestra may be obvious (Fig. 3.6). Soft tissue swelling, loss of fascial planes and increased soft tissue density are also features.

Laboratory features
Culture of the organism is useful for confirmation of the diagnosis and providing antimicrobial drug sensitivities for treatment. Most animals do not show an obvious leucocytosis or shift to the left.

Treatment
Treatment of bacterial osteomyelitis is often a combination of surgical drainage and antibiotic therapy. In acute osteomyelitis, drainage may be necessary to release exudate. Surgical drains can be inserted, and in some cases multiple drill holes are made through the bone cortex to allow drainage from the medullary cavity. The drain may be protected against contamination from

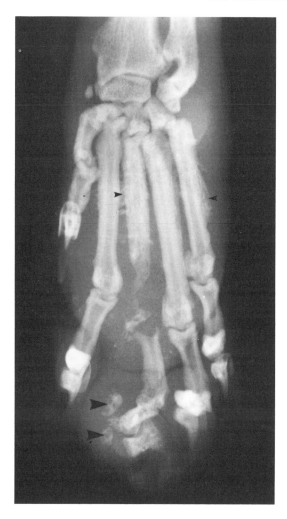

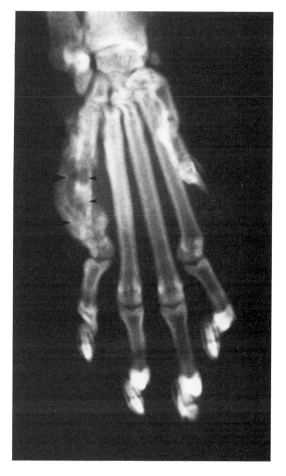

Fig. 3.6 Craniocaudal radiograph of the left forefoot showing osteomyelitis of the metacarpus of digit 5. There is a sequestrum (small arrows) associated with periosteal new bone forming a bridge (large arrows) alongside the sequestrum.

Fig. 3.5 Craniocaudal radiograph of the right forefoot showing osteomyelitis following a penetrating bite wound. There is obvious destruction of the distal end metacarpal bone of digit 3. Extensive periosteal new bone is present on all the metacarpal bones (small arrows). Soft tissue calcification is seen within the digital pad of digit 3 (large arrows). There is gross soft tissue swelling of the foot.

the surroundings by bandaging. Inserted drains also allow local irrigation with saline and antibiotic solutions. Enforced rest of the animal is important, even to the extent of hospitalization and immobilization of the affected limb by bandage or cast. The antibiotic of choice should be based on laboratory culture and sensitivity. However, treatment should always be started whilst awaiting the laboratory results. Most organisms are susceptible to ampicillin, clindamycin, cephaloridine and the amoxycillin/clavulanic acid combination. Some Gram-negative organisms only respond to gentamycin or kanamycin. Anaerobic infections usually respond to lincomycin, ampicillin, chloramphenicol, metronidazole and cephaloridine. The drugs are given systemically (preferably orally) and locally if possible. Systemic administration is often necessary for several weeks. Surgical drains are normally only left in the tissues for 4–7 days.

The treatment of chronic osteomyelitis may be similar to that of acute osteomyelitis. In addition, areas of dead bone, or sequestra, must be surgically removed. Surgical implants may also need to be removed. The insertion of drains is recommended. Chronic osteomyelitis may resolve completely with treatment although some cases may fail to respond. Some cases apparently resolve but are subject to periodic relapses of the osteomyelitic process, presumably associated with residual quiescent infection becoming activated, possibly by some stress factor. Some cases that do not clear may be treated by limb amputation or local resection of the diseased bone and the insertion of a replacement bone graft. Infected nail beds with osteomyelitis of the digital bones are often better treated by amputation of the digit – care should be taken to distinguish osteomyelitis and carcinoma of the digit (see below).

Treatment of a compound fracture should be by immediate local antisepsis, systemic antibiotics and support bandaging of the limb. The fracture may be repaired a few days later and antibiotic therapy continued for 3–4 weeks. Potentially infected fractures must be rigidly fixed, and compression techniques or the external fixator offer the best approach.

Non-suppurative osteomyelitis

Mycotic infection of bone, sometimes associated with infection of other tissues, has been reported in the cat.

Coccidioidomycosis
Coccidioides immitis is endemic in the southwestern USA. It is believed that most infections are contracted from soil and dust. Granulomatous lesions can occur in many different organs, for example lung, liver, kidney, lymph nodes, skin. In one case reported by Reed *et al.* (1963) there was radiographical and pathological evidence of fungal spread to bone. Biopsy and culture

are necessary for a definitive diagnosis although serological tests are also used. Treatment necessitates the use of antifungal drugs, for example amphotericin B.

Cryptococcosis
Infection with the yeast-like fungus *Cryptococcus neoformans* is the commonest systemic fungal disease of cats. The organism is widely distributed in nature, although pigeon faeces are the most frequently reported source. Four main clinical syndromes are reported in the cat: respiratory, neurological, cutaneous and ocular. The organism is regarded as an opportunist invader in animals that are compromised by immunodeficiency, debility, malnutrition, etc. Lytic bony lesions of the head and sinuses have been documented (Rutman *et al.*, 1975). Diagnosis depends on finding the organisms in material from infected tissues or in discharges. Immunological tests are also available. Antifungal agents are used in treatment (Wilkinson, 1984a).

Blastomycosis
Blastomyces dermatitis is rare in the cat. It is endemic in certain areas of North America and has been isolated from the soil. It may cause just pulmonary disease, skin disease, CNS and ocular disease although some cases have had widespread systemic involvement. Skeletal lesions may develop via haematogenous spread or by extension from a subcutaneous nodule (Horne, 1964). Oedema, pain and occasionally draining tracts are found in the affected area. There is radiographic evidence of bone destruction with resulting periosteal new bone. Biopsy and culture are necessary for a definitive diagnosis.

Histoplasmosis
This disease is caused by the yeast-like fungus *Histoplasma capsulatum*. It is a disease mainly of the reticuloendothelial system and two forms have been described: a benign form involving the lungs and associated lymph nodes, and a disseminated form involving several organs including liver, spleen, intestine, bone and lung. Mahaffey *et al.* (1977) described joint lesions characterized

by a soft tissue thickening and, in some cases, by bony destruction within the joint. Discharging sinuses were related to some infected joints. Goad and Roenick (1983) described a disseminated case in a 1-year-old domestic short-hair cat that had multiple osteomyelitis lesions. Successful treatment is unlikely.

Aspergillosis

Aspergillus fumigatus infection may cause either a necrotizing or a granulomatous disease, usually affecting the lung and intestine. Infection can localize to the frontal sinuses and cause local bone destruction (Wilkinson, 1984a). Diagnosis is made from a biopsy or serological examination. Treatment with thiabendazole-type drugs can be attempted.

Streptomyces

A streptomycete infection involving the scapula of a cat has been reported (Lewis *et al.*, 1972). The infection was apparently introduced by gunshot. Surgical resection of the lesion was unsuccessful.

METABOLIC BONE DISEASES

Nutritional secondary hyperparathyroidism in kittens (nutritional osteopenia, juvenile osteopenia)

Aetiology and pathogenesis

This disease is characterized by a reduced mineralization of the skeleton and is normally seen in young kittens, particularly of the Siamese breed, fed a meat-rich diet (Krook *et al.*, 1963; Bennett, 1976a,b). Meat is rich in phosphorus but has a low calcium content; for example horsemeat has a Ca:P ratio of 1:10, liver 1:50 and heart 1:50. The feeding of a diet low in calcium and/or rich in phosphorus leads to a transient hypocalcaemia. This stimulates the release of parathyroid hormone which acts on bone, kidney and intestine to help restore calcium levels to normal. Resorption of bone to release calcium into the bloodstream is an important homeostatic mechanism, but after prolonged release of parathyroid hormone, the skeleton becomes significantly weakened. The

bone turnover is greatly increased with resorption occurring faster than formation. Resorbed bone tends to be replaced, to a limited extent, by fibrous tissue. The parathyroid glands become hyperplastic showing enlargement, increased cellularity and the presence of increased numbers of light chief cells and 'water clear' cells.

The most significant aetiological factor is the feeding of calcium-deficient diets to the young cat. Meat, cereal, grain, fruit and nuts are all deficient in calcium, and excessive phosphorus in the diet is also a problem since it will interfere with the normal absorption of calcium. Other factors can interfere with calcium absorption, for example gastrointestinal disease, thyroid disease, vitamins A and D, renal insufficiency, magnesium, phytate and fluorine. The rate of growth is probably important too, the faster growing kittens being more susceptible, and there may be other genetic predisposing factors to explain why only certain kittens in a litter may be clinically affected. Certainly, there are obvious differences between individual cats in their ability to retain calcium and utilize it on a low intake (Scott, 1984). The Siamese breed may be more often affected because they tend to be fed meat-rich diets with little or no milk, and the breeding queens tend to have large litters which may result in inadequate calcium supplies to the very young kittens. It is important to note that a genetic bone disease (osteogenesis imperfecta) with similar clinical features to nutritional secondary hyperparathyroidism occurs in the cat and usually has a very poor prognosis.

Clinical signs

Young kittens of a few weeks or months of age are affected. Lameness is often the presenting sign and this may be due to apparent musculoskeletal pain or to pathological fractures of the bones. The latter often show little displacement. Pathological fractures of the vertebrae can occur and may cause profound neurological disturbances, for example paraplegia, urinary retention and overflow, and provide a hopeless prognosis.

Bone weakness may cause obvious bending of the limbs and it is common to have deformity of

the thoracic wall, sternum and pelvis. Epiphyseal growth is usually stunted and sometimes
dcformcd, and normal tooth development and
maintenance can be adversely affected. There is
often apparent weakness and laxity of joints and
a 'flat-footed' appearance.

Radiography
The most obvious feature is a loss of bone density
(Figs. 3.7 & 3.8). The contrast between bone and
soft tissue is poor. The cortices appear very thin.
Pathological fractures are usually obvious and
may show as 'folding' fractures (Fig. 3.7). There
may be evidence of healing fractures that were
not detectable clinically. The growth plates are of
normal dimensions. There is often an area of
increased mineralization within the metaphysis,
an area of preferential mineralization. Deformity
of bones may be assessed on radiography and it is
often worth while radiographing the pelvis and
thorax as routine to check for any deformities,
since they can affect the prognosis. Any cat showing paraplegia or paraparesis should have careful
spinal evaluation (Fig. 3.8).

Laboratory features
Blood calcium and phosphorus levels are usually
in the normal range (Krook, 1971) except in
extreme cases. Urinary calcium and phosphorus
levels are also of limited help in aiding diagnosis,
although a reduced urinary calcium level may be
seen. Radioimmunoassay of circulating parathyroid hormone levels is a useful test but, is not
routinely available for the cat.

Treatment and prognosis
The feeding of a meat-rich diet should be terminated and a nutritionally balanced diet substituted.
Calcium and phosphorus supplementation is recommended. Sterilized bonemeal is the most
commonly used, but will not readily correct an
abnormal dietary Ca:P ratio and must thus be
used with a balanced diet. Calcium lactate and
borogluconate can be used to provide calcium
without phosphorus, but relatively large amounts
are necessary. The use of a calcium preparation
with aluminium carbonate gel will provide cal-

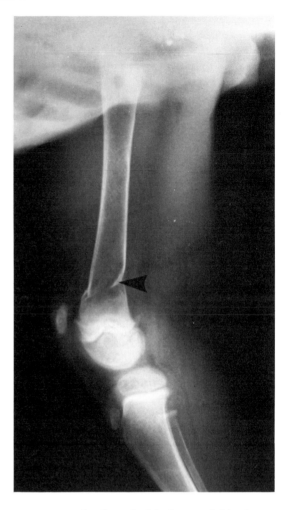

Fig. 3.7 Lateral radiograph of the femur and tibia of a cat
with nutritional secondary hyperparathyroidism. The
cortices are thin and the contrast between bone and soft
tissue is poor. There is a 'folding' fracture of the distal
femur (arrow).

cium and help remove excess phosphorus (Miller,
1969).

Cage rest of the affected animal is helpful and
analgesics may be necessary. In many cases, the
animals will respond within a short time. There
may be residual stunting and deformity and pelvic
collapse can lead to defaecatory and obstetrical
problems, and thoracic deformity may cause
respiratory problems. Surgical treatment of the

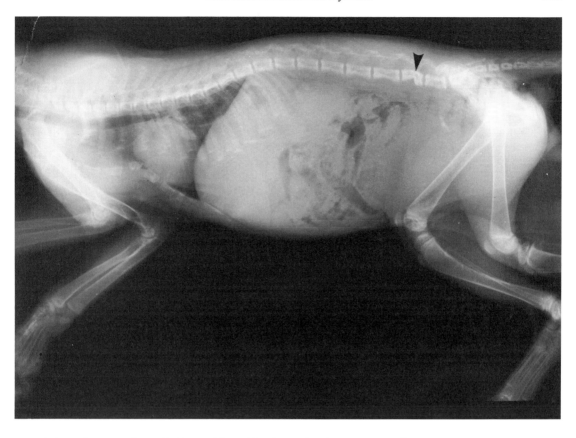

Fig. 3.8 Lateral survey radiograph of a cat with nutritional secondary hyperparathyroidism. The cortices of the long bones are thin and there is a pathological fracture of L6 (arrow). The cat was paraparetic.

pelvic and thoracic deformities is possible, but often difficult and unrewarding. Pathological fractures often require no treatment other than rest, although intramedullary pinning and external fixator techniques are sometimes advantageous and fractures affecting the lower limbs can be externally supported. Fractures of the vertebral column often have a poor prognosis; euthanasia of the cat is necessary if the neurological deficit is severe.

Osteodystrophy of mature cats

The exact aetiology and pathogenesis of this disease is unknown. It is described in the American literature (Riser *et al.*, 1968; Herron, 1983). It is possibly associated with long-term meat- or liver-rich diets fed to confined cats. Bone demineralization occurs, possibly as a result of secondary hyperparathyroidism. Bone cortices become thinned, but periosteal new bone along the shafts of the long bones is a feature. This hyperostosis is difficult to explain; it may be an effect of excess vitamin A although the pattern of bony overgrowth differs from that normally seen in hypervitaminosis A (see below). Affected cats are sluggish, and may present with constipation due to a narrowed pelvic canal caused by pelvic collapse. Treatment is to correct the diet. Medicinal or surgical treatment may be required for the constipatory problem.

Rickets (osteomalacia)

Rickets, although often confused with nutritional secondary hyperparathyroidism, is virtually unknown in the cat. The exact aetiology of rickets is uncertain although dietary deficiency of vitamin D and a deficiency of phosphorus and/or calcium are important. There is some evidence that high-cereal, low-meat diets are rachitogenic, not just because of a mineral/vitamin imbalance. The feeding of such diets to cats is very unusual.

The main pathological feature of rickets is a failure of bone and cartilage matrix to calcify. Clinically, in the young animal, the epiphyseal line becomes very much widened because of the failure of the growing cartilage to calcify and ossify. There is poor skeletal mineralization. Secondary hyperparathyroidism is also involved in the pathogenesis.

The clinical signs are similar to those of nutritional hyperparathyroidism. Radiography reveals poorly mineralized bones and, in the young animal, widening of growth plates. Treatment includes the provision of a balanced diet and vitamin D supplementation, for example 80 IU/day. Excess vitamin D can easily reach toxic levels resulting in soft tissue calcification and even more serious effects, and thus supplementation should be carefully controlled and never used as a routine measure in young kittens.

Hypervitaminosis A

Aetiology and pathogenesis

The daily vitamin A requirement of cats is relatively high, 1600–2000 IU (Gershoff *et al.*, 1957; Moore *et al.*, 1963; Scott, 1964). The reasons for this are the poor absorption of carotene, the precursor of vitamin A, from the intestine and the limited conversion of carotene to vitamin A. It is probably the awareness of this potential deficiency problem that has encouraged owners to supplement cats' diets with vitamin A, usually in the form of liver. Unfortunately, cats enjoy liver and become habituated to it. The feeding of excess liver, particularly to the exclusion of anything else, causes hypervitaminosis A (Seawright *et al.*, 1967; Baker & Hughes, 1968; Fry, 1968; Lucke *et al.*, 1968; Bennett, 1976a,b).

The effects of excess vitamin A vary according to the age of the cat, the chronicity, and possibly the actual level of vitamin intake. Basically, there appears to be a disturbance in osteoblastic and osteoclastic functions. In young cats, there is a suppression of osteoblast activity and degenerative changes in the cartilaginous epiphyseal plates, and the appositional and longitudinal growth of long bones is reduced (Clark & Seawright, 1968; Clark *et al.*, 1970; Clark, 1970, 1971a). Exostoses in ligaments and tendons, particularly affecting the cervical/thoracic spine, but also the limb joints, are more characteristic of a less acute toxicity in the mature cat. In addition to skeletal changes, there is extensive lipid infiltration of parenchymatous organs, which might predispose the animal to secondary disease (Clark, 1971b).

A liver-rich diet in the immature cat also leads to nutritional secondary hyperparathyroidism.

Clinical signs

The most typical case is the adult cat, presented 1–5 years after starting a virtually all-liver diet. The initial signs may be lameness, stiffness and pain. The cats are obviously uncomfortable and become reluctant to move. The spine is often partly ankylosed and the cats can sometimes be held 'like a board'. The neck shows reduced motion. Affected limb joints may be enlarged, painful and show a reduced range of motion. Occasionally, a foreleg lameness can be associated with a neurological deficit, due to spinal exostoses compressing the peripheral nerves to the forelimb. Pathological changes may be confined to just the spine or just limb joints, or may affect both together.

Occasionally, the owners present the animal complaining of an unkempt coat. This is a result of spinal ankylosis, the cat being unable to turn its head sufficiently for grooming. The animals are sometimes obese through inactivity, although anorexia and weight loss can occur. The teeth often show a yellow discoloration and gum problems are not uncommon.

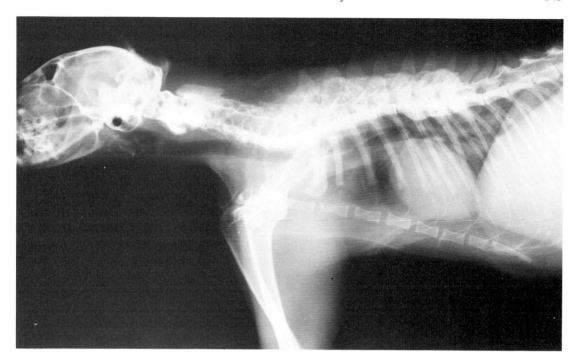

Fig. 3.9 Lateral radiograph of the cervical and thoracic spine of a cat with hypervitaminosis A. There is a typical bony proliferation along the spine.

Radiography

Radiography of the spine will show the typical exostoses affecting the cervical and thoracic vertebrae (Fig. 3.9). Exostoses can also be seen in affected limb joints, the bony proliferation often confining itself to ligaments and joint capsules (Fig. 3.10). In the young kitten, radiographic features might include poor mineralization, bony deformity and uneven growth of epiphyseal plates.

Treatment

Dietary liver should be stopped although, in practice, this is difficult to achieve since the cat often refuses to eat anything other than liver. The bony exostoses will not resolve, but pain relief and clinical improvement do occur. Bone deformities in the kitten are likely to persist. Analgesics can be tried and surgical removal of exostoses is possible in certain limb joints, but any resultant damage to the ligaments, etc. must be corrected.

Hypovitaminosis A

Scott (1964) reported that hypovitaminosis A is 'fairly common' in cats, though often unrecognized. Certainly, as discussed above, the feline requirement for vitamin A is comparatively high.

A deficiency of vitamin A again causes an imbalance between bone production (osteoblastosis) and resorption (osteoclastosis). The disease is seen mainly in young kittens, particularly if the maternal supply of the vitamin is deficient. There is distortion and malformation of long bones, cranial bones and vertebral column (Mellanby, 1941, 1950). The bones become bulky and with the cranial and vertebral bones, this results in a reduced size of the vertebral canal, cranial vault and various foraminae, through which pass nerves and blood vessels.

The overall result is pressure on the brain,

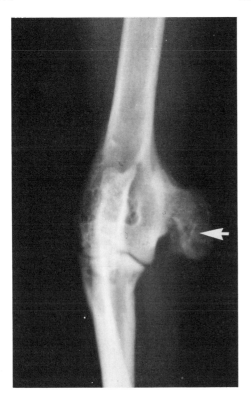

Fig. 3.10 Craniocaudal radiograph of the elbow joint of a cat with hypervitaminosis A. There is extensive bony proliferation involving the collateral ligament (arrow).

spinal cord, cranial nerves and spinal nerves, causing a variety of neurological symptoms. Scott (1964) states that skull and vertebral changes develop at about the fifth week of life. Gershoff *et al.* (1957) failed to show changes in the skeletal and nervous tissues of experimentally deficient cats, but did report squamous metaplasia of various epithelial structures, for example, respiratory tract, conjunctivae, salivary glands and endometrium. Corneal vascularization and ulceration, retinal degeneration, poor reproductive function, anorexia, weight loss, muscular weakness and ocular discharge are also documented (Gershoff *et al.*, 1957; Scott, 1964).

The deformed cranial and vertebral bones may cause difficult parturition as well as interfering with the hearing, sight and survival of the kitten. Radiography of the skull bones will show increased thickness of bones, especially those surrounding the posterior fossa of the brain. The long bones may show deformities, and the shaft may not show an obvious compact cortex and the endosteum may be indistinct.

Dietary supplementation with vitamin A is the treatment, up to 2000 IU/day.

Renal secondary hyperparathyroidism

Aetiology and pathogenesis

This bone disease is related to chronic renal insufficiency. The underlying renal lesion is variable and may be acquired, for example chronic nephritis, glomerulonephritis, nephrosclerosis, amyloidosis, or congenital, for example polycystic kidneys. Once the renal disease causes reduction in the glomerular filtration rate, phosphorus is retained and hyperphosphataemia develops; there is a compensatory fall in blood calcium which stimulates the release of parathyroid hormone, which causes bone breakdown and the release of calcium into the blood. The renal damage may also interfere with production of 1,25-dihydroxycholecalciferol, the active metabolite of vitamin D, thus resulting in an effective deficiency of vitamin D which could interfere with normal calcium absorption from the gut, and also lead to osteomalacia.

Clinical signs

It is often the old cat which is affected. Signs related to the renal dysfunction are often present, for example vomiting, polydipsia, dehydration, weight loss and depression. Signs of skeletal demineralization may not be apparent although softened jaw bones, loose teeth, generalized stiffness and lameness, and even pathological fractures, may be present. Affected jaw bones are susceptible to fracture during dentistry.

Radiography

Poor bone mineralization may be seen. Resorption of alveolar socket bone and loss of the lamina dura dentes are fairly typical. Soft tissue calcification may also be seen.

Laboratory features

Laboratory tests for impaired renal function are useful. Serum analysis for calcium and phosphorus levels is often unrewarding although the latter may be elevated. Urinary excretion of calcium and phosphorus is usually decreased. Alkaline phosphatase is often elevated in the blood and increased levels of parathyroid hormone may be detectable.

Treatment

Ideally, the aim of treatment is to halt the progression of the renal disease. Often this is not feasible. Realistically, treatment is directed towards reducing the excretory load of the kidneys and to provide substances that the kidney is failing to conserve. A low-protein diet is recommended, although this is often not acceptable to the cat. Calcium should be provided as the gluconate or lactate and vitamin D supplementation may be helpful, even as the active metabolite (see Chapters 5 and 24).

Primary hyperparathyroidism

Primary hyperparathyroidism has been attributed to a primary hyperplasia or to a neoplastic change of the parathyroid glands (adenoma or carcinoma). Primary hyperparathyroidism is very rare in the cat; a case of hyperplasia was described by Blunden *et al.* (1986). The cat presented with lethargy, reluctance to move and pain along the back. Radiological examination revealed multifocal and polyostotic lesions, particularly of the axial skeleton.

Primary hypoparathyroidism

Forbes *et al.* (1990) described primary hypoparathyroidism in a 1-year-old cat. The clinical features included anorexia, muscle spasms, lethargy and mild tetany of the hindlimbs. There was hypocalcaemia and hyperphosphataemia. Histological examination of the left excised thyroid and parathyroid glands suggested a diagnosis of lymphocytic parathyroiditis of possible autoimmune origin. Successful treatment includes initial intravenous and subcutaneous calcium, followed by oral calcium lactate and vitamin D. Although mobilization of calcium from the skeleton is reduced in this condition, the effect on the skeleton itself is of no consequence.

Iatrogenic primary hypoparathyroidism can also develop as a sequel to injury or removal of the parathyroid glands at the time of thyroid surgery, e.g. in hyperthyroid cats after bilateral thyroidectomy.

ARTHRITIS

Although the term 'arthritis' literally means inflammation of a joint it is used in a broader sense to cover a number of well-defined joint diseases which may be characterized by both inflammatory and degenerative changes. Traditionally, arthritis is broadly divided into the degenerative arthropathies (traumatic, osteoarthritis) and the inflammatory arthropathies (infective, immune-based) according to which pathological process is most in evidence. The feline species is now known to suffer many different types of arthritis (Fig. 3.11). Table 3.2 summarizes the main features of arthritis in the cat. Haemophilic arthropathy is not reported in the cat although haemophilia has been (Cotter *et al.*, 1978).

Traumatic arthritis

This type of arthritis follows a single acute injury to the joint. The trauma may result from traffic accidents, fights with other animals, abuse from man, awkward falls and excessive stresses on joints, or from gunshot wounds.

The articular damage caused is variable. There may be just a mild inflammation of the joint capsule or ligaments, the so-called 'sprain', or more severe damage may be evident, for example, intra-articular bony or cartilage fractures, torn or

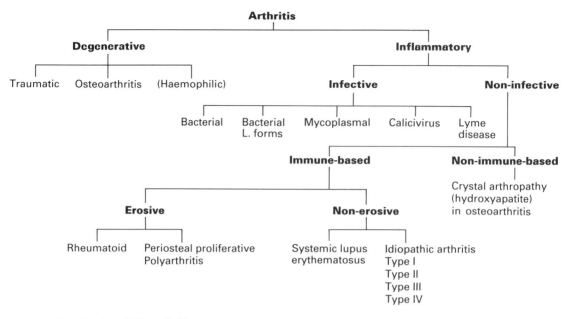

Fig. 3.11 Classification of feline arthritis.

stretched ligaments, lacerated joint capsule and displaced or torn menisci.

There is usually a synovitis, which may be localized, and haemorrhage or increased synovia present within the joint cavity. The synovitis is characterized by hyperplasia and hypertrophy of the lining layer, and a few inflammatory cells within the supporting layer, and areas of haemorrhage and haemosiderin deposits within the synovium.

The animal is presented with an obvious lameness and there is pain and swelling associated with the affected joint. Care must be taken to check for any serious bone or ligament damage; radiography may be helpful for this. A synovial fluid sample from a traumatized joint may contain blood; it usually shows some loss of viscosity, a normal mucin clot and a normal or slightly elevated white cell count, most of which are mononuclear cells.

Treatment depends on the severity of the injury. Some cases may necessitate surgical intervention, for example fracture repair, ligament replacement or support bandaging for a few days.

Milder cases may only require restricted exercise and/or anti-rheumatic drugs. Low doses of corticosteroids are helpful in cases of traumatic arthritis. Traumatic arthritis can predispose a joint to bacterial infective arthritis, the infection usually developing a few days after the initial trauma. Such cases can be difficult to diagnose without examining a synovial fluid sample. Osteoarthritis can also follow a traumatic arthritis, especially after repeated traumatic episodes.

Osteoarthritis

Osteoarthritis is defined as a disorder of moveable joints characterized by deterioration and abrasion of articular cartilage and by the formation of new bone at the articular margins. There are two main forms of the disease, primary and secondary. Secondary osteoarthritis is thought to be the more common and in this form the disease is secondary to some other joint disorder. In the cat it is thought to follow repeated joint trauma, perhaps associated with their agile lifestyle. Osteoarthritis secondary to articular

Table 3.2 A summary of the main diagnostic features of feline arthritis.

Type of arthritis	Clinical features	Radiographic features	Laboratory features
Traumatic	Single joint. History of trauma	Increased soft tissue density. Fractures. Ligament damage	Synovial fluid viscous. Normal or increased white cells, mainly mononuclear. May contain blood
Osteoarthritis	Usually single joint	Osteophyte development. Increased soft tissue density	Synovial fluid viscous. Normal or increased white cells, mainly mononuclear
Bacterial infective	Usually single joint	Increased soft tissue density. Loss of bone. Periosteal new bone. Soft tissue calcification	Synovial fluid watery. Increased quantity. Increased white cells, mainly polymorphonuclear. Culture organism from synovial fluid and/or membrane.
Infective bacterial L forms	Multiple joints, subcutaneous abscesses	Increased soft density. Bone destruction	Synovial fluid watery, increased in quantity. Increased numbers of polymorphonuclear cells. Difficult to culture organism
Mycoplasmal	Multiple joints	Increased soft tissue. Bone destruction	Synovial fluid watery, increased in quantity. Increased numbers of polymorphonuclear cells. May see organisms in synovial fluid smear. Difficult to culture. Evidence of immunosuppression
Calicivirus	One or more joints. May follow primary vaccination in young kitten. Spontaneous recovery	Very little. Soft tissue changes	Synovial fluid increased in quantity. Increased white cells
Lyme disease (borreliosis)	One or more joints. Other signs. History of tick infestation. Rapid response to antibiotic therapy	Increased soft tissue density	Synovial fluid increased in quantity. Increased numbers of polymorphonuclear cells. Positive serum titre to *Borrelia burgdorferi*. Difficult to culture
Rheumatoid	Multiple joints, bilaterally symmetrical	Increased soft tissue density. Loss of bone, erosions, generalized loss of mineral. Periosteal new bone	Synovial fluid watery. Increased quantity. Increased white cells, mainly polymorphonuclear. Rheumatoid factor in blood in some cases
Systemic lupus erythematosus	Multiple joints, bilaterally symmetrical. Other features of a multisystemic disease	Mainly increased soft tissue density	Synovial fluid watery. Increased white cells, mainly polymorphonuclear. Antinuclear antibody in blood
Periosteal proliferative polyarthritis	Multiple joints, bilaterally symmetrical. Mainly carpi and hocks	Very extensive periosteal new bone. Also erosive changes. Increased soft tissue density	Synovial fluid watery. Increased quantity. Increased white cells, mainly polymorphonuclear.

continued on p. 148

Table 3.2 *Continued*

Type of arthritis	Clinical features	Radiographic features	Laboratory features
Idiopathic arthritis	Multiple joints, bilaterally symmetrical. Type I: uncomplicated Type II: infection elsewhere in the body Type III: gastrointestinal disease Type IV: neoplastic disease – usually myeloproliferative disease	Increased soft tissue density. Slight periosteal new bone in some cases	Synovial fluid watery. Increased white cells, mainly polymorphonuclear

fractures, ligament tears and joint luxation/subluxation is also recognized. Osteoarthritis of the shoulders and elbows is most common in the older cat. Osteoarthritis is generally regarded as a final common pathway of joint failure rather than as a distinct disease entity.

Pathological features

Degeneration of articular cartilage is an important part of osteoarthritis. This may be seen grossly as an increase in dullness accompanied by a colour change from white to white-grey or yellow. The surface may appear fissured and disrupted and there may be obvious erosion or ulceration. Histologically, cartilage degeneration is seen as a loss of the superficial layers, horizontal flaking and fibrillation, and vertical splits. There is a loss of metachromatic staining. Ultimately, cartilage may be sheared off exposing the underlying subchondral bone, which often responds by becoming thickened. Cartilage degeneration is associated with certain well-defined biochemical changes, for example increased hydration of articular cartilage, increased galactosamine–glucosamine ratio and a greater extractability of proteoglycan aggregate with high molarity calcium chloride (McDevitt, 1973; McDevitt & Muir, 1976).

The other main feature of osteoarthritis is the production of osteophytes or bony outgrowths, which occur principally at the marginal zone, where articular cartilage and synovium meet, and at the attachment of joint capsule and ligaments.

These osteophytes initially develop outside the epiphysis of the joint but with time can become an integral part of the joint, such that the joint takes on a completely different shape. This process of remodelling is an important feature of osteoarthritis and is thought to be the mechanism by which the joint is trying to cope with altered stresses placed upon it.

Hypertrophy and hyperplasia of the lining layer of the synovial membrane is regularly seen in osteoarthritic joints; accumulations of mononuclear inflammatory cells are often seen, but the degree of inflammatory change is usually mild (Fig. 3.12).

Subchondral cysts are sometimes seen; they arise from the replacement of bony trabeculae and marrow by mixed connective tissue. Degeneration of intra-articular menisci and vascular abnormalities are also features of osteoarthritis.

Clinical signs

Lameness is the usual presenting sign although many joints affected with osteoarthritis are asymptomatic. Generally, the lameness is of a chronic nature, of insidious onset, and there is usually a progressive deterioration with time. Lameness and stiffness often follow periods of exercise and will initially clear with rest. As the disease progresses, stiffness becomes more pronounced following rest. Cold and damp weather will often exacerbate the lameness. A sudden onset lameness may occur with established osteo-

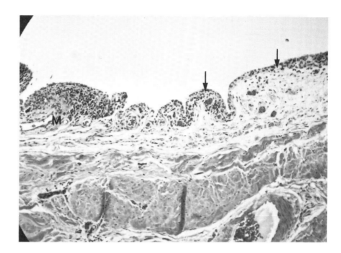

Fig. 3.12 Photomicrograph of a synovial membrane biopsy from an osteoarthritic joint. The lining layer shows hyperplasia and hypertrophy (arrows). There is a small accumulation of mononuclear inflammatory cells (M) within the supporting layer (H&E) (×50).

arthritis – this can be due to a joint sprain since osteoarthritic joints are susceptible to trauma, or to an exacerbation of the synovitis caused by, for example, the release of cartilage breakdown products or hydroxyapatite crystals into the articular cavity.

Affected joints may be obviously enlarged due to osteophyte formation, bony remodelling and joint capsule fibrosis. Increased synovial fluid within the articular cavity may be evident. Pain and crepitus are sometimes appreciated and reduced joint motion is often a feature.

In cases of secondary osteoarthritis, clinical signs referable to the underlying predisposing joint disorder may also be apparent.

Radiography
The most typical feature is the presence of new bone deposits, referred to as osteophytes, spurs, exostoses or as a 'lipping' of the joint margin. They are visualized as an irregularity or roughening of the bony outline, as obvious masses of bone protruding from the normal bone margin, or as irregular densities of bone where the deposits are superimposed on the normal osseous architecture (Figs. 3.13 & 3.14). Sclerosis of subchondral bone may be seen in long-standing cases and subchondral cysts are sometimes seen as discrete radiolucent defects.

Narrowing of the joint space is a feature indicative of articular cartilage loss, but such narrowing is difficult to appreciate without weight-bearing films, and the technical problems of obtaining these are obvious.

Intra- or peri-articular calcification may be seen in osteoarthritic joints: such calcification occurs within the synovial membrane, ligaments, tendons or menisci (Fig. 3.15). However, calcification particularly within the menisci of the stifle joint, is commonly seen in the cat in joints that are otherwise normal and in which there is no clinical problem (Fig. 3.16).

Radiography is also useful in assessing joint remodelling and in assessing other joint disease which might be initiating the osteoarthritis.

Laboratory features
Synovial fluid is often increased in quantity, and has reduced viscosity. The white cell count may be slightly elevated (Table 3.2) and the majority of cells are macrophages and lymphocytes. Synovial lining cells and cartilage cells, and very occasionally bone cells, may be seen. The fluid does not clot on exposure to air, and the mucin clot test is normal.

Treatment

GENERAL
It is difficult to organize a cat's exercise regime, but it is desirable to keep exercise regular as

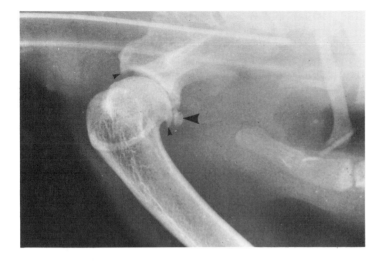

Fig. 3.13 Lateral radiograph of the left shoulder joint showing advanced osteoarthritis. There is osteophyte development on the caudal humeral head and tuber scapula (small arrows) and there appears to be a separate ossicle at the caudal margin of the glenoid (large arrow).

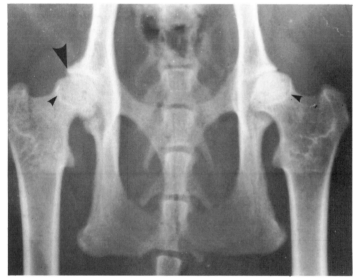

Fig. 3.14 Ventrodorsal radiograph of the pelvis, showing bilateral osteoarthritis of the hip joints. There is a collar of new bone on each femoral neck (small arrows) with new bone on the cranial effective acetabular rim (large arrow). There is slight dysplasia.

much as possible, i.e. to try to encourage the cat to exercise at certain set times of the day. If the clinical problem is particularly bad at any time, strict rest for a few days is desirable.

NON-STEROIDAL ANTI-RHEUMATIC DRUGS
The use of anti-rheumatic drug therapy is restricted because of the many toxicity problems that occur. Many drugs that are used in the dog and man are untried in the cat and it is unwise to experiment with these drugs. Phenylbutazone has been used in the cat (English & Seawright, 1964).

However, toxicity was seen in an experimental study at a daily dose of 44 mg/kg bodyweight. The cat showed progressive loss of appetite, decrease in bodyweight, dehydration, depression and death (Carlisle *et al.*, 1968). Degenerative changes in the kidney were seen histologically. It is suggested that if phenylbutazone is used in the cat, the dose should be 6–12 mg/kg bodyweight in a divided dose and that continuous, prolonged therapy should be avoided. Aspirin at a dose of 25 mg/kg every 24 hours can also be used in the cat (Davis & Westfall, 1972). There is also a study suggesting

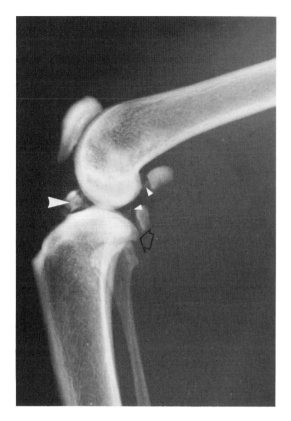

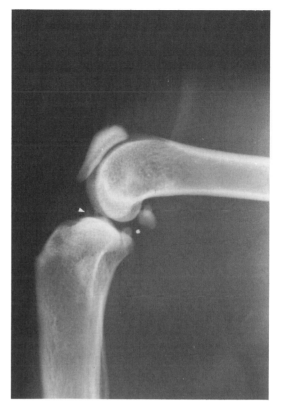

Fig. 3.15 Lateral radiograph of the stifle joint showing extensive calcification with the cranial cruciate ligament (large arrow). There is also calcification within the soft tissues of the joint on the caudal aspect of the femorotibial joint (small arrows). There is new bone production on the caudal aspect of the tibia (open arrow). This cat was not lame.

Fig. 3.16 Lateral radiograph of the stifle joint showing calcification within the joint space (arrow). An anteroposterior view suggested this was within the medial meniscus. This is a common incidental finding in the feline knee joint.

that flunixin* may be used in the cat at a dose of 1.0 mg/kg once a day (Lees & Taylor, 1991) although no clinical trials involving repeated dosing have been done. Ketaprofen† at a dose of 1 mg/kg daily for 5 days, is also recommended for the cat.

CORTICOSTEROIDS
There is much argument as to the value of corticosteroids in the treatment of osteoarthritis.

* Finadyne; Scherine-Plough Animal Health, Mildenhall, Suffolk, UK.
†Ketofen; Rhône Mérieux Ltd., Spire Green Centre, Harlow, Essex UK.

They are, of course, safe to use in the cat and can produce obvious clinical improvement, even at relatively low doses, for example 0.1–0.5 mg prednisolone/kg bodyweight. There is some evidence that high doses of corticosteroids promote cartilage degeneration and can thus speed up the osteoarthritic process. Short courses are preferable and should only be repeated if the clinical problem is particularly severe. Corticosteroids are useful in those joints showing acute flare-ups of lameness.

ANALGESIC DRUGS
The opiate, dextropropoxyphene, can be used in the cat at a daily dose rate of up to 32 mg *per os*, or 2.2 mg/kg by intramuscular injection (Davis &

Donnelly, 1968). There is a human formulation of this drug, with paracetamol (Distalgesic), which has been used, although paracetamol toxicity causing death is reported in the cat (Leyland & O'Meara, 1974). It is suggested that an adult cat should not receive more than 300 mg of paracetamol per day (see also Chapter 27).

Morphine is the potent analgesic of choice in the cat. However, it is seldom required for the treatment of osteoarthritis, although it may be used in other types of arthritis; the dose should not exceed 0.1 mg/kg bodyweight by subcutaneous or intramuscular injection (Davis & Donnelly, 1968; Yoxall, 1978). Similarly, pethidine is rarely used in osteoarthritis; it is much less toxic than morphine but doses in excess of 100 mg may cause excitement and chronic convulsions (Wilkinson, 1968).

SODIUM HYALURONATE
The intra-articular injection of sodium hyaluronate* is recommended for treating osteoarthritis. The dose is 0.1 ml and the injection can be combined with surgery. It is difficult to evaluate the usefulness of this drug in small animal patients.

POLYSULPHATED GLYCOSAMINOGLYCANS
The intra-articular injection of polysulphated glycosaminoglycans† (dose 0.1 ml once a week for 4 weeks) can be used in the cat. The drug can help cartilage repair and improve synovial fluid viscosity. The subcutaneous injection of pentosan sulphate‡ at a dose of 3 mg/kg bodyweight is an alternative treatment; a course of four injections is given at weekly intervals.

Surgical treatment

CORRECTION OF ANY UNDERLYING CAUSE AND DEBRIDEMENT
In cases of secondary osteoarthritis, correction of the underlying cause may be possible, for

* Hyartil-Vet.; Pharmacia Ltd., Hounslow, Middlesex, UK.
†Adequan; Janssen Animal Health, Wantage, Oxon, UK.
‡Cartrophen-Vet; Univet Ltd., Bicester, Oxon, UK.

example the insertion of a prosthetic ligament into an unstable joint. In some cases, debridement of the joint is feasible, and includes the removal of osteophytes (cheilectomy) or loose bodies.

EXCISION ARTHROPLASTY
The destruction of a joint by removing one of the bony components can often help in producing a pain-free articulation, for example femoral head resection or condylectomy of the mandible.

REPLACEMENT ARTHROPLASTY
The replacement of a diseased joint with a prosthetic one has been used in the cat, but technical and financial restrictions are significant.

ARTHRODESIS
Surgical fusion of an arthritic joint can be helpful in removing pain. Obviously joint motion is lost and therefore the animal has a stiff limb. Most of the major limb joints of the cat can be arthrodesed — elbow, carpus, stifle and hock joints. The main reason for arthrodesis is chronic instability of the joint associated with extensive ligament damage and osteoarthritis.

Infective arthritis

Infective arthritis is defined as an inflammatory arthropathy caused by a microbial agent, which can be isolated from the joint.

Bacterial arthritis (septic arthritis)
Bacteria may enter a joint via a penetrating wound, or by extension of infection from surrounding tissues, including bone and soft tissue, or by haematogenous localization. The commonest type in the cat is penetrating bite wounds sustained during fights with other cats. Any joint can be affected although the carpus is most commonly involved.

Haematogenous spread is associated with an infected focus elsewhere in the body from which the organisms originate, for example oral, respiratory, genitourinary and skin infections. Single joint involvement is usual. Bacterial endocarditis, although rare in the cat, is another possible source of infection and may involve several joints. In young kittens, an infective arthritis can be associated with an infected umbilicus or postparturient uterine and mammary gland infections of the queen. In these cases, several different joints of the kitten can become infected. Joint abscessation may be evident and severe joint destruction can occur, in which case euthanasia is often necessary. Haematogenous infection is more likely to localize to a joint that has been traumatized and thus an initial lameness due to a 'sprain' may become complicated by infection within a few days. Osteoarthritis also predisposes a joint to infection. Spinal joints can become infected (see below).

Various organisms can be involved, including *Staphylococcus* spp., *Streptococcus* spp., *Pasteurella* spp., coliforms and anaerobes.

CLINICAL SIGNS

Generally only a single joint is affected and the joint is usually swollen, hot and painful. There may be loss of joint movement and crepitus, if present, generally indicates extensive bony and cartilage damage. Systemic illness may be present, but not in all cases. Other signs may be present in specific cases, for example skin wounds with penetrating bites.

RADIOGRAPHY

Soft tissue swelling is the most obvious feature in the early stages. The joint capsule may be obviously thickened or distended, causing displacement of fascial planes. Intra-articular fat pads may lose their radiolucency as exudate accumulates. The joint space may be widened although changes in joint space are difficult to assess without weight-bearing radiographs. Periosteal new bone, which can often be extensive, is another feature (Figs. 3.17 & 3.18). Destruction of articular cartilage may be seen as a loss of joint space. Bony destruction will also occur with time; this may be seen as an erosive change or as a more obvious loss of bone with an irregular widening of the joint space (Figs. 3.17 & 3.18). Periarticular calcification is sometimes seen.

Ligament damage can be a complication to

infective arthritis and may be appreciated on radiography. Secondary osteoarthritic changes may also occur. Advancing osteomyelitis in adjacent bones is sometimes also apparent (Figs. 3.17 & 3.18). Sclerosis of bone adjacent to the infection may be seen and sometimes bony ankylosis occurs.

LABORATORY FEATURES

A leucocytosis may or may not be present. Mild anaemia is often a feature. Aspiration of synovial fluid from the affected joint is a useful procedure for diagnostic confirmation. The fluid is increased in quantity, turbid and watery, and sometimes bloody. The mucin clot is poor and the fibrinogen clot often positive. White cells are increased in number and the majority are polymorphs. The presence of toxic, ruptured and degranulated neutrophils is often associated with bacterial arthritis.

The synovial fluid can be cultured for bacterial organisms and antibiotic sensitivity testing performed. However, in some cases the organisms cannot be grown from the fluid, although culture of a synovial membrane biopsy will yield the organism.

TREATMENT

Systemic antibiotic administration, preferably based on sensitivity testing, is the treatment of choice. Treatment for several weeks (2–6 weeks) is generally the rule. In some cases, a drainage tube can be inserted into the joint to allow drainage and local instillation of antibiotics (Fig. 3.19). Soluble ampicillin can be given intra-articularly; a combination of amoxycillin and clavulanic acid* and clindamycin are useful systemic antibiotics for joint infections.

If articular damage is severe, surgical treatment may be necessary, for example arthrodesis, excision arthroplasty or even amputation.

Once the infection has been cleared, any residual lameness can be treated with short-term corticosteroids, since some cases of bacterial in-

* Synulox; Smith Kline Beecham Animal Health, Tadworth, Surrey, UK.

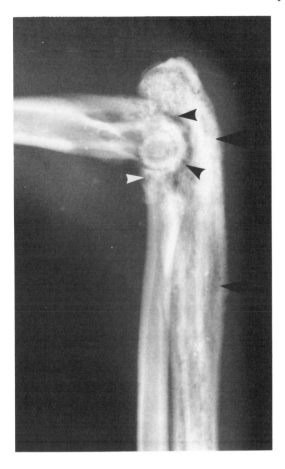

Fig. 3.17 Lateral radiograph of the left elbow illustrating a bacterial infective arthritis. There is a widened, irregular humero-ulnar joint space (small black arrows); an erosive destruction of bone in the radial head (white arrow); and extensive periosteal new bone deposited along the ulnar shaft (large black arrows).

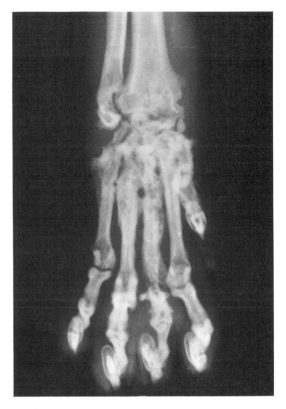

Fig. 3.18 Craniocaudal radiograph of the left carpus and foot illustrating a bacterial infective arthritis of the carpus. The carpal bones show obvious destruction. There is periosteal new bone on the distal radius and ulna and along the metacarpal bones. The infection has obviously extended the length of metacarpal bone 3 and into the metacarpophalangeal joint causing its destruction.

fective arthritis are complicated by a persisting synovitis associated with non-viable microbial antigens. Corticosteroids can control this inflammation. These drugs may also help to reduce soft tissue swelling and joint stiffness.

Arthritis associated with bacterial L-forms

Three cats with pyogenic subcutaneous abscesses and arthritis associated with a probable bacterial L-form (i.e. a cell wall-deficient bacterium) were described by Carro *et al.* (1989). The infection spread locally and haematogenously to involve

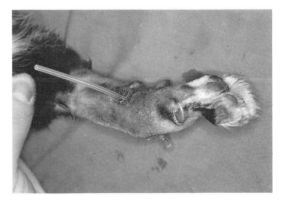

Fig. 3.19 Photograph showing a drainage tube inserted into an infected carpus.

other joints and subcutaneous sites. Joint destruction was evident on radiography of some joints. Although the infection was resistant to many broad-spectrum antibiotics, it was readily susceptible to tetracycline. These organisms are very difficult to grow in the laboratory and routine cultures of the abscesses and joints will be negative.

Mycoplasmal arthritis

There are several different feline isolates of mycoplasmas, and most are found naturally in the upper respiratory and urogenital tracts of healthy cats. A case of *Mycoplasma gateae* infection in a cat has been reported (Moise *et al.*, 1983). The cat suffered a polyarthritis and tenosynovitis and there were bone and cartilage erosions. There was evidence that the cat was immunosuppressed, i.e. lowered gammaglobulin levels in the blood. Pedersen *et al.* (1983b) also reported a single case in an old debilitated cat being treated with surgery and radiation for an oral squamous cell carcinoma. *M. felis* was isolated from a young cat with a fibrinopurulent polyarthritis and tenosynovitis and, again, there were thought to be underlying immunodeficiencies (Hooper *et al.*, 1985).

The synovial fluid is thin and cloudy and contains large numbers of white cells, most of which are neutrophils. The neutrophils are not toxic, degranulated or ruptured. The organisms can be cultured on special media or sometimes visualized in the fluid by using Wright–Leishmann or Giemsa stains. Mycoplasmal arthritis can be treated with tylosin, gentamycin, erythromycin or tetracycline.

Calicivirus arthritis

A fleeting stiffness, soreness and lameness with high fever has been reported in young kittens, 6–12 weeks of age, possibly caused by certain strains of calicivirus infection (Pedersen *et al.*, 1983a). The kittens are often ill for 2–4 days and demonstrate pain when muscles and joints are manipulated. During the acute phase of illness, calicivirus can be recovered from the blood, and at least one strain has not been neutralized by antibodies produced by the more commonly used vaccine strains. The condition can therefore occur in kittens vaccinated with some calicivirus vaccines. The prognosis is good, as the disease seems self-limiting.

An experimental study with two strains of calicivirus (FCV-2280 and FCV-LLIC) has produced a transient 'limping' syndrome in young kittens (Pedersen *et al.*, 1983a). Joints appeared to be painful on manipulation, but examination of synovial fluid and synovial membrane did not show an active arthritis. Fluorescent antibody techniques also failed to demonstrate a virus within the joints. The author has also produced arthritis and lameness in cats experimentally infected with field strains of calicivirus, and has cultured live virus from the diseased joint (Dawson *et al.*, 1993).

A transient, sometimes protracted inflammatory (poly)arthropathy occurs as an uncommon complication to vaccination (Dawson *et al.*, 1992). The component of the multivalent vaccines that is responsible is calicivirus, since calicivirus antigens have been demonstrated within synovial macrophages of vaccinated cats (Bennett *et al.*, 1989). Treatment is usually unnecessary, although corticosteroids can be given in persistent cases. This form of polyarthritis is similar to Type II idiopathic polyarthritis, as discussed below. Calicivirus can certainly produce an acute arthritis in the cat either following natural infection or live virus vaccination, and this may be associated with intra-articular live virus or non-viable virus antigens, suggesting that calicivirus can produce a true infectious viral arthritis and also an immune-based arthritis. In most cases the arthritis is short-lived. The role of calicivirus in chronic arthritis is uncertain.

Lyme disease

Lyme disease as first described in man is a multisystemic illness associated with infection by the tick-borne spirochaete *Borrelia burgdorferi*. The term borreliosis, Lyme borreliosis and Lyme arthritis are also used to describe the disease attributed to *B. burgdorferi*. The infection appears widespread and has been described in many domestic animals (e.g. dogs, cats, horses and

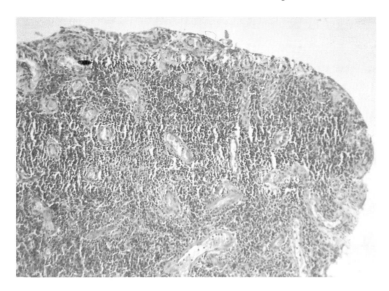

Fig. 3.20 Photomicrograph of a synovial membrane biopsy from a cat with periosteal proliferative polyarthritis. There is an extensive mononuclear cell infiltrate (H&E) (×50).

cattle) as well as man in the USA, Europe and Asia. Magnarelli *et al.* (1990) reported that 10 of 71 serum samples taken from cats which had been infected with ticks were positive for *B. burgdorferi* antibodies. They also reported that of two larvae and 20 nymphs removed from cats, one larva and two nymphs were infected with the spirochaete. Jacobson and Saidla (1990) reported seropositivity in 15% of feline sera samples submitted for *B. burgdorferi* titres. Although cats can become infected and seroconvert, there is disagreement as to whether they suffer clinical disease. The clinical signs reported in domestic animals, especially the dog, include fever, anorexia, lethargy, lymphadenopathy and lameness. The lameness is generally, but not always, localized to one or more joints, which may be swollen, hot and painful on manipulation. Muscle disease, meningitis, carditis, renal disease and neurological disease have also been reported. Because the clinical signs can be somewhat vague and because infection can occur without clinical disease, it is difficult to diagnose Lyme disease accurately. The criteria for diagnosis are discussed in a review by Bennett *et al.* (1992), but basically these should be:

1 History of exposure to ticks
2 Clinical disease consistent with borreliosis
3 Laboratory features consistent with clinical disease
4 Positive serological test for *Borrelia* antibodies
5 Prompt response to antibiotic therapy in most cases
6 Exclusion of other possible diagnoses.

Culture of the organism from disease tissues would confirm the diagnosis but the organism is very fastidious and difficult to grow in the laboratory.

Immune-based arthritis

The classification of feline immune-based arthritis is shown in Fig. 3.11. There are several different types and, in all, the main pathological feature is a chronic active synovitis (Fig. 3.20) generally affecting several joints in a bilaterally symmetrical fashion. The aetiology of all these types of arthritis is unknown, and although infection may be suspected, no microorganisms can be cultured from the joint; they are referred to as the non-infective inflammatory polyarthropathies.

They can be distinguished from other types of arthritis because of their multiple joint involvement, the presence of watery synovial fluid within affected joints containing large numbers of polymorphonuclear cells, and the radiographic features (Table 3.2). As a group, they are rare and this makes accurate descriptions difficult. The following account is based on the author's cases (Bennett & Nash, 1985), and those reported by Pedersen *et al.* (1980), Wilkinson and Robins (1979), Moise and Crissman (1982) and Robertson (1982). They can be subdivided into two broad groups according to whether or not there are destructive changes visible on the radiographs. Where such changes are present the arthritis is referred to as an erosive type, if not as a non-erosive type.

Erosive types

RHEUMATOID ARTHRITIS (RA)

This may be defined as a chronic, progressive and destructive polyarthritis. The criteria used to standardize the diagnosis of this disease are based on those used in human rheumatology.

1 Stiffness after rest.
2 Pain or tenderness on motion of at least one joint.
3 Swelling of at least one joint.
4 Swelling of one other joint within a 3-month period.
5 Symmetrical joint swelling.
6 Subcutaneous nodules (not yet reported in the cat).
7 Radiographic changes suggestive of rheumatoid arthritis.
8 Serological evidence of rheumatoid factor.
9 Abnormal synovial fluid.
10 Characteristic histological changes in the synovium.
11 Characteristic histological changes in subcutaneous nodules.

To diagnose classical rheumatoid arthritis, seven criteria must be fulfilled and five fulfilled to diagnose definite rheumatoid arthritis. In addition, two of criteria 7, 8 and 10 should be satisfied. Also with criteria 1–5, they should be present for at least 6 weeks.

Rheumatoid arthritis is classed as an autoimmune disease because of the presence of rheumatoid factor (RF), an autoantibody against immunoglobulin, although RF is not always de-tectable and can occur in other joint diseases. The pathogenesis of the synovitis involves immune complex formation within the joint, which involves RF.

PERIOSTEAL PROLIFERATIVE POLYARTHRITIS (PPP)

This disease is characterized by extensive periosteal new bone around affected joints, mainly the hocks and carpii (Fig. 3.21). Erosive changes in the joints usually occur, and pathology also occurs at the attachment of ligaments and tendons (enthesopathies).

The pathogenesis of the synovitis is uncertain although it is believed to involve immune complexes. Pedersen *et al.* (1980, 1983b) have related the aetiology of the disease to feline leukaemia virus and feline syncytia-forming virus infections. They suggest leukaemia virus produces immunosuppression and allows syncytia-forming virus to multiply in the joints of certain genetically predisposed individuals to cause the disease. However, the incidence of leukaemia virus in affected cats is no greater than a control population of hospital cats (Bennett, unpublished data) and feline syncytia-forming virus has not been successful in producing the disease experimentally (Pedersen *et al.*, 1980). This virus is regularly cultured from the tissues of normal cats, including the joints, and it may be that an inflamed joint, containing many actively dividing cells, is an ideal environment for the virus to grow.

Non-erosive types

ARTHRITIS ASSOCIATED WITH SYSTEMIC LUPUS ERYTHEMATOSUS (SLE)

This is a non-erosive symmetrical polyarthritis and is one feature of a multisystemic disease. The three criteria used to diagnose this disease are listed below.

1 There should be multisystem involvement: the common manifestations are polyarthritis, autoimmune haemolytic anaemia, immune mediated thrombocytopenia, leucopenia, pyrexia, glomerulonephritis, skin disease and meningitis. It can be several weeks before multisystem in-

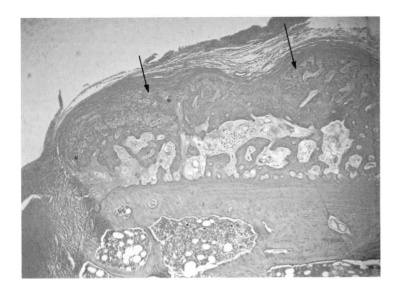

Fig. 3.21 Photomicrograph of a joint with periosteal proliferative polyarthritis. Extensive new bone is present (arrows) (×35).

volvement is apparent. It is rare to have more than two body systems involved at any one time.

2 Antinuclear antibody (ANA) should be detectable in the blood.

3 The immunopathological features consistent with the clinical involvement should be demonstrable: for example antibodies against red cells, platelets and white cells should be shown in cases with anaemia, thrombocytopenia and leucopenia; and immunoglobulin and complement deposits should be shown in tissue biopsies of synovium, kidney and skin in cases showing arthritis, glomerulonephritis and dermatitis.

Criteria 1 and 2 must always be satisfied; if only 1 and 2 are fulfilled, then probable SLE is diagnosed; if all three are satisfied, definite SLE is diagnosed.

SLE is an autoimmune disease because of the presence of autoantibodies, which play an important role in the pathogenesis of the disease – antibodies against red blood cells, platelets and white cells and against nuclear antigens. Complexes of antinuclear antibody, nuclear antigens and complement are thought to produce disease by a Type III hypersensitivity reaction, i.e. arthritis, glomerulonephritis, dermatitis.

IDIOPATHIC ARTHRITIS

All cats with polyarthritis that do not satisfy the criteria for RA, PPP or SLE are included in this broad classification. Idiopathic arthritis is subdivided into four subtypes:

Type I: Uncomplicated polyarthritis, i.e. uncomplicated by the associations described in other subtypes.

Type II: Polyarthritis associated with infection elsewhere in the body, for example conjunctivitis, respiratory tract infection, urinary tract infection, skin infection.

Type III: Polyarthritis associated with gastrointestinal disease.

Type IV: Polyarthritis associated with neoplastic disease, for example myeloproliferative disease.

These types of arthritis are thought to be mediated by immune complex hypersensitivity reactions. Other organs can be involved in the immune complex hypersensitivity, for example kidneys (glomerulonephritis), eyes (uveitis, retinitis) and skin (dermatitis), and thus these cats with multisystemic involvement can resemble cases of SLE, but they are consistently negative for ANA.

The significance of the associations described above is not clear. They may just be coincidental or part of the same disease process. Alternatively, they may represent antigenic foci for immune complex formation.

Clinical signs

The features of cats with polyarthritis are very similar, no matter which type. Rheumatoid arthritis is more chronic in both its onset and clinical course. These cats usually show a generalized stiffness of increasing severity over several months. Reluctance to jump and exercise becomes apparent. The joints may be swollen and painful on manipulation and crepitus and reduced movement are common. In some cases, joint laxity is appreciated and some cats have obvious joint deformities. Any age of cat can be affected. The periosteal proliferative polyarthritis is, again, often chronic in nature and is more commonly seen in male and male-castrate cats. The cats are stiff, and may show periods of inappetence and lethargy. The affected joints (mainly hocks and carpi) become very thickened.

The arthritis of SLE and of the idiopathic types generally has a more rapid onset. The cats are often very uncomfortable and appear sore all over. They become unwilling to exercise and may favour particular limbs. They resent being handled and can become uncooperative. Fever, malaise and stiffness may be present. In many cases, joints are obviously swollen and painful, although in some cases it can be difficult to appreciate either periarticular swelling or synovial distension. SLE and idiopathic polyarthritis are more common in young adult cats.

Cats with SLE and with the idiopathic forms of arthritis may show other signs of immune complex disease, for example skin disease, glomerulonephritis and retinitis. The idiopathic Type II cats will also show signs related to infection elsewhere in the body, for example conjunctivitis, respiratory disease. The author has seen lame cats associated with a chlamydial conjunctivitis (*Chlamydia psittaci* infection), and prolonged treatment of the conjunctivitis with local and oral tetracyclines will resolve the lameness. Chlamydia can be cultured from diseased conjunctiva or the presence of antigens can be demonstrated in conjunctival smears. Chlamydial serum antibodies

are generally increased in cats with chlamydial conjunctivitis (Wills *et al.*, 1988). The Type III cats will have gastrointestinal signs, for example bloody diarrhoea. Loss of bodily condition can occur. The Type IV cats may have signs related to the neoplastic lesion. All cats seen by the author with idiopathic Type IV polyarthritis have had myeloproliferative disease, which can be diagnosed by a bone marrow biopsy examination.

Radiography

The radiographic signs of the different types of inflammatory polyarthropathy can be very similar. Rheumatoid arthritis is characterized typically by bony destructive changes, which can show as obvious erosions in the joint margin, as an increased, often irregular joint space or as an overall loss of mineralization of the bones of the joint (Fig. 3.22). Destructive changes are also seen in periosteal proliferative polyarthritis but are usually less extensive. This form of arthritis is characterized particularly by extensive 'fluffy' deposits of periosteal new bone (Figs. 3.23 & 3.24). These new bone deposits usually extend beyond the confines of the joint. Bony deposits and, sometimes, cortical erosion of bone may also occur where muscles, ligaments and tendons insert, e.g. the triceps brachii attachment on the olecranon and the gastrocnemius tendon on the os calcis (Fig. 3.25). In some cases, extensive new articular bone may develop causing partial or even complete ankylosis (Figs. 3.26 & 3.27).

Periosteal new bone does occur in the other inflammatory arthropathies, but to a lesser extent.

Soft tissue changes may be seen in all cases of polyarthritis and include periarticular thickening, distension of joint capsule and loss of intraarticular fat shadows (Fig. 3.28). These changes are often the only ones seen in systemic lupus erythematosus and idiopathic polyarthritis, but they do consistently occur in other forms and, indeed, in the early stages of rheumatoid and periosteal proliferative polyarthritis, soft tissue changes may be all that are evident, the bony changes occurring later.

Repeated radiography of joints is helpful in

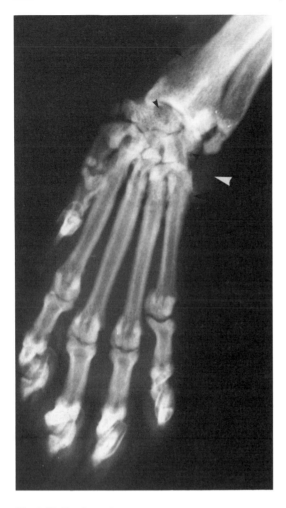

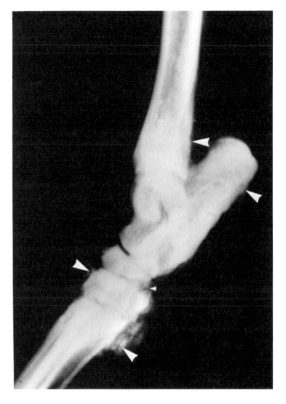

Fig. 3.22 Craniocaudal radiograph of the right carpus of a cat with rheumatoid arthritis. There are obvious erosions within the radial and ulnar carpal bones (small arrows). There is some periosteal new bone production on the radius and proximal metacarpus (large black arrows). There is also obvious increased soft tissue density and swelling (large white arrow).

Fig. 3.23 Lateral radiograph of the left hock joint of a cat with periosteal proliferative polyarthritis. There is an erosive change within the distal intertarsal joint (small arrow). There is an extensive 'fluffy' periosteal deposition of new bone (large arrows) involving all the tarsal bones, distal tibia and proximal metatarsus. The reaction extends well beyond the confines of the hock joint, and is very different to the osteophyte development seen in osteoarthritis.

monitoring the progression of the arthritis. With time, secondary osteoarthritic changes may become apparent as joints become damaged and unstable. Radiography of other body systems may be relevant in some cases, for example evidence of respiratory tract infections.

Laboratory features

Some cases show anaemia, leucocytosis or leucopenia. Serum globulin levels are generally increased, either absolutely or relatively. Blood enzymes (alkaline phosphatase, alanine transaminase, aspartate transaminase) may be increased.

Synovial fluid analysis is useful to confirm an inflammatory arthropathy. The fluid is generally watery and turbid. There is a poor mucin clot and a high white cell count, most of which are polymorphonuclear cells (Table 3.2). The fibrino-

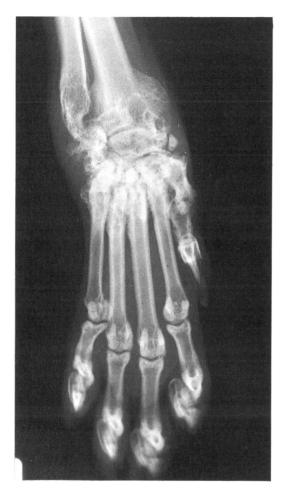

Fig. 3.24 Craniocaudal radiograph of the carpus of a cat with periosteal proliferative polyarthritis. There is extensive new bone formation. Some of the joint spaces appear widened and irregular, consistent with bony destruction.

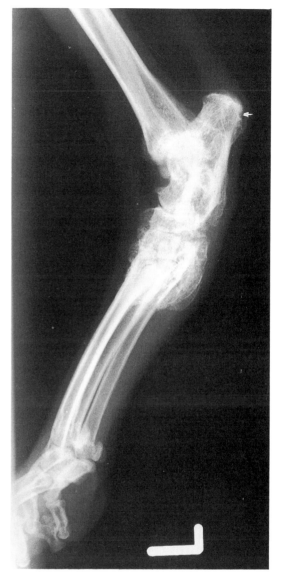

Fig. 3.25 Lateral radiograph of the hock joint of a cat with periosteal proliferative polyarthritis. There is a great deal of new bone production on the tarsal bones, metatarsus and distal tibia. There is new bone on the tuber calcis, together with a small erosion (arrow), consistent with an erosive enthesopathy.

gen clot test may be positive, i.e. the sample may clot on standing if not collected in anticoagulant. Microbiological examination of synovial fluid or synovial membrane samples is negative.

Cats with rheumatoid arthritis may show rheumatoid factor in the blood; this is detected by the modified Rose–Waaler test or by ELISA. Antinuclear antibody must be shown in cats with systemic lupus erythematosus. An indirect immunofluorescence test is generally used (Fig.

3.29). The LE-cell test can also be used to demonstrate antinuclear antibodies in the cat (Fig. 3.30).

Cats with systemic lupus erythematosus may

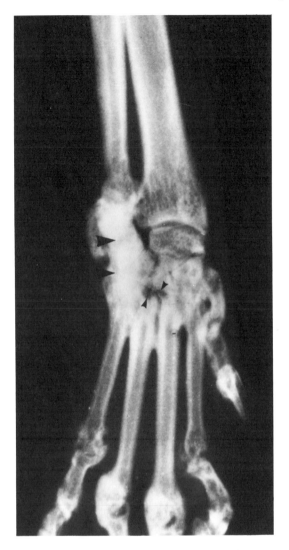

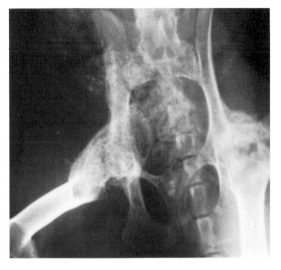

Fig. 3.27 Ventrodorsal radiograph of the pelvis of the same cat as in Fig. 3.26. There is extensive bony proliferation around both hip joints resulting in almost total ankylosis. There was also ankylosis of the left sacroiliac joint of this cat.

Fig. 3.26 Craniocaudal radiograph of the carpus of a cat with periosteal proliferative polyarthritis. There is ankylosis of some joints (large arrows) and destructive changes are also present (small arrows). The metacarpophalangeal joints also show destruction and bony proliferation.

show red blood cell autoantibodies and these can be detected by the direct Coombs' (antiglobulin) test. Autoantibodies against platelets may be shown by the PF-3 test or by ELISA, and against leucocytes by the antiglobulin consumption test.

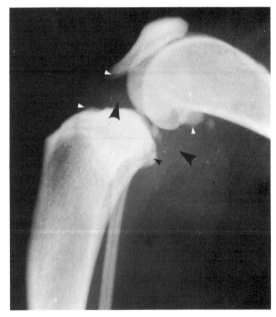

Fig. 3.28 Lateral radiograph of the stifle joint of a cat with idiopathic polyarthritis. There is some loss of the intra-articular fat shadow and distension of the joint capsule on the caudal aspect (large arrows). There are slight secondary osteoarthritic changes (small arrows).

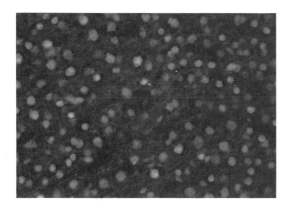

Fig. 3.29 Photomicrograph showing fluorescence of nuclei indicating the presence of antinuclear antibody in a case of systemic lupus erythematosus. Indirect immunofluorescence test, substrate rat liver, anti-feline IgG, FITC (×900).

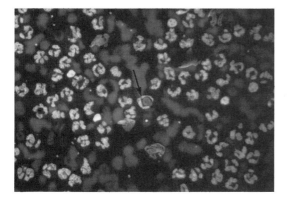

Fig. 3.30 Photomicrograph of a blood smear showing a LE-cell (arrow). Fluorescent-Feulgen stain (×900).

Treatment

Glucocorticoids are the drugs of choice and prednisolone is the most commonly used. For the acute onset cases a dose of between 2 and 4 mg/kg bodyweight is used, and after 2 weeks the dose is gradually reduced. The dose is reduced over a period of 6–8 weeks, providing clinical remission persists. In some cases the drug can be stopped completely, in others a low maintenance dose is necessary. Ideally, alternate day therapy should be used in the latter. If remission does not occur or occurs only at high doses of steroids, then a combination of cytotoxic drugs and prednisolone should be tried. Cyclophosphamide is the most commonly used cytotoxic drug, at a dose of 2.0–2.5 mg/kg bodyweight. The dose is given orally, once daily on four consecutive days of each week. Corticosteroids are used at an anti-inflammatory dose (0.1–0.5 mg/kg).

Complete blood cell counts are done each week whenever an animal is receiving cytotoxic drugs. If the white cell count falls below 6000/mm^3, the dose is decreased by one-quarter; if it falls below 4000/mm^3, the drug should be discontinued for 1 week and then reinstituted at one-half of the original dose. Cytotoxic drugs are stopped 1 month after complete remission is achieved, although steroids may be continued for longer. Cyclophosphamide should not be used for longer than 4 months because of the potential bladder complications. Cats receiving steroids and cytotoxic drugs should be protected, as far as possible, from infections, which could be fatal for an immunosuppressed patient. For example, cats should receive frequent vaccination boosters (dead vaccines only), despite the likelihood of a poor response, and they should be confined in the home environment as much as is practical, and during re-examinations at the surgery care should be taken to minimize exposure to possible pathogens.

With the chronic erosive rheumatoid and periosteal proliferative arthritis cases, it is often better to treat these cats with low-dose prednisolone for short periods when the animal is particularly bad.

In case of idiopathic polyarthritis of Types II, III and IV, treatment of the infective, gastrointestinal or neoplastic process is relevant. If these can be successfully treated, the arthritic problem may resolve without anti-inflammatory or immunosuppressive therapy. If not, these drugs have to be instituted.

Other drugs can be used to help control the articular pain; these have been discussed under osteoarthritis. Gold injections (sodium aurothiomalate*) have been used in human and canine

* Myocrisin; May and Baker Ltd., Dagenham, Essex, UK.

patients and although the author has no experience with this drug in the feline species, it has apparently been used without toxicity problems (Brown, 1964). There is now an oral preparation of gold (auranofin*) and, although it has been used successfully in the dog, there are no data for its use in the cat.

The prognosis of immune-based arthritis in cats is variable, and some cases will not respond very well. Since affected cats can be depressed and miserable, euthanasia is often requested by the owner, although many cats can cope with their disability and retain a reasonable quality of life.

NEOPLASTIC AND NEOPLASTIC-LIKE LESIONS

The classification of bone and joint neoplasms is fraught with confusion due to differences in histopathological assessment by different pathologists. The following classification is based on published reports and the author's accumulated cases.

Osteocartilaginous exostoses (osteochondromatosis)

These lesions occur in a solitary form (solitary osteocartilaginous exostoses or solitary osteochondromatosis) or as a multiple disease (multiple osteocartilaginous exostoses or feline osteochondromatosis (Pool, 1981). The solitary lesions are benign, slow-growing tumours of cartilage origin, and have a cartilaginous cap that gives rise to cancellous bone by endochondral ossification (Turrel & Pool, 1982). They occur at the ends of bones (generally the long bones), most frequently in mature cats, and will cause lameness. The exostoses are seen on radiography; they appear dense and have a slightly irregular but clearly defined border. Treatment is by surgically removing the exostosis; the prognosis is good, although local regrowth can occur. Malignant transformation can sometimes occur (to osteosar-

---

* Ridaura; Bridge Pharmaceuticals, Welwyn Garden City, Herts, UK.

coma, juxtacortical osteosarcoma or chondrosarcoma), and this may necessitate amputation.

The multiple lesions have been reported in the cat by Jubb and Kennedy (1963), Riddle and Leighton (1970), Brown *et al.* (1972), Pool and Carrig (1972), Pool and Harris (1975) and Hubler *et al.* (1986). Most cases have been seen in the Siamese breed although the domestic short hair has also been affected. The lesions are partially ossified protuberances arising from the cortex of bones. Initially the histological features are similar to the solitary form, but eventually they become more like a sarcoma than an osteochondroma. They occur over the scapulae, sternum, ribs, pelvis and cervical lumbar vertebrae and less often affect the limb bones. Radiography shows these to be extensive calcified masses. A retrovirus infection has been suggested as an aetiology for the multiple disease since C-type virus particles have been found in the tumour, and several cats have been FeLV positive. The progress with feline osteochondromatosis is poor, most cats surviving for less than a year after the onset of clinical signs (enlarging masses over the skeleton, lameness, paresis). There is no helpful treatment.

Osteosarcoma

Osteosarcoma is the commonest primary bone neoplasm of the cat (Purdy, 1961; Schmidt & Langham, 1967; Engle & Brodey, 1969; Jacobson, 1971; Liu *et al.*, 1974). Osteosarcoma tends to occur in aged, female domestic short-hair cats — the average age is about 11 years with a range of 2–20 years (Cotchin, 1956, 1957, 1984) although Bitetto *et al.* (1987) reported it more commonly in castrated males. The sites of localization of limb bone tumours are not so sharply defined as in the dog. The humerus, femur and tibia are commonly affected (Cotchin, 1984; Bitetto *et al.*, 1987); the tumour may localize in any particular part of the affected bone although some authors report a predilection in the metaphyses (Bitetto *et al.*, 1987). Most limb bones can be affected as can the sacrum, coccyx, pelvis, ribs and skull. Osteosarcoma associated with a previous fracture has been reported in the cat (Bennett *et al.*, 1979).

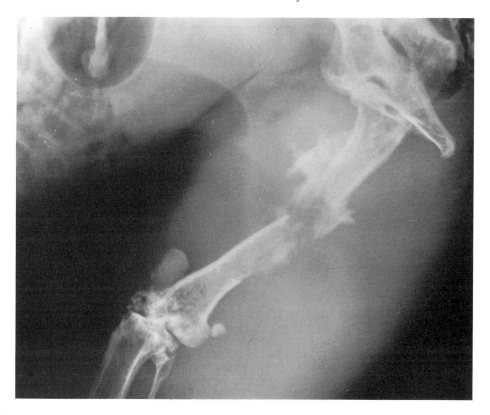

Fig. 3.31 Lateral radiograph of the left femur showing an osteosarcoma which had apparently arisen from a previous fracture site. There is obvious destruction of bone with a small amount of periosteal new bone. Increased soft tissue density is evident. The stifle joint shows calcified masses within the soft tissues (incidental finding).

Clinically, the cats are usually presented with obvious lameness. Swelling over the neoplasm is a consistent feature. Pain over the area and reduced movement in the associated joints is common. The radiographical features are variable (Liu *et al.*, 1974). There may be predominant osteolysis, characterized by radiolucency of the bone, with thinning and loss of the cortices, and this is most likely with tumours of the appendicular skeleton (Figs. 3.31 & 3.32). Sunbursting and periosteal new bone, including the Codman's triangle phenomenon may be seen. In other cases, the tumours appear very radiodense and the radiodensity extends into the soft tissues with an irregular outline (Fig. 3.33). Pathological fractures are not uncommon. Confirmation of the diagnosis may be made by the histological examination of a biopsy.

In general, osteosarcomas metastasize slowly in cats, although spread to the lungs, regional lymph nodes and kidneys has been reported. Treatment by surgical excision of the mass or amputation of the affected limb has been apparently successful, with no sign of metastatic disease (Liu *et al.*, 1974; Bitetto *et al.*, 1987).

Extraskeletal osteosarcoma

Extraskeletal osteosarcomas have been defined as malignant bone-forming tumours arising from somatic soft tissue without connection to any osseous structures. They are extremely rare neoplasms and only one case is reported in the cat (Arnone *et al.*, 1984).

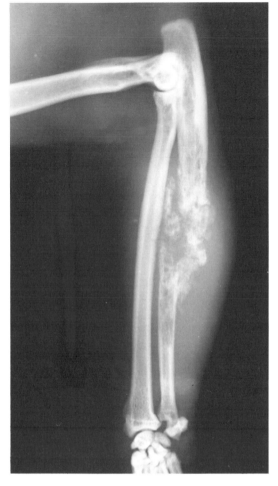

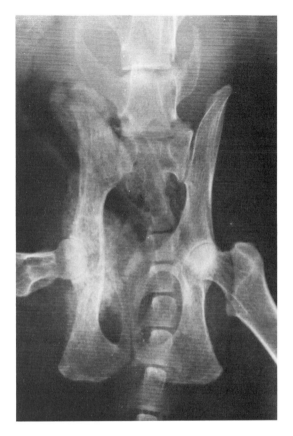

Fig. 3.33 Ventrodorsal radiograph of the pelvis showing an osteosarcoma arising from the vicinity of the acetabulum. There is extensive new bone production which has an irregular border.

Fig. 3.32 Lateral radiograph of the lower limb showing an osteosarcoma of the mid-shaft ulna. There is obvious bone destruction with minimal periosteal new bone. Soft tissue swelling is obvious.

Extraskeletal osteoma

A benign osseous neoplasm was described in the foreleg of an 8-year-old spayed female cat (Jobora & Paton, 1984). It was described as an osteoma and was surgically excised. A similar lesion described by Jacobson (1971) was classified as an ossifying fibroma-osteoma; this tumour recurred after local excision.

Parosteal osteoma
(feline osteoma, parosteal osteosarcoma, juxtacortical osteosarcoma)

This is a rare tumour in the cat – it arises from the outer surface of the cortex of bones. Four cases were reported by Liu *et al.* (1974); three developed in the frontal bone and one in the mandible. Jacobson (1971) and Banks (1971) reported the tumour in limb bones. Bitetto *et al.* (1987) reported one case affecting the distal humerus, and Cottril *et al.* (1987) described the tumour affecting both orbits in an eight-year-old cat. Clinically, a hard mass can be palpated and is firmly attached to the bone. The owners usually notice the developing mass. Radiography shows irregular, poorly defined masses of variable mineral density. They are usually attached to the underlying bone cortex but in some planes may appear not to contact the regional bone. The neoplasms appear not to metastasize and thus surgical excision or debulking may be attempted.

Chondrosarcoma

Chrondrosarcoma was reported in three cats by Liu *et al.* (1974). The neoplasms were located in the right ramus of the mandible, the left proximal tibia and the right posterior scapula. The obvious clinical feature was a firm, fixed mass involving bone. The two cats with limb bone involvement were lame. Radiography demonstrated a lobulated, radio-opaque mass which had destroyed portions of the affected bones. Metastases are unlikely and thus radical local excision or limb amputation may be considered. An intranasal chondrosarcoma was reported by Straw *et al.* (1986) and was treated unsuccessfully by radiotherapy.

Osteoma

Osteomas are benign tumours of osteoblastic origin, and have been reported arising from the zygoma, mandible (Knecht & Greene, 1977) and at the dorsum sellae turcicae of the skull (Liu *et al.*, 1974). The masses are firm, non-painful and slow growing. On radiography they appear well circumscribed and radiopaque, with a smooth border. They may be treated by local excision.

Osteoid osteoma

This tumour is composed of a small core or nidus of osteoid tissue surrounded by a mantle of sclerotic bone. Only one case has been reported in the cat (Liu *et al.*, 1974). The tumour occurred in the tenth thoracic vertebra of a 14-year-old cat. The clinical features included pain and inability to jump and groom. Radiography revealed a densely radio-opaque vertebral body that contained a rounded zone of increased radiodensity. This dense nidus was demarcated by a thin radiolucent zone in the otherwise sclerotic body of the vertebra. The mass had expanded and was impinging on the spinal cord.

Multilobular chondromas (chondroma rodens)

These are locally invasive mesenchymal tumours that usually arise from the flat bones of the skull. They are characterized by multiple lobules, each possessing a mature fibrous outer layer, a poorly differentiated mesenchymal middle layer and a central core of cartilage or bone. There are two reports of these tumours affecting the skull of the cat (Jacobson, 1971; Morton, 1985). They can be excised if surgical access allows. Malignant transformation can occur and there is one example of a chondrosarcoma arising from a multilobular chondroma in the cat (Morton, 1985).

Osteoclastoma

Osteoclastoma (giant cell tumours) have been described in the cat; for example, affecting the distal femur in a 1-year-old cat (Howard & Kenyon 1967), the distal tibia of an 8-year-old white Persian (McClelland, 1941), the radius of a 6-year-old cat (Crocker, 1919) and the ulna of a 12-year-old domestic short hair (Bennett & Duff, 1983).

The clinical features include lameness, which may not be severe, and swelling over the affected bone. Pain on pressure is another feature. Radiography shows osteolysis of bone. The lesions appear expansile with thinning of the cortices. Fine bony trabeculae may be seen within the radiolucent area giving a so-called 'soap bubble' appearance (Fig. 3.34). Periosteal bone reaction is generally absent.

Osteoclastomata are usually slow growing and the degree of malignancy is variable. Secondary spread of the tumour to the lungs and kidneys has been reported (Howard & Kenyon, 1967). The case reported by Bennett and Duff (1983) was successfully treated by resection of the lower two-thirds of the ulna. The remaining proximal ulna

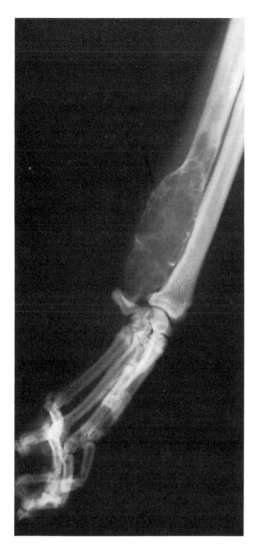

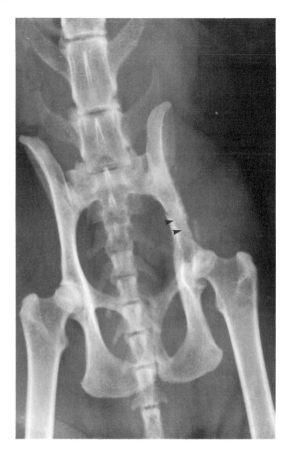

Fig. 3.35 Ventrodorsal radiograph of the pelvis showing a giant cell sarcoma of the ilium. There is bony destruction with some periosteal new bone and soft tissue calcification. A pathological fracture is present (arrow). Osteoarthritis of the hip joints is present (incidental finding).

Fig. 3.34 Lateral radiograph of the lower limb showing an osteoclastoma of the distal ulna. There is an expansile lesion forming a radiolucent defect in which there are several bony trabeculae giving a 'soap-bubble' appearance. The ulnar cortices are thinned.

was fixed to the radius and a bone graft was inserted at the carpus to replace the styloid process of the ulna. The graft was fixed to the distal radius, and was used to anchor the ulnar carpal ligament and a reinforcing prosthetic wire ligament.

Giant cell sarcoma

Two giant cell sarcomas of periosteal origin were reported in the pelvis of two cats; the left ilium of one cat and the left ischium of the other (Bennett, 1975). Radiography showed irregular destructive changes in the ilium together with periosteal new bone; a pathological fracture was also evident (Fig. 3.35). Bony destruction was also visible in the ischium and again a pathological fracture was present (Fig. 3.36).

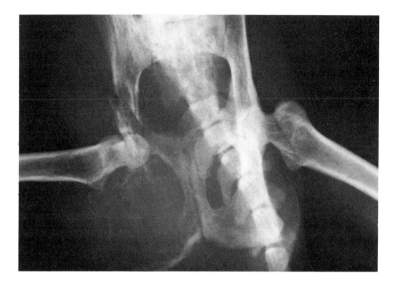

Fig. 3.36 Ventrodorsal radiograph of the pelvis showing a giant cell sarcoma involving the ischium and ilium. There is extensive bony destruction. A pathological fracture of the ilium is present.

Spindle cell sarcoma

A spindle cell sarcoma of periosteal origin was reported in the right ilium of a cat (Bennett, 1975). Radiography revealed a very dense, oval, calcified mass with an irregular border, replacing a large area of the ilium (Fig. 3.37). Secondary tumour deposits were present in the lungs.

Fibrosarcoma

A primary intraosseous (medullary) fibrosarcoma was reported in the olecranon of a 1½-year-old cat (Levitt & Doige, 1989). Radiography revealed osteolysis with minimal new bone production. Amputation of the limb was carried out and although local venous and lymph node metastases were present, the cat was well at a one year follow-up. A similar lesion was reported in the distal ulna of a 9½-year-old cat by Tischler and Owens (1986).

Synovioma

Synovioma is a rare neoplastic lesion of the cat (Nielsen, 1952; Hulse, 1966; Davies & Little, 1972; Thoday & Evans, 1972). The tumours tend to occur in the distal limbs and are intimately associated with the tendon sheaths from which they presumably arise. Local recurrence is com-

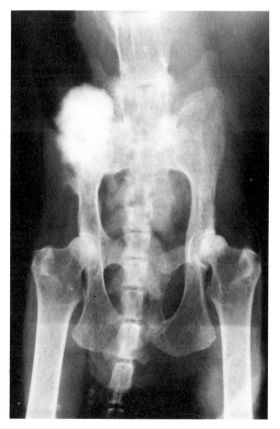

Fig. 3.37 Ventrodorsal radiograph of the pelvis showing a spindle cell sarcoma of the ilium. There is a very dense mass of new bone.

mon and thus amputation of the limb proximal to the lesion is probably the best treatment, although local resection has been successful (Thoday & Evans, 1972). Metastatic spread is rare.

Synovial sarcoma

The synovial sarcoma or malignant synovioma is a very rare neoplasm of the cat. Gresti (1975) reported two cases, both of which were bilateral. The tumours are particularly destructive and radiography reveals soft tissue swelling and bone destruction within the joint with an irregular periosteal response. These tumours rapidly metastasize and thus the prognosis is poor. Limb amputation may be attempted.

Aneurysmal bone cyst

This is a benign lesion of bone characterized by blood-filled spaces and solid areas with spindle cell stroma, containing osteoid and multinucleated giant cells (Spjut *et al.*, 1971). Jacobson (1971) reported a single case and Liu *et al.* (1974) reported three cases in domestic short-hair cats. In the latter series, the lesions arose from the sacrum, coccygeal vertebrae and wing of the left ilium. Swelling and tenderness were the obvious clinical features. Radiographically, the lesion was characterized by a circumscribed eccentrically located 'blown out' rarefaction in the affected bone. The cortex was thin but remained intact. In some radiographs, a lobulated 'soap-bubble'-like trabecular structure extended into the rarefied area. Euthanasia of all three cats was carried out. A case reported in the ribs of a 3½-year-old domestic short-hair cat was treated by surgical resection (Biller *et al.*, 1987) and another case in the scapula of a 15-month-old domestic short-hair cat by amputation (Walker *et al.*, 1975).

Fibrous dysplasia

Fibrous dysplasia is a developmental abnormality of bone characterized by the presence of immature osseous trabeculae in a fibrous matrix

(Jaffe, 1958). The lesion was described in the right ramus of the mandible of an 11-year-old cat and in the distal ulna of a 3-year-old cat (Liu *et al.*, 1974). The mandibular swelling was painless, but was associated with difficulty in opening the mouth. The other cat was lame on the affected foreleg. Radiographically, the affected bone showed a marked homogeneous radiodensity. There was also periosteal new bone formation affecting the ulna. Excision of the mandibular lesion and amputation of the distal ulna were carried out with no recurrence reported.

A generalized congenital case has been seen by the author in a 9-week-old male DSH kitten (Bennett & Kelly, 1984), and was named 'striped bone disease' after the radiographic appearance. The cat was presented with a watery nasal discharge and generalized stiffness and an obvious right foreleg lameness. There was pain on pressure of the long bones and on manipulation of some of the joints. The cat held its lower jaw partly open. The kitten was undersized for its age.

Radiography showed a bizarre striped appearance to all the bones of the skeleton, both axial and appendicular (Fig. 3.38). Multiple bone biopsies showed woven bone covering mature lamellar bone. Intertrabecular fibrous connective tissue was conspicuous and varied in density throughout the biopsies. All biopsies were similar in appearance, suggesting some form of dysplasia, bearing some resemblance to human fibrous dysplasia of bone. The cat was negative for leukaemia virus, and blood analyses were unremarkable except for a very high ESR. No treatment was given. The cat managed reasonably for a month and then suddenly died; permission for a postmortem examination was refused.

Metastatic neoplasms of bone and joints

Secondary spread of primary soft tissue neoplasms to the skeletal system seems to be rare in the cat (Russell & Walker, 1983). They include mammary gland carcinoma (Kas *et al.*, 1970) and bronchial carcinoma (Gustafsson & Wolfe, 1968; Pool *et al.*, 1974; Pollack *et al.*, 1984; May &

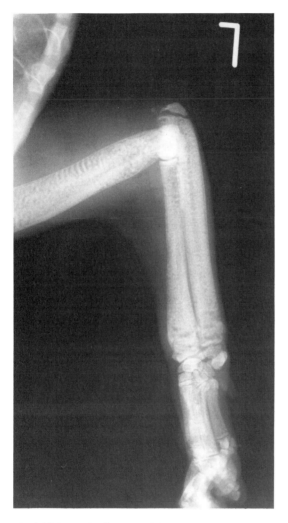

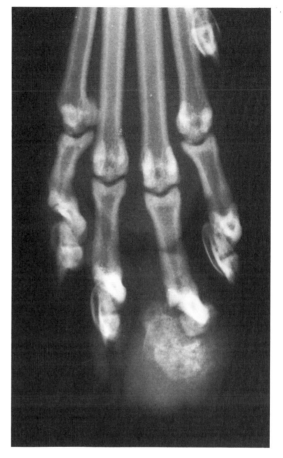

Fig. 3.39 Craniocaudal radiograph of the foot of an 8-year-old cat with a bronchial carcinoma metastasis to digit 3. The digital pad is swollen and there is extensive calcification within the soft tissues. The 3rd phalanx shows local osteolysis.

Fig. 3.38 Lateral radiograph of the forelimb of a 9-week-old kitten with 'striped' bone disease. There is a bizarre appearance of the long bones. The cortices are thickened and there are areas of radiolucency and radiodensity often giving a 'striped' appearance. There are several irregular areas of radiolucency in the distal radius and ulna.

Newsholme, 1989). Metastasis of pulmonary carcinoma to the digits is an interesting syndrome; metastases generally affect multiple digits (Pool *et al.*, 1974; Pollock *et al.*, 1984; May & Newsholme, 1989). The pulmonary lesion may be very small and difficult to identify even at postmortem examination and certainly can be present

without respiratory signs (May & Newsholme, 1989). These cats with digital involvement present with multiple digital swelling and painful lameness and frequently a permanent exsheathment of the claw of the affected digit. Radiography shows bone loss of the 3rd (and sometimes 2nd) phalanx with irregular mineralisation and obvious soft tissue opacity (Fig. 3.39). These pulmonary carcinomas can metastasize to other sites, e.g. muscle, kidney, heart, skin (Schmitz, 1978; May & Newsholme, 1989); metastasis to the muscle also produces a painful lameness.

The difficulty of identifying the primary pulmonary lesion may indicate that some cases of 'primary' digital carcinoma (Brown *et al.*, 1985) may in fact have been misdiagnosed. Lymphosarcoma affecting the tarsi of the cat has been reported (Barclay, 1979) and presumably represented a metastatic spread.

Direct extension of neoplasms to bone

Fibrosarcoma
Liu *et al.* (1974) reported 11 cases where a fibrosarcoma had invaded local bone, for example maxilla, frontal bone, mandible, humerus, digital bones, carpus and ribs. The tumour invades and causes lysis of the bone. Many cases do not metastasize and local resection can be successful. With mandibular involvement, partial resection of the lower jaw is feasible (Penwick & Nunamaker, 1987; Withrow & Holmberg, 1983). Despite expectations, the cosmetic and functional results of mandibulectomy are surprisingly good. Similarly, premaxillectomy and maxillectomy have also been used in the cat to treat oral neoplasms involving bone (Salisbury *et al.*, 1986), although recurrence with some tumours is likely (Emms & Harvey, 1986).

A neoplastic syndrome characterized by multicentric subcutaneous fibrosarcomas has been reported (Hardy, 1976; Susanek, 1983). These tumours are fast growing, developing in cats less than 5 years old, and are associated with a C-type oncornavirus (feline sarcoma virus). Metastases of these tumours to muscle and lung as well as local invasion of bone can occur. The prognosis is poor.

Carcinomas
Of eight cats with squamous cell carcinoma involving bone, invasion of the skull bones occurred in six cases and the bones of the digits in two (Liu *et al.*, 1974). Radiography shows loss of bone mineralization with erosion and soft tissue swelling. Periosteal new bone is also sometimes evident. Oral carcinomas involving the bones of the skull have also been reported by Emms and Harvey (1986), Salisbury *et al.* (1986) and Straw *et al.* (1986).

Other neoplasms
Lymphosarcoma, lymphoma, rhabdomyosarcoma, melanoma, haemangiosarcoma, reticulum cell sarcoma and meningiosarcoma have all been associated with bony involvement (Liu *et al.*, 1974; Straw *et al.*, 1986). A mandibular epidermoid carcinoma associated with extensive bony proliferation has been reported in the cat (Miller *et al.*, 1969). In young cats, fibromeloblastoma is generally invasive into the maxilla, and has been reported in Siamese and short-hair cats (Engle & Brodey, 1969; Dubielzig *et al.*, 1979). Neurofibrosarcoma (Brown *et al.*, 1978), fibromatous epulis (Salisbury *et al.*, 1986) and malignant fibrous histiocytoma (Gleiser *et al.*, 1979) are other examples of soft tissue neoplasms invading adjacent bone.

Synovial cyst

A subcutaneous synovial cyst was recently described in a 16½-year-old spayed DSH cat (Prymak & Goldschmidt, 1991). It was located over the medial aspect of the elbow joint and was surgically excised without complications or recurrence. Synovial cysts are benign lesions which originate from the synovium of joints, bursae or tendon sheaths. These are usually noticed as a developing mass although they can occasionally result in skin ulceration. They should be included in a differential diagnosis of tumours in the subcutaneous tissues of the extremities. Their exact pathogenesis is unknown.

Synovial osteochondrometaplasia

This condition (also called synovial osteochondromatosis) is characterized by osseous and cartilaginous masses formed by hyperplastic metaplasia of synovial cells (Freund, 1937). The cartilaginous masses often undergo calcification. The bony and cartilaginous lesions are found embedded within the synovial layer. The disease is most often monoarticular and can cause lameness particularly in the later stages. It has been reported in metacarpal joints (Pool, 1981) and in the stifle and elbow (Hubler *et al.*, 1986). The lesions are readily apparent on radiography and often have the appearance of being free joint bodies. However, because they are within the synovium they are very difficult to remove surgically. Surgical stripping of the synovium with the lesions is possible but surgical access will always be limited. Synovial osteochondrometaplasia has been linked to osteochondromatosis (multiple cartilaginous exostoses) (Hubler *et al.*, 1986).

INHERITED, CONGENITAL AND DEVELOPMENTAL DISORDERS

Osteogenesis imperfecta

This is an inherited bone disease characterized by poor mineralization and excessive bone fragility. Although this term was commonly used in the early literature to describe poor bony mineralization in young cats and dogs, most of these cases were purely nutritional in aetiology (nutritional secondary hyperparathyroidism) and thus the term was incorrectly used. However, the author has seen cases of osteopenia in kittens not related to nutrition which could be classified as osteogenesis imperfecta. Such cases usually present with bone pain, sometimes associated with pathological fractures. The cats are usually stunted, reluctant to move and often have periods of depression and inappetence. The diet is satisfactory (a low-calcium, high-phosphorus diet will exacerbate the clinical signs) and blood calcium and phosphorus levels are normal. Radiography reveals a poorly mineralized skeleton and evidence of pathological fractures. There are two forms of this disease – osteogenesis imperfecta congenita, which is the more serious, and osteogenesis imperfecta tarda. The former is often complicated by other signs such as thin ('blue') sclera, translucent teeth, thoracic abnormalities, thin skin, herniae, deafness and wormian bones visible on skull radiographs. Treatment of these

conditions is often unrewarding and euthanasia is generally necessary. Supplementation of the diet with bonemeal is necessary to help skeletal mineralization and the bone pain has to be controlled with either non-steroidal anti-inflammatory drugs or with low doses of corticosteroids (corticosteroids may inhibit skeletal mineralization). The author has only seen cases which would fit the osteogenesis imperfecta tarda category and this is the only type described elsewhere (Gehring, 1975; Jezyk, 1985; Cohn & Meuten, 1990).

Juvenile idiopathic osteoporosis or osteopenia is a similar disorder of decreased skeletal density which differs from osteogenesis imperfecta only in that the prognosis is good (the animals improve as they mature) and there are no abnormalities seen on the skull radiographs.

Manx cat

Absence of a tail in the Manx breed is inherited as a dominant trait and Manx homozygotes die prior to birth. The Manx gene is apparently semi-lethal in that females are in preponderance.

There are four expressions of the Manx gene which are controlled by modifying polygenes (Wilkinson, 1984c). The 'rumpy' is the true Manx cat without tail vertebrae. The 'rumpy-riser' has a small number of coccygeal vertebrae forming a usually immobile upright projection. The 'stumpy' has a longer, usually mobile tail, although it is often kinked, knobbly and deformed. The rarer 'longie' has a longer but still short tail of normal appearance. The gene produces effects throughout the vertebral column varying from a slight decrease in length of individual vertebrae in the cranial spine to a decrease in number and fusion of more caudal vertebrae. Pelvic and sacral bones are also involved and there may be spina bifida, which may cause neurogenic incontinence and defaecatory problems. The latter is made worse by the reduced lumen of the pelvic canal (see also Chapter 2).

Kinked tail

A kink between the coccygeal vertebrae has been reported as a recessive trait in domestic cats (Catcott, 1964; Saperstein *et al.*, 1976).

Polydactylia

The presence of extra digits on one or more feet is not uncommon (Danforth, 1947a,b; Chapman & Zeiner, 1961; Sis & Getty, 1968). The forefeet are most often affected and usually five toes are present in addition to the dew claws. The condition is inherited as an autosomal, single dominant trait, the probable effect of which is to incite some change in the pre-axial (i.e. medial) part of the limb bud causing an excess of growth in that area (Sis & Getty, 1968); the gene has variable expressivity. Affected cats can normally cope although regular trimming of the nails is often necessary. Amputation of extra digits is sometimes indicated if secondary complications occur, for example recurrent interdigital infections or recurrent traumatic injury.

Ectrodactylia

The congenital absence of one or more toes or parts of a digit is rare in the cat (Searle, 1952; Schneck, 1974a). Schneck (1974a) described a kitten with only two toes on the left forefoot.

Syndactylia

Fusion of the digits in a cat has been reported (Hays, 1917); it is rare.

Amelia and hemimelia

The congenital absence of a limb or limbs (amelia) and the congenital absence of the whole or part of the distal limb (hemimelia) occur occasionally in kittens (Catcott, 1964; Lewis & Van Sickle, 1970; Schneck, 1974b; Jezyk, 1985). Radial and ulnar hemimelia are most often seen. Agenesis of the rear limb is described as peromelus ascelus and is very rare.

Arrested development of the long bones of the forelimbs

A congenital failure of the forelimb bones to grow to their natural length has been reported in the cat (Williams-Jones, 1944; Robinson, 1971). Such cats are referred to as 'kangaroo cats'.

Mandible ramus aplasia

Abnormal ossification of the mandible resulting in micrognathia has been reported in the cat (Ingham, 1970).

Congenital duplication

Various types of duplication have been described (Saperstein *et al.*, 1976).

Arthrogryposis

A 2-month-old domestic short-hair cat was presented with an inability to flex and extend its joints (Saperstein *et al.*, 1976). There was marked fatty atrophy of all the limb muscles. The cat was euthanased.

Chondrodysplasia

The Scottish fold-ear cat arises from a single dominant gene, which if homozygous results in the ear fold, accompanied by skeletal abnormalities of the tail and lower extremities (Jackson, 1975). The tail is short and stumpy due to the gross reduction in length of coccygeal vertebrae with expansion of the epiphyseal plates. There is also shortening of the feet due to decreased length of metacarpal, metatarsal and phalangeal bones. Certain bones tend to fuse and a large easily recognized tarsal exostosis is formed. These deformities can be avoided and the fold-ear retained by always mating fold-ear to normal prick-ear cats.

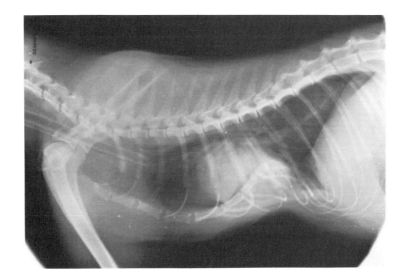

Fig. 3.40 Lateral radiograph of the thoracic cavity of a cat with pectus excavatum. The caudal sternebrae are displaced dorsally, causing displacement of the heart and trachea. The cat was presented with chronic coughing and tachypnoea.

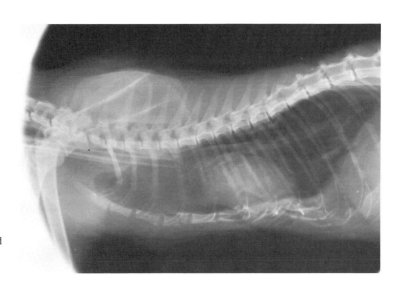

Fig. 3.41 Lateral radiograph of the thoracic cavity of the cat shown in Fig. 3.40. Surgical resection of the deformed sternebrae has been carried out. The heart and trachea are better positioned.

Achondroplasia

Another form of dwarfism associated with a lysosomal storage disease of the liver has been described in the cat (Hegreberg & Norby, 1973; Hegreberg *et al.*, 1974). Such cats die between 1 and 4 months of age. In addition to the dwarfism, there is muscle weakness, particularly of the rear limbs, and enlarged liver, spleen and lymph nodes with ascites. The disease is inherited as an autosomal recessive trait.

Congenital hypothyroidism

This is rare in the cat. Affected kittens show disproportionate dwarfism, lethargy, constipation and a juvenile hair coat. Mental retardation may be a feature as may hydrocephalus. Radiographically there is delayed closure of fontanelles, delayed appearance of epiphyses, which when they do appear are irregular and fragmented, and cortical thickening of the long bones.

Maxillofacial compression

Shortening of the maxilla and mandible as in the Persian, Angora and Himalayan breeds has been exaggerated by in-breeding of lines of breeding cats with brachycephalic traits. The condition predisposes to respiratory, pharyngeal and ocular disease. This deformity is also referred to as 'peke face' or 'dish face' (Catcott, 1964).

Craniofacial malformation in Burmese kittens

This malformation affects the brain, cranial cavity and face (Anon, 1982). The cranial cavity is enlarged and the cerebral hemispheres are duplicated. The eyes may be missing or small and there may be no nostrils or nasal cavities. The upper jaw and palate may be partially duplicated.

Pectus excavatum

This condition refers to a deformity of the sternum where the sternebrae are displaced dorsally such that the diameter of the thoracic cavity is reduced (Fig. 3.40). The deformity has been associated with nutritional secondary hyperparathyroidism and mucopolysaccharidosis, although some cases seem to represent a distinct entity. One such case, reported by Bennett (1973), showed chronic respiratory disease, presumably due to long-term displacement of the heart, lungs and trachea. The diagnosis is easily confirmed by thoracic radiography. The case was successfully treated by surgical resection of the deformed sternum (Fig. 3.41). The condition has also been reported by Grenn and Lindo (1968).

Other skeletal abnormalities

The presence of 14 thoracic vertebrae, 14 pairs of ribs and nine sternebrae segments has been documented (Lindsay, 1968). This was associated with a caudal displacement of the heart. Fusion of the cervical spine associated with neurological manifestations (Klippel–Feil anomaly) has been described (Jezyk, 1985).

Mucopolysaccharidosis

Aetiology and pathogenesis

The mucopolysaccharidoses are a group of diseases due to inborn errors of mucopolysaccharide metabolism; they are classed as lysosomal storage diseases (Jezyk, 1985). At least 12 specific forms are recognized in man, each due to a defect in a different lysosomal enzyme concerned with the degradation of glycosaminoglycans. There is incomplete degradation of mucopolysaccharides, which accumulate or are stored in lysosomes. Only two forms have been described in the cat: mucopolysaccharidosis Type I and Type VI (Cowell *et al.*, 1976; Jezyk *et al.*, 1977; Langweiler *et al.*, 1978). Skeletal deformities are seen in both diseases, but are only one of several types of abnormality present. Mucopolysaccharidosis Type VI has been reported in Siamese and Siamese-cross cats, and Type I in white domestic short-hair cats. Both Types I and VI have been shown to be autosomal recessive diseases. Type I is characterized by a deficiency of the enzyme α-L-iduronidase such that the normal degradation of dermatan and heparin sulphates is interrupted. Type VI is characterized by a deficiency of aryl-sulphatase B, again involved in the breakdown of dermatan sulphate.

Clinical signs

In Type I there is deformity of the skull bones; the head appears broad with a short maxilla, frontal bossing, depressed nasal bridge and small ears. The corneas are cloudy. The animal has a crouched gait with the stifles abducted and the forelegs widely placed, and a wheelbarrow posture of the hindlegs during locomotion has been observed. The sternum is concave and the dorsal neck skin thickened. Manipulation of the head, neck and joints may be painful. Skeletal abnormalities include wide and asymmetrical cervical vertebrae, which may be partly fused, subluxation of the hip joints and pectus excavatum. Chronic upper respiratory tract infection, ocular discharges and chronic diarrhoea may be present.

Type VI mucopolysaccharidosis may also be associated with a short, broad head. Drooping and swelling of the upper eyelids and absence of the lower incisor teeth are also documented. A crouching gait is again common; abduction of the stifles and pain and crepitus in several joints is reported. The epiphyseal and metaphyseal areas of the long bones are enlarged and irregularly shaped. Neck manipulation is painful and there is increased muscle tone in some limbs. Neurological deficits may be present suggesting multifocal disease in the brain/stem and cervical/thoracic spinal cord. Slight diffuse corneal clouding, retinal atrophy, and deformity of the vertebrae with bony proliferation and fusion are all recorded; bony proliferation around limb joints is also a feature. Thoracic deformity (pectus excavatum) and hip subluxation are also reported. Radiography often shows a variable generalized osteopenia with sclerosis of the vertebral endplates and articular facets; the long bones have marked epiphyseal dysplasia accompanied by severe degenerative joint disease. The animals may be several months of age or even young adults when first presented.

Radiography

Radiography will demonstrate the various bony deformities as discussed above. Radiography of the cervical/thoracic spine and limb joints may show bony proliferation – the appearance can be similar to hypervitaminosis A.

Laboratory features

In Type VI, examination of a blood smear may help in the diagnosis since the majority of neutrophils contain excessive coarse metachromatic granular material and 3% of leucocytes are large cells containing basophilic granules. The urine of affected cats shows the presence of excessive amounts of the mucopolysaccharides dermatan sulphate and sometimes chondroitin sulphate in both Types I and VI; this is readily demonstrated by allowing a drop of urine to dry on a microscope slide and then staining the mucopolysaccharide with toluidine blue. Actual levels of mucopolysaccharide can be measured and compared with controls; affected animals have much higher levels.

Deficiencies of the specific lysosomal enzymes may be demonstrated, i.e. arylsulphatase B (Langweiler *et al.*, 1978) and α-L-iduronidase (Haskins *et al.*, 1979).

Treatment

There is no specific therapy. The aim is to alleviate symptoms – these animals may live comfortably as pets if symptomatic treatment is given.

Patellar luxation

Congenital medial patellar instability has been reported in the cat (Flecknell & Gruffydd-Jones, 1979). It has been suggested that instability may not be uncommon, although clinical lameness is rare. The Devon Rex may show a susceptibility, but it has been seen in other breeds, including the domestic short hair. Lateral patellar luxation has also been recognized, but is less common (Schrader & Sherding, 1989).

The clinical features include intermittent 'locking' of the stifle, followed by extension of the joint to release the patella, plus abnormal gait and carriage of the limb. Some cases show deformity of the stifle, for example a shallow trochlear groove and rotation of the tibial tuberosity, although the severe angular and torsional deformities of the femur and tibia seen in the dog are very rare in the cat. Cats can also suffer a traumatic luxation of the patella and the femoropatellar joint can also luxate or subluxate secondary to a hip dislocation. Traumatic patellar luxation may be more likely to occur if there is an underlying congenital instability of the femoropatellar joint, insufficient to cause a clinical problem until trauma, which may be comparatively mild, aggravates the joint. Patellar luxation/subluxation will cause secondary osteoarthritis in time.

Surgical correction of a medial patellar luxation can be tried if the clinical problem is severe enough. A capsular overlap technique may be tried, or even a tibial tuberosity relocation if there is obvious displacement of the tuberosity. Deepening of the trochlear groove is also feasible.

Hip dysplasia

Radiographical features of hip dysplasia are often seen in the cat (Fig. 3.14), but they are usually incidental findings, not associated with a hindleg lameness. The disease can produce secondary osteoarthritis. The radiographical features have been reported by several authors (Riser, 1964; Carlson, 1967; Kolde, 1974; Peiffer *et al.*, 1974; Holt, 1978) and are similar to those of the dog; for example, widening of lateral and medial joint space, subluxation of the femoral head, shallow acetabulae and osteophyte development.

Clinical signs can sometimes be severe, and include a crouching hindleg gait, howling with pain, inability to climb stairs, reluctance to defaecate, and pain and crepitus in the hip joints. The condition is said to be more common in the Siamese breed (Riser 1964; Peiffer *et al.*, 1974).

Treatment has included resection of the pectineus muscle (Kolde, 1974; Peiffer *et al.*, 1974) and femoral head resection (Holt, 1978). Mild cases may respond to rest (confinement) and analgesics.

Osteochondrosis

Osteochondrosis is defined as an idiopathic disease characterized by a disturbed endochondral ossification in the young animal. It is a common disease of the larger breeds of dog. A case of osteochondrosis dissecans of the humeral head has been reported in a 9-month-old male Burmese kitten (Butcher & Beasley, 1986), although it is possible that the lesion was an osteochondral fracture. The kitten responded to surgical excision of the cartilage flap.

Other congenital abnormalities

Boehringer (1975) described a 1½-year-old tortoiseshell domestic short-hair queen with abnormal development of an extremity. The phalanges of digits 2 and 3 were enclosed in a common skin, the 2nd and 3rd phalanges were fused and two claws arose from the common stump. The phalanges of digit 4 were absent.

MUSCLE DISEASE

Myositis

Bacterial myositis can often result from bite or gunshot wounds and local abscessation may occur. Treatment includes drainage, local antisepsis and systemic antibiotics. Occasionally, foreign bodies including teeth, claws and airgun pellets may be lodged in the tissues and require surgical removal. Foreign bodies are likely to be associated with non-healing sinuses and radiography can help in assessing these cases.

Other causes of myositis, such as parasitic and immune-based, are not well documented in the cat. Cases of *Spirocerca lupi* infection of the oesophagus are reported in cats in Africa and the southern USA. Such lesions are nodular and cause vomiting and regurgitation; treatment is by surgical excision.

Localized myositis ossificans

This is characterized by heterotopic non-neoplastic bone formation in a single muscle or group of muscles or other soft tissue (Dahlin, 1967). The ossification may be associated with trauma. Liu *et al.* (1974) described a case in a 2-year-old cat. The cat was presented with firm nodules palpable on the medial aspect of both elbows. Radiography revealed a calcified mass proximal to each olecranon. The adjacent bones did show periosteal proliferation. Surgical resection of the lesions proved an effective treatment. The lesions consisted of proliferated fibrous and osteoid tissue in the muscle; there were well-formed calcified osseous trabeculae with more mature osseous tissue disposed peripherally. Figure 3.42 shows the radiographic appearance of myositis ossificans in a 6-year-old domestic short-haired.

Generalized myositis ossificans (fibrodysplasia ossificans)

This is a rare disorder of interstitial connective tissue, in which widespread muscle degeneration results from excessive fibrous tissue development

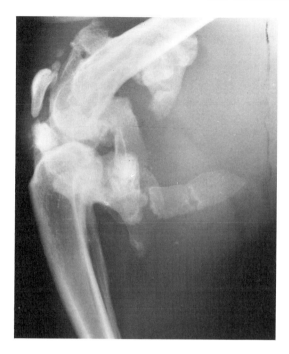

Fig. 3.42 Lateral radiograph of the stifle area of a cat with localized myositis ossificans. There are extensive bony deposits within the muscles and soft tissues around the joint.

with dystrophic calcification and ossification. The disease may be a primary connective tissue defect affecting initially the epimyseal connective tissue. Atrophy and displacement of muscles, entrapment of nerves and progressive immobility occur. It is not an inflammatory disease. A suspected case has been described in a 10-month-old cat (Norris *et al.*, 1980). The cat was presented with stiffness and progressive posterior paresis. Several firm nodules were palpable in the limb muscles. The muscles, especially those of the hindquarter, were swollen and firm. There was marked reduction in flexion and extension of the hip and stifle joints; the forelegs were bowed and movement of the elbow and shoulder joints restricted.

Widespread fibrosis and ossification of skeletal muscles was noted, most of which contained bony spicules, which in the semi-membranosus had organized into a second femoral shaft com-

plete with marrow cavity. A bridge of mineralized connective tissue fused the scapulae to the ribs dorsally. Histologically, there was extensive replacement of muscle fibres by mature dense fibrous tissue with bony trabeculae forming within the connective tissue. In adjacent areas, there was acute swelling and hyaline degeneration of muscle fibres. Only skeletal muscle was affected. Other cases have been reported by Warren and Carpenter (1984).

Aortic thromboembolism

Iliac thrombosis is a well-known syndrome in the cat, the animal presenting with an inability to stand on its hindlegs. There is an absence of femoral pulses. The resultant ischaemia of the hindlegs has an important effect on peripheral nerves and muscles (Griffiths & Duncan, 1979). In cases reported, motor function was markedly reduced distal to the stifle, particularly in the cranial tibial muscles. Improvement occurred in 2–3 weeks and complete recovery of motor function occurred in some cases. Affected muscles were often hard and painful on palpation.

Many peripheral nerves had myelin defects to varying degrees; most demonstrated obvious degeneration but a few survived the ischaemia. Regeneration of damaged nerve fibres was demonstrated. Infarction of the cranial tibial muscles was common.

The prognosis of these cases is good providing further ischaemic episodes do not occur and providing respiratory involvement is not present.

Treatment is based on prevention of extension of the clot and further primary thrombosis (heparin) and prevention of the effects of clot breakdown factors (5HT antagonists, e.g. cyproheptadine, and α blockade, e.g. acepromazine) and, in chronic cases, the use of drugs to reduce platelet aggregation (aspirin). Embolectomy is also possible (see also Chapter 11).

Myasthenia gravis

This disease is associated with a failure of normal neuromuscular transmission. Signs include generalized muscle weakness, dyspnoea, muscle tremor, ataxia and collapse when the animal is exercised (Dawson, 1970; Mason, 1976). A change in voice and difficulty in prehension and swallowing of food are also reported. The aetiology is unknown although cases can either be congenital or acquired. Autoimmunity is thought to be involved in the latter type, where antibodies against acetylcholine receptors can be demonstrated. Both types have been described in the cat (Indrieri *et al.*, 1983). One case of autoimmune myasthenia gravis was associated with a thymoma (Scott-Moncrieff *et al.*, 1990).

Diagnosis is based on a dramatic response to anticholinesterase drugs, for example edrophonium* (2.5–5.0 mg IV). Electrophysiological testing can also help with diagnosis.

Treatment is with oral pyridostigmine bromide or neostigmine; the maintenance dose will vary between individual animals. Prednisolone therapy and possible surgical thymectomy should be considered if autoimmunity is thought to be involved.

Hypokalaemic polymyopathy (muscle weakness syndrome; sporadic feline hypokalaemic polymyopathy)

This was widely reported in the USA in the mid-1980s but seems rare in the UK (Hopkins, 1989). The presenting signs include acute onset of severe muscle weakness, characterized clinically by ventral flexion of the neck, reluctance to walk, stiff gait, easy fatigability and apparent muscle pain (Dow *et al.*, 1987a,b). There is a severe hypokalaemia associated with the clinical signs. Serum creatine phosphokinase levels are increased and electromyographic abnormalities are reported (e.g. excessive insertional activity, spontaneous activity including positive sharp waves and fibrillation potentials, bizarre high-frequency discharges). Muscle biopsies most often show no abnormalities. Prolonged excessive uri-

* Tensilon, Roche Products Ltd., Welwyn Garden City, Herts, UK.

nary potassium losses were thought to have caused the potassium depletion associated with renal dysfunction and evidence of the latter was generally found on routine blood examination. The potassium loss was compounded by insufficient dietary potassium. It has been concluded that the potassium requirement for cats receiving a 33% protein diet is at least 0.3%; in kittens fed 0.2% potassium diets signs of potassium deficiency will occur (Hills *et al.*, 1982). The feeding of an acidifying diet may also increase potassium depletion (Dow *et al.*, 1987b) and certain drugs may accelerate renal potassium losses (e.g. diuretics, corticosteroids). The hypokalaemia, although secondary to renal disease, will itself cause further renal pathology. Most manufacturers have now increased the potassium content of their diets and levels of 0.5–0.7% are not uncommon. Muscle weakness and hypokalaemia have also been seen secondary to renal tubular acidosis (Drazner, 1980) and in a cat with primary hyperaldosteronism (Eger *et al.*, 1983).

The treatment of these cats is with oral potassium, preferably as potassium gluconate at a dose of 5–10 mmol/cat/day, given in two divided doses. Once clinical improvement has occurred and serum potassium levels are back to normal, the oral potassium supplement can be reduced; maintenance supplements of 2–6 mmol potassium/day may be necessary. Intravenous potassium therapy is best avoided but is sometimes necessary if the hypokalaemia is severe. The potassium should be administered at a rate of 0.5–1.0 mmol/kg/h. Potassium chloride should be diluted in a balanced electrolyte solution such as lactated Ringers' solution and administered via an infusion pump since highly concentrated potassium-containing solutions must be infused carefully to avoid phlebitis and potentially fatal hyperkalaemia. During such infusion serum potassium must be monitored together with ECG recording. Fluids that do not contain concentrations of potassium that are capable of replacing the deficit rapidly should not be used since they may actually worsen the hypokalaemia by a dilution effect. An alternative to administering highly concentrated potassium solutions is to infuse dopamine (0.5 µg/kg/min) which causes translocation of potassium from the intracellular to the extracellular fluid.

Burmese sporadic myopathy

This was described as an inherited disease by Mason (1988). The age of onset of signs varied from 4 to 10 months with an average of 7.4 months. The affected cats would develop ventro-flexion of the neck with the chin pressing on the anterior sternum; this could occur during rest or when walking. When walking, the head would rhythmically nod up and down as though co-ordinated with limb movement. The forelimbs were stiff, straight and hypermetric, while the hindlimbs would flex normally but were wide-spread and ataxic. Pupil dilation and claw protru-sion occurred with handling, stress or fright. Affected animals could only walk short distances. Convulsions were also reported. The animals would improve and show complete normality be-fore relapsing days or weeks later. The original problem was likened to thiamine deficiency and treatment of some cases with thiamine was thought to help reduce the severity of the signs. However, it is now thought to be a hypokalaemic polymyopathy and the Burmese breed has an inherited predisposition (Blaxter *et al.*, 1986; Jones & Alley, 1988). Treatment with potas-sium replacement as discussed above is generally successful.

Tetanus

The cat is particularly resistant to tetanus but several case reports have appeared (e.g. Baker *et al.*, 1988). The tetanus or muscle rigidity may initially be localized to the area of the wound if present. This can progress to generalized muscle stiffness and rigidity. The tonic contraction of the muscles may prevent ambulation; if the animal can walk they will have a very stiff gait. Severely affected animals lie on their sides with rigidly outstretched limbs and tails curved dorsally. Opisthotonus is common. Ears are drawn closely together with wrinkling of the skin of the fore-head. Spasms of the extraocular muscles cause intermittent enophthalmos and protrusion of the third eyelids. Spasms of facial and masticatory muscles result in narrowed palpebral fissures, curling of the lips (risus sardonicus) and inability to open the mouth (trismus). Treatment is with tetanus antitoxin, antibiotics and supportive care and recovery can occur. The muscle spasms can be controlled with phenothiazine, barbiturates and diazepam.

Fibrotic myopathy

Fibrous replacement of the semitendinosus muscle has been described in the cat (Lewis, 1988). The lameness was characterized by an abnormal gait, where there was marked flexion of the hip, stifle and hock as the leg was advanced with an abruptly shortened anterior stride. The muscle was felt as a taut band on the caudo-medial aspect of the thigh, which limited the extent of abduction. The cause, like fibrotic myopathies in other species, was not determined. Surgical lengthening of the muscle abolished the lameness immediately postoperatively but the clinical signs returned later.

Dystrophy-like myopathies

Vos *et al.* (1986) described two cases of feline myopathy characterized by varying muscle fibre diameter, internal nuclei, moderate degeneration and necrosis of solitary muscle fibres and slight to moderate endomysial and perimysial fibrosis. Very few regenerating muscle fibres were present. Only one of the cats showed a locomotor dis-order, characterized by inability to jump and a 'kangaroo-like' gait; chronic vomiting was also a feature. Hulland (1970) reported two young litter-mate Siamese cats with weakness ultimately re-sulting in an inability to support body weight. Muscle histology included irregular atrophy and hypertrophy of muscle fibres, individual muscle fibres showing degenerative and fragmentation with aggregation of histiocyte cells and lack of muscle fibre regeneration.

Other myopathies

Gershoff and Norkin (1962) described degenerative myopathy in cats fed vitamin E-deficient diets, not containing unsaturated fatty acids. A clinical case of vitamin E deficiency was described in a cat fed a very unusual diet (Dennis & Alexander, 1982). The animal presented with swollen muscles in fore and hindlegs associated with difficult and painful movement. Histological examination of the muscle revealed several degenerative changes, e.g. pale swollen myofibres, loss of cross-striations, hyaline degeneration and necrosis with flocculation granules and myophagia by macrophages. Some swollen myofibres showed proliferation of sarcolemmal nuclei and occasional centralization of the nuclei but no giant cell formation within myofibre cylinders. Chronic inflammatory change was also present.

A myopathy of unknown origin was reported by Joshua (1965). There was extensive myonecrosis, replacement fibrosis and muscle regeneration. The clinical signs included malaise, lameness and emaciation with hardening and contracture of both triceps brachii muscles and biceps femoris in the right hindleg.

A histological myonecrosis was described in a cat by Gardner (1967). The affected muscle showed swelling, coagulation and fragmentation of the sarcoplasm in the necrotic fibres, which were interspersed with normal fibres. The cause of the myonecrosis was unknown and the cat did show other lesions such as ecchymoses, icterus and pulmonary oedema.

Contracture of the gastrocnemius muscle/tendon

A bilateral contracture of the gastrocnemius muscles/tendons with hyperextension of both tarsal joints was described in a 5-month-old kitten (Rengel *et al.*, 1977). The clinical signs were severe overextension of the hocks with heavy callus formation on the cranial surface of the tarsi, which were in contact with the ground. The case was treated successfully by surgical lengthening of the gastrocnemius tendons. A unilateral case in a 3-month-old kitten, seen by the author, had severe secondary bony changes within the hock joint. Two transarticular Kirschner wires were used to hold the hock joint in flexion. These were later removed and the kitten retained a normal foot posture.

DISEASES OF THE VERTEBRAL COLUMN

Intervertebral disc protrusions

King and Smith (1960a,b) found that dorsal disc protrusions occurred mainly in old cats over 15 years of age, where they were common and often multiple. These protrusions had occurred without noticeable clinical signs. Any part of the column could be affected, although the more severe varieties of protrusion were slightly more common in the cervical region.

Cases of disc protrusion associated with clinical disease have been reported in the cat (Heavner, 1971; Hoerlein, 1978; Seim & Nafe, 1981; Littlewood *et al.*, 1984), but such cases are rare. The diagnosis and prognosis have largely depended upon a detailed clinical examination. Plain radiography is seldom of help. Calcification of prolapsed intervertebral discs is rare in the cat (King *et al.*, 1958). A protruded disc should give a disc space which appears narrower than its neighbours, but King and his co-workers also found that disc spaces that appeared narrow on radiographs often contained normal discs and protruded discs were often associated with normal width disc spaces. Myelography will help to localize disc lesions.

Corticosteroids are often used for treatment. Dorsal decompressive laminectomy and disc removal has been reported (Seim & Nafe, 1981).

Disc explosions do occur in the cat, and like the dog are associated with episodes of major trauma, for example a road traffic accident. The damage to the spinal cord is caused by an impact injury. Prognosis depends on the severity of clinical disease. Corticosteroids may be tried for treatment; decompression of the spine is seldom indicated.

Spondylosis deformans
and ankylosing hyperostosis

Osteophyte development on the vertebral bodies of the spine has been described in the cat (Pommer, 1933; Beadman *et al.*, 1964; Read & Smith, 1968). It is often an incidental finding, not associated with clinical signs, and its incidence increases with age (Read & Smith, 1968). Vertebral osteophytes are also seen in hypervitaminosis A and mucopolysaccharidosis.

Bacterial discospondylitis

Bacterial infections very occasionally localize to the spinal joints of the cat, particularly the intervertebral discs, where a discospondylitis results. The clinical signs are mainly stiffness and a painful back or neck. A neurological deficit may also result (Norsworthy, 1979). The infection is presumed to be blood-borne and the urinary tract is a possible source of infection.

Radiography may help in confirming the diagnosis, although the changes can be subtle. There may be destruction of vertebral bone on either side of the disc space, giving the space an irregular and widened appearance. Sclerosis of the vertebral bodies on either side of the lytic area may be seen and a spondylotic reaction may also be present. Alternatively, little more than a narrowing of the affected disc space will be apparent.

Treatment involves long-term systemic antibiotics, possibly in conjunction with surgical curettage of the lesion. In cases with obvious neurological deficits, more sophisticated spinal surgery may be required, for example decompressive laminectomy. Penetrating bite wounds at the tail base have been associated with an infective spondylitis of the coccygeal vertebrae.

Atlantoaxial subluxation

Hypoplasia of the odontoid process with subluxation of the atlantoaxial joint has been described in an 11-month-old Siamese cat (Shelton *et al.*, 1991). The cat presented with progressive ataxia, tetraparesis and proprioceptive deficits.

The atlantoaxial joint was stabilized by Kirschner wires inserted across the articular facets of C1 and C2.

MISCELLANEOUS DISEASES

Hypertrophic pulmonary osteoarthropathy

This is very rare in the cat. It is a disease characterized by periosteal proliferation of new bone along the shafts of the limb bones. In most cases the disease is associated with an intrathoracic mass.

The aetiology of the condition is not understood, but it is generally accepted that there is a rapid increase in peripheral blood flow in the extremities, which is followed by excessive formation of highly vascular connective tissue and subsequent periosteal bone formation. About seven cases have been reported in the domestic cat. Richards (1977) reported a case in a 1½-year-old cat associated with a thymoma, and Roberg (1977) described a case in an 11-year-old cat associated with bronchiolar carcinoma. In both cases, the forelimbs were more affected than the hindlimbs and the phalanges were unaffected. The bony reaction was more extensive and less regular than seen in other species. Other cases have included pulmonary tuberculosis and a case with no intrathoracic abnormalities but with a renal papillary adenoma (Nafe *et al.*, 1981). Treatment is aimed at removal of the thoracic disease. Removal of solitary intrathoracic masses may result in regression of the bony changes. If neoplastic disease is involved then the prognosis is often poor due to recurrence or metastatic spread. There is always the possibility that the thoracic mass is itself a metastatic spread from a primary focus elsewhere in the body. Unilateral intrathoracic vagotomy (on the side of the lesion), incision of periosteal pleura, subperiosteal rib resection and bilateral cervical vagotomy have been associated with resolution of the bony lesion in other species (Brodey, 1980). Analgesics may also help.

Clinically, the animals are presented with lameness, which may be shifting, associated with swollen painful limbs. Radiography is a helpful aid to diagnosis.

Disuse osteopenia

This is a bony loss in an individual bone or limb or in the entire skeleton, caused by a lack of weight-bearing and normal body stress. It is most often seen in a limb not being used because of fracture healing. External support of a limb by, for example, a plaster cast will cause bone loss over a period of time. Radiographically, the affected bones appear obviously osteopenic. Pathological fracture is always a possible untoward sequel.

The aetiology is unknown although reduced blood supply through the bone due to muscular inactivity, etc. will cause blood stagnation and increase $p(CO_2)$ levels, which will stimulate osteoclastosis (Little, 1973). Affected animals may show elevated blood calcium and phosphorus and may excrete increased levels of urinary calcium. The process is reversible and normal bone will be reformed when the normal stresses are reapplied to the bone.

Osteopetrosis

Osteopetrosis is a descriptive term and refers to a generalized skeletal sclerosis or a generalized increase in skeletal mass. It has been seen by the author as a congenital problem and as an acquired problem and presumably reflects an imbalance in bone turnover. The difference between the terms osteosclerosis and osteopetrosis is not precisely defined. However, osteopetrosis is a generalized condition and the radiographic increase in skeletal mass is always striking. Two acquired cases, one in a 3-year-old cat and the other in an 8-year-old were reported by Kramers *et al.* (1988). Radiography of both cats showed a generalized massive increase of bone density in the vertebrae, a marked cortical thickening in the long bones with loss of normal trabecular structure, especially in the subchondral areas, and additional irregular osseous structures within the medullary cavity of the long bones. One cat was severely anaemic.

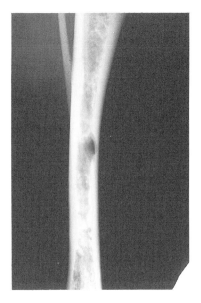

Fig. 3.43 Radiographs of the bone of a 6-week-old kitten with congenital osteopetrosis. Note the thickened cortices and the areas of increased bone density within the medullary cavities. Pathological fractures are often present, because of increased brittleness of the bones.

There are a number of different aetiopathogenetic mechanisms incriminated in acquired osteopetrosis although many cases go unexplained.

Congenital (possibly inherited) osteopetrosis has been seen in one kitten by the author (Fig. 3.43). The whole skeleton was affected and pathological fractures were seen (although the bone is very dense it is brittle and susceptible to fracture). Skeletal pain, stunted growth and poor appetite were all features. Some cases of congenital osteopetrosis can be cured by transplantation of spleen or bone marrow cells from normal littermates to provide a population of functionally competent osteoclasts.

Myelofibrosis-osteosclerosis syndrome

Myelofibrosis is characterized by fibroblastic proliferation and varying degrees of collagen deposition in the marrow cavity. Primary (idiopathic) myelofibrosis is defined as a chronic myeloproliferative disease associated with myeloid metaplasia of the liver, spleen and lymph nodes and abnormal growth of haematopoietic cells in bone marrow. Secondary myelofibrosis occurs as a non-specific, reactive change following prolonged bone marrow damage (Weiss & Armstrong, 1985). Osteosclerosis may occur in some cases of myelofibrosis although it may not be apparent radiographically. Hoover and Kociba (1974) reported varying degrees of medullary osteosclerosis in neonate cats with anaemia induced by inoculation of feline leukaemia virus. Both bone formation and resorption were inhibited but the latter more so. Flecknell and co-workers (1978) similarly reported osteosclerosis associated with leukaemia virus infection, and Ward *et al.* (1969) described osteosclerosis as a terminal development in cats with naturally occurring erythroleukaemias.

Feline hyperaesthesia syndrome

This syndrome refers to those cats which present with apparent pain or hyperaesthesia on handling, especially over the lumbar spine. A

Table 3.3 Differential diagnoses of the feline hyperaesthesia syndrome

Trauma e.g. fracture pelvis, fracture/dislocation coccyx
Bite wounds-especially base of tail
Osteomyelitis
Myositis
Dermatitis
Pansteatitis
Feline infectious peritonitis
Abdominal pain
Aortic thromboembolism
Polyarthritis
Myeloproliferative disease
Hip dysplasia
Osteopetrosis
Hyperparathyroidism
Intervertebral disc disease
Discospondylitis
Spondylosis deformans
Ankylosing hyperostosis
Spinal tumours e.g. lymphosarcoma
Idiopathic

number of possible diagnoses need to be considered (Table 3.3), but there are many cases of 'idiopathic hyperaesthesia' where no diagnosis is established. Such cases may respond to corticosteroid therapy although some require euthanasia.

Plasma cell pododermatitis

Various skin lesions, particularly of the feet, can cause lameness in the cat. Plasma cell pododermatitis is a rare condition, characterized by swelling and softening of multiple footpads with ulceration sometimes occurring (Gruffydd-Jones *et al.*, 1980; Taylor & Schmeitzel, 1990) (see Chapter 1). Once ulceration occurs, haemorrhage, which can be recurrent and persistent, will result. Histopathologically the lesions are characterized by extensive infiltrates of lymphocytes and plasma cells. The aetiology of the condition is unknown although it is considered to be immune

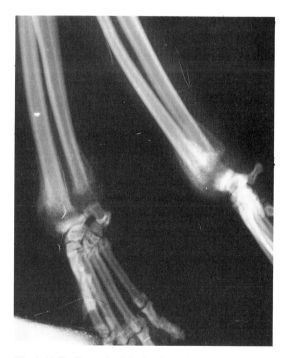

Fig. 3.44 Radiograph of the forefeet of a cat with metaphyseal osteopathy. Note the areas of radiolucency within the distal metaphyses of both radii and ulnae. New bone is also present, extending along the diaphyses.

based and hence treatment with corticosteroids can help. Surgical closure of the ulcers to control the haemorrhage is advisable (Taylor & Schmeitzel, 1990).

Other skin lesions of the feet include bacterial and mycotic infections, viral infections (Cooper & Sabine, 1972; Flecknell *et al.*, 1979), foreign bodies, neoplasia, irritant exposure, eosinophilic granuloma and autoimmune skin diseases amongst others (Scott, 1980; Taylor & Schmeitzel, 1990).

Feline metaphyseal osteopathy

This disease is characterized by bony resorption from the metaphyses, generally resulting in pathological fractures. It most often affects the proximal femoral metaphyses, but can affect others, and there may be multiple lesions (Fig. 3.44). Both adults and kittens can be affected. The aetiology of this disease is unknown, although metaphyseal necrosis has been produced by intravenous inoculation of herpesvirus (Hoover & Greismer, 1971).

REFERENCES

Anon (1982) Craniofacial malformation in Burmese kittens. *Feline Pract.* **12**(6), 32–3.

Arnone B., Labanti G. & Bolletino T. (1984) Extraskeletal osteosarcoma in a cat: clinical and histopathological aspects. *Associazione Italiano Veterinari per Piccoli Animal* **23**(4), 217–20.

Baker J.L., Waters D.J. & de LaHunta A. (1988) Tetanus in two cats. *J. Am. Anim. Hosp. Ass.* **24**, 159–64.

Baker J.R. & Hughes I.B. (1968) A case of deforming cervical spondylosis in a cat associated with a diet rich in liver. *Vet. Rec.* **83**, 44–5.

Banks W.C. (1971) Parosteal osteosarcoma in a dog and a cat. *J. Am. Vet. Med. Ass.* **158**, 1412–5.

Barclay S.M. (1979) Lymphosarcoma in tarsi of a cat. *J. Am. Vet. Med. Ass.* **175**, 582.

Beadman R.M., Smith R.N. & King A.S. (1964) Vertebral osteophytes in the cat. *Vet. Rec.* **76**, 1005–7.

Bennett D. (1973) Successful surgical correction of pectus excavatum in a cat. *Vet. Med./Small Anim. Clin.* **68**(9), 936.

Bennett D. (1975) Orthopaedic disease affecting the pelvic region of the cat. *J. Small Anim. Pract.* **16**, 723–38.

Bennett D. (1976a) Nutrition and bone disease in the dog and cat. *Vet. Rec.* **98**, 313–20.

Bennett D. (1976b) Nutrition and bone disease in the cat. *Feline Advisory Bureau Bulletin* **15**(4), 5–7.

Bennett D. & Campbell J.R. (1976) Mechanical interference with lower jaw movement as a complication of skull fractures. *J. Small Anim. Pract.* **17**, 747–51.

Bennett D. & Duff S.I.R. (1980) Transarticular pinning as a treatment for hip luxation in the dog and cat. *J. Small Anim. Pract.* **21**, 373–9.

Bennett D. & Duff S.I.R. (1983) Giant cell tumour of the ulna in a cat. *J. Small Anim. Pract.* **24**, 341–5.

Bennett D. & Kelly D.F. (1984) Unpublished data.

Bennett D. & Nash A.S. (1988) Feline immune-based polyarthritis – a study of 31 cases. *J. Small Anim. Pract.* **29**, 501–23.

Bennett D., Campbell J.R. & Brown P. (1979) Osteosarcoma associated with healed fractures. *J. Small Anim. Pract.* **20**, 13–8.

Bennett D., Gaskell R.M., Mills A., Knowles J., Carter S.D. & McArdle F. (1989) Detection of feline calicivirus antigens in the joints of infected cats. *Vet. Rec.* **124**, 329–32.

Bennett D., May C. & Carter S.D. (1992) Lyme disease. In Raw M.-E. & Parkinson T.J. (eds) *Veterinary Annual*, vol. 32. Butterworth Scientific Ltd., Surrey.

Berg J.N., Fales W.H. & Scanlan C.H. (1979) Occurrence of anaerobic bacteria in diseases of the dog and cat. *Am. J. Vet. Res.* **40**, 876–81.

Biller D.S., Johnson G.C., Birchard S.S. & Fingland R.B. (1987) Aneurysmal bone cyst in a rib of a cat. *J. Am. Vet. Med. Ass.* **190**, 1193–5.

Bitetto W.V., Patnaik A.K., Schraeder S.C. & Mooney S.G. (1987) Osteosarcoma in cats: 22 cases (1974–1984). *J. Am. Vet. Med. Ass.* **190**, 91–3.

Blaxter A.C., Lieverley P., Gruffydd-Jones T. & Wotton P. (1986) Periodic weakness in Burmese kittens. *Vet. Rec.* **118**(22), 619–20.

Blunden A.S., Wheeler S.J. & Davies J.V. (1986) Hyperparathyroidism in the cat of probable primary origin. *J. Small Anim. Pract.* **23**, 791–8.

Boehringer B.T. (1975) Foot deformity in a cat. *Feline Pract.* **5**(3), 50.

Brodey R.S. (1980) Hypertrophic osteoarthropathy. In *Spontaneous Animal Models of Human Disease.* Academic Press Inc., New York.

Brown N.O., Patnaik A.K., Mooney S., Hayes A., Harvey H.J. & MacEwen E.G. (1978) Soft tissue sarcomas in the cat. *J. Am. Vet. Med. Ass.* **173**, 744–9.

Brown P.J., Hoare C.M. & Rochlitz I. (1985) Multiple squamous cell carcinoma of the digits in two cats. *J. Small Anim. Pract.* **26**, 323–8.

Brown R.J., Trevethan W.P. & Henry V.L. (1972) Multiple osteochondroma in a Siamese cat. *J. Am. Vet. Med. Ass.* **160**, 433–5.

Brown W. (1964) cited by English & Seawright (1964) (See reference).

Butcher R. & Beasley K. (1986) Osteochondritis dissecans in a cat. *Vet. Rec.* **118**(23), 646.

Carlisle C.H., Penny R.H.C., Prescott C.W. & Davidson H.A. (1968) Toxic effects of phenylbutazone on the cat. *Br. Vet. J.* **124**, 560–8.

Carlson W.D. (1967) *Veterinary Radiology*, Ballière Tindall, London, p. 429.

Carro T., Pedersen N.C., Beaman B.L. & Munn R. (1989) Subcutaneous abscesses and arthritis caused by a probable bacterial L-form in cats. *J. Am. Vet. Med. Ass.* **194**, 1583–8.

Carter H.E. (1964) The clinical approach to fractures in small animals. *Vec. Rec.* **76**, 1412–7.

Catcott E.J. (1964) *Feline Medicine and Surgery*. American Veterinary Publications, Wheaton, Illinois.

Chapman V.A. & Zeiner F.N. (1961) The anatomy of polydactylism in cats with observations on genetic control. *Anat. Rec.* **141**, 205–17.

Clark L. (1970) The effect of excess vitamin A on long bone growth in kittens. *J. Comp. Path.* **80**, 625–34.

Clark L. (1971a) Mid-diaphyseal bone turnover during and after vitamin A toxicosis in kittens. *J. Comp. Path.* **81**, 365–71.

Clark L. (1971b) Hypervitaminosis A: a review. *Aust. Vet. J.* **47**, 568–71.

Clark L. & Seawright A.A. (1968) Skeletal abnormalities in the hindlimbs of young cats as a result of hypervitaminosis A. *Nature* **217**, 1174–6.

Clark L., Seawright A.A. & Hrdlicka J. (1970) Exostoses in hypervitaminosis A cats with optimal calcium-phosphorus intakes. *J. Small Anim. Pract.* **11**, 553–61.

Cohn L.A. & Meuten D.J. (1990) Bone fragility in a kitten: an osteogenesis imperfecta-like syndrome. *J. Am. Vet. Med. Ass.* **197**, 98–100.

Cooper L.M. & Sabine M. (1972) Paw and mouth disease in a cat. *Aust. Vet. J.* **48**, 644.

Cotchin E. (1956) Further examples of spontaneous neoplasms in the domestic cat. *Brit. Vet. J.* **112**, 263–72.

Cotchin E. (1957) Neoplasia in the cat. *Vet. Rec.* **69**, 425–36.

Cotchin E. (1984) Neoplasia. In Wilkinson G.T. (ed) *Diseases of the Cat and Their Management*, Chapter 15. Blackwell Scientific Publications, Oxford.

Cotter S.M., Bremmer R.M. & Dodds W.J. (1978) Hemophilia A in three unrelated cats. *J. Am. Vet. Med. Ass.* **172**, 166–8.

Cottrill N.B., Carter J.D., Pechman R.D., Dubielzig R.R. & Waldron D.R. (1987) Bilateral orbital parosteal osteoma in a cat. *J. Am. Anim. Hosp. Ass.* **23**(4), 405–8.

Cowell K.R., Jezyk P.F., Haskins M.E. & Patterson D.F. (1976) Mucopolysaccharidosis in a cat. *J. Am. Vet. Med. Ass.* **169**, 334–9.

Crocker W. (1919) Osteoclastoma in cat foreleg. *Cornell Vet.* **9**, 142.

Dahlin D.C. (1967) *Bone Tumors*, 2nd edn. C.C. Thomas, Springfield, Illinois.

Danforth C.H. (1947a) Heredity of polydactyly in the cat. *J. Hered.* **38**, 107–12.

Danforth C.H. (1947b) Morphology of the feet in polydactyl cats. *J. Anat.* **80**, 143–71.

Davies J.D. & Little N.R.F. (1972) Synovioma in a cat. *J. Small Anim. Pract.* **13**, 127–33.

Davis L.E. & Donnelly E.J. (1968) Analgesic drugs in the cat. *J. Am. Vet. Med. Ass.* **153**, 1161–7.

Davis L.E. & Westfall B.A. (1972) Species differences in biotransformation and excretion of salicylate. *Am. J. Vet. Res.* **33**, 1253–62.

Dawson J.R.B. (1970) Myasthenia gravis in a cat. *Vet. Rec.* **86**, 562–3.

Dawson S., Bennet D., Carter S.D., Bennett M., Meanger J., Turner P.C., Carter M.J., Milton I. & Gaskell R.M. (1993) Acute arthritis of cats associated with feline calicivirus infection. *Res. Vet. Sci.* (in press).

Dawson S., McArdle F., Bennett D., Carter S.D., Bennett M., Ryvou R. & Gaskell R.M. (1992) Investigation of vaccine reactions and breakdowns following feline calicivirus vaccination. *Vet. Res.* **132**, 346–350.

Dennis J.M. & Alexander R.W. (1982) Nutritional myopathy in a cat. *Vet. Rec.* **111**, 195–6.

Dow S.W., Fettman M.J., Le Couteur R.A. & Hamar D.W. (1987a) Potassium depletion in cats: renal and dietary influence. *J. Am. Vet. Med. Ass.* **191**, 1569–75.

Dow S.W., Le Couteur R.A., Fettman M.J. & Spurgeon T.L. (1987b) Potassium depletion in cats: hypokalaemic polymyopathy. *J. Am. Vet. Med. Ass.* **191**, 1563–8.

Drazner F.H. (1980) Distal renal tubular acidosis associated with chronic pyelonephritis in a cat. *Calif. Vet.* **34**, 15–21.

Dubielzig A.R., Adams W.M. & Brodey R.S. (1979) Inductive fibroblastoma – an unusual dental tumor of young cats. *J. Am. Vet. Med. Ass.* **174**, 720–2.

Eger C.E., Robinson W.R. & Huxtable C.R.R. (1983) Pituitary aldosteronism (Conn's syndrome) in a cat: a case report and review of comparative aspects. *J. Small Anim. Pract.* **24**, 293–307.

Emms S.G. & Harvey C.E. (1986) Preliminary results of maxillectomy in the dog and cat. *J. Small Anim. Pract.* **27**(5), 291–306.

Engle G.G. & Brodey R.S. (1969) *J. Am. Anim. Hosp. Ass.* **5**, 21.

English P.B. & Seawright A.A. (1964) Deforming cervical spondylosis of the cat. *Aust. Vet. J.* **40**, 376–81.

Flecknell P.A. & Gruffydd-Jones T.J. (1979) Congenital luxation of the patellae in the cat. *Feline Pract.* **9**(3), 18–20.

Flecknell P.A., Gibbs C. & Kelly D.F. (1978) Myelosclerosis in a cat. *J. Comp. Path.* **88**, 627–31.

Flecknell P.A., Orr C.M., Wright A.L., Gaskell R.M. & Kelly D.F. (1979) Skin ulceration associated with herpes virus in cats. *Vet. Rec.* **104**, 313–5.

Forbes S., Nelson R.W. & Guptill L. (1990) Primary hypoparathyroidism in a cat. *J. Am. Vet. Med. Ass.* **196**, 1285–7.

Freund E. (1937) Chondromatosis of joints. *Arch. Surg.* **34**, 670.

Fry P.D. (1968) Cervical spondylosis in the cat. *J. Small Anim. Pract.* **9**, 59–61.

Gardner D.E. (1967) Skeletal myonecrosis in a cat. *New. Z. Vet. J.* **15**, 211–3.

Gehring V.H. (1975) Osteogenesis imperfecta bei der katze. *Kleintierpraxis* **20**, 205.

Gershoff S.N. & Norkin S.A. (1962) Vitamin E deficiency in cats. *J. Nutr.* **77**, 303–8.

Gershoff S.N., Andrus S.B., Hegsted D.M. & Lentini E.A. (1957) Vitamin A deficiency in the cat. *Lab. Invest.* **6**, 227–40.

Gleiser C.A., Rawlston R.L., Jardine J.H. & Gray K.N. (1979) Malignant fibrous histiocytoma in dogs and cats. *Vet. Path.* **16**(2), 199–208.

Goad M.E.P. & Roenick W.J. (1983) Osseous histoplasmosis in a cat. *Feline Pract.* **13**(2), 32–6.

Grenn H.H. & Lindo D.E. (1968) Pectus excavatum (funnel chest) in a feline. *Can. Vet. J.* **9**, 279–92.

Gresti A. (1975) Occurrence of bilateral articular synoviomas in two cats. *Clin. Vet.* **98**, 156.

Griffiths I.R. & Duncan I.D. (1979) Ischaemic neuromyopathy in cats. *Vet. Rec.* **104**, 518–22.

Gruffydd-Jones T.J., Orr C.M. & Locke V.M. (1980) Footpad swelling and ulceration in cats: a report of five cases. *J. Small Anim. Pract.* **21**, 381–9.

Gustafsson P. & Wolfe D. (1968) Bone-metastasizing lung carcinoma in a cat. *Cornell Vet.* **58**, 425–30.

Hardy W.D. (1976) The aetiology of canine and feline tumours. *J. Am. Anim. Hosp. Ass.* **12**, 313–34.

Haskins M.E., Jezyk P.F., Desnick R.J., McDonough S.K. & Patterson D.F. (1979) Mucopolysaccharidosis in a domestic short-haired cat – a disease distinct from that seen in the Siamese cat. *J. Am. Vet. Med. Ass.* **175**, 384–7.

Hays G.P. (1917–1918) A case of syndactylous cat. *Morphol.* **30**, 65–82.

Heavner J.E. (1971) Intervertebral disc syndrome in the cat. *J. Am. Vet. Med. Ass.* **159**, 425–7.

Hegreberg G.A. & Norby D.E. (1973) An inherited storage disease of cats. *Fed. Proc.* **32**, 821.

Hegreberg G.A., Norby D.E. & Hamilton M.J. (1974) Lysosomal enzyme changes in an inherited dwarfism of cats. *Fed. Proc.* **33**, 598.

Herron M.R. (1983) The musculoskeletal system. In Pratt P.W. (ed) *Feline Medicine*, Chapter 13. American Veterinary Publications Inc., Drawer K.K., Santa Barbara.

Hill F.W.G. (1977) A survey of bone fractures in the cat. *J. Small Anim. Pract.* **18**, 457–63.

Hills D.L., Morris J.G. & Rogers Q.R. (1982) Potassium requirement of kittens as affected by dietary protein. *J. Nutr.* **112**, 216–22.

Hoerlein B.F. (1978) *Canine Neurology*. W.B. Saunders, Philadelphia, p. 551.

Holt P.E. (1978) Hip dysplasia in a cat. *J. Small Anim. Pract.* **19**, 273–6.

Hooper P.T., Ireland L.A. & Carter A. (1985) Mycoplasma polyarthritis in a cat with probable severe immune deficiency. *Aust. Vet. J.* **62**, 352.

Hoover E.A. & Griesemer R.A. (1971) Bone lesions produced by feline herpes virus. *Lab. Investigation* **25**, 457–64.

Hoover E.A. & Kociba G.J. (1974) Bone lesions in cats with anaemia induced by feline leukaemia virus. *J. Nat. Cancer Inst.* **53**, 1277–84.

Hopkins A.L. (1989) Sporadic feline hypokalaemic polymyopathy. *Vet. Rec.* **125**, 17.

Horne R. (1964) Feline systemic mycoses: an up-to-date review. *Mod. Vet. Pract.* **45**(1), 39–46.

Howard E.B. & Kenyon E.B. (1967) Malignant osteoclastoma (giant cell tumor) in the cat with associated mast cell response. *Cornell Vet.* **57**, 398–409.

Hubler M., Johnson K.A., Burling R.T., Francis D.F. & Ratcliffe R.C.C. (1986) Lesions resembling osteochondromatosis in two cats. *J. Small Anim. Pract.* **27**(3), 181–7.

Hulland T.J. (1970) Muscle. In Jubb K.V.F. & Kennedy P.C. (eds) *Pathology of Domestic Animals*, vol. II, 2nd edn. Academic Press, New York, pp. 453–74.

Hulse E.V. (1966) A benign giant-cell synovioma in a cat. *J. Path. Bact.* **91**, 269–71.

Indrieri R.J., Creighton S.R., Lambert E.H. & Lennon V.A. (1983) Myasthenia gravis in two cats. *J. Am. Vet. Med. Ass.* **182**, 57–60.

Ingham B. (1970) Dysplasia of a ramus of the mandible in a cat. *Br. Vet. J.* **126**, iii–iv.

Jackson O.F. (1975) Congenital bone lesions in cats with fold-ears. *Bulletin Feline Advisory Bureau* **14**(4), 2–4.

Jacobsen R.H. & Saidla J.E. (1990) Update on feline Lyme disease. *Feline Health Topics for Veterinarians* **5**, 1–8. Cornell University.

Jacobson S.A. (1971) *Comparative Pathology of the Tumors of Bone*. C.C. Thomas, Springfield, Illinois.

Jaffe H.L. (1958) *Tumors and Tumorous Conditions of the Bones and Joints*. Lea & Febiger, Philadelphia.

Janssens L.A.A., Janssens G.O. & Janssens D.L. (1991) Anterior cruciate ligament rupture associated with cardiomyopathy in three cats. *Vet. Comp. Orthop. Traumat.* **4**, 35–7.

Jezyk P.E. (1985) Constitutional disorders of the skeleton in dogs and cats. In Newton C.D. & Nunamaker D.M. (eds) *Textbook of Small Animal Orthopaedics*, Chapter 57. J.B. Lippincott, Philadelphia.

Jezyk P.F., Haskins M.E., Patterson D.F., Mellman W.J. & Greenstein M. (1977) Mucopolysaccharidosis in a cat with arylsulfatase B deficiency: A model of Maroteaux–Lamy syndrome. *Science* **198**, 834–6.

Jobora A.G. & Paton J.S. (1984) Extraskeletal osteoma in a cat. *Aust. Vet. J.* **61**, 405–7.

Jones B.R. & Alley M.R. (1988) Hypokalaemic myopathy in Burmese kittens. *New Zeal. Vet. J.* **36**, 150–1.

Joshua J.O. (1965) *The Clinical Aspects of Some Diseases of Cats*. William Heinemann Medical Books, London.

Jubb K.J.F. & Kennedy P.C. (1963) *Pathology of Domesticated Animals*. Academic Press, New York, pp. 12, 56.

Kas N.P., Van der Heul R.O. & Misdorp W. (1970) Metastatic bone neoplasms in dogs, cats and a lion (with some comparative remarks on the situation in man). *Zentralbl. Veterinaer Med.* **17**, 909–19.

King A.S. & Smith R.N. (1960a) Disc protrusion in the cat: distribution of dorsal protrusions along the vertebral column. *Vet. Rec.* **72**, 335–7.

King A.S. & Smith R.N. (1960b) Disc protrusion in the cat: age incidence of dorsal protrusion. *Vet. Rec.* **72**, 381–3.

King A.S., Smith R.N. & Kon V.M. (1958) Protrusion of the intervertebral disc in the cat. *Vet. Rec.* **70**, 509–12.

Knecht C.D. (1978) Fractures in cats; a survey of 100 cases. *Feline Pract.* **8**(3), 43–6.

Knecht C.D. & Greene J.A. (1977) Osteoma of the zygomatic arch in a cat. *J. Am. Vet. Med. Ass.* **171**, 1077.

Kolde D.L. (1974) Pectineus tenectomy for treatment of hip dysplasia in a domestic cat: a case report. *J. Am. Anim. Hosp. Ass.* **10**, 564–5.

Kramers P., Fluckiger M.A., Rahn B.A. & Cordey J. (1988) Osteopetrosis in cats. *J. Small Anim. Pract.* **29**, 153–64.

Krook L. (1971) In Kirk R.W. (ed) *Current Veterinary Therapy*, 4th edn. W.B. Saunders, Philadelphia.

Krook, L., Barrett R.B., Usui K. & Woolke R.E. (1963) Nutritional secondary hyperparathyroidism in the cat. *Cornell Vet.* **53**, 224–40.

Langweiler M., Haskins M.E. & Jezyk P.F. (1978) Mucopolysaccharidosis in a litter of cats. *J. Am. Anim. Hosp. Ass.* **14**, 748–51.

Lees P. & Taylor P.M. (1991) Pharmacodynamics and pharmacokinetics of flunixin in the cat. *Br. Vet. J.* **147**, 298.

Levitt L. & Doige C.E. (1989) Pulmonary intraosseus fibrosarcoma in a cat. *J. Am. Vet. Med. Ass.* **194**, 1601–3.

Lewis D.D. (1988) Fibrotic myopathy of the semitendinosus muscle in a cat. *J. Am. Vet. Med. Ass.* **193**, 240–1.

Lewis G.E., Fidler W.J. & Crumrine M.H. (1972) Mycetoma in a cat. *J. Am. Vet. Med. Ass.* **161**, 500–3.

Lewis R.E. & Van Sickle D.C. (1970) Congenital hemimelia (agenesis) of the radius in a dog and cat. *J. Am. Vet. Med. Ass.* **156**, 1892–7.

Leyland A. & O'Meara A.F. (1974) Probable paracetamol toxicity in a cat. *Vet. Rec.* **94**, 104–5.

Lindsay F.E.F. (1968) Skeletal abnormalities of a cat thorax. *Br. Vet. J.* **124**, 306–8.

Little K. (1973) *Bone Behaviour*. Academic Press, London.

Littlewood J.D., Herrtage M.E. & Palmer A.C. (1984) Intervertebral disc protrusion in a cat. *J. Small Anim. Pract.* **25**, 119–27.

Liu S.-K., Dorfman H.D. & Patnaik A.K. (1974) Primary and secondary bone tumors in the cat. *J. Small Anim. Pract.* **15**, 141–56.

Lucke V.M., Baskerville A., Bardgett P.L., Mann P.G.H. & Thompson S.Y. (1968) Deforming cervical spondylosis in the cat associated with hypervitaminosis A. *Vet. Rec.* **82**, 141–2.

McClelland R.B. (1941) A giant cell tumor of the tibia in a cat. *Cornell Vet.* **31**, 86–7.

McDevitt C.A. (1973) Biochemistry of articular cartilage; nature of proteoglycans and collagen of articular cartilage and their role in ageing and osteoarthritis. *Ann. Rheum. Dis.* **32**, 364–78.

McDevitt C.A. & Muir H. (1976) Biochemical changes in the cartilage of the knee in experimental and natural osteoarthritis in the dog. *J. Bone. Jt. Surg.* **58B**, 94.

Magnarelli L.A., Anderson J.F., Levine H.R. & Levy S.A. (1990) Tick parasitism and antibodies to *Borrelia burgdorferi* in cats. *J. Am. Vet. Med. Ass.* **197**, 63–6.

Mahaffey E., Gabbert N., Johnson D. & Guffey M. (1977) Disseminated histoplasmosis in three cats. *J. Am. Anim. Hosp. Ass.* **13**, 46–51.

Mason K. (1988) A hereditary disease in Burmese cats manifested as an episodic weakness with head nodding and neck ventroflexion. *J. Am. Anim. Hosp. Ass.* **24**, 147–51.

Mason K.V. (1976) A case of myasthenia gravis in a cat. *J. Small Anim. Pract.* **17**, 467–72.

May C. & Newsholme S.J. (1989) Metastasis of feline pulmonary carcinoma presenting as multiple digital swelling. *J. Small Anim. Pract.* **30**, 302–10.

May C., Bennett D. & Downham D.Y. (1991) Delayed physeal closure associated with castration in cats. *J.*

Small Anim. Pract. **32**, 326–8.

Mellanby E. (1941) Skeletal changes affecting the nervous system produced in young dogs by diets deficient in vitamin A. *J. Physiol.* **99**, 467–86.

Mellanby E. (1950) *A Story of Nutritional Research: the Effect of Some Dietary Factors on Bones and the Nervous System.* Williams & Wilkins, Baltimore.

Miller A.S., McCrae M. & Rhodes W.H. (1969) Mandibular epidermoid carcinoma with reactive bone proliferation in a cat. *Am. J. Vet. Res.* **30**, 1465–8.

Miller R.M. (1969) Nutritional secondary hyperparathyroidism. *Vet. Med./Small Anim. Clin.* **64**, 400–8.

Moise N.S. & Crissman J.W. (1982) Chronic progressive polyarthritis in a cat. *J. Am. Anim. Hosp. Ass.* **18**, 965–9.

Moise N.S., Crissman J.W., Fairbrother J.F. & Baldwin C. (1983) Mycoplasma gateae arthritis and tenosynovitis in cats: case report and experimental reproduction of the disease. *Am. J. Vet. Res.* **44**, 16–21.

Moore T., Sharman I.M. & Scott P.P. (1963) Vitamin A in the kidney of the cat. *Res. Vet. Sci.* **4**, 397–403.

Morton D. (1985) Chondrosarcoma arising in a multilobular chondroma in a cat. *J. Am. Vet. Med. Ass.* **186**(8), 804–6.

Nafe L.A., Herron A.J. & Burke R.L. (1981) Hypertrophic osteopathy in a cat associated with renal papillary adenoma. *J. Am. Anim. Hosp. Ass.* **17**, 659.

Nielson S.W. (1952) Extraskeletal giant cell tumor in a cat. *Cornell Vet.* **42**, 304–11.

Norris A.M., Pallett L. & Wilcock B. (1980) Generalized myositis ossificans in a cat. *J. Am. Anim. Hosp. Ass.* **16**, 659–63.

Norsworthy G.D. (1979) Discospondylitis as cause of posterior paresis. *Feline Pract.* **9**(1), 39–40.

Pedersen N.C., Pool R.R. & O'Brien T. (1980) Feline chronic progressive polyarthritis. *Am. J. Vet. Res.* **41**, 522–35.

Pedersen N.C., Laliberte L. & Ekman S. (1983a) A transient febrile limping syndrome of kittens caused by two different strains of feline calici virus. *Feline Pract.* **13**(1), 26–35.

Pedersen N.C., Pool R.R. & Morgan J.P. (1983b) Joint diseases of dogs and cats. In Ettinger S.J. (ed) *Textbook of Veterinary Internal Medicine, Diseases of the Dog and Cat*, 2nd edn., chap. 84. W.B. Saunders, Philadelphia.

Peiffer R.L. Jr, Young W.O. Jr & Blevins W.E. (1974) Hip dysplasia and pectineus resection in the cat. *Feline Pract.* **4**(3), 40–3.

Penwick R.C. & Nunamaker D.M. (1987) Rostral mandibulectomy: a treatment for oral neoplasia in the dog and cat. *J. Am. Anim. Hosp. Ass.* **23**, 19–25.

Pollack M., Martin R.A. & Diters R.W. (1984) Metastatic squamous cell carcinomas in multiple digits of a cat: case report. *J. Am. Anim. Hosp. Ass.* **20**, 835–9.

Pommer A. (1933) *Wein tierärztl. Mschr.* **20**, 129–46.

Pool R.R. (1981) Osteochondromatosis. In Bojrab M.J. (ed) *Pathology in Small Animal Surgery*. Lea & Febiger, Philadelphia, pp. 641–9.

Pool R.R. & Carrig C.B. (1972) Multiple cartilaginous exostoses in a cat. *Vet. Path.* **9**, 350–9.

Pool R.R. & Harris J.M. (1975) Feline osteochondromatosis. *Feline Pract.* **5**(2), 24–30.

Pool R.R., Bodle J.E., Mantos J.J. & Ticer J.W. (1974) Primary lung carcinoma with skeletal metastases in the cat. *Feline Pract.* **4**(4), 36–41.

Prymak C. & Goldschmidt M.H. (1991) Synovial cysts in five dogs and one cat. *J. Am. Anim. Hosp. Ass.* **27**, 151–4.

Purdy J.G. (1961) Osteogenic sarcoma in a cat. *Canad. Vet. J.* **2**, 156.

Read R.M. & Smith R.N. (1968) A comparison of spondylosis deformans in the English and Swedish cat and in the English dog. *J. Small. Anim. Pract.* **9**, 159–66.

Reed R.E., Hoger R.S. & Trautman R.J. (1963) Coccidioidomycosis in two cats. *J. Am. Vet. Med. Ass.* **143**, 953–6.

Rengel M.F., Farrow C.S., Leighton R.L. & Rose R.L. (1977) Contracted gastrocnemius tendons: a surgical approach toward correction. *Feline Pract.* **7**(1), 14–23.

Richards C.D. (1977) Hypertrophic osteoarthropathy in a cat. *Feline Pract.* **7**(2), 41–3.

Riddle W.E. & Leighton R.L. (1970) Osteochondromatosis in a cat. *J. Am. Vet. Med. Ass.* **156**, 1428–30.

Riser W.H. (1964) In Catcott E.J. (ed) *Feline Medicine and Surgery*. American Veterinary Publications Inc., Illinois, p. 296.

Riser W.H., Brodey R.S. & Shirer J.F. (1968) Osteodystrophy in mature cats: A nutritional disease. *J. Am. Vet. Radiol. Sol.* **9**, 37–46.

Roberg J. (1977) Hypertrophic pulmonary osteoarthropathy in a cat. *Feline Pract.* **7**(6), 18–22.

Robertson J.L. (1982) Chronic progressive polyarthritis in a cat. *Carnation Research Digest* **18**, 8–15.

Robinson R. (1971) *Genetics for Cat Breeders*. Pergamon Press, Oxford, p. 170.

Russell R.G. & Walker M. (1983) Metastatic and invasive tumors of bone in dogs and cats. *Vet. Clin. N. Am.* **13**(1), 163–80.

Rutman M.A., Rickards D.A. & Chandler F.W. (1975) Feline cryptococcosis. *Feline Pract.* **5**(3), 36–43.

Salisbury S.K., Richardson D.C. & Lantz G.C. (1986) Partial maxillectomy and premaxillectomy in the treatment of oral neoplasia in the dog and cat. *Vet. Surg.* **15**, 16–26.

Saperstein G., Harris S. & Leipold H.W. (1976) Congenital defects in domestic cats. *Feline Pract.* **6**(4), 18–43.

Schmidt R.E. & Langham R.F. (1967) A survey of feline

neoplasms. *J. Am. Vet. Med. Ass.* **151**, 1325–33.

Schmitz J.A. (1978) Bronchogenic carcinoma in a cat presenting as rear leg lameness. *Feline Pract.* **8**(3), 18–22.

Schneck G.W. (1974a) A case of ectrodactylia in a cat. *Bulletin Feline Advisory Bureau* **14**(1), 27.

Schneck G.W. (1974b) Two cases of congenital malformation (peromelus ascelus and ectrodactyly) in cats. *Vet. Med. Small Anim. Clin.* **69**, 1025–6.

Schrader S.C. & Sherding R.G. (1989) Disorders of the skeletal system. In Sherding R.G. (ed) *The Cat. Disease and Clinical Management*, chap. 46. Churchill Livingstone, New York, pp. 1247–92.

Schrauwers E. & Appeldoorn A. (1991) Anterior cruciate ligament rupture associated with cardiomyopathy in three cats. *Vet. Comp. Orthop. Traumat.* **4**, 158.

Scott D.W. (1980) Feline dermatology. 1900/1978 a monograph. *J. Am. Anim. Hosp.* **16**, 331–459.

Scott P.P. (1964) Nutritional Requirements and Deficiencies. In Catcott E.J. (ed) *Feline Medicine and Surgery*. American Veterinary Publications Inc., Wheaton, Illinois.

Scott P.P. (1984) Nutrition. In Wilkinson G.T. (ed) *Diseases of the Cat and Their Management*, 2nd edn., chap. 1. Blackwell Scientific Publications, Oxford.

Scott-Moncrieff J.C., Cook J.R. & Lant Z. (1990) Acquired myasthenia gravis in a cat with thymoma. *J. Am. Vet. Med. Ass.* **196**, 1291–3.

Searle A.G. (1952–1953) Hereditary 'split-hand' in the domestic cat. *Annals of Eugenics* **17**, 274–82.

Seawright A.A., English P.B. & Gartner R.J.W. (1967) Hypervitaminosis A and deforming cervical spondylosis of the cat. *J. Comp. Path.* **77**, 29–39.

Seim H.B. & Nafe L.A. (1981) Spontaneous intervertebral disc extrusion with associated myelopathy in a cat. *J. Am. Anim. Hosp. Ass.* **17**, 201–4.

Shelton S.B., Bellah J., Chrisman C. & McMullen D. (1991) Hypoplasia of the odontoid process and secondary atlantoaxial luxation in a Siamese cat. *Progr. Vet. Neurol.* **2**, 209–11.

Sis R.F. & Getty R. (1968) Polydactylism in cats. *Vet. Med. Small Anim. Clin.* **63**, 948–51.

Spjut H.J., Dorfman H.D., Fechner R.E. & Ackerman L.V. (1971) *Tumors of Bone and Cartilage*. Armed Forces Institute of Pathology, Washington.

Straw R.C., Withrow S.J., Gillette E.L. & McChesney A.E. (1986) Use of radiotherapy for the treatment of intra-nasal tumours in cats: six cases (1980–1985). *J. Am. Vet. Med. Ass.* **189**, 927–9.

Sullivan M. (1989) Temporomandibular ankylosis in the cat. *J. Small Anim. Pract.* **30**, 401–5.

Susanek S.J. (1983) Feline skin tumours. *Compend. Contin. Educ. Pract. Vet.* **5**, 251–8.

Taylor J.E. & Schmeitzel L.P. (1990) Plasma cell pododermatitis with chronic footpad hemorrhage in two cats. *J. Am. Vet. Med. Ass.* **197**, 375–7.

Thoday K.L. & Evans J.G. (1972) Synovioma in a cat. *J. Small Anim. Pract.* **13**, 399–402.

Tischler S.A. & Owens J.M. (1986) Ulnar fibrosarcoma in a cat. *Mod. Vet. Pract.* **67**, 39.

Turrel J.M. & Pool R.R. (1982) Primary bone tumour in the cat. A retrospective study of 15 cats and a literature review. *Vet. Radiol.* **23**, 152.

Vos J.H., van der Linde-Sipman J.S. & Goedegebrurure S.A. (1986) Dystrophy-like myopathy in the cat. *J. Comp. Path.* **96**, 335–41.

Walker M.A., Duncan R., Shaw J.W. & Chapman W.W. (1975) Aneurysmal bone cyst in a cat. *J. Am. Vet. Med. Ass.* **167**, 933–4.

Walker R.W., Richardson D.C., Bryant M.J. & Draper C.S. (1983) Anaerobic bacteria associated with osteomyelitis in domestic animals. *J. Am. Vet. Med. Ass.* **182**, 814–6.

Ward J.M., Sodikoff C.H. & Schalm O.W. (1969) Myeloproliferative disease and abnormal erythrogenesis in the cat. *J. Am. Vet. Med. Ass.* **155**, 879–88.

Warren H.B. & Carpenter J.L. (1984) Fibrodysplasia ossificans in three cats. *Vet. Pathol.* **21**, 495.

Weiss D.S. & Armstrong P.F. (1985) Secondary myelofibrosis in three dogs. *J. Am. Vet. Med. Ass.* **187**, 423–5.

Wilkinson G.T. (1968) A review of drug toxicity in the cat. *J. Small Anim. Pract.* **9**, 21–32.

Wilkinson G.T. (1984a) Mycotic diseases. In Wilkinson G.T. (ed) *Diseases of the Cat and Their Management*, 2nd edn., chap. 18. Blackwell Scientific Publications, Oxford.

Wilkinson G.T. (1984b) Diseases of the locomotor system. In Wilkinson G.T. (ed) *Diseases of the Cat and Their Management*, 2nd edn., chap. 8. Blackwell Scientific Publications, Oxford.

Wilkilson G.T. (1984c) Diseases of the reproductive system. In Wilkinson G.T. (ed) *Diseases of the Cat and Their Management*, 2nd edn., chap. 10. Blackwell Scientific Publications, Oxford.

Wilkinson G.T. & Robins G.M. (1979) Polyarthritis in a young cat. *J. Small Anim. Pract.* **20**, 293–7.

Williams-Jones H.E. (1944) Arrested development of the long bones of the forelimbs in a female cat. *Vet. Rec.* **56**, 449.

Wills J.M., Howard P.G., Gruffydd-Jones T.J. & Wathes C.M. (1988) Prevalence of Chlamydia psittaci in different cat populations in Britain. *J. Small Anim. Pract.* **29**, 327–39.

Withrow S.J. & Holmberg O.L. (1983) Mandibulectomy in the treatment of oral cancer. *J. Am. Anim. Hosp. Ass.* **19**, 273–86.

Yoxall A.T. (1978) Pain in small animals – its recognition and control. *J. Small Anim. Pract.* **19**, 423–38.

Chapter 4 / The Blood and Haemopoietic System

R. J. EVANS

Disorders of the blood and haemopoietic system are particularly common in the cat and are often fatal. The two retroviruses, feline leukaemia virus (FeLV) and feline immunodeficiency virus (FIV) in large part account for the high incidence of blood disorders. These viruses and the epidemiology, pathogenesis and control of infection are discussed in Chapters 15 and 16. The aim of this chapter is to provide a concise overview of the normal features of feline blood and the differential diagnosis of the major blood disorders in the cat. A brief atlas of normal and abnormal appearances of feline blood cells is presented as Plates 4.1–4.16.

SAMPLE COLLECTION AND ROUTINE HAEMATOLOGICAL DETERMINATIONS

Collection of blood samples of good quality and of adequate volume from cats can be difficult. Cats are resentful of sampling from the cephalic vein and collapse of the vessel and poor blood flow render this an unsatisfactory site for venepuncture. The jugular vein is the site of choice and many cats are tolerant of sampling from this site, particularly if they are held inverted, a technique illustrated by Evans and Gruffydd-Jones (1984). Rough handling of the cat should be avoided since physiological leucocytosis results. Anaesthesia or sedation may induce marked and unpredictable changes in haematological values. Feline red cells shrink in the presence of excess concentrations of EDTA. Care should be taken to fill sample bottles to the correct volume. Haematological samples for diagnosis should be collected before any therapy since resultant blood changes may render diagnosis unnecessarily difficult. Representative reference values for cats are given in Table 4.1. These are to orientate the reader, but should not be used in the interpretation of laboratory results. Always refer to the reference ranges from the laboratory performing the investigations. Reference ranges for haematological parameters in the cat are wide. This may be due to failure to recognize the effects of breed variation, physiological variations and subclinical disease. Reference to previous determinations in the same individual aids meaningful interpretation as does the making of repeated determinations so that trends with time are made apparent as disease develops.

Haemoglobin
Haemoglobin determinations give artefactually high values when substantial numbers of Heinz or erythrocyte refractile (ER) bodies are present. The lysate should be centrifuged to sediment these before the reading is taken.

Red cell count
Feline red cells are relatively small (mean cell volume 40–55 fl). When using an electronic counter segregating cells by size the instrument must have variable thresholds and these should be appropriately set otherwise marked errors arise. There will be underestimation of the red cell count and overestimation of mean cell volume (MCV) and mean cell haemoglobin (MCH),

Table 4.1 Normal haematological values in adult cats.

PCV	0.30–0.45 l/l
RBC	4.7–9.2 × 10^{12}/l
Hb	9.0–15.5 g/dl
MCHC	30–36.5 g.dl^{-1}
MCV	40–55 fl
WBC	5.5–22.0 × 10^9/l
Bands	0–0.3 × 10^9/l
Neutrophils	3.2–13.4 × 10^9/l
Lymphocytes	2.6–6.8 × 10^9/l
Monocytes	0–0.85 × 10^9/l
Eosinophils	0–3.2 × 10^9/l
Basophils	0.1 × 10^9/l
Platelets	200–600 × 10^9/l
Plasma protein	55–85 g/l
Bleeding time	1.5–5 min
Whole blood clotting time	3–5 min
Kaolin-cephalin clotting time ⎫	Test system variable: compare with
Activated partial thromboplastin time ⎬	plasma from normal animal on
One-stage prothrombin time ⎭	each occasion

and of mean cell haemoglobin concentration (MCHC) when this is calculated on the basis of a notional haematocrit derived from cell count and MCV.

Reticulocyte enumeration

Morphologically distinguishable classes of reticulocyte are found in the cat. These have variously been divided into two or three types (Cramer & Lewis, 1972; Fan *et al.*, 1978; Jain, 1986). The author regards classification into three types as difficult to sustain. The two types are heavily reticulated cells and cells with a much finer punctate reticulum. The latter are older cells and therefore seen later in a marrow response: the reticulocyte in the cat has a prolonged maturation period. Coarsely reticulated cells (aggregate reticulocytes) are well correlated with the current marrow response and with polychromatic red cell numbers on Romanowsky-stained smears (Alsaker *et al.*, 1977). A polychromatic red cell count is therefore an easier way of assessing marrow response. The peak response occurs from 5–6 days after the acute induction of anaemia, reflecting the timespan of reticulocyte production from stem cells. Finely reticulate cells may

achieve much higher numbers than the coarsely reticulated (aggregate) cells and being relatively mature are a reflection of earlier bone marrow activity. Their count peaks at 10–12 days. Counts as high as 12% may be found in normal cats and up to 50% in anaemias with a marrow response.

Platelet enumeration

Platelet counting by electronic methods is unreliable. Spontaneous platelet aggregation is common as are shift platelets. Feline platelet counts are best performed by the visual method using a haemocytometer chamber.

Bone marrow aspiration

Bone marrow aspiration is indicated in pancytopenia, non-responsive anaemia, leucopenia, thrombocytopenia, suspected myeloid dysplasia, leukaemia or polycythaemia. It provides information about marrow activity and pathological infiltration.

Bone marrow aspiration may be performed from the iliac crest or from the shaft of the femur via the inter-trochanteric fossa. The author prefers the former site, but prepares a sufficiently large area so that the latter may be used if there is need. In cats bone marrow aspiration is best performed under general anaesthesia or heavy sedation.

The pattern of bone marrow needle is not critical, but it should be short, around 19 gauge and have a stylet and adjustable stop. It must be sterile. A sterile syringe, sterile-filtered 3.8% trisodium citrate or acid citrate dextrose (ACD) solution and trays of acid-alcohol washed slides are also required.

The area overlying the iliac crest and the head of the femur are shaved. The animal is laid on the opposite side. The skin is surgically prepared and the area draped. With a back and forth rotating movement, the needle is advanced into the lateral aspect of the iliac crest, aiming for a point some 0.25 cm inside its border, and being careful to keep the needle at 90° to the surface of the bone as it curves up towards the skin. Care should be exercised: with undue force the iliac crest may fragment. Once the needle has been felt to enter the marrow cavity, the stylet is removed and the syringe, containing approximately 0.2 ml of citrate solution or ACD, is attached. A short, sharp withdrawal of the plunger should result in a drop of viscous marrow flowing into the barrel. This is all that is required: excess suction results in dilution with blood and results in poor films. The material collected is discharged onto a number of slides. Sharply tapping one edge of a slide on a hard surface will cause excess blood to drain away. The flecks of marrow which remain are spread using another slide, laid face down upon them, drawn along with the minimum pressure. If no marrow is obtained, the attempt should be repeated before inserting the stylet, removing the needle and repositioning it elsewhere in the crest. If several attempts are unsuccessful, collection from the trochanteric fossa may be attempted. Detailed description of bone marrow cytology is outside the scope of this chapter. It is advised that smears are submitted to specialist laboratories for staining and interpretation. Individuals with experience of bone marrow cytology in the dog will find that of the cat broadly similar. The reader is referred to Schryver (1963), Gilmore *et al.* (1964), Penny *et al.* (1970) or Schalm (1972) for accounts of feline marrow cytology.

THE RED CELLS

Feline red blood cells are smaller and more nearly spherical than those of the dog, having a mean corpuscular volume (MCV) in the range 40–55 fl. The spherical form of the cells renders the area of central pallor indistinct and makes detection of pathological spherocytosis impossible. Slight anisocytosis is a normal feature. Howell–Jolly bodies are common in normal cats; some individuals have them in 1% of red cells (Hammon, 1940; Penny *et al.*, 1970). They are stained deep purple or blue-black in Romanowsky preparations, being residual nucleoprotein following nuclear expulsion. In many normal cats erythrocyte refractile (ER) bodies are present in up to 10% of cells, generally at or near their periphery. ER bodies have been recorded in up to 50% of erythrocytes in normal individuals (Beritic, 1965). The author has not encountered such high frequencies. ER bodies are unstained in Romanowsky smears but are stained by new methylene blue and are indistinguishable from Heinz bodies formed in the presence of oxidant intoxicants. Endogenous Heinz body formation is increased in diabetes mellitus, hyperthyroidism and lymphoma (Christopher, 1989). Red cell crenation is a common artefact in films prepared from cat blood. The red cell lifespan in the cat is relatively short compared with that in other species, ranging from 66 to 80 days in normal animals (Marion & Smith, 1983a). Some immature red cells stain in a stippled fashion with Romanowsky stains and such basophilic stippling is occasionally present in a few percent of red cells of apparently normal cats. It is, however, commonly encountered in anaemias with a marrow response.

In newborn kittens the packed cell volume, red cell count, haemoglobin concentration and mean corpuscular haemoglobin concentration are all low relative to adult values, but the mean corpuscular volume is increased. The haematocrit, haemoglobin concentration and MCV subsequently fall, reaching their lowest values at 4–6 weeks of age as a consequence of marginal iron status of the milk (Weiser & Kociba, 1983a).

Feline haemoglobins

Two major types of haemoglobin, haemoglobin A (HbA) and HbB, have been identified in cats, which have identical α- but differing β-chains. HbA and HbB coexist but show great variability of the ratio in which they are found in normal individuals (Lessard & Taketa, 1969; Taketa *et al.*, 1978). Three minor subtypes of HbB, known as HbB_1, HbB_2 and HbB_3, are also found (Taketa, 1974). HbA and HbB are of lower oxygen affinity than many other mammalian haemoglobins and this may be expected to enhance oxygen delivery to the tissues. HbB_1, HbB_2 and HbB_3 subtypes have higher binding affinities for oxygen than the major types. The oxygen affinity of feline HbA, but not HbB, is regulated by red cell 2,3-diphosphoglycerate (2,3-DPG); the concentration at which this is normally present in feline red cells is unusually low.

Feline haemoglobin is extremely susceptible to oxidative damage, manifested, for example, in paracetamol poisoning, and this is probably due to the large number of susceptible disulphydryl bonds in feline globins.

Feline red cell antigens

Recent evidence suggests that there is only a single important blood group antigen system borne by feline red cells. This system has two antigens, A and B, and three phenotypes, A, B and AB (Auer & Bell, 1981; Giger, 1992). The mode of inheritance of these antigens is somewhat unusual: A and B are alleles at a single gene locus with B behaving as recessive to A. It therefore appears that the AB phenotype is due to the existence of a third allele. The A antigen generally occurs with higher frequency than the B antigen, whilst AB is rare. There is, however, wide breed and geographical variation in the relative frequencies of the A and B alleles (see Giger, 1992, for a detailed discussion). The differing blood group substances are determined by the form of neraminic acid expressed on red cell membrane gangliosides and glycoproteins (Andrews *et al.*, 1992). Cats have naturally occurring allo- or isoantibodies to these blood group substances with haemagglutinating and haemolytic activity. The former activity is due to IgM and the latter to IgG plus IgM (Wilkerson *et al.*, 1991). Titres for both activities are higher in cats with type B cells than those with type A, and there are no antibodies in cats with the AB phenotype. These alloantibodies are responsible for the occurrence of transfusion reactions and haemolytic disease of the newborn.

Red cell abnormalities

Anaemia

Anaemia is a common and frustrating clinical problem. Cats generally present late in the course of the disease and by then the prognosis is poor. Anaemia is to be regarded as a clinical sign; it is not a diagnosis. The cause of anaemia must always be sought.

PATHOPHYSIOLOGY

The major physiological effect of anaemia is upon the oxygen-carrying capacity of the blood. The degree of impairment of the function of individual tissues by the consequent hypoxia depends upon their normal oxygen requirement. Signs related to the central nervous system, the musculoskeletal system and the cardiovascular system are prominent. As the haemoglobin concentration falls, cardiovascular compensatory mechanisms increase cardiac output and decrease peripheral resistance. Blood volume is kept constant by plasma volume expansion. There is diversion of blood flow from those tissues with low oxygen demand. The changes in haemoglobin types and oxygen affinity that occur in the anaemic cat are unusual and their adaptive value is difficult to predict. In anaemia, HbA concentrations are unchanged but HbB_1, HbB_2 and HbB_3 are increased at the expense of HbB. Concentrations of 2,3-DPG increase considerably and further reduce the inherently low oxygen affinity of HBA. Thus the diversity of haemoglobin oxygen affinities is increased in anaemia.

INVESTIGATION OF THE ANAEMIC PATIENT

The first step is to obtain clinical evidence and laboratory confirmation of anaemia. If this is present the type of anaemia should then be identified as a prerequisite to investigation of its cause. It is useful to separate these three elements of the investigation as an aid to logical analysis. An approach to investigation of feline anaemias has been presented as a flow diagram by Evans & Gruffydd-Jones (1984).

Clinical features

The signs which are present in an anaemic patient may be due:

1 to the anaemia itself,

2 to the compensatory adjustments

3 to the disorder causing the anaemia.

The balance of these varies from case to case depending on the degree of anaemia and the nature and the severity of the cause. The haemoglobin concentration at which signs develop depends on: the rate of fall in PCV; the degree of compensatory adjustment; and on exertional demand. Signs appear at higher haemoglobin concentrations in rapidly developing anaemias and in aged patients since compensatory changes are less marked. As cats can regulate their lifestyle to minimize exertion, and since owner's demands of an animal are often minimal, anaemia may be profound before illness is suspected.

Signs found include:

1 Lethargy and generalized weakness are the most common early signs.

2 Anorexia and weight loss are also common.

3 Pallor of mucous membranes is a cardinal sign but effects of cardiovascular function and reactivity on the appearance of the mucous membranes must be borne in mind. Absence of pallor does not preclude the presence of mild or moderate anaemia, nor does its presence establish anaemia.

4 Cold sensitivity and heat-seeking.

5 Cardiovascular signs. The high output state is the main source of cardiovascular signs, but pre-existing heart disease may be exacerbated. Tachycardia is common. Haemic murmurs are difficult to resolve in the cat. Radiography or electrocardiography may reveal cardiac enlargement.

6 Tachypnoea and dyspnoea on exertion are common. They are rarely noted at rest, until anaemia becomes severe.

7 Pyrexia is usually due to the underlying disorder or, in animals with concomitant leucopenia, to secondary infection, but fever spikes may accompany haemolysis.

8 Retinal haemorrhages may be noted in severe anaemia (Fischer, 1970).

9 Pica.

Establishing the presence of anaemia

The historical and clinical features of anaemia are non-specific. Other causes of lassitude, weakness, dyspnoea and hyperdynamic circulation must be considered. They may also accompany or underlie anaemia. The presence of anaemia and its degree can be established only by measuring blood haemoglobin concentration (or PCV). It should be noted that in the first 8 hours after acute haemorrhage or in severely dehydrated animals these values will be misleadingly high.

Discriminating the types of anaemia

The type of anaemia is determined from a full blood count, determination of the derived red cell indices and examination of a well-made, well-stained blood smear (Table 4.2).

Identifying the cause of the anaemia

The cause of the anaemia is the key to treatment and prognosis. Determination of the cause requires:

1 History and clinical examination.

2 Blood examination.

3 Special investigations.

Features of the history which are of particular relevance in determining the cause of anaemia are listed below.

1 The rate of onset. Rapid onset suggests acute haemorrhage, haemolysis or acute leukaemia.

2 Recurrent infections suggest accompanying agranulocytosis, which in turn may be due to bone marrow aplasia or myeloproliferative disease. Alternatively, they may be due to lym-

Table 4.2 Differentiation of acquired feline anaemia.

A Orderly marrow response (reticulocytosis, polychromasia, anisocytosis, increased MCV of appropriate magnitude)

1 Evidence of external or internal bleeding: haemorrhagic anaemia
2 No evidence of blood loss. Evidence of haemolysis (Heinz bodies, schistocytes, icterus, free haemoglobin, haemoglobinuria, methaemoglobinaemia) may or may not be present: haemolytic anaemia
   (a) Red cell parasites present: FIA or other parasitic anaemia
   (b) Heinz bodies increased in number and/or methaemoglobinaemia present: oxidative haemolysis
   (c) Evidence of haemolysin ingestion (e.g. saponin-containing plants): physicochemical haemolysis
   (d) Autoagglutination and/or positive antiglobulin (Coombs') test, ANA or LE-cell test: immune-mediated haemolysis
   (e) Red cell agglutination in the cold: cold-agglutinin disease
   (f) Schistocytes present, antiglobulin test negative, evidence of DIC or of cavernous tumour: mechanical haemolysis
   (g) FeLV-positive, antiglobulin test negative: FeLV-related haemolysis
   (h) None of the above: idiopathic haemolysis

B Disorderly marrow response (inappropriate macrocytosis and or NRBC present with reticulocytopenia. Abnormal cells from other lineages may or may not be present)

1 Myelophthisis, myeloid dysplasia and/or FeLV-positivity detected: dyserythropoietic anaemia

2 Evidence of lead ingestion and/or marked basophilic stippling. Blood lead levels increased: anaemia of lead poisoning

C No marrow response

1 Normochromic normocytic anaemia. Bone marrow hypocellular with normal or increased myeloid/erythroid ratio, or acellular. No systemic disease detected: marrow hypoplasia or aplasia
2 Normochromic normocytic anaemia. Bone marrow hypocellular with normal or increased myeloid/erythroid ratio, or acellular. FeLV or FIV positive: FeLV- or FIV-related marrow hypoplasia or aplasia
3 Normochromic normocytic anaemia. Bone marrow normocellular or hypocellular and possibly infiltrated; iron store may be increased. Neoplasia, chronic renal failure, chronic inflammation or other systemic disease detected: anaemia of systemic disease

D Marrow response absent or inadequate

1 Normochromic normocytic anaemia, or hypochromic microcytic anaemia. Bone marrow normocellular or hypercellular maturation arrest at late normoblast stage. Evidence of iron deficient-diet or chronic blood loss: iron deficiency anaemia.

phopenia. Lymphopenia is an important feature of FIV infection whilst granulocytopenia is encountered in FeLV infection.

3 Pyrexia may be due to infection, acute haemolysis, immunopathology or neoplasia.

4 Blood loss may be due to trauma, local bleeding lesions or haemostatic disorders.

5 Urinary system signs. Polyuria, polydipsia or uraemic episodes suggest that the anaemia is associated with renal disease.

6 A history which establishes any drug administration and exposure to toxins is essential.

7 Diet. The diet should be ascertained in all cases. It is particularly relevant in kittens since iron deficiency is most common at around the time of weaning.

Clinical examination for signs of underlying disease is essential. It cannot be assumed that laboratory examination will reveal the cause of the anaemia.

1 Skin. The skin should be examined for petechiation, ecchymoses and the skin lesions of systemic lupus erythematosus (see Chapter 1). In leucopenic animals, indolent ulceration or discharging sinuses may be present.

2 Mucous membranes. Evidence of icterus and

of a haemorrhagic tendency should be sought. The absence of icterus does not rule out haemolytic anaemia. Cyanosis or a muddy-brown discoloration may be present in anaemia due to oxidant poisons.

3 Superficial lymph nodes. Enlargement of lymph nodes suggests lymphosarcoma, tumour metastasis or local or generalized infection (including FeLV viraemia), but may also be due to extramedullary haemopoiesis.

4 Eye. Uveitis, choroiditis or retinal infiltration may be associated with leukaemic infiltration or with systemic disease, particularly feline infectious peritonitis, toxoplasmosis or tuberculosis.

5 Mouth and pharynx. Gingivitis or severe ulceration may be encountered in leucopenic animals, but the common occurrence of these signs reduces their value in the cat. Mouth ulcers may also be present in uraemia. Tonsillar enlargement may indicate infection, lymphosarcoma or tonsillar carcinoma.

6 Abdomen and gastrointestinal tract. Hepatomegaly and splenomegaly should be sought. These rarely reflect extravascular haemolysis. They are more likely to be due to leukaemic infiltration of these organs or to extramedullary haemopoiesis. Intra-abdominal masses may involve the lymph nodes, gastrointestinal tract, reproductive system, kidney and bladder and should be sought by palpation and, if necessary, by radiography.

7 Musculoskeletal system. Generalized or shifting lameness is moderately common and is often associated with FeLV positivity, leucopenia or immune-mediated polyarthropathy.

8 Urinary system. Haematuria may be due to urinary tract lesions or haemostatic defects. Proteinuria (>1 g/l) due to glomerular involvement is associated with systemic lupus erythematosus.

Special investigations

All anaemic cats merit investigation of their FeLV and FIV status. Bone marrow aspiration is indicated in cases where there is leucopenia, thrombocytopenia, dyshaemopoiesis or no marrow response. If there is icterus, total and direct bilirubin, bile acids and serum alanine transaminase and alkaline phosphatase levels should

be measured to assess liver function and status. For details of evaluation of the liver the reader is referred to Chapter 8 and to Evans and Heath (1988).

Causes of anaemia

Anaemia will be considered using the following categories:

1 Anaemia due to excessive red cell breakdown: haemolytic anaemia
2 Haemorrhagic anaemia
3 Iron-deficiency anaemia
4 Aplastic and hypoplastic anaemia
5 Anaemia associated with FeLV or FIV infection
6 Anaemia associated with other systemic disorders

ANAEMIA DUE TO EXCESSIVE RED CELL BREAKDOWN: HAEMOLYTIC ANAEMIA

It is unusual to suspect haemolytic anaemia on clinical grounds. Occasionally there may be muddy coloration of the mucous membranes associated with oxidant intoxicants. When haemolysis is exceptionally rapid and intravascular, icterus and haemoglobinuria may be seen. Haemolytic anaemias are characterized, once established, by reticulocytosis, anisocytosis, polychromasia and increased mean cell volume. These reflect the marrow response. Nucleated red blood cells may appear in the blood and the number of Howell–Jolly bodies increases. There may also be neutrophilia and a left shift. The bone marrow response takes several days to develop. Animals with acute haemolysis may therefore present before there is evidence of regeneration.

Feline infectious anaemia (FIA)

Anaemia associated with infection by *Haemobartonella felis* is relatively common. Many such cats are infected with FeLV or FIV or are otherwise immunosuppressed. The prognosis is such cases is much worse than in primary haemobartonellosis. It is therefore essential to investigate cats fully in which *Haemobartonella* infection is detected before deciding upon advice to the owner and a plan of management. Haemobartonellosis is discussed fully in Chapter 22.

Immune-mediated haemolytic anaemia

Immune-mediated haemolytic anaemia is increasingly being recognized in the cat (Werner & Gorman, 1984). Many cases are associated with FeLV-positivity or with myeloproliferative or lymphoproliferative disease (Gorman & Evans, 1987). Often the onset is insidious and animals present at an advanced stage: occasionally an intravascular haemolytic crisis with icterus or haemoglobinuria may be seen. One or more of hepatomegaly, splenomegaly, lymphadenopathy and pyrexia may be noted. Often autoagglutination of erythrocytes is detectable on the blood film. The total and differential white cell counts are variable. Diagnosis requires demonstration of anti-red cell antibodies or of erythrocyte-bound C3 by the direct antiglobulin test (direct Coombs' test). Alternatively serum anti-erythrocyte antibodies may be demonstrated by the indirect antiglobulin test. Care is needed in interpretation. Some apparently normal individuals give positive results. Autoimmunity to red cells may be associated with systemic lupus erythematosus. A positive Coombs' test may be found in haemobartonellosis, myeloproliferative and lymphoproliferative disease but the contribution of immune-mediated erythrocyte destruction to these anaemias is unclear. It is therefore essential to investigate thoroughly for underlying disease before assuming that primary immune-mediated haemolysis has been identified.

Neonatal haemolytic disease

There is no transplacental transfer of immunoglobulin in cats. Neonatal haemolytic disease (neonatal isoerythrolysis) arises due to colostral transfer of anti-erythrocyte antibodies from nursing queens to kittens. This can occur even with first litters in the cat because of the high levels of alloantibodies, particularly in type B queens (Giger, 1992). Giger (1992) suggests that this may be sufficiently common as to be a major cause of the fading kitten syndrome. Severe intravascular haemolysis results with marked haemoglobinuria, icterus, and associated lethargy developing within 1 to 2 days after birth (Cain & Suzuki, 1985; Hubler *et al.*, 1987). Death may ensue within a day of signs developing. Less severely affected kittens may cease suckling and fail to thrive. In animals that survive several days or manifest very mild disease necrosis of the tail tip may be seen. Incompatible matings should be avoided whenever possible. If a queen is pregnant following a known or suspected incompatible mating, the condition can be prevented by removing the kittens before they take colostrum and fostering or hand-rearing them. Kittens that become affected following suckling should be removed from the dam for at least 2–3 days and fostered on a dam of appropriate blood type or fed milk replacer by hand.

Systemic lupus erythematosus

Immune-mediated anaemia, leucopenia or thrombocytopenia may occur as part of the autoimmune syndrome of systemic lupus erythematosus (SLE). Some cases are associated with propylthiouracil therapy for hyperthyroidism (Peterson *et al.*, 1984), but spontaneous cases are seen. Haematological manifestations can occur alone or in combination with other signs. Persistent or recurrent mild fever with associated lethargy and inappetence is common. Skin involvement is seen, as is glomerulonephritis which results in proteinuria and may progress to renal failure; polyarthropathy gives rise to lameness, which shifts or may be difficult to localize; meningeal involvement results in deranged behaviour and seizures (see Chapters 1 and 2). Diagnosis rests upon the presence of an appropriate constellation of clinical and haematological features together with the presence of anti-nuclear antibody (ANA) or a positive LE cell test. Positive ANA or LE cell tests in the absence of clinical signs of SLE are not uncommon and can be associated with FeLV infection. Demonstration of hypocomplementaemia is a useful confirmatory finding but few UK labs presently offer assays for feline C3. Immunohistochemical demonstration of immune complexes and/or complement associated with glomerular or skin basement membrane is helpful.

Cold agglutinin disease

Anti-erythrocyte antibodies of the IgM class may give rise to cold agglutinin disease (Schrader &

Hurvitz, 1973). In this condition haemolysis is usually absent or minimal and the anaemia is mild. Significant haemolysis occasionally occurs. On exposure to cold, erythrocyte agglutination occurs in peripheral vessels leading to microvascular occlusion and poor perfusion. Cyanosis and gangrene of the digits, the tips of the pinnae, the tail and occasionally the eyelids or the apex of the nose result and the affected parts may slough. The animal should be kept in a warm environment.

Paracetamol, methylene blue and other
oxidant intoxicants
Intoxication of cats with paracetamol (acetaminophen) is common and is discussed in Chapter 27. Intravascular haemolysis is an important component of the resulting syndrome. This is due to oxidative damage to haemoglobin with the formation of methaemoglobin, giving the blood a chocolate brown colour, and the precipitation of oxidatively denatured haemoglobin as Heinz bodies. The susceptibility of cats to such oxidant intoxicants is a function of the large number of reactive sulphydryl groups in feline globin compared to that of other species (Taketa, 1967, 1974) and low activity of methaemoglobin reductase. The mechanisms and approaches to treatment have been reviewed (Hjelle & Grauer, 1986; Evans, 1988) and the reader is referred also to Chapter 27. Urinary antiseptics containing methylene blue have been administered to cats from time to time. Methylene blue is an oxidant compound and there is marked Heinz body formation and methaemoglobinaemia, accompanied by severe intravascular haemolysis (Schechter *et al.*, 1973). Cats that survive the acute effect develop a bone-marrow response. Methionine, phenazopyridine or benzocaine also induce haemolytic anaemia with methaemoglobinaemia and Heinz body formation (Harvey & Kornick, 1976; Maede *et al.*, 1985; Wilkie & Kirby, 1988).

Congenital haemolytic anaemia
Congenital erythropoietic porphyria has been reported in the cat and appears to be inherited in an autosomal dominant fashion (Glenn *et al.*,

1968; Giddens *et al.*, 1975). There is defective biosynthesis of porphyrin precursors of haem, haemolytic anaemia and pinkish-brown staining of teeth and bones due to pigment accumulation. The anaemia is macrocytic but hypochromic since haemoglobin synthesis is reduced. Poikilocytosis and target cells are noted. Porphyrins are excreted in the urine, which is dark and fluoresces in ultraviolet light. Affected animals also show marked photosensitivity and severe renal disease. A spontaneous haemolytic anaemia associated with haemoglobin crystalloid formation has been recorded in Siamese kittens. The biochemical defect has not been characterized (Altman, 1974).

Haemolytic anaemia of unknown aetiology
Cases of haemolytic anaemia having no identifiable cause are encountered from time to time. Often autoagglutination of erythrocytes is detectable on the blood film and this may be immune-mediated but gives false-negative Coombs' test results. The total and differential white cell counts are rather variable. If the toxic causes of haemolysis, feline infectious anaemia and haemorrhage have all been ruled out, administration of prednisolone using the regimen for immune-mediated disease may produce transient improvement but the prognosis remains poor in the long term.

HAEMORRHAGIC ANAEMIA
Haemorrhage due to trauma is a frequent occurrence. Acute haemorrhagic anaemias due to other causes are distinctly uncommon (apart from those due to bleeding disorders see p. 216). It must be remembered that, in the absence of fluid therapy, it may be 12 hours or more after bleeding commences before fluid shifts and haemodilution restore the circulating blood volume. Measurements of red cell parameters during this time give no index of the severity of blood loss. At this stage, signs of circulatory compromise due to volume depletion, particularly pallor of mucous membranes, poor capillary refill, increasing pulse rate coupled with decreasing pulse volume, are better indicators of the extent of blood loss and of response to

therapy. These should be monitored regularly as a guide to treatment required and its effectiveness. Once the PCV has fallen it may be another 2–3 days before the marrow response is apparent and extramedullary haemopoiesis becomes established. Once this has occurred the anaemia is macrocytic but normochromic or hypochromic, with reticulocytosis resulting in polychromasia and anisocytosis. Howell–Jolly bodies may be increased in number and nucleated red blood cells may be found in the circulating blood.

In cases where bleeding occurs internally there is no depletion of red cell constituents, there may be an extremely active erythropoietic response and hypochromasia is rare. Chronic blood loss is usually secondary to other disorders and results in a less obviously responsive picture. Blood may be lost through chronic bleeding lesions in the gastrointestinal or urinary tract. These and exceptionally heavy flea burdens may produce anaemia, as may coccidiosis in kittens. Depletion of iron stores may result with the consequent hypochromasia. Severe iron depletion may result in abrupt marrow aplasia. Haemostatic disorders are discussed on p. 216.

IRON DEFICIENCY: HYPOCHROMIC ANAEMIA
Iron deficiency anaemia due to simple dietary insufficiency is rare in adult cats. Mild normocytic normochromic or microcytic hypochromic anaemia is encountered in suckling kittens. The iron deficiency is rarely sufficient to present as a clinical problem but occasional litters or, more commonly, a few individuals in a litter have lower haemoglobin levels and fail to thrive. Treatment is then required and iron supplements should be given (see p. 203).

ANAEMIA OF REDUCED RED CELL
PRODUCTION: HYPOPLASTIC ANAEMIA,
RED CELL APLASIA, APLASTIC ANAEMIA
AND PANCYTOPENIA
Anaemia due to reduced red blood cell production is extremely common in the cat. In a proportion of such cases the aetiology is apparent. Feline leukaemia virus (FeLV) infection, chronic inflammatory disease, chronic renal failure or toxic agents may be responsible. Other forms of anaemia may progress to aplastic anaemia as a consequence of bone marrow exhaustion. In many cases of marrow hypoplasia or aplasia, however, the aetiology remains obscure. Reduced cell production by the bone marrow commonly affects all cell series producing pancytopenia. Since this is secondary to the primary marrow disorder, the conditions are correctly termed marrow hypoplasia or aplasia. The anaemia of marrow hypoplasia is normochromic and normocytic and reticulocytes are absent. Blood platelets and granulocytes have considerably shorter lifespans than do red cells, so that animals may present with recurrent or overwhelming infection or with bleeding before anaemia is well developed. Bone marrow aspiration confirms the diagnosis. There may be a dry or bloody tap and trephine biopsy may be required. The marrow is hypocellular, commonly with reduction in all cell series. If only the red cell series is affected pure red cell aplasia results, with normochromic normocytic anaemia but normal white cell and platelet numbers. In all these conditions the prognosis is poor.

ANAEMIA ASSOCIATED WITH FeLV AND
FIV INFECTION

Anaemias associated with FeLV infection
These, in aggregate, are the most commonly encountered symptomatic anaemias; indeed, up to 70% of anaemic cats are found to be FeLV positive. Cats of any age and either sex may be affected, but most commonly they are young adult animals and there is a preponderance of males (Cotter, 1979).

Non-responsive anaemia is the most common form encountered in FeLV-infected cats. The non-responsive anaemias associated with FeLV-infection may be divided into two classes. In many cases the anaemia is normochromic but macrocytic (Weiser & Kociba, 1983b). Many non-anaemic FeLV-positive cats also show macrocytosis. Reticulocyte counts are low but nucleated red blood cells may be present in the peripheral blood indicating dyshaemopoiesis. Many animals are lymphopenic and/or neutropenic but oc- casionally there is neutrophilia. The platelet count is normal or increased but large bizarre platelets are often present. A small proportion of animals are thrombocytopenic. It has been suggested that these cases represent a response to haemolysis (Weiser & Kociba, 1983b). That, however, seems unlikely in most cases. Rather, the evidence of deranged haemopoiesis involving the myeloid and megakaryocytic lineages in ad- dition to the erythroid precursors indicates that these are to be regarded as cases of myelodys- plastic syndrome (see below). The bone marrow shows changes typical of myeloid dysplasia. In the remainder the anaemia is aplastic or hypo- plastic and thus normochromic and normocytic. The platelet and leucocyte counts may be normal or there may be pancytopenia. Bone marrow aspiration reveals a marrow ranging from nor- mocellular to severely hypocellular with hypo- plasia or aplasia of all series or pure aplasia of the erythroid series.

Haemolytic anaemia occurs in a small propor- tion of anaemic FeLV-positive cats. There is a marrow response which is orderly and there may be jaundice. There is an increased MCV, reticulocytosis appropriate for the degree of anaemia, polychromasia, anisocytosis and in some cases mild splenomegaly or lymphaden- opathy. Such cats often show no evidence of infection with *Haemobartonella felis* or of other FeLV-related disease. Some but not all of these cats are Coombs' test-positive and it is not clear why the remainder haemolyse. The anaemia is of moderate severity and rarely life-threatening but the animal is debilitated. A few have a transient haemolytic episode with spontaneous recovery. More commonly, there is a persistent anaemia with recurrent haemolytic episodes. Others show inexorable slow haemolysis, which is eventually fatal. In some cases lymphoproliferative or myeloproliferative disease or non-responsive anaemia may supervene. The long-term prognosis in all cases of FeLV associated anaemia is grave.

Anaemia associated with FIV infection

The anaemia associated with FIV infection is commonly normochromic, normocytic and non- regenerative. Erythroid dysplasia or myelodys- plastic syndrome with maturation arrest in the erythroid series and Coombs'-positive anaemias also occur while haemolytic anaemia due to co- infection with *Haemobartonella felis* is a relatively common finding (Sparger, 1990; Shelton *et al.*, 1990a).

ANAEMIA ASSOCIATED WITH OTHER
SYSTEMIC DISEASES

Anaemia which is a sign of another medical dis- order is commonly encountered in the cat. These anaemias do not conform readily to any single or simple description of haematological type and signs of the primary disorder are often the key to diagnosis.

Lead poisoning

Lead poisoning is rarely reported in cats (see Chapter 28), although this low incidence may represent under-reporting. Old paint is the usual source. Gastrointestinal and central nervous signs are predominant. Although anaemia is a common feature of lead poisoning in man, the dog and a number of other species, only three feline cases appear to have shown anaemia (Holzworth, 1956; Jacobs, 1979). In these the anaemia was mild, normochromic and normocytic, with accom- panying leucopenia and little evidence of a marrow response. In two cases basophilic stippl- ing was marked and many nucleated red cells were found; in the third only occasional cells with basophilic stippling were noted. Diagnosis is by means of blood lead determinations and treat- ment should be with calcium edetate (see Chapter 28).

Chronic renal failure

Normochromic normocytic anaemia is common in chronic renal failure, but may be masked by dehydration unless attention is also paid to the plasma protein concentration. There is no reticulocytosis but nucleated red blood cells may be encountered. The total white cell count is usually normal or mildly elevated although this may mask neutrophilia accompanied by lym-

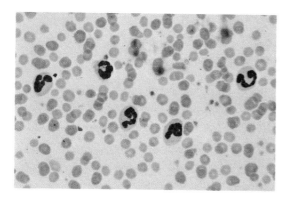

Plate 4.1 Blood film showing normal feline red cells. Note the very apple-shaped form of the red cells with a minimal area of central pallor and a much smaller diameter than canine red cells. Also present are a number of platelets. These are the small anucleate bodies with purple granulation. Five mature neutrophils, with segmented nuclei and containing fine dust-like pale pink granules are seen. This cat had a marked neutrophilia. In the cytoplasm of one neutrophil there is an angular blue body; this is a Döhle body.

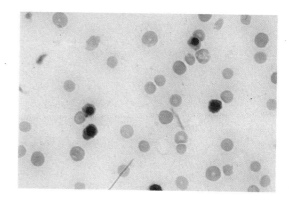

Plate 4.3 Four nucleated red blood cells with highly pyknotic nuclei present in an haemoglobinized cytoplasm are seen in this film. The remainder of the red cells show marked variation in size (anisocytosis) and a number of larger cells have a bluish tint to the cytoplasm (polychromasia). These large polychromatic cells correspond to coarse reticulocytes and are an index of recent marrow erythropoietic activity. This animal had an anaemia with a marrow response and the MCV was increased.

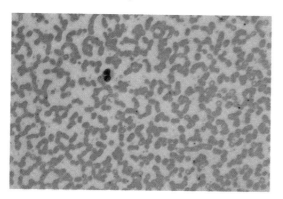

Plate 4.2 Many of the red cells contain discrete round basophilic inclusions varying between 0.2 and 0.5 μm in diameter. These are Howell–Jolly bodies. The red cells are also stuck together in clumps; this is autoagglutination and was not reversed by dilution with saline.

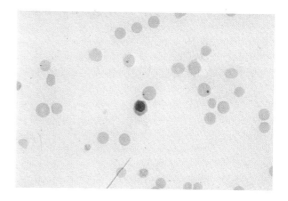

Plate 4.4 Another anaemia with a marrow response. A nucleated red cell and a number of Howell–Jolly bodies are to be seen. Polychromasia and anisocytosis are very marked.

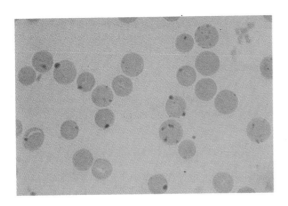

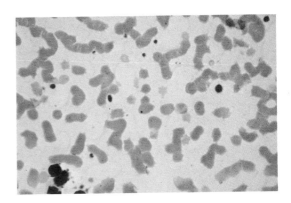

Plate 4.5 This cat had inadvertently been given par-acetamol by its owner and had developed dyspnoea and muddy cyanosis. The bulk blood sample was chocolate brown in colour. The blood was stained supravitally with new methylene blue before the film was made. The discrete blue-green round submembrane bodies at the periphery of many of the red cells are Heinz bodies which consist of oxidatively degraded haemoglobin. In addition four reticulocytes (immature red cells) with punctate or chain-like staining in the cytoplasm are present. The stained material is messenger RNA and polyribosomes, precipitated by the stain.

Plate 4.7 There are two discrete basophilic Howell–Joly bodies present in this film. Many of the red cells however bear reddish-purple coccoid or coccobacillary bodies which are substantially smaller than the Howell–Joly bodies and in places form chains. These bodies are *Haemobartonella felis* the causative organism of feline infectious anaemia (FIA). Auto-agglutination is also present. This is common in FIA and probably reflects the presence of secondary anti-red cell antibodies.

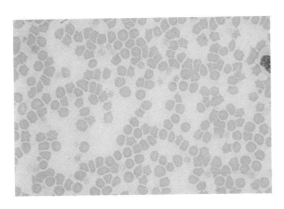

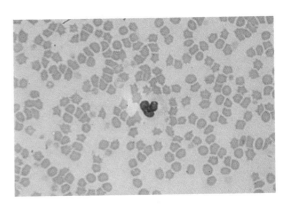

Plate 4.8 A neutrophil showing marked toxic vacuolation and a small number of basophilic toxic granules in its cytoplasm.

Plate 4.6 This film is from a kitten with iron deficiency. The MCHC was reduced and the cells are flatter and show a larger area of central pallor than do normally haemoglobinized cells. This film also demonstrates crenation, a drying artefact to which feline red cells are particularly susceptible.

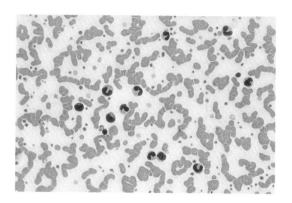

Plate 4.9 This film from a case of severe pyothorax shows a marked neutrophilia with a severe left shift (a leukaemoid reaction). Marked reactive neutrophilias such as this one can be extremely difficult to differentiate from myeloid leukaemia. Abundant band neutrophils are present as well as a rather small metamyelocyte and a plasma cell. The neutrophils show toxic vacuolation. Numerous large (poikilocytes) and small (schistocytes) angular red cell fragments produced by mechanical damage to red cells are present.

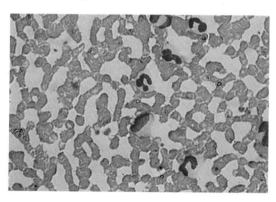

Plate 4.10 Neutrophils, bands and monocytes in the peripheral blood in a case of chronic myeloid leukaemia.

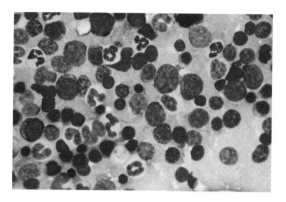

Plate 4.11 Bone marrow in a case of chronic granulocytic leukaemia. The marrow is hypercellular and dominated by abnormal granulocytic precursor cells. These cells are maturing through to bands and segmented cells.

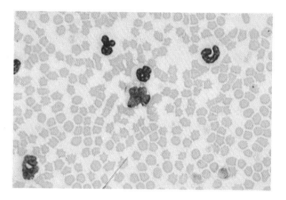

Plate 4.12 The large nucleated cell in the centre of the field is a monocyte. It has an irregular nucleus with skein-like chromatin. The cytoplasm is slatey blue-grey with abundant phagocytic vacuoles` and scant azurophilic granules.

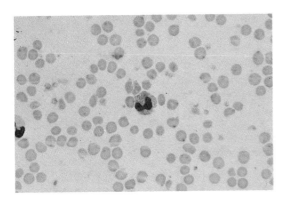

Plate 4.13 The nucleated cell is a normal eosinophil and contains abundant dull red, rod-shaped granules which almost fill the pale blue cytoplasm.

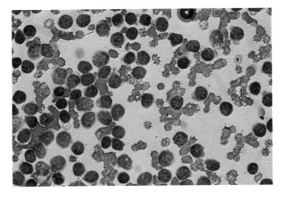

Plate 4.15 The peripheral blood in a case of lymphoid leukaemia. Vast numbers of abnormal prolymphocytes and lymphoblasts are present.

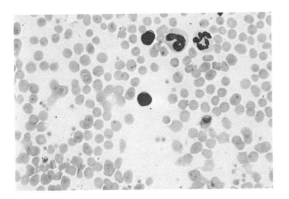

Plate 4.14 Two lymphocytes are present in the midline of this field, the nuclei are round with very condensed chromatin and only a thin crescent of Royal blue cytoplasm is visible. Two neutrophils are present, one with a very mature segmented nucleus, the other with an immature nucleus which is barely segmented. Several of the red blood cells contain Howell–Jolly bodies.

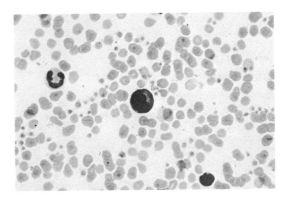

Plate 4.16 The nucleated cell in the centre of the field is a plasma cell. It has intensely stained plum-purple cytoplasm and an excenteric semilunar nucleus with lumpy peripheral condensation of the chromatin. Adjacent to the nucleus is the pale cytoplasmic zone (Hoff) corresponding to the Golgi apparatus.

phopenia. The platelet count is usually normal but bleeding may occur, resulting from platelet dysfunction induced by uraemic toxins. Often the anaemia is not sufficiently marked for there to be clinical signs directly referable to it but the severity tends to increase with progression of the renal failure. Bone marrrow aspiration may yield normocellular, hypocellular or mildly hypercellular marrrow. The erythroid series is hypoplastic and the myeloid to erythroid ratio is elevated. The anaemia is predominantly due to depression of erythropoiesis. Marrow depression, reduced renal erythropoietin production, reduced red cell survival, haemorrhage and reduced iron recycling may all contribute to the pathogenesis of the anaemia.

Anaemia of inflammatory disease
Mild to moderate normochromic normocytic anaemia is often seen in inflammatory or chronic diseases. It is encountered in feline infectious peritonitis, prolonged abscessation, pyometra, pleuritis and with many neoplasms. The anaemia closely resembles that of chronic renal failure, but there is great variability in leucocyte count depending on the inciting cause. Increased red cell destruction, reduced serum iron levels and impaired erythropoiesis contribute to the pathogenesis of the anaemia (Weiss & Krehbiel, 1983; Weiss *et al.*, 1983). Signs are rarely referable to the anaemia.

Management of anaemia
The general approach to the management of anaemia is as follows.
1 To treat the disorder causing the anaemia wherever possible.
2 Administration of specific haematinic agents where indicated.
3 Administration of bone marrow stimulants where indicated.
4 Symptomatic and supportive treatment.

TREATMENT OF THE UNDERLYING DISORDER
Unfortunately, as will be apparent from the preceding discussion, many of the causes of feline anaemia are not readily amenable to treatment.

However, the following steps are crucial to any management strategy:
1 Arrest blood loss if present. The risk in acute haemorrhage is from volume depletion and circulatory collapse rather than from reduced oxygen transport capacity, except in the worst cases. Circulatory volume should be maintained by infusion of crystalloids and colloids; blood transfusion is only required if the PCV falls rapidly or more than 25% of blood volume is lost.
2 Relieve systemic disease if possible:
 (a) In anaemia of inflammation treatment of the primary disorder is the important consideration. Infection should be aggressively treated with appropriate antimicrobial agents.
 (b) In chronic renal failure uraemic toxin molecules contribute to marrow depression. Treatment of the metabolic abnormalities and careful conservative management may therefore produce a little improvement in haemopoiesis. Treatment with androgenic steroids or haematinic agents (see below) may be attempted but is of limited value.
 (c) Known or suspected toxicants should be withdrawn and specific therapy initiated where possible (see Chapter 28).
 (d) In immune-mediated disorders treatment is initiated with immunosuppressive doses of prednisolone (2–4 mg/kg daily in two doses) until the PCV starts to rise, usually within 5 days. The dose of prednisolone is then progressively reduced at 14–21-day intervals. Once 0.25 mg/kg daily is reached alternate-day therapy is given before stopping if that is possible. It is important to monitor the anaemia: some animals may need maintenance therapy. Prednisolone is contraindicated in carriers of haemobartonellosis since it can precipitate recrudescence (Harvey & Gaskin, 1978): it is wise to check for this.

ADMINISTRATION OF SPECIFIC HAEMATINIC AGENTS
Haematinic agents should not be administered before an adequate haematological examination has been completed since the effects may obscure the diagnosis. Neither should haematinic agents

be administered unless there is a specific indication for so doing. This is rare in the cat, the major indication being for correction of hypochromasia, usually in kittens. Most commonly iron-dextran (25 mg/kg weekly) is used, but this preparation is painful to administer and ferrous sulphate tablets (28.5–57 mg/kg daily) may therefore be preferred. Iron administration is not indicated in normochromic anaemias with the sole exception of anaemia following haemorrhage, when there may be some depletion of marrow iron stores even in the absence of evidence of under-haemoglobinization. Treatment of the anaemia of inflammation is of doubtful value although in an experimental study haematinic agents did induce a response (Weiss *et al.*, 1983). It should be remembered that iron may exacerbate bacterial infections, and excessive administration can lead to intoxication.

ADMINISTRATION OF BONE MARROW STIMULANTS

Nandrolone and other androgenic steroids have a specific stimulant action on erythropoiesis, probably mediated via increased erythropoietin levels. They are therefore of some value in marrow aplasia or hypoplasia. A dose at the upper limit of the therapeutic range should be given once weekly for 6 weeks. Regular monitoring of peripheral blood and re-examination of bone marrow aspirates are helpful in assessing response. Unfortunately, this is often poor in cats. In other anaemias nandrolone is contra-indicated since over-stimulation may itself bring about marrow failure.

RECOMBINANT ERYTHROPOIETIN

Recombinant human erythropoietin is now relatively readily available and may have a role in the therapy of some feline anaemias (Cowgill, 1992). It may be expected to be of value in the anaemia of chronic renal failure since in this case circulating erythropoietin concentrations are subnormal. Giger (1993) suggests 75–150 IU/kg s.c. three times weekly followed by tapering down of the dose once the PCV increases to 0.3 l/l to avert the possibility of excessive red cell formation.

It is possible that development of antibodies to erythropoietin may occur, in which case the PCV is likely to drop despite continued administration of erythropoietin. It may also be of use to increase red cell mass prior to presurgical collection of blood for subsequent autotransfusion. Other, speculative, indications include FeLV- and tumour-associated anaemias, and the minimization of the toxicity of cytotoxic chemotherapy.

SUPPORTIVE THERAPY

Blood transfusion

Blood transfusion is indicated when the packed cell volume falls rapidly or drops below about 0.14 l/l. It may also be indicated in haemostatic insufficiency due to thrombocytopenia or DIC, inherited coagulation defects (haemophilia, factor IX deficiency and von Willebrand's disease) or the acquired defect following ingestion of anti-coagulant rodenticides. In circumstances where restoration of platelet count and function is required, freshly drawn blood is essential, whereas in coagulopathies fresh-frozen plasma may be preferred. For red cell replacement, feline blood collected in acid citrate-dextrose solution (ACD) can be stored at 4°C for 3 weeks (Marion & Smith, 1983b) or citrate-phosphate-dextrose (CPD) for 4 weeks, but this is rarely done and blood is often collected immediately prior to use. The jugular vein is the site of choice for blood collection and the technique illustrated by Evans & Gruffydd-Jones (1984) may conveniently be employed for collection of up to 75 ml of blood from a donor. Cats used as donors should be free of FeLV, FIV and *Haemobartonella felis* infection. Unmatched blood should not be used and test doses of blood should not be given since 1 ml of mismatched blood can result in a fatal reaction. The donor and the recipient should be blood-typed and/or crossmatching performed since transfusion reactions are likely to occur even on first transfusion due to the presence of preformed alloantibodies (Auer *et al.*, 1982; Giger, 1992). Typing and cross-matching can be easily and reliably performed using slide agglutination techniques (Giger, 1992; Norsworthy, 1992). For detecting A-positive cells in typing, anti-A antiserum from a type B cat can be used, while for detecting type B cells *Triticum vulgaris* lectin is a convenient reagent. For recipients of the AB type, blood from A-type donors can safely be used for transfusion since AB cats have no alloantibodies. It is recommended that stored blood be warmed by passing it through coiled tubing lying in a bath of water at 37°C. Use of an in-line filter is recommended. Administration should be at 0.5 ml/min or slower and therefore bags (transfer bags may conveniently be used) and drip sets are to be preferred for large transfusions.

When they do occur, transfusion reactions have an initial phase characterized by agitation and crying, hypotension, apnoea or hypopnoea and bradycardia with atrioventricular block followed by depression, recumbency, urination, vomiting and hypersalivation (Auer *et al.*, 1982; Giger, 1992). Death may occur in the first 1–3 minutes or the animal may survive and develop tachycardia and tachypnoea. Subsequently the consequences of intravascular haemolysis become apparent as haemoglobinaemia, haemoglobinuria and hyperbilirubinaemia. Blood transfusion is best avoided in immune-mediated disease unless the anaemia is life-threatening, in view of the great risk of a haemolytic crisis.

Other measures
Other supportive therapy may be helpful: in particular vitamins and a high-protein diet may be of some value. If fluid therapy is considered it must be appreciated that haemodilution will exaggerate the anaemia and its effect.

Polycythaemia
Polycythaemia is an increase in red cell mass. The differential diagnosis of polycythaemia requires the discrimination of polycythaemia vera, which is a myeloproliferative disorder (see below), from secondary reactive polycythaemia.

Secondary polycythaemia may arise because of anoxia due to cardiopulmonary disease or high altitude. A feline case has been reported in association with Fallot's tetralogy (Kirby & Gillick,

1974). In man it also occurs as a consequence of erythropoietin-producing renal tumours. Causes of secondary polycythaemia should be eliminated before diagnosing polycythaemia vera.

Polycythaemia vera is characterized by excessive uncontrolled production of red cells. There are a small number of reports of feline polycythaemia vera (Reed *et al.*, 1970; Duff *et al.*, 1973; Theilen & Madewell, 1979). Affected animals may be presented because of markedly congested mucous membranes or the consequences of blood hyperviscosity, most commonly transient and variable neurological signs due to poor brain perfusion. The PCV is markedly elevated (often 70–85 l/l) but plasma protein concentration is normal. The platelet and white cell counts may also be elevated. Bone marrow aspiration reveals a markedly hypercellular marrow with a decreased myeloid:erythroid ratio dominated by maturing erythroid cells. The author is not aware of any attempt to treat a feline case of the disease.

WHITE BLOOD CELLS

White blood cell counts
The total white cell count is variable: for instance, it is readily elevated by stress and breed variations probably exist; moreover, subclinical disease may go unrecognized. The differential count is also inconstant. Absolute values are more meaningful and more easily interpreted than percentages. In kittens, lymphocytes constitute up to two-thirds of the white cells, while in adults 85% may be neutrophils and the absolute white blood cell count is somewhat higher. Rather high eosinophil counts are found in many ostensibly normal cats which may relate to substantial helminth burdens.

Morphology of feline white blood cells
The morphology of feline white cells stained by Romanowsky methods will be described briefly. The author uses the May–Grünwald–Giemsa variant as giving the most subtle gradations of staining and thus facilitating cell differentiation. For additional information on the form and

function of feline leucocytes the reader is re-fered to Jain (1986). For discussion of the cyto-chemistry of feline white cells see Jain (1986) and Facklam and Kociba (1986).

Neutrophils

Feline neutrophils have relatively large nuclei, which are rather irregular and less commonly show pronounced lobulation than do those of the dog. There is irregular chromatin condensation. The cytoplasm is pale with a fine faint-pink granulation. In females, 4–11% of neutrophils may have a nuclear drumstick appendage (sex-chromatin lobe) compared with up to 1.9% of cells in males (Loughman *et al.*, 1970). Band (immature) neutrophils have a smooth U-shaped or sigmoid nucleus with reticular chromatin showing areas of slight condensation. Bands con-stitute less than 2% of the peripheral blood white cells in the healthy cat.

Monocytes

The monocyte is the largest feline leucocyte and has a nucleus which is commonly angularly and irregularly bi- or trilobed but occasionally round or bean-shaped. The chromatin shows little con-densation and has skein-like strands. The cyto-plasm is dull blue-grey with a ground-glass appearance. Azurophilic granulation is uncom-mon in feline monocytes. Phagocytic vacuoles may be present.

Eosinophils

Feline eosinophils usually have a bilobed, 'spectacle'-shaped nucleus. Their granules are fine, rod-shaped and reddish-orange, lacking the obvious refractility seen in other species. The granules almost completely fill the cytoplasm.

Basophils

Feline basophils lack the prominent granulation seen in other species. The cytoplasm is greyish and it contains many small, faint-staining, round, variously grey and pinkish-purple granules. The nucleus is weakly lobulated.

Lymphocytes and plasma cells

The lymphocytes of peripheral blood are pre-dominantly small. They have a round or slightly indented nucleus with variable chromatin con-densation. The cytoplasm forms a narrow rim and is intensely blue. Small numbers of azurophilic cytoplasmic granules are occasionally found.

The feline plasma cell has relatively more cyto-plasm, which is intensely basophilic with a pale Golgi zone adjacent to the nucleus. The nucleus is eccentric, has clumps of condensed chromatin and is round or occasionally bean-shaped. Plasma cells are rarely encountered in peripheral blood.

Abnormalities of white cells

Leucopenia

Leucopenia is a moderately common haemato-logical finding in cats and is often severe and persistent. It is important because severe secondary infection in consequence may be life-threatening and because it invariably indicates serious underlying disease. Leucopenia is often associated with infection with FeLV or with FIV (Hopper *et al.*, 1989). Marked leucopenia is most commonly due to neutropenia but may be due to severe lymphopenia or to panleucopenia. The importance of lymphopenia as a reason for leucopenia has been brought into prominence by the recognition of FIV, in which it is a common feature (Pedersen *et al.*, 1987; Harbour *et al.*, 1988; Hopper *et al.*, 1989; Yamomoto *et al.*, 1989; Shelton *et al.*, 1990a). Lymphopenia is a relatively frequent finding in cats; it is sometimes due to exogenous or endogenous glucocorticoids or to stress. FeLV infection in young kittens may give rise to thymic atrophy with lymphopenia and immuno-incompetence. A reduced lymphocyte count may be seen in the early stages of lym-phosarcoma and those lymphoid cells present are often lymphoblasts. Pure deficiencies of single cell lines may also arise without severely de-pressing the total white cell count. Eosinopenia unaccompanied by a decrease in the other granulocytes is usually due to endogenous or exogenous glucocorticoids.

Leucopenia may be due to increased cell de-

Table 4.3 Causes of leucopenia.

Decreased cell production
  FeLV infection
  FIV infection
  Feline enteritis virus infection
  Feline infectious peritonitis (infrequently: leucocytosis
    is more common)
  Marrow aplasia or hypoplasia
  Myeloproliferative disease (myelodysplastic syndromes,
    acute leukaemia or myelofibrosis)
  Myelophthisis
  Therapy with cytotoxic drugs

Cell sequestration
  Endotoxic or septic shock
  Anaphylaxis

Increased cell utilization
  Gram-negative septicaemia
  Endotoxic or septic shock
  Viraemia
  Severe pyogenic infection
  Toxoplasmosis (in a proportion of cases in the subacute
    and chronic phases)
  Viraemia

Increased cell destruction
  Gram-negative septicaemia
  Endotoxic or septic shock
  Disseminated intravascular coagulation
  Hypersplenism

struction or utilization, to sequestration or to decreased white cell production. Absolute values for all the white cell series should therefore be inspected. Causes of leucopenia are classified in Table 4.3. The common causes are: FeLV or FIV infection; myeloproliferative disease; marrow aplasia; and myelophthisis. From the study of Chickering *et al.* (1985), there is little evidence that immune-mediated leucopenia occurs in cats, but in view of its regular occurrence in other species it seems likely that it will be documented in the cat.

CLINICAL FEATURES ASSOCIATED WITH
LEUCOPENIA
The signs with which leucopenic animals may present are rather variable and reflect failure to control infection and immuno-incompetence.

One can, however, recognize a number of typical syndromes.

1 Acute presentation is not uncommon with severe leucopenia. There are four main clinical forms:
  (a) Severe, often haemorrhagic gastroenteritis.
  (b) Overwhelming Gram-negative septicaemia; this is often associated with (a).
  (c) Overwhelming disseminated pyogenic infection.
  (d) Cellulitis or localized pyogenic infection.
2 Chronic moderate leucopenia is more often seen. This is rather variable in presentation but frequently the cat has shown general malaise and anorexia and failed to thrive for days, weeks or months and there is often a mild to moderate lymphadenopathy which may be localized or generalized. There will usually be evidence of increased susceptibility to infection, which may take the form of:
  (a) Recurrent or persistent pyrexia.
  (b) Chronic skin disease, recurrent abscessation or discharging sinuses.
  (c) Chronic stomatitis, gingivitis or periodontitis.
  (d) Chronic diarrhoea.
  (e) Rhinitis.
  (f) Ocular discharge, often with associated conjunctivitis or keratitis.
  (e) Chronic internal infection such as uterine stump or ovarian ligature abscesses or granulomas, or low-grade but persistent peritonitis following spaying.

THE APPROACH TO THE LEUCOPENIC PATIENT
The approach to the patient presenting with signs suggestive of leucopenia in many ways resembles that employed with the anaemic patient. Thus, the approach may be divided into three elements:
1 Establishing whether the patient is leucopenic.
2 Establishing which cell series is/are affected.
3 Investigating the underlying cause.

History and examination
A detailed medical history should be taken, as for an anaemic patient, and with emphasis on evidence of chronic or recurrent infection and of the

underlying cause. Examination also parallels that of the anaemia patient. Evidence of localized or generalized lymphadenopathy, of splenomegaly or hepatomegaly should be sought carefully, as should evidence of localized or generalized infection. Petechiation or bleeding tendencies may be significant since thrombocytopenia may accompany agranulocytosis, particularly if it is due to marrow dysfunction. Thoracic and abdominal radiography may be of value in supporting suspicions of effusion associated with infectious processes and confirming liver and spleen size.

Laboratory investigation

A full haematological examination will show whether the patient is leucopenic and which cell series is involved. Concurrent non-regenerative anaemia and thrombocytopenia suggest bone marrow involvement as does evidence of dys-haemopoiesis. Toxic granulation and a profound left-shift may suggest overwhelming infection, as may the presence of schistocytes and regenerative anaemia. The latter may also be present in agranulocytosis accompanying autoimmune haemolytic anaemia or systemic lupus erythematosus. Lymphopenia suggests a viral cause, particularly FIV or FeLV, a subleukaemic condition, or toxoplasmosis.

Further investigations

Blood examination is rarely fully diagnostic and other investigations will be required to confirm or extend haematological findings.
1 The FIV and FeLV status of all leucopenic cats should be determined.
2 If there is pyrexia or other evidence of infection, blood culture or culture of samples from other appropriate sites may be indicated.
3 If there is evidence to suggest bone marrow pathology, bone marrow aspiration is indicated.
4 Biopsy of enlarged lymph nodes, spleen and liver may also be helpful.
In a proportion of cases these investigations are not diagnostic. It is then necessary to support the patient, to observe and to reinvestigate after several days or weeks depending upon the progress of the condition.

CONDITIONS UNDERLYING LEUCOPENIA

Feline panleucopenia virus infection (feline infectious enteritis)

The profound panleucopenia associated with the parvovirus of feline panleukopenia is discussed in Chapter 13. Parvovirus infection should always be considered when a leucopenic animal is presented but it should be borne in mind that FeLV infection can result in a syndrome closely resembling acute feline infectious enteritis.

Leucopenia associated with FeLV infection

Leucopenia due to FeLV infection may present in several ways. The association between FeLV and a syndrome of acute enteritis closely resembling panleucopenia is well recognized. This often follows some stress and runs a peracute course with severe depression, dehydration, hypothermia, collapse and death. The faeces are heavily tinged with bloody mucus or frank blood may be passed. Haematological examination reveals features closely resembling panleucopenia. Some aid in differentiation is provided by their incidence. Panleucopenia is a highly infectious disease and if a susceptible colony is infected a number of cases are likely to be seen in a short period of time. In contrast, FeLV-related acute enteritis is a sporadic problem.

Leucocyte disturbances associated with FIV infection

A number of leucocyte abnormalities are associated with FIV infection (Pedersen *et al.*, 1987; Harbour *et al.*, 1988; Hopper *et al.*, 1989; Shelton *et al.*, 1990a). Lymphopenia is common as is neutropenia, and the two may coexist. In other cases the neutrophil and lymphocyte counts are at the bottom of their reference ranges. Mild monocytosis is frequently present. Uncommonly lymphocytosis may be noted. FIV and FeLV infection may occur together in which case the leucopenia is worse and the animals die at an earlier age than cats affected only with FIV (Ishida *et al.*, 1989; Shelton *et al.*, 1990a). Very severe neutropenia may arise when FIV-positive cats are treated with griseofulvin (Shelton *et al.*, 1990b).

Gram-negative septicaemia

Gram-negative septicaemia may give rise to profound leucopenia, often with severe toxic granulation and a degenerative left-shift (Schalm *et al.*, 1975).

Reduced granulocyte production

Reduced output of granulocytes from the bone marrow may arise in a number of conditions. Bone marrow aplasia due to drugs or toxins may be selective or may involve all cell series. Such agranulocytosis may also be idiopathic (Swenson *et al.*, 1988). Neutropenia is a common finding in myelodysplastic syndromes and acute leukaemias (Blue *et al.*, 1988) due to replacement of normal bone marrow by abnormal cells and interference with normal haemopoiesis (see below).

MANAGEMENT OF LEUCOPENIC ANIMALS

The management of leucopenic animals has three major components.

1 Treatment of the underlying disorder if that is possible.

2 Administration of marrow stimulants where appropriate.

3 Provision of supportive therapy.

Treatment of the underlying disorder

Only bacterial infections, autoimmune causes and hormonal causes of leucopenia are readily amenable to treatment. Incriminated drugs and toxins should be withdrawn in cases of failure of granulopoiesis or of lymphopenia.

Administration of marrow stimulants

In agranulocytosis due to marrow failure of idiopathic origin, or due to drugs or toxins, administration of nandrolone plus prednisolone, may have limited effect in stimulating granulopoiesis. Antimicrobial cover is essential.

Supportive therapy

It is not possible significantly to raise the white cell count by whole blood transfusion and it is rarely practical to provide leucocyte concentrates for this purpose even in referral centres. Aggressive antimicrobial therapy of established infections is essential. The antimicrobial regime must be effective against Gram-negative and Gram-positive organisms. Ampicillin or co-amoxiclav plus gentamicin is a useful combination. The patient's water and electrolyte balance must be maintained.

PROGNOSIS

The prognosis in all leucopenic animals is grave. A small proportion of animals with FeLV-induced leucopenia recover, but are at risk of succumbing to other FeLV-related disease later.

Leucocytosis

Leucocytosis is an increase in the number of leucocytes; it may be either physiological or pathological. Physiological leucocytosis is a common occurrence in the cat and may partly explain the wide normal range of white blood cell counts. The great majority of cases of pathological leucocytosis are inflammatory in origin and predominantly due to an increase in neutrophil polymorphs.

PHYSIOLOGICAL LEUCOCYTOSIS

Physiological leucocytosis is catecholamine-induced. It is a frequent occurrence in cats and is particularly marked in young animals and those which are not accustomed to being handled. It may occur with fear, excitement, rough handling, in strange surroundings or with seizures or exercise. It is apparent within 2–5 minutes and usually persists for 20 minutes to 1 hour. All the white cells are increased, usually to values around the upper limit of their normal range or slightly higher, with neutrophilia and lymphocytosis being prominent features of the response. The lymphocyte count may come to exceed that for neutrophils.

STRESS LEUCOCYTOSIS

Stress leucocytosis occurs as a consequence of increased circulating glucocorticoids of exogenous or endogenous origin. There is a neutrophilia but no left shift; lymphopenia and eosinopenia are observed and there may be monocytosis but it is a less consistent finding than in other species and tends to arise late in the response (Jain, 1986). Stress leucocytosis is relatively uncommon in the cat, but may be seen following surgery, in trauma and painful conditions, in other non-inflammatory disorders including neoplasia, and in spontaneous or iatrogenic Cushing's disease. The response develops within 6 hours after the insult begins and, depending upon whether the cause is transient or persistent, may wane over the course of 24 hours or may be long-lasting.

INFLAMMATORY LEUCOCYTOSIS
Neutrophilia, with a left-shift, is the principal feature of inflammatory leucocytosis. In this circumstance the left-shift is known as regenerative. The white cell count is commonly in the range $20–40 \times 10^9/l$ and only infrequently exceeds $75 \times 10^9/l$ (Schalm, 1962; Jain, 1986). Toxic changes are a frequent finding in feline neutrophils and are non-specific. These changes include the presence of pale-blue angular cytoplasmic inclusions (Döhle bodies), diffuse cytoplasmic basophilia and vacuolation, and variably sized purple cytoplasmic granules. Döhle bodies are a particularly common finding; toxic vacuolation is seen with moderate frequency but toxic granulation is rare. Inflammatory leucocytosis is seen in infection, trauma, necrosis, hypersensitivity, haemorrhage and haemolysis. The most severe responses, with the neutrophilia and left-shift both being marked, are associated with localized acute pyogenic processes.

INAPPROPRIATE LEUCOCYTE RESPONSES
From time to time in severe pyogenic infections or Gram-negative septicaemias inappropriate responses may be seen:
1 Bands may exceed polymorphs in number (degenerative left-shift).
2 There may be left-shift with neutropenia (see above).
3 There may be profound leucocytosis with an extreme left-shift including metamyelocytes, myelocytes and even promyelocytes (a leukaemoid reaction). Profound monocytosis

and monoblastosis may also be present.

A leukaemoid reaction can be difficult to differentiate from granulocytic (myeloid) leukaemia. Anaemia accompanies the latter but may also be present in leukaemoid reactions. The presence of markedly abnormal myeloblasts may allow diagnosis of malignancy with certainty. If this is not the case, bone marrow aspiration is indicated even when infection is present since this may be secondary to the white cell abnormalities rather than the cause. The marrow aspirate is usually diagnostic since the changes in a leukaemoid reaction are usually not sufficiently marked to suggest leukaemia. In rare cases, however, the distinction cannot be made until post-mortem examination.

Eosinophilia may be a marked feature of hypereosinophilic syndrome in which there is infiltration of a variety of tissues and organs with eosinophils (McEwen *et al.*, 1985). The infiltration commonly involves the liver, spleen, gut and lymph nodes but other sites may also be affected. Despite recurring suggestions to the contrary (see, for example, Verhaert *et al.*, 1987) this condition is quite discrete from eosinophilic leukaemia.

Congenital morphological abnormalities of white cells
Abnormal granulation of neutrophils is seen as an autosomal recessive inherited trait in Birmans (Hirsch & Cunningham, 1984), and granulation abnormalities of a wide range of cell types, including platelets and granulocytes, are observed in Chediak–Higashi syndrome (see p. 220). Metachromatic granules are seen in granulocytes, lymphocytes and monocytes in mucopolysaccharidosis VI (Jezyk *et al.*, 1977). In mannosidosis there is vacuolation of lymphocytes and monocytes (Alroy *et al.*, 1989) Nuclear hyposegmentation (Pelger–Huët anomaly) has also been recorded (Latimer *et al.*, 1985).

HAEMOPOIETIC NEOPLASIA AND DYSPLASIA

Haemopoietic neoplasms are extremely common in the cat; indeed, they account for nearly one-third of all feline neoplasia (Neilsen, 1969). Few other species have such a high prevalence of spontaneous neoplastic disease of the haemopoietic system. This is largely because of the frequency of FeLV infection. Haemopoietic neoplasms may arise from any blood cell lineage. They have classically been divided into those originating from the lymphoid lineages, the lymphoproliferative conditions, and those arising from the bone marrow stem cells responsible for the genesis of red cells, leucocytes and megakaryocytes, known as the myeloproliferative conditions. But the occasional coexistence of lymphoid and myeloid neoplasms in the same animal and cases of lymphoblastic leukaemia supervening in myeloid dysplasia suggest that the distinction may be somewhat illusory. The lymphoproliferative conditions may be divided into leukaemic conditions, with neoplastic cells arising predominantly in the bone marrow, and solid tumours, with cell proliferation occurring predominantly at other sites. Approximately 80–90% of all feline haemopoietic neoplasms are localized lymphomas, strongly associated with FeLV. FeLV positivity is a feature of many animals with other haemopoietic disorders, including neoplasia and dysplasia. FIV has been implicated in the induction of feline neoplasms but its role is presently uncertain (Hopper *et al.*, 1989).

The term 'myeloid dysplasia' is used to describe a complex of conditions in which there is disordered proliferation and maturation of haemopoietic cells in bone marrow, but in which proliferation has not become entirely autonomous (Linman & Bagby, 1978; Blue *et al.*, 1988). The classification and nomenclature of leukaemias and myelodysplastic disorders is still the subject of considerable controversy. Until recently the classification of such disorders has been based on subjective criteria which have made comparison between reports and the consistent study of the natural history and response to therapy of these conditions unsatisfactory. The growing recognition that myelodysplastic changes commonly precede acute myelogenous leukaemia has contributed much to the concepts of leukaemiogenesis and to improvements in classification. Attempts to apply the now well-developed French-American British (FAB) classification of human

leukaemic and preleukaemic conditions (Bennett *et al.*, 1976, 1982; Mufti *et al.*, 1985) to the domestic animals are leading to considerable advances in the understanding and classification of the bone marrow disorders in a number of species, including the cat (Grindem *et al.*, 1985a; Evans & Gorman, 1987; Blue *et al.*, 1988). The concept that dysplastic and neoplastic conditions of the haemopoietic system are stem cell disorders and that they may thus affect any haemopoietic lineage and commonly involve more than one lineage is central to this new understanding. Indeed it has been suggested that all the manifestations of marrow dysplasia and haemopoietic neoplasia may represent elements in the spectrum of a single disorder (Linman & Bagby, 1978). The concept that there is a progression of changes which may evolve from normality, through myelodysplastic syndromes (MDS) to acute leukaemia or marrow failure is consonant with the belief that the induction of neoplasia is a multistep event. Linman and Bagby (1978) termed the dysplastic changes and associated clinical features preleukaemic syndrome. The terms 'myeloid dysplasia' or 'myelodysplastic syndrome(s)' have recently been preferred because of the natural history of the conditions. Many patients with a myelodysplastic syndrome will progress to acute leukaemia but other outcomes are well recognized. The majority of feline cases will progress to overt haemopoietic neoplasms within weeks or months; others remain stable; some have slowly but progressively worsening severity of dysplasia; yet others show a waxing and waning course without becoming frankly leukaemic; and a proportion die of bone marrow failure (Grindem *et al.*, 1985a; Evans & Gorman, 1987; Blue *et al.*, 1988).

Myelodysplastic syndromes

The conditions generally recognized as myelodysplastic syndromes in man are refractory anaemia (RA); refractory anaemia with ringed sideroblasts (RARS); refractory anaemia with excess blasts (RAEB); chronic myelomonocytic leukaemia (CMML); and RAEB in transformation (Bennett *et al.*, 1982). Of these RAEB (Baker & Valli,

1986) and CMML (Raskin & Krehbiel, 1985) have been recognized in the cat, as has an analogue of RARS but with irregular haemosiderin disposition in sideroblasts (Blue *et al.*, 1988). Some authors also regard chronic granulocytic leukaemia, polycythaemia vera and aplastic anaemia as myelodysplastic conditions with considerable justification.

The animal with a myelodysplastic syndrome usually presents with the consequence of a cytopenia affecting one or more marrow lineages. Most of the cases previously classified as smouldering, or subleukaemic leukaemias are now best regarded as being examples of myeloid dysplasia. Many cats with myeloid dysplasia are FeLV-positive (Grindem *et al.*, 1985a; Baker & Valli, 1986; Evans & Gorman, 1987; Blue *et al.*, 1988). Animals with myelodysplastic syndromes are best left untreated apart from appropriate supportive therapy for the consequences of the cytopenias.

Acute leukaemias

A variety of disorders in which more than 30% of the cells in the bone marrow are blast cells are encountered in the cat. These are the acute leukaemias. Formerly they have been classified as acute myeloid (granulocytic) leukaemia, monocytic leukaemia, acute myelomonocytic leukaemia, erythroleukaemia, erythraemic myelosis, reticuloendotheliosis, megakaryocytic myelosis and acute lymphoid (lymphoblastic) leukaemia on subjective criteria. These descriptive terms are difficult to apply consistently or rigorously and the terminology and objective criteria of the FAB classification are to be preferred (Grindem *et al.*, 1985a; Evans & Gorman, 1987; Blue *et al.*, 1988). The categories of acute myelogenous leukaemias within the FAB classification are: acute myelogenous leukaemia without maturation (M1); acute myelogenous leukaemia with maturation (M2); hypogranular promyelocytic leukaemia (M3); acute myelomonocytic leukaemia (M4); acute monocytic leukaemia (M5); erythroleukaemia (M6); and megakaryoblastic leukaemia (M7). Three variants of acute lymphoblastic leukaemia are recognized: L1, in which the cells are small

with scanty cytoplasm and inconspicuous nucleoli; L2, with a heterogeneous population but with many large cells with abundant cytoplasm and prominent nucleoli in a quarter or more of the cells; and L3, with a homogeneous population of large cells with prominent nucleoli and moderate amounts of deeply basophilic vacuolated cytoplasm. Of these, M2, M4, M5, M6, L1, L2 and L3 have been identified in cats by strict application of the FAB criteria (Grindem *et al.*, 1985; Blue *et al.*, 1988).

Myelofibrosis

Contrary to previous belief it has now been demonstrated that the fibroblasts of bone marrow are not derived from the haemopoietic stem cell (Golde *et al.*, 1980). Fibroblast proliferation with fibrosis of the marrow cavities is, however, a feature of acute myelogenous leukaemia and myelodysplastic syndromes as well as idiopathic myelofibrosis in man. In the cat myelofibrosis has been associated with acute myelogenous leukaemias and myelodysplastic syndromes (Blue, 1988) and FeLV infection (Sodikoff & Schalm, 1968; Hoover & Kociba, 1974; Flecknell *et al.*, 1978; Onions *et al.*, 1982). The fibrosis is probably secondary to megakaryocytic dysplasia and release of platelet- and megakaryocyte-derived growth factor (Castro-Malaspina, 1984).

Other haemopoietic neoplasms

Chronic haemopoietic neoplasms have not yet been related to the acute leukaemias and myelodysplastic syndrome although, as noted above, some have been tentatively included in classification schemes and there are growing arguments that they may be regarded as part of the same spectrum of conditions. Amongst cats the chronic malignancies are much rarer than myelodysplastic syndrome and acute leukaemias.

Polycythaemia vera

Polycythaemia vera is probably to be regarded as a form of myeloid dysplasia. It is discussed on p. 205.

Chronic granulocytic leukaemias

Well-differentiated chronic granulocytic leukaemias comparable to those seen in man appear to be uncommon in the cat. Most cases of granulocytic leukaemia in the literature fall into the more acute variants discussed above. Rarely cats with similar clinical features to those noted above are encountered and prove to have high mature neutrophil counts and hypercellular well-ordered marrow. Some of these may be chronic granulocytic leukaemias although there is often infection present and therefore difficulty arises in separating them from leukaemoid leucocytosis. Eosinophilic leukaemia is rare and must be carefully differentiated from the hypereosinophilic syndromes (Jain, 1986). There are few case reports of basophilic leukaemia (Saar & Reichel, 1983).

Chronic lymphoid leukaemia

Uncommonly, chronic lymphocytic leukaemia is encountered (Holzworth, 1960a; Thrall, 1981) and the total white cell count may reach $200 \times 10^9/l$. The cells are predominantly small lymphocytes and many are 'smudged' on blood and marrow aspirate smears.

Plasma cell myeloma

Myelomas are neoplasms of plasma cells which often produce sufficient immunoglobulin to produce a detectable elevation of serum globulins with a discrete monoclonal peak of myeloma protein on electrophoresis. There are many reports of feline multiple myeloma although it is a relatively rare neoplasm in cats (MacEwan & Hurvitz, 1977). There is focal proliferation of plasma cells, which may involve only the bone marrow or which may be seen in the parenchymatous organs and lymph nodes also. Plasma cells are rarely seen in the blood. In most cases the presentation is non-specific with depression, anorexia and weight loss, together with marked anaemia as presenting signs and the hypergammaglobulinaemia is discovered incidentally. Marrow infiltration may result in granulocytopenia and thrombocytopenia in addition to anaemia. Susceptibility to infection and haemostatic abnormalities result. More specific manifestations such as hyperviscosity syndrome or multiple erosions of bone cortices with bone pain and pathological fractures are relatively uncommon in the cat although both do arise. Bence-Jones proteinuria is also less common in affected cats than dogs, although it can occur, and renal amyloidosis may develop. Diagnosis is by serum electrophoresis coupled with the identification of large numbers of neoplastic plasma cells in aspirates from bone marrow or a peripheral mass.

Malignant mastocytosis

The origin of mast cells remains uncertain. Mast cell neoplasms may not be of haemopoietic origin and do not appear to be related to FeLV infection (Hayes, 1976; Muller, 1983). They may occur as focal masses or with diffuse proliferation of mast cells. Focal tumours are the more common form and are often cutaneous although they may occur elsewhere. Diffuse infiltration may involve the spleen, liver, lymph nodes, bone marrow and lungs. Affected animals may develop disturbed gastrointestinal function or gastric ulceration due to histamine release from the neoplastic cells. Heparin release may result in coagulopathy. Cutaneous and visceral involvement may be found in the same animal. In approximately half of cats with the diffuse form, neoplastic cells are present in the blood and/or the bone marrow. Mast cells may be distinguished from basophils by their larger size, round nuclei and larger granules.

Investigation of suspected haemopoietic dysplasia or neoplasia

Clinical examination should be essentially as outlined for the investigation of anaemia. Animals may present with one or more clinical features related to primary or secondary effects of the neoplasm. Although the presence of haemopoietic dysplasia or neoplasia may be suspected on clinical grounds, it is frequently an incidental finding on laboratory investigation because of the non-specific nature of the signs. The prognosis and management will depend upon whether the animal is suffering from a myelodysplastic syndrome or whether there is frank leukaemia.

However, similar clinical features are encountered in both. Diagnosis and decisions about management therefore rest heavily upon the examination of peripheral blood and of bone marrow aspirates.

Clinical features
The clinical features outlined below should alert the clinician to the possibility of haemopoietic dysplasia or neoplasia and collection of blood and bone marrow for examination should then be a high priority:
1 Anaemia: an extremely common finding in these conditions. It is often severe, macrocytic and refractory.
2 Cachexia: marked loss of condition and weakness, often coupled with loss of appetite, are prominent findings.
3 Recurrent infection/pyrexia: leucopenia or functional abnormalities of the circulating white cell population predispose to infection. Septicaemia, recurrent bacteraemia, disseminated or recurrent localized infections may be seen.
4 Pyrexia: recurrent or persistent pyrexia is a common presenting feature. It may be associated with infection but in many cases no infective process can be identified. In such cases pyrogen release from neoplastic cells or immune-mediated processes may be responsible.
5 Lymphadenopathy: mild to moderate discrete or generalized lymphadenopathy is commonly encountered. It may be due to neoplastic infiltration, extramedullary haemopoiesis or reaction to infection.
6 Splenomegaly and hepatomegaly: these may arise singly or together. They may be due to infiltration by neoplastic cells, to extramedullary haemopoiesis or to sequestration of abnormal or opsonized cells.
7 Bleeding tendency: disordered haemostasis may be encountered as a consequence of thrombocytopenia, platelet dysfunction, coagulopathy or of disseminated intravascular coagulation (see p. 222).
8 Uveitis: uveitis may be noted if there is infiltration of the iris and ciliary body by neoplastic cells. The iris is dull and swollen and there is aqueous flare. There may also be hypopyon,

hyphaema or keratitic precipitates. The involvement may be unilateral or bilateral.
9 Skin lesions: nodular skin lesions may be present in mastocytosis, and in cutaneous lymphosarcoma.

Radiography
Radiography has value in the investigation of such cases. Abdominal radiographs may confirm suspicions of hepatomegaly and splenomegaly. In severe cases of myelofibrosis (see p. 212) radiography of a long bone may reveal decreased size and decreased radiolucency of the marrow cavity. Localized lytic lesions of bone, osteoporosis or compression fractures may be seen in plasma cell myeloma, due to invasion of bone by malignant cells from the marrow.

Haematological examination
The peripheral blood features accompanying lymphoproliferative and myeloproliferative disease are varied. In myelodysplastic syndromes the animal may show anaemia, granulocytopenia, thrombocytopenia or any combination of these. These cytopenias are commonly transient and recurrent. Anaemia is most commonly nonresponsive and normochromic but macrocytic, although some cases are normocytic or microcytic. Nucleated red cells may be present despite reticulocytopenia, and this and macrocytosis in the absence of a response indicate dyserythropoiesis. Haemolytic anaemias which may be Coombs'-positive or unexplained are also encountered and rarely there is haemorrhagic anaemia secondary to thrombocytopenia and bleeding. There is generally evidence of granulocytic and megakaryocytic dyspoiesis manifest by the presence of morphologically abnormal cells in the blood. Large, atypically granulated platelets and giant neutrophils showing disparities in nuclear and cytoplasmic maturity, abnormal nuclear or granular morphology or monocytoid features are common. Circulating micromegakaryocytes may be present. In the acute leukaemias severe anaemia is usually present. The total white cell count is often normal or reduced although it can be markedly elevated by circulating lymphoid cells.

Bone marrow aspiration and trephine biopsy

Bone marrow aspiration should be undertaken. Dry or bloody taps are not uncommon. In such cases histological examination of core biopsies may also be helpful. In myelodysplastic syndromes bone marrow examination usually reveals an inappropriately hypercellular marrow for the blood counts, and disordered maturation of one or more lineages with an excess of immature cells but less than 30% of cells being blasts. However, in some cases the marrow may be hypoplastic. Small, mononuclear megakaryocytes and other abnormalities of megakaryocytic nuclear morphology and maturation are a frequent feature. Refractory anaemia with an excess of blast cells, in some cases with siderocytes, is also a common finding (Baker & Valli, 1986; Blue *et al.*, 1988). In acute leukaemias more than 30% of the marrow cells will be blasts and their identity as determined from their morphology, cytochemistry and ultrastructure will determine whether the condition is an acute lymphoid leukaemia (L1–3) or an acute myelogenous leukaemia (M1–7) and the subcategory into which it falls (Grindem *et al.*, 1985a,b; Facklam & Kociba, 1986). Biopsy of enlarged lymph nodes, or of the liver or spleen if enlarged, may also be of value in identifying leukaemic infiltration in the acute leukaemias, but must be undertaken with great caution. Cytogenetic analysis may prove diagnostically helpful (Grindem & Buoen, 1989).

Other investigations

Culture of specimens from localized areas of infection is of value, as is blood culture if bacteraemia or septicaemia is suspected.

Post-mortem examination

The detailed post-mortem findings differ from condition to condition, but commonly there is a firm, fleshy bone marrow. The lymph nodes, spleen and liver may all be enlarged and firm in consistency. The spleen and liver may be pale or distinctly mottled. Changes in other organs are variable. Histological examination reveals the infiltration of affected organs by neoplastic cells. In myelofibrosis there is a hypocellular bone marrow with mild to marked reticulin fibrosis (Blue, 1988).

Management

Few of the feline haemopoietic dysplastic and neoplastic conditions are amenable to effective treatment. In myelodysplastic syndromes chemotherapy is not indicated and supportive treatment is given to minimize the consequences of secondary effects such as infection. The prognosis is poor. Although cats with myelodysplastic syndromes may survive as long as 18 months, many undergo transformation to acute leukaemia within a few weeks of diagnosis. The acute myelogenous leukaemias are rapidly fatal and treatment has thus far proved ineffective. The chemotherapy of acute lymphoblastic leukaemia, chronic lymphocytic leukaemia, myeloma and mastocytosis are discussed in Chapter 27.

HAEMOSTASIS

The physiological termination of bleeding involves the interaction of three components:

1 The vascular wall
2 The blood platelets
3 The coagulation system of the plasma

Within a few minutes of injury, vascular constriction and the formation of a plug of aggregated blood platelets lead to arrest of the escape of blood (the primary haemostatic response). The platelet plug, which would otherwise break down after a few hours, is then stabilized by the formation of fibrin by the coagulation system (the secondary haemostatic response). The normal platelet count in the cat is $200–600 \times 10^9/l$. The mean platelet volume is $11–18\,fl$ (Weiser & Kociba, 1984). On the Romanowsky stained blood film the platelets have a pale-blue cytoplasmic rim surrounding a denser purple granular nucleoid. Clot retraction, which is an index of platelet function, usually occurs within 2 hours.

Platelet morphology resembles that of man and platelet aggregation is induced by adenosine diphosphate, collagen, pig plasma, and proteolytic snake venom but not by thrombin (Lewis, 1981).

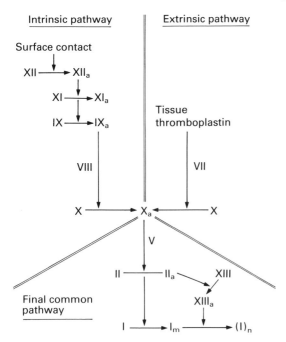

Intrinsic pathway   Extrinsic pathway

Surface contact

Final common
pathway

Key (suffix 'a' denotes the activated form of a clotting
factor):

I   Fibrinogen, I_m fibrin monomer, $(I)_n$ fibrin
         polymer
II   Prothrombin, II_a thrombin
V   Labile factor
VII   Stable factor
VIII   Antihaemophilic globulin
IX   Christmas factor
X   Stuart–Prower factor
XI   Plasma thromboplastin antecedent
XII   Hageman factor
XIII   Fibrin-stabilizing factor
PK   Prekallikrein (Fletcher factor),
         KK kallikrein
HMWK   High molecular weight kininogen

Fig. 4.1 The blood coagulation system and its three
component pathways.

The normal coagulation system of the cat is of the
classical mammalian form indicated in Fig. 4.1,
having a slow high-amplification intrinsic pathway
and a fast low-amplification extrinsic pathway,
which converge on the final common pathway at
the level of factor X. There are, however, some
significant differences from the pattern in man:
factors V and VIII are present at much higher
activity, factors VII, IX, X, XI and XII at slightly

higher levels, and Fletcher factor (prekallikrein)
activity is extremely low (Lewis, 1981). As in
other species factor VIII coagulant protein circu-
lates as a complex with factor VIII-related antigen,
a discrete protein derived from an autosomal
gene. Factor VIII-related antigen is involved in
platelet interactions with damaged endothelium.
The fibrinolytic system is present in cat plasma
(Lewis, 1981), as is progressive antithrombin
activity.

Haemostatic disorders

Disordered haemostasis may be encountered as a
consequence of thrombocytopenia, platelet dysfunction, coagulopathy or of disseminated intravascular coagulation. Bleeding disorders may be
congenital or acquired.

Investigation of a suspected bleeding disorder
The history and clinical evaluation should:
1 Eliminate a local lesion as the cause of bleeding.
2 Confirm an abnormal tendency to bleed.
3 Establish whether the defect involves the primary haemostatic system (platelets and blood
vessel) or the secondary response (blood
coagulation).
4 Identify whether the defect is long-standing/
congenital (and therefore likely to be inherited)
or acquired.
5 Elucidate the mode of inheritance if the condition appears to be hereditary.
6 Identify underlying disease if the condition is
acquired.

HISTORY
To distinguish normal from abnormal bleeding it
is essential to document carefully the time of
onset, frequency, extent, duration and site of
bleeding or bruising, together with the nature and
severity of any inciting causes. Abnormal bleeding occurs in two clinically discrete ways:
1 Spontaneous bleeding, often from unusual sites.
2 Prolonged bleeding after obvious injury.

Spontaneous bleeding
Bleeding associated with platelet and vessel wall
defects is characteristically superficial involving

the skin and mucous membranes. It takes the form of petechiation, purpura, ecchymoses or epistaxis. Bleeding from visceral mucous membranes may cause haematemesis, melaena or haematuria. The cat's fastidious habits often result in owners overlooking melaena or haematuria. Spontaneous bleeding due to coagulation abnormalities is uncommon in cats and ocurs only in marked defects, but when noted it is often deep and severe. It may be into skeletal tissues, joints or other body cavities. Sudden-onset bleeding with mixed features may occur in warfarin intoxication, in von Willebrand's disease with a marked deficit, and in severe disseminated intravascular coagulation (see below).

Bleeding following injury (including surgery and dentistry)

When bleeding follows injury, the salient points are the time of onset in relation to the injury and the duration. With platelet or vessel defects, bleeding is prolonged, with no evidence of cessation. In coagulation defects the bleeding may stop as if normal, as a platelet plug forms, but it restarts some hours later as the platelet-plug breaks down. To be significant, traumatic wounds must divide the full skin thickness and must gape. Searching for scars may help remind owners of incidents that they cannot otherwise recall. The most useful information about post-surgical bleeding is that it may relate to simple procedures in which little is done to secure haemostasis from the smaller vessels, for example castration and dental extractions. Surgery in which the wound is carefully sewn up in layers may be survived by patients with severe haemostatic abnormalities.

FAMILY HISTORY

The breed and sex of the affected individual should be noted. Inquiries should be made as to whether similar abnormalities have been noted in related animals. If the condition is heritable, it is probable that the signs and severity will be similar in affected members of a kindred. Dissimilar bleeding patterns may usually be disregarded. Similar patterns increase the evidence for a genuine abnormality and the inheritance pattern is of diagnostic value. Factor VIII deficiency (haemo-

philia A) and factor IX deficiency (haemophilia B) are sex-linked traits.

CLINICAL EXAMINATION

The clinical examination has three main objects:
1 To identify any local lesion or systemic disease that may explain an observed bleeding tendency.
2 In the absence of evidence of localized or generalized disease producing bleeding, to confirm the presence of a clinically significant abnormality.
3 To discover whether the defect affects the platelet and vascular components of haemostasis, the coagulation component, or both.
Evidence of superficial or of deep bleeding should be sought (see above) and a search made for a causative local lesion or underlying general disease.

If the history and/or clinical examination support the possibility of a bleeding disorder, further investigation is indicated.

The bleeding time should be measured three times. An ear pinna is shaved on its outer surface, preferably the day before the determination. The skin is swabbed with alcohol and allowed to dry. A lancet is used to produce a gaping skin wound remote from a major vessel. A stopwatch is started at the moment the wound is made. The emerging blood is gently absorbed onto the edge of a filter paper every 15 seconds. The bleeding time is the time taken for blood to stop issuing from the wound. In the cat this is normally 1.5–5 minutes; a bleeding time over 7 minutes can be considered abnormal. A prolonged bleeding time indicates a platelet or vascular wall abnormality.

LABORATORY INVESTIGATION

The laboratory examination should comprise the following:
1 A red blood cell evaluation, including examination of a blood film.
2 A white cell evaluation, including examination of a blood film.
3 Enumeration and morphological assessment of the platelets.
4 A whole blood clotting time (WBCT: screening test of the intrinsic system) followed by evaluation of clot retraction (crude test of platelet function).
5 An activated partial thromboplastin time

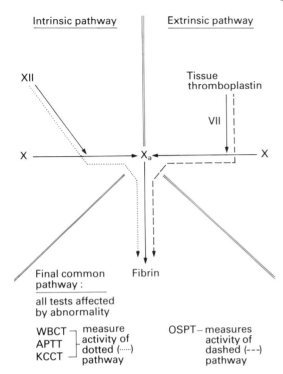

Intrinsic pathway   Extrinsic pathway

The WBCT, APTT and KCCT measure activity of the dotted pathway (··········). The OSPT measures activity of the dashed pathway (-------). In conditions affecting the final common pathway results of all four of these tests are abnormal.

Fig. 4.2 Diagram of the relationship of screening tests to the three components of the clotting system (see Fig. 4.1).

(APTT) or a kaolin cephalin clotting time (KCCT) (a more sensitive index of the intrinsic system and final common pathway) (Fig. 4.2).

6 Determination of the one-stage prothrombin time (OSPT: an assessment of the extrinsic system and final common pathway) (Fig. 4.2).

The interpretation of the laboratory findings is summarized in Table 4.4. If only the intrinsic tests are abnormal this relates the abnormality to this pathway; conversely if only the one-stage prothrombin time is abnormal the extrinsic pathway is implicated. If both extrinsic and intrinsic pathway tests are affected, there may be abnormality of the final common pathway. Alternatively, there may be multiple abnormalities as in warfarin poisoning and disseminated intravascu-

lar coagulation (DIC). If there is clinical evidence of systemic disease, or thrombocytopenia with co-agulation disturbance, DIC should be suspected. If DIC is suspected fibrin degradation products (FDP) should be determined. All the above determinations can be performed in a practice laboratory and commercial reagents are available. A normal animal should always be tested at the same time as a patient to provide a control value since the biological reagents used are rather variable. Examples of reference values for screening tests have been given by Killingsworth *et al.* (1985) but for the above reason they should only be used for orientation not for the interpretation of results.

Further investigation requires single factor assays. For these the animal should be referred to a specialist laboratory. However, the diagnosis can often be extrapolated with a substantial degree of certainty from the history, clinical signs and screening test results.

Quantitative disorders of platelets

THROMBOCYTOPENIA

Thrombocytopenia is an acquired abnormality and may occur as the result of decreased platelet production (in marrow hypoplasia, haemopoietic neoplasms, idiopathic thrombocytopenia, cyto-toxic therapy or irradiation, infection with FeLV or FIV), increased destruction (in immune-mediated thrombocytopenia), sequestration (in hypersplenism) or increased utilization (in DIC). Thrombocytopenia may accompany viral or Gram-negative bacterial infections.

Idiopathic thrombocytopenia

In idiopathic thrombocytopenia only platelet production is decreased, whereas in other circumstances resulting in reduced production all marrow lineages are commonly involved. Bone marrow aspiration is diagnostic.

Immune-mediated thrombocytopenia

Immune-mediated thrombocytopenia occurs as a primary disease (Joshi *et al.*, 1979) in the cat and in association with other conditions. It has been

Table 4.4 Laboratory diagnosis of bleeding disorders.

Disorder	Platelet count	Bleeding time	WBCT	KCCT APTT	OSPT	Fibrinogen level	FDP
Platelet disorders							
Thrombocytopenia	▼	▲	N	N	N	N	N
von Willebrand's disease	N	▲	N or ▲	N or ▲	N	N	N
Functional defects	N	▲	N	N	N	N	N
Vessel abnormalities	N	▲	N	N	N	N	N
Coagulation defects							
Liver disease	N	N	[▲]	[▲]	▲	N	N
Haemophilia A (Factor VIII deficiency)	N	N	▲	▲	N	N	N
Haemophilia B (Factor IX deficiency)	N	N	▲	▲	N	N	N
Factor XII (Hageman factor) deficiency	N	N	▲	▲	N	N	N
Coumarin intoxication	N	N	[▲]	[▲]	▲	N	N
Combined platelet and coagulation defect							
DIC	▼	▲	▲	▲	▲	▼	▲

Key: WBCT = whole blood clotting time, KCCT = kaolin-cephalin clotting time, APTT = activated partial-thromboplastin time, OSPT = one-stage prothrombin time, FDP = fibrin degradation products, N = normal, ▲ = increased, ▼ = decreased, [ ] = test of low sensitivity.

noted as a component of systemic lupus erythematosus (Jain & Switzer, 1981). The identification of antiplatelet antibody is best performed by demonstrating platelet- or megakaryocyte-bound immunoglobulin by indirect immunofluorescence since the platelet factor 3 (PF3) assay is extremely capricious and lacks specificity for immunoglobulin binding. Treatment is with immunosuppressive doses of prednisolone (2–4 mg/kg daily in two divided doses) tailed off once the platelet count has started to rise significantly, usually after 2–7 days. Vincristine (0.03 mg/kg, i.v., per week) may be of value as an additional treatment if there is no response to glucocorticoids since as well as being immunosuppressive it results in platelet release from the marrow. Splenectomy should only be considered if there is no response to glucocorticoids plus vincristine, other causes of thrombocytopenia have been ruled out and there is splenomegaly.

THROMBOCYTOSIS

A transient and moderate elevation in platelet count may follow haemorrhage. Abnormally large shift platelets may also be present. Bone marrow examination reveals increased numbers of normal megakaryocytes which are actively budding platelets. This is a transient physiological response which must be distinguished from the persistent elevation of platelet count in the haemopoietic neoplasm thrombocythaemia. In cases of doubt, repeated marrow aspiration is required.

Functional abnormalities of platelets

Few functional abnormalities of platelets have been documented in the cat. Congenital platelet dysfunction is seen in von Willebrand's disease as a consequence of the reduced level of factor VIII-related antigen and there is no intrinsic abnormality of the platelets (see below). Platelet dysfunction is generally acquired. In uraemia platelet aggregation is inhibited by a dialysable factor which accumulates in plasma. Thus petechiation and ecchymosis formation is not uncommon in advanced renal failure. Otherwise acquired dysfunction is usually due to exogenous chemicals, the most important of which are non-steroidal anti-inflammatory drugs (NSAIDs), particularly aspirin (Penny *et al.*, 1967), although aspirin does of course have therapeutic application in feline thromboembolism. NSAIDs are discussed further in Chapter 27. Many other drugs interfere with platelet function, and although such effects are often suspected, none is well documented in cats.

CHEDIAK–HIGASHI SYNDROME

The Chediak–Higashi syndrome is a congenital abnormality inherited in an autosomal recessive fashion. It is manifested as abnormal granulation of many cell types, including granulocytes and blood platelets, due to a dysgenesis of lysosomal and other intracellular membranes. The condition has been reported in a line of Persian cats with yellow eyes and 'blue-smoke' hair (Kramer *et al.*, 1975, 1977; Collier *et al.*, 1979). The affected animals show a bleeding tendency consistent with a platelet abnormality, as well as a tendency to recurrent infection. They have an increased bleeding time (Parker *et al.*, 1988).

Congenital coagulation abnormalities

HAEMOPHILIA (HAEMOPHILIA A, FACTOR VIII DEFICIENCY) AND VON WILLEBRAND'S DISEASE

Haemophilia has been recorded in DSH, LH and Devon Rex cats. Haemophilia is a congenital condition, inherited in a sex-linked recessive fashion, in which the level of factor VIII coagulant

activity is reduced. The signs are typical of a coagulopathy (see above), with excessive bleeding, particularly following surgery. Spontaneous bleeding appears to be relatively uncommon even in severely affected cats. The severity of signs varies with the level of factor VIII in the individual. The whole blood clotting time and kaolin-cephalin clotting time are increased while the one-stage prothrombin time is normal (Cotter, 1978; Littlewood, 1986). Factor VIII-related antigen levels are normal or increased. This and the inheritance pattern rule out a diagnosis of von Willebrand's disease. In von Willebrand's disease, which is an autosomal trait, factor VIII-related antigen is reduced with a parallel lowering of factor VIII coagulant activity in consequence. von Willebrand's disease, with undetectable factor VIII-related antigen and low levels of factor VIII coagulant activity, has been reported in a Himalayan cat (French *et al.*, 1987).

Prophylactic maintenance therapy of haemophilia is not practicable. Drugs interfering with platelet function should be avoided: they exacerbate the bleeding tendency. When bleeding occurs, factor VIII replacement therapy is indicated. This may be achieved in a number of ways. If bleeding has led to severe anaemia, then transfusion of fresh whole blood is appropriate. In the absence of severe anaemia, intravenous infusion of fresh plasma or of purified factor VIII is indicated. If blood or plasma are used, it is crucial that these are fresh since factor VIII is labile. In the event that it is wished to breed from a queen belonging to an affected line screening to ascertain whether she is a carrier of the trait is advisable.

FACTOR IX DEFICIENCY (HAEMOPHILIA B, CHRISTMAS DISEASE)

Factor IX deficiency is a sex-linked recessive trait with clinical signs characteristic of a coagulopathy. The same pattern of abnormalities is seen in screening tests as for haemophilia A and the two conditions can be distinguished only by correction tests or by specific assay of factor VIII and factor IX. Prophylactic therapy is not practicable. Treatment of bleeding episodes should be by transfusion of fresh blood or plasma or by infusion of factor IX concentrates. The same cautionary comments about antiplatelet drugs apply as for haemophilia A.

HAGEMAN FACTOR (FACTOR XII) DEFICIENCY
Hageman factor is responsible for contact activation of the intrinsic pathway. One might expect that this would be a key factor and that its absence would lead to severe disease. Paradoxically, this is not the case, probably because platelet activities can substitute for activated factor XII. The cats reported to have this condition have no bleeding tendency (Didisheim *et al.*, 1959; Lewis, 1981). The condition has been shown to be inherited in an autosomal recessive manner in the cat, as in man (Kier *et al.*, 1980).

Combined deficiencies of factors VIII and XII (Littlewood & Evans, 1990) and of factors IX and XII (Dillon & Boudreaux, 1988) have been reported in kindreds of cats. The author has recorded a multi-factor deficiency in Devon Rex cats in the UK involving the factors comprising the prothrombin complex (Evans, 1985), and subsequently Maddison *et al.* (1990) have recorded a similar coagulopathy with reduced levels of factors II, VII, IX and X.

Acquired coagulation abnormalities

INTOXICATION WITH WARFARIN AND
RELATED COUMARIN OR INDANDIONE
ANTICOAGULANTS
It is popularly believed that cats are fastidious feeders and will not eat bait or poisoned vermin and that poisoning with warfarin and similar agents does not arise. This is certainly untrue: the author has encountered a number of such cases in cats. The most common presenting sign in cats appears to be pulmonary haemorrhage, but bleeding from other sites occurs and there may be superficial as well as deep bleeding.

The synthesis of coagulation factors II, VII, IX and X occurs in the liver and is vitamin K-dependent, Warfarin and related compounds antagonize vitamin K producing a deficiency of these factors. Both the intrinsic and the extrinsic pathways are affected, but the best laboratory test to confirm the clinical suspicion is the one-stage prothrombin time. Treatment is directed to restoring haemostatically adequate levels of factors II, VII, IX and X. Antagonism of the intoxicant by administration of vitamin K_1 (phytomenadione) is essential. Vitamin K_1 should be administered intravenously at a dose of 2–5 mg/kg and a further prothrombin time performed 8–24 hours later to check for correction before changing to oral administration of 2–5 mg/kg daily. If the prothrombin time has not been normalized intravenous administration should be repeated. The timespan for which oral administration of phytomenadione needs to be maintained is dependent upon the persistence of the agent involved. Second-generation anticoagulant rodenticides such as brodifacoum, bromadiolone, difenacoum and flocoumafen are extremely long-lasting and treatment for 4 weeks is required. The one-stage prothrombin time should be checked 3 days after stopping treatment and therapy re-initiated for a further 14 to 21 days if necessary. It must be remembered that it takes up to 6 hours to achieve a clinical response to the first dose of vitamin K_1. During this interval physical measures should be taken to control bleeding if necessary. The patient should be protected from impact and pressure, kept warm and may need sedation. Factor-replacement therapy may also be valuable during this period, and may be achieved by administering fresh plasma (or fresh platelet-rich plasma in centres able to prepare this). If blood loss has been substantial, transfusion of whole blood is indicated. Provided the condition is recognized early and therapy is intensive and adequately maintained, the prognosis is good. If death occurs, widespread haemorrhage and petechiation is seen at post-mortem examination: there are no specific diagnostic features. It should be noted that many modern rodenticides incorporate the long-acting coumarin derivatives and/or calciferol (see Chapter 28).

OTHERS
A vitamin K-responsive coagulopathy has been reported in association with a case of exocrine pancreatic insufficiency (Perry *et al.*, 1991).

ACQUIRED INHIBITORS

There is one case report of a cat with a plasma factor which inhibited factor XI (Feldman *et al.*, 1983).

Platelet and coagulation abnormalities in combination: disseminated intravascular coagulation (DIC)

In DIC, generalized activation of the haemostatic and fibrinolytic systems leads to excessive consumption of platelets and clotting factors with diffuse microvascular thrombosis or microembolism but also a haemostatic defect. DIC is variable in severity, duration and spectrum depending on the initiating stimulus. There may be mild to florid abnormal bleeding, shock, microvascular obstruction with tissue necrosis and consequent dysfunction of single or multiple organs. The syndrome may be precipitated by septicaemia, endotoxinaemia or viraemia, release of thromboplastin from tumours, from red cells by haemolysis or from other tissues following surgery, trauma or burns. DIC may also be initiated by antigen-antibody complexes. DIC has been recognized in the cat associated with mesothelioma and hepatitis (Schaer & Meyer, 1988) as a component of panleucopenia, of the FeLV-induced panleucopenia-like syndrome and of feline infectious peritonitis (Weiss *et al.*, 1980), but has not yet been widely sought or documented in this species. The condition should be suspected when an animal shows abnormal bleeding with combined features of coagulant and platelet defects; when a moribund animal is ostensibly warm and well perfused or when an animal's condition deteriorates suddenly, particularly if shock or major haemorrhage supervene.

LABORATORY INVESTIGATION OF DIC

The laboratory findings may change rapidly during the development and progression of DIC. Frequent assessments must be made and interpreted in the light of the changing clinical situation. Diagnosis of DIC requires demonstration of consumption of clotting factors and platelets and the consequences of activation of the fibrinolytic system. The whole blood clotting time and the platelet count are useful screening tests. An increased whole blood clotting time with accompanying thrombocytopenia is presumptive evidence of DIC. This may be confirmed by showing clotting factor depletion and the presence of fibrin degradation products (FDP) as a consequence of fibrinolytic activation. Routine haematology is an important component of the investigation. The presence or absence of anaemia must be ascertained and the plasma examined for haemoglobin. The blood film may show angular red cell fragments (schistocytes), which may be formed in DIC as red cells pass through a mesh of fibrin. The white cell count is of considerable significance. It is essential to determine whether leukaemia is present. In infection, the absence of leucocytosis, resulting in a normal or low white blood cell count, will suggest endotoxin release or Gram-negative septicaemia.

MANAGEMENT AND PROGNOSIS

Whenever possible the disorder underlying DIC should be treated aggressively. This is often sufficient to reverse the haemostatic abnormality. If there is no bleeding and the laboratory tests indicate mild abnormality, fluid, electrolyte and acid–base imbalances should be corrected. If significant bleeding is occurring, infusion of fresh plasma or fresh frozen plasma is indicated. If these are not available fresh blood may be employed but there is some risk of haemolysis which may aggravate the situation. Plasma replenishes not only depleted clotting factors, but also their inhibitors. If despite all these measures, clinical or laboratory observation reveals a rapidly worsening situation, heparin therapy is indicated. Heparin administration may appear paradoxical in the face of a haemorrhagic crisis. The aim is to stop the continuing coagulation, allowing synthesis or infusion to replace clotting factors and inhibitors; to allow the marrow response to restore platelet levels; and to enable fibrinolysis and clearance to remove deposited fibrin and anticoagulant FDP. Heparin should be administered 4- to 12-hourly at a dose level of 50 IU/kg. Alternatively, 7–40 IU/kg/h can be given by continuous infusion. Frequent laboratory monitoring of the platelet count and fibrinogen titre is essential. Heparin administration should be stopped when clinical and laboratory investigations show that the DIC has been arrested. In early or mild cases the prognosis is fair and some animals may make a full recovery. In severe or advanced cases the prognosis is grave.

Thrombosis

Thrombus formation and thromboembolism associated with cardiomyopathy and giving rise to ischaemic neuromyopathy is discussed in Chapters 2 and 11.

REFERENCES

Alroy J., Freden G.O., Goyal V., Raghavan S.S. & Schunck K.L. (1989) Morphology of leukocytes from cats affected with alpha-mannosidosis and mucopolysaccharidosis VI (MPS VI). *Vet. Pathol.* **26**, 294–302.

Alsaker R.D., Laber J., Stevens J. & Perman V. (1977) A comparison of polychromasia and reticulocyte counts in assessing erythrocyte regenerative response in the cat. *J. Amer. Vet. Med. Assoc.* **170**, 39–41.

Altman N.H. (1974) Intraerythrocytic crystalloid bodies in cats and their comparison with hemoglobinopathies in man. *Ann. N.Y. Acad. Sci.* **241**, 589–93.

Andrews G.A., Chavey P.S., Smith J.E. & Rich L. (1992) Feline blood group A and B antigens are determined by the form of neuraminic acid expressed on gangliosides and glycoproteins of the erythrocyte membrane. *Vet. Clin. Pathol.* **21**, 30.

Auer L. & Bell K. (1981) The AB blood group system of cats. *Anim. Blood Groups Biochem. Genet.* **12**, 287.

Auer L. & Bell K. (1983) Transfusion reactions in cats due to type AB blood group incompatibility. *Res. Vet. Sci.* **35**, 145–52.

Auer L., Bell K. & Coates S. (1982) Blood transfusion reactions in the cat. *J. Amer. Vet. Med. Assoc.* **180**, 729–30.

Baker R.J. & Valli V.E.O. (1986) Dysmyelopoiesis in the cat: a disorder resembling refractory anaemia with excess blasts in man. *Canad. J. Vet. Res.* **50**, 3–6.

Bennett J.M., Catovsky D., Daniel M.T., Flandrin G., Galton D.A.G., Gralnick H.R. & Sultan C. (1976) Proposals for the classification of acute leukaemias. *Brit. J. Haematol.* **33**, 451–8.

Bennett J.M., Catovsky D., Daniel M.T., Flandrin G., Galton D.A.G., Gralnick H.R. & Sultan C. (1982) Proposals for the classification of the myelodysplastic syndromes. *Brit. J. Haematol.* **51**, 189–99.

Beritic T. (1965) Studies on Schmauch bodies: I The incidence in normal cats (*Felis domestica*) and the morphologic relationship to Heinz bodies. *Blood* **25**, 999–1008.

Blue J.T. (1988) Myelofibrosis in cats with myelodysplastic syndrome and acute myelogenous leukaemia. *Vet. Pathol.* **25**, 154–60.

Blue J.T., French T.W. & Kranz J.S. (1988) Non-lymphoid haematopoietic neoplasia in cats: a retrospective study of 60 cases. *Cornell Vet.* **78**, 21–42.

Braend M. & Andersen A.E. (1980) Blood polymorphisms is cats. *Anim. Blood Groups Biochem. Genet.* **11**, Suppl. 63.

Cain G.R. & Suzuki Y. (1985) Presumptive neonatal isoerythrolysis in cats. *J. Amer. Vet. Med. Assoc.* **187**, 46–8.

Castro-Malaspina H. (1984) Pathogenesis of myelofibrosis: role of ineffective megakaryopoiesis and megakaryocyte components. In Castro-Malaspina H. & Wasserman L.R. (eds) *Myelofibrosis and the Biology of Connective Tissue.* Alan R. Liss, New York, pp. 307–22.

Chickering W.R., Prasse K.W. & Dawe D.I. (1985) Development and clinical application of methods for detection of antineutrophil antibody in serum of the cat. *Amer. J. Vet. Res.* **46**, 1809–14.

Christopher M.M. (1989) Relation of endogenous Heinz bodies to disease and anaemia in cats: 120 cases (1978–87). *J. Amer. Vet. Med. Assoc.* **194**, 1089–95.

Collier L.L., Bryan M.G. & Prieur D.J. (1979) Ocular manifestations of the Chediak–Higashi syndrome in four species of animals. *J. Amer. Vet. Med. Assoc.* **175**, 587–95.

Cotter S.M. (1978) Haemophilia A in three unrelated cats. *J. Amer. Vet. Med. Assoc.* **172**, 166–8.

Cotter S.M. (1979) Anaemia associated with feline leukaemia virus infection. *J. Amer. Vet. Med. Assoc.* **175**, 1191–4.

Cotter S.M. (1982) Blood transfusion reactions in cats. *J. Amer. Vet. Med. Assoc.* **181**, 5–6 (correspondence).

Couto C.G. (1989) Oncology. In Sherding R.G. (ed) *The cat: Diseases and Clinical Management.* Churchill-Livingstone, New York, pp. 589–647.

Cowgill L.D. (1992) Application of recombinant human erythropoietin in dogs and cats. In Kirk R.W. & Bonagura J.D. (eds) *Current Veterinary Therapy: Small Animal Practice XI.* W.B. Saunders, Philadelphia, pp. 484–7.

Cramer D.V. & Lewis R.M. (1972) Reticulocyte response in the cat. *J. Amer. Vet. Med. Assoc.* **160**, 61–7.

Didisheim P., Hattori K. & Lewis J.H. (1959) Haematologic and coagulation studies in various species. *J. Lab. Clin. Med.* **53**, 886–75.

Dillon A.R. & Boudreaux M.K. (1988) Combined factors IX and XII deficiencies in a family of cats. *J. Amer. Vet. Med. Assoc.* **193**, 883–4.

Duff B.C., Allan G.S. & Howlett C.R. (1973) A presumptive case of polycythaemia vera in a cat. *Austr. Vet. Pract.* **3**, 78–9.

Evans R.J. (1988) Toxic hazards for cats. *Vet. Ann.* **28**, 251–60.

Evans R.J. & Gorman N.T. (1987) Myeloproliferative disease in the dog and cat: Definition, classification and diagnosis. *Vet. Rec.* **121**, 437–42.

Evans R.J. & Gruffydd-Jones T.J. (1984) Anaemia in cats. *In Practice* **6**, 168–79.

Evans R.J. & Heath M.F. (1988) The laboratory assessment of hepatobiliary damage and dysfunction. In Chandler E.A. (ed) *Advances in Small Animal Practice*, vol. 1. Blackwell Scientific Publications, Oxford, pp. 30–59.

Eyquem A. & Podliachouk L. (1954) Les groupes sanguine des chats. *Ann. Inst. Pasteur.* **87**, 91–4.

Eyquem A., Podliachouk L. & Millot P. (1962) Blood groups in chimpanzees, horses, sheep, pigs and other mammals. *Ann. N.Y. Acad. Sci.* 320–8.

Facklam N.R. & Kociba G.J. (1986) Cytochemical characterization of feline leukemic cells. *Vet. Pathol.* **25**, 155–61.

Fan L.C., Dorner J.L. & Hoffman W.E. (1978) Reticulocyte response and maturation in experimental acute blood loss in the cat. *J. Amer. Anim. Hosp. Assoc.* **14**, 219–24.

Feldman B.F., Soares C.J., Kitchell B.E. & Brown C.C. (1983) Haemorrhage in a cat caused by inhibition of factor XI (plasma thromboplastin antecedent). *J. Amer. Vet. Med. Assoc.* **182**, 589–91.

Fischer C.A. (1970) Retinopathy in anaemic cats. *J. Amer. Vet. Med. Assoc.* **156**, 1415–27.

Fleckneu P.A., Gibbs C. & Kelly D.F. (1978) Myelosclerosis in a cat. *J. Comp. Pathol.* **88**, 627–31.

French T.W., Fox L.E., Randolph J.F. & Dodds W. (1987) A bleeding disorder (von Willebrand's disease) in a Himalayan cat. *J. Amer. Vet. Med. Assoc.* **190**, 437–9.

Giddens W.E. Jr., Labbe R.F., Swango J.L. & Padgett G.A. (1975) Feline congenital erythropoietic porphyria associated with severe anaemia and renal disease. Clinical morphologic and biochemical studies. *Amer. J. Pathol.* **80**, 367–86.

Giger U. (1993) *Proc. Soc. Vet. Clin. Pharm. Therap.* (In press).

Giger U. (1992) The feline AB blood group system and incompatibility reactions. In Kirk R.W. & Bonagura J.D. (eds) *Current Veterinary Therapy: Small Animal Practice*, XI. W.B. Saunders Company, Philadelphia, pp. 470–4.

Gilmore C.E., Gilmore V.H. & Jones T.C. (1964) Bone marrow and peripheral blood of cats: technique and normal values. *Pathol. Vet.* **1**, 18–40.

Glenn B.L., Glenn H.G. & Omtvedt I.T. (1968) Congenital porphyria in the domestic cat (*Felis catus*); pre-

liminary investigation on inheritance pattern. *Amer. J. Vet. Res.* **29**, 1653–7.

Golde D.W., Hocking W.G., Quan S.G., Sparkes R.S. & Gale R.P. (1980) Origin of human bone marrow fibroblasts. *Brit. J. Haematol.* **44**, 183–7.

Gorman N.T. & Evans R.J. (1987) Myeloproliferative disease in the dog and cat: Clinical presentations, pathophysiology and treatment. *Vet. Rec.* **121**, 490–6.

Grindem C.B. (1985) Ultrastructural morphology of leukaemic cells in the cat. *Vet. Pathol.* **22**, 147–55.

Grindem C.B. & Buoen L.C. (1989) Cytogenetic analysis of nine leukemic cats. *J. Comp. Pathol.* **101**, 21–30.

Grindem C.B., Perman V. & Stevens J.B. (1985a) Morphological classification and clinical and pathological characteristics of spontaneous leukaemia in 10 cats. *J. Amer. Anim. Hosp. Assoc.* **21**, 227–36.

Grindem C.B., Stevens J.B. & Perman V. (1985b) Cytochemical reactions in cells from leukaemic cats. *Vet. Clin. Pathol.* **14**, 6–12.

Hammon W.D. (1940) Cellular blood elements of normal kittens. *Anat Rec.* **76**, 259–67.

Harbour D.A., Williams P.D., Gruffydd-Jones T.J., Burbidge J. & Pearson G.R. (1988) Isolation of a T-lymphotropic lentivirus from a persistently leucopenic domestic cat. *Vet. Rec.* **122**, 84–6.

Harvey J.W. & Gaskin J.M. (1978) Feline haemobartonellosis: attempts to induce relapses of clinical disease in chronically infected cats. *J. Amer. Anim. Hosp. Assoc.* **14**, 453–6.

Harvey J.W. & Kornick H.P. (1976) Phenazopyridine toxicosis in the cat. *J. Amer. Vet. Med. Assoc.* **169**, 327–31.

Hayes A., Mastrota F., Mooney S. & Hurvitz A. (1982) Safety of transfusing blood in cats. *J. Amer. Vet. Med. Assoc.* **181**, 4–5 (correspondence).

Hirsch V.M. & Cunningham T.A. (1984) Hereditary anomaly of neutrophil granulation in Birman cats. *Amer. J. Vet. Res.* **45**, 2170–4.

Hjelle J.J. & Grauer G.F. (1986) Acetaminophen induced toxicosis in dogs and cats. *J. Amer. Vet. Med. Assoc.* **188**, 742–6.

Holmes R. (1953) The occurrence of blood groups in cats. *J. Exp. Biol.* **30**, 350–7.

Holzworth J. (1956) Anemia in the cat. *J. Amer. Vet. Med. Assoc.* 471–88.

Hoover E.A. & Kociba J.G. (1974) Bone lesions in cats with anaemia induced by feline leukaemia virus. *J. Natl. Cancer Inst.* **53**, 1277–84.

Hopper C.D., Sparkes A.H., Gruffydd-Jones T.J., Crispin S.M., Muir P., Harbour D.A. & Stokes C.R. (1989) Clinical and laboratory findings in cats infected with feline immunodeficiency virus. *Vet. Rec.* **125**, 341–6.

Hubler M., Kaelin S., Hagen A., Fairburn A., Canfield P. & Ruesch P. (1987) Feline neonatal isoerythrolysis in two litters. *J. Small Anim. Pract.* **28**, 833–8.

Ishida T., Washizu T., Toriyabe K., Motoyoshi S., Tomoda I. & Pederson N.C. (1989) Feline immunodeficiency virus infection in cats in Japan. *J. Amer. Vet. Med. Assoc.* **194**, 221–5.

Jain N.C. (1986) *Schalm's Veterinary Hematology*, 4th edn. Lea & Febiger, Philadelphia.

Jain N.C. & Switzer J.W. (1981) Autoimmune thrombocytopenic purpura in dogs and cats. *Vet. Clin. N. Amer. (Small Anim. Pract.)* **11**, 421–34.

Jarrett W.F.H. & Mackey L.J. (1974) International histological classification of tumours of domestic animals. Neoplastic diseases of the haematopoietic and lymphoid tissues. *Bull. World Health Org.* **50**, 21–34.

Jezyk P.F., Haskins M.E., Patterson D.F., Mellman W.J. & Greenstein M. (1977) Mucopolysaccharidosis in a cat with arylsulfatase b deficiency: a model of Maroteaux–Lamy syndrome. *Science* **198**, 834–6.

Joshi B.C., Raplee R.G., Powell A.L. & Hancock F. (1979) Autoimmune thrombocytopenia in a cat. *J. Amer. Anim. Hosp. Assoc.* **15**, 585–8.

Keir A.B., Bresnahan J.F., White F.J. & Wagner J.E. (1980) The inheritance pattern of factor XII (Hageman) deficiency in domestic cats. *Canad. J. Compar. Med.* **44**, 309–14.

Killingsworth C.R., Weiss D.J., Eyster G.E., Bartlett P. & Bell T.G. (1985) Screening coagulation tests in the cat: reference values based on direct venipuncture and cathetized samples. *Vet. Clin. Pathol.* **14**, 19–23.

Kirby D. & Gillick A. (1974) Polycythaemia and tetralogy of Fallot in a cat. *Can. Vet. J.* **15**, 114–8.

Kramer J.W., Davis W.C. & Prieur D.J. (1977) The Chediak–Higashi syndrome of cats. *Lab. Invest.* **36**, 554–62.

Kramer J.W., Davis W.C., Prieur D.J., Baxter J. & Norsworthy G.D. (1975) An inherited disorder of Persian cats with intracytoplasmic inclusions in neutrophils. *J. Amer. Vet. Med. Assoc.* **166**, 1103–4.

Latimer K.S., Rakich P.M. & Thompson D.F. (1985) Pelger–Huët anomaly in cats. *Vet. Pathol.* **22**, 370–4.

Lessard J.L. & Taketa F. (1969) Multiple hemoglobins in fetal newborn and adult cats. *Biochim. Biophys. Acta.* **175**, 441–4.

Lewis J.H. (1981) Comparative haematology: studies on cats including one with factor II (Hageman) deficiency. *Comp. Biochem. Physiol.* **68A**, 355–60.

Linman J.W. & Bagby G.C. (1978) The perleukaemic syndrome (haemopoietic dysplasia). *Cancer* **42**, 854–64.

Littlewood J.D. (1986) Haemophilia A (Factor VIII) deficiency in the cat. *J. Small Anim. Pract.* **27**, 541–6.

Littlewood J.D. & Evans R.J. (1990) A combined deficiency of factor VIII and a contact activation defect in a family of cats. *Brit. Vet. J.* **146**, 30–5.

Loughman W.D., Frye F.L. & Condon T.B. (1970) XY/ XXY mosaicism in three male tricolor cats. *Amer. J. Vet. Res.* **31**, 307–14.

MacEwan S.A. & Hurvitz A.I. (1977) Diagnosis and management of monoclonal gammopathies. *Vet. Clin. N. Amer. (Small Anim. Pract.)* **7**, 119–32.

McEwen S.A., Valli V.E.O. & Hulland T.J. (1985) Hypercosinophilic syndrome in cats: a report of three cases. *J. Amer. Anim. Hosp. Assoc.* **21**, 735–9.

Mackey L.J., Jarrett W.F.H., Jarrett O. & Laird H.M. (1975) Anaemia associated with feline leukaemia virus infection in cats. *J. Nat. Cancer Inst.* **54**, 209.

Maddison J.E., Watson A.D.J., Eade I.G. & Exner T. (1990) Vitamin K-dependent multifactor coagulopathy in Devon Rex cats. *J. Amer. Vet. Med. Assoc.* **197**, 1496–7.

Madewell B.R. & Feldman B.F. (1980) Characterisation of anaemias associated with neoplasia in small animals. *J. Amer. Vet. Med. Assoc.* **176**, 419.

Maede Y., Hoshino T., Inaba M. & Namioka S. (1985) Methionine-induced haemolytic anaemia with methaemoglobinaemia and Heinz body formation in erythrocytes in cats. *J. Japan Vet. Med. Assoc.* **38**, 568–71.

Marion R.S. & Smith J.E. (1983a) Survival of erythrocyte after autogenous and allogeneic transfusion in cats. *J. Amer. Vet. Med. Assoc.* **183**, 1437–9.

Marion R.S. & Smith J.E. (1983b) Post-transfusional viability of feline erythrocyte stored in acid citrate-dextrose solution. *J. Amer. Vet. Med. Assoc.* **183**, 1459–60.

Mauk A.G., Whelan M.T., Putz G.R. & Taketa F. (1970) Anemia in domestic cats: effect on hemoglobin components and whole blood oxygenation. *Science* **185**, 447–9.

Mufti G.J., Stevens J.R., Oscier D.G., Hamblin T.J. & Machin D. (1985) Myelodysplastic syndromes: a scoring system with prognostic significance. *Brit. J. Haematol.* **59**, 425–33.

Neilsen S.W. (1969) Spontaneous haematopoietic neoplasms of the domestic cat. In *Comparative Morphology of Haematopoietic Neoplasms*. Nat. Cancer Inst. Monograph No. 32, pp. 73–90.

Onions D.E., Jarrett O., Testa N., Fassoni F. & Toth S. (1982) Selective effect of feline leukaemia virus on early erythroid precursors. *Nature* **296**, 156–8.

Parker M.T., Collier L.L., Keir A.B. & Johnson G.S. (1988) Oral mucosa bleeding times of normal cats and cats with Chediak–Higashi syndrome or Hageman trait (factor XII deficiency). *Vet. Clin. Pathol.* **17**, 9–12.

Pedersen N.C., Ho E.W., Brown M.L. & Yamamoto J.K. (1987) Isolation of a T-lymphotropic virus from domestic cats with an immunodeficiency-like syndrome. *Science* **235**, 790–3.

Penny R.H.C., Carlisle C.H., Prescott C.W. & Davidson H.A. (1967) Effect of aspirin (acetylsalicylic acid) on the haemopoietic system of the cat. *Brit. Vet. J.* **123**, 151–61.

Penny R.H.C., Carlisle C.H. & Davidson H.A. (1970) The blood and marrow picture of the cat. *Brit. Vet. J.* **126**, 459–64.

Perry L.A., Williams D.A., Pidgeon G.L. & Boosinger T. (1991) Exocrine pancreatic insufficiency with associated coagulopathy in a cat. *J. Amer. Anim. Hosp. Assoc.* **27**, 109–14.

Raskin R.E. & Krehbiel J.D. (1985) Myelodysplastic changes in a cat with myelomonocytic leukemia. *J. Amer. Vet. Med. Assoc.* **187**, 171–4.

Reed C., Ling J.V., Gould D. & Kaneko J.J. (1970) Polycythaemia vera in a cat. *J. Amer. Vet. Med. Assoc.* **157**, 85–91.

Saar C. & Reichel C. (1983) Einige besondere Leukoseformen bei einer katze. *Prakt. Tierartz.* **5**, 443–50.

Schaer M. & Meyer D. (1988) Benign mesothelioma, hyperthyroidism, non-suppurative hepatitis and disseminated intravascular coagulation in a cat. *J. Amer. Vet. Med. Assoc.* **24**, 195–202.

Schalm O.W. (1972) Interpretations in feline bone marrow cytology. *J. Amer. Vet. Med. Ass.* **161**, 1418–25.

Schalm O.W., Jain N.C. & Carroll E.J. (1975) *Veterinary Hematology*, 3rd edn. Lea & Febiger, Philadelphia.

Schechter R.D., Schalm O.W. & Kaneko J.J. (1973) Heinz body hemolytic anaemia associated with the use of urinary antiseptics containing methylene blue. *J. Amer. Vet. Med. Assoc.* **162**, 37–44.

Schrader L.A. & Hurvitz A.I. (1983) Cold agglutinin disease in a cat. *J. Amer. Vet. Med. Assoc.* **183**, 121–2.

Schryver H.F. (1963) The bone marrow of the cat. *Amer. J. Vet. Res.* **24**, 1012–7.

Shelton G.H., Abkowitz J.L., Linenberger M.L., Russell R.G. & Grant C.K. (1989) Chronic leukopenia associated with feline immunodeficiency virus infection in cats. *J. Amer. Med. Assoc.* **194**, 253–5.

Shelton G.H., Linenberger M.L., Grant C.K. & Abkowitz J.L. (1990a) Hematological manifestations of feline immunodeficiency virus infection. *Blood* **76**, 1104–9.

Shelton G.H., Grant C.K., Linenberger M.L. & Abkowitz J.L. (1990b) Severe neutropenia associated with griseofulvin therapy in cats with feline immunodeficiency virus infection. *J. Vet. Intern. Med.* **4**, 317–9.

Sodikoff D.H. & Schalm O.W. (1968) Primary bone marrow disease in the cat. III. Erythremic myelosis and myelofibrosis – a myeloproliferative disorder. *Calif. Vet.* **23**, 16–20.

Sparger E.E. (1991) Feline immunodeficiency virus. Chapter 27 In August J.R. (ed) *Consultations in Feline Internal Medicine* W.B. Saunders Co. Philadelphia. pp. 543–50.

Swenson C.L., Kociba G.J. & Arnold P. (1988) Chronic idiopathic neutropenia in a cat. *J. Vet. Intern. Med.* **2**, 103–7.

Taketa F. (1967) Studies on cat hemoglobin and hybrids with human hemoglobin. *Biochemistry* **6**, 3809–14.

Taketa F. (1974) Organic phosphates and hemoglobin structure–function relationships in the feline. *Ann. N.Y. Acad. Sci.* **241**, 524–37.

Taketa F., Chen J.Y. & Palosaari N. (1968) Hemoglobin A and B of the cat: occurrence in the same cell. *Hemoglobin.* **3**, 371–8.

Theilen G.H. & Madewell B.R. (1979) *Veterinary Cancer Medicine*. Lea & Febiger, Philadelphia.

Verhaert L., Maenhout T., De Geest J., van der Stock J., de Schepper J. & Hoorens J.K. (1987) Hypereosinofiel syndroom bij de kat: een onderdeel van het leuemie complex? *Vlaams Diergen. Tijds.* **56**, 128–34.

Weiser M.G. & Kociba G.J. (1983a) Sequential changes in erythrocyte volume distribution and microcytosis associated with iron deficiency in kittens. *Vet. Pathol.* **20**, 1–12.

Weiser M.G. & Kociba G.J. (1983b) Erythrocyte macrocytosis in feline leukaemia virus associated anemia. *Vet. Pathol.* **20**, 687–97.

Weiser M.G. & Kociba G.J. (1984) Platelet concentration and platelet volume distribution in healthy cats. *Amer. J. Vet. Res.* **45**, 518–22.

Weiss D.J. & Krehbiel J.D. (1983) Studies of the pathogenesis of anemia of inflammation: erythrocyte survival. *Amer. J. Vet. Res.* **441**, 1830–1.

Weiss R.C., Dodds W.J. & Scott F.W. (1980) Disseminated intravascular coagulation in experimentally induced feline infectious peritonitis. *Amer. J. Vet Res.* **41**, 663–71.

Weiss D.J., Krehbiel J.D. & Lund J.E. (1983) Studies of the pathogenesis of anemia of inflammation: mechanisms of impaired erythropoiesis. *Amer. J. Vet. Res.* **441**, 1832–5.

Werner L.L. & Gorman N.T. (1984) Immune-mediated disorders of cats. *Vet. Clin. N. Amer. (Small Anim. Pract.)* **14**, 1039–64.

Wilkerson M.J., Meyers K.M. & Wardrop K.J. (1991) Anti-A isoagglutinins in two type B cats are IgG and IgM. *Vet. Clin. Pathol.* **20**, 10–14.

Wilkie D.A. & Kirby R. (1988) Methemoglobinaemia associated with dermal application of benzocaine cream in a cat. *J. Amer. Vet. Med. Assoc.* **192**, 85–6.

Yamomoto J.K., Hansen H., Ho E.W., Morishita T.Y., Okuda T., Sawa T.R., Nakamura R.M. & Pederson N.C. (1989) Epidemiological and clinical aspects of feline immunodeficiency virus infection in cats from the continental United States and Canada and possible mode of transmission. *J. Amer. Vet. Med. Assoc.* **194**, 213–20.

Chapter 5 / The Urinary System

C. J. GASKELL

INTRODUCTION

Conditions affecting the urinary tract form an important part of feline medicine, making up in one survey in Britain at least 4% of cases seen by veterinary surgeons (Fennell, 1975). They can be divided into those affecting the upper urinary tract, i.e. the kidneys, and those causing disease of the lower urinary tract, i.e. the bladder and urethra. Disease of the feline ureter is rare.

DISEASES OF THE KIDNEY

The incidence of clinically significant renal disease in cats is not known, but it is undoubtedly common, and recent surveys of cases of chronic renal disease have collated some demographic and clinical information (DiBartola et al., 1987). Renal insufficiency or failure, the inability of the kidneys to excrete metabolites and maintain ionic and pH homeostasis, is frequently diagnosed in older cats without the type of renal disease being established. Indeed, the precise diagnosis in the individual cat may not be important as treatment is often, at present, symptomatic. Lucke (1968) and DiBartola et al. (1987) have reviewed the morphological diagnoses in chronic renal disease but there is otherwise a dearth of data on the relative importance of different causes of renal failure. The management and prevention of renal failure in the future should be based on a greater understanding of the diseases and their predisposing causes.

Another manifestation of renal disease recognized in cats is the nephrotic syndrome, the result of a protein-losing glomerulopathy. These two clinically, though not necessarily aetiologically distinct entities will be considered separately, following a resumé of the recognized causes of pathology of the feline kidney.

Causes of renal disease

Congenital renal disease

Congenital renal abnormalities are uncommon in the cat, but a number, including agenesis, renal fusion and polycystic kidneys, have been described with and without clinical signs of renal dysfunction. Polycystic kidneys are recorded in long-haired cats, and cases in related individuals have been reported (Rendano & Parker, 1976; Northington & Juliana, 1977; Crowell et al., 1979). Renal parenchyma is replaced by variable numbers of cysts and signs of renal failure are usually seen in the first years of life, though occasionally individuals may appear normal for some years. The kidneys are usually palpably enlarged and characteristically have a cystic appearance on intravenous urography (Fig. 5.1). Occasionally, individual renal cysts are found incidentally and have been seen associated with the presence of biliary cysts.

Chronic interstitial nephritis

Chronic interstitial nephritis (CIN) is recognized in the cat as one of the commoner causes of end-stage or shrunken, scarred kidneys (Lucke, 1978). In a survey of 74 cases of chronic renal disease, 54% were diagnosed as chronic tubulointerstitial

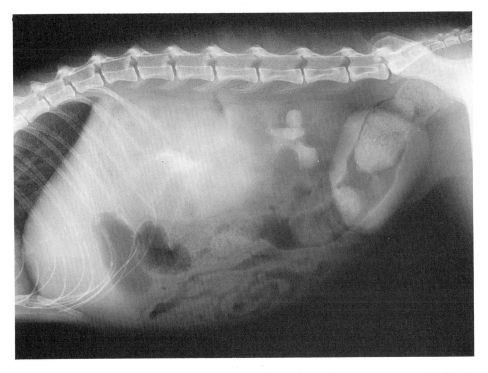

Fig. 5.1 Lateral abdominal radiograph of a long-haired cat made 1 hour after an intravenous urogram. Both kidneys are enlarged and polycystic. Congenital polycystic kidneys were confirmed at post-mortem examination.

nephritis (DiBartola *et al.*, 1987). Certainly many cats with terminal renal failure have small, scarred kidneys, but it is often difficult at this stage to determine the underlying pathology, which may or may not be CIN. The cause, or causes, of CIN are not known. Serological surveys for evidence of leptospirosis have shown only a small percentage of all cats to be positive, and there is no evidence that a leptospire is a cause of CIN in cats (Lucke & Crowther, 1965). Other suggestions include immune-mediated disease.

A pre-mortem diagnosis of CIN can only be made by renal biopsy and is of little value clinically. A better understanding of the aetiology and pathogenesis of CIN would be of value in preventing or recognizing the disease at an early stage.

Bacterial infection of the kidney

The incidence of bacterial infection of the kidneys, or pyelonephritis, is not known, nor is the importance of chronic pyelonephritis as a cause of chronic end-stage kidneys and renal failure. Chronic pyelonephritis accounted for approximately 10% of 74 cases of chronic renal disease in one series (DiBartola *et al.*, 1987), though in end-stage disease morphological diagnosis may be difficult and infection may have been eliminated from the kidney. Acute pyelonephritis, with pyrexia, depression and sublumbar pain is rarely diagnosed and in the chronic stage the clinical findings are similar to other causes of chronic renal disease. Even the demonstration of bacteria in urine will not distinguish upper from lower urinary tract infection, and the two may well coexist. The source of infection is not known; evidence in other species suggests that ascending infection may be important and that urinestasis following obstruction may predispose to infection. It has been shown that pyelonephritis can be established experimentally in the cat by the haematogenous route in temporarily obstructed

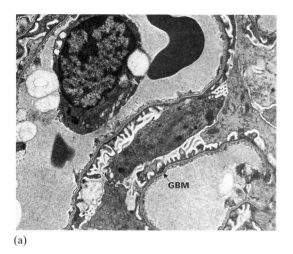
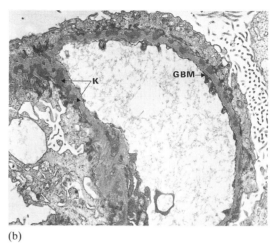

(a)   (b)

Fig. 5.2 Electron microscopic appearance of normal feline glomerulus (a) and a glomerulus from a cat with membranous glomerulonephritis (b). In (b) the basement membrane (GBM) is thickened and contains electron-dense immune complex deposits (K). There is also fusion of the foot processes (FP). (×7140)

kidneys (Kelly *et al.*, 1979). Where a diagnosis of pyelonephritis is suspected on the basis of clinical signs and urine analysis, antibiotic treatment based on urinary bacterial culture and sensitivity is indicated. A variety of organisms, including *E. coli*, *Proteus* spp. and *Staphylococcus* spp. have been isolated from cases of feline pyelonephritis. Distal renal tubular acidosis has been reported in cats with pyelonephritis (Watson *et al.*, 1986).

Renal abscesses have been recorded in the cat, usually demonstrated only at post-mortem examination. Renal calculus disease, often associated with bacterial infection in other species, is rare in the cat.

Glomerulonephritis

Glomerular disease, specifically membranous glomerulonephritis (MGN), is well recognized in cats as a cause of nephrotic syndrome (Nash *et al.*, 1979; Lucke, 1982; Nash & Wright, 1983). It is associated with the deposition of antibody-antigen complexes in the basement membrane (Fig. 5.2) and the subsequent activation of complement and inflammatory reaction, together with increased vascular permeability, activation of coagulation cascade and kinin generation.

Both immunoglobulin, usually IgG, and complement can be demonstrated in the basement membrane using immunofluorescent or immuno-chemical techniques (Arthur *et al.*, 1984). The identity of the antigen or antigens in the immune complexes is not usually known, though immune-complex glomerulonephritis has been produced experimentally in cats following repeated injections of bovine albumin (Nash *et al.*, 1990). Feline leukaemia virus (FeLV) has been associated experimentally with glomerulonephritis in the cat (Anderson & Jarrett, 1971), but clinically cases are invariably FeLV-negative.

The damage to the glomerular basement membrane leads to an increased permeability to low molecular weight proteins such as albumin and the development of the nephrotic syndrome (see below). Where glomerular damage is severe, subsequent scarring may lead to complete loss of function of the glomerulus and its dependent tubule. If widespread, this loss may be appreciated clinically as chronic renal failure, and morphological evidence of MGN may be present in a significant proportion of 'end-stage' kidneys in older cats. Such cats may or may not have shown previous episodes of nephrotic syndrome.

Nephrotic syndrome associated with membranous glomerulonephritis is recognized most frequently in young adult cats. There is some suggestion that males may be more commonly affected, but there appears to be no breed predilection. The long-term prognosis for cases is variable; those with evidence of renal failure do not do well, while those showing nephrotic syndrome fare better, with in one series survival up to 6 years (Arthur *et al.*, 1986).

Other forms of glomerulonephritis appear to be rare in cats. Glomerulonephritis associated with autoimmune disease, such as systemic lupus erythematosus, has been recognized. Cases of the periosteal proliferative form of chronic progressive polyarthritis may show histological evidence of glomerulonephritis (Pedersen *et al.*, 1980). Comparisons with the dog might suggest a reversible glomerulonephritis associated with pyometritis, but none has yet been demonstrated in cats. Renal amyloidosis, while it may affect the glomeruli, is more usually a tubular disease in cats.

Renal neoplasia
Primary renal tumours are rare in the cat, and little information is available on their behaviour and clinical presentation. In a review of reported cases, the majority were histologically malignant (Caywood *et al.*, 1980). A diagnosis of renal neoplasia might be considered where renal enlargement is found, and treatment by surgical removal contemplated where involvement is unilateral and there is no evidence of metastatic disease.

Lymphosarcoma is by far the commonest tumour affecting the kidney of the cat. Involvement is usually bilateral: the kidneys may be the major organs affected and the cat may show signs of renal insufficiency, or alternatively the involvement of the kidneys may be of minor clinical importance compared to other sites. The kidneys may be diffusely or focally involved and thus enlargement may be regular or irregular. An increase in size can often be appreciated by abdominal palpation or abdominal radiographs (Fig. 5.3). Not all cases of renal lymphosarcoma will be viraemic or antigenaemic (see Chapter 15)

and confirmation of the diagnosis may be made by biopsy of the kidney or other affected sites or at post-mortem examination. Treatment of renal lymphosarcoma may be attempted; Mooney *et al.* (1987) reported good response in 17 of 28 cases (see Chapter 15).

The involvement of the feline kidney in metastatic disease other than lymphosarcoma is rare.

Amyloidosis
Amyloid is a glycoprotein thought to be produced by the reticuloendothelial system in response to prolonged antigenic stimulation, such as occurs in chronic inflammatory or neoplastic disease. It has been suggested that amyloid deposits may be related to hypervitaminosis A (Clark & Seawright, 1968). The accumulation of amyloid in the kidneys is recognized as a cause of renal failure in cats (*c.* 10% of cases in one series; DiBartoli *et al.*, 1987). Unlike the dog, where the clinical signs are usually related to glomerular damage, renal amyloid in cats is usually deposited in the tubules, leading to signs of renal insufficiency. The disease is chronic by nature and signs may be gradual in onset, though in some cats the clinical course is rapid. Clinical deterioration may well be associated with necrosis of the renal papilla, a not uncommon feature of renal amyloidosis in the cat and presumed to be due to vascular obstruction. Such necrosis may be indicated clinically as haematuria. The kidneys are often relatively normal or even slightly enlarged on clinical examination. Amyloidosis is recognized most frequently in middle-aged to older cats and may well be more common than is generally thought. No successful treatment of amyloidosis has been reported in cats. Renal amyloidosis has been reported in a number of Abyssinian cats in the USA, some of whom were closely related (Chew *et al.*, 1982, DiBartola *et al.*, 1986). The amyloid in these cats is the reactive, or AA, type and its distribution may not be restricted to the kidneys. Affected animals may present in renal failure between 1 and 5 years of age, or deposits may be slight and not clinically significant; females are more commonly affected than males.

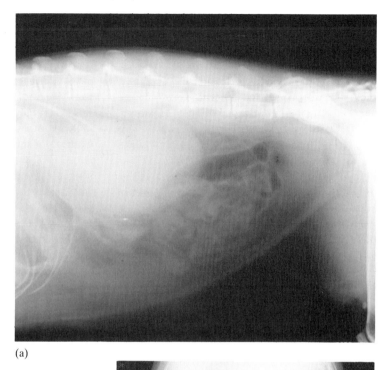

(a)

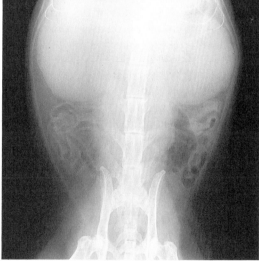

(b)

Fig. 5.3 (a) Lateral and (b) ventrodorsal radiographs of a 7-year-old Siamese cat with bilateral renal enlargement due to lymphosarcoma.

Other renal disease

FELINE INFECTIOUS PERITONITIS (FIP)

The kidneys are commonly affected in the dry or atypical form of FIP, along with involvement of the central nervous system and uveal tract. Renal failure may be the presenting syndrome. The kidneys are irregularly involved, and may feel enlarged on abdominal palpation and be impossible to distinguish clinically from renal lymphosarcoma. The diagnosis and management of FIP are discussed in Chapter 17.

TOXIC OR CHEMICAL RENAL DISEASE

While many substances, such as heavy metals, and a number of drugs, such as the aminoglycoside antibiotics (e.g. gentamycin), amphotericin B, doxorubicin and non-steroidal anti-inflammatory agents are known to be nephrotoxic, there are few well-documented cases in the cat. However, nephrotoxic agents should always be considered, particularly when signs of failure are sudden in onset, and care should be taken in azotaemic cats to avoid the use of drugs known to damage the kidneys of other species. The metabolites of ethylene glycol, a constituent of antifreeze, are also nephrotoxic: poisoning may be suspected by the presence of calcium oxalate crystals in the urine.

HYDRONEPHROSIS

Dilation of the renal pelvis following obstruction to urine flow leads to hydronephrosis, gross enlargement of the kidney and reduction in renal parenchyma. In an individual case the cause of the obstruction may not be clear, though congenital abnormalities of the ureter, or acquired defects such as calculi, obstructing masses or surgical trauma (e.g. following neutering) should be considered. Loss of function in affected kidneys may be complete but unilateral involvement does not usually lead to overall renal insufficiency. In these cases, the diagnosis is suggested by palpation of the grossly enlarged kidney, often following an impression of abdominal enlargement. Treatment is aimed either at removing the cause of the obstruction, whereby some function may be saved or restored, or removing the kidney when hydronephrosis is of long standing and remaining renal parenchyma is minimal. Hydronephrotic kidneys are said to be prone to bacterial infection and occasionally may present as foci of infection, i.e. pyrexia, depression, neutrophilia and evidence on urine analysis of bacterial infection. Whenever removal of one kidney is contemplated the status of the other kidney should be assessed first, by measurement of blood urea or creatinine and possibly by intravenous urography. In long-standing unilateral hydronephrosis the unaffected kidney may show compensatory hypertrophy.

PERIRENAL PSEUDOCYSTS

Perirenal or perinephric pseudocysts are accumulations of fluid around one or both kidneys, either subcapsular or extracapsular. They are uncommon, and present usually as slowly progressive renal or abdominal enlargement without other signs of renal disease. Their pathogenesis is unknown and management consists of drainage and ablation of the cyst(s) (Brace, 1983).

RENAL CALCULUS DISEASE

The presence of calculi, of uroliths, in the renal pelvis is rare in cats though struvite, urate and oxalate stones have been recorded. The signs associated with such calculi range from none to renal failure. Treatment may include measures to combat bacterial infection, dietary management and surgical removal.

RENAL AND URETERIC TRAUMA

Intrarenal and subcapsular haemorrhage are the most common sequelae to upper urinary tract trauma, but may often go undiagnosed following general abdominal trauma. Haemorrhage is generally self-limiting in these sites, requiring only supportive treatment. Damage or tearing of the renal arteries or veins may lead to serious retroperitoneal haemorrhage and hypovolaemia, but it is difficult to diagnose. Signs of continuing loss of blood despite supportive therapy, and particularly with blood also present in the peritoneal cavity, suggest the need for exploratory surgery. Abdominal radiographs to demonstrate a loss of fat contrast in the dorsal, retroperitoneal part of the abdomen may be helpful. Ureteric damage, either following trauma or iatrogenic following surgery, and leading to urine leakage or obstruction, may be demonstrated by intravenous urography.

Clinical aspects of renal disease

Renal failure

Renal insufficiency is only apparent clinically when overall renal function is impaired to a point where the kidneys fail to prevent the build-up of metabolites; this usually follows the loss of some 75% of renal functional mass. Classically, renal failure is divided into pre-renal, renal and post-renal causes and the division is clinically useful. Any condition leading to reduced renal perfusion may lead to pre-renal failure. Dehydration is the commonest cause, and a degree of renal insufficiency also occurs in left-sided heart failure associated, for instance, with cardiomyopathy. Pre-renal factors may also exacerbate, or clinically unmask, insufficiency of renal origin. The commonest cause of post-renal failure is urethral obstruction, discussed under lower urinary tract conditions. The various types of renal disease leading to failure have been discussed above, but regardless of the underlying pathology, the clinical signs, management and prognosis are often similar.

The division of cases of renal failure into acute or chronic may be helpful in terms of prognosis, but is frequently difficult to achieve. Renal disease due to an acute insult is much less common than chronic renal disease despite the often precipitous nature of the clinical history.

CLINICAL SIGNS

Anorexia or inappetence, depression and lethargy, and weight loss are the signs most frequently seen in cats with renal insufficiency (DiBartola *et al.*, 1987). Vomiting is a less consistent sign and polydipsia and polyuria are reported by owners less often in the cat than in the dog, probably due to differences in habits between the species. Gingivitis with ulceration, particularly of the edges of the tongue; pallor of the mucous membranes due to a non-regenerative anaemia; and secondary hyperparathyroidism with softening of the facial bones are all less common, but may be striking features in individual cases. Uraemic breath may be present but is often lost in a general halitosis. Palpation of the kidneys may reveal changes in renal shape and size, most commonly the marked reduction with an irregular outline of end-stage kidneys, but occasionally, as with lymphosarcoma or feline infectious peritonitis, enlargement. Chronic renal failure is typically seen in older cats and the presence of intercurrent disease such as neoplasia should also be assessed.

Differentiation of cases of renal failure into acute and chronic can sometimes be based on the duration of signs, particularly weight loss, poor appetite and anaemia or hyperparathyroidism. However, this may be misleading as extra-renal factors such as intercurrent disease or dehydration may lead to an acute onset of signs in a cat with pre-existing chronic renal disease.

Some cats may remain inappetent, thin and polyuric in so-called compensated renal failure for some time. If decompensation occurs, the signs may progress rapidly to complete loss of appetite, dehydration, profound depression, coma and death with, in some cases, uraemic convulsions terminally.

DIAGNOSIS

A diagnosis of renal failure may be suspected from the clinical signs. These may, however, be non-specific: the presenting signs of depression or lethargy, inappetence and weight loss are commonly seen in a variety of disease conditions. Confirmation of the diagnosis, usually with laboratory data, is always advisable.

LABORATORY TESTS

The laboratory confirmation of renal failure is based on the demonstration of elevated levels of metabolites, normally urea (or urea nitrogen) and creatinine in the blood. Both these parameters are useful indicators of renal function and glomerular filtration rate (GFR); blood urea (BU) is used more frequently, though creatinine is strictly speaking a better indicator, being unaffected by diet and the level of protein metabolism. For this reason, creatinine is also of more value in following the progress of renal disease and function. More accurate measures of GFR are obtained by assessment of the creatinine clearance, obtained by measuring the volume and creatinine concentration of urine passed over a 24-hour period and correlating this with serum creatinine levels, or more accurately still by measuring the clearance of an exogenous substance such as inulin. These tests are infrequently practicable. The degree of elevation of BU or creatinine associated with clinical signs is variable, probably because these products, while used as a measure of the build-up of other toxic waste metabolites, are not particularly toxic in themselves. It is also difficult to prognosticate merely on the level of BU. However, signs of inappetence and lethargy are generally seen with BU levels of greater than 25 mmol/l (normal 5–10 mmol/l) and by 40 mmol/l the cat will be anorexic and markedly depressed. Failure to drink and maintain hydration adds a pre-renal component to the renal failure, which will be reflected in a further rise in creatinine and BU. In the absence of any post-renal component, for example urinary tract obstruction, BU levels of greater than 60 mmol/l carry a very poor prognosis. Elevations in BU may be seen associated merely with pre-renal factors, though generally it does not rise above 20 mmol/l in these circumstances; in these cases renal insufficiency is generally associated with the production of concentrated urine.

Failure to excrete inorganic phosphorus leads to an elevation in blood levels in renal insufficiency and a tendency for blood calcium levels to fall. However, increased parathyroid activity and the mobilization of calcium from the skeleton generally ensures that hypocalcaemia is not evident until the later stages of renal failure. The mobilization of calcium in the presence of high phosphorus leads to mineralization of soft tissue; where this involves the kidney tubules renal function is further impaired. Cats in renal failure show alterations in sodium and potassium homeostasis, and a number show hyponatraemia and/or hypokalaemia (DiBartola *et al.*, 1987). The relationship between renal disease and sodium and potassium balance in cats remains an area of debate: clinically important potassium depletion associated with renal disease and low dietary levels has been reported in a number of cats (Dow *et al.*, 1987), and in association with distal renal tubular acidosis (Watson *et al.*, 1986).

Cats with glomerular disease will show varying degrees of hypoalbuminaemia and hypercholesterolaemia. Cats with CRF typically show a non-regenerative anaemia, due presumably to reduced production of erythropoietin by the kidney and a reduced lifespan for circulating red cells. Urine analysis may be useful in assessing renal function, but is not uniformly so. Urine specific gravity (SG) or osmolarity is usually low (<1015) in chronic renal failure, of value in distinguishing chronic insufficiency from pre-renal or acute renal failure, where more concentrated urine is produced. However, some cats in CRF may produce urine of SG in the order of 1030. Urine pH is of limited value in renal disease; urinary tract infection may be associated with a higher than normal pH but other evidence should be looked for in the sediment for confirmation. The presence of bacteria, red blood cells and inflammatory cells is indicative of infection in the urinary tract; if casts are present it is suggestive of upper urinary tract disease. Casts of different types may be seen in renal disease of various aetiology, but are not reliably present. Levels of proteinuria are also variable, though cases associated with glomerular disease will continue to lose albumin in the urine.

Radiography is not often of major value in the diagnosis of renal disease. Plain radiographs may demonstrate the size and shape of the kidneys, but the poor excreting ability of the kidneys in the presence of renal insufficiency produces little concentration of contrast in the renal mass following intravenous urography. Where hyperparathyroidism is marked, reduction in bone density, particularly of the maxilla, may be appreciated radiographically, as may calcification of soft tissues (Fig. 5.4), although this is said to occur less frequently than in the dog. In congenital renal disease, where the kidneys may be polycystic, urography may be diagnostic, but in most cases of renal failure the kidneys are either not enhanced by contrast or are shown to be small and irregular, merely confirming a clinical or plain radiographic finding. Renal arteriography would be more useful, particularly for localized renal disease, but is rarely practicable. Ultrasonography is useful in the evaluation of cystic and other changes within the kidneys.

Renal biopsy is the only way to attempt a definitive diagnosis of the underlying pathology in a case of renal failure (see p. 235). However, where the disease has progressed to the point of failure, the changes are often non-specific and frequently irreversible, and thus the information

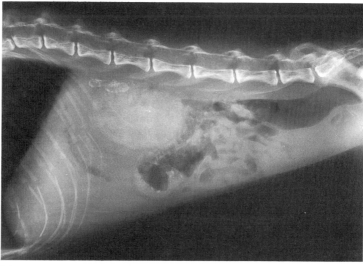

(a)

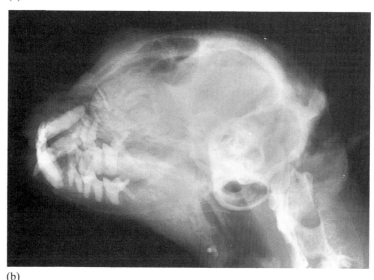

(b)

Fig. 5.4 Radiographs of a 6-year-old cat in chronic renal failure. (a) The lateral abdominal radiograph shows widespread calcification of soft tissues including kidneys, aorta and femoral arteries. Calcification of the adrenals, while marked in this case, is a not uncommon finding in older cats. (b) The lateral oblique radiograph of the skull shows marked reduction in bone density, particularly in the mandible. Congenital polycystic kidneys were found at post-mortem examination.

gained at biopsy may be of little value in terms of management. For this reason, renal biopsy is not frequently employed in such cases.

MANAGEMENT

A diagnosis of renal failure is most often made without a clear understanding of the underlying cause and thus specific treatment may not be possible. Supportive therapy and management may improve the condition of the cat, but by the time the animal is presented even this may be difficult. Thus the prognosis for an individual case is variable and not always easy to assess at initial presentation.

Management of renal failure may be broadly divided into those cases where the cat is still drinking and those where the severity of failure is greater and the animal is depressed, has stopped drinking and is dehydrated. For the former, the primary objective is to ameliorate the effects of renal insufficiency by maintaining a high fluid intake, restricting dietary protein and phosphorus, using anabolic steroids and antiemetics where necessary and giving vitamin supplementation. It is sometimes possible through such measures to slow the progression of the disease. Fluid turnover is encouraged by giving ready access to liquid, and encouraging the cat to drink by keeping the supply fresh and offering milk and gravy if these prove palatable. The addition of salt (sodium chloride) to the diet will increase the total fluid turnover in the cat but is felt to be unhelpful due to the effect of high salt intake on blood pressure. Hypertension is known to accelerate the progression of renal disease in other species through its affect on the remaining glomeruli. This is probably true for the cat, and hypertension and the clinical consequences such as retinal detachment have been seen in cases of feline CRF (Krawiec & Gelberg, 1989). Diets for CRF should therefore be moderately restricted in salt, and any remaining hypertension managed using drugs such as diuretics (e.g. frusemide: 2–4 mg/kg bodyweight every 8 or 12 hours), β-blockers (e.g. propranolol; 2.5–5 mg every 8–12 hours) or vasodilators (e.g. captopril*; 0.5–2 mg every 8 hours).

The manipulation of dietary protein and phosphorus in chronic renal failure in the cat can be achieved using either specially formulated proprietary foods or home-produced foods. The objective is to provide protein of high biological value and useful amino acid composition at levels no higher than maintenance requirements, thus reducing to a minimum urea and other nitrogenous products of protein catabolism. The calorie requirement is provided by fats, particularly those of animal origin, and to a lesser extent by carbohydrates. However, few data are available on the dietary requirements of the cat in naturally occurring CRF and given the peculiar and particular needs of the normal cat in terms of total protein levels and specific amino acid requirements (see Chapter 24), extrapolation from other species such as the dog may not be very helpful. The cat, too, is often a fastidious feeder, especially when unwell, and may not take readily to dietary manipulation. This, together with de-

bate as to the appropriate time in the progression of renal disease to institute dietary protein restriction makes the management of individual cases of CRF a matter of judgment. Reduced levels of dietary phosphorus are used to help control the hyperphosphataemia of CRF; the use of agents such as aluminium hydroxide to bind dietary phosphorus within the bowel can be attempted but these products are not very acceptable to cats. Hypocalcaemia is best managed through reduction in blood phosphorus levels: supplementation of the diet with calcium can be used at doses of *c.* 20 mg/kg BW.

Supplementation of the diet with the B vitamin complex is also recommended, as cats in CRF fail to conserve water-soluble vitamins. Anabolic steroids may also be helpful in stimulating protein anabolism and red blood cell production in uraemic cats, although their effectiveness clinically is often difficult to assess. Glucocorticoids are contraindicated as they increase protein breakdown. Antibiotics are of value in the presence of bacterial infection in the urinary tract; the choice of antibiotic is influenced by its concentration in the urinary tract and the avoidance of potentially nephrotoxic agents. Clinically some cats respond to such therapy, suggesting a role in some cases for bacterial infection, possibly superimposed on other pathology. Vomiting, associated either with uraemic gastritis or the central effect of the azotaemia, appears to be less common in the cat than the dog. Where it occurs control can be attempted using metaclopramide† (0.2–0.4 mg/kg BW every 8 hours *per os*), cimetidine‡ (5 mg/kg BW every 8 hours *per os*) or acetylpromazine (0.05–0.2 mg/kg BW by injection).

In those cases of chronic renal disease where the cat has stopped drinking, dehydration rapidly ensues leading to so-called uraemic crisis. In such cases the restoration of fluid volume and thus glomerular filtration is of primary importance, together with the correction of the resultant acidosis. The recognition and management of any intercurrent and possibly precipitating extra-

* Capoten, E.R. Squibb & Sons Ltd., Hounslow, Middx, UK.

† Emequell, SmithKline Beecham, Animal Health, Tadworth, Surrey, UK.

‡ Tagamet, SmithKline Beecham, Welwyn Garden Gty, Herts, UK.

renal disease is also important. The choice of replacement fluid is based on the knowledge that electrolyte loss, particularly sodium and chloride, and to a lesser extent potassium, is marked in animals with CRF and thus in the absence of specific information on blood levels, a balanced electrolyte solution such as lactated Ringer's is indicated. The lactate is of value in combating the acidosis. Direct measurement of plasma pH and bicarbonate concentration is necessary to define the degree of acidosis accurately, but in their absence it is useful to estimate the probable bicarbonate required, based on the general condition of the cat. Between 2 and 6 mmol/kg BW as sodium bicarbonate may be necessary, of which half should be given slowly intravenously and the remainder in intravenous fluids over the next 6–8 hours.

Most cases of CRF will respond to correction of dehydration, and diuresis can be maintained, if necessary, by further administration of fluid therapy. The failure of the cat to produce urine following fluid replacement is an indication for the use of osmotic diuretics such as glucose or mannitol; these are generally preferred to agents such as frusemide. While frusemide is simple to use, it does produce further chloride and sodium loss and is more likely to result in hypovolaemia. Glucose, administered as a 20% solution intravenously, has the added advantage of being inexpensive and also of providing calories, and a step-by-step technique for glucose diuresis has been suggested previously (Low, 1971).

1 Fluid deficits are corrected with lactated Ringer's, and the animal weighed and the bladder emptied.
2 A 20% dextrose solution is given intravenously at a rate of 2 ml/min for 10–15 minutes, preferably through a central line, and then at a rate of 1 ml/min; the total amount given is between 25 and 65 ml/kg bodyweight.
3 Urine is tested for glucose to assess the efficacy of the diuresis, and if present should be followed by a urine flow of 1–2 ml/min. If urine flow is not adequate by the time 15–20 ml/kg bodyweight of glucose has been given, the infusion must be stopped to avoid over-hydration and hyperosmolarity.

4 Once all the glucose has been administered, the cat should be reweighed to assess loss in bodyweight and any deficit made up with lactated Ringer's.
5 Such a regime may be repeated two or three times in 24 hours and the cat re-evaluated for improvement in general condition and blood urea/creatinine levels. Plasma electrolye levels, particularly potassium, should be monitored if diuresis is protracted and supplementation provided if necessary.

Where the cat fails to produce urine following such a regime, other diuretics such as frusemide may be tried, but the prognosis is very poor. Peritoneal dialysis has been described in the dog for the maintenance of animals in acute, potentially reversible renal shutdown, and the same technique could be applied to the cat (Osborne *et al.*, 1972). Haemodialysis is rarely feasible. Renal transplantation has been successfully carried out in a small number of cats, using cyclosporin to suppress rejection (Gregory & Gourley, 1992). Once urine flow has been established and a reduction in the azotaemia achieved, the methods described above to maintain a cat with chronic renal insufficiency can be implemented.

Good nursing, including the provision of warmth, cleanliness and attention, is of very considerable importance at all stages in the management of renal failure in cats. The minimizing of stress and the risk of intercurrent disease is also important and in the context of intercurrent disease, it is always worth considering that superimposed disease may have precipitated renal decompensation in a previously compensated cat, and recognition and treatment of any such condition is clearly of importance.

Owners of such cats should be advised to seek early veterinary attention for conditions, e.g. mild gastroenteritis, which in uncompromised cats would invariably be self-limiting.

Nephrotic syndrome

Nephrotic syndrome is well recognized in cats and in the great majority of cases is associated with a membranous glomerulonephritis (MGN) (see above). The damage to the glomerular basement membrane leads initially to a loss of protein, mainly the smaller molecular weight albumin, into the glomerular filtrate. In those cases of MGN where severe hypoalbuminaemia develops, clinical signs of nephrotic syndrome may be appreciated. Such signs are not always present and cannot be related directly to the level of plasma albumin. In some cases, glomerular damage and subsequent sclerosis leads to a loss of glomerular and dependent tubular function and to renal insufficiency.

CLINICAL SIGNS

The nephrotic syndrome is characterized by the development of subcutaneous oedema, most obvious in dependent areas such as the limbs, ventral abdomen and thorax and, to a lesser extent, in the neck and face (Fig. 5.5). Transudate may also accumulate in the peritoneal, pleural and pericardial cavities. Although oedematous, the cat may remain quite bright, though in severe cases the animal may become inappetent and depressed. Diarrhoea may develop in some cases, due presumably to bowel oedema. The kidneys are usually normal on abdominal palpation.

The presence of clinical signs in an individual cat is often intermittent with recurrence common. In some cases, signs of chronic renal failure may develop as tubular function is lost below damaged glomeruli; the signs of failure in these individuals are the same as with any cause of renal insufficiency.

DIAGNOSIS

The diagnosis of nephrotic syndrome is based on the clinical signs and confirmed by the demonstration of large amounts (>10 g/l) of albumin in the urine and a hypoalbuminaemia (<20 g/l). Confirmation that the syndrome is due to a membranous glomerulonephritis can only be achieved by renal cortical biopsy (see above). Other laboratory values that may be altered include plasma cholesterol, which for reasons not clearly understood is frequently raised, and plasma globulin, which may also be raised. Urine specific gravity is usually high (>1040) and a mild anaemia is some-

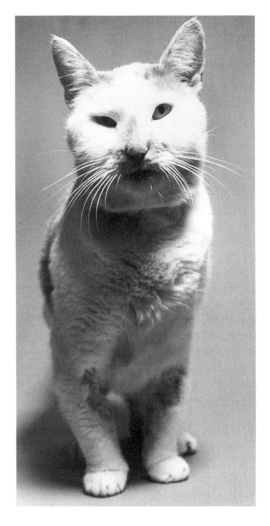

Fig. 5.5 A cat with nephrotic syndrome due to membranous glomerulonephritis, showing typical oedematous swelling of the feet, ventral chest and neck, and face.

times present. Blood urea and creatinine levels are usually normal or slightly elevated due to reduced renal perfusion. These parameters are markedly raised in those cases of glomerulonephritis where renal damage is severe enough to cause insufficiency. In these cases, however, the diagnosis is usually one of renal failure, as at this stage protein loss and hence proteinuria may not be severe enough to implicate glomerular disease specifically.

TREATMENT

The management of the nephrotic syndrome is aimed at reducing the oedema using diuretics such as frusemide (2–4 mg/kg bodyweight twice a day) and attempting to increase blood albumin levels by feeding high-protein diets or supplementing with protein hydrolysates, though the latter is contentious due to the effect of high protein levels on glomerular blood flow and damage. The feeding of a low-salt diet to minimize sodium and water retention is theoretically useful, but control is more practically achieved using diuretics. In those cases where blood volume is reduced, as shown by haemoconcentration, plasma expanders may be useful to overcome the reduction in natural osmolarity.

The control of the underlying glomerulopathy is more difficult. The antigen in the immune complex is invariably unknown and hence cannot be controlled. Suppression of the immune response using corticosteroids, for example prednisolone at 1–2 mg/kg bodyweight/day, may be beneficial in some cases, but their overall usefulness is unclear. No information is available on the use of other immunosuppressive agents such as cyclophosphamide or combinations of such drugs in the cat for this purpose.

The majority of cases appear to respond clinically to supportive treatment and cage rest with or without corticosteroid therapy, and thus the short-term prognosis is good. Proteinuria frequently persists, however, and a percentage of cases show recurrence of the nephrotic syndrome over a period of months or years (Arthur *et al.*, 1986). In a number of animals the renal lesions progress until renal failure occurs. Some cats, though, show only one or two episodes of oedema, and at present it is not possible to distinguish between these animals and those that will show frequent recurrence, nor to offer advice or treatment to influence the recurrence rate. It is suggested that immunohistological examination of renal biopsy material may give a guide to prognosis, with those cats showing IgM and IgA deposits having a poorer outlook (Arthur *et al.*, 1986).

DISEASES OF THE URETERS

Diseases of the ureters are rare in the cat. Congenital defects such as ectopic ureters, with the ureter emptying distal to the bladder, have been reported in the cat but are very uncommon (for example Bebko *et al.*, 1977; Biewenga *et al.*, 1978). Urinary incontinence is the major sign, of which perineal scalding due to constant soaking is a useful indicator. In the few cases that have been recorded, males and females are equally represented and most cases have shown signs since birth or weaning. Individuals with unilateral ectopia may also urinate normally. Diagnosis is made by contrast radiography, the course of the ureters being demonstrated following an intravenous urogram against a pneumocystogram. Surgical relocation of the ectopic ureters into the bladder is the treatment of choice, with any secondary bacterial infection being treated before surgery. Damage to ureters has been reported following uterine surgery, leading to the development of a ureterovaginal fistula and incontinence (Allen & Webbon, 1980).

LOWER URINARY TRACT DISEASE

Cases of lower urinary tract disease are common in feline practice, presenting with signs which include haematuria, increased frequency or difficulty in urination, obstruction to urine flow or, rarely, incontinence. While a number of conditions are recognized, the most important entity is the feline urological syndrome.

Feline urological syndrome (FUS)

The feline urological syndrome (FUS, urolithiasis, urethral obstruction, 'blocked cat') is the most important lower urinary tract condition of cats. It is characterized by haematuria and dysuria, with or without urethral obstruction. Such a definition may include any condition of the lower urinary tract, and this together with the lack of a defined cause for the syndrome makes it important to rule out other, albeit less common, causes of such signs. The incidence of FUS has been assessed by a number of surveys in Britain and the USA as about 0.5% of the population per annum, though up-to-date data are not available and it is a clinical impression in the United Kingdom that the incidence has fallen in recent years.

Urethral obstruction with a mixture of struvite crystals and a proteinaceous matrix occurs, for purely anatomical reasons, almost invariably in the male: cystitis is seen with equal frequency in both sexes. Despite initially conflicting data, neutered cats appear to be at greater risk. There is no clear explanation of this; it does not appear to be related to urethral development and diameter. FUS is uncommon in cats less than 1 year of age, and shows no marked breed incidence though it may be seen more frequently in long-haired cats. Recurrence is common in unmanaged cats, varying between 30 and 50% in different series.

Pathogenesis and aetiology

The pathogenesis of the 'clinical' stages of FUS is fairly clear, though the sequence of events prior to the development of signs is poorly understood. The urethral obstruction seen in the male, and very occasionally in the female, is due to the accumulation of struvite ($Mg.NH_4.PO_4.6H_2O$) crystals in a proteinacious matrix in the urethra, typically at the tip of the penis or at the level of the bulbo-urethral glands. Occasionally, the obstructing material may be predominantly crystalline, and less commonly it may be sabulous in nature. Similar material may be found in the bladder (Fig. 5.6). The effect of the urethral obstruction is to reduce and eventually stop glomerular filtration, leading to a rapid build-up of waste metabolites such as urea, and a failure of kidneys to maintain ionic and acid–base balance. Failure of renal function, and particularly the development of hyperkalaemia, leads to coma and death in 48–92 hours.

The aetiology of FUS is not known although it is clear that various factors may predispose an individual cat to the disease. A number of these factors were identified in epidemiological studies

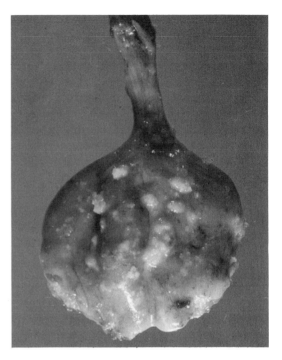

Fig. 5.6 Post-mortem specimen showing the accumulation of sabulous material in the bladder of a cat that died following urethal obstruction.

carried out in Europe and the USA in the 1970s; they included inactivity, as assessed by access to and time spent out-of-doors, neutering, being overweight, eating dry food and having a low fluid intake. These and other factors may also act synergistically, the possession of more than one predisposing factor giving more than additive risk value.

It is interesting to note that a number of these factors had been identified as early as 1925 (Kirk): some have been the subject of very considerable recent investigation. Suggestions that diet may have a crucial role in FUS through its effect on urinary environment have been frequently made: possible factors have included the level of ash in the diet and more recently dietary magnesium concentrations, the feeding of low-moisture or dry cat foods (DCF), and the influence of diet on urinary pH. However, the feeding of high-ash diets does not in itself appear to be important and while the disease can be produced by feeding high levels of dietary magnesium, such levels are considerably higher than those found in commercial cat foods and the effect is influenced significantly by other dietary ions. An increased risk of FUS has been associated with the feeding of low-moisture or dry cat foods, most marked when these foods form a high proportion of the diet. This increased risk of FUS on DCF compared to other types of diet (e.g. canned) may be associated in part with the effect on the cat's total fluid intake. The related factor of extra-food fluid intake has also been shown to influence the risk of disease, those cats drinking less than a saucerful of fluid daily being significantly more likely to develop FUS. It has been shown that cats have a lower total fluid intake, lower urinary volume and more concentrated urine when fed an experimental diet in a dry form (i.e. 90% dry matter) than when the same food is fed in a higher moisture (i.e. 10% dry matter) form. The manner of feeding may also influence the effect, for the kinetics of fluid balance in cats fed specific meals of DCF may differ considerably from those in animals fed on an *ad libitum* basis.

Feeding patterns, as well as the composition of the diet, will also influence urinary pH, an important role for which has been identified in FUS. Urine of low pH, <6.8, reduces the incidence of struvite crystalluria and hence the risk of urethral obstruction. The effect of urinary pH on the level of struvite crystalluria and hence on the incidence of FUS is thought to be more important than that of magnesium levels. This observation, together with the role of dietary ionic composition, has formed the basis of the dietary recommendations for the management of the condition which have been developed in recent years.

These various factors, while important, are clearly not the cause of FUS, since they are present in many healthy cats and absent in some cases of the disease. Some, such as the formulation of commercial foods, have been influenced by modifications implemented since the epidemiological studies were carried out.

The underlying aetiology remains obscure. A role for viral agents was suggested by US workers in the early 1970s, following their isolation of a calicivirus (Manx strain) and subsequently a second, cell-associated feline herpesvirus. Other workers have been unable to confirm these findings and it seems unlikely that the primary cause of FUS is viral. Recent work with the original US herpesvirus isolate has not been conclusive, but has shown a close relationship between the virus and a bovine herpesvirus (BHV 4). It is generally accepted that bacterial infection, though it may be present, has no primary role in FUS.

FUS is clearly a multifactorial disease problem. Epidemiology, while not suggesting a cause, has produced a profile of the cat most likely to develop FUS, and thereby suggests logical approaches to management. The increased ability to manipulate the pathogenesis of the condition by altering the urinary environment through diet is valuable, particularly for cats known to be predisposed, but the lack of understanding of the underlying aetiology of the condition remains. The role and importance of the protein component of the obstructing material is particularly poorly understood.

Clinical signs

The clinical signs associated with FUS are haematuria, increased frequency of urination, and dysuria or anuria. Within this broad description, the syndrome can be divided into cats with cystitis/urethritis and no obstruction to urine flow, and those with partial or complete urethral obstruction. In the latter group, the presence of obstruction leads to increasing attempts to urinate, abdominal discomfort, licking of the perineum and progression to depression, coma and death from renal failure within 48–72 hours. In the early stages, owners may confuse the signs with those of constipation (Fig. 5.7). On clinical examination the bladder of obstructed cats is large, tense and painful; care should be taken to prevent bladder rupture, which may occasionally occur spontaneously. In cases of cystitis the bladder is small, firm and painful.

Diagnosis

Diagnosis of FUS is usually uncomplicated and based on clinical signs, but the lack of a definitive

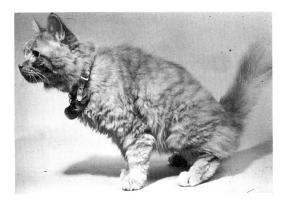

Fig. 5.7 Male cat with urethral obstruction in the typical crouching position.

diagnostic test and the potential confusion with other causes of lower urinary tract disease make the use of urinalysis and culture/sensitivity and, on occasions, radiography, essential in those cases which are not typical or fail to respond.

Management

URETHRAL OBSTRUCTION

The treatment of cats with urethral obstruction should be regarded as an emergency. Management is based on an understanding of the pathogenesis of clinical signs and consists of not only the relief of the obstruction, but also the correction of the systemic effects of the renal failure. While in many cases of recent obstruction the systemic effects are limited, in some cats their correction is the priority. In such cases relief of bladder pressure by cystocentesis should be followed by stabilization before clearance of the obstruction is attempted. The prevention of recurrence both in the immediate post-obstruction period and in the long term is also an important consideration.

Relief of the obstruction
The aim of treatment is to clear the obstruction with a minimum of additional trauma to the urethra, and hence the lowest risk of subsequent scarring and narrowing. Treatment with

antispasmodics, for example atropine, pancreatic extract, or with tranquillizers is rarely successful although it has the advantage of being atraumatic. Occasionally, and where the obstruction is at the tip of the penis, the white gritty material may be milked from the urethra by gentle massage of the lubricated penis. The use of manual pressure on the bladder to force the obstructing material out is rarely helpful and carries the considerable risk of rupturing the bladder. In a large number of cases, urethral irrigation and catheterization are necessary to clear the obstruction. This should be carried out, in all but the most depressed animals, under general anaesthesia. Following extrusion and cleaning of the penis, initial irrigation is best achieved using a blunt-ended lacrimal duct needle (Fig. 5.8). Sterile water, saline or sodium acetate/acetic acid buffer (Walpole's solution) should be used to flush the urethra repeatedly in an attempt to break down or dissolve the obstructing material. Once the penile urethra has been cleared, a plastic tom-cat catheter may be passed and irrigation continued where a higher obstruction is present. Some obstruction to the passage of the catheter will usually be appreciated in the normal cat with the penis extruded as the urethra passes over the ischium, and this should not be confused with pathological obstruction; release of the penis and caudal traction on the prepuce will allow the urethra to straighten and the catheter to pass into the pelvic urethra. Repeated lavage is often required before the obstructing material is removed. Wherever possible, such material should be flushed clear, since forcing the catheter past the obstructing plug will traumatize the urethral wall and predispose to later stricture formation. Reintroduction of the metal stylet with the catheter in the urethra should also be avoided as the stylet may well pass through the side holes and damage the urethra. Once the catheter has been passed, the bladder is emptied by syringe suction; lavage of the bladder with sterile water or buffer, or the instillation of antibacterial agents is of doubtful value, unless a bacterial cystitis is present. Where urethral catheterization is not achieved, cystocentesis may be helpful in removing resistance to back-flushing.

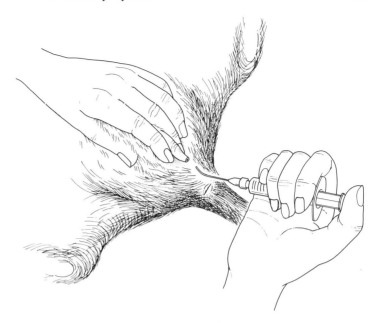

Fig. 5.8 Extrusion of the penis for urethral catheterization. A lacrimal needle is used to irrigate the distal portions.

Failure to relieve the obstruction is an indication for immediate urethrostomy, although this technique, if needed at all, is better carried out as an elective procedure when the urethra and the cat have recovered from the acute obstructive episode.

Correction of systemic effects of obstruction
The depression seen in cats with complete obstruction for longer than *c.* 24 hours is associated with an acidosis, raised plasma potassium levels and azotaemia. Blood urea levels, often >60 mmol/l, may indicate the severity of the renal failure, which is life-threatening but invariably reversible. Together with the restoration of urine flow, treatment should include intravenous fluid therapy with a balanced electrolyte solution such as lactated Ringer's; the small amount of potassium in these fluids is probably insignificant. In the absence of immediate laboratory results or blood gas analysis as a basis for treatment, an ECG trace is of value: a loss of P waves and spiked T waves are a good marker of hyperkalaemia and an indication for intravenous sodium bicarbonate at a rate of 1–3 mEq/kg bodyweight, by slow intravenous injection and by the addition of a

similar amount to the intravenous fluid. This dose of bicarbonate may be repeated as necessary. Such cats are frequently hypothermic, and warmth as well as general nursing is important. The use of intravenous insulin together with glucose to lower the elevated levels of blood potassium rapidly has been described but is rarely indicated, particularly if sodium bicarbonate is used.

Management in the post-obstruction period
The maintenance of urine flow immediately following relief of the obstruction is important both to maintain urethral patency and to monitor urine production, and is often best achieved by placing an indwelling urinary catheter. A catheter is secured to the prepuce by three or four loose stitches and the resultant incontinence may be controlled in severely depressed cats by attaching tubing, for example from an intravenous administration set, to the catheter, carrying the urine away to a bottle. An Elizabethan collar is often necessary to prevent the cat interfering with the catheter or tubing. Any obstruction of the catheter may be cleared by retrograde flushing. The disadvantages of an indwelling catheter,

namely the predisposition to ascending bacterial infection and the continuous damage to the urethral mucosa, must be weighed against the advantages of control of urethral patency and the decompression of the bladder. The latter is of particular value where the bladder has been chronically distended and tone is poor. In cases where relief of obstruction is straightforward and the cat is systemically well, the use of an indwelling catheter is rarely indicated; where an indwelling catheter is used, it should be for as short a time as possible. The use of antibiotics to prevent secondary bacterial infection is controversial, and should ideally only follow culture and sensitivity. Nephrotoxic antibiotics (e.g. aminoglycosides) should be avoided. Prophylactic use in the presence of an indwelling catheter may merely encourage resistant infections. Urinary antiseptics containing methylene blue cause haemolytic anaemia in cats and should be avoided. Cats which have recently been obstructed should not be given urinary acidifiers.

A number of cats undergo a marked diuresis following the relief of the obstruction; this may last for 2 or 3 days, or in some cases up to 10 days, and is believed to be due both to the clearance of accumulated metabolites and a temporary inability of the renal tubules to concentrate urine effectively. Fluid therapy, either subcutaneous or intravenous, is necessary to maintain hydration in these animals. Initially, a balanced electrolyte solution is appropriate, but in a small number of cats continued diuresis may lead to excessive loss of ions, and supplementation, particularly with potassium, may be necessary. The potential for both dehydration and hypokalaemia in these cats should be recognized.

LONG-TERM MANAGEMENT

Recurrence of urethral obstruction is common in FUS; in one UK series some 30% of cats surviving the obstructive episode had further episodes within 6 months. Owners should be made aware of this and warned to look for the early signs of obstruction. Prevention of recurrence is hampered by a poor understanding of the underlying cause or causes, but it is logical to attempt to control these factors which have been recognized as predisposing to FUS. Low fluid intake is known to be associated with the condition; thus dry cat foods should be avoided and the cat may be encouraged to take in more fluid by adding water to the food, adding salt to the food and offering palatable fluid such as gravy where this is accepted. Fresh water should always be available. Diets should be chosen which are low in magnesium (<2% on a dry matter basis) and which give a low urinary pH (6.0–6.5), best measured during the period of alkaline tide some 4 hours post-prandial. Commercial prescription diets are available with these objectives for both the weeks immediately post-obstruction and in the long term; evidence for the efficacy of such regimes in preventing recurrence of naturally occurring FUS over prolonged periods is still being accumulated. Overweight and low levels of activity are also associated with FUS, but are less easy to manipulate. A clean litter tray or ready access to outside should always be provided. Urinary acidifiers may be valuable in the long term; not all are useful in consistently reducing pH, but ammonium chloride has been shown to be effective. Acidifiers are best given with food to offset the effect of the alkaline tide.

Recurrence of urethral obstruction in the male cat may be prevented by the surgical removal of the distal, narrow portion of the urethra, the most commonly employed techniques being perineal or prepubic urethrostomy. Of these two techniques, the former is favoured by most, and has been very adequately described in the literature (Johnston, 1974; Long, 1977; Gaskell *et al.*, 1978). Such surgery should be reserved for those cases where repeated obstruction occurs despite the use of dietary measures; such recurrences are often associated with a degree of stricture formation. The prognosis following urethrostomy is good, though surgery does not control the underlying problem of FUS and recurrent sterile cystitis may occur. It has also been well demonstrated that ascending bacterial cystitis is common following perineal urethrostomy. Urethral stricture and urinary incontinence have both been recorded as postoperative problems but are not common following uncomplicated surgery.

Cystitis

Relatively little attention has been given to the recurrent, bacteriologically sterile cystitis seen in both sexes as part of the feline urological syndrome. Such cases usually resolve spontaneously after a few days; therapy, including urinary acidifiers and antibiotics, is frequently recommended though the true value of such treatment is difficult to assess. Advice aimed at increasing fluid intake and reducing the dietary levels of magnesium should be given: fresh water and a clean litter tray should be readily available, exercise 'encouraged' and bodyweight controlled. Care must be taken, particularly in view of the sometimes recurrent nature of the condition, to distinguish the idiopathic cystitis of FUS from that associated with a bacterial cystitis, the presence of true calculi, or the rare cases of neoplasia of the urinary bladder. Cystitis associated with the use of the cytotoxic drug cyclophosphamide is well recognized in a number of species and has been reported in cats (Stanton & Legrende, 1986). Administration of the drug should be ceased immediately and diuresis initiated.

Lower urinary tract infection

Bacterial infection of the lower urinary tract is recognized in cats, though it is less common than in dogs. The reasons for this are not clear but may include the higher osmolarity of feline urine. Bacterial infection is uncommon as a primary entity, occurring almost invariably as a secondary phenomenon following other forms of lower urinary tract disease, e.g. recurrent FUS, or in cats with an indwelling urinary catheter. The clinical signs are those of increased frequency, dysuria and/or haematuria; the cat is rarely systemically unwell and mild infections may cause no clinical signs at all. Diagnosis is based on the presence of red blood cells, epithelial and inflammatory cells, and bacteria in the urine. Bacterial culture is best carried out on urine obtained by cystocentesis and should demonstrate significant

numbers of organisms ($>1 \times 10^4$/ml). Samples obtained at catheterization or from voided urine may be useful diagnostically but are of less value for culture. Cystocentesis can be carried out easily and safely in most cats (see below). If the bladder is not palpable the cat is caged until sufficient urine has been formed. Bacterial sensitivity will indicate the appropriate therapy, and treatment for at least 14 days is usually advisable, with longer courses necessary in cases of chronic cystitis. Penicillins or potentiated sulphonamides are the most useful drugs in the first instance. A diagnosis of bacterial cystitis, particularly if there is a failure to respond to treatment or there is a rapid recurrence of signs, should prompt further investigations into a possible underlying cause. Fungal infection of the lower urinary tract is rare but has been reported, usually due to *Candida albicans*, after repeated antibacterial therapy. It appears to be difficult to eradicate.

Viral infection of the urinary tract has been proposed as a component of feline urological syndrome (see above). Feline calicivirus (FCV) and feline syncytium-forming virus (FeSFV) may be isolated from the urine of cats but no clinical significance has been associated with their presence.

Parasitic infestation of the feline bladder due to *Capillaria feliscati* occurs in certain parts of the world, e.g. Australia (Waddell, 1968). Infection is not usually associated with clinical signs; diagnosis is based on the demonstration of eggs in the urine, and fenbendazole (25 mg/kg BW twice daily for 3–10 days) is suggested as treatment (Brown & Prestwood, 1986).

Calculus disease

Discrete cystic calculus formation, as opposed to the accumulation of struvite crystals in a sabulous protein matrix seen in FUS, is uncommon. The majority of affected cats are over 1 year of age, and there does not appear to be any sex or breed predisposition. Struvite (magnesium ammonium phosphate) calculi are by far the most frequent type encountered; they are often flat and discoid in appearance or may appear as multiple

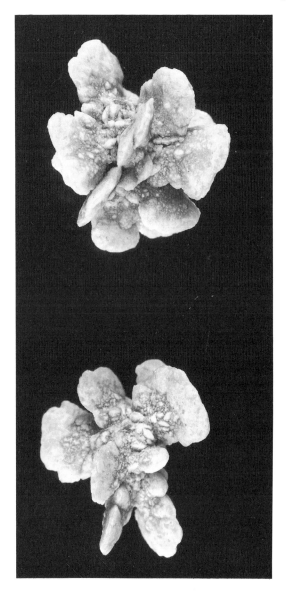

Fig. 5.9 Phosphatic calculi from the bladder of a female cat. Calculi may be single or multiple 'discs'.

calculi are also recorded but in large series each type generally makes up less than 5% of the total. Calculi in the renal pelvis in cats do occur but are rare. The presence of bladder calculi should be suspected where cystitis is persistent or recurrent. Radiographic demonstration, using plain and contrast cystography, may be difficult and confirmation of the diagnosis may only be achieved at cystotomy.

Traditional management has been surgical, but the successful use of diets which create an acidic, low magnesium and dilute urinary environment in which cystic struvite calculi dissolve over a period of 4–6 weeks has been described (Osborne *et al.*, 1989). Such prescription diets are commercially available. Appropriate antibiotic therapy is indicated where urine culture reveals bacterial infection. The prevention of recurrence of sterile struvite uroliths may be attempted by the feeding of diets low in magnesium and producing an acidic pH. Alternatively, urinary acidifiers, such as methionine (*c.* 1 g/day) or ammonium chloride (*c.* 0.8 g/day), may be given at mealtimes to control the normal post-prandial alkaline tide in urine. Proven medical regimes for the control of other types of urolith formation have yet to be devised.

Neoplasia

Tumours of the feline bladder are rare, and those of the ureters and urethra very rare (Schwarz *et al.*, 1985; Brearley *et al.*, 1986). Transitional cell carcinoma is the most frequent tumour type. Benign tumours occur very infrequently. Malignant bladder tumours are seen typically in older animals (two-thirds are aged between 8 and 13 years) and cause haematuria and dysuria, which is unresponsive to treatment for cystitis. Secondary bacterial infection may be present. Diagnosis may be made on contrast cystography and laparotomy (Fig. 5.10); surgical treatment is rarely feasible due to the infiltrative nature of the tumours and the frequently late presentation. Cystectomy, with translocation of the trigone or ureters into portions of the gastroenteric tract, has not proved a successful technique.

'discs' (Fig. 5.9). Unlike the dog the majority are bacteriologically sterile, though a small number of 'struvite' calculi are associated with infection and may be a mixture of struvite and other components, e.g. calcium phosphate, urate. Calcium oxalate, calcium phosphate and ammonium urate

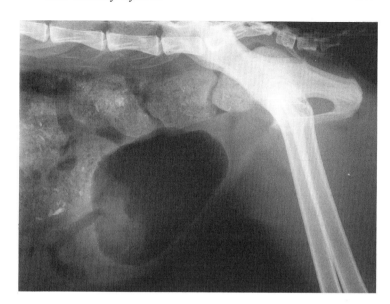

Fig. 5.10 Pneumocystogram in a cat with transitional cell carcinoma of the bladder.

Trauma

Rupture of the bladder may occur as the result of trauma. Inability to palpate the bladder after some hours without urination suggests bladder rupture, which may be confirmed by contrast radiography. Unmanaged cases will develop post-renal azotaemia. Treatment is by surgical repair when the cat has recovered from the immediate effects of the trauma, during which time an indwelling urethral catheter may allow urine to drain from the bladder to the outside, rather than pass into the peritoneal cavity.

Trauma to the urethra may result from pelvic fracture but is seen less commonly than in the dog. The most frequent cause of urethral injury arises from attempts to clear urethral obstruction due to crystalline deposits (see FUS above). Severe urethral trauma or rupture is an indication for urethrostomy.

Urinary incontinence

Urinary incontinence in the cat is uncommon. Ureteric disease, such as ectopia, is rare and has been discussed earlier. Acquired urinary incon-tinence, associated with overflow of urine from a distended bladder, is seen occasionally with fractures of the sacrococcygeal region, where the tail is often flaccid also, and as a feature of some cases of feline dysautonomia (Key–Gaskell syndrome). In both, faecal incontinence and/or constipation may also be present. Treatment consists of manual emptying of the bladder and the use of bethanecol* (1.25–2.5 mg *per os* twice daily), although the prognosis for neurologically induced bladder dysfunction is guarded. Care should be taken with the use of parasympathomimetics such as bethanecol and side-effects such as lacrimation, salivation and abdominal cramps treated with atropine. Urinary and faecal incontinence has also been reported associated with extreme vertebral abnormalities in Manx cats (see also Chapters 2 and 3). Prolonged distension of the bladder due to urethral obstrution (FUS) may leave a bladder with poor tone and overflow incontinence in the immediate post-obstruction period.

Urethral incompetence has been described in cats, which urinate normally but also dribble urine

* Myotonine, Glenwood Laboratories, Canterbury, Kent, UK.

(Barsanti & Downey, 1984). Phenylpropano-lamine, an adrenergic agonist, has been used at doses of 12.5 mg *per os* b.i.d. or 7 mg *per os* t.i.d. An equivalent to the hormone-responsive incontinence that is recognized in neutered bitches does appear to be seen in cats (Barsanti & Downey, 1984).

INVESTIGATIVE TECHNIQUES IN URINARY DISEASE

Urine sampling

The technique used for obtaining a urine sample depends to some extent on the tests to be applied. A fresh sample obtained from a clean box with no litter is satisfactory for basic urine analysis, i.e. specific gravity, pH and crude assessment of protein levels. A sample for bacterial culture requires a sterile technique and a number of procedures are available.

Mid-stream sample

A mid-stream sample can be obtained from most, but not all, cats by the application of steady, but not excessive, pressure on the bladder through the abdominal wall. There is little point, and some danger, in increasing the pressure in a cat that is unwilling to release urine. Such cats often urinate naturally as soon as they are returned to the cage.

Urethral catheterization

Urethral catheterization in the cat requires heavy sedation or general anaesthesia if damage to the urethral wall as a result of spasm or struggling is to be avoided. A tom-cat catheter with a stylet can be used in both sexes. In the male the penis is extruded manually and the well-lubricated catheter introduced into the urethral orifice. The catheter will pass easily for the first 2 cm or so, but resistance is frequently encountered at the brim of the pelvis; release of the extruded penis will allow the urethra and catheter to move cranially into the pelvic cavity and the catheter can be advanced. In the female the urethral orifice does not protrude above the floor of the vagina,

and may be catheterized by running the tip of the catheter blind along the floor of the vagina. If this is not successful, an auroscope may be useful to identify the urethral opening.

Cystocentesis

Urine obtained by direct puncture of the bladder through the abdominal wall is the most satisfactory sample for urine culture. The procedure is no more stressful than routine blood sampling and provided restraint is adequate to prevent sudden movement, this can be done without sedation or anaesthesia. The cat is restrained in lateral recumbency and a small area of the ventral midline just cranial to the pubis shaved and cleaned. The bladder is held against the ventral abdominal wall and a needle (23 gauge) introduced through the abdominal wall into the bladder and urine removed. The slight trauma to the bladder wall may lead to the presence of a few red blood cells in the sample.

Urine analysis

Detailed descriptions of urine analysis may be found in clinical pathology texts, but certain features of normal feline urine are worthy of brief comment. The concentration of feline urine, as assessed by specific gravity, is variable but may be of high (>1045) in cats fed low-moisture or dry foods. Urinary pH is also variable and, while typically acidic on a meat-based diet, will vary with dietary composition. Urine retained for a long time in the bladder tends to become more alkaline.

Urine produced in the hours following a meal is also alkaline, though such fluctuations in pH level out in most cats that urinate only infrequently. Urinary protein levels are generally higher in the cat than the dog and the presence of slight or moderate proteinuria, as assessed by dipstick techniques, does not of itself indicate significant urinary tract disease. The presence of lipid droplets in feline urine is a normal finding and is related to the large amount of lipid present in normal renal tubules of all members of the Felidae. Phosphate, or struvite, crystals are also a normal component of feline urinary sediment, particularly in alkaline urine. Whether such crystalluria is an accurate reflection of bladder urine composition is debatable, as crystals may be seen forming in freshly voided urine on a microscope slide. The tendency for cats to show stress hyperglycaemia is sometimes reflected in glycosuria in otherwise normal animals.

Renal biopsy

Biopsy of the diseased kidney is often the only way of making a definite diagnosis. A biopsy may be obtained either as a wedge tissue taken from the greater curvature of the kidney at laparotomy, or more conveniently by using a percutaneous biopsy needle (e.g. Trucut*).

A needle biopsy is most easily taken from the left kidney. The cat is anaesthetized and a small area of the left flank over the kidney prepared surgically. The kidney is then raised by external manipulation to a subcutaneous position and held there. A small incision in the skin is made over the caudal pole and the biopsy needle introduced into the renal cortex parallel to the long axis of the kidney, taking care to keep the needle within the cortex of the kidney. The manipulation of the needle to take the biopsy is best done by an assistant who slides back and then re-advances the cutting cover of the needle before withdrawing the whole needle plus biopsy specimen. Digital pressure is then applied over the caudal pole of the kidney for a few minutes to minimize bleeding and a single stitch is then placed in the skin wound. Nash (1983, 1986) has examined the potential problems and suggested modifications to the technique, emphasizing the importance of avoiding major arcuate vessels within the kidney to avoid haemorrhage and the creation of areas of infarction. Some subcapsular haemorrhage is probably common following biopsy. The needle biopsy specimen, which can be divided, should be fixed or stored immediately for light or electron microscopy, immunochemistry, etc. as appropriate. Alternatively a wedge biopsy can be taken at laparotomy. This has the advantage of allowing inspection of the kidney and providing a larger specimen, but is more invasive and potentially more damaging to the kidney.

Radiography

Radiography of the urinary tract is a useful adjunct to diagnosis and the various techniques are briefly discussed here. Radiology textbooks should be consulted for further details. All investigations of the urinary tract should be preceded by 12 hours' starvation and the administration of an enema to ensure the removal of overlying intestinal contents. All contrast studies are best carried out under heavy sedation or general anaesthesia.

Kidneys

PLAIN RADIOGRAPHS
The kidneys are frequently well seen on plain lateral and ventrodorsal radiographs outlined by retroperitoneal fat. Both feline kidneys are relatively mobile compared to the dog; the left is more caudal than the right and both are approximately 2½ times the length of the second lumbar vertebra. It is worth noting that mineralization of the adrenal glands, situated at the cranial poles of the kidneys, is occasionally seen in older cats as an incidental finding.

INTRAVENOUS UROGRAM (IVU)
Intravenous contrast agents using iodine compounds such as sodium or meglumine iothalamate† or diatrizoate‡ may be used in the cat to demonstrate the presence, position, shape and to some extent function of the kidneys, though it is true that in the majority of cases of renal disease this information is often already available from other techniques. High-dose urography (2 ml/kg bodyweight of 7% w/v) given as a rapid bolus,

* Trucut disposable biopsy needle; Travenol laboratories Ltd., Thetford, Norfolk, UK.

† Conray 420, May & Baker Ltd., Dagenham, Essex, UK.
‡ Hypaque 45, Bayer UK Ltd., Bury St Edmunds, Suffolk, UK.

preferably into the jugular vein, gives the best results. A radiograph, most usefully a ventro-dorsal view, made as the injection is completed may show an arteriogram, while a film made some 60 seconds later will show a nephrogram, i.e. with contrast in the arterioles and tubules. The renal pelvis will be opacified in the normal cat at about 5 minutes post-injection. Routinely, subsequent films may be made at 10 and 20 minutes depending on the information required. Renal concentration of contrast may be very poor in azotaemic cats.

RENAL ARTERIOGRAPHY

This technique, whereby contrast is introduced into the aorta at the level of the renal arteries or selectively into one renal artery, produces good renal outlines and is particularly useful in non-functioning kidneys. However, the practicalities are such that it is rarely employed.

Ureter

The ureters are not normally seen on plain radiographs, but may be demonstrated by contrast agents as an extension of an intravenous urogram. Abdominal pressure to produce increased ureteric filling is of little value in the cat.

Bladder

The urinary bladder is usually identifiable on plain radiographs in the well-nourished cat with good abdominal contrast. Contrast cystography may be used to identify an unseen bladder or in an attempt to demonstrate cystic or local disease. Negative or positive contrast agents are introduced into an empty bladder through a urethral catheter, 30 ml usually being adequate for bladder distension. Where double-contrast cystography is to be used, a technique most useful for ulcerating lesions of the bladder wall, a small amount of positive contrast (approximately 5 ml) is introduced to coat the bladder wall, followed by sufficient negative contrast agent to distend the bladder. While air is the negative contrast agent invariably used, carbon dioxide is theoretically preferable as the risk of gas embolism, particularly following trauma, has been demonstrated

in man and is reduced by the more soluble CO_2.

Positive contrast is best provided by the iodinated compounds used for intravenous contrast studies, diluted 1:10 with sterile water or saline. Though not essential, it is good practice to remove the agents from the bladder following cystography.

ULTRASOUND

The use of ultrasound to obtain images of the urinary tract can be valuable. The advantages over radiography are those of safety and the ability to investigate fluid spaces, such as cystic kidneys or the bladder, without resort to contrast techniques (Barr, 1990).

REFERENCES
AND FURTHER READING

Allen W.E. & Webbon P.M. (1980) Two cases of urinary incontinence in cats associated with acquired vagino-ureteral fistula. *J. Small Anim. Pract.* **21**, 367–71.
Anderson L.J. & Jarrett W.F.H. (1971) Membranous glomerulonephritis associated with leukaemia in cats. *Res. Vet. Sci.* **12**, 179–80.
Arthur J.E., Lucke V.M., Newby T.J. & Bourne J. (1984) An immunohistological study of feline glomerulonephritis using the peroxidase-antiperoxidase method. *Res. Vet. Sci.* **37**, 12–7.
Arthur J.E., Lucke V.M., Newby T.J. & Bourne J. (1986) The longterm prognosis of feline idiopathic membranous glomerulonephritis *J. Am. Anim. Hosp. Assoc.* **22**, 731–7.
Barr F. (1990) *Diagnostic Ultrasound in the Dog and Cat.* Blackwell Scientific Publications, Oxford.
Barsanti J.A. & Downey R. (1984) Urinary incontinence in cats. *J. Am. Anim. Hosp. Assoc.* **20**, 979.
Bebko R.L., Prier J.E. & Biery D.N. (1977) Ectopic ureters in a male cat. *J. Am. Vet. Med. Ass.* **171**, 738–40.
Biewenga W.J., Rothhuiyen J. & Voorhant G. (1978) Ectopic ureters in the cat – a report of two cases. *J. Small Anim. Pract.* **19**, 531–7.
Bohonowych R.O., Parks J.L. & Greene R.W. (1978) Features of cystic calculi in cats in a hospital population. *J. Am. Vet. Ass.* **173**, 301–3.
Brace J.J. (1983) Perirenal cysts (pseudocysts) in the cat. In Kirk R.W. (ed) *Current Veterinary Therapy*, vol. VIII. W.B. Saunders, Philadelphia, p. 980.
Brearley M.J., Thatcher C. & Cooper J.E. (1986) Three cases of transitional cell carcinoma in the cat and a

review of the literature. *Vet. Rec.* **118**, 91.

Brown S.A. & Prestwood A.K. (1986) Parasites of the urinary tract. In Kird R.W. (ed) *Current Veterinary Therapy IX*. W.B. Saunders, Philadelphia.

Burrows C.F. & Bovee K.C. (1978) Characterisation and treatment of acid–base and renal defects due to urethral obstruction in cats. *J. Am. Vet. Med. Ass.* **172**, 801–5.

Caywood D.D., Osbourne C.A. & Johnston G.R. (1980) Neoplasms of the canine and feline urinary tracts. In Kirk R.W. (ed) *Current Veterinary Therapy VII*. W.B. Saunders, Philadelphia.

Chew D.J., Dibartola S.P., Boyce J.T. & Gasper P.W. (1982) Renal amyloidosis in related Abyssinian cats. *J. Am. Vet. Med. Assoc.* **181**, 139–42.

Clark L. & Seawright A.A. (1968) Amyloidosis associated with chronic hypervitaminosis A in cats. *Aust. Vet. J.* **44**, 584.

Cromwell W.A., Hubbell J.J. & Riley J.C. (1979) Polycystic renal disease in related cats. *J. Am. Vet. Med. Ass.* **175**, 286.

Dibartola S.P., Rutgers H.C., Zack P.M. & Tarr M.J. (1987) Clinicopathologic findings associated with chronic renal disease in cats: 74 cases (1973–1984). *J. Am. Vet. Med. Assoc.* **190**, 1196–202.

DiBartola S.P., Tarr M.J. & Benson M.D. (1986) Tissue distribution of amyloid deposits in Abyssinian cats with familial amyloidosis. *J. Comp. Path.* **96**, 387.

Dow S.W., Fettman M.J., Lecouteur R.A. & Hamar D.W. (1987) Potassium depletion in cats: renal and dietary influences *J. Amer. Vet. Med. Ass.* **191**, 1569–75.

Fabricant C. (1977) Herpesvirus-induced urolithiasis in specific pathogen-free male cats. *Amer. J. Vet. Res.* **38**, 1837.

Fabricant C. & Gillespie J.M. (1974) Identification and characterisation of a second feline herpesvirus. *Inf. Immun.* **9**, 460.

Fennell C. (1975) Some demographic characteristics of the domestic cat population in Great Britain with particular reference to feeding habits and the incidence of the feline urological syndrome. *J. Small Anim. Pract.* **16**, 775–83.

Gaskell C.J. (1979) Studies on the feline urological syndrome. PhD Thesis, University of Bristol.

Gaskell C.J., Denny H.R., Jackson O.F. & Weaver A.D. (1978) Clinical management of the feline urological syndrome. *J. Small Anim. Pract.* **19**, 301–14.

Gaskell R.M., Gaskell C.J., Page W., Dennis P. & Voyle C.A. (1979) Studies on a possible viral aetiology for the feline urological syndrome. *Vet. Rec.* **105**, 243–7.

Gregory C.R. & Gourley I.M. (1992) Renal transplantation in clinical veterinary medicine. In Kirk R.W. & Bonagura J.D. (eds) *Current Veterinary Therapy XI*. W.B. Saunders, Philadelphia. pp. 870–75.

Jackson O.F. (1975) The case against a viral aetiology in feline urolithiasis. *Vet. Rec.* **96**, 70.

Johnston D.E. (1974) Feline urethrostomy – a critique and new method. *J. Small Anim. Pract.* **15**, 421.

Kelly D.F., Lucke V.M. & McCullagh K.G. (1979) Experimental pyelonephritis in the cat. *J. Comp. Path.* **89**, 25–139.

Kirk H. (1925) *The Diseases of the Cat*. Baillicrc Tindall and Cox, London. p. 261.

Long P.D. (1977) A technique for perineal urethrostomy in the cat. *J. Small Anim. Pract.* **18**, 407.

Low D.G. (1971) Osmotic diuresis in the treatment of uraemia. In Kirk R.W. (ed) *Current Veterinary Therapy IV*. W.B. Saunders, Philadelphia, pp. 725–7.

Lucke V.M. (1978) Renal disease in the cat. *Vet. Rec.* **102**, 301–3.

Lucke V.M. (1982) Glomerulonephritis in the cat. In Grunsell C.S. & Hill F.W.G. (eds) *The Veterinary Annual*. Scientechnica, Bristol, pp. 270–8.

Lucke V.M. & Crowther S.T. (1965) The incidence of leptospiral agglutination titres in the domestic cat. *Vet. Rec.* **77**, 647.

Mooney S.C., Hayes A.A., Matus R.E. & MacEwen E.G. (1987) Renal lymphoma in cats: 28 cases (1977–1984). *J. Am. Vet. Med. Assoc.* **191**, 1473–7.

Nash A.S. (1986) Renal biopsy in the normal cat: development of a modified disposable biopsy needle. *Res. Vet. Sci.* **40**, 246–51.

Nash A.S. & Wright N.G. (1983) Membranous nephropathy in sibling cats. *Vet. Rec.* **113**, 180–2.

Nash A.A., Wright N.G., Spencer A.J., Thompson H. & Fisher E.W. (1979) Membranous nephropathy in the cat; a clinical and pathological study. *Vet. Rec.* **105**, 71–7.

Nash A.S., Boyd J.S., Minto A.W. & Wright N.G. (1983) Renal biopsy in the normal cat: an examination of the effects of single needle biopsy *Res. Vet. Sci.* **34**, 347–56.

Northington J.W. & Juliana M.M. (1977) Polycystic kidney disease in a cat. *J. Small Anim. Pract.* **18**, 663–6.

Osborne C.A., Low D.G., Perman V. & Barnes D.M. (1968) Neoplasms of the canine and feline urinary bladder; incidence, etiologic factors, occurrence and pathologic features. *Am. J. Vet. Res.* **29**, 2041–55.

Osborne C.A., Low D.G. & Finco D.R. (1972) *Canine and Feline Urology*. W.B. Saunders, Philadelphia.

Osborne C.A., Polzin D.J., Kruger J.M., Lulich J.P., Johnston G.R. & O'Brien T.D. (1989) Relationship of nutritional factors to the cause, dissolution and prevention of feline uroliths and urethral plugs. *Vet. Clin. North Amer.* **19**, 561–81.

Pedersen P.C., Pool R.R. & O'Brien T.R. (1980) Feline progressive polyarthritis. *Amer. J. Vet. Res.* **41**, 522.

Reif J.S., Bovee K., Gaskell C.J., Batt R.M. & Maguire T.E. (1977) Feline urethral obstruction; a case-control study. *J. Amer. Vet. Med. Ass.* **170**, 1320.

Rendano V.T. & Parker R.B. (1976) Polycystic kidneys and peritoneo-pericardial diaphragmatic hernia in the cat: a case report. *J. Small Anim. Pract.* **17**, 479–85.

Rich L.J. & Fabricant C. (1969) Urethral obstruction in male cats; transmission studies. *Can. J. Comp. Med.* **33**, 164.

Rich L.J. & Fabricant C. (1971) Experimental production of urolithiasis in male cats. *J. Am. Vet. Med. Ass.* **158**, 974.

Schaer M. (1975) The use of regular insulin in the treatment of hyperkalaemia in cats with urethral obstruction. *J. Am. Anim. Hosp. Ass.* **11**, 106.

Schwarz P.D., Greene R.W. & Patnaik A.K. (1985) Urinary bladder tumors in the cat: a review of 27 cases. *J. Am. Anim. Hosp. Assoc.* **21**, 237.

Stansbury R.Z. & Truesdail R.W. (1955) Occurrence of vesicular calculi in cats receiving different diets. *N. An. Vet.* **36**, 841.

Stanton M.E. & Legrende A.M. (1986) Effects of cyclophosphamide in dogs and cats. *J. Am. Vet. Med. Assoc.* **188**, 1319.

Waddell A.H. (1968) Further observation on capillaria felis-cati infections in the cat. *Aust. Vet. J.* **44**, 33.

Walker A.D., Weaver A.D., Anderson R.S., Crighton G.W., Fennell C., Gaskell C.J. & Wilkinson G.T. (1977) An epidemiological survey of the feline urological syndrome. *J. Small Anim. Pract.* **18**, 283.

Watson A.D.J., Culvenor D.J., Middleton D.J. & Rothwell T.L.W. (1986). Distal renal tubular acidosis in a cat with pyelonephritis. *Vet. Rec.* **119**, 65–8.

Willeberg P. (1975) Diets and the feline urological syndrome: a retrospective case-control study. *Nord. Vet. Med.* **27**, 1.

Willberg P. (1981) Epidemiology of the feline urological syndrome. *Adv. Vet. Sci. Comp. Med.* **25**, 311–44.

Chapter 6 / The Respiratory System

C. J. GASKELL

INTRODUCTION

The investigation of disease of the respiratory tract is based, as in many other body systems, upon the identification of the portion primarily involved. Disease of the upper respiratory tract (URT) is dominated by viral infections; the clinical signs of the acute disease, the epidemiology and the management of these infections are dealt with in Chapter 14, while the chronic sequelae are discussed below. Conditions affecting the trachea and lung are relatively uncommon, while the pleura is not infrequently involved in disease of both respiratory and non-respiratory origin.

DISEASES OF THE UPPER RESPIRATORY TRACT

The nostrils

Ulceration of the external nares, particularly the nasal septum, is not infrequently seen with feline calicivirus infection and is usually self-limiting. Persistent ulceration is seen associated with eosinophilic granuloma (the so-called 'rodent' ulcer) and with squamous cell carcinoma (SCC) (Fig. 6.1) (see also Chapter 1). Differentiation between these two may be suspected on appearance, the squamous cell carcinoma often being more extensive, but confirmation of the diagnosis rests on biopsy. Squamous cell carcinoma is locally malignant but responds well to cryosurgery or radiation therapy, often leaving surprisingly little facial distortion. Eosinophilic granuloma may be treated in the same way, though medical treatment with corticosteroids given systemically or injected intralesionally may also be effective. Successful treatment with megestrol acetate* has also been reported. The use of local medication is of little use as it is rapidly licked off and the rough surface of the tongue may make the lesion worse.

Distortion of the nostrils due to wounds may occur, though is rarely of anything but cosmetic importance; congenital defects of the nostrils would seem to be rare.

The nasal cavity

Chronic rhinitis ('chronic snuffles')
Chronic bacterial rhinitis is invariably a sequel to viral upper respiratory tract (URT) disease. The condition is not uncommon in cats due to a combination of the frequency of URT disease, the compact nature of the feline nose and the changes in the epithelium provoked by the particular viral infections. The presence of feline immunodeficiency virus (FIV) in some cases of chronic rhinitis (Yamamoto *et al.*, 1989) suggests that immunological factors may also play a role. Affected animals show a chronic bilateral mucopurulent nasal discharge with intermittent sneezing. Such cats may show periodic inappetence, but are frequently systemically well. Obstruction to the drainage of the frontal sinuses due to diseased turbinate tissue leads to a secondary sinusitis and the condition is often erroneously referred to as chronic sinusitis. Diagnosis is based on a history of initial viral URT disease and the exclusion,

* Ovarid, Pitman-Moore Ltd., Crewe, UK.

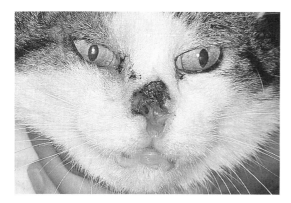

Fig. 6.1 Squamous cell carcinoma on the external nares.

where possible, of other causes of nasal discharge such as fungal rhinitis or neoplasia. Radiographs of the nasal cavity will show bilateral loss of radiolucency in the nasal cavity (seen best using an intra-oral/occlusal film); lateral radiographs may demonstrate soft-tissue filling of the two superimposed frontal sinuses while a dorsoventral view will allow some comparison of the left and right frontal sinuses (Fig. 6.2) (Coulson, 1988). The 'skyline' view of the frontal sinuses, frequently used in the dog, is not useful in the cat due to the anatomy of the skull.

The management of cases of chronic rhinitis and sinusitis is problematic, and the best form of treatment is prevention by the adequate use of broad-spectrum antibiotic therapy in the acute URT infection. Once permanent damage to the nasal mucosa has occurred, control of repeated opportunist bacterial infection may be extremely difficult. The persistence of clinical signs is not necessarily associated with a persistence of viral excretion, though viral carriers, particularly carriers of feline viral rhinotracheitis (FVR) virus, may show signs of nasal discharge and conjunctivitis on viral recrudescence (see Chapter 14). The FIV status of the cat should be assessed, though its role in an individual case will not always be clear. Antibiotic therapy in the chronic phase should be based on bacterial culture and sensitivity and should be maintained over some weeks. However, signs frequently recur when treatment is stopped and in certain cases the con-

tinuous use of low-dose antibiotic therapy may be necessary to achieve some measure of control. Mucolytics (e.g. bromhexine*) may also help to control the clinical signs. The results of treatment with autogenous bacterial vaccines have been disappointing.

More aggressive, surgical treatment for chronic rhinitis and sinusitis has been described, but should be reserved for refractory cases (Lane, 1982). Trephining of the frontal sinuses, with drainage, flushing and the local instillation of antibiotics, may give temporary relief in those cases when the sinuses are involved but does little for the underlying rhinitis.

The placement of drainage tubes and subsequent flushing of the sinuses and nasal cavities, such as might be carried out in the dog, causes considerable distress to the cat and should not be undertaken lightly. Rhinotomy with removal of the diseased turbinate tissue and the establishment of adequate sinus drainage is also poorly tolerated by cats. Postoperative care, including the use of tracheostomy and pharyngostomy tubes (see Chapter 8), is important. The results of surgery are often disappointing and even where an improvement occurs, nasal discharge may persist for some weeks postoperatively. However, the combination of such a surgical approach with the use of fat implants to obliterate the frontal sinus has been reported to be effective (Anderson, 1987).

Some cases of chronic rhinitis show considerable improvement on being housed out-of-doors, but this is not always practicable.

Nasal mycoses
Mycotic infection of the nose is an uncommon cause of persistent nasal discharge in the cat. The discharge may be unilateral or bilateral, and in long-standing cases there may be destruction of the nasal bones and facial distortion (Fig. 6.3). Diagnosis may be made by examination of a stained smear of the discharge, biopsy or on culture. *Cryptococcus neoformans* is the fungal

* Bisolvon, Boehringer Ingelheim Ltd., Bracknell, Berks, UK.

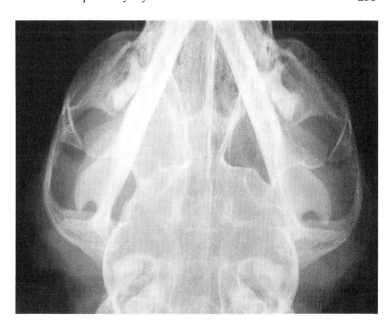

Fig. 6.2 Dorsoventral radiograph of the skull of a cat showing opacification of the right frontal sinus.

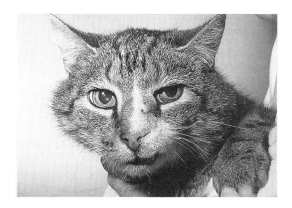

Fig. 6.3 Nasal and facial distortion due to nasal mycotic infection (maduromycosis).

organism most frequently implicated in the nasal mycoses in cats, and involvement of the skin, central nervous system or the eyes may be seen in addition to the nasal cavities. As with all unusual infections in the cat it is prudent to check the FIV and FeLV status of the animal. Treatment of choice would seem to be ketoconazole (10–15 mg/kg BW twice daily *per os* with food for up to 60 days) (Legrende *et al.*, 1982), but the use of amphotericin B (0.3 mg/kg bodyweight injected intravenously three times a week) has been reported despite its nephrotoxicity. The oral antifungal agent 5-fluorocytosine (flucytosine) (125 mg/kg bodyweight per day in four divided doses for 4–6 weeks) has also been used successfully in feline cryptococcosis, alone or in combination with amphotericin B or autogenous vaccines (Wilkinson, 1979; Wilkinson *et al.*, 1983) (see Chapter 23). Other mycotic infections, for example maduromycosis, are occasionally encountered. Nasal aspergillosis is rare in cats and is usually associated with other infections or chronic disease; treatment is similar to that for cryptosporidiosis.

Nasal neoplasia

Neoplasia of the nasal cavity is uncommon, but is seen occasionally in the older cat. Lymphosarcoma and adenocarcinoma both cause persistent nasal discharge (usually unilateral and frequently blood-stained) and facial swelling. Diagnosis may be suspected from the radiographic appearance but is confirmed by biopsy, usually obtained through the nostril using a

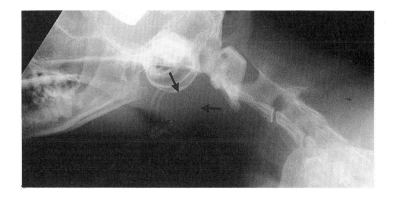

Fig. 6.4 Lateral radiograph of the pharyngeal region of a cat with a nasopharyngeal polyp, showing loss of nasopharyngeal airway and compression of oropharynx.

needle (e.g. Trucut*) or forceps. Treatment is not usually feasible; in the case of lymphosarcoma other areas of the body, for example the kidneys, are frequently involved and local recurrence is said to be common with adenocarcinoma. The nasal cavities are occasionally the site for sarcomas (e.g. osteosarcoma or fibrosarcoma).

Nasopharyngeal polyps
Benign polyps are occasionally seen in the nasopharynx of young cats, causing mucopurulent nasal discharge, respiratory embarrassment and dysphagia (Bedford *et al.*, 1981; Lane *et al.*, 1981; Bradley *et al.*, 1985). The origin of these polyps is the subject of some discussion, but they are inflammatory lesions, most probably the result of ascending bacterial infection of the middle ear or Eustachian tube. If polyps are present in the middle ear, the cat may show otorrhoea and signs of otitis interna (see Chapter 10). Inspection of the pharynx *per os* may reveal the caudal portion of the mass or depression of the soft palate; examination of the caudal portion of the nasopharynx using a dental mirror may also be helpful. Lateral radiographs of the nasopharynx will demonstrate the presence of polyps (Fig. 6.4) and open-mouth views of the tympanic bullae should be taken whether or not signs of ear disease are present. Treatment is by surgical removal *per os* by traction on the polyp and section of the stalk as it emerges

* Trucut Disposable Biopsy Needle, Travenol Laboratories Ltd., Thetford, Norfolk, UK.

from the eustachian tube. Care must be taken during the induction of anaesthesia due to the respiratory embarrassment caused by the nasopharyngeal mass. The response to removal of the polyp is good and while recurrence may occur when removal is simply by section of the stalk, more radical surgery involving bulla osteotomy and curettage of the bulla may lead to complications such as Horner's syndrome, though this is usually temporary.

Other causes of rhinitis
Trauma to the head not infrequently causes splitting of the hard palate, often associated with a mandibular symphyseal fracture, and may lead to chronic rhinitis and nasal discharge due to the passage of food into the nasal cavity. Treatment is by surgical repair of the defect and appropriate antibiotic treatment of any secondary bacterial rhinitis. Cleft palate is a congenital defect giving signs seen early in life. Trauma and distortion of intranasal structures may also lead to chronic nasal discharge, with or without secondary infection. Foreign bodies such as grass seeds are a possible, though uncommon, cause of nasal discharge in the cat.

Discharge is usually unilateral and treatment involves their removal through nasal flushing, and antibiotic treatment. The extension of dental disease into the nasal cavity may also cause rhinitis. Any condition, such as megoesophagus, which causes persistent regurgitation or vomiting of food may potentially cause secondary rhinitis but, again, this is uncommon. Nasopharyngeal stenosis has been reported as a cause of chronic snuffling and difficulty in breathing in cats; the presence of the membrane in the nasopharynx is probably due to chronic inflammation (Mitten, 1988).

Nasal sinuses

The major sinuses of the domestic cat are the frontal sinuses; the maxillary and sphenoid sinuses are merely shallow recesses of the nasal cavity (other felids have different nasal sinus anatomy). The size of the frontal sinuses varies considerably between breeds of domestic cat. Primary disease of the frontal sinuses is rare, infection invariably being secondary to rhinitis, and the management of sinuses has been considered with that of rhinitis. Dullness of percussion of diseased sinuses in the cat is difficult to appreciate due to their size, and disease is best appreciated radiographically (Coulson, 1988).

The larynx

For all its subtleties of anatomy and function, disease of the larynx is recognized only rarely in the cat. Cases of feline viral rhinotracheitis may have a component of laryngitis and occasional cases show severe ulceration of the larynx. The larynx may be involved in generalized lymphosarcoma, or occasionally with thyroid tumours arising from ectopic thyroid tissue. Laryngeal paralysis is rare in the cat but has been described as a cause of dyspnoea, changes in voice and purring, and coughing due to aspiration (Hardie *et al.*, 1981). Experience of treatment is limited but is similar to that used in dogs where the condition is more commonly recognized. Laryngeal spasm in cats, usually associated with manipulation of the larynx under too light a plane of anaesthesia, is well recognized and may be prevented by the application by spray of local anaesthetic. The spasmodic coughing shown by some cats in the absence of other signs and often attributed to groomed hair 'caught in the throat' may be due to episodic and self-limiting laryngospasm (Knowlen, 1991). Laryngeal oedema is occasion-

ally seen following the use of the anaesthetic agent alphaxalone* and if severe enough to cause dyspnoea should be treated with corticosteroids.

Laryngeal foreign bodies are rare due to the fastidious nature of the cat, but occasionally needles or bones may become lodged in the pharyngeal and laryngeal region causing acute discomfort, dysphagia and/or dyspnoea.

DISEASES OF THE LOWER RESPIRATORY TRACT

The trachea

Specific conditions of the trachea are rare in cats. Inflammation, and associated coughing, is sometimes seen with URT viral and chlamydial infections, and tracheitis may also occur due to inhalation of food following regurgitation or overzealous force-feeding. Tracheal collapse, stenosis and hypoplasia are either very rare or unrecorded in the cat and tracheal tumours are similarly almost unknown. Compression of the trachea with dyspnoea may occur at the thoracic inlet due to anterior mediastinal lymphosarcoma or other tumours, e.g. thymoma. Tracheal trauma may result from, for example, a fight. Where penetration of the trachea has occurred, this may be complicated by the presence of subcutaneous emphysema appreciated on palpation by the crackling sensation of the cat's skin. Subcutaneous emphysema and associated pneumomediastinum is very occasionally seen due to leakage of air from a major bronchus, a rare complication of severe upper respiratory tract infection. Treatment of such emphysema is usually not necessary, though obvious defects in the trachea should be closed. Tracheal neoplasia is very rare, though individual cases of tracheal lymphosarcoma, adenocarcinoma and squamous cell carcinoma have been reported (e.g. Beaumont, 1982). Tracheal disease can be investigated using a small fibre-optic or rigid endoscope. In cases of chronic tracheobronchitis, washings can be taken for

---

* Saffan, Pitman-Moore Ltd., Crewe, UK.

culture and cytology. In an anaesthetized cat a sterile male dog urinary catheter is passed through a sterile endotracheal tube to the tracheal bifurcation and 1–2 ml of sterile saline are injected and then aspirated into a large syringe. The injection of saline may be repeated two or three times in order to get sufficient aspirate. The endotracheal tube can also be swabbed for bacterial culture.

Bronchial disease

Bronchial disease without involvement of other parts of the respiratory tract is uncommon, and while chronic bronchitis is occasionally recognized, it is not as commonly seen in cats as in dogs. Infection, such as that due to upper respiratory tract viruses and secondary bacteria, foreign material, food, medication and inhaled irritants or allergens may all cause inflammation of the bronchi with coughing and dyspnoea. Radiological examination may be helpful in longstanding disease, with a pattern of thickened bronchial walls being seen. Cytology and culture of bronchial washings may also be helpful.

Feline bronchial asthma

The most frequently recognized primary disease of the bronchi is feline bronchial asthma. This syndrome, also referred to as allergic bronchitis, is characterized by recurrent episodes of sudden onset, paroxysmal, dry coughing and expiratory dyspnoea. Open-mouthed breathing and cyanosis may be seen in severe cases and wheezing, crackling noises may be heard on auscultation. Radiographs of the chest may appear normal or may show increased radiolucency and flattening of the diaphragm due to trapping of air and overdistension of the lung fields. Haematology reveals a marked eosinophilia (15–20% of the white cell count) in the majority of cases. The aetiology of feline asthma is thought to be allergic and while the offending allergen is rarely found, it may be worth questioning the owner for an obvious source, for example sprays or cat litter. Acute episodes respond promptly to the use of corticosteroids, initially given intramuscularly (prednisolone, 2 mg/kg bodyweight), followed by oral dosage over about one week; recurrent episodes are common.

Lungs

Pneumonia

Although pneumonia is uncommon in the cat, many possible aetiologies have been recorded and, whenever the diagnosis is suspected, efforts should be made to identify the underlying cause. Cats with pneumonia typically show pyrexia, depression, inappetence and weight loss with coughing and dyspnoea. On auscultation, increased lung sounds are heard associated with the accumulation of secretions within the airways. Radiographs of the chest are useful to demonstrate the distribution, nature and extent of the pneumonia, which will vary with the underlying cause.

Viral pneumonia associated with upper respiratory tract virus infection may occur, specifically with certain strains of calicivirus. In kittens such pneumonia may be acute and fatal, but disease in older animals generally involves secondary bacterial infection. Bacteria are indeed frequently involved in the pneumonic process. They are invariably secondary to another insult or injury to the lungs, though it has been suggested that *Bordetella bronchiseptica* may be a primary pathogen in young kittens (Willoughby *et al.*, 1991). Rarely, bacterial infection will lead to discrete lung abscess formation. Chlamydial infection may also involve the lungs but in general other infectious agents are rare causes of pneumonia. Tuberculosis in cats is uncommon since the control of *Mycobacterium bovis* but is potentially important due to the zoonotic risk. The alimentary form is the most common (Orr *et al.*, 1980) but the respiratory tract may be involved. Diagnosis is based on the demonstration of acid-fast organisms in secretions. Treatment is unlikely to be successful, and is usually discouraged (see Chapter 23). *Toxoplasma gondii* has also been reported as a cause of interstitial pneumonia, though infection is usually asymptomatic (see Chapter 25). Mycotic infections, including histoplasmosis, blastomycosis, coccidioidomycosis and crypto-

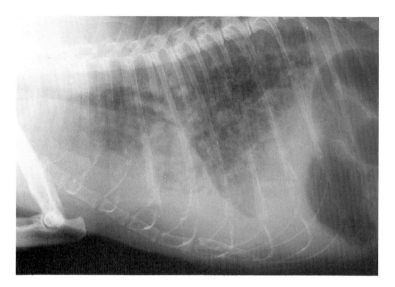

Fig. 6.5 Lateral radiograph of a cat with pulmonary carcinoma, showing multiple densities throughout the lung fields and pleural fluid.

mycosis have also been recorded as causing pneumonia in isolated cases. Where obscure types of infectious pneumonia occur it is relevant to investigate the immune status of the animal, particularly the presence of FIV or FeLV infection.

Inhalation pneumonia may follow the aspiration of foreign bodies or food and is seen as a complication in oesophageal disease, for example megoesophagus, oesophageal stricture, feline dysautonomia, and other causes of dysphagia, persistent regurgitation or vomiting. Radiographically the signs of loss of pulmonary radiolucency with air bronchograms are typically seen in the ventral portions of the cranial and middle lobes. Occasionally over-zealous force-feeding or administration of medication or barium may lead to an inhalation pneumonia. This is a particular risk when administering liquid paraffin in, for example, the management of constipation or hairballs, the smooth nature of the medication making aspiration and a resultant lipid pneumonia a potential problem.

Treatment in most cases of pneumonia is aimed at the control of secondary bacterial infection and the identification and attempted removal of the underlying cause. Antibiotic therapy should ideally be based on culture and sensitivity of organisms isolated by tracheal or bronchial swabs or aspirates, but where this is not feasible, such therapy should be broad-spectrum, for example tetracyclines. Mucolytics, such as bromhexine, may also be helpful in breaking down bronchial and pulmonary exudate. The prognosis in individual cases depends on the underlying cause and the severity of lung involvement.

Neoplasia

Neoplastic disease of the lungs may be primary or secondary. Primary lung tumours are rare, invariably malignant and mostly adenocarcinoma in type (Carpenter *et al.*, 1987). While some cases present as solitary nodules, most primary lung tumours show a multiple, nodular distribution throughout the lungs, often with the formation of pleural fluid (Gruffydd-Jones & Flecknell, 1978; Moulton *et al.*, 1981) (Fig. 6.5). In some cases, however, widespread metastatic disease may give rise to signs before respiratory function is impaired (Moore & Middleton, 1982) and a number of cases have been described where metastases have occurred in multiple digits (May & Newsholme, 1989) (see Chapter 3). The accumulation of the pleural fluid leads to tachypnoea and dyspnoea (see 'pleural neoplasia', p. 268). The lungs may also be involved in multicentric neoplastic disease, for example lymphosarcoma, or metastatic disease from tumours such as mammary carcinoma. Radiographic examination of the chest is the most useful aid to diagnosis but is insensitive in the early stages of metastatic disease. Treatment of lung tumours, with the exception of the rare solitary primary tumours where lobectomy might be considered, is not possible and the prognosis is unfavourable. However, where clinical signs are minimal, or due to potentially manageable secondary bacterial infection, immediate euthanasia may not be indicated. Hypertrophic pulmonary osteoarthritis (HPOA) has been recorded in the cat, but is extremely rare.

Parasitic disease

ALEUROSTRONGYLUS

Infection with the bronchiolar metastrongyle *Aleurostrongylus abstrusus* is common but often asymptomatic and self-limiting; in some cases, however, heavy infestation causes coughing. More rarely, superimposed bacterial infection may lead to severe pneumonia and associated pleural effusion has been reported. A transport host, for example a rodent, is usually part of the life cycle and thus the infection is seen in young 'outdoor' cats; older cats are rarely affected. The diagnosis is made on the demonstration of first-stage larvae in the faeces (see Chapter 25). Radiographs of the chest in clinically affected cats may reveal multiple small nodules but are not diagnostic, and haematological examination frequently shows neutrophilia and eosinophilia.

Most cases recover without treatment but, where signs warrant it, therapy with fenbendazole (20 mg/kg bodyweight daily for 5 days) can be used. Levamisole (25 mg/kg bodyweight divided daily and given every other day over 10 days) has also been used but care must be taken as the drug is poorly tolerated by cats.

PARAGONIMIASIS

The lung fluke *Paragonimus* is reported in cats in the USA but not in Britain. Adult flukes and ova in the airways cause coughing and occasionally dyspnoea, and localized pulmonary inflammation and occasionally pneumothorax may develop.

Diagnosis is by demonstration of the eggs in faeces; radiographs may be helpful, typically showing cavitated opacities in the lungfields representing encysted adult flukes (Pechman, 1976). Fenbendazole is reported to be an effective treatment.

DIROFILARIASIS

Infection of cats with the heartworm *Dirofilaria immitis* is recognized in endemic areas of the world and causes a range of clinical signs including coughing and dyspnoea. Diagnosis may be difficult and treatment, as in dogs, is not without risk (Rawlings, 1986).

Pulmonary oedema

Pulmonary oedema is most frequently the result of congestive cardiac failure associated with cardiomyopathy (see Chapter 11). Clinically the cat shows progressive dyspnoea, with mouth breathing and cyanosis particularly when stressed. Radiographically pulmonary oedema may be difficult to differentiate from other infiltrative conditions of the lungs such as pneumonia, but other clinical and radiographic features may be diagnostic. Other potential but unusual causes of pulmonary oedema include toxin ingestion (e.g. paraquat) and smoke inhalation.

Pleural cavity

The loss of thoracic cavity due to disease of the pleural cavity and accumulation of pleural fluid, is a common cause of tachypnoea and dyspnoea in cats. Affected animals often show a remarkable ability to cope with severely impaired pulmonary volume at rest but often show severe dyspnoea when stressed by clinical, or more particularly, by radiographic examination. Considerable caution must therefore be taken when handling these cats. Radiography is an important diagnostic aid in such cases, but initially only dorsoventral or erect lateral views may be possible, and on no account should a ventrodorsal radiograph be made before the cause and extent of the dyspnoea have been assessed.

The presence of fluid within the pleural cavity

is a common component or sequel to pleural disease and thus thoracentesis is an important technique in both diagnosis and treatment. General anaesthesia in such cases is frequently contraindicated and the procedure is best carried out under local anaesthesia, with the cat gently restrained in sternal recumbency. An area over the ventral third of the seventh intercostal space is surgically prepared and the skin, intercostal muscles and pleura of the seventh intercostal space infiltrated with local anaesthetic approximately one-third of the way up the chest wall. The decision on which side of the chest to approach should be guided by clinical or radiological evidence of the distribution of the pleural fluid; if the distribution is even, the right side is usually chosen. A needle (20/21 gauge), butterfly needle or preferably an over-the-needle catheter, is introduced through the skin just behind the intercostal space, moved slightly cranial (to create a flap effect on withdrawal) and introduced through the intercostal space on the cranial edge of the rib into the pleural cavity. When a needle and catheter are used, a small nick in the skin should be made with a scalpel blade to prevent rucking up of the leading edge of the catheter. A syringe or stop-cock should be attached to the needle before introduction to prevent aspiration of air into the chest.

The differential diagnosis of pleural fluid in the cat is shown in Table 6.1, together with the salient features of the radiographic appearance and pleural fluid (Gruffydd-Jones & Flecknell, 1978).

Rupture of the diaphragm

Rupture of the diaphragm is invariably traumatic in origin and a history of recent trauma or the presence of other signs such as skin abrasions, split claws or bone fractures is helpful. Congenital peritoneopericardial hernias also occur from time to time. Auscultation and percussion of the chest may reveal areas of dullness and, more useful, displacement of the heart sounds; borborygmi from prolapsed bowel are unusual. The abdomen may feel empty on palpation and elevation of the front part of the body may give some relief from the dyspnoea. Elevation of the rear end is contraindicated as it may precipitate fatal respiratory embarrassment. In some cases of diaphragmatic rupture, however, especially those where a piece of liver has been incarcerated in the chest through a relatively small defect, clinical signs may not be apparent for some weeks, or even months, after the original trauma. When signs do develop they are associated with the accumulation of fluid, a modified transudate, in the pleural cavity.

Radiographs of the chest are invaluable in confirming the diagnosis. In long-standing cases pleural fluid may mask radiographic evidence of a ruptured diaphragm and should be removed by thoracentesis and/or diuresis and the animal radiographed again. Where the position of abdominal

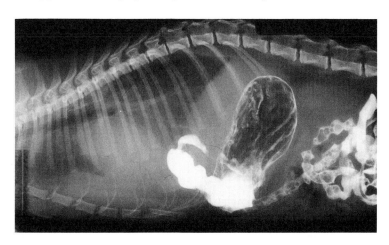

Fig. 6.6 Lateral radiograph of the chest and abdomen of a cat following the administration of barium. The pylorus is displaced cranially beyond the line of the diaphragm (partially obscured by pleural fluid) indicating rupture of the diaphragm.

Table 6.1 Appearance and laboratory characteristics of pleural fluid in different thoracic conditions, together with the associated radiographic appearance.

	Pleural fluid				
	Appearance	Protein levels	Cytology	Bacterial culture	Radiographic appearance
Exudative pleurisy	Variable, including: blood-stained, creamy, floccular, purulent	Moderate	Neutrophils	Positive in some, but not all cases	Pleural fluid uni- or bilateral
Anterior mediastinal lymphosarcoma	Clear, blood-tinged (occasionally lactescent)	Moderate	Lymphocytes + immature blast forms	Sterile	Loss of lucency in anterior thorax Caudal displacement of the heart/carina Dorsal displacement of trachea ± pleural fluid ± dilation of cervical oesophagus
Acquired cardiac disease	Clear	Low	(Unhelpful)	Sterile	Bilateral pleural fluid Cardiomegaly
Pulmonary carcinoma	Clear	Moderate	(Unhelpful)	Sterile	Bilateral pleural fluid Multiple small opacities in lung parenchyma
Ruptured diaphragm	Clear (blood-tinged)	Low	(Unhelpful)	Sterile	Loss of thoracic lucency Loss of diaphragm line Displacement of abdominal organs Displacement of heart/carina ± pleural fluid
Chylothorax	Lactescent	(Unsuitable)	Lymphocytes (chylomicrons)	Sterile	Bilateral pleural fluid
Feline infectious peritonitis	Yellow, tacky (may form clot on standing)	High (globulin)	(Unhelpful)	Sterile	Bilateral pleural fluid ± peritoneal fluid

organs, for example the stomach and bowel, cannot be readily identified, or where tachypnoea makes a still radiograph difficult, the careful administration of a small amount (10 ml) of barium can be helpful (Fig. 6.6).

The displacement of stomach or bowel, identified by their contents of ingesta or air, the loss of diaphragm line, the displacement of thoracic organs and the loss of thoracic radiolucency are all radiographic signs of rupture of the diaphragm.

The replacement of the abdominal organs in the peritoneal cavity and surgical repair of the diaphragmatic defect should be carried out as soon as practicable. Occasionally, prolapse of the stomach into the chest and subsequent gastric tympany may lead to rapidly progressive dyspnoea and necessitate thoracentesis to relieve gastric distension; surgical correction should follow as soon as possible. The management of anaesthesia is crucial. Pre-anaesthetic oxygenation is valuable and induction should be rapid, with an endotracheal tube introduced immediately to assist respiration. Intermittent positive-pressure ventilation is necessary when the peritoneal cavity, and hence the pleural cavity, is opened and reinflation of the lungs after replacement of the displaced organs in the abdomen should be gradual. The surgical pneumothorax should be reduced during or following closure of the diaphragm, though reinflation of the lungs must be carried out cautiously as pulmonary oedema would seem to be a significant postoperative problem (Garson *et al.*, 1980). The risk of hypothermia during and following surgery should also be recognized.

Pneumothorax

The presence of free air within the pleural cavity is usually associated with trauma due to a penetrating wound of the chest, rib fractures or spontaneous rupture of the lung. A mild pneumothorax may cause no obvious respiratory embarrassment, though greater amounts of free air will cause dyspnoea and tachypnoea, often compounded by the pain of the thoracic trauma. Auscultation and percussion reveal increased thoracic resonance dorsally, and radiographs show a characteristic lifting of the base of the heart in the lateral recumbent view, with partial collapse and 'leafing' of lung lobes seen in both lateral and dorsoventral views. In a standing lateral view taken with a horizontal beam, air accumulates in the dorsal part of the chest.

A decision to aspirate the air rather than to wait for natural absorption depends on the clinical condition and progress of the cat. When necessary aspiration should be carried out, with the animal in sternal recumbency, in the dorsal third of the seventh or eighth intercostal space using a 23 or 21 gauge needle. Local anaesthesia may not be necessary where a fine gauge needle is used. Aspiration may need to be repeated and in rare instances, where rapid recurrence of pneumo-

thorax occurs, an indwelling catheter may be necessary. Such a catheter requires fairly constant observation to prevent the cat from dislodging it. Tension pneumothorax, where air continues to enter the pleural cavity during inspiration but cannot be removed at expiration, requires rapid relief and closure of the defect. Pneumothorax has also been reported with *Paragonimus* (lung fluke) infestation (see above). Occasionally pneumothorax may be accompanied by pneumomediastinum and extension to subcutaneous emphysema, particularly where leakage occurs from a major airway.

Haemothorax

Haemothorax is usually associated with trauma and the clinical signs of tachypnoea and collapse may be due as much to the hypovolaemia as to loss of lung volume. Auscultation of the chest reveals dullness ventrally with some muffling of heart sounds and the radiological appearance is that of any free fluid in the pleural cavity (see 'Exudative pleurisy', below), though there may be other evidence of trauma, for example fractured ribs or intrapulmonary haemorrhage. The diagnosis is confirmed by the finding of non-clotting blood on thoracentesis. Other causes of haemothorax include bleeding tumours or disorders of haemostasis.

Treatment is largely supportive and consists of fluid therapy and warmth. The free blood in the pleura is resorbed over a few days, though rapid or continuous haemorrhage may necessitate exploratory thoracotomy.

Anterior mediastinal (thymic) lymphosarcoma

Anterior mediastinal, or thymic, lymphosarcoma is a manifestation of feline leukaemia virus (FeLV) infection and is typically seen in young cats between 8 months and 3 years, particularly of the oriental breeds (Gruffydd-Jones *et al.*, 1979) (see Chapter 15). Dyspnoea and regurgitation of food are the most common clinical signs, caused by the formation of pleural fluid and by the compression of the trachea and oesophagus by the tumour mass. Anorexia, depression and weight loss may also occur but anaemia, a com-

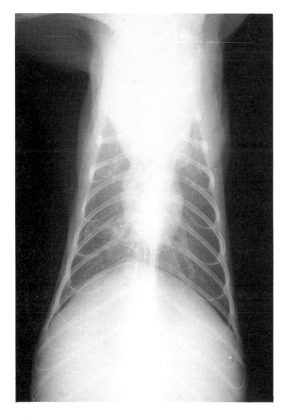

Fig. 6.7 Dorsoventral radiograph of the chest of a cat with anterior mediastinal lymphosarcoma, showing a mass cranial to the heart.

mon feature of other manifestations of FeLV infection, is not usually seen in this form. Evidence of lymphosarcoma elsewhere, for example peripheral lymph nodes, may also be present. On auscultation, the heart sounds are displaced caudally and are frequently muffled; palpation of the cranial part of the chest reveals a marked reduction in the normal compressibility or spring of the rib cage.

Radiographs of the chest are often diagnostic, showing in the dorsoventral (Fig. 6.7) and in the recumbent lateral view the presence of an anterior mediastinal soft tissue mass, and in the latter view elevation and sometimes compression of the trachea, caudal displacement of the heart, as judged by the position of the carina, and occasionally dilation of the cervical oesophagus with air (Fig. 6.8). Some two-thirds of cases show evidence of a variable amount of pleural fluid and in a smaller number evidence of bronchial or abdominal lymphadenopathy may be seen radiographically. Thoracentesis may be used to confirm the clinical and radiographic impression; the fluid in the majority of cases is a blood-stained modified transudate though it may occasionally be chylous. Cytological examination shows the presence of malignant lymphoblasts.

Treatment of anterior mediastinal lymphosarcoma can be attempted with good short-term

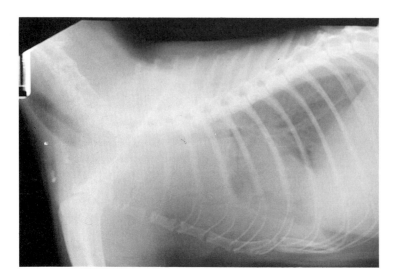

Fig. 6.8 A recumbent lateral radiograph of the chest of a cat with anterior mediastinal lymphosarcoma, showing elevation of the trachea, caudal displacement of the carina, pleural fluid and dilation of the cervical oesophagus with air.

results in some cases (see Chapter 15). The implications of FeLV infection should be considered in a cat from a colony; the great majority of cases of anterior mediastinal lymphosarcoma are positive on virus isolation and may be a source of infection to cats in close contact.

It is important to be aware of the occasional occurrence of thymomas in the anterior mediastinum in older cats; the prognosis for this tumour is fair and hence differentiation from lymphosarcoma is important (see below).

Exudative pleurisy (pyothorax, empyema)

The accumulation of purulent material in the pleural cavity is a well-recognized entity in the cat. The underlying cause is often not clear and while penetrating wounds of the chest, spread of subcutaneous infection, extension of pneumonia and perforating wounds of the oesophagus have all been suggested, such factors are frequently absent in individual cases. The clinical signs are variable; some cats show just tachypnoea or dyspnoea, often of fairly sudden onset despite the apparent chronicity of the condition, while other cases may be markedly depressed with pyrexia and weight loss. Typically fluid is present on both sides of the chest, though unilateral pyothorax occasionally occurs, particularly when the fluid is viscid. Auscultation and percussion reveal thoracic dullness, especially ventrally, with some muffling of heart sounds.

Radiographs are valuable in identifying the presence, the distribution and the amount of pleural fluid. In the recumbent lateral view, this fluid displaces the dorsal borders of the diaphragmatic or caudal lung lobes ventrally from the thoracic vertebrae and leads to a loss of contrast within the ventral portion of the chest. A dorsoventral view shows loss of radiolucency laterally due to fluid density, and interlobular fissures may be seen (Fig. 6.9). In some cases where the fluid is fibrinous the visceral pleura may become thickened and restrictive, causing rounding of lung margins, a finding which bodes ill for the successful reinflation of lung fields and control of the pleural infection.

Confirmation of the diagnosis is made by

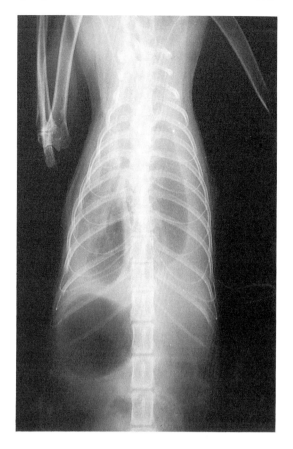

Fig. 6.9 Dorsoventral radiograph of the chest of a cat with exudative pleurisy, showing fluid density lateral to the lung fields.

thoracentesis and the gross appearance, cytology and bacterial culture of the fluid obtained. Such fluids vary in appearance from a reddish-brown, watery exudate to creamy-yellow, inspissated material. Smears of the fluid reveal large numbers of leucocytes, and Gram-stained smears usually show the presence of organisms. However, bacterial culture, which should be carried out aerobically and anaerobically, may fail to identify the organisms. A large number of bacteria have been cultured from pleural exudate, including *Bacteroides* spp., streptococci, staphylococci and *Pasteurella multocida*. Nocardial infection, one of the more common causes of exudative pleurisy in the dog, would seem to be less important in the cat.

Treatment is based on the removal of the underlying cause of the pleural infection, though this may well not be identified; the removal of the pleural fluid; the control of the infection; and the prevention of recurrence of fluid formation. Pleural fluid is initially removed by thoracentesis using a needle, or preferably a catheter. The gauge of needle or catheter and the ease with which the fluid may be withdrawn depends upon the nature and viscosity of the fluid; the decision on which side of the chest to drain should be taken on the radiographic evidence of the distribution of the fluid. Unilateral accumulations of pleural exudate are seen, but in most cases the fluid is bilateral and while the mediastinum is not usually intact in such cases, thoracentesis from both left and right pleural cavities may be necessary to remove all the fluid present. Treatment with systemic antibiotics should be initiated, preferably chosen following culture and sensitivity testing of organisms from the pleural fluid. The use of antibiotics introduced into the pleural cavity has been advocated. A small number of cases will recover following a single removal of fluid, but generally repeated drainage of fluid is necessary. While the prognosis in such cases is often said to be poor, persistence with thoracentesis and appropriate and prolonged antibiotic treatment may well be rewarded, particularly where the condition is recognized early. A more aggressive approach to management involving the use of an indwelling chest drain is indicated in some cases, particularly where the fluid is viscid or initial response to therapy is poor (Sherding, 1979).

A rubber indwelling chest drain or thoracic trocar catheter is introduced under anaesthesia through the chest wall in the seventh or eighth intercostal space. A small skin incision is made about 1 cm caudal to this point and the drain/catheter tunnelled forwards subcutaneously before penetrating the chest wall. The drain is introduced using curved artery forceps to grip the tip of the tube. The drain or catheter should be stitched to the skin by means of tape, bandaged firmly in place against the body wall and

suitably occluded when not in use. Management of the chest drain requires care; it may be poorly tolerated by some cats and an Elizabethan collar may be needed. Such a drain allows repeated aspiration of pleural fluid and the use of pleural lavage. Lavage may be carried out using sterile isotonic fluids containing soluble antibiotics, about 50–100 ml being introduced at body temperature slowly at one time and aspirated about 1 hour later.

Lavage is carried out twice daily and continued until only small quantities of fluid are being produced, largely due to the presence of the tube itself. The tube is usually in place for some 4–7 days. Antibiotic therapy is continued for a further period of time.

Occasionally a constricting pyogenic membrane may form on the visceral pleura: while surgical removal has been described, this is rarely attempted and the prognosis for these cases is poor.

A specific form of exudative pleurisy is associated with feline infectious peritonitis (FIP) (see Chapter 17). While the majority of cases of typical or wet FIP show ascites, about 20% also have pleural fluid and in a small number of cases it may predominate and be of clinical significance. The clinical signs are referable to the presence of pleural fluid, with weight loss, inappetence and anaemia also frequently seen. Thoracentesis reveals a characteristic straw-coloured, tenacious fluid which clots on standing and is high in protein. While temporary improvement may follow removal of the fluid, no effective treatment is currently available and the prognosis is hopeless.

Chylothorax

The accumulation of chyle or chylous effusions in the pleural cavity of the cat is uncommon. Chyle may leak from the thoracic duct following trauma or surgery, or following infection or neoplastic disease involving the duct, and causes progressive tachypnoea. Radiographs of the chest will provide information on the distribution of the fluid and on the presence of other pleural disease, for example anterior mediastinal lymphosarcoma. The fluid is milky with a high proportion of small lymphocytes

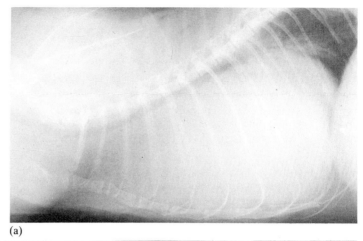

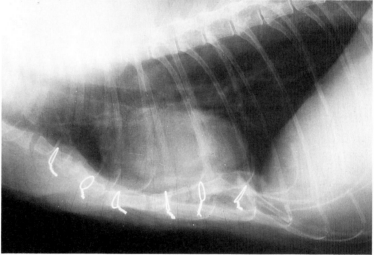

Fig. 6.10 Thymoma: lateral radiographs of a 9-year-old DSH cat. (a) Showing a large anterior mediastinal mass. (b) A postoperative radiograph following surgical resection of a thymoma through a sternal approach.

(a)

(b)

on cytological examination; the milky appearance, due to the presence of chylomicrons, will clear with ether and on a smear the fat droplets will stain with Sudan orange.

Initial management is conservative. Fat-restricted diets and repeated drainage of the chyle by thoracentesis, often necessary over many weeks, may lead to resolution, presumably due to natural repair of the duct. Surgical ligation or repair of the duct has been described but is difficult to achieve. Palliative pleurodesis using tetracycline may be attempted if other methods fail to achieve resolution. A detailed review of the literature and relevant anatomy has been given by Lindsay (1974).

Cardiomyopathy
The congestive heart failure associated with cardiomyopathy in cats is characterized by pleural fluid and pulmonary oedema, and the resulting tachypnoea and dyspnoea may be confused with that caused by other pleural diseases. The specific diagnosis and treatment of cardiomyopathy is discussed in Chapter 11.

Neoplasia

Neoplasia of the pleural cavity, apart from anterior mediastinal lymphosarcoma, is rare in the cat. Pulmonary carcinoma is seen occasionally in older cats and may cause tachypnoea and dyspnoea due to the accumulation of pleural fluid. Radiographs will demonstrate this fluid and the presence of multiple and mottled radiodensities in the lung fields (Fig. 6.5). Thoracentesis reveals a modified transudate, the cytology of which is unhelpful. Diuresis may provide temporary relief, but the prognosis is hopeless. Thymomas are occasionally seen in cats; these tumours typically occur in older animals and are benign and slow growing. They may be associated with pleural fluid and present with dyspnoea or regurgitation due to pressure on the oesophagus. An association with myasthenia gravis has been made in other species. Surgical resection may be curative or at least palliative (Fig. 6.10) and hence differentiation from anterior mediastinal lymphosarcoma is important. Mesotheliomas appear to be rare in cats.

REFERENCES
AND FURTHER READING

Anderson G.I. (1987) The treatment of chronic sinusitis in six cats by ethmoid conchal curettage and autogenous fat graft sinus ablation. *Vet. Surg.* **16**, 131–4.

Beaumont P.R. (1982) Intratracheal neoplasia in two cats. *J. Small Anim. Pract.* **23**, 29–35.

Bedford P.G.C., Carlson A., Sharp N.J.H. & Longstaffe J.A. (1981) Nasopharyngeal polyps in the cat. *Vet. Rec.* **109**, 551–3.

Bradley R.L., Noone K.E., Saunders G.K. & Patnaik A. (1985) Nasopharyngeal and middle ear polypoid masses in 5 cats. *Vet. Surg.* **14**, 141.

Carpenter J.L., Andrews L.K. & Holzworth J. (1987) Tumors and tumor-like lesions. In Holzworth J. (ed) *Diseases of the Cat; Medicine and Surgery.* W.B. Saunders, Philadelphia, p. 468.

Coulson A. (1988) Radiography as an aid to diagnosis of nasal disorders in the cat. *Vet. Ann.* **28**, 150–8.

Garson H.L., Dodman N.H. & Barker G.J. (1980) Diaphragmatic hernia: analysis of fifty-six cases in dogs and cats. *J. Small Anim. Pract.* **21**, 469–81.

Gruffydd-Jones T.J. & Flecknell P.A. (1978) The prognosis and treatment related to the gross appearance and laboratory characteristics of pathological thoracic fluids in the cat. *J. Small Anim. Pract.* **19**, 315–28.

Gruffydd-Jones T.J., Gaskell C.J. & Gibbs C. (1979) Clinical and radiological features of anterior mediastinal lymphosarcoma in the cat: a review of 30 cases. *Vet. Rec.* **104**, 304–7.

Hardie E.M., Kolata R.J., Stone E.A. & Steiss J.E. (1981) Laryngeal paralysis in three cats. *J. Am. Vet. Med. Assoc.* **19**, 879.

Knowlen G.G. (1991) The coughing cat. In August J.R. (ed) *Consultations in Feline Medicine.* W.B. Saunders, Philadelphia, p. 171.

Lane J.G. (1982) *ENT and Oral Surgery of the Dog and Cat.* J. Wright, Bristol.

Lane J.G., Orr C.M., Lucke V.M. & Gruffydd-Jones T.J. (1981) Nasopharyngeal polyps arising from the middle ear of the cat. *J. Small Anim. Pract.* **22**, 511–22.

Legrende A.M., Gomph R. & Bone D. (1982) Treatment of feline cryptococcosis with ketoconazole. *J. Am. Vet. Med. Ass.* **181**, 1541–2.

Lindsay F.E.F. (1974) Chylothorax in the domestic cat – a review. *J. Small Anim. Pract.* **15**, 241–58.

May C. & Newsholme S.J. (1989) Metastasis of feline pulmonary carcinoma presenting as multiple digital swelling. *J. Small Anim. Pract.* **30**, 302–10.

Mitten R.W. (1988) Nasopharyngeal stenosis in four cats. *J. Small Anim. Pract.* **29**, 341–5.

Moore A.S. & Middleton D.J. (1982) Pulmonary carcinoma in three cats with non-pulmonary signs only. *J. Small Anim. Pract.* **23**, 501–9.

Moulton J.E., Tscharner C. & Schneider R. (1981) Classification of lung carcinomas in the dog and cat. *Vet. Pathol.* **18**, 513–28.

Orr C.M., Kelly D.F. & Lucke V.M. (1980) Tuberculosis in cats; a report of four cases. *J. Small Anim. Pract.* **21**, 247–53.

Pechman R.D. (1976) The radiographic features of pulmonary paragonimiasis in the dog and cat. *J. Am. Vet. Radiol. Soc.* **17**, 182.

Rawlings C.A. (1986) Heartworm disease in cats. In *Heartworm Disease in Dogs and Cats.* W.B. Saunders, Philadelphia, pp. 295–310.

Sherding R.G. (1979) Pyothorax in the cat. *Compend. Contin. Educ. Practicing Veterinarian* **1**, 247.

Wilkinson G.T. (1979) Feline cryptococcosis; a review and seven case reports. *J. Small Anim. Pract.* **20**, 749–68.

Wilkinson G.T., Bate M.J., Robins G.M. & Croker A. (1983) Successful treatment of four cases of feline cryptococcosis. *J. Small Anim. Pract.* **24**, 507–14.

Willoughby K., Dawson S., Jones R.C., Symons M., Daykin J., Payne-Johnson C., Gaskell R.M., Bennett M. & Gaskell C.J. (1991) Pneumonia in kitten caused by *Bordetella bronchiseptica. Vet. Rec.* **129**, 407–8.

Chapter 7 / The Genital System
and Paediatrics

T. J. GRUFFYDD-JONES

THE GENITAL SYSTEM

Introduction

The tremendous increase in the number of cats kept as pets in the UK has been accompanied by an increased interest in pedigree cats and their breeding. This has led to greater demands on the veterinary surgeon to advise on breeding management and to investigate reproductive failure. Requests of this type are now commonplace but there is relatively little information on reproduction in cats, particularly with respect to infertility, on which to base such advice.

Normal reproduction

Cats living under natural conditions are seasonally polyoestrous. However, provision of artificial lighting will abolish the anoestrous period, which normally occurs from September to December, and most cats confined indoors will display sexual activity throughout the year. There is considerable variation in the age of puberty and oestrous cycle patterns within breeds of cats, but particularly between breeds (Jemmett & Evans, 1977; Povey, 1978). In general, the Oriental cats (Siamese, Burmese and foreign short-haired cats) tend to mature much earlier than other breeds. They may first display oestrus well before 6 months of age, whilst long-haired and British short-haired cats may not mature until over 1 year of age. Long-haired cats may cycle only once or twice a year and the period of oestrus may last only a few days. In contrast, oestrus in Oriental cats may last 10 days or more and

the inter-oestrus interval may be as short as 1 week. Oriental queens may sometimes develop a permanent display of oestrous behaviour if not mated. Oestrus is termed 'calling' by cat breeders. It is characterized by restlessness, continual squirming and rubbing, increased sociability, vocalization and adoption of the oestrous posture. In adopting the true oestrous posture, the queen crouches on her front legs, and extends and paddles with her hindlegs causing spinal lordosis, whilst deflecting her tail to one side. She presents herself in this way to other cats or humans. There is considerable individual variation in the extent of the oestrous display in individual cats, but it is generally more marked in Oriental queens. This behaviour is often mistaken as an indication of back pain by owners unfamiliar with the normal oestrous posture. Changes in the external genitalia are unusual during oestrus although occasionally a scant mucoid discharge may be observed. In most cats no distinctive period of pro-oestrus can be recognized and oestrus is characterized by a sudden adoption of oestrous behaviour, followed by an equally abrupt cessation. Queens will continue to display oestrus and accept mating after ovulation has occurred and the corpora lutea have begun to secrete significant amounts of progesterone.

One of the unusual features of reproduction in cats is the phenomenon of induced ovulation. Mating is generally required for successful ovulation. In unmated cycles the follicles fail to ovulate and form corpora lutea but simply undergo atresia. The mechanism of induced ovulation depends on vaginal receptors that are stimulated by the male(tom)cats' penis during coitus. These cause the hypothalamus to release gonadotrophin-releasing factor, which in turn causes the pituitary gland to release luteinizing hormone (LH). The mechanism of LH release in cats has been a subject of considerable interest in recent years and there is now a good understanding of the factors which influence this process (Gruffydd-Jones, 1989).

1 Number of matings – a single mating may not be adequate to induce ovulation and the critical factor appears to be overcoming a threshold for stimulation of the pituitary gland to release LH. In queens that fail to ovulate a barely detectable increase in LH occurs after mating, but if any marked increase has been achieved ovulation will be triggered. Ovulation is generally an 'all or nothing' phenomenon with all ripe follicles ovulating together. The time course for LH release is quite short with peak concentrations being achieved within 90 minutes after mating and therefore it is important that the multiple matings take place in quick succession. If cats are allowed to mate at will this will invariably occur, several matings following the first mating within 30 minutes or so.

2 Day of oestrus – oestrogens are thought to be important in priming the release of LH and queens may not be fully 'primed' early in oestrus. The optimum day for mating is probably around days 2 to 4 of oestrus.

3 Individual variability – the receptivity of queens to mating-induced ovulation may show some individual variability. There are many instances in which ovulation has been demonstrated in queens that have had no opportunity to mate. Receptors similar to those found in the vagina are also found in the lumbar area; in particularly receptive queens it is possible that stroking over this area or mounting by another queen (which is not unusual behaviour in groups of breeding queens) may provide sufficient stimulation to induce LH release.

These factors clearly have practical implications in the management of cats at mating to optimize the chances of ovulation occurring at the appropriate time.

During mating the tom mounts the queen and grabs the scruff of her neck with his teeth. The actual period of coitus lasts only a few seconds and as the tom's penis enters her vagina, the queen will cry out. Immediately after coitus the tom dismounts and retires a short distance while the queen displays her post-coital 'rage-reaction'. This frequently involves lashing out at the tom followed by frantic rolling and licking at the vulva. The absence of this typical post-coital reaction suggests that coitus has not occurred.

Ovulation occurs 24–36 hours after mating and the eggs spend a further 4 days travelling down the oviduct. Implantation begins approximately 2 weeks after mating. The corpora lutea are not essential for the maintenance of pregnancy during its latter stages and ovariectomy after 50 days will not cause abortion. The factors involved in controlling luteal lifespan are not fully understood. The role of prostaglandins is uncertain, but they do not appear to have a straightforward luteolytic action in cats. The duration of gestation is very variable. Most pregnancies last 63–65 days, but parturition before 60 days or after 70 days is not considered abnormal. It is also not uncommon to encounter split births, with some kittens being born on one day and the remainder being born 24–48 hours later.

There is also considerable variation in litter size. Oriental queens tend to have large litters, occasionally in excess of ten, while long-haired cats may average only two or three kittens in each litter. A small proportion of queens will display oestrous behaviour during pregnancy. Some of these will mate and ovulate successfully giving rise to the phenomenon of superfetation – the simultaneous development of two sets of fetuses of differing ages within the same uterus.

Some queens will display a post-partum oestrus within a fortnight of parturition. However, this will usually only occur if the litter is removed at birth and the queen is not allowed to feed her kittens.

Passage of 'liver-like' pieces of tissue at parturition along with normal litters is common and these represent partially resorbed or mummified fetuses that have died *in utero*. They are particularly common in large litters and probably result from overcrowding in the uterus.

Unsuccessful, sterile matings will lead to formation of corpora lutea and pseudopregnancy. This does not usually entail lactation and nesting behaviour, as in the bitch, but more subtle changes in behaviour suggestive of pregnancy and weight gain may be noted. The duration of pseudopregnancy is variable but usually lasts approximately 6 weeks, which leads to an extended inter-oestrus interval.

Pregnancy diagnosis
Pregnancy diagnosis is vital in the assessment of reproductive failure. It is most successfully performed by abdominal palpation from 3 to 4 weeks after mating when each conceptus is palpable as a tense, spherical swelling. Care must be taken not to confuse faecal boluses or kidneys with the conceptuses, particularly in the event of a small litter. Repeated abdominal palpation on successive days is valuable in doubtful cases. The conceptual swellings become softer, elongate and merge from 5 weeks onwards. They are then difficult to palpate until the last week or so of pregnancy, when fetal heads can be identified. Abdominal distension usually becomes prominent from about 5 weeks onwards.

Cat breeders use the phenomenon of 'pinking up' as an indication of pregnancies. This refers to a hyperaemia of the teats, which occurs 3–4 weeks after mating. It is a progesterone-dependent change and also occurs in pseudopregnancy.

Radiography and ultrasound may also be used for pregnancy diagnosis. Ultrasonography is now more widely available in practice and has the advantage over manual palpation of indicating fetal viability, which may be of particular value in assessing queens with a history of gestational failure. Fetal skeletal calcification does not become readily recognizable on radiography until the last fortnight of pregnancy by which time the presence of fetuses can generally be detected readily by other means. It may be of value after parturition to check for retained fetuses if fetal maceration is suspected. Pregnancy diagnosis can be performed by radiography early in pregnancy by identifying the presence of uterine swellings but radiographic exposure is probably best avoided at this stage.

Mismating
Oestrogens given shortly after mating will block oviductal transport and oestradiol administered at a dosage of 0.25 mg 40 hours after mating has been used for mismating (Herron & Sis, 1974). However, such high dosage with oestrogens may lead to subsequent reproductive complications. Cats are also very sensitive to toxic effects of marrow suppression and hepatotoxicity with oestrogens. Their use is therefore questionable.

As mentioned above, prostaglandins do not have a clear-cut luteolytic action and are therefore unsuitable as abortifacients during the early stages of pregnancy.

The best policy following mismating is either to spay the cat 2–3 weeks later if the queen is not required for future breeding or to allow her to carry the litter to term.

Oestrus suppression
A number of progestational agents are available for the control of oestrus in cats. The most widely used drug is megestrol acetate. This may be used to prevent a single oestrous period by administration of 5 mg for three consecutive days on the first day that oestrous behaviour is observed. However, it is more frequently used at a dosage of 1.25 mg twice weekly to indefinitely postpone oestrus. There is considerable individual variation in response to this drug and it is advisable to determine the minimum effective dosage for each queen.

The two other progestagens most commonly used for oestrus control in cats are medroxyprogesterone acetate and proligesterone. They are usually used in injectable form for more prolonged suppression of oestrous. Their major disadvantage is their lack of flexibility compared to oral preparations.

Certain side-effects may arise with the use of

these drugs through their inherent progestational action. They may modify behaviour and increase appetite, leading to weight gain. More serious side-effects are predisposition to endometritis, adrenal suppression and development of diabetes mellitus (see Chapter 12). Mammary hyperplasia is an uncommon side-effect (see below). The pathogenesis of endometritis (discussed below) is complex but the key factor is progestational dominance of the uterus. The use of progestagens will therefore increase the risk of endometritis developing in queens with a predisposition to this disorder. The diabetogenic potential of progestagens has only recently been recognized. This may be partly dose related, the risk increasing with prolonged usage. Certain individuals appear to have a predisposition for showing this side-effect and overt diabetes mellitus may develop after only a relatively short period of treatment. The underlying mechanism by which the progestagens induce diabetes mellitus is complex and it has been suggested that the different progestagens vary in their diabetogenic potential. In some cases the diabetes mellitus will resolve if progestagen therapy is withdrawn (which creates a significant disadvantage in the use of depot preparations) but in others the condition persists despite withdrawal of the drug.

Nevertheless, oestrous suppression is desirable in certain circumstances:

1 In queens that have reached puberty at a very early age and are not considered sufficiently mature to breed.

2 For planning and spacing of litters throughout the year.

3 To enable queens to regain condition after their litters have been weaned.

The appetite is often reduced during oestrus and if the queen is allowed to call incessantly, she may lose condition. In addition, some breeders claim that they have difficulty in breeding from queens allowed to call repeatedly without mating.

Alternative methods are available to pharmacological suppression of oestrus. Vaginal swabbing or mating with a vasectomized tom will induce pseudopregnancy, although care must be taken to prevent a fertile mating during the same oestrous period. This will extend the inter-oestrus interval to around 5–9 weeks.

Reproductive failure

Queens

Reproductive failure in queens can be divided into several types, according to the stage at which the problem arises and following a practical approach to their differentiation and diagnosis.

FAILURE TO CALL

Sufficient time should be allowed for a young queen to mature, bearing in mind her breed, before considering a failure of puberty. Weight is an important determinant of puberty and small queens may mature relatively later. In addition, the season at the time of birth influences puberty. Queens born in the autumn will usually mature the following spring, but kittens born in the spring may not call until the following year.

Social contacts with other cats have an important effect on oestrous behaviour in queens. Failure of puberty frequently occurs in a single pet queen denied contact with other cats. Such queens may display oestrus if housed either with other breeding queens or in close proximity to a stud tom. In contrast, oestrus may occasionally be suppressed in timid queens maintained in a group. Determination of serum oestradiol concentrations generally show that normal follicular activity is taking place but that oestrous behaviour is inhibited (Shille *et al.*, 1979). These individuals will generally call if housed alone.

If failure of oestrus develops in previously proven queens the possibility of pseudopregnancy should be investigated. This is a common occurrence if neutered toms are housed with the breeding queens. Neutered toms, even if castrated prepubertally, will frequently mount and mate breeding queens. They do not have penile spines, which develop as a testosterone-dependent secondary male characteristic, but these are not essential to stimulate the vagina adequately to induce ovulation. If queens are introduced to the tom (or neutered toms) during the inter-oestrus period, oestrous behaviour is often not observed

Table 7.1 Treatment regimes for inducing oestrus in cats.

Equine chorionic gonadotrophin (eCG)
  Days 1 & 2   100 IU
  Days 3, 4 & 5   50 IU

Follicle stimulating hormone (FSH)
  2 mg daily for up to 5 days or until signs of oestrus
  develop

---

although a subsequent pregnancy confirms that oestrus has taken place. It is possible that mating early in oestrus and the opportunity to mate at will, may inhibit development of the oestrous display. A similar situation may arise if neutered toms are housed with the queens. Serum progesterone estimations will readily identify if pseudopregnancy is occurring and the problem is easily rectified by separating breeding queens and neutered toms.

Hormonal induction of oestrus is possible and regimes using either equine chorionic gonadotrophin (eCG) or follicle stimulating hormone (FSH) have been described as outlined in Table 7.1 (Gruffydd-Jones, 1990).

The response to treatment is very variable, particularly in pedigree queens, and there is a danger of under- or overdosing. Underdosing will be ineffectual and overdosing may cause superovulation or development of ovarian cysts. This approach to failure of oestrus should therefore be kept as a final resort.

FAILURE TO MATE

This is not a common problem in cats. Occasionally oestrus is inhibited in nervous queens that travel to the stud tom for mating. These queens may mate successfully if they are moved some time before oestrus in order to allow them to become familiar with their new surroundings.

Characteristic changes occur in the cellular appearance of vaginal smears throughout the reproductive cycle. However, vaginal cytology is not a very suitable technique for identifying oestrus and pinpointing the optimum time for mating, since the vaginal stimulation that occurs

during the collection of the vaginal smear may prematurely induce ovulation.

FAILURE TO PRODUCE LIVE KITTENS AFTER MATING

Ovulation failure
Pregnancy failure is the most likely explanation of failure to produce kittens after mating; however, ovulation failure is occasionally encountered. The latter can be identified by the collection of a blood sample within 3–10 days of mating for progesterone assay. Progesterone concentrations will not rise above the baseline level of 3–4 nmol/l in queens failing to ovulate, but will be considerably higher than this following successful ovulation.

In cases of apparent ovulation failure the first step should be to investigate the mating management. It is important to establish that coitus is occurring and that the tom is not simply mounting the queen. Failure of the queen to display the typical post-coital behaviour should be considered an indication that coitus is not taking place. It is also important to ensure that the mating management is arranged to optimize the chances of mating-induced ovulation, i.e. multiple matings are taking place in quick succession on each day of oestrus.

Hormonal induction of ovulation can be achieved using human chorionic gonadotrophin (hCG). This should be given at a dosage of 200 IU intravenously or subcutaneously as close to mating as possible. Although this treatment may be successful the advisability of using in a breeding programme a queen which can ovulate successfully only after exogenous hormonal manipulation should be considered carefully.

Fertilization failure and pre-implantation loss
Fertilization is very efficient in cats and this largely reflects the phenomenon of induced ovulation, which ensures that fresh sperm will be awaiting the ova following ovulation. Pre-implantation losses are also generally minimal in cats. Fertilization failure and pre-implantation loss are therefore relatively unimportant causes of repro-

ductive failure in cats. Their investigation is complex and generally necessitates attempted recovery of the eggs at laparotomy within the first 6 days of mating. The procedure for egg collection requires specialized techniques and is not usually feasible in practice.

Pregnancy failure
Abortion and particularly resorption are the most important forms of pregnancy failure in cats. These occur after implantation and can therefore be differentiated from earlier problems of fertilization failure and pre-implantation loss by positive pregnancy diagnosis. Resorption is often accompanied by a sudden reduction in abdominal size with a bloody vaginal discharge and may be mistaken for abortion.

NUTRITIONAL DEFICIENCIES
Although various extreme nutritional deficiencies can give rise to reproductive failure these are rare in practice with the possible exception of taurine deficiency. The importance of taurine as an essential component of the diet of cats has been recognized only relatively recently and previous minimum requirements for taurine are now considered to have been too low. The association of taurine deficiency with retinal disease and dilated cardiomyopathy is well established. However, in experimentally induced studies of taurine deficiency, various reproductive problems have been encountered including the birth of stillborn kittens and reductions in litter size (Sturman *et al.*, 1986). The importance of taurine deficiency as a cause of naturally occurring resorptions is not known. Reputable pet food manufacturers now ensure that the taurine content of their feline diets allows a considerable margin of safety and deficiency is unlikely to occur if such foods constitute a major part of the diet. However, a deficiency is possible if breeders compile their own diets and the dietary management should be investigated in all cases of reproductive failure.

HORMONAL FACTORS
No convincing evidence exists that hormonal imbalances are a significant cause of reproductive failure in cats. There are anecdotal reports of progesterone deficiency causing habitual resorption or abortion, which can be rectified by progesterone supplementation. The postulated mechanism in this disorder is premature regression of the corpora lutea leading to a critical drop in progesterone levels. This would therefore be expected to occur before around day 40–45 of pregnancy, after which pregnancy can be maintained by fetoplacental production of progesterone. Serial estimations of serum progesterone concentrations to demonstrate abnormally low levels in the first two-thirds of pregnancy would be the only reliable method of diagnosing this problem. Abnormally low concentrations of progesterone have rarely been demonstrated in queens at our clinic. In one queen progesterone supplementation with a progesterone implant resulted in a successful pregnancy despite a history of habitual resorptions, although the progesterone deficiency occurred late in pregnancy and probably resulted from inadequate fetoplacental production of progesterone, since only one or two kittens were subsequently produced.

Ovarian cysts are common in cats but these are of a simple histological appearance and there is no evidence that they are endocrinologically active or cause reproductive failure. Most of them probably represent developmental abnormalities.

INFECTIOUS DISEASES

Feline leukaemia virus (FeLV)
FeLV has been considered an important cause of pregnancy failure in the past. However, the prevalence of this virus in pedigree cats has been dramatically reduced by breeders using the test and removal system, and FeLV infection is now relatively uncommon in pedigree breeding catteries.

FeLV-related reproductive failure most often appears as resorption at around 5–7 weeks of pregnancy with passage of a pink vaginal discharge. Abortion is seen less frequently and if infected cats are rebred, reproductive failure may occur progressively earlier with each subsequent pregnancy. The underlying mechanism of the reproductive failure is not known. Although most

FeLV-infected queens are likely to be infertile, if they do breed successfully, congenital infection of the kittens occurs. However, genetic transfer of FeLV does not appear to occur and this implies that there is transplacental infection of the fetuses. This has led in turn to the suggestion that resorption results from fetal death induced by the virus. However, chronic endometritis is common in FeLV-infected infertile queens and this, which may be predisposed by FeLV-related immunosuppression, may account for the reproductive failure.

Chlamydia psittaci

Chlamydia spp. cause infertility in other species and there is strong circumstantial evidence to incriminate *Chlamydia psittaci* in reproductive failure in cats. Chlamydias are frequently isolated from infertile cats, or high antibody titres are found indicating recent or active infection. There may also be a history of conjunctivitis suggestive of chlamydial infection in catteries with infertility problems. In addition, the organism can be readily isolated from the vagina of infected queens and occasionally from aborted fetuses. Despite this strong circumstantial evidence, no direct cause and effect has been demonstrated.

The reproductive failure appears as abortion around the 5th to 7th week of pregnancy. If chlamydial infection is suspected to be responsible for the infertility, a prolonged course of oxytetracycline is indicated. This may lead to a successful return to breeding.

Feline panleucopenia virus

Feline panleucopenia virus (feline infectious enteritis virus) has a trophism for rapidly developing cells and if a pregnant queen is infected, transplacental spread of the virus occurs leading to fetal infection and death. However, most breeding cats are regularly vaccinated and in practise this is a rare cause of infertility.

Other infectious agents

The role of other infectious agents in infertility is unclear. Any infection which causes significant illness, particularly if associated with pyrexia,

may lead to abortion as a non-specific result. The respiratory viruses may therefore be associated with abortion in the acute stage of infection but there is no evidence that carrier status is associated with any reproductive problems. Feline immunodeficiency virus (FIV) infection has been demonstrated in some cats with a history of recent abortion, but since the virus is so prevalent, this may be a coincidental finding. Abortion has been observed in some experimentally infected cats in the primary phase of FIV infection.

Reproductive failure has been linked with feline infectious peritonitis (FIP). This is difficult to substantiate in view of the problems in diagnosing FIP virus infection and the uncertainty in identifying carrier status. It is possible that concurrent infection with FeLV may be the explanation for infertility in some catteries with endemic FIP.

Toxoplasmosis causes abortion in some species. However, there is little evidence to incriminate this as a cause of infertility in cats and attempts to induce reproductive failure by challenge of pregnant queens have been unsuccessful (Dubey & Hoover, 1977).

Mycoplasma species have been reported as a relatively common isolate from vaginal swabs but are generally not considered to be significant pathogens in cats.

CHRONIC ENDOMETRITIS

Chronic endometritis is one of the most common causes of reproductive failure in cats and can occur in a variety of different forms. In mild cases the problem may be manifested as the birth of stillborn kittens but as the severity increases it progresses to resorption and eventually early embryonic death.

The cause of chronic endometritis is complex and multifactorial, although the primary factor is the hormonal milieu which leads to endometrial changes of cystic hyperplasia and leaves the uterus vulnerable to secondary infection. Repeated and prolonged progesterone dominance is the key factor and this may arise through successive luteal phases in the absence of pregnancy (i.e. pseudopregnancy, which may be influenced by management factors – see 'Failure of oestrus') or the use of progestagens. A variety of opportunist bacteria may cause secondary infection, including *E. coli*, β-haemolytic streptococci, *Staphylococcus aureus*, *Proteus* spp. and occasionally anaerobes. These bacteria are part of the normal vaginal flora in cats and therefore the significance of their isolation from vaginal swabs collected from queens with suspected endometritis is difficult to assess.

Endometritis should be suspected in any queen with a history of a vaginal discharge unrelated to parturition or abortion. However, by no means every queen with endometritis will have shown a vaginal discharge and diagnosis in these cases is difficult, depending on histological examination of uterine biopsies. Full-thickness wedge biopsies are obtained at laparotomy and this also provides the opportunity to examine the uterus grossly. If the uterus is severely thickened the prospects for future breeding are poor and spaying should be considered.

Histological examination allows assessment of the severity of endometrial changes and is important in prognosis. Severe changes are likely to be irreversible but mild cases may respond to treatment. Subsequent management is probably the most important factor in achieving resolution and successful breeding. In the first instance the queen should be allowed one or two calls unmated in the hope that the uterine infection will resolve under oestrogen dominance. Subsequently progestational dominance, unless during pregnancy, should be avoided. No progestagens should be used and the breeding management should be arranged to avoid both prolonged periods of calling without breeding and possible factors which may induce pseudopregnancy, such as mating or mounting by neutered toms. Prostaglandins are not significantly luteolytic in cats but their ecbolic effect may be beneficial in the acute phase (Arnberg & Flagstad, 1985). Antibiotics are frequently given but their value is questionable.

Some cases may progress to pyometra with a continual heavy purulent vaginal discharge. The accumulation of uterine exudates can be very extensive leading to gross abdominal distension.

'Closed' pyometras are relatively common in cats. Affected individuals are often surprisingly well and do not show the secondary toxaemic changes seen in bitches with pyometra, but uterine enlargement, readily detectable on abdominal palpation, will point to the diagnosis.

FAILURE OF PARTURITION
This is not a common problem in queens and in most cases results from uterine inertia. Oxytocin may be administered if the cervix is open and there is no obstruction to the passage of the kittens. However, if this is unsuccessful, Caesarean section will be necessary. Queens that have undergone Caesarean section may not nurse their litters satisfactorily and there may be a failure of milk let-down.

Toms
Requests to investigate reproductive failure in toms are seldom encountered. In most cases requests are to investigate lack of libido or failure to produce kittens in a previously proven tom.

LACK OF LIBIDO
The most important factors in causing an otherwise healthy young entire male to show lack of libido are psychological. This most often occurs in toms that have been first used at a very young age. Such animals may initially appear keen to mate but withdraw from the queen at the last moment. It may be possible to trace the problem to a mating with an uncooperative queen who has displayed a particularly marked post-coital 'rage reaction' or some other stress. Attempts to improve the tom's confidence by selecting tractable queens may prove successful. A recent illness may also cause a temporary loss of libido.

FAILURE TO PRODUCE KITTENS
It is important to establish that several queens of proven fertility have been successfully mated and that no conceptual swellings have subsequently been identified at pregnancy diagnosis before considering a diagnosis of infertility in a tom.

Semen can be collected from toms by use of an artificial vagina or electro-ejaculation, but this is seldom feasible in practice. A cruder approach to confirming the presence or absence of sperm in the semen is to collect a vaginal smear from an oestrous queen allowed to mate with the tom. Sperm can readily be identified after staining the air-dried smear with Leishman's or methylene blue. An attempt may also be made to determine the morphology of the sperm, although motility and sperm counts cannot be assessed by this method.

No specific treatment is likely to be of value in stimulating spermatogenesis. However, temporary aspermia may follow a recent illness, which may be subclinical, and fertility may be regained after a period of up to several months or more.

There are no specific infections that are recognized as a cause of reproductive failure in toms. Orchitis is sometimes seen as a feature of feline infectious peritonitis, but affected cats invariably die.

Other conditions of the genital tract

Neoplasia
Tumours of the testicles, ovaries and uterus are rare in cats. Occasionally uterine tumours may cause a persistent bloody vaginal discharge.

Uterine prolapse
This is a rare sequel to parturition. It may be possible to reduce the prolapse, but hysterectomy may be required. The prognosis is guarded since affected queens are usually in severe shock.

Uterine torsion
This condition is also rare in cats. It is notable for two reasons. First, it is one of the few causes of genuinely sudden death in previously healthy adult cats. Second, it may lead to uterine rupture and a possible explanation for some of the occasional bizarre cases of extrauterine fetuses.

Conditions of the mammary glands

Neoplasia
Tumours of the mammary glands are quite common in old cats and a large proportion of these are malignant. Mammary tumours tend to metastasize, particularly to the lungs. Surgical excision should therefore not be undertaken unless chest radiographs are clear.

Mammary hypertrophy
This condition is seen either as an uncommon complication following the use of progestagens in cats of both sexes, whether entire or neutered, or occasionally in pregnant queens (Hinton & Gaskell, 1977). It is characterized by massive hypertrophy of the mammary glands. All the mammae are usually involved and there may be considerable oedema of the overlying skin. Ulceration may occur in time. In cats receiving progestagens, the condition resolves following withdrawal of the drug. It may necessitate ovariohysterectomy in pregnant cats. The main importance of this condition is in its similarity of appearance to neoplasia. However, it can be readily differentiated on histological examination of a biopsy.

Mastitis
Mastitis occasionally occurs during lactation. In acute cases the queen will be severely depressed, inappetent, dehydrated and pyrexic. One or more mammary glands are swollen, hot and painful. Occasionally they may abscessate. There is a good response to antibiotics and poulticing of the affected glands. It is vital to remove the litter, both to prevent further spread of infection and trauma of the mammary glands and to prevent the kittens from ingesting the infected milk.

In cases of chronic or mild mastitis, the queen may show no clinical signs, with the condition manifesting itself as gastrointestinal disturbances and death in the kittens.

Other conditions

LACTATIONAL TETANY (ECLAMPSIA)
Lactational tetany is an uncommon complication following parturition in cats. Despite its name, it may occasionally occur during pregnancy. It is characterized by ataxia, tremors and twitching of the muscles. This will progress to fits if untreated.

The condition responds rapidly to slow intra-venous injection of 5–10 ml of 20% calcium borogluconate. Five percent solution may be administered subcutaneously and the diet should be supplemented with a suitable source of calcium. Collocal D* or bone flour are suitable for this purpose.

PAEDIATRICS

Introduction

Prior to birth, fetal kittens live in an ideal environment directly receiving the major requirements for life from the queen via the placenta. Important physiological adjustments must occur to some of the major body functions, particularly the cardiopulmonary system, around the time of birth to enable the kittens to survive. Kittens are very vulnerable for the first few weeks of life and still depend on their dams for some of the most important requirements for life. This is therefore the period which carries the highest risk of mortality.

Care of breeding queens and young kittens

The most important factor in determining survival in the neonatal period is the adjustment of the cardiopulmonary system and initiation of breathing to ensure that the oxygen supply is maintained to body tissues. This is greatly aided by an uncomplicated parturition and to this end the queen should be established in the kittening quarters some time before parturition is anticipated to ensure that she has adequate time to settle in her new environment. Individual preference of the queen should be accommodated as far as possible. Most queens tend to be secretive about kittening and prefer a quiet environment. Other more highly socialized queens resent being separated at kittening and this provides a conflict with the requirement of isolation to assist in disease prevention for the young litter.

* Collocal D; C Vet Ltd., Bury St. Edmunds, Suffolk.

The queen should be attended throughout parturition particularly if she is an inexperienced maiden queen. If the queen is very secretive and resents interference during this period it is necessary to organize some arrangement to allow her to be observed without causing intrusion. This ensures that any difficulties in parturition are recognized early and rectified with the minimum of delay. It is also then possible to ensure that the kittens are cleaned correctly after birth. Ideally this duty should be left to the queen as her cleaning actions will both aid bonding and stimulate breathing. However, it is vital that obstruction to breathing does not occur and if necessary the amniotic sac and any discharges should be cleaned away.

Neonates are relatively tolerant of hypoxia and, in addition, their haemoglobin type maximizes the efficiency of oxygen transfer. It is therefore worth while persisting for some time in efforts to revive any kittens which appear reluctant to breathe.

Kittens have little thermoregulatory control over the first few weeks of life and depend on the warmth provided by their mother's body and a dry, warm nesting environment. Chilling will soon lead to depression of the suckling reflex with consequent hypoglycaemia and death. Most queens have very strong maternal instincts and make good, attentive mothers. If a cosy nest box is provided the queen's body heat will ensure that the immediate nesting environment temperature is adequate. Again, it is important that the queen is settled in the nest box. If not she may constantly be moving the kittens, which can lead to chilling. Nest boxes should be made of material that can be suitably disinfected or discarded after use.

Regular suckling, particularly immediately after parturition, is vital. Neonates are vulnerable to hypoglycaemia and regular feeding is necessary to ensure this does not occur. Hypoglycaemia leads to suppression of the suckling reflex which accentuates the hypoglycaemia and will rapidly end in death. Suckling in the first few days of life is also important to ensure that good levels of maternally derived immunity (MDI) are achieved. Negligible levels of antibodies are usually obtained by placental transfer prior to parturition and kittens depend on colostrum for MDI (Scott *et al.*, 1970). Although colostral transfer may continue for up to 72 hours, most occurs within the first 24 hours and it is therefore vital that the kittens suckle well during this period. Regular use of vaccine boosters for the queen, preferably just prior to mating, will also assist in ensuring that good levels of MDI are achieved.

Contented kittens spend around 90% of their time sleeping for the first few weeks of life. They are born blind and their eyes begin to open 7–10 days after birth. From around 3 weeks of age they become more adventurous, emerge from the nest box and begin to feed themselves, often sharing some of the queen's solid food before they learn to lap fluids. The kittens are usually weaned at about 6–8 weeks of age, although earlier weaning is possible. The kittens should not be moved from isolation to the main colony until they have been fully vaccinated. This may conflict with advice from behaviourists that it is important that kittens should be socialized as early as possible, but priority should be given to measures which minimize the risk of infectious disease. The author is convinced from personal experience and extensive discussion with cat breeders that such an approach does not have any serious deleterious effect on development of normal behaviour.

Artifical rearing

Occasionally queens fail to rear their litter satisfactorily, particularly after Caesarean section, and it is necessary either to foster or to rear the kittens artifically. It may also be desirable to remove the kittens at birth in certain circumstances – for example if the queen is a respiratory virus carrier or is affected by certain disorders such as mastitis or eclampsia. Fostering should be considered if another queen is available with kittens within one week of the age of those to be fostered. The maternal instincts of queens are so strong that it is unlikely that there will be any problems in the acceptance of new kittens. If no suitable foster queen is available, hand-rearing should be considered. This is extremely time-consuming and should not be attempted without careful thought. Cat's milk is very rich and is much higher in protein and fat than the milk of most other species (Baines, 1981). A milk substitute formulated specifically for cats (such as Cimicat*) should therefore be used. Cow's milk and baby milk substitutes are not satisfactory. For the first few days of life the kittens will require feeds of 1–2 ml every 2–3 hours, but by the second week they will be able to last most of the night without feeding. Specially designed feeding bottles are available (e.g. Catac† feeding bottle), but in an emergency a small syringe can be used. The kittens can also be fed using a fine plastic stomach tube introduced orally or intranasally. The tube should be introduced to a depth corresponding to the distance from the nose to the last rib. The milk should be warmed to 37°C before feeding. By 8 weeks of age the kittens will require four meals a day of up to 12 ml. A cosy nest box should be provided and the ambient temperature must be maintained at about 30°C. After feeding, the anogenital region should be gently massaged to stimulate urination and defecation.

Recognizing problems in young kittens

The critical nature of the neonatal period has been emphasized above, and certain losses are inevitable over this period, even with optimum neonatal management. It is important, therefore, in investigating kitten mortality in a cattery to establish the extent and pattern of losses, and to assess whether these losses are acceptable. Extensive databases on kitten mortality exist for cat colonies, but much less information is available for breeding catteries. An acceptable maximum figure for mortality rates up to weaning is probably around 10%, half of this representing stillbirths. Average birthweights of mixed breed, colony-maintained cats are around 100 g. However, much lower normal birthweights should be

---

* Cimicat; Hoechst Ltd., Walton, Milton Keynes, UK.
† Catac Products, Newnham Street, Bedford, UK.

expected for some pedigree kittens, particularly of the lighter framed Oriental breeds, which tend to have much larger litters.

Regular weighing of the kittens can provide a useful assessment of performance and has the added advantage of accustoming the kittens to handling from a young age. Colony-maintained cross-bred kittens will gain up to 30 g daily, but weight gains may be much more modest for pedigree kittens, particularly for kittens from large litters.

There are limited ways in which young kittens demonstrate distress, irrespective of the underlying cause. They may be much more restless than normal, fail to sleep contentedly for prolonged periods as should normally occur and may cry excessively. They tend to wander aimlessly predisposing themselves to chilling. The queen may appear to neglect sick kittens and they may be found away from the nest box. They cease feeding and the suckling reflex becomes depressed. In view of the limited range of clinical signs sick kittens display, clinical examination is generally unrewarding. In many cases a diagnosis can be made only at post-mortem examination and this will often reveal infections and congenital abnormalities which would otherwise pass unnoticed. This may enable preventative action to protect the remainder of the litter or may provide useful information on which to base future breeding plans.

The major causes of death in young kittens are environmental and managemental factors, maternal factors, infections and congenital conditions.

Environmental and management factors

Post-mortem examination fails to reveal a clear cause of death in a large proportion of kittens which die within the first few days of life. Undoubtedly environmental and management factors, particularly chilling and failure to suckle, considered above, are responsible for many of these. The loss of occasional kittens may simply reflect inattentive queens, but major losses in the first few days of life suggest some basic mismanagement problem. This can be investigated satisfactorily only by visiting the cattery, by detailed study of the normal husbandry measures and by assessment of breeding records.

Maternal factors

Management of the queen is crucial in the general management over the neonatal period and some of the ways in which this can influence chilling, etc. have already been stressed.

A wide range of dietary factors may potentially contribute to neonatal problems, but many of these arise only with gross imbalances unlikely to arise in practice. The most important potential dietary factor is taurine deficiency. Taurine is an essential amino acid for cats and it is clear that earlier recommendations for taurine levels underestimated the requirement, which led to some cases of deficiency. Retinal disease and dilated cardiomyopathy are well recognized as consequences of taurine deficiency, but in experimentally induced deficiencies various breeding problems, including the birth of weakly or stillborn kittens, occur (Sturman *et al.*, 1986). The importance of taurine deficiency in naturally occurring neonatal morbidity is not known but it is likely to be a factor in at least some catteries. Taurine concentrations of reputable brands of cat foods are now maintained at considerably higher levels and deficiency should be considered in catteries in which nutritional needs depend largely on a home-formulated diet.

Maternal factors may also play an important role in infectious problems either through contributing to protection or predisposing to infection. The queen is the major source of early protection against infectious agents in the form of MDI derived from colostrum. However, the queen may also predispose to infectious disease by acting as a source of infection as a consequence of her carrier status or development of mastitis. She may also play a role in umbilical infections (see below).

Bacterial infections

An important route of infection in newborn kittens is the umbilicus. The kitten may be infected by vaginal organisms during birth or by opportunist organisms in the environment after birth.

Infection may track up the umbilical vessels to cause a liver abscess or it may lead to peritonitis. Several kittens in the litter, or frequently the complete litter, may be affected. Close examination of the umbilicus will sometimes reveal slight discoloration or swelling. Antibiotics are indicated for treatment, but the response in established cases is poor.

Another quite common source of infection in pre-weaning kittens is infected milk from mastitis in the queen. In acute mastitis the queen will show clinical signs, but in chronic mastitis the queen may seem well and her mammary glands may appear normal. Mastitis leads to gastroenteritis in the kittens, with diarrhoea and occasionally vomiting. The kittens must be separated from their mother and hand-reared.

Viral and chlamydial infections
Viruses are a major cause of disease in young kittens in breeding catteries. Kittens are most vulnerable between 3 and 10 weeks of age when maternally derived immunity is waning. Panleucopenia, the respiratory viruses and chlamydioses are the most important infections in kittens.

Panleucopenia virus infection is generally successfully prevented in breeding catteries by vaccination. However, the virus is very stable, and if introduced into a cattery can survive in the environment for at least one year. There is therefore a danger of infection in young kittens during the critical period between the waning of maternally derived immunity and vaccination. Infection may cause sudden death in young kittens with no premonitory signs. It may also cause vomiting, diarrhoea, depression, dehydration and intussusception. The problem can be controlled by serially vaccinating kittens from a young age, ensuring that at least one vaccination is received at 12 weeks of age or older (see Chapter 13).

Although the mortality rate in young kittens infected with respiratory viruses is lower than with panleucopenia, the morbidity rate in catteries where the viruses are endemic is high. Long-term sequelae such as chronic ocular problems and chronic rhinitis are also common in recovered individuals. Infection is usually derived from a carrier mother. In the case of feline herpesvirus (FHV) the stress of parturition and lactation may induce excretion in a latent carrier.

Recurrent infection of young litters causing conjunctivitis at around 5–8 weeks-of-age can be a serious problem in catteries with endemic *Chlamydia psittaci* infection. This is distinct from the viscous ocular discharge which sometimes affects kittens during the first week or two of life, around the time that their eyes open, and which is probably of bacterial origin. The clinical signs may be very persistent, lasting for 2 months or more. The epidemiology of *Chlamydia psittaci* is not clear but it appears to follow the same pattern as seen with respiratory viruses in young litters. The organism has little ability to survive in the environment and therefore carriers are likely to be crucial to the spread of infection, although carrier status has not been demonstrated unequivocally. A vaccine is available to protect against chlamydiosis and control depends largely on this and on systemic treatment of the kittens with oxytetracycline, or treatment of all the cats in the cattery prior to breeding in an attempt to eliminate the organism. Side-effects of oxytetracycline treatment, particularly discoloration of the teeth of kittens, must be considered in treating kittens or pregnant queens.

Respiratory virus, *Chlamydia psittaci* infections and their control are discussed fully in Chapters 14 and 21.

Thymic atrophy leading to early death has been reported in young kittens experimentally infected with feline leukaemia virus (FeLV). However, this does not appear to be an important naturally occurring problem and any breeding problems related to FeLV infection are more likely to be manifested as infertility.

Kittens infected with feline infectious peritonitis (FIP) virus may develop FIP-related disease, most often the effusive form, around the time of weaning. Disease in such young kittens raises the possibility of congenital infection although this has not been convincingly demonstrated. Frequently a large proportion or all of the kittens in a litter may develop disease. It is also common for kittens to develop signs of FIP shortly after rehoming and this may be related to stress, which is considered an important trigger factor for the disease. If a litter has shown FIP at an early age, there is a high chance of FIP developing in subsequent litters from the same queen. It is therefore unwise to rebreed from such queens. It has been postulated that FIP may be linked with significant early mortality problems in some catteries in the absence of clinical signs or postmortem findings characteristic of the disease. This is a tenuous link, based merely on evidence that FIP is endemic in some such catteries. Further investigation is hampered by the unavailability of suitable screening tests for diagnosing infection and identifying carriers. Coronavirus serology is of no value in such cases.

It is essential that if viral diseases are to be successfully controlled in a cattery queens should kitten and rear their litters in strict isolation. Communal raising of litters exposes the kittens to any carriers present in the household, but in isolation the mother is the only possible source of infection provided that sensible management is practised. Kittens can then be sold without ever having contact with adult cats in the cattery, or can be vaccinated when old enough and before introduction to the main cattery.

Parasitic infections
Parasitic infections may be particularly severe in young kittens, causing significant clinical disease. Ectoparasite infections, mainly involving fleas, may lead to anaemia and may contribute to the spread of certain other infectious agents.

Prenatal infection does not occur with *Toxocara cati*, the major nematode of cats. However, infection is spread via the milk and kittens should effectively be considered infected from birth. It is therefore important that a regular treatment for nematodes is implemented by breeders for all kittens.

Coccidiosis is uncommon as a cause of disease in adult cats but can become a significant problem in young kittens, particularly if hygiene is poor and concurrent disease problems are present. This leads to weight loss and diarrhoea, sometimes containing blood.

Fungal infections
Ringworm infection can become a major problem in breeding catteries and infection is particularly severe in young kittens. This is considered more fully in Chapter 1.

Miscellaneous disorders
Young kittens are very vulnerable to trauma and this is an important cause of death. External injuries may not be obvious, but recent trauma may become evident on post-mortem examination.

Neonatal isoerythrolysis. This has been reported in several countries including Australia (Hubler *et al.*, 1987). High levels of naturally occurring antibodies against blood group antigens are seen frequently in cats. These may be secreted in the milk of nursing queens and absorbed by neonatal suckling kittens. If there is incompatibility between the blood group of the queen and kittens a haemolytic reaction may result in jaundice, haemoglobinuria and death. This situation may arise if the queen is blood group B, which is often associated with the presence of a potent anti-A haemolysin, and has produced group A kittens when mated to an group A tom. Most case reports have involved Colourpoint or long hair (LH) cats.

Congenital abnormalities
There are many congenital abnormalities of cats which may become apparent during the first few months of life and some of these may cause death of young kittens (Saperstein *et al.*, 1976; Robinson, 1977). Some will be discovered on casual examination of the kittens, but in other cases a post-mortem examination will be required to reveal their presence. Many inborn errors of metabolism are recognized in man and other species, and these can only be diagnosed in life, often requiring sophisticated laboratory investigation. A few such congenital defects of metabolism have been recognized in cats, but they have received little consideration in this species and it is likely that they may account for some of the occasional losses encountered in young kittens.

Once a congenital deformity has been recognized, it is the responsibility of the veterinary surgeon to advise the breeder of the most appropriate course of action. Information about the possible involvement of genetic factors and the mode of inheritance is required for such advice, but unfortunately this is not available for many congenital deformities. In some cases a breed predisposition is recognized, but although suggestive, this in itself is not proof of hereditary transmission. Decisions concerning the most appropriate advice can also be complicated by the possibility of either a hereditary or a non-genetic, developmental basis for the same congenital abnormality. A number of factors may help to differentiate between these two possibilities (Gruffydd-Jones & Evans, 1984).

1 Previous cases of the same abnormality in kittens produced by either of the parents mated to other cats or to each other, or related cats.
2 Evidence of a breed predisposition.
3 The presence of multiple abnormalities in the same kitten or littermates.
4 Exposure to possible teratogens such as infectious agents, drugs, etc.

The first two factors are suggestive of a hereditary problem, the second two of a non-genetic, developmental abnormality.

Infection of fetuses by panleucopenia virus resulting from placental transfer from the dam or infection during the first few days of life can lead to cerebellar damage. This causes ataxia in young kittens and is discussed in more detail in Chapter 13. Pregnant queens should therefore not be vaccinated with live virus vaccines and unless information has been provided to confirm their safety, all other live vaccines should be avoided during pregnancy.

Griseofulvin is known to be teratogenic in cats and various deformities including cleft palate, umbilical hernia and anophthalmia have been seen in kittens following its use in pregnancy (Gruffydd-Jones & Wright, 1977). Very little is known about the teratogenic potential of other drugs in cats and therefore they should be avoided in pregnancy if possible.

If insufficient information is available to eliminate the possibility of a hereditary basis to the defect, the breeder should be advised either to perform a test mating programme or neuter both parents and all littermates. Any related cats should also be considered as potential carriers of the trait.

Some congenital conditions have already been discussed in earlier chapters. A number of congenital cardiac abnormalities occur in cats. These may cause sudden death in the first few months of life and some, such as fibroelastosis, are known to be hereditary. Of the congenital neurological conditions, several may be inherited, for example lysosomal storage disease and hydrocephalus, whilst congenital ataxia or cerebellar hypoplasia associated with the teratogenic effect of panleucopenia virus has already been mentioned. Three congenital deformities – primary megoesophagus, pyloric dysfunction and megoesophagus secondary to a vascular ring stricture – may cause persistent regurgitation or vomiting of food in young kittens. They often first become apparent when the affected kittens are weaned onto solid foods. Radiography is required for their differentiation. Pyloric dysfunction occurs most commonly in Siamese kittens and is probably hereditary.

Congenital spinal deformities, including spina bifida, are seen in cats carrying the Manx gene, but are also encountered in other breeds. They may result in neurological abnormalities leading to ataxia, incontinence, etc. Pericardio-peritoneal diaphragmatic hernia is usually associated with dyspnoea in young cats but can lead to early death. It is seen mainly in long-haired (LH) cats. A range of congenital ocular abnormalities (Fig. 7.1) has been recorded in cats and these are described in Chapter 9.

Multiple congenital renal cysts occur occasionally in LH cats. They result in bilaterally enlarged, irregular kidneys and interfere with renal function although this is not usually sufficiently compromised to result in clinical signs until adulthood has been reached. The noticeable preponderance in LH cats suggests the possibility of a hereditary basis to the condition.

Several of the more common congenital abnormalities deserve special mention.

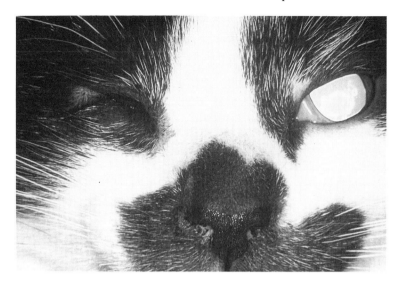

Fig. 7.1 Unilateral anophthalmia in a kitten associated with the teratogenic effect of griseofulvin.

CLEFT PALATE

Cleft palate is probably the most common congenital deformity of cats and is a significant cause of neonatal mortality in some catteries (Fig. 7.2) (Loevy & Tenyes, 1968). Affected kittens are unable to suckle efficiently and milk may pass into the trachea, leading to an aspiration pneumonia. The kittens usually die within the first few days of life. Cleft palate may be inherited, but may also arise as a result of a non-genetic developmental influence and has been seen following the administration of griseofulvin to pregnant queens.

UMBILICAL HERNIA

Another common congenital deformity of cats is umbilical hernia, but it may also be seen in combination with other gross anomalies in the same kitten or in others from the same litter, strongly suggesting a non-genetic developmental origin (Henricson & Burnstein, 1965). The extent of the lesion is extremely variable. In mild cases there is simply a temporary, easily reducible prolapse of fat, but in the most severe cases there is complete failure of formation of the ventral abdominal wall, often with associated agenesis of the gastrointestinal tract. Care must be taken not to confuse this condition with traumatic damage to the umbilicus caused by an over-zealous queen during severing of the cord.

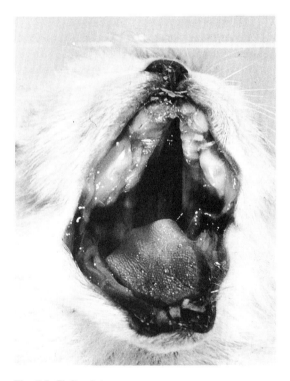

Fig. 7.2 Cleft palate.

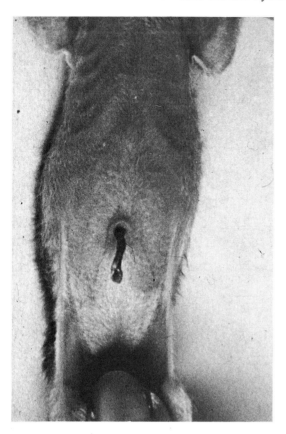

Fig. 7.3 A Burmese kitten with a flattened rib cage. There is a dorsoventral compression of the thorax which has led to prominent, increased angulation of the costochondral junctions.

FLATTENED RIB CAGE ('FLAT-CHESTED' KITTENS)

This deformity is usually not evident at birth and is first noted at 2–6 weeks of age. There is extreme dorsoventral compression of the thorax leading to exaggerated angulation of the costochondral junctions (Fig. 7.3). The deformity leads to dyspnoea and in severe cases there may be cardiac failure resulting from severe compression of the heart. Affected kittens do not thrive well. They have poor coats and do not gain weight as rapidly as their unaffected littermates. There may also be a marked lordosis in the thoracic vertebral column and a peculiar frog-like gait due to inability of the kittens to raise their bodies from the ground normally. A more localized depression of the sternum, termed pectus excavatum or 'funnel chest', may also be seen. It is not clear whether this is related to flattened rib cages or is a separate entity. No treatment of flat-chested kittens is possible, but in most kittens the chest deformity becomes less noticeable at 3–4 months of age and the kittens rapidly put on weight. The deformity has been seen in most breeds of cats but is particularly common in the Burmese breed.

Recently, skeletal deformities, resembling flattened rib cages, have been reported in kittens born to queens receiving a taurine-deficient diet (Sturman *et al.*, 1986). The role of taurine deficiency in naturally occurring flattened rib cages is not clear.

Treatment of sick young kittens

Every attempt should be made to determine the underlying cause of illness in young kittens, and to treat this. However, specific treatment of the underlying cause is not possible for certain problems, particularly the viral infections, and general supportive treatment is crucial. This approach is also necessary in the early management of neonatal diseases before a specific diagnosis is made, which may not be possible until laboratory investigations, including post-mortem examination, have been undertaken.

Prevention of chilling is important and if the kittens have been separated from their mother, an ambient temperature of around 30°C should be maintained. Artifical feeding is vital to combat dehydration and hypoglycaemia, to which kittens are particularly vulnerable. Initally oral rehydration fluids containing glucose should be used, administered by stomach tube. Once the kitten's condition has stabilized milk replacements may be introduced (as described under 'Artifical rearing' above). Administration of oxygen can be valuable particularly in the first day or two of life when respiratory function may be compromised by physiological immaturity.

Particular care is necessary in antibiotic therapy (Davis, 1984). Hepatic enzyme systems, required for metabolism of many antibiotics, are poorly developed in kittens and as a consequence certain antibiotics such as tetracyclines and possibly sulphonamides are better avoided. Synthetic penicillins or cephalosporins are the preferred choice in most situations. Higher dosages are required initially than the normal dose for weight based on adult cats, but the frequency of treatment should be reduced.

REFERENCES AND FURTHER READING

Arnberg J. & Flagstad A. (1985) Prostaglandin $F_{2\alpha}$ treatment of feline open pyometra. *Nor. Vet. Med.* **37**, 386.

Baines F.M. (1981) Milk substitutes and the hand-rearing of orphan puppies and kittens. *J. Small Anim. Pract.* **22**, 555.

Cline E.M., Jennings L.L. & Sojka N.J. (1980) Breeding laboratory cats during artificially induced oestrus. *Lab. Anim. Sci.* **29**, 338.

Davis L.E. (1984) Drug disposition in neonatal animals. *J. Am. Vet. Med. Ass.* **184**, 1161.

Dubey J.P. & Hoover E.A. (1977) Attempted transmission of Toxoplasma gondii infection from pregnant cats to their kittens. *J. Am. Vet. Med. Ass.* **170**, 538.

Gruffydd-Jones T.J. (1989). Some aspects of reproduction in cats. *Adv. Small Anim. Pract.* **1**, 79.

Gruffydd-Jones T.J. (1990) Reproductive endocrinology of the cat. In Hutchison M. (ed) *Manual of Small Animal Endocrinology*, chap. 8. BSAVA Publications.

Gruffydd-Jones T.J. & Evans R.J. (1984) What to do if your cat produces deformed kittens. *Bull. Feline Advisory Bureau* **21**(5), 4.

Gruffydd-Jones T.J. & Wright A.I. (1977) Deformed kittens. *Vet. Rec.* **100**, 206.

Henderson R.T. (1984) Prostaglandin therapeutics in the bitch and queen. *Aust. Vet. J.* **61**, 317.

Henricson B. & Burnstein S. (1965) Hereditary umbilical hernia in cats. *Vet. Bull.* **35**, 453.

Herron M.A. & Sis R.F. (1974) Ovum transport in the cat and the effect of estrogen administration. *Am. J. Vet. Res.* **35**, 1277.

Hinton M. & Gaskell C.J. (1977) Non-neoplastic mammary hypertrophy in the cat associated either with pregnancy or with oral progestagen therapy. *Vet. Rec.* **100**, 277.

Hubler, M., Kaelin S., Hagen A., Fairburn A., Canfield P. & Ruesch P. (1987) Feline neonatal isoerythrolysis in two litters. *J. Small Anim. Pract.* **28**, 833.

Jemmett. J.E. & Evans J.M. (1977) A survey of sexual behaviour and reproduction of female cats. *J. Small Anim. Pract.* **18**, 31.

Loevy H. & Tenyes V.L. (1968) Spontaneous cleft palate in a family of Siamese cats. *Cleft Palate J.* **5**, 57.

Povey R.C. (1978) Reproduction in the female cat. A study of breeders. *Can Vet. J.* **19**, 207.

Robinson R. (1977) *Genetics for Cat Breeders*, 2nd edn. Pergamon Press, Oxford.

Saperstein G., Harris S. & Leipold H.W. (1976) Congenital defects in domestic cats. *Feline Practice* **6**(4), 18.

Scott F.W., Csiza C.K. & Gillespie J.H. (1970) Maternally derived immunity to feline panleukopenia. *J. Am. Vet. Med. Ass.* **156**, 439.

Shille V.M., Lundstrom K. & Stabenfeldt G.H. (1979) Follicular function in the domestic cat as determined by levels of estradiol-17β in plasma and related to estrous behaviour and cornification of exfoliated vaginal epithelium. *Biol. Reprod.* **21**, 953.

Sturman J.A., Gargano A.D., Messing J.M. & Imaki H. (1986) Feline maternal taurine deficiency: effect on mother and offspring. *J. Nutr.* **116**, 655.

Wildt D.E., Kinney G.M. & Seager S.W.J. (1978) Gonadotrophin induced reproductive cyclicity in the domestic cat. *Lab. Anim. Sci.* **28**, 301.

Chapter 8 / The Alimentary System

H. C. RUTGERS

INTRODUCTION

Gastrointestinal disease is a common presenting complaint in the cat, with vomiting and diarrhoea the two most frequent signs. However, feline gastroenterology is still a relatively unexplored field wherein much has been derived from canine and human medicine, even though cats have a different anatomy, physiology, biochemistry and dietary habits.

Diseases of the oropharynx and stomach are relatively common, while oesophageal, colonic and pancreatic disease are rare. Diseases of the small intestine and liver were considered uncommon until recently, but these are now being recognized with increasing frequency. Since clinical signs of gastrointestinal disease may closely mimic those of diseases of other body systems, a thorough physical examination and diagnostic evaluation are important. However, knowledge of feline gastrointestinal disease is hampered by the lack of specific and sensitive diagnostic tests applicable to this species, which is especially the case for small intestinal and pancreatic disorders. In the future, improved diagnostic methods will undoubtedly lead to a better recognition of the manifold conditions that may affect the cat's alimentary system.

DISEASES OF THE OROPHARYNX

Oropharyngeal diseases are common in feline medicine and may represent primary localized disorders or manifestations of systemic disease. Presenting signs frequently include halitosis, in-appetence or dysphagia, ptyalism, bleeding from the mouth and signs of pain. In early stages, decreased appetite and a change in chewing pattern may be the only signs noticed by the owner.

A thorough history and physical examination are important in all cats with oropharyngeal disease, particularly since it can be associated with disease of other body systems. For instance, mucopurulent oculonasal discharges may indicate underlying viral respiratory disease, and lesions on other mucocutaneous junctions can point toward immune-mediated disorders such as pemphigus vulgaris. A complete oral examination will often require sedation or general anaesthesia. Laboratory evaluation is indicated in cats with signs of systemic disease and in otherwise healthy cats with non-responsive stomatitis, and should include haematology, a check for feline leukaemia virus (FeLV) and feline immunodeficiency virus (FIV), and a biochemical profile (specifically for blood glucose and urea/creatinine). The value of oral bacterial cultures is questionable in view of the many bacteria normally present in the mouth. Virus isolation in cats with chronic stomatitis may help to shed light on the aetiology, but has no direct bearing on the diagnosis and clinical outcome. Radiographs may demonstrate neoplastic disease, and biopsy of specific lesions may help to differentiate inflammatory disease from neoplasia.

Diseases of the lips

Eosinophilic granuloma complex
Eosinophilic ulcers, plaques and granulomas can occur in the oral cavity. Eosinophilic ulcer occurs

most frequently and is usually found on the upper lip (Plate 8.1). It is a chronic, slowly progressive lesion appearing as a firm, well-circumscribed, red-brown, ulcerated midline swelling ('indolent ulcer'). It is a disease of adult cats, seen most commonly in females. The aetiology is unknown. Suggested causes are constant irritation (e.g. due to licking with the cat's rough tongue), low-grade bacterial infection or chronic allergy; however, none of these has been substantiated (Scott, 1980). Occasionally, lip ulcers are precancerous and undergo transformation into squamous cell carcinoma or fibrosarcoma. The lesion's location and appearance are usually sufficient for a presumptive diagnosis, but in atypical cases biopsy may be necessary to differentiate it from neoplasia. Eosinophilic granulomas and plaques are found less frequently and may occur anywhere in the mouth.

The treatment of choice is early and aggressive use of systemic glucocorticoids, such as oral prednisolone or subcutaneous methylprednisolone acetate* (20 mg/cat every 2 weeks until the lesion is gone). Recurrent lesions may require long-term alternate-day glucocorticoid treatment. Oral progestagens (megestrol acetate†, 2.5 mg every 2–3 days) may be effective in some cases instead of glucocorticosteroids, but their indiscriminate use is not recommended because of side-effects (Scott, 1980). Non-specific immunomodulators such as mixed bacterial vaccine or levamisole (5 mg/kg three times a week) have also been used with some success (Rosenkrants, 1989). Other modes of therapy that have been advocated are intralesional corticosteroids, surgical excision, cryotherapy and radiotherapy. No treatment is effective in all cases, and residual scarring and recurrence are common.

Other diseases

Inflammation of the lips, uncommon in the cat, may be associated with trauma, dental tartar, dermatitis and autoimmune disease. Ulceration of the lip has also been reported with cowpox virus infection (Martland *et al.*, 1983).

* Depo-Medrone; Upjohn Ltd., Crawley, West Sussex.
† Ovarid; Coopers Pitman-Moore, Crewe, Cheshire.

Squamous cell carcinoma may occur on the lips but is seen more frequently in the oral cavity. Biopsy may be required to distinguish it from eosinophilic granuloma. Treatment is with surgical excision or cryosurgery, but recurrence is common.

Congenital malformations include harelip, which may occur alone or in combination with a cleft palate. Surgical correction may be possible if the lesion is not too extensive (Harvey, 1987).

Diseases of the oral cavity

Gingivitis/stomatitis

Inflammation of the oral mucosa is a common problem in cats, and may range from localized inflammation of the gums (gingivitis) to generalized inflammation of the whole oral cavity (stomatitis). There are many possible causes, such as physical, chemical or thermal injury, infection, periodontal disease, systemic disease and immunological disorders; however, frequently the aetiology remains unclear and treatment difficult. Complete laboratory evaluation is often necessary to rule out underlying disease. Treatment for many types of stomatitis is prolonged, and frequently the condition cannot be cured but is at best controlled through continuous use of medication (Harvey, 1991).

VIRAL INFECTIONS

Infection with the upper respiratory viruses, especially feline calicivirus, is an important cause of acute mouth ulceration in cats. There are many different strains of calicivirus, some of which produce mouth ulcers only, while other strains cause an upper respiratory disease syndrome with associated mouth ulceration. Ulcers are most commonly seen on the rostral dorsolateral margin of the tongue, but they may also occur on the rhinarium or palate. Feline herpesvirus infections are usually accompanied by oral ulcers only when there are severe signs of upper respiratory infection; when present, ulcers tend to be more extensive and severe. Treatment is primarily supportive and symptomatic, consisting of antibiotics to combat secondary bacterial infections, fluids with added B vitamins to correct dehydration, cleansing of nose and eyes, and general nursing care. Cats may be reluctant to eat or be anorexic, necessitating management with soft and sloppy food or tube feeding.

Feline leukaemia virus (FeLV)-infected cats often have chronic gingivitis-stomatitis, probably due to immune suppression (Cotter *et al.*, 1975). Cats with chronic non-responsive gingivitis-stomatitis should therefore be tested for the presence of FeLV; however, a recent study showed a low FeLV prevalence in a survey of cats with chronic stomatitis (Knowles *et al.*, 1989). Control is mainly aimed at improving oral hygiene (brushing, chlorhexidine mouth rinses). In addition, short-term use of antibiotics may be useful. Feline immunodeficiency virus (FIV) may also be associated with chronic gingivitis-stomatitis in cats (Pedersen *et al.*, 1987; Knowles *et al.*, 1989), but further isolation studies are required to clarify its role in this disease complex. It is likely that FIV-induced immunosuppression may predispose to development of oral lesions, but that there is no direct aetiological relationship between FIV and gingivitis-stomatitis in the cat (Harvey, 1991).

Oral lesions have occasionally been described with feline panleucopenia virus infection, and include necrotic gingivitis, severe ulceration of tongue and palate, and sloughing of the soft palate. Usually, gastrointestinal signs predominate.

CHEMICAL IRRITATION AND TRAUMA

Cats are usually fastidious eaters and irritant substances are ingested infrequently, usually during grooming or playing. Dieffenbachia house plants can cause severe oral irritation and ulceration, and in some cases pharyngeal oedema. Antihistaminics and tube feeding may be required for a few days until lesions resolve. Similarly, poinsettia house plants can cause stomatitis and gastroenteritis. Strong acids or bases which are licked from the cat's fur can cause mucosal ulceration. Treatment consists of removal of the agent from the hair and skin, flushing of oral lesions, and fluid and nutritional support until the oral tissues heal.

PERIODONTAL DISEASE (see also p. 290)

Plaque-induced periodontal disease may be the most common chronic oral disease in cats (Gaskell *et al.*, 1988). Bacterial plaque and minerals combine to form calculus, found mostly on the teeth surfaces close to the gum margins, resulting in gingivitis and retraction of the gingival margin, formation of gingival pockets, periodontitis, and loosening and loss of teeth. However, gingivitis and periodontitis may also occur unassociated with plaque. Uniquely in the cat, severe periodontal inflammation may result in external root resorption, with progressive, resorptive lesions at the cemento-enamel junction of teeth, often referred to as 'neck lesions' (Reichart *et al.*, 1984). Therapy includes hand or ultrasonic scaling, removal of severely affected teeth, curettage of periodontal pockets, tooth polishing to remove residual deposits, and local application of 0.1% chlorhexidine solution. Home care is important for plaque control and includes routine teeth cleansing and feeding of a hard dry food. Gingivitis and periodontitis are further managed with antibiotics, such as metronidazole, and local antiseptics, such as chlorhexidine.

SYSTEMIC DISEASE

Chronic renal failure may be accompanied by gingivitis and halitosis, due to urea-splitting microorganisms converting salivary urea into ammonia, causing mucosal erosions and the typical 'uraemic' smell. Similarly, in diabetes mellitus the elevated salivary glucose level may lead to oral bacterial infection and gingivitis. Immune suppression in general, as can be found with many chronic diseases, may also predispose to gingivitis. Oral ulcerations are often a feature of the autoimmune diseases pemphigus vulgaris and systemic lupus erythematosus, uncommon in the cat. Nutritional disorders such as hypervitaminosis A also occasionally result in chronic gingivitis.

IDIOPATHIC CHRONIC STOMATITIS

Chronic non-specific gingivitis and stomatitis is a common and often intractable problem in cats. Clinical signs usually are halitosis, difficulty in eating, pawing of the face, and drooling of saliva, which may be blood-stained. Examination of the mouth may reveal a spectrum of changes including hyperaemia and swelling of the gingival margins, vesiculation and ulceration of the oral mucosa (often at the angle of the jaw), and gingival hyperplasia around the premolars and molars (Plate 8.2). Affected areas bleed easily when traumatized. There is considerable variation between cases, with the whole spectrum present in some cats, while in others only ulceration of the fauces is found. There is no age, breed or sex predisposition, although there may be a possible subgroup of young kittens with mild transient gingival hyperaemia (Gaskell *et al.*, 1988).

The cause of the condition is unknown. Viral involvement has been suggested based on the frequent isolation of calicivirus from oropharyngeal swabs from cats with chronic stomatitis and the high prevalence of antibody to FIV in these cats; however, chronic stomatitis cannot be reproduced following experimental infection, suggesting a multifactorial aetiology (Knowles *et al.*, 1989). An immune-mediated component has been suspected in cats in the USA in which oral biopsy was consistent with lymphocytic-plasmacytic gingivitis (Johnessee & Hurvitz, 1983) (Plate 8.3).

Diagnosis is made by ruling out all other possible causes. Treatment is symptomatic and supportive only. Dental plaque and calculus, if present, should be removed, and teeth which are loose or show extensive external root resorption should be removed. In some recurrent cases, extraction of all teeth except the canines has provided long-term benefit, but this should be considered a last resort measure. Marked proliferative tissue should also be removed, since this is easily traumatized during feeding. Local antiseptics such as chlorhexidine are probably of value only immediately after tooth cleaning. Antibiotics may be of short-term benefit by restoring appetite and reducing discomfort, even though bacteria do not appear to play a primary role in this disease process. Empirically, a broad-spectrum combination of ampicillin (50 mg t.i.d.) and metronidazole (50 mg b.i.d.) given for at least 3 weeks has proven useful (Knowles *et al.*, 1989; Harvey, 1991). Paediatric drops are easiest to

administer. However, recurrence is common after antibiotics are stopped, and while repeated courses may alleviate signs, this may not maintain control of the disease. Systemic corticosteroids may reduce inflammation but inhibit healing and allow for proliferation of bacteria; however, they may be useful in combination with antibiotics in badly affected cats, and they have been used when all else failed in refractory cases. Megestrol actetate has also been used to suppress inflammation, but has no advantages over corticosteroids. Other treatments suggested include cryosurgery, oral vitamins and antiseptics, but their value is debatable. Nursing care is very important, especially the frequent offering of soft and tempting food. Nevertheless, the management of these cases often remains frustrating and unrewarding.

Oral neoplasia

The most common tumour is squamous cell carcinoma, which usually occurs sublingual caudal to the frenulum or on the upper or lower gingivae (Cotter, 1981) (Plate 8.4). It is locally invasive and tends to recur following surgical excision. Early stages are often asymptomatic and may resemble eosinophilic granuloma, granulation tissue or even trauma, necessitating biopsy. Distant metastasis is rare. Prognosis is generally poor; complete surgical excision is often impossible, and radiation or chemotherapy are usually unsuccessful. If the lesion has not spread, mandibulectomy may be effective (Harvey, 1986). The second most common oropharyngeal tumour is fibrosarcoma, occurring most frequently on the gingivae. Non-malignant mass lesions in the cat's mouth include eosinophilic granuloma, foreign body reaction and gingival hyperplasia/periodontal disease.

Disorders of teeth

DENTAL CALCULUS
Calculus (or tartar) – bacterial plaque combined with mineral hydroxyapatite – is seen most commonly in older cats, particularly those fed soft foods. Accumulation of calculus may lead to gingivitis and periodontitis. Treatment consists of

removal of calculus and extraction of affected teeth when periodontitis or root resorption is severe. Antibiotic therapy may be indicated in severe cases, to be instituted just prior to dental treatment. Prophylaxis includes routine teeth cleansing and feeding of a hard dry food.

DENTAL CARIES, ABSCESSES AND FRACTURES
Dental caries is rare in the cat, but is seen occasionally affecting molar teeth. Treatment is usually by extraction (Lane, 1982). Abscessation around the roots of the teeth is uncommon and may lead to radiographically visible osteolysis. The affected tooth should be extracted. In some cases, biopsy may be necessary to differentiate osteomyelitis from tumour involving facial bones.

Fractures of the teeth are uncommon and usually due to trauma. Endodontic therapy (root canal procedure) can be performed to salvage such teeth, but is difficult in the cat.

Oral trauma and foreign bodies
Road traffic accidents and the 'high rise syndrome' (falling from a window or balcony) are not uncommon causes of severe oral injuries in the cat. The most common oral injury is mandibular symphyseal separation, which is usually managed by simple circum-mandibular wiring. With comminuted fractures, this may be combined with figure-eight wiring around the canine teeth. Other common injuries are fractures of the mandible and/or maxilla and avulsion of the lower lip from the mandibular symphysis. Fractures of the horizontal ramus can be managed by applying a loose muzzle for 3 weeks or by intramedullary wire placement.

Electrical cord injury can cause burns in any part of the mouth, but the hard palate, tongue and commissures of the lip are most commonly affected. The extent of the burns may not be visible for several days; tissue and bone sloughs necessitating deep debridement and reconstructive surgery may be necessary in some cases.

The most common oral foreign bodies in the cat are string, thread and needles. String and thread are usually found below the tongue and may become embedded in the tongue base.

Needles can lodge in the tongue, cheek or oropharynx. Other possible causes are bone and grass fragments. Treatment consists of removal of the foreign body and topical and supportive treatment.

Palate defects
Congenital midline defects of the hard and soft palate are occasionally seen in kittens. Clinical signs are nasal regurgitation of milk, failure to thrive, and aspiration pneumonia. Surgical correction of cleft palate usually is possible if the patient can survive until large enough for anaesthesia and surgery, usually performed between 2 and 4 months of age (Harvey, 1987).

Acquired splitting of the hard palate in cats is usually due to trauma, such as a fall from a height. Fresh midline lacerations may not need surgical repair if there is no bubbling through the defect from the nose, but larger defects need suturing with or without use of mucoperiosteal flaps. Acquired defects between the nasal and oral cavities may also be associated with periodontal disease or tooth extraction (oronasal fistula), neoplasms and severe chronic infections.

Diseases of the salivary glands

Salivary gland disease is rare in the cat. Salivary mucocele is managed as in the dog with resection of the affected gland and drainage of the mucocele (Wallace *et al.*, 1972). Neoplasia of the mandibular gland is occasionally seen in old cats, presenting with a firm, non-painful swelling in the neck. Surgical removal is curative if there is no metastasis. Hypersalivation is a common sign of hepatic encephalopathy in cats with congenital portosystemic shunts (see below).

Diseases of the pharynx

Pharyngitis
Pharyngitis is usually an extension of oral or upper respiratory disease. It is commonly seen in association with viral upper respiratory tract disease and as part of the feline plasma cell gingivitis-pharyngitis complex (Johnessee & Hurvitz, 1983). Clinical signs are gagging, coughing and anorexia.

Pharyngitis and tonsillitis have also been attributed to chronic vomiting and reflux of acidic gastric contents (Reindel *et al.*, 1987).

Nasopharyngeal polyps
Nasopharyngeal polyps are well-circumscribed masses on a narrow stalk extending from the middle ear down the eustachian tube into the pharynx. They usually form in reaction to otitis media and extend more commonly into the external ear canal than into the nasopharynx. In the nasopharynx they cause stertorous breathing, sneezing and dysphagia. The mass usually can only be visualized with the cat anaesthetized by pulling the soft palate anteriorly. The polyp is then removed by gently pulling and twisting so that the entire stalk is removed. Treatment must also be directed at the underlying otitis media.

Pharyngeal foreign bodies
Pharyngeal foreign bodies such as bones or needles are seen occasionally. Diagnosis is by direct visualization or radiography. Treatment is by surgical removal.

Neoplasia
Neoplasia of the pharynx is uncommon. Squamous cell carcinoma of the tonsil is seen occasionally; prognosis is poor since these tumours tend to metastasize widely, in contrast to squamous cell carcinomas arising in the oral cavity.

Pharyngostomy tube
Pharyngostomy tube placement allows for enteral hyperalimentation of cats with gastrointestinal or respiratory tract disease and a temporary inability or unwillingness to eat. This technique involves placement, under local or general anaesthesia, of a rubber or polyethylene tube into the pharynx distal to the hyoid apparatus and immediately rostral to the origin of the oesophagus (Lane, 1982; Crowe, 1990). The tube can be left in place for up to 3 weeks, and is preferable to protracted force-feeding or repeated gastric intubation. However, its use has been associated with development of oesophagitis and, in some cats, with vomiting and aspiration of vomitus; for

this reason, nasogastric tube feeding or tube gastrostomy are generally preferred for long-term enteral hyperalimentation.

DISEASES OF THE OESOPHAGUS

Oesophageal disease occurs relatively infrequently in the cat. The main presenting clinical sign is usually regurgitation; other signs may include dysphagia, repeated swallowing movements and excessive salivation. Regurgitation, the passive return of fluid or food from the oesophagus, must be differentiated from vomiting, the active expulsion of contents from the stomach and duodenum; this is important in order to distinguish oesophageal from gastrointestinal disease. Regurgitation may occur immediately after eating, as with proximal oesophageal disease or complete oesophageal obstruction, or it can be delayed for several hours, as with oesophageal dilatation, which provides a reservoir for fluid and food. The regurgitated material usually consists of white foam (mucus and saliva) and undigested food which may be tubular-shaped, and has a near neutral pH. Coughing, dyspnoea and fever associated with secondary aspiration pneumonia may accompany oesophageal signs; occasionally, these are the only complaint of the owner.

Diagnosis of oesophageal disease
Physical examination is often unrewarding but may reveal evidence of an underlying systemic disorder such as feline dysautonomia, or of secondary disease such as aspiration pneumonia.

Radiography is the most important technique in the diagnosis of oesophageal disorders. The oesophagus is not normally seen on plain radiographs of neck and chest but may be visualized when it contains air, fluid, food or foreign material. Chest radiographs may also show complications such as aspiration pneumonia and oesophageal perforation (mediastinitis, pneumomediastinum or pneumothorax, and pyothorax). Oesophageal contrast studies are best performed using barium sulphate paste (Microtrast*). The

*Microtrast; Nicholas Laboratories, Slough, Berks, UK.

normal feline oesophagus has prominent transverse folds in the caudal third creating a characteristic 'herringbone' appearance. To demonstrate an oesophageal motility disorder, partial obstruction or stricture, liquid barium (e.g. Micropaque*) can be administered mixed with food. Oesophageal motility disorders are best evaluated using fluoroscopy, but its use is limited due to the cost of the equipment. When chemical restraint is necessary, deep sedation or anaesthesia should be avoided, since this may result in artificial oesophageal flaccidity or dilatation.

Endoscopy of the oesophagus with either rigid or flexible fiberoptic instruments allows for direct visualization of mucosal lesions, tissue biopsy and foreign body removal (Plate 8.5). Oesophageal biopsies may also be obtained non-invasively using a peroral suction biopsy capsule†.

Oesophageal diseases

Megaoesophagus

Megaoesophagus refers to a disease syndrome characterized by a diffuse severe oesophageal motility disorder resulting in a large flaccid oesophagus. Both in cats and in dogs megaoesophagus is a primary neuromuscular oesophageal disorder; this is in contrast to humans, where it is often secondary to failure of the distal oesophageal sphincter to relax (achalasia). Achalasia has not been reported in the dog and cat.

Megaoesophagus is much less common in the cat than in the dog. It may be congenital or acquired. Congenital megaoesophagus is rare. Inheritance via a recessive non-sex-linked trait has been suggested for primary megaoesophagus found in four related kittens (Clifford *et al.*, 1971). Signs occurred around the time of weaning and included regurgitation of solid food, poor growth and in some cases aspiration pneumonia. Megaoesophagus in association with a concurrent gastric emptying disorder has been reported in young Siamese cats presented with persistent projectile vomiting (Pearson *et al.*, 1974). Clini-

cal signs were primarily due to delayed gastric emptying and improved in some cases following pyloromyotomy; however, the relationship between the abnormalities is not well understood. Suspected congenital megaoesophagus was recently reported in two cats; dietary management with upright feeding was successful in controlling signs for 6 years in one of these (Hoenig, 1990).

Acquired megaoesophagus occurs most commonly as a component of feline dysautonomia. The majority of these cats have radiographic evidence of oesophageal dilatation, although this may be clinically asymptomatic in some cases (Fig. 8.1). Other clinical signs associated with this syndrome include persistent pupillary dilatation, decreased lacrimal and nasal secretions, bradycardia and constipation (Sharp *et al.*, 1984). Megaoesophagus occurs occasionally in cats with systemic muscular diseases such as polymyositis and polymyopathy; it is a rare complication of myasthenia gravis, in contrast to the situation in dogs. Megaoesophagus has also been reported as a result of a lead-associated neuropathy in a cat with severe lead toxicosis (Maddison & Allen, 1990). However, in many cases the cause of megaoesophagus is not understood.

Diagnosis of megaoesophagus is usually based on routine and contrast radiography. In cases with subtle changes or segmental hypomotility, fluoroscopy may be necessary. If a systemic neuromuscular disorder is suspected, additional testing may be indicated, such as a Tensilon response test for myasthenia gravis, measurement of serum muscle enzymes for polymyositis, and electromyography and nerve conduction testing for neuromuscular disease.

Management of megaoesophagus consists of frequent feedings of small semi-liquid meals with the cat in an upright position. It may be helpful to keep the cat in this position for 10–15 minutes after the meal, for instance by carrying it around on one's shoulders, so that food may pass by gravity into the stomach. Antibiotics may be needed in case of secondary aspiration pneumonia. If an underlying disorder can be identified, specific treatment of the primary condition may

* Micropaque; Nicholas Laboratories, Slough, Berks, UK.
† Watson Capsule; Ferraris Development and Engineering Co., Edmonton, London, UK.

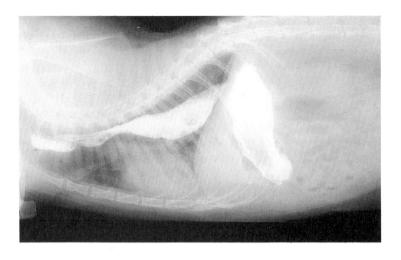

Fig. 8.1 Lateral thoracic radiograph of a 2½-year-old domestic short-haired cat with feline dysautonomia and megaoesophagus 5 minutes after barium administration. The cat was not regurgitating.

lead to improvement of oesophageal dysfunction. However, in many cases the megaoesophagus is permanent and the long-term prognosis poor.

Vascular ring anomalies

Congenital vascular ring anomalies of the great vessels constrict the oesophagus at the base of the heart resulting in dilatation of the cervical and cranial thoracic oesophagus. The most common anomaly is a persistent right aortic arch, although other rare anomalies have been reported (McCandlish *et al.*, 1984; Wheaton *et al.*, 1984). Affected cats usually are presented because of regurgitation of solid food since the time of weaning and failure to thrive. Radiography will demonstrate marked oesophageal dilatation cranial to the heart base; the caudal thoracic oesophagus often remains normal, which differentiates it from a megaoesophagus. The treatment of choice for a persistent right aortic arch is surgical ligation and transection of the constricting ligament. Supportive management with upright feeding of a semi-liquid diet is necessary pre- and postoperatively. Prognosis is usually good if surgery is performed at an early age before irreversible oesophageal dilatation has occurred.

Oesophagitis

Primary oesophagitis is rare and may be seen as a consequence of trauma or ingestion of caustic materials. Severe oesophagitis and stricture were described in a cat after licking undiluted benzalkonium chloride, which had been used as an electrocardiographic conductant, from the skin (Bilbrey *et al.*, 1989). A chronic inflammatory oesophagitis with secondary papilloma formation has been described in a young cat (Wilkinson, 1970). Rarely, oesophageal ulceration may be a complication of calicivirus infection. More commonly, oesophagitis occurs secondary to gastro-oesophageal reflux following general anaesthesia, persistent vomiting or hiatal hernia, and is due to pooling of gastric contents in the oesophagus (Pearson *et al.*, 1978). Conversely, oesophagitis itself may further predispose to gastro-oesophageal reflux, since inflammation of the distal oesophagus lowers the pressure of the gastro-oesophageal sphincter. Consequently, treatment for gastro-oesophageal reflux is often indicated whenever oesophagitis is present.

Clinical signs of oesophagitis are regurgitation, hypersalivation and dysphagia. When oesophagitis is due to hiatal hernia or persistent vomiting, both regurgitation and vomiting may be seen. A tentative diagnosis of oesophagitis is based upon the history, particularly if there has been a recent anaesthesia, and clinical signs. Radiographs are usually normal but may occasionally reveal a hiatal hernia as a predisposing cause. Endoscopy may show mucosal erythema, erosions or ulceration, and mucosal biopsy may confirm the diagnosis.

Mild oesophagitis may resolve spontaneously once an underlying cause such as a foreign body has been removed, but severe oesophagitis may require complete oesophageal rest, e.g. by placement of a gastrostomy tube. Additional symptomatic therapy includes frequent small feedings of a soft, bland food, and antibiotics to control secondary mucosal bacterial invasion. With severe discomfort, liquid antacids (5 ml orally every 2–4 hours) or local anaesthetic gels (Mucaine*, 0.25 ml orally 3 times daily) can be given. Reflux oesophagitis is treated by reducing the amount and acidity of gastric acid refluxed into the oesophagus. Metoclopramide (Emequell†) decreases gastro-oesophageal reflux by increasing the pressure of the gastro-oesophageal sphincter and promotes gastric emptying, and is given at 0.2–0.4 mg/kg orally 3 times daily. Antacids have to be given very frequently in order to lower gastric acidity; instead, the H_2-receptor blocker cimetidine (Tagamet‡, 5 mg/kg 3 times daily orally) is preferred. In cats with severe oesophageal ulceration, prednisolone (0.25–0.5 mg/kg/day) may be used to prevent stricture formation.

Oesophageal foreign bodies
Cats may acquire foreign bodies while hunting or playing. Common foreign bodies are string, fish-hooks, needles, bones and hair balls (Plate 8.6), which generally lodge at the thoracic inlet, heart base or oesophageal hiatus. Clinical signs are usually acute and include repeated swallowing or regurgitaton, painful dysphagia, hypersalivation and anorexia. Depression, fever and dyspnoea may be seen with oesophageal perforation or secondary aspiration pneumonia. Plain radiographs of chest and/or neck are usually diagnostic; however, oesophagoscopy is indicated to assess the

extent of oesophageal damage and to remove the object. The management of oesophageal foreign bodies is an emergency, since the incidence of complications increases with time. Under general anaesthesia, a rigid or flexible endoscope can be used to either remove the foreign body using grasping forceps, or to push it in the stomach, from which it can be removed via gastrotomy. Bone foreign bodies are digested by acid in the stomach and may not need surgery. When a conservative approach fails, oesophagotomy is required to remove the foreign body; however, this is associated with a high complication rate. Following removal of the object, the cat should be treated with antibiotics, soft food frequently, and fluids if needed. Small perforations may be managed medically with antibiotics, a pharyngostomy or gastrostomy tube, and fluid support, but larger lesions will require surgical repair.

Oesophageal stricture
Stricture formation is a possible complication of severe oesophageal ulceration. In the cat, it is most commonly associated with reflux oesophagitis after general anaesthesia, and also with irritants and foreign bodies. Signs of stricture formation following general anaesthesia are first seen between 3 days and 2 weeks after the procedure (Pearson *et al.*, 1978). Gradually increasing dysphagia and regurgitation of especially solids are the predominant signs. A stricture is usually diagnosed with contrast radiography and confirmed endoscopically. The treatment of choice involves the gradual stretching of the stricture by bouginage, which is the use of progressively larger tapered probes under general anaesthesia to break down the fibrous scar tissue. Alternatively, urinary catheters of increasing size or balloon catheters may be used (Zawie, 1987). Oesophageal dilatation is repeated at 1- to 2-week intervals as needed, and may have to be repeated periodically for several months. Prednisolone (0.5–1.0 mg/kg/day) is given concurrently to prevent re-formation of scar tissue. Surgery may be required when dilatation is unsuccessful or the stricture too tight.

* Mucaine; Wyeth Laboratories, Maidenhead, Berks, UK.
† Emequell; Beecham Animal Health, Brentford, Middx, UK.
‡ Tagamet; Smith Kline & French Laboratories, Welwyn Garden City, Herts, UK.

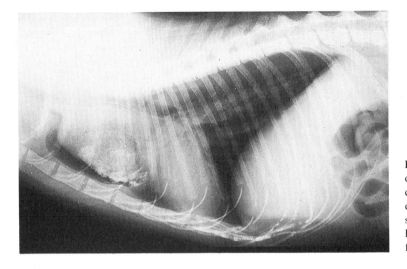

Fig. 8.2 Survey thoracic radiograph of a 4-year-old Persian cat with a congenital oesophageal diverticulum. Note the increased soft tissue density cranial to the heart, representing the fluid- and food-filled diverticulum.

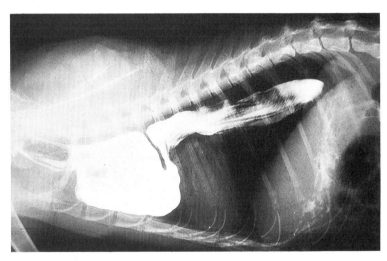

Fig. 8.3 Lateral chest radiograph of the cat in Fig. 8.2 following administration of barium, confirming that the soft tissue density is an oesophageal diverticulum. There is also moderate generalized megoesophagus.

Oesophageal diverticula

Diverticula are congenital (Figs. 8.2 & 8.3) or acquired sac-like evaginations of one or more layers of the oesophageal wall, and are rare in the cat. Acquired diverticula are generally secondary to oesophageal disease and usually occur in the distal oesophagus; signs are due to local impaction of ingesta and ulceration of the mucosa. Treatment is symptomatic as for oesophagitis, but surgery may be required for large diverticula.

Oesophageal neoplasia

Neoplasms of the oesophagus are uncommon. Squamous cell carcinoma is the most common primary malignant tumour, occurring in old cats with chronic and progressive regurgitation, weight loss and anorexia (Happe *et al.*, 1978; Vernon & Roudebush, 1980). Diagnosis is made with contrast radiography, showing filling defects in usually the distal oesophagus, and confirmed via endoscopy and biopsy. Oesophageal compression due to perioesophageal neoplasia is most commonly due to mediastinal lymphosarcoma, usually seen

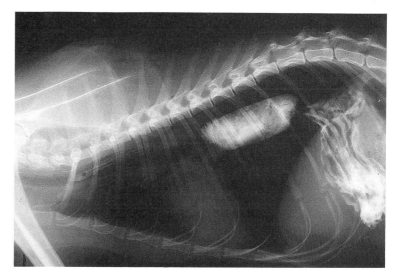

Fig. 8.4 Lateral chest radiograph of a 2-year-old domestic short-haired cat with a hiatal hernia immediately after barium administration. The stomach is seen protruding cranial to the diaphragm. There is also mild megaoesophagus, which was confirmed on follow-up radiographs. This cat had signs of vomiting as well as regurgitation.

in young cats (Gruffydd-Jones *et al.*, 1979). Apart from regurgitation, other findings may include dyspnoea (due to pleural fluid) and a non-compressible thorax. Diagnosis is based on radiography and, where appropriate, thoracentesis and cytology of pleural fluid. Prognosis for oesophageal squamous cell carcinoma is poor, but mediastinal lymphosarcoma may be managed with combination chemotherapy.

Hiatal hernia

A hiatal hernia is a protrusion of a structure (usually the distal oesophagus and stomach) through the oesophageal hiatus of the diaphragm into the chest. A sliding hiatal hernia, with intermittent cranial displacement of the abdominal part of the oesophagus and part of the stomach, is the most common form (Bright *et al.*, 1990). Clinical signs are related to reflux oesophagitis and include hypersalivation, gagging, regurgitation and vomiting shortly after eating, and in severe cases anorexia and weight loss (Peterson, 1983; Ellison *et al.*, 1987); in cats, signs are usually mild and intermittent. Rarely, if large portions of the stomach are herniated, there may be acute signs of gastric obstruction. The diagnosis is made radiographically, and is easiest when the hernia is persistent (Fig. 8.4). Small intermittent hernias

may be demonstrated following application of pressure to the abdomen during radiography, or with fluoroscopy. Treatment is as for reflux-oesophagitis, with surgery (tightening of the hiatus, and gastropexy; anti-reflux procedures such as fundoplication are optional) reserved for symptomatic hiatal hernias that are unresponsive to medical therapy (Prymak *et al.*, 1989; Bright *et al.*, 1990; Waldron *et al.*, 1990).

Naso-oesophageal and oesophagostomy tubes

Naso-oesophageal tubes are easily placed and are very useful for short-term nutritional support. They are preferred to nasogastric tubes because they do not traverse the cardia and thus cause less problems with gastric reflux. Commercially available infant feeding tubes made of polyvinyl chloride, 3½ to 6 French in size, are most commonly used. After 2% lidocaine has been instilled in the nostril the lubricated tube is passed through the ventral nasal meatus and the tip is advanced until it ends in the distal oesophagus; it is then sutured in place. An Elizabethan collar and extension tube are used if necessary.

Placement of oesophagostomy tubes has recently been reported as a fast and convenient alternative to the pharyngostomy tube (Crowe, 1990). These can be placed either surgically or percutaneously using an intravenous jugular vein catheter. Early results have been promising. Principles of enteral hyperalimentation have been discussed elsewhere (Crowe, 1990; Carnevale *et al.*, 1991; Abood & Buffington, 1992).

DISEASES OF THE STOMACH

Gastric disease is relatively common in the cat. Vomiting is the main sign, but it has to be remembered that vomiting may also be associated with intestinal disease and many disorders outside the gastrointestinal tract, such as liver and renal disease, pancreatitis, peritonitis, hypoadrenocorticism, ketoacidotic diabetes mellitus, drugs/toxins and neurological disorders. Other signs associated with gastric disease may include anorexia, nausea, pica and weight loss. The composition of the vomitus can be a clue to the underlying cause, e.g. when it contains hair balls. Melena (black tarry stools) may be seen with bleeding in the stomach or upper small intestine.

Diagnosis of gastric disease

Physical examination is frequently normal in cats with gastric disease, although occasionally gastric masses and foreign bodies may be palpated. The mouth should be examined carefully for string trapped under the tongue base, which may be a clue to the presence of a string foreign body as the cause of vomiting (Felts *et al.*, 1984).

In cats with severe or chronic vomiting, haematological and biochemical evaluation and urinalysis are recommended to rule out other conditions that mimic gastric disease, and to assess the metabolic complications that may arise with vomiting, such as dehydration and electrolyte depletion (especially hypokalaemia). The stool should also be examined for parasites such as ascarids which may cause vomiting in cats. Rarely, microscopic analysis of vomitus may reveal the gastric parasite *Ollulanus tricuspis* (Hargis *et al.*, 1983a).

Plain abdominal radiographs allow for assessment of gastric position, foreign bodies and wall abnormalities. Following a 12-hour fast, the stomach is usually empty; retention of material in the stomach might suggest a foreign body or delayed gastric emptying due to an outflow obstruction or motility disorder. Complete evaluation usually requires contrast studies and distension of the stomach, e.g. using air or liquid barium (10–15 ml/kg given via stomach tube). In most cats, the stomach is empty in 60 minutes. A gastric retention abnormality is best evaluated by giving barium mixed with food; the stomach should be empty in 10–12 hours. Double contrast gastrography (3 ml/kg barium sulphate suspension given via stomach tube followed by distension with air) allows for optimal evaluation of the gastric mucosal surface (Evans & Biery, 1983).

Endoscopy is the preferred method for further evaluation of gastric disease, allowing for direct visualization of the gastric mucosa, biopsy and foreign body removal (Plate 8.7). Small flexible fiberoptic endoscopes (outside diameter 7.9–10.0 mm) are most suitable. Gastric biopsies may also be obtained via laparotomy. At surgery, the stomach can be fully examined and a full-thickness biopsy taken, while foreign bodies and masses can be removed and outflow obstructions corrected. Biopsies should always be taken even when no gross abnormalities are found, because there may be major histological abnormalities without any gross changes. Since in the cat vomiting can be the only sign of small intestinal disease, the intestine should also be biopsied (duodenum during endoscopy, jejunum at laparotomy) when obtaining stomach biopsies in a chronically vomiting cat.

Gastritis

Acute gastritis is not as common in the cat as in the dog, probably due to the more fastidious nature of cats. Possible aetiologies are dietary indiscretion, ingestion of foreign material (e.g. plants, drugs, toxins) and infectious agents such as enteric viruses and parasites (ascarids, *Ollulanus tricuspis*). Signs include acute onset of vomiting, depression and possibly diarrhoea when there is concurrent intestinal involvement. Diagnosis is usually based on history and clinical signs, and is supported by response to symp-

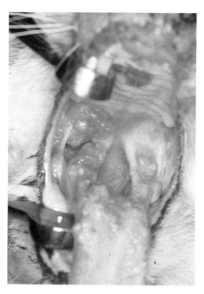

Plate 8.1 Eosinophilic granuloma of the upper lip and oral cavity in an adult domestic short-haired cat.

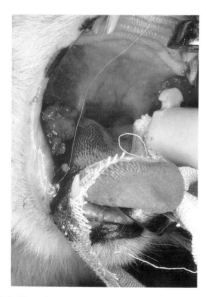

Plate 8.2 Chronic stomatitis in an adult domestic short-haired cat.

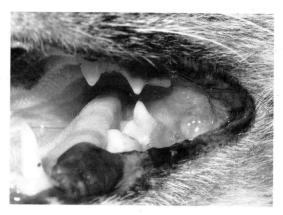

Plate 8.3 Lymphocytic-plasmacytic gingivitis in a 13-year-old domestic short-haired cat: proliferative changes in the angle of the jaw.

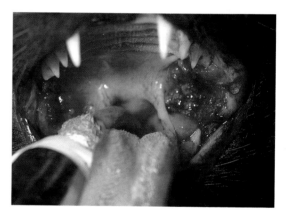

Plate 8.4 This 10-year old domestic short-haired cat had proliferative plasma cell gingivitis at the left glossopalatine arch, and squamous cell carcinoma at the right side.

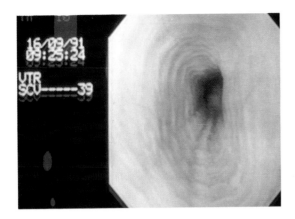

Plate 8.5 Endoscopic view of a normal feline oesophagus. Note the typical herringbone pattern.

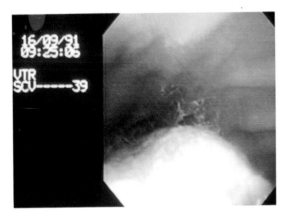

Plate 8.6 Furball in the oesophagus of a cat with mega-esophagus.

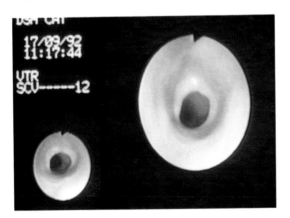

Plate 8.7 Endoscopic view of a normal cat stomach, showing the pyloric canal and the pylorus. The pylorus is wide open, and through it one can see the first part of the normal-looking duodenum.

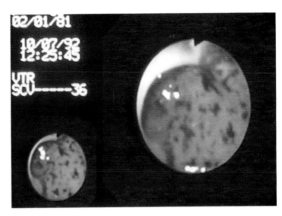

Plate 8.8 Endoscopic view of the stomach of a cat with haemorrhagic gastritis, the cause of which was unknown. The cat responded well to symptomatic treatment.

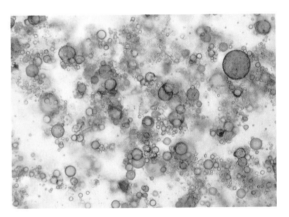

Plate 8.9 Refractile orange fat droplets in stool stained with Sudan III following addition of 36% acetic acid and heating; ×10. This is indicative of an excess of split fats, as may be found in small intestinal malabsorptive disorders. (Reprinted from Rutgers H.C. (1989) Diarrhoea in the cat. *In Practice* **11**, 139, with permission.)

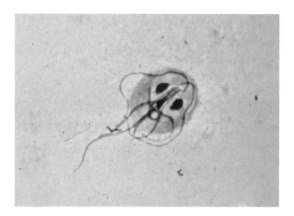

Plate 8.10 *Giardia* trophozoite in a Giemsa-stained faecal smear; ×100. (Reprinted from Rutgers H.C. (1989) Diarrhoea in the cat. *In Practice* **11**, 139, with permission.)

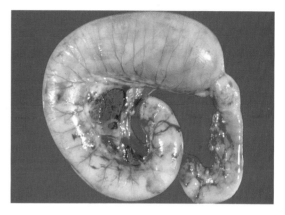

Plate 8.12 Resected small intestine of the cat of Fig. 8.7, showing progressive dilation of the bowel with abrupt termination due to an annular constricting adenocarcinoma. (Reprinted from Rutgers H.C. (1989) Diarrhoea in the cat. *In Practice* **11**, 139, with permission.)

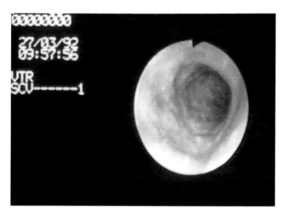

Plate 8.11 Endoscopic view of the duodenum of a cat with lymphocytic-plasmacytic enteritis. Note the irregular aspect of the mucosa.

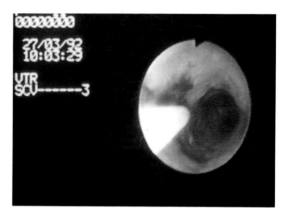

Plate 8.13 Aspiration of duodenal juice through a plastic tube which is passed through the biopsy channel of the endoscope. This is the same cat as in Plate 8.11.

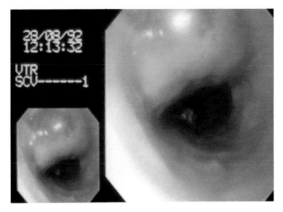

Plate 8.14 Colonoscopy in a cat presented because of recurrent rectal prolapse showing a mass in the dorsal rectal wall. Mucosal biopsy was non-diagnostic, and full-thickness biopsy and resection was required in this case.

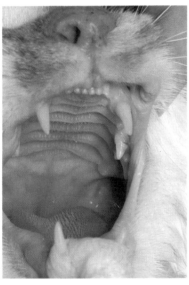

Plate 8.15 Yellow mucous membranes in a jaundiced cat with cholangiohepatitis.

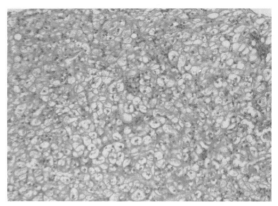

Plate 8.16 Liver biopsy obtained percutaneously with a Menghini needle from an 8-year-old domestic short-haired cat with idiopathic hepatic lipidosis. There is severe distension of hepatocytes with lipid, causing distortion of hepatic cords and sinusoids.

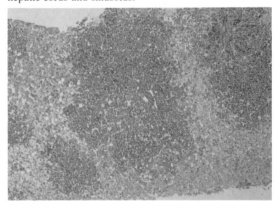

Plate 8.17 Liver biopsy obtained percutaneously with a Menghini needle of the cat of Fig. 8.12, showing invasion of the hepatic parenchyma with dark-coloured clusters of lymphocytes. Histological diagnosis was lymphosarcoma.

tomatic therapy (fasting followed by frequent small feedings of a bland food, and fluid support if needed). Central-acting anti-emetics such as metoclopramide (Emequell, 0.2–0.4 mg/kg 3 times daily) or chlorpromazine (Largactil*, 0.5 mg/kg subcutaneously 1–3 times daily) can be used in case of profuse vomiting, while antacids and broad-spectrum antibiotics are indicated with severe mucosal damage.

Chronic gastritis may occur with long-standing foreign bodies, in association with inflammatory bowel disease and hyperthyroidism, or, less commonly, on its own. The aetiology is often unclear; immune mechanisms and chronic irritation due to dietary sensitivities or plants have been implicated. Severe chronic fibrosing gastritis has been reported in cats infected with *Ollulanus tricuspis* (Hargis *et al.*, 1982), while the role of gastric *Chlamydia* infection needs further clarification (Hargis *et al.*, 1983b). A hyperplastic gastropathy has been described in a young Siamese cat with chronic intermittent vomiting and weight loss, in which radiological and gastroscopic examination revealed enlarged gastric rugae (Dennis *et al.*, 1987). Medical and surgical treatment in this case were unsuccessful. In general, signs of chronic gastritis are vague, mainly consisting of chronic intermittent vomiting, and definitive diagnosis requires gastric mucosal biopsy, either via endoscopy (Plate 8.8) or via laparotomy. Treatment consists of removing the cause, if possible, and dietary manipulations with small frequent feedings of low-allergenic foods (e.g. homemade chicken- or lamb-based diets). Empirical treatment with prednisolone (0.5–1.0 mg/kg/day for 4 weeks, then tapering) may be helpful in non-responding cases.

Gastric foreign bodies
With the exception of hair balls, gastric foreign bodies are uncommon in the cat, although small toys, sewing needles and thread, and fishhooks occasionally occur. Accumulation of small amounts of hair in the stomach which is then vomited up is compatible with normal grooming behaviour.

Occasionally, large hair concretions accumulate in the stomach, especially in long-haired cats, where they may cause a mechanical gastritis or outflow obstruction. Periodic administration of lubricants such as liquid paraffin will usually facilitate passage of accumulated hair, but large concretions may have to be removed surgically. Recurrent hair ball formation may be a consequence of underlying gastrointestinal disease, and in these cases biopsies of stomach and intestine should be obtained. Most other foreign bodies will require removal via surgery or endoscopy.

Gastric ulceration
Any cause of acute or chronic gastritis may result in gastric ulcers if damage is severe enough. Specific causes include administration of ulcerogenic drugs (e.g. aspirin), stress, malignant mast cell tumours, gastrin-secreting tumours, liver disease and renal failure. Mastocytomas produce histamine which may result in excessive gastric hydrochloric acid production; however, clinically evident ulceration is uncommon. Gastric and duodenal ulcers, which were thought to be due to gastrin production by the tumour, have been reported in a cat with pancreatic gastrinoma (Middleton & Watson, 1983). Uraemic gastritis and ulceration, due to uraemic toxins and hypergastrinaemia, is not as common in the cat as in the dog. Gastric ulceration may also be superimposed upon gastric neoplasia. Signs include vomiting with either fresh or digested blood, anorexia and depression. Acute shock may be seen with gastric perforation. Chronic gastric blood loss may result in iron-deficiency anaemia. Barium contrast radiography may demonstrate large ulcers, but endoscopy or laparotomy are often necessary to identify smaller ulcers or gastric erosions. Medical management includes removal of the cause if identified and reduction of gastric acid production using antacids or cimetidine (5 mg/kg 3–4 times daily). Another useful drug is sucralfate (Antepsin*, 1/8 to 1/4 of a 1 g tablet 3–4 times daily), a coating agent which binds to the ulcer site; it may be used in combination with

---

* Largactil; May & Baker Ltd., Dagenham, Essex, UK.

* Antepsin; Wyeth Laboratories, Maidenhead, Berks, UK.

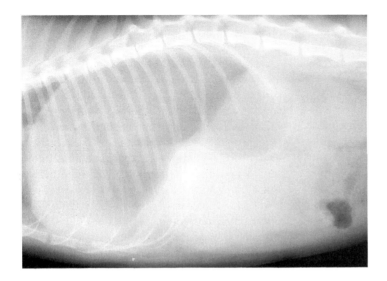

Fig. 8.5 Lateral radiograph of a 16-month-old domestic short-haired cat with a diaphragmatic hernia and herniation of the stomach into the chest.

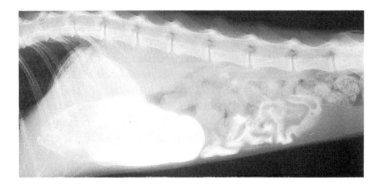

Fig. 8.6 Lateral abdominal radiograph of a 1-year-old domestic short-haired cat with delayed gastric emptying 5 hours after barium administration. Gastric hair balls obstructing the pylorus were found on surgery.

cimetidine if given 1 hour earlier, since it is less effective at higher pH. In chronic and severe cases, surgical resection of a localized bleeding ulcer may be necessary (Moreland, 1988).

Gastric neoplasia

Gastric tumours are rare in the cat. Benign polyps or leiomyomas are occasionally encountered and usually do not cause clinical signs. Lymphosarcoma is the most common malignant tumour, and presents as an ulcerated mass or diffuse infiltration (Turk *et al.*, 1981). Gastric adenocarcinomas are uncommon, and carcinoid tumours are very rare. Signs are related to gastric ulceration with or without outlet obstruction, and frequently also include anorexia and weight loss.

Diagnosis is usually by open surgical biopsy. Prognosis for malignant neoplasia is generally poor, although combination chemotherapy may be attempted for lymphosarcoma.

Delayed gastric emptying

This may be due to a gastric outflow obstruction or a motility disorder. Outflow obstructions in the cat may be associated with either mechanical lesions, such as foreign bodies, tumours, mucosal hypertrophy or gastric herniation (Fig. 8.5), or with pyloric dysfunction (Fig. 8.6). Pyloric stenosis is usually seen in young cats, and there may be an increased incidence in the Siamese breed (Twaddle, 1971; Pearson *et al.*, 1974). Signs include persistent projectile vomiting post-weaning, gastric distension and stunted growth. Radiographic examination demonstrates delayed passage of contrast medium and gastric retention, and, in some cases, megoesophagus. The pylorus of these cats appears normal at surgery, yet there is often clinical improvement following pyloromyotomy or pyloroplasty.

Gastric motility disorders have not yet been reported in the cat, but may be a cause of chronic vomiting (Twedt & Tams, 1989). Signs usually are those of gastric retention in the absence of other demonstrable abnormalities, and management consists of frequent feedings of a liquid meat-based diet, and metoclopramide (0.2–0.5 mg/kg 2–3 times daily) to increase gastric and proximal small intestinal contractility, to relax the pylorus, and to act as a central antiemetic.

Tube gastrostomy

Tube gastrostomy in the cat is well tolerated and allows for effective enteral hyperalimentation. Both operative (Crane, 1980) and percutaneous methods of tube placement using a flexible endoscope (Bright, 1989; Fulton & Dennis, 1992) have been described. The tube can be left in place for several weeks to allow for feeding of gruel and water, and its use has been associated with fewer complications than seen with pharyngostomy tubes. After use they can be simply pulled out while the tube is occluded to prevent leakage from its tip into the wound.

DISEASES OF THE
SMALL BOWEL

Small intestinal disease is commonly recognized by the presence of diarrhoea. Sometimes, accompanying signs such as anorexia, vomiting and weight loss are more prominent features, since, due to the fastidious habits of cats, diarrhoea may not be noticed by the owner. In some cats, vomiting may be the only sign of small intestinal disease.

Diagnosis

History-taking is important to assess duration and severity, to localize the problem to the small or large bowel, to evaluate for underlying extraintestinal disease (e.g. renal failure) and to identify predisposing factors (e.g. diet, environment). Malabsorption syndromes usually cause bulky stools, while large bowel disease tends to result in scant faeces containing fresh blood and mucus, associated with tenesmus and urgency. Physical examination may reveal evidence of underlying systemic disease (e.g. hyperthyroidism) or secondary complications. Abdominal palpation is particularly useful in the cat and may reveal abnormalities such as fluid or gas-filled bowel loops, neoplasms, intussusception, plication of intestine (linear foreign body), enlarged mesenteric lymph nodes or ascites. In cats with chronic diarrhoea, faeces should be examined for endoparasites and cultured for enteropathogens, while Sudan III stains may be helpful to detect steatorrhoea (Plate 8.9). Haematology may reveal anaemia (associated with chronic disease, malnutrition or blood loss), leucopenia (as with panleucopenia, FeLV-associated panleucopenia-like syndrome and sepsis) and eosinophilia (eosinophilic gastroenteritis, endoparasitism). A serum biochemical profile and urinalysis can help rule out metabolic disorders such as renal failure and liver disease. Serological tests include an FeLV- and FN-test, toxoplasma titre and thyroid hormone determination. Few procedures are available for further assessment of small bowel diarrhoea in the cat, except for the oral fat tolerance test which can be used as a preliminary screening test for EPI. Plain abdominal radiographs may reveal signs compatible with intussusception, obstructive bowel disease or ascites in the case of protein-losing enteropathy. Upper GI barium series (8–10 ml liquid barium sulphate per kg) may demonstrate neoplastic, granulomatous and severe infiltrative disease. Endoscopy of stomach and duodenum allows for visual inspection and biopsy. However, in cats with chronic small bowel diarrhoea, it is frequently necessary to obtain biopsies via laparotomy to obtain a specific diagnosis of chronic small intestinal disease. It is important to biopsy the intestine at multiple sites, minimally including duodenum, jejunum and ileum, even if no lesions are visible by gross inspection. Response to therapy may also be used in some cases to help establish tentative diagnoses, for example trial-and-error test diets in dietary intolerance, while occult giardiasis may be excluded by response to an anti-giardial drug such as metronidazole.

Treatment of diarrhoea

GENERAL PRINCIPLES

Acute diarrhoea in cats is often self-limiting. Supportive or symptomatic treatment may be necessary in the more severely affected cases, and consists of replacement of fluid and electrolyte deficits as needed, dietary restriction and modification, and sometimes short-term symptomatic treatment with anti-diarrhoeal drugs. Cats with chronic diarrhoea, however, usually require a specific diagnosis for appropriate treatment.

DRUG THERAPY

Symptomatic anti-diarrhoeal therapy with drugs that affect intestinal motility or secretion is infrequently indicated in the cat. The use of motility modifiers such as anticholinergics and opiates is limited because of their side-effects (ileus and excitation, respectively) (Willard, 1985), and the efficacy of oral protectants is doubtful. Corticosteroids are often used in the treatment of chronic inflammatory bowel disease because of their immunosuppressive and anti-inflammatory effect. Oral prednisolone is preferred because it has fewer side-effects, while dosages can be adapted instantaneously as needed. Antimicrobial therapy is only indicated in specific bacterial gastrointestinal infections (e.g. *Salmonella*, *Campylobacter* or *Giardia*) or when there is severe mucosal damage and a high risk of secondary sepsis or endotoxaemia. Antibiotics may also be considered in cats with chronic diarrhoea in which small intestinal bacterial overgrowth is suspected.

DIETARY MANAGEMENT

Rest of the gastrointestinal tract is of major importance in the treatment of cats with acute as well as chronic diarrhoea. In acute diarrhoea, this can be done by total restriction of oral food intake for 24 hours or more. In chronic problems, this is done to a certain extent by feeding controlled diets.

Intestinal inflammation due to any cause has the potential to increase gastrointestinal permeability, resulting in increased absorption of gut antigens such as food proteins, which may generate a secondary dietary hypersensitivity. Feeding of a controlled diet as an adjunct to medical treatment is therefore important in the initial management of many cats with both acute and chronic diarrhoea. The ideal controlled diet should consist mostly of a highly digestible, high biological-value animal protein (e.g. poultry, lamb or fish) and should contain a minimum of starch, lactose or additives (Kronfeld, 1983). Cats, unlike dogs, have a low tolerance for starch, especially when they have diarrhoea, and should be fed a protein-based rather than a carbohydrate-based diet. The diet should be as hypoallergenic as possible and have good palatability, while frequent feeding of small amounts should be possible to avoid overload of intestinal absorptive capacity. Restriction of dietary fat, to ameliorate steatorrhoea, is not as important in the cat as in the dog; some diarrhoeic cats actually seem to do better when fed a relatively high-fat diet. Vitamin and mineral supplementation is especially important in cats with chronic diarrhoea since poor body stores, decreased intake and increased loss can lead to rapid depletion. Home-made diets can be formulated by the owner, e.g. boiled lamb or chicken and cooked white rice. Animal fat or fish oil should be added if the diet is given on a long-term basis, since cats need a dietary source of animal fat to provide arachidonic acid (Kronfeld, 1983).

Infectious diseases

Viral enteritis

Feline panleucopenia virus has a predilection for rapidly dividing cells, particularly for intestinal crypt epithelium, resulting in enteritis, but also for haematopoietic tissue, resulting in panleucopenia. As a result of vaccination, panleucopenia is less common than in the past, but individual cases still occur. Clinical signs initially consist of anorexia, depression, fever and vomiting, followed by severe dehydration and diarrhoea, which is often bloody (Pollock, 1984). Diagnosis is usually based on signs and haematological demonstration of panleucopenia. Successful treatment involves antibiotics, intensive fluid therapy and antiemetics. Intermittent or chronic diarrhoea may remain a problem in some cats which recover from panleucopenia, presumably due to severe, irreversible damage during the acute phase of the disease.

A feline enteric corona virus that is closely related but not identical to the virus of feline infectious peritonitis (FIP) may cause a clinical enteritis of varying severity in recently weaned kittens (Pedersen *et al.*, 1981). Diarrhoea is usually mild and self-limiting, but severe cases may occasionally need fluid and antibiotic support. This coronavirus is not pathogenic in adult cats, but derives its significance from the fact that it cross-reacts in serological tests currently used in the diagnosis of FIP.

There may be more primary enteric viruses playing a role in the pathogenesis of acute diarrhoea in the cat; for example, rotavirus and astrovirus have been described in young kittens with transient diarrhoea. However, these are likely to be of minor importance, causing at most mild self-limiting diarrhoea. A viral aetiology has also been postulated for the syndrome of nictitating membrane protrusion and diarrhoea, based on the isolation of a torovirus-like agent from the stool of these cats (Muir, 1990). This disease may affect several cats simultaneously and is usually self-limiting, although clinical signs may persist for several weeks.

The intestines may also be involved as part of a generalized viral infection. The feline leukaemia virus (FeLV)-panleucopenia-like syndrome occurs in stressed or debilitated FeLV-positive cats and may be associated with anaemia and thrombocytopenia. It is seen most commonly as one of the problems in an FeLV-infected colony, and diagnosis is based on demonstration of FeLV-positive status in an adequately vaccinated cat. Treatment is supportive only, and prognosis is poor. About 15% of cats infected with feline immunodeficiency virus (FIV) are presented because of chronic enteritis, usually manifested by chronic diarrhoea, weight loss, anorexia and dehydration (Ishida *et al.*, 1989; Yamamoto *et al.*, 1989). The actual incidence of bowel disease in FIV may be higher since many cats with FIV have histological evidence of diffuse enterocolitis, even if they have not had clinical signs of enteritis. Opportunistic infections (e.g. *Cryptosporidium*, *Giardia*) may also occur. The feline infectious peritonitis (FIP) virus may cause granulomatous enteritis or serositis in the course of 'dry' FIP.

Bacterial enteritis

Bacteria are frequently implicated as a cause of diarrhoea in cats, but their importance is overestimated. Certain bacteria such as *Escherichia coli* are part of the normal gut flora, and can be normally isolated from the faeces. No specific serotypes of *E. coli* have been found in association with feline diarrhoea, and abundant growth of *E. coli* on stool culture is thought to be the result of the intestinal disturbance rather than the cause. The possible occurrence of enteropathogenic *E. coli* needs further study. An additional problem is that many potential enteropathogens, such as *Campylobacter jejuni*, may also be found in the faeces of clinically healthy cats.

Infection with *Salmonella* spp. may cause an acute gastroenteritis, especially in young and debilitated animals, often with clinical signs of lower bowel involvement (enterocolitis). Salmonellosis in cats may also present as a more chronic, nonspecific febrile illness, often without concurrent signs of gastrointestinal involvement (Dow *et al.*, 1989). The use of antibiotics in salmonellosis is controversial, since they may prolong faecal shedding of organisms, resulting in a chronic carrier state. Antibiotic treatment should be instituted only when there is systemic illness, and is best based on the results of faecal culture and sensitivity testing. Initial empirical treatment of a cat with suspected salmonellosis can be with ampicillin (or amoxycillin) or a trimethoprim-sulphonamide combination (Dow *et al.*, 1989). Occasionally, healthy cats are asymptomatic carriers of *Salmonella* spp.; their role in the perpetuation of the disease is uncertain. Excretion of organisms is usually short-lived in cats, but owners should be warned of the zoonotic potential.

Campylobacter jejuni has been recognized as a cause of acute, chronic or intermittent diarrhoea, mostly in kittens. It also may be concomitant with other intestinal disease agents, suggesting a synergistic or opportunistic mode of action (Dillon *et al.*, 1987). The diarrhoea is often watery and may contain blood. Other signs of infection may include fever, nausea and vomiting. Diagnosis is based on isolation of the organism from fresh stool. *Campylobacter* requires microaerophilic conditions for growth, and false negatives may occur if proper techniques for sampling and culturing are not followed. Antibiotic treatment (e.g. erythromycin 40 mg/kg/day for 5–10 days) is indicated only when infection is associated with clinical disease. The disease is a potential zoonosis, although concurrent infection of pet and owner is more likely to be the result of the exposure of both to a common source.

Other bacteria may sporadically cause intestinal disease and diarrhoea in cats. *Bacillus pisiformis*, the cause of Tyzzer's disease (a rare but fatal haemorrhagic enterocolitis associated with multifocal hepatic necrosis), has been reported in immunosuppressed kittens (Bennett, 1977). *Yersinia pseudotuberculosis*, a common organism in small mammals and wild birds, may cause diarrhoea, weight loss and mesenteric lymphadenopathy in cats following oral infection (Obwolo & Gruffydd-Jones, 1977). The alimentary form of tuberculosis has been described in cats fed infected milk, causing diarrhoea, emaciation and mesenteric lymphadenopathy, resembling intestinal lymphosarcoma (Orr *et al.*, 1980).

Parasites

Infections with helminths rarely cause diarrhoea, although occasionally kittens with heavy roundworm infestations develop signs. Infection with the protozoan parasite *Giardia* spp. is a relatively common, frequently underdiagnosed cause of intermittent or continuous chronic diarrhoea (Kirkpatrick, 1986). Stools are loose or watery

and occasionally contain mucus. Chronic infection may cause weight loss. Some cats are asymptomatic carriers. Diagnosis can be difficult due to the periodicity in the excretion of the organism in the faeces, therefore multiple stool specimens should be examined if the first is negative. Fresh direct saline smears may reveal the motile trophozoites (Plate 8.10) while the small oocysts (12 μm) are best detected following zinc sulphate flotation and microscopic examination under oil immersion. Treatment is with oral metronidazole (50 mg/kg once daily for 5 days).

Recently, cryptosporidia have also been recognized as potential enteropathogens in the cat (Bennett *et al.*, 1985); FeLV-induced immunocompromise may be a predisposing factor (Goodwin & Barsanti, 1990; Monticello *et al.*, 1987). Diagnosis may be difficult since routine detection of *Cryptosporidium* sp. in faecal samples is hampered by the small size (4–5 μm) of the oocysts and the need for special concentration techniques. Identification of organisms is facilitated by use of an acid-fast stain (cryptosporidia stain red) of a feacal smear, or by faecal flotation using Sheather's sugar solution. Infection is usually self-limiting in immunocompetent individuals; however, cryptosporidiosis is now recognized as a zoonosis, and cats positive for cryptosporidiosis should be considered a potential source for human infection, in particular for immunocompromised individuals.

Cats may harbour other coccidia, but their clinical sigificance is unclear. Coccidial infections usually are well-tolerated, but heavy infections in young kittens may result in diarrhoea and dehydration with copious fluid, mucoid and often bloody faeces. Conditions of poor hygiene or high-density housing as in catteries may lead to outbreaks of coccidiosis, as may the stress of weaning, travel and exposure to cold. Treatment is with sulphonamides (50 mg/kg/day for 7–21 days).

Small bowel inflammatory disease

These are diseases of unknown aetiology characterized by diffuse infiltration of the intestinal mucosa by various populations of inflammatory cells, which may involve the small intestine only or the stomach and/or colon as well. Pathological classification is based on the predominant cell type present. In some cases, the inflammatory reaction may represent a non-specific pathological response of the gut to intraluminal irritants, such as infectious agents (e.g. *Giardia*, bacterial overgrowth), toxins or food allergy (Nelson *et al.*, 1984; Rutgers *et al.*, 1988). In most cats, the disease is idiopathic; an immune pathogenesis is suspected, which is supported by the steroid responsiveness of many of these diseases.

Lymphocytic-plasmacytic enteritis

This is being diagnosed with increasing frequency as a cause of chronic intermittent vomiting and diarrhoea in cats (Willard *et al.*, 1985; Tams, 1986a). Vomiting is often a predominant initial clinical sign, slowly increasing in frequency, and later accompanied by soft or occasionally watery diarrhoea, inappetence and weight loss. Laboratory findings and contrast radiography usually are normal. Diagnosis is by intestinal biopsy, either by endoscopy (Plate 8.11) or via laparotomy, and histological examination. Other diseases have to be ruled out, since lymphocytic-plasmacytic infiltrates in the gut wall may also occur as a nonspecific response to a variety of intestinal irritants such as food allergy, giardiasis and bacterial overgrowth. Corticosteroids are the initial treatment; mild cases respond to prednisolone at a dose of 1–2 mg/kg daily for 2–4 weeks and then gradually decreasing until clinical signs resolve, while severe cases often require higher dosages and long-term therapy. Cats that fail to respond may be given adjunct metronidazole at 10–20 mg/kg twice daily; its beneficial effect might be due to an inhibition of cell-mediated imunity. If remission is not maintained on this combination, the immunosuppressive drug azathioprine* may be used at a dose of 0.3 mg/kg on alternate days. Hypoallergenic diets may provide supportive treatment but are unlikely to be effective alone.

* Imuran; Wellcome Medical Division, Crewe, Cheshire, UK.

Feline eosinophilic enteritis

This may either present as a relatively mild form of inflammatory bowel disease, characterized by moderate eosinophilic infiltrates in the intestinal wall and a good response to treatment with corticosteroids, or it may be part of the hypereosinophilic syndrome (Hendricks, 1981; Tams, 1986b). The eosinophilic syndrome is an uncommon, distinct entity in middle-aged cats, characterized by anorexia, vomiting, diarrhoea (often bloody), marked diffuse thickening of the small bowel wall due to infiltration with eosinophils, and peripheral eosinophilia. Eosinophilic infiltrates in other organs are common, and may result in hepatosplenomegaly and mesenteric lymphadenopathy. Diagnosis is by biopsy of the small or large intestine, and treatment is with high levels of steroids. In contrast to the dog, long-term prognosis for these cats is often poor.

Granulomatous enteritis

This is rare, and is characterized by granulomatous inflammation of the ileum and colon resulting in mass-like thickening of a region of the bowel wall (Van Kruiningen, 1983). Surgical resection and corticosteroid treatment have met with variable success.

Intestinal neoplasia

Adenocarcinoma and lymphosarcoma are the most common intestinal tumours in cats (Patnaik *et al.*, 1976; Turk *et al.*, 1981), followed by mast cell tumours. Clinical signs are vague, insidious and progressive, and include anorexia, weight loss, vomiting and, less frequently, diarrhoea.

Adenocarcinomas are seen predominantly in older animals (>11 years), most frequently in the ileum and jejunum. Siamese cats appear to be predisposed (Birchard *et al.*, 1986). Adenocarcinoma often grows inwards, producing an annular constriction and partial obstruction with minimal outward enlargement. It may also cause segmental thickening within the bowel wall and act like an expanding mass. Mucosal ulceration is common and may result in blood loss anaemia. This tumour is often not palpable, and barium radiographs showing a partial obstruction and

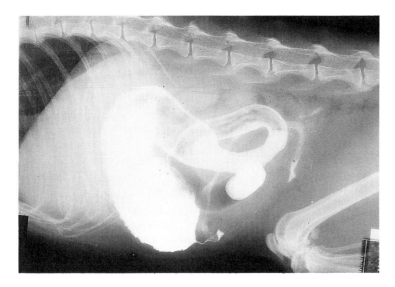

Fig. 8.7 Lateral abdominal radiograph, 3 hours after barium administration, of an old domestic short-haired cat with intestinal adenocarcinoma. Note the narrowed lumen at the site of obstruction and the dilation proximal to it.

laparotomy are required for the diagnosis (Fig. 8.7 & Plate 8.12). Treatment is by surgical resection of the affected intestine. Prognosis is generally poor, although a 28-month survival time following surgery has been reported (Patnaik *et al.*, 1981).

Gastrointestinal lymphoma in the cat can originate anywhere in the small bowel, but it is most common at the ileocaecocolic junction when localized. It usually causes segmental thickening of the intestinal wall, which may occur at multiple sites. A diffuse form, causing marked thickening of the entire small intestine, is less common (Tams, 1986b). Mucosal ulceration may occur. Cats with these tumours are usually older than cats with other forms of lymphoma, averaging 8 years, and most are FeLV-negative. On physical examination the bowel may feel thickened or a distinct mass may be palpated, while palpation may also reveal hepatosplenomegaly, enlarged mesenteric lymph nodes or peripheral lymphadenopathy. Laboratory findings are variable, and abdominal contrast radiography may reveal infiltration or nodularity of the bowel wall. The diagnosis is made by intestinal biopsy. Several chemotherapeutic protocols have been used, but the prognosis is generally poor.

Intestinal mast cell tumours present as segmental intestinal thickening or enlargement without ulceration, and are palpable in about 50% of the cases (Alroy *et al.*, 1975). Treatment is by wide surgical resection, but metastasis at the time of diagnosis is common.

Benign conditions include mucosal polyps, which have been described in both the small and the large intestine (Orr *et al.*, 1980; Van Niel, 1989). Polyps may be single or multiple, and vary in size. Clinical signs range from asymptomatic to diarrhoea (often with blood) and partial obstruction due to stricture formation.

The gut may also be affected secondarily by non-intestinal tumours. Gastroduodenal ulceration is found in cats with mast cell tumours elsewhere or with disseminated mastocytosis, presumably due to chronic hypersecretion of gastric acid due to histamine released from the tumour. A rare cause of duodenal ulceration is gastric hypersecretion (Zollinger–Ellison syndrome) associated with pancreatic gastrinoma (Middleton & Watson, 1983; van der Gaag *et al.*, 1988).

Metabolic and endocrine disorders

Many metabolic and endocrine disorders affect the small intestine indirectly and may cause diarrhoea. Cats with chronic renal failure may show diarrhoea as well as polyuria, polydipsia and weight loss, and diarrhoea has also been described in association with diabetes mellitus. Usually, diarrhoea is a minor component, and signs of the primary disease predominate. Hyperthyroidism, however, may have prominent gastrointestinal signs such as increased frequency of defecation and volume of faeces as well as frank diarrhoea, in addition to its classical symptoms of polyphagia, weight loss and hyperactivity. Some cats may have steatorrhoea and malabsorption. Signs resolve following treatment of the underlying thyroid disorder.

Small intestinal bacterial overgrowth (SIBO)

The incidence and importance of SIBO in the cat is not yet known, although SIBO is now recognized as an important cause of diarrhoea and weight loss in dogs (Batt & Hall, 1989). Furthermore, it recently has been shown that normal cats may harbour large numbers of bacteria in the proximal small intestine (Johnston *et al.*, 1993). SIBO in the cat can be suspected circumstantially on the basis of clinical signs and response to antibiotics, but definitive diagnosis can only be made by quantitative bacterial culture of duodenal juice obtained endoscopically (Plate 8.13) or via laparotomy ($>10^5$ organisms/ml). Treatment is with oral antibiotics (tetracycline, metronidazole, tylosin), while underlying causes (e.g. motility disorders, gastrointestinal stasis and immunodeficiency) should be identified and treated if possible.

Diet and intestinal pathology

The role of diet in the aetiology of feline diarrhoea is as yet uncertain; diet is often suggested as a possible cause, but few specific examples can be quoted (Walton & Parish, 1968; Nelson *et al.*, 1984). Intolerance to cow's milk is the best recognized dietary cause of diarrhoea in the cat and has been attributed to a lactose intolerance, although it may also be an allergy to bovine milk protein.

Adverse reactions to food include food allergy (with a proven immunological basis), food intolerance (mechanism unknown), and dietary indiscretions (Strombeck & Guildford, 1990). Clinical signs of food allergy or intolerance can be gastrointestinal (vomiting and diarrhoea), cutaneous (pruritus, miliary dermatitis), and/or on occasion respiratory (bronchoconstriction). Signs often occur suddenly after months or years of eating the offending foodstuff. Diagnosis is made by feeding a hypoallergenic diet exclusively for at least 3 weeks and observing resolution of clinical signs, with recrudescence of signs when the original diet is reintroduced. Hypoallergenic diets should consist of a single protein and carbohydrate source in a 1:2 ratio, e.g. lamb and boiled white rice, chicken and rice, or cottage cheese and rice. Avoidance of the offending foodstuff is curative. Individual foodstuffs can be evaluated one at a time for a 7-day test period to identify those that elicit a reaction versus those that can be incorporated into a maintenance diet.

Intestinal obstruction

Specific causes of intestinal obstruction in cats include foreign bodies (Fig. 8.8), intussusception, tumours, strictures or adhesions, bowel herniation, abscesses or granulomas, and congenital abnormalities such as diverticular malformations (Ablin *et al.*, 1991). High obstructions are associated with more severe signs, such as acute onset of vomiting, depression, anorexia, abdominal pain and collapse. Abdominal palpation and radiography usually suggest a tentative diagnosis of intestinal obstruction, warranting exploratory surgery. Linear foreign bodies sometimes may be managed conservatively if a sublingually fixed string can be cut; however, surgery is necessary if clinical signs persist or worsen, or if there are signs of peritonitis (Felts *et al.*, 1984). In all cases, preoperative stabilization of the patient, and maintenance of fluid, electrolyte and acid–base homeostasis during and after surgery are crucial.

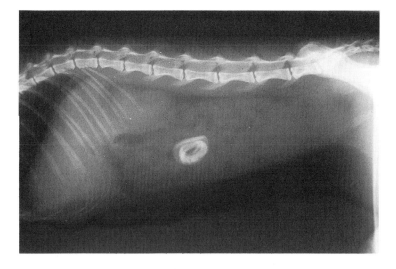

Fig. 8.8 Foreign body in the small intestine of a young cat presented for chronic vomiting. At surgery it was found to be part of a glass syringe.

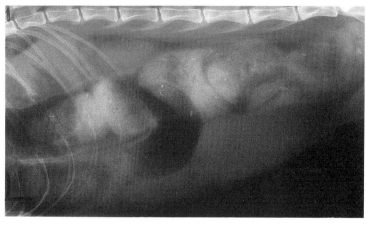

Fig. 8.9 Lateral abdominal radiograph of a 3-year-old domestic short-haired cat with obstipation, showing distension of the colon with impacted faeces.

DISEASES OF THE LARGE BOWEL

Large bowel disease in the cat may result in signs of colitis or in constipation. Colitis usually causes frequent defecation of small volumes of stool containing mucus and/or fresh blood, which is often associated with tenesmus and urgency. Constipation is characterized by failure to defecate and/or frequent unsuccessful attempts to defecate. Some cats may pass small amounts of liquid faeces after a lot of straining. In unobserved cases, the cat may be presented only because of secondary signs such as depression, anorexia and vomiting.

Colitis

Colitis appears to be much rarer in the cat than in the dog. Colonic disease may occur in combination with small bowel inflammatory disease or on its own (Van Kruiningen *et al.*, 1983). Infectious causes of colitis may include enteropathogenic bacteria (e.g. *Salmonella*, *Campylobacter*), fungi (e.g. *Aspergillus*) or protozoa (e.g. *Giardia*, coccidia). Abrasive colitis may be associated with ingestion of excessive hair or other foreign material (Sherding, 1989). In many cases the aetiology is unknown, although dietary allergy has been implicated in some cats with lymphocytic-plasmacytic colitis (Nelson *et al.*, 1984). A tentative diagnosis of colitis is usually based on clinical signs, but definitive diagnosis depends on results of faecal parasitology and culture, blood haematology and biochemistry, and colonic biopsy. Large bowel biopsies can be obtained relatively easily using a small rigid colonoscope or with a paediatric suction biopsy capsule.

When infectious and abrasive causes have been eliminated, treatment with sulphasalazine* (25 mg/kg or 250 mg once daily) may be indicated (Leib *et al.*, 1986). This drug, often effective in the treatment of chronic colitis in the dog, needs to be used with caution in the cat because of the potential toxicity of the salicylate portion. In cases that fail to respond, additional treatment with prednisolone or metronidazole may be necessary. Cats with lymphocytic-plasmacytic colitis may also respond to dietary management with hypoallergenic diets such as lamb and rice (Nelson *et al.*, 1984).

Constipation

Constipation is common in the cat, presumably because of the grooming behaviour and infrequent defaecation of this species, and is usually due to impaction of the colon with a mixture of faeces and ingested foreign material, especially hair. Constipation may also occur secondary to mechanical obstruction (caused by rectal or colonic tumours, strictures or extraluminal masses), painful anorectal and orthopaedic conditions, and neurological diseases (lumbosacral spinal cord abnormalities, feline dysautonomia). Chronic recurrent constipation (obstipation) may lead to megacolon. Congenital megacolon, due to the absence of myenteric ganglion cells, is rare in the cat. Idiopathic megacolon has been described in middle-aged to older cats, and may be due to acquired degenerative neuromuscular disease, leading to colonic hypomotility, dilatation and obstipation (Rosin *et al.*, 1988). Diagnosis is usually based upon physical examination. Neurological examination and abdominal radiography may be required to rule out underlying causes

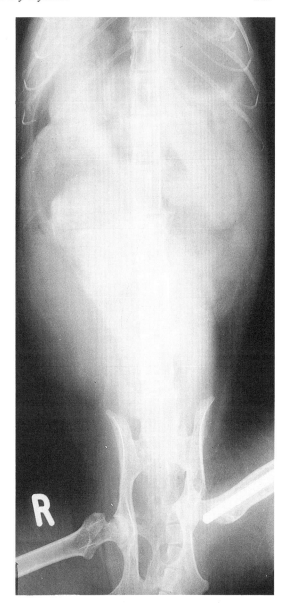

Fig. 8.10 Ventrodorsal abdominal radiograph of the cat of Fig. 8.9, showing that the obstipation is associated with narrowing of the pelvic canal due to an old pelvic fracture. Also note the intramedullary pin in the left femur.

* Salazopyrin; Pharmacia GB Ltd., Milton Keynes, Bucks, UK.

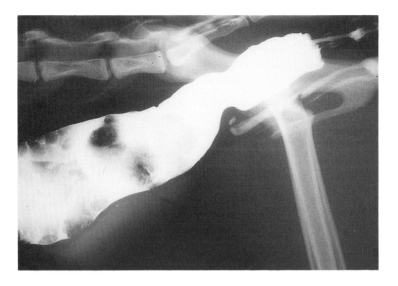

Fig. 8.11 Barium enema in a 1-year-old female spayed domestic short-haired cat demonstrating a rectal stricture. The cat had developed progressive straining to defaecate after being spayed. At surgery, spay adhesions constricting the rectum were found.

such as neurological disease, healed pelvic fractures (Fig. 8.10) or neoplasms (Plate 8.14).

Initial treatment consists of gentle removal of the impacted material using stool softeners and enemas (warm water with or without a mild soap; or 5–10 ml mineral oil; or osmotic laxatives such as Micralax*). Phosphate enemas should not be used since these are toxic for cats. In severe cases, manual removal under general anaesthesia may be required. The underlying cause of constipation should be corrected and recurrences should be prevented using regular grooming, dietary management, stool softeners and laxatives as needed. Bulking diets may include brown bread, bran (1 tablespoon/day), or bulk-forming laxatives such as Isogel† (one 5 ml spoonful daily with food), while milk may be added to the diet to effect. Lubricant laxatives such as liquid or white soft paraffin (Katalax‡, ½–1 inch of paste 1–2 times daily) or mineral oil (2–5 ml/day) may also be given as required. With chronic therapy, cats should be supplemented with vitamins since these laxatives may interfere with the absorption of fat-

soluble vitamins. Mineral oil should have flavouring added since it is tasteless and easily aspirated, which may lead to lipid pneumonia. Stimulant laxatives are useful on a short-term basis only. Subtotal colectomy has proven useful in some cats with severe chronic obstipation or megacolon unresponsive to medical treatment (Webb, 1985; Rosin et al., 1988).

Anorectal disease
Rectal prolapse occasionally results from severe straining due to feline urological syndrome, colitis or constipation. The most common cause is severe enteritis/proctitis due to endoparasites in young kittens. It is usually self-limiting with management of the underlying condition, although gentle repositioning and temporary placement of a pursestring suture in the anus may be necessary. Rarely, surgical treatment via colopexy is required.

Rectal stricture may be associated with chronic proctitis, trauma or neoplasia. Diagnosis is based on signs of tenesmus, ribbon-shaped stool and constipation, and on rectal palpation of a stricture; in equivocal cases a barium enema may be performed (Fig. 8.11). Dietary management with stool softeners can help in mild cases, but otherwise a rectal pull-through surgical procedure may be necessary.

* Micralax; Smith Kline & French Laboratories, Welwyn Garden City, Herts, UK.
† Isogel; Allen & Hanburys Ltd., Greenford, Middx, UK.
‡ Katalax; C-Vet Ltd., Bury St. Edmunds, Suffolk, UK.

Diseases of the anus and anal sacs are not common in the cat. Impaction or abscessation of the anal sacs is seen infrequently, and managed with expression, infusion if infected, and in rare cases surgical excision. Congenital deformities such as atresia ani and urethrorectal fistulas are reported occasionally in newborn kittens (Van den Broek *et al.*, 1988). Surgical correction is possible, but the prognosis is guarded.

DISEASES OF THE EXOCRINE PANCREAS

Feline pancreatic disease is difficult to recognize due to the vagueness of signs and the lack of specific diagnostic tests. However, subclinical chronic inflammation of the pancreatic ducts is a not uncommon autopsy finding in older cats (Owens *et al.*, 1975), suggesting that the actual incidence of pancreatic disease may be underestimated.

Pancreatitis

Chronic pancreatitis is more common than acute pancreatitis, but distinction on clinical symptoms alone is difficult. Chronic pancreatitis in the cat is often subclinical and signs may be seen only during acute exacerbations of the disease. Possible causes are coexisting cholangitis/ cholangiohepatitis, trauma and toxoplasmosis (Kelly *et al.*, 1975; Garvey & Zawie, 1984). In the USA and tropical countries, chronic pancreatic fibrosis and inflammation have been associated with pancreatic infection with parasites (*Eurytrema procyonis*, liver flukes). Clinical signs are vague and variable, and usually include weight loss, depression, anorexia and, less frequently, vomiting (Schaer, 1979). Cats with acute pancreatitis may have abdominal pain and an anterior abdominal mass (Kitchell *et al.*, 1986). Laboratory data may show moderate elevation of liver enzymes (due to concurrent cholangiohepatitis, toxic hepatitis or bile duct compression), hyperglycaemia and neutrophilia. Serum amylase and lipase are often normal or only mildly increased. Abdominal radiography may show loss of contrast and displacement of organs and the duo-

denum in the right cranial abdomen. However, most cases are diagnosed via exploratory laparotomy. Treatment is mostly supportive, including restriction of oral intake, i.v. fluid therapy and prophylactic antibiotics. Occasionally, loss of pancreatic tissue is severe, leading to diabetes mellitus and/or exocrine pancreatic insufficiency.

Exocrine pancreatic insufficiency (EPI)

EPI is rare in the cat, and is mostly seen in older animals as a result of chronic pancreatitis. Signs are non-specific, and include polyphagia, weight loss, diarrhoea and steatorrhoea (Duffell, 1975; Hoskins *et al.*, 1982; Garvey & Zawie, 1984). A vitamin K-responsive coagulopathy has been described in a young cat with EPI and severe steatorrhoea (Perry *et al.*, 1991). Diagnosis is difficult in the cat, due to the lack of specific sensitive tests. Faecal smears stained with Sudan III may reveal steatorrhoea, predominantly due to unsplit fat; however, microscopic tests for undigested food are insensitive assays. The plasma turbidity test has been advocated as a crude screening test for in practice but is subjective and insensitive, while intestinal malabsorption cannot be ruled out with a negative result. The serum trypsinogen-like immunoreactivity (TLI) test, of value in the diagnosis of EPI in the dog (Williams & Batt, 1983), has yet to be validated for the cat. Quantitative assay of proteolytic activity determined by azocasein hydrolysis or radial-enzyme diffusion in at least three faecal samples appears to be more reliable (Williams, 1987; Williams & Reed, 1989). Signs of EPI in the cat closely mimic those of hyperthyroidism and inflammatory bowel disease, and these diseases have to be excluded (Watson *et al.*, 1981). Finally, response to therapy may help with the diagnosis. Treatment consists of pancreatic enzyme replacement (Pancrex powder*, 1 tsp per 10 kg bodyweight in food 2 or 3 times daily).

Neoplasia

Pancreatic neoplasia is uncommon. Adenocarcinoma occurs in older cats and leads to weight

* Pancrex V Powder; Paines & Byrne Ltd., Greenford, Middx, UK.

loss, anorexia, vomiting and occasionally ascites or obstructive jaundice due to common bile duct compression (Garvey & Zawie, 1984). Some cats have a palpable cranial abdominal mass. The diagnosis is generally made at laparotomy. Prognosis is poor, since widespread metastases often exist prior to diagnosis. There are also single reports of a malignant foregut carcinoid arising from the pancreatic enterochromaffin cells (Carakostas et al., 1979), with signs resembling those of pancreatic adenocarcinoma, and gastrinomas, with signs due to duodenal ulceration (Middleton & Watson, 1983; Van der Gaag et al., 1988).

DISEASES OF THE LIVER

Cats have certain unique features of hepatic metabolism and anatomy which are important for the understanding of feline liver disorders. Metabolic features are a relative deficiency of glucuronyl transferase, affecting the liver's ability to metabolize drugs and chemicals, and an inability to synthesize arginine, an important part of the hepatic urea cycle, which predisposes cats to hyperammonaemia during periods of inadequate food intake or anorexia. An anatomical feature is that the major pancreatic duct joins the common bile duct before its entry into the duodenum, which may explain the frequent coexistence of pancreatic and biliary tract disease in the cat.

Diagnosis of liver disease
Clinical signs of feline liver disease are typically chronic, vague and non-specific, and include anorexia, vomiting, diarrhoea and weight loss. Hepatomegaly and jaundice (Plate 8.15) are more specific findings which may be noticed on physical examination. In general, cats with liver disease present with large rather than small livers.

Laboratory evaluation is essential for diagnostic evaluation and to rule out other metabolic illnesses; findings may include bilirubinuria (always significant in the cat, since this species has a high renal threshold for bilirubin), hyperbilirubinaemia, elevated serum alkaline phosphatase (which has a short half-life in the cat, so that even a mild increase is indicative of cholestasis), and elevated serum transaminases (indicative of

hepatic parenchymal damage) (Meyer & Center, 1986). Liver function tests of value in the assessment of non-hyperbilirubinaemic liver disease include the sulphobromophthalein (BSP) retention test, indocyanine green (ICG) clearance, ammonia tolerance, and serum bile acid analysis (Center et al., 1983, 1986). Because of its sensitivity and convenience, the preferred liver function test is measurement of serum bile acid levels during fasting and 2 hours postprandial.

Abdominal radiography gives an indication of liver size and shape. Ultrasonography is a more sensitive method for evaluation of hepatic parenchymal changes, vasculature and the biliary tree. Mesenteric venography is performed in cases of suspected portosystemic shunts (Fig. 8.13). This technique involves laparotomy and cannulation of a mesenteric vein using a catheter of the largest possible diameter (e.g. 19-gauge, 8-inch), after which 5–15 ml of an aqueous contrast medium is manually injected as rapidly as possible and a radiograph taken at the end of injection. However, in most cases of suspected primary liver disease a liver biopsy (percutaneous, keyhole, via laparoscopy or during laparotomy) will be necessary to establish a specific diagnosis, a prognosis and an appropriate therapeutic regimen. A coagulation profile should be evaluated prior to biopsy, especially when done percutaneously.

General treatment of feline liver disease
Medical management of feline hepatobiliary disorders is dependent on the type and severity of the underlying liver disease, but generally includes parenteral fluid therapy as needed, feeding of a balanced diet with moderate to high levels of high biological value protein, and vitamin supplementation (Center, 1986). It may be necessary to force-feed the cat or administer nutrients via nasogastric, pharyngostomy or stomach tube, to ensure adequate caloric (80–100 kcal/kg/day), fluid and vitamin intake. Hepatic encephalopathy may be managed by feeding a restricted protein diet, with daily lactulose* (0.5–2.5 ml orally 3 times daily) added as required; in severe cases, antibiotics capable of reducing intestinal am-

---

* Duphalac; Duphar Laboratories Ltd., Southampton, UK.

monia production and absorption, such as neo-mycin or metronidazole, are given concurrently. Coagulopathies may be managed initially with vitamin K_1 (5 mg subcutaneously once or twice daily) for 2–4 days to rule out vitamin K deficiency secondary to cholestasis; if there is no response, bleeding is likely to be due to hepatocellular failure and a fresh blood or plasma transfusion to replenish clotting factors may be required.

Several systemic infectious and metabolic ill-nesses, such as septicaemia, feline infectious per-itonitis (FIP), diabetes mellitus, hyperthyroidism, myeloproliferative disorders and hypoxia may lead to secondary hepatic involvement and ab-normal liver tests. Consequently, a thorough clinical and laboratory evaluation is necessary to help determine the primary cause of hepatic changes.

Cholangitis/cholangiohepatitis complex
(Plate 8.15)
Cholangiohepatitis is a disease complex consist-ing of cholangitis, cholangiohepatitis and biliary cirrhosis, and is characterized by the nature of the inflammatory infiltrate within and around the bile ducts. Lymphocytic cholangitis, a common cause of feline liver disease in the UK, is thought to have an immune-mediated aetiology, possibly subsequent to suppurative inflammation resulting in immune-mediated self-perpetuating inflam-mation. Suppurative cholangitis probably results from bacterial invasion of the bile duct by enteric bacteria (Hirsch & Doige, 1983). There often is concurrent interstitial pancreatitis (Kelly *et al.*, 1975). Biliary cirrhosis, characterized by exten-sive fibrosis and chronic inflammation, is the un-common final stage. Clinical signs are vague and recurrent in the early stages and may include intermittent anorexia, fever, lethargy, vomiting and jaundice. Cats with lymphocytic cholangitis may be polyphagic in the early stages, and are frequently presented because of ascites and/or jaundice (Lucke & Davies, 1984).

In the early stages, biochemical testing shows mild to moderate increases in serum ALP, GGT, ALT and AST activities. Hyperbilirubinaemia and raised globulins develop later. Lymphocytic cholangitis may be difficult to distinguish from FIP when ascites is present. Cats with FIP usually have more severe signs of anorexia, depression and weight loss, while the ascitic fluid has a higher protein content. FIP titres may also assist in the diagnosis. However, definitive diagnosis of cholangiohepatitis must be based upon liver biopsy and bile culture. For the suppurative form, systemic antibiotics (e.g. ampicillin, amoxycillin, or based on sensitivity) should be administered for at least 1–2 months. The lymphocytic form requires immunosuppressive treatment with prednisolone (2–4 mg/kg/day tapering to 1 mg/kg every other day) to control the signs. Sludging and inspissation of bile is a common complication and may lead to choleliths and biliary obstruction requiring surgery. Prognosis is very variable, and the aim of treatment is more to control than to cure the disease. Intermittent therapy may be necessary as the disease activity waxes and wanes. Successful treatment of suppurative chol-angiohepatitis using cholecystojejunostomy and prolonged antibiotic therapy has been reported (Shaker *et al.*, 1991).

Toxic hepatopathy
There are many causes of hepatotoxicity in the cat, including bacterial, fungal and plant toxins, drugs (e.g. acetaminophen), heavy metals and other environmental chemicals. The clinical course may vary from a chronic debilitating ill-ness to acute liver failure. Elevated serum trans-aminases and bilirubin are common laboratory findings. Liver biopsy may reveal a characteristic pattern of zonal necrosis suggesting toxicity; how-ever, the actual cause is often not ascertained (Zawie & Garvey, 1984). Cats that do not die from acute liver failure often recover with supportive care, which should include fluid and antibiotic therapy with vitamin and glucose supplementation. Parenteral antibiotics are recommended because of the increased risk of septicaemia and endotoxaemia associated with reduced hepatic reticuloendothelial activity.

Feline hepatic lipidosis (Plate 8.16)
Fatty infiltration of the liver may occur with ob-esity, endocrine disorders such as diabetes mel-

litus, various toxins and hypoxia. In the cat, hepatic lipidosis is often idiopathic and characterized by extreme accumulation of triglycerides due to a disruption in hepatic lipid metabolism, resulting in severe liver dysfunction (Barsanti *et al.*, 1977; Thornburg *et al.*, 1982; Jacobs *et al.*, 1989). This syndrome is very common in cats in North America but has not yet been reported as a specific entity in the UK. The aetiology is unknown, but obesity, chronic anorexia, protein–calorie imbalance and amino acid deficiency have been implicated (Rogers & Cornelius, 1985).

Common clinical signs are anorexia of several weeks' duration, progressive weight loss, jaundice, hepatomegaly and, less frequently, hepatic encephalopathy. Obesity is a predisposing factor. Many cats have a history of vomiting. Liver biochemistries are characterized by hyperbilirubinaemia and a marked elevation of ALP, consistent with severe intrahepatic cholestasis. Serum GGT activity, however, usually remains within the normal range or it becomes only mildly elevated, in contrast to other feline liver disorders wherein the magnitude of increase in GGT parallels that of ALP. Definitive diagnosis requires a liver aspirate or biopsy (Plate 8.16), demonstrating obvious hepatocellular cytosolic vacuolation. Supportive care and long-term force-feeding of a balanced cat food diet are the most important aspects of therapy, and it is frequently necessary to place a nasogastric or gastrostomy tube to facilitate force-feeding. The nasogastric tube is less comfortable than a gastrostomy tube, and the latter is therefore used for long-term nutritional management at home. Prognosis used to be guarded to poor, but recently a 65% survival rate was described following weeks to months of intensive nutritional support via a surgically placed gastrostomy tube (Jacobs *et al.*, 1989).

Neoplasia

Primary hepatic tumours are uncommon in the cat. Hepatocellular carcinoma, bile duct carcinoma and carcinoids have been reported, causing progressive weight loss, jaundice, intermittent vomiting and sometimes a palpable abdominal mass (Feldman *et al.*, 1976; Alexander & Kock, 1982; Post & Patnaik, 1992). Ultrasonography is valuable in indicating whether hepatic involvement is focal or diffuse. Diagnosis is by biopsy. Prognosis is poor unless focal tumour resection is possible.

More commonly, the liver is the site of metastatic neoplasia or it is involved in systemic neoplasia (e.g. lymphosarcoma, disseminated mastocytosis) (Fig. 8.12, Plate 8.17). While primary hepatic lymphosarcoma is rare, the liver is often involved in multicentric lymphosarcoma along with the spleen and lymph nodes. Myeloproliferative disorders and systemic mast cell disease are also common. Combination chemotherapy is possible for lymphosarcoma and mastocytosis.

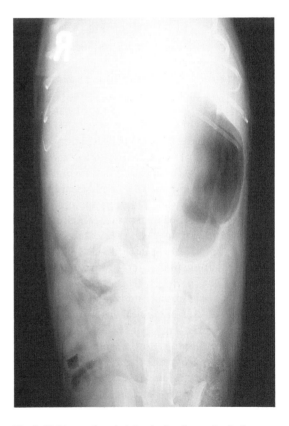

Fig. 8.12 Ventrodorsal abdominal radiograph of a 6-year-old domestic short-haired cat with marked right-sided liver enlargement due to hepatic lymphosarcoma.

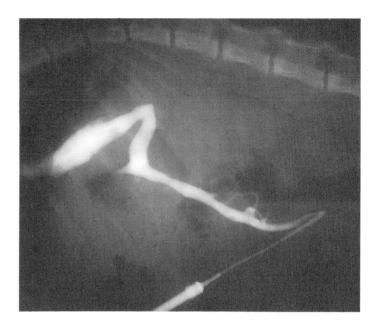

Fig. 8.13 Lateral abdominal radiograph during contrast mesenteric venography of a young cat with an extrahepatic portosystemic shunt. (Reprinted with permission, Rutgers 1993.)

Congenital portosystemic shunts

Congenital portosystemic shunts in cats are becoming more frequently recognized (Rothuizen *et al.*, 1982; Berger *et al.*, 1986; Scavelli *et al.*, 1986; Blaxter *et al.*, 1988). Most cats with congenital shunts demonstrate neurobehavioural signs from a young age, with first signs appearing around the age of 3 months. Clinical signs are mostly related to hepatic encephalopathy and include intermittent ptyalism, anorexia, depression, amaurosis (apparent blindness), behavioural changes and occasionally seizures. Neurological signs may or may not be associated with meals. Non-specific signs are anorexia or polyphagia, diarrhoea, vomiting and polydipsia. Common findings on physical examination are small body size, prominent kidneys and a typical copper-coloured iris (Center & Magne, 1990). Elevated blood ammonia and bile acid concentrations are the most consistent laboratory findings. Liver enzyme activities may be mildly elevated. Urinary ammonium biurate crystals occur less frequently than in the dog. Liver size is usually normal on radiographs. Ultrasonography can sometimes demonstrate the presence of a shunt, but mesenteric venography is usually performed to confirm the diagnosis and locate the anomalous vessel (Fig. 8.13). Surgical correction by partial or complete ligation of the anomalous vessel is the treatment of choice (Birchard, 1984; Birchard & Sherding, 1986). Most congenital portosystemic shunts in cats are extrahepatic and are therefore amenable to surgical management, although occasionally intrahepatic shunts are accessible for ligation. Medical treatment before surgery primarily involves minimizing signs of hepatic encephalopathy, using low protein diets, lactulose, and neomycin or metronidazole, and has to be continued for variable amounts of time following surgery while the liver regenerates. In some cases, recurrence of neurological signs was associated with recanalization of the shunt (Blaxter *et al.*, 1988). If surgical ligation is not possible, conservative treatment may be continued; prognosis for these cases has been variable.

Bile duct obstruction

Extrahepatic bile duct obstruction may be due to sludged bile associated with the cholangiohepatitis complex, bile pigment stones, neoplasia, compression of the common bile duct by pancreatitis, or bile duct strictures. Clinical signs vary dependent upon the underlying cause but usually include anorexia, vomiting, fever and weight loss. Jaundice is seen with complete biliary obstruction. Serum bilirubin, cholesterol and ALP activity are generally markedly increased, while transaminase activities vary. Serum bile acid concentrations are usually very high. With complete bile duct obstruction, stools may become acholic, and there may be bleeding tendencies that are responsive to vitamin K administration. Ultrasonography is the most useful technique to evaluate the biliary tree for obstruction. Choleliths, which are usually composed of cholesterol, bilirubin and calcium, are usually radiolucent and do not show up on plain abdominal radiographs (Heidner & Campbell, 1985). Surgical intervention will be necessary in the majority of cases, and may involve a cholecystectomy and bile culture in case of choleliths, or more radical biliary diversion procedures in case of strictures or neoplasia. Cholelithiasis is often associated with cholangitis, necessitating long-term antibiotic therapy postoperatively.

Miscellaneous liver diseases
Infection with liver flukes (*Platynosonum* spp.) has been described in cats in North America and tropical regions (Bielsa & Greiner, 1984; Lewis *et al.*, 1991). Signs are often mild, and diagnosis is difficult since the eggs are only sporadically found on faecal examination. Hepatic involvement in toxoplasmosis is rare, although acute hepatitis associated with a *Toxoplasma gondii* infection has been reported in a young adult cat (Dubey *et al.*, 1990).

Biliary cysts are occasionally found and may be associated with pancreatic or renal cysts. They rarely give clinical problems, although large cysts may cause progressive abdominal enlargement and discomfort. Surgical excision is curative. Congenital biliary atresia with associated multiple large biliary cysts has been reported in a kitten with signs of jaundice and hepatomegaly (Hampson *et al.*, 1987).

DISEASES OF THE PERITONEUM

Peritoneal disease may be suspected when there is abdominal effusion or pain, or a history of acute abdominal trauma. Physical examination and abdominal radiography help to distinguish abdominal effusion from other causes of abdominal enlargement, such as pregnancy, pyometra, increased liver or kidney size, and neoplasia (Fig. 8.14). Differentiation among types of effusion is based on clinical presentation, radiographic or ultrasonographic findings, and the results of peritoneal fluid analysis.

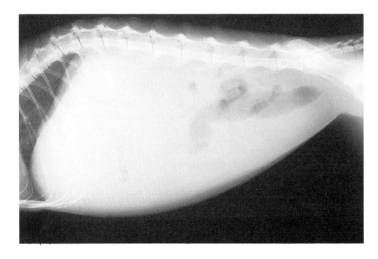

Fig. 8.14 Lateral abdominal radiograph of a 2-year-old domestic short-haired cat with ascites. Laparotomy and liver biopsy were consistent with lymphocytic cholangitis.

Table 8.1 Characteristics of peritoneal effusions.

Parameter	Transudate	Modified transudate	Exudate
Total protein (g/l)	<25	25–50	>30
Specific gravity	< 1.018	1.010–1.030	≫ 1.018
Number of cells ($\times 10^9$/l)	≪ 0.5	0.5–5.0	> 5.0

Abdominal effusion

Abdominal midline paracentesis using a 21 gauge needle and syringe is performed following radiographic confirmation, usually with the animal in lateral recumbency. Fluid samples should be collected aseptically and used for laboratory evaluation (cell count, specific gravity, total protein content and cytology) and, if indicated, bacterial culture. Classification of effusions into transudates, modified transudates or exudates is based on the physicochemical characteristics of the effusion (see Table 8.1). Further subclassification is based on the cytological features.

Aetiology of peritoneal effusions

Pure transudates are thin and clear, have low protein values, and contain few, mononuclear cells. They result from hypoalbuminaemia (usually less than 10 g/l) due to glomerulonephropathies, protein-losing enteropathies and, rarely, severe liver disease.

Modified transudates are thin, often serosanguinous, and contain more protein and cells, which are predominantly mononuclear. They are found with portal hypertension, abdominal neoplasia, chylous effusion (rare, and usually associated with neoplasia), and occasionally with congestive heart failure. Cardiac disease in the cat usually results in pleural effusion only. Liver disease in the cat rarely results in ascites, except for lymphocytic cholangitis which may be accompanied by a high-protein effusion very similar to the fluid seen with FIP.

Exudates are cloudy, and the colour varies from reddish-brown to yellow. Protein content and cell count are high because of increased number of inflammatory cells. If the inflammatory effusion is septic, degenerated neutrophils will be present, and bacteria may be seen. Septic exudates occur with intestinal perforation, penetrating wounds, ruptured pyometra or abscesses, and bacterial peritonitis. Non-septic inflammation is seen with leakage of bile or urine, FIP and circulatory compromise (e.g. thrombosis or torsion).

Haemoabdomen is rare in the cat, but may occur with traumatic injury, neoplasia (haemangiosarcoma, vascular tumour) and bleeding disorders (Warfarin, thrombocytopenia). Chylous abdominal effusion is seen occasionally, usually in association with intra-abdominal neoplasia affecting lymphatics.

Peritonitis

Primary peritonitis is rare in the cat, except for FIP. Secondary peritonitis is more common and usually develops following abdominal trauma, surgery, or necrosis and rupture of intra-abdominal viscera. Chemical peritonitis, due to leakage of bile, urine or pancreatic enzymes, often progresses with time into septic peritonitis.

Clinical signs include vomiting, anorexia, depression, pyrexia, abdominal pain or distension, and in severe cases shock. Radiographs are seldom diagnostic but may reveal gastrointestinal ileus, loss of serosal detail, abdominal fluid, and free gas in case of a ruptured viscus. Laboratory examination usually reveals a neutrophilic leucocytosis with left shift; in acute peritonitis, however, neutropenia will occur. Abdominal paracentesis, cytology and culture of abdominal fluid are essential for the diagnosis.

Early treatment is important to prevent complications, and consists of fluid (and plasma) replacement, broad-spectrum antibiotics and removal of the underlying cause if identified.

Except for FIP, peritonitis usually warrants exploratory laparotomy to locate and correct the source of infection.

REFERENCES

Ablin L.W., Moore F.M., Shields Henney L.H. & Berg J. (1991) Intestinal diverticular malformations in dogs and cats. *Compend. Cont. Educ. Pract. Vet.* **13**, 426–30.

Abood S.K. & Buffington C.A.T. (1992) Enteral feeding of dogs and cats: 51 cases (1989–1991). *J. Am. Vet. Med. Assoc.* **201**, 619–22.

Alexander R.W. & Kock R.A. (1982) Primary hepatic carcinoid (APUD cell carcinoma) in the cat. *J. Small Anim. Pract.* **23**, 767.

Alroy J., Leav I., Delellis R. & Weinstein R. (1975) Distinctive intestinal mast cell neoplasia of domestic cats. *Lab. Invest.* **33**, 159.

Barsanti J.A., Jones B.D., Spano J.S. & Taylow H.W. (1977) Prolonged anorexia associated with hepatic lipidosis in three cats. *Feline Pract.* **7**, 52–7.

Batt R.M. & Hall E.J. (1989) Chronic enteropathies in the dog. *J. Small Anim. Pract.* **30**, 3.

Bennett A.M. (1977) Tyzzer's disease in cats experimentally infected with feline leukemia virus. *Vet. Microbiol.* **2**, 49.

Bennett M., Baxby D., Blundell N., Gaskell C.J., Hart C.A. & Kelly D.F. (1985) Cryptosporidiosis in the domestic cat. *Vet. Rec.* **116**, 73–4.

Berger B., Whiting P.G., Breznock E.M., Bruhl-Day R. & Moore P.F. (1986) Congenital feline portosystemic shunts. *J. Am. Vet. Med. Assoc.* **188**, 517–20.

Bielsa L.M. & Greiner E.C. (1984) Liver flukes (*Platynosonum concinnum*) in cats. *J. Am. Anim. Hosp. Assoc.* **21**, 269–74.

Bilbrey A., Dulisch M.I., & Stallings B. (1989) Chemical burns caused by benzalkonium chloride in eight surgical cases. *J. Am. Anim. Hosp. Assoc.* **25**, 31–4.

Birchard S.J. (1984) Surgical management of portosystemic shunts in dogs and cats. *Compend. Cont. Educ. Pract. Vet.* **6**, 795–800.

Birchard S.J. & Sherding R.G. (1992) Feline portosystemic shunts. *Compend. Cont. Educ. Pract. Vet.* **14**, 1295–300.

Birchard S.J. Couto C.G. & Johnson S. (1986) Nonlymphoid intestinal neoplasia in 32 dogs and 14 cats. *J. Am. Anim. Hosp. Assoc.* **12**, 307.

Blaxter A.C., Holt P.E., Pearson G.R., Gibbs C. & Gruffydd-Jones T.J. (1988) Congenital portosystemic shunt in the cat: a report of 9 cases. *J. Small Anim. Pract.* **29**, 631–45.

Bright R.M. & Bauer M.S. (1989) Surgery of the digestive system. In Sherding R.G. (ed) *The Cat. Diseases and Clinical Management*, vol. 2. Churchill Livingstone, New York, p. 1047.

Bright R.M., Sackman J.E., Denovo C. & Toal S. (1990) Hiatal hernia in the dog and cat: a retrospective study of 16 cases. *J. Small Anim. Pract.* **31**, 244.

Carakostas M.C., Kennedy G.A. & Kittleson M.D. (1979) Malignant foregut carcinoid in a domestic cat. *Vet. Pathol.* **16**, 607.

Carnevale J.M., Kallfelz F.A., Chapman G. & Meguid M.M. (1991) Nutritional assessment: guidelines to selecting patients for nutritional support. *Compend. Cont. Educ. Pract. Vet.* **13**, 115–21.

Center S.A. (1986) Feline liver disorders and their management. *Compend. Cont. Educ. Pract. Vet.* **8**, 889–902.

Center S.A. & Magne M.L. (1990) History, physical examination, and clinicopathologic features of portosystemic vascular anomalies in the dog and cat. *Sem. Vet. Med. Surg. (Sm. Anim.)* **5**, 83–93.

Center S.A., Bunch S.E., Baldwin B.H., Hornbuckle W.E. & Tennant B.C. (1983) Comparison of sulfobromophthalein and indocyanine green clearances in the cat. *Am. J. Vet. Res.* **44**, 727–30.

Center S.A., Baldwin B.H. & Erb H. (1986) Bile acid concentrations in the diagnosis of hepatobiliary disease in the cat. *J. Am. Vet. Med. Assoc.* **189**, 891–6.

Clifford D.H., Soifer F.K. & Wilson C.F. (1971) Congenital achalasia of the oesophagus in four cats of common ancestry. *J. Am. Vet. Med. Ass.* **158**, 1554.

Cotter S.M. (1981) Oral-pharyngeal neoplasms in the cat. *J. Am. Anim. Hosp. Assoc.* **17**, 917–20.

Cotter S.M., Hardy W.D. & Essex M. (1975) Association of feline leukaemia virus with lymphosarcoma and other disorders in the cat. *J. Am. Vet. Med. Ass.* **166**, 449–54.

Crane S.W. (1980) Placement and maintenance of a temporary feeding tube gastrostomy in the dog and cat. *Compend. Cont. Educ. Pract. Vet.* **10**, 770.

Crowe D.T. (1990) Nutritional support for the hospitalized patient: an introduction to tube feeding. *Compend. Cont. Educ. Pract. Vet.* **12**, 1711–20.

Dennis R., Herrtage M.E., Jefferies A.R. & Matic S. (1987) A case of hyperplastic gastropathy in a cat. *J. Small Anim. Pract.* **28**, 491.

Dillon A.R., Boosinger T.R. & Blevins T.W. (1987) Campylobacter enteritis in dogs and cats. *Compend. Cont. Educ. Pract. Vet.* **9**, 1176.

Dow S.W., Jones R.L., Henik R.A. & Husted P.W. (1989) Clinical features of salmonellosis in cats: six cases (1981–1986). *J. Am. Vet. Med. Ass.* **194**, 1464.

Dubey J.P., Zajac A., Osofsky S.A. & Tobias L. (1990) Acute primary toxoplasmic hepatitis in an adult cat shedding Toxoplasma gondii oocysts. *J. Am. Vet. Med. Ass.* **197**, 1616–8.

Duffell S.J. (1975) Some aspects of pancreatic disease in

the cat. *J. Small Anim. Pract.* **16**, 365.

Ellison G.W., Lewis D.D., Philips L. & Tarvin G.B. (1987) Esophageal hiatal hernia in small animals: Literature review and a modified surgical technique. *J. Am. Anim. Hosp. Assoc.* **23**, 391.

Evans S.M. & Biery D.N. (1983) Double contrast radiography in the cat. *Vet. Radiol.* **24**, 3.

Feldman B.F., Strafuss A.C. & Gabbert N. (1976) Bile duct carcinoma in the cat. Three case reports. *Feline Pract.* **6**, 33.

Felts J.F., Fox P.R. & Burk R.L. (1984) Thread and sewing needles as gastrointestinal foreign bodies in the cat: a review of 64 cases. *J. Am. Vet. Med. Assoc.* **184**, 56.

Fulton R.B. & Dennis J.S. (1992) Blind percutaneous placement of a gastrostomy tube for nutritional support in dogs and cats. *J. Am. Vet. Med. Assoc.* **201**, 697–700.

Garvey M.S. & Zawie D.A. (1984) Feline pancreatic disease. *Vet. Clin. North. Am. (Sm. Anim. Pract.)* **14**, 1231.

Gaskell C.J., Knowles J.O. & Gaskell R.M. (1988) Chronic stomatitis in the cat. In Grunsell C.S.G., Raw M.E. & Hill F.W.H. (eds), *The Veterinary Annual*, vol. 28. Scientechnica, London, pp. 246–50.

Goodwin M.A. & Barsanti J.A. (1990) Intractable diarrhea associated with intestinal cryptosporidiosis in a domestic cat also infected with feline leukemia virus. *J. Am. Anim. Hosp. Assoc.* **26**, 365–8.

Gruffydd-Jones T.J., Gaskell C.J. & Gibbs C. (1979) Clinical and radiographic features of anterior mediastinal lymphosarcoma in the cat; a review of thirty cases. *Vet. Rec.* **104**, 304.

Hampson E.C.G.M., Filippich L.J., Kelly W.R. & Evans K. (1987) Congenital biliary atresia in a cat: a case report. *J. Small Anim. Pract.* **28**, 39–48.

Happe R.P., Van der Gaag I. & Wolvekamp W.T.C. (1978) Oesophageal squamous cell carcinoma in two cats. *Tijdschr. Diergeneesk.* **103**, 1080.

Hargis A.M., Prieur D.J. & Blanchard J.L. (1982) Chronic fibrosing gastritis associated with Ollulanus tricuspis in a cat. *Vet. Pathol.* **19**, 320.

Hargis A.M., Prieur D.J. & Blanchard J.L. (1983a) Prevalence, lesions, and differential diagnosis of Ollulanus tricuspis infection in cats. *Vet. Pathol.* **20**, 71.

Hargis A.M., Prieur D.J. & Gaillard E.T. (1983b) Chlamydial infection of the gastric mucosa in twelve cats. *Vet. Pathol.* **20**, 170.

Harvey C.E. (1986) Oral surgery: radical resection of maxillary and mandibular lesions. *Vet. Clin. North. Am.* **16**, 983.

Harvey C.E. (1987) Palate defects in dogs and cats. *Compend. Cont. Educ. Pract. Vet.* **9**, 404–18.

Harvey C.E. (1991) Oral inflammatory diseases in cats. *J.*

Am. Anim. Hosp. Assoc. **27**, 585–91.

Heidner G.L. & Campbell K.L. (1985) Cholelithiasis in a cat. *J. Am. Vet. Med. Assoc.* **186**, 176–7.

Hendrick M. (1981) A spectrum of hypereosinophilic syndromes exemplified by six cats with eosinophilic enteritis. *Vet. Pathol.* **18**, 188.

Hirsch V.M. & Doige C.E. (1983) Suppurative cholangitis in cats. *J. Am. Vet. Med. Assoc.* **182**, 1223–6.

Hoenig M., Mahaffey M.B., Parnell P.G. & Styles M.E. (1990) Megaesophagus in two cats. *J. Am. Vet. Med. Assoc.* **196**, 763–5.

Hoskins J.D., Turk J.R. & Turk M.A. (1982) Feline pancreatic insufficiency. *Vet. Med. Small Anim. Clin.* **77**, 1745.

Ishida T., Washizu T. & Toriyabe K. (1989) Feline immunodeficiency virus in cats from Japan. *J. Am. Vet. Med. Assoc.* **194**, 221.

Johnessee J.S. & Hurvitz A.I. (1983) Feline plasma cell gingivitis. *J. Am. Anim. Hosp. Assoc.* **19**, 179–81.

Johnston K., Lamport A.S. & Batt R.M. (1993) An unexpected bacterial flora in the proximal small intestine of normal cats. *Vet. Rec.* **132**, 302–303.

Kelly D.F., Baggott D.G. & Gaskell C.J. (1975) Jaundice in the cat associated with inflammation of the biliary tract and pancreas. *J. Small Anim. Pract.* **16**, 163.

Kirkpatrick C.E. (1986) Feline giardiasis: a review. *J. Small Anim. Pract.* **27**, 69.

Kitchell B.E., Strombeck D.R., Cullin J. & Harrold D. (1986) Clinical and pathological changes in experimentally induced acute pancreatitis in cats. *Am. J. Vet. Res.* **47**, 1170.

Knowles J.O., Gaskell R.M., Gaskell C.J., Harvey C.E. & Lutz H. (1989) Prevalence of feline calicivirus, feline leukaemia virus and antibodies to FIV in cats with chronic stomatitis. *Vet. Rec.* **124**, 336–8.

Kronfeld D.J. (1983) Feeding cats and feline nutrition. *Compend. Cont. Educ. Pract. Vet.* **5**, 419.

Lane J.G. (1982) *ENT and Oral Surgery of the Dog and Cat.* John Wright, Bristol.

Leib M.S., Sponenberg D.P., Wilcke J.R. & Loar A.S. (1986) Suppurative colitis in a cat. *J. Am. Vet. Med. Ass.* **188**, 739.

Lewis D.T., Malone J.B., Taboada J., Hribernik T.N., Pechman R.D. & Dean P.W. (1991) Cholangiohepatitis and choledochectasia associated with Amphimerus pseudofelineus in a cat. *J. Am. Anim. Hosp. Assoc.* **27**, 156–61.

Lucke V.M. & Davies J.D. (1984) Progressive lymphocytic cholangitis in the cat. *J. Small Anim. Pract.* **25**, 249–60.

McCandlish I.A.P., Nash A.S. & Peggram A. (1984) Unusual vascular ring in a·cat: left aortic arch with right ligamentum arteriosum. *Vet. Rec.* **114**, 338.

Maddison J.E. & Allan G.S. (1990) Megaesophagus attributable to lead toxicosis in a cat. *J. Am. Vet. Med. Ass.* **188**, 739.

Martland M.F., Fowles S., Poulton G.J. & Baxby D. (1983) Poxvirus infection of a domestic cat. *Vet. Rec.* **112**, 171–2.

Meyer D.J. & Center S.A. (1986) Approach to the diagnosis of liver disorders in dogs and cats. *Compend. Cont. Educ. Pract. Vet.* **8**, 880–8.

Middleton D.J. & Watson A.D.J. (1983) Duodenal ulceration associated with gastrin secreting pancreatic tumor in a cat. *J. Am. Vet. Med. Ass.* **183**, 461.

Monticello T.M., Levy M.G., Bunch S.E. & Fairley R.A. (1987) Cryptosporidiosis in a feline leukemia virus-positive cat. *J. Am. Vet. Med. Ass.* **191**, 705.

Moreland K.J. (1988) Ulcer disease of the upper gastro-intestinal tract in small animals: pathophysiology, diagnosis, and management. *Compend. Cont. Educ. Pract. Vet.* **10**, 1265.

Muir P. (1990) Isolation of a novel virus from cats with nictitating membrane protrusion and diarrhoea. *Proc. Ann. Meet. Am. Anim. Hosp. Assoc.* p. 669.

Nelson R.W., Dimperio M.E. & Long G.G. (1984) Lymphocytic-plasmacytic colitis in the cat. *J. Am. Vet. Med. Ass.* **184**, 1133.

Obwolo M.J. & Gruffydd-Jones T.J. (1977) Yersinia pseudotuberculosis in the cat. *Vet. Rec.* **100**, 424.

Orr C.M., Kelly, D.F. & Lucke V.M. (1980a) Tuberculosis in cats. A report of two cases. *J. Small Anim. Pract.* **21**, 247.

Orr C.M., Gruffydd-Jones T.J. & Kelly D.F. (1980b) Ileal polyps in Siamese cats. *J. Small Anim. Pract.* **21**, 669.

Owens J.M., Drazner F.H. & Gilbertson S.R. (1975) Pancreatic disease in the cat. *J. Am. Anim. Hosp. Assoc.* **11**, 83.

Patnaik A.K., Liu S.K. & Johnson G.F. (1976) Feline intestinal adenocarcinoma. A clinicopathologic study of 22 cases. *Vet. Pathol.* **13**, 1.

Patnaik A.K., Johnson G.F. & Greene R.W. (1981) Surgical resection of intestinal adenocarcinoma in the cat with survival of 28 months. *J. Am. Vet. Med. Assoc.* **178**, 479.

Pearson J.C., Gaskell C.G., Gibbs C. & Waterman A. (1974) Pyloric and oesophageal dysfunction in the cat. *J. Small Anim. Pract.* **15**, 487–501.

Pederson N.C., Boyle J.F., Floyd K., Fudge A. & Barker J. (1981) An enteric corona virus infection of cats and its relationship to feline infectious peritonitis. *Am. J. Vet. Res.* **42**, 368.

Pederson N.C., Ho E.W. & Brown M.L. (1987) Isolation of a T-lymphotropic virus from domestic cats with an immunodeficiency-like syndrome. *Science* **235**, 790–3.

Perry L.A., Williams D.A. & Pidgeon G. (1989) Feline exocrine pancreatic insufficiency associated with a coagulopathy. *Proc. 7th Ann. Meeting Am. Coll. Vet.*

Int. Med. San Diego, p. 134.

Perry L.A., Williams D.A., Pidgeon G.L. & Bosinger T.R. (1991) Exocrine pancreatic insufficiency with associated coagulopathy in a cat. *J. Am. Anim. Hosp. Assoc.* **27**, 109–14.

Peterson S.L. (1983) Esophageal hiatal hernia in a cat. *J. Am. Vet. Med. Assoc.* **183**, 325.

Pollock R.V.H. (1984) The parvoviruses. Part I. Feline panleukopenia virus and mink enteritis virus. *Compend. Cont. Educ. Pract. Vet.* **6**, 227.

Post G. & Patnaik A.K. (1992) Nonhematopoietic hepatic neoplasm in cats: 21 cases (1983–1988). *J. Am. Vet. Med. Assoc.* **210**, 1080–2.

Prymak C., Saunders H.M. & Washabau R.J. (1989) Hiatal hernia repair by restoration and stabilization of normal anatomy: an evaluation in 4 dogs and 1 cat. *Vet. Surg.* **18**, 386–91.

Reichart P.A., Durr U.M., Triadan H. & Vickendey G. (1984) Periodontal disease in the domestic cat. *J. Periodont. Res.* **19**, 67–75.

Reindel J.F., Trapp A.L., Armstrong P.J. & Stickle R.L. (1987) Recurrent plasmacytic stomatitis-pharyngitis in a cat with esophagitis, fibrosing gastritis, and gastric nematodiasis. *J. Am. Vet. Med. Assoc.* **190**, 65–7.

Rogers K.S. & Cornelius L.M. (1985) Feline icterus. *Compend. Cont. Educ. Pract. Vet.* **7**, 391.

Rosenkrantz W. (1989) Eosinophilic granuloma complex (confusion). *Vet. Focus.* **1**, 29.

Rosin E., Walshaw R., Mehlhaff C., Matthiesen D., Orsher R. & Kusba J. (1988) Subtotal colectomy for treatment of chronic constipation associated with idiopathic megacolon in cats: 38 cases (1979–1985). *J. Am. Vet. Med. Ass.* **193**, 850.

Rothuizen J., Van den Ingh T.S.G.A.M., Voorhout G., Van der Luer R.J.T. & Wouda W. (1982) Congenital portosystemic shunts in sixteen dogs and three cats. *J. Small Anim. Pract.* **23**, 67–81.

Rutgers H.C. (1993) Diagnosis and management of portosystemic shunts in the dog and cat. *In Practice* **15**, 175.

Rutgers H.C., Batt R.M. & Kelly D.F. (1988) Lymphocytic-plasmacytic enteritis associated with bacterial overgrowth in a dog. *J. Am. Vet. Med. Ass.* **192**, 1739.

Scavelli T.D., Hornbuckle W.E., Roth L., Rendano V.T., De Lahunta A., Center S.A., French T.W. & Zimmer J.F. (1986) Portosystemic shunts in cats: seven cases (1976–1984). *J. Am. Vet. Med. Ass.* **189**, 317–25.

Scott D.W. (1980) Feline dermatology 1900–1978: A monograph. *J. Am. Anim. Hosp. Assoc.* **16**, 331.

Schaer M.S. (1979) A clinicopathologic survey of acute pancreatitis in thirty dogs and five cats. *J. Am. Anim. Hosp. Assoc.* **15**, 681.

Shaker E.H., Zawie D.A., Garvey M.S. & Gilbertson S.R. (1991) Suppurative cholangiohepatitis in a cat. *J.*

Am. Anim. Hosp. Assoc. **27**, 148–50.

Sharp N.J.H., Nash A.S. & Griffiths I.R.G. (1984) Feline dysautonomia (the Key–Gaskell syndrome): A clinical and pathological study of forty cases. *J. Small Anim. Pract.* **25**, 599.

Sherding R.G. (1989) Diseases of the intestines. In Sherding R.G. (ed) *The Cat. Diseases and Clinical Management*, vol. 2. Churchill Livingstone, New York, p. 955.

Strombeck D.R. & Guildford W.G. (1990) Adverse reactions to food. In Strombeck D.R. & Guildford W.G. (eds), *Small Animal Gastroenterology*, 2nd edn. Stonegate Publishing, Davis, Calif., p. 344.

Tams T.R. (1986a) Chronic feline inflammatory bowel disorders. Part I. Idiopathic inflammatory bowel disease. *Compend. Cont. Educ. Pract. Vet.* **8**, 371.

Tams T.R. (1986b) Chronic feline inflammatory bowel disorders. Part II. Feline eosinophilic enteritis and lymphosarcoma. *Compend. Cont. Educ. Pract. Vet.* **8**. 464.

Thornburg L.P., Simpson S. & Diglio K. (1982) Fatty liver syndrome in cats. *J. Am. Anim. Hosp. Assoc.* **18**, 397.

Turk M.A.M., Gallina A.M. & Russell T.S. (1981) Non-hematopoietic gastrointestinal neoplasia in cats: a retrospective study. *Vet. Pathol.* **18**, 614.

Twaddle A.A. (1971) Congenital pyloric stenosis in two kittens corrected by pyloroplasty. *New Zeal. Vet. J.* **19**, 26.

Twedt D.C. & Tams T.R. (1989) Diseases of the stomach. In Sherding D.G.(ed) *The Cat. Diseases and Clinical Management*, vol. 2. Churchill Livingstone, New York, p. 929.

Van den Broek A.H.M., Else R.W. & Hunter M.S. (1988) Atresia ani and urethrorectal fistula in a kitten. *J. Small Anim. Pract.* **29**, 91.

Van der Gaag I., Van den Ingh T.S.G.A.M., Lamers C.B. & Lindeman J. (1988) Zollinger–Ellison syndrome in a cat. *Vet. Quart.* **10**, 151.

Van Kruiningen H.J., Ryan M.J. & Shindel N.M. (1983) The classification of feline colitis. *J. Comp. Path.* **93**, 275.

Van Niel M.H., Van der Gaag I. & Van den Ingh T.S.G.A.M. (1989) Polyposis of the small intestine in a young cat. *Zentralbla. Veterinarmed.* **36**, 161.

Vernon F.F. & Roudebush P. (1980) Primary oesophageal carcinoma in a cat. *J. Am. Vet. Med. Ass.* **16**, 547.

Waldron D.R., Moon M., Leib M.S., Barber D. & Asbury M.A.Y.S. (1990) Oesophageal hiatal hernia in two cats. *J. Small Anim. Pract.* **31**, 259.

Wallace L.J., Guffy M.M., Gray A.P. & Clifford J.H. (1972) Anterior cervical sialocele (salivary cyst) in a domestic cat. *J. Am. Anim. Hosp. Assoc.* **8**, 74.

Walton G.S. & Parish W.E. (1968) Spontaneous allergic dermatitis and enteritis in a cat. *J. Small Anim. Pract.* **83**, 35.

Watson D.J., Church D.B., Middleton D.J. & Rothwell T.L.W. (1981) Weight loss in cats which eat well. *J. Small Anim. Pract.* **22**, 473–82.

Webb S.M. (1985) Surgical management of acquired megacolon in the cat. *J. Small Anim. Pract.* **26**, 399.

Wheaton L.G., Blevins W.E. & Weirich W.E. (1984) Persistent right aortic arch associated with other vascular anomalies in two cats. *J. Am. Vet. Med. Ass.* **184**, 848.

Wilkinson G.T. (1970) Chronic papillomatous oesophagitis in a young cat. *Vet. Rec.* **87**, 355.

Willard M.D. (1985) Newer concepts in treatment of secretory diarrheas. *J. Am. Vet. Med. Ass.* **186**, 86.

Willard M.D., Dalley J.B. & Trapp A.L. (1985) Lymphocytic-plasmacytic enteritis in a cat. *J. Am. Vet. Med. Ass.* **186**, 181.

Williams D.A. (1987) New tests of pancreatic and small intestinal function. *Compend. Cont. Educ. Pract. Vet.* **9**, 1173–1176.

Williams D.A. & Batt R.M. (1983) Diagnosis of canine exocrine pancreatic insufficiency by the assay of serum trypsin-like immunoreactivity. *J. Small Anim. Pract.* **24**, 583–8.

Williams D.A. & Reed S.D. (1989) Evaluation of pancreatic function in cats by assay of faecal proteolytic activity – comparison of two methods. In *Proc. World Sm. Anim. Vet. Assoc. Congress, Harrogate. England*, p. 199.

Yamamoto J.K., Hansen H. & Ho E.W. (1989) Epidemiology and clinical aspects of feline immunodeficiency virus infection in cats from the continental United States and possible modes of transmission. *J. Am. Vet. Med. Assoc.* **194**, 213.

Zawie D.A. (1987) Medical diseases of the oesophagus. *Compend. Cont. Educ. Pract. Vet.* **9**, 1146.

Chapter 9 / The Eye

J. SANSOM

CLINICAL EXAMINATION

An ophthalmoscopic examination may be carried out in isolation or as part of a general clinical examination. This can be particularly relevant in the neonate where the eye and adenexa should be examined for the presence of congenital and inherited defects. When examining the eyes the general health of the patient should always be considered. Some eye conditions may cause systemic signs, and likewise systemic disease may manifest as an ocular condition. A detailed case history should be obtained, and the breed, age and sex may be particularly relevant in ocular disease.

An ophthalmoscopic examination should always be carried out in a room capable of being darkened. Patients should first be observed with as little restraint as possible. This may mean allowing the animal to wander free or be gently restrained on a table. This allows the clinician to compare both eyes and observe any obvious differences or abnormalities between them. Sedation or general anaesthesia should be avoided, as it will cause enophthalmos, third eyelid protrusion, globe rotation and miosis, complicating ophthalmoscopic examination and possibly leading to misdiagnosis. After a gross examination of both eyes has been performed, a more detailed examination should be carried out. For this purpose good illumination and instrumentation are necessary. The form of examination is often a matter of personal preference. However, the eye should be examined in a logical sequence, so that a whole eye examination is

performed. It is often helpful to examine both eyes under diffuse illumination first. The pupillary light reflex should also be tested at this stage. The room should then be darkened, a mydriatic used when necessary and the eyes examined under focal illumination. By carrying out an examination in this order the possibility of missing abnormalities is avoided.

Diffuse illumination

An overhead examination light or pen torch can be used for this purpose. The beam of light is directed onto the surface of the eye and adnexa, through the anterior chamber and onto the iris and the surface of the lens, in order to detect any abnormalities. This approach is an excellent screening procedure and allows comparison between the two eyes before a more detailed examination is performed. The pupillary light reflex can also be assessed at this stage (see 'Visual assessment' below).

Direct ophthalmoscopy

The direct ophthalmoscope has a light source that is almost parallel with the examiner's line of vision. The area of illumination and the selection of lenses, apertures and filters, will vary between the different makes of ophthalmoscopes. It is important to select an ophthalmoscope that offers a wide area of illumination, with as little corneal reflection as possible. A range of lenses from -5 to $+20$ is desirable but there is little indication for anything outside this range.

Direct ophthalmoscopy requires a moderate

amount of practice and skill but offers a very detailed examination of the whole eye. The image is real, erect and magnified ($\times 15$). It is possible to assess the depth or height of lesions on a dioptre scale (3 dioptres = 1 mm). Direct ophthalmoscopy has the disadvantage of a small field of vision at any one time.

Procedure

Direct ophthalmoscopy should be carried out in a room capable of being darkened. It may be necessary, particularly in the cat, to dilate the pupils with a mydriatic (Mydriacyl*), which should be instilled in the eye about 10–15 minutes before examination. The dilated pupil will make an ophthalmoscopic examination of the fundus easier but is not essential in all cases. Animals that are apprehensive or frightened often have widely dilated pupils.

1 The ophthalmoscope is set at zero and held against the examiner's eye. The examiner must learn not to accommodate. The other hand is used to steady the patient's head and direct the eye towards the beam of illumination. If necessary the lids can be retracted. Undue pressure should not be put onto the eyes as this may increase intra-ocular pressure and change the appearance of the retinal vasculature.

2 Distant direct ophthalmoscopy is performed at a distance from the patient of about 60 cm (24 in). The tapetal reflex can be seen at the centre of the field of vision; the pupil, lens, the iris and the cornea will also be visible. Any opacities at this distance will be retro-illuminated and appear as dark or blackened areas.

3 The examiner should then move to within 3–5 cm (1–2 in) of the eye. The fundus should appear in focus. After the fundus has been examined the positive lenses are used to examine from fundus to cornea and adnexa.

Indirect ophthalmoscopy

There are several ways of examining the eye by indirect ophthalmoscopy. The simplest method is

* Mydriacyl (tropicamide), Alcon Laboratories, Watford, UK.

to have a light source such as a pen torch or ophthalmoscope near the examiner's eyes and a 20 dioptre lens held near the patient's eye. Mydriasis is essential for this type of examination. A large area of the fundus can be examined at any one time. The image is inverted and reversed. The degree of magnification is in the region of $\times 2$ to $\times 4$ and in contrast to the $\times 15$ magnification provided by the direct ophthalmoscope. There are two types of indirect ophthalmoscope available, monocular and binocular.

Monocular indirect ophthalmoscope

The monocular indirect ophthalmoscope is probably the easiest of all ophthalmoscopes to use. It gives a good upright view of the fundus and can also be focused onto the anterior segment of the eye. However, it will have the disadvantage of any indirect ophthalmoscope in that it does not provide any satisfactory degree of magnification which is particularly important in examining the anterior chamber and adnexa.

Binocular indirect ophthalmoscope

The binocular indirect ophthalmoscope is a difficult instrument to master. It is essential to have a dark room and dilated pupil. This instrument provides an inverted and reversed image of the fundus with a $\times 4$ magnification and a field of vision in the region of 8 to 14 disc diameters. This large field of vision in combination with stereopsis allows for fast funduscopic examination of patients. The instrument also has a very bright light source giving a great depth of field and a better image when the eye is not optically clear, e.g. with diseased cornea or aqueous and vitreal opacities.

Biomicroscopy

The biomicroscope or slit-lamp provides focal or diffuse illumination with a variable degree of magnification ($\times 25$). The light beam is intense and can be varied in height and depth across the field of the objective. By this means it renders visible suspended particles (Tyndall phenomena). Any pathological changes in the normal transparency of ocular structures will also be detected. Diffuse illumination allows for a quick examination of the eyes. Direct focal illumination in the form of a slit-beam provides a three-dimensional view of the transparent ocular media. The beam of light can be altered to provide either an optical block of light or a narrow optical section or line. This can give detailed information as it passes through tissues such as the cornea and the lens. As with the direct ophthalmoscope the slit-lamp can be used to retro-illuminate tissues. This means that the observed feature is viewed in the pathway of reflected light. The object will appear as one colour in direct illumination and another colour when retro-illuminated. For instance, a small cataract when retro-illuminated will appear as a dark spot in the lens, but when directly illuminated will appear grey to white in colour. With the biomicroscope one can focus on structures from the adnexa to the vitreous.

Visual assessment

In animals it is difficult to assess defective vision. A history is useful as animals often manage well in familiar surroundings but when removed to a different environment defective vision becomes apparent. One way of assessing vision is to let the cat wander around the consulting room, first in bright artificial light and then in subdued lighting. An obstacle course can be created. The light from an ophthalmoscope can be directed onto the floor and moved about in a darkened room; this will often attract the animal's attention, and when vision is normal the animal will fix onto the moving light and follow it about. Cotton wool balls can be dropped from a height in front of the animal in order to assess vision. The pupillary light reflex and the menace reflex are helpful in establishing the integrity of the retina, the optic nerve and the descending neurological pathways.

Pupillary light reflex
The pupillary light reflex assesses the function of the retina, optic nerve, oculomotor nerve and iris sphincter muscles. The term 'direct pupillary light reflex' refers to the response that occurs in the

eye which receives the direct light stimulus. However, a pupillary response will occur in the contralateral eye due to the decussation of optic nerve fibres at the optic chiasma. This is the indirect or consensual light reflex.

Pathology involving the retina, optic nerve, optic chiasma, oculomotor nerve and iris will result in a change in the pupillary light response. Whilst blinding conditions such as progressive retinal atrophy or retinal detachment may result in a poor to absent reflex, it should be remembered that a good light reflex is not synonymous with vision. The pupillary light reflex is a subcortical reflex.

Menace reflex
The menace reflex involves a similar pathway to the pupillary light reflex; however, the visual cortex is also involved. The response of animals to this reflex is variable and they may over- or under-react. The stimulus is provided by a menacing gesture to the side of the face. Care should be taken to avoid creating air currents over the eye.

THE ORBIT

The eye in the cat, like the dog, is contained within an incomplete bony orbit. It is incomplete because the dorsolateral wall is formed by a collagenous orbital ligament which often becomes ossified in the cat. Inferiorly the floor of the orbit is mainly soft tissue consisting of the medial and lateral pterygoid muscle and a small bony shelf arising from the maxillary bone which lies above the molar teeth. This anatomical arrangement allows access to the orbit from the mouth through the pterygopalatine fossa, which lies just behind the last upper molar tooth. The bony components to the orbit are formed by the frontal, palatine, lacrimal, maxillary, zygomatic and presphenoid bones. Medially the bony wall is thinner and this may allow extension of infection from the nasal cavity or sinuses. Connective tissue (periorbita) surrounds the eye and orbital contents. These consist of the globe, the extraocular muscles, the retractor oculi muscle, cranial nerves II, III,

IV, V and VI, autonomic nerves, blood vessels, smooth muscle and fat and the zygomatic salivary gland. The orbit in the cat is compact and usually deeply set. Proptosis is therefore an uncommon condition in the cat and is usually the result of severe orbital trauma.

Exophthalmos

Exophthalmos is the protrusion of a normal sized globe from its orbit due to disease or a space-occupying lesion. It should not be confused with hydrophthalmos, which is a chronic enlargement of the globe due to glaucoma. At its extreme proptosis results when the globe is totally displaced from the orbit. The incompleteness of the bony orbit in the cat allows a space-occupying lesion to be present for some time before exophthalmos may become apparent. In arriving at a clinical diagnosis of exophthalmos the following signs should be noted:

1 A globe that is exophthalmic is of a normal size, i.e. the same size as the other eye assuming that the control eye is normal. The corneal diameters of both eyes will be the same.
2 The globe that is exophthalmic will be more prominent. This is due to displacement and may be more obvious when viewed from above.
3 Retropulsion is a valuable diagnostic tool. In the presence of a space-occupying lesion it becomes difficult to push the exophthalmic globe back towards the orbital apex.
4 The intraocular pressure is normal in cases of exophthalmos.
5 Deviation of the globe may occur depending on the position of the space-occupying lesion. The third eyelid may also be protruded.

It is important that a very careful examination is conducted as it is relatively easy to make a misdiagnosis. The exophthalmic globe is invariably visual and has little or no ocular pathology in the early stages. With time an exposure keratitis, conjunctivitis and uveitis and even retinal detachment may develop.

Diagnostic procedures

1 Under general anaesthesia the pterygopalatine fossa of the affected orbit should be examined.

Investigation of this area is performed by inserting a haemostat towards the orbit after making a small incision. This procedure should be undertaken with care and it is inadvisable to irrigate the area. Using a 20 gauge needle it may be possible to obtain a sample for cytology.
2 Radiography of the skull and orbit may be helpful. Contrast angiography and venography have been found useful in the presence of orbital vascular tumours. Orbitography and ultrasonography are also helpful in cases of neoplasia.
3 Surgical exploration of the orbit may be indicated if the above procedures are inconclusive. Several approaches are possible (Blogg, 1980).

Causes of exophthalmos

ORBITAL INFECTION AND INFLAMMATION
Infection and inflammation of the orbit can be caused by bite wounds, penetrating conjunctival or oral foreign bodies, dental disease and frontal sinusitis. Haematogenous spread of pyogenic and fungal infections is also possible. The incomplete bony orbit is a predisposing factor. Foreign bodies may lodge in the mouth behind the last upper molar and penetrate the oral mucosa to lodge in the orbital space. They may also penetrate this area through the facial tissues. Upper molar tooth root abscessation may also cause orbital inflammation and infection. The condition may be acute or chronic. The presenting signs are usually unilateral, with swelling of the periorbital area, conjunctival inflammation, chemosis, blepharitis and uveitis. The third eyelid may be protruded and the eye deviated. There may be pain on opening of the mouth due to inflammation of the pterygoid muscle. Retropulsion of the globe will cause discomfort. Pain over the affected side of the head may be obvious and pyrexia may also be present. Bilateral exophthalmos has been reported with mycotic infections (Whitley, 1984). Nutritional steatitis has also been reported to cause orbital inflammation in the cat (Peiffer, 1981).

Diagnosis
1 Investigation of the pterygopalatine fossa may reveal the presence of a purulent discharge if

there is abscess formation. In the presence of a cellulitis investigation of this area is unrewarding, but the response to medication is dramatic and diagnostic.

2 The cardinal signs of orbital infection are pain, pyrexia, heat and swelling over the periorbital areas. The condition is usually acute and unilateral.

3 Haematology will demonstrate a leucocytosis.

Treatment

With prompt treatment the condition should rapidly resolve.

1 Drainage should be provided through the pterygopalatine fossa. This can be achieved using a No. 15 surgical blade to make a small incision in the oral mucosa. A closed haemostat is then used to create a drainage pathway through the pterygoid muscles. Flushing of the retrobulbar space is sometimes advocated but is generally not considered to be a very safe procedure. Any offending molar teeth should be extracted.

2 Systemic antibiotics should be given for a period of up to 10 days.

3 Diuretics may be helpful if there is marked chemosis.

4 False tear preparations should be applied frequently to the exposed globe to prevent an exposure keratitis.

5 Analgesics may be indicated.

ORBITAL TRAUMA

Orbital trauma is usually the result of extensive blunt trauma to the head. This is most likely to be the result of a road traffic accident. There is often severe subconjunctival haemorrhage and chemosis. The eyelids may become oedematous and the third eyelid may be protruded. The globe may become exophthalmic due to retrobulbar haemorrhage. Fractures of the frontal sinuses will lead to subconjunctival emphysema.

Limited orbital trauma may be due to violent recovery from general anaesthesia or following difficult removal of the upper molar teeth. Exophthalmos will be due to retrobulbar haemorrhage but this usually resolves within 24 hours.

Diagnosis

Where the patient has been involved in a road traffic accident it is obviously necessary to assess the cardiovascular and neurological status and stabilize the patient before dealing with the orbital trauma. The orbit should be palpated for the presence of fractures or crepitus. Where possible an ophthalmoscopic examination should be performed. Radiography and ultrasonography may be indicated.

Treatment

Treatment should be aimed at preventing further swelling and retrobulbar haemorrhage. The use of cold compresses or a padded bandage may be of value. Sedation may be necessary. The following drugs may be helpful.

1 Lubricants, e.g. methylcellulose, should be applied to the cornea to prevent an exposure keratitis.

2 Anti-inflammatories such as corticosteroids may help to reduce orbital swelling.

3 Diuretics may also be helpful to prevent additional swelling.

4 Mydriatics are indicated if a uveitis is present.

5 Antibiotics should be given both topically and systemically to prevent infection.

6 Exploratory orbitotomy may be indicated at a later date if there is a recurrent cellulitis or fistula formation, as this may indicate the presence of a sequestrum or a foreign body.

If orbital trauma is severe then the prognosis must be guarded as strabismus, facial asymmetry and cranial nerve damage may be permanent sequelae.

ORBITAL NEOPLASIA

See section on neoplasia below.

Phthisis bulbi

Phthisis bulbi is an atrophy of the globe as the result of severe ocular trauma or infection. It results from a failure of aqueous production and subsequent shrinking of the globe. Deposition of osteoid tissue and sarcoma formation can occur long after the initial insult (see 'Neoplasia' below).

The phthitic globe is also prone to recurrent infection. Enucleation is the treatment of choice.

Enophthalmos

Enophthalmos is the retraction of the normal globe into the orbit. It must be differentiated from microphthalmos and phthisis bulbi. The enophthalmic globe is of a normal size with no sign of any gross pathology, nystagmus or deviation. Retraction of the globe may be an active process due to corneal or conjunctival discomfort which can be abolished by local anaesthesia – a useful diagnostic test. Passive retraction of the globe will result from a loss of supporting orbital tissue. Enophthalmos is frequently accompanied by prominence of the nictitating membrane.

Causes of enophthalmos

1 Loss of retrobulbar fat. This may be due to localized orbital inflammation leading to a unilateral enophthalmos. Wasting diseases and senility will lead to bilateral enophthalmos which is not uncommon in the geriatric patient.
2 Chronic orbital abscessation will result in a myositis followed by atrophy of the retrobulbar muscles.
3 Horner's syndrome (Plate 9.4).
4 Congenitally large orbit.
5 Tetanus is a cause of bilateral enophthalmos due to spasm of the retractor oculi muscles.
6 Orbital neoplasia – although more likely to cause exophthalmos orbital neoplasia has been reported to cause enophthalmos (Pentlarge *et al.*, 1989).

Treatment

Treatment relies on an accurate diagnosis in order to identify the underlying cause where possible.

Microphthalmos

Microphthalmos is an abnormally small globe often associated with multiple ocular anomalies such as persistent pupillary membranes, cataract and ocular nystagmus. This type of nystagmus indicates that the blindness is of a congenital origin. Microphthalmos may be unilateral or bilateral. Frequently it is associated with a small palpebral fissure. The condition should be differentiated from phthisis bulbi and enophthalmos. The aetiology often remains obscure; in the dog there appears to be a hereditary factor. The administration of griseofulvin to pregnant queens has been reported to cause microphthalmos (Scott *et al.*, 1974).

Congenital ocular dysplasia

This condition is seen in the Burmese cat (Koch, 1979). It encompasses a multitude of craniofacial anomalies including an absence of the globe. Kittens from an affected litter may, however, have normal eyes, eyelid and corneal dermoids, or multiple anomalies.

Hydrophthalmos (buphthalmos, megaloglobus)

Hydrophthalmos is a chronic enlargement of the globe in response to an increase in intraocular pressure which causes a stretching of the cornea and the sclera. Accompanying features may be a low intraocular pressure, episcleral injection, corneal oedema, mydriasis, lens luxation, and retinal and optic atrophy. The condition must be differentiated from exophthalmos. Enucleation is indicated if the eye is painful or neoplasia is suspected.

Proptosis

The Persian and other brachycephalic skulls are predisposed to proptosis. Trauma is the commonest cause. The degree of displacement will vary with the severity of the trauma. The proptosed eye rapidly becomes desiccated, and the constriction of the eyelids behind the globe leads to ischaemic necrosis. The extraocular muscles become stretched or ruptured and the optic nerve may be avulsed. Rapid replacement of the globe under local or general anaesthesia is imperative. The prognosis must be guarded. Accompanying hyphaema and mydriasis carry a poor prognosis, whilst a miotic pupil carries a better prognosis. However, if the globe is hypotonic (indicating globe rupture) or the optic nerve is ruptured, then enucleation should be performed.

Treatment

Patients should first be assessed for shock and then if possible a general anaesthetic given while replacing the globe. The eye should be irrigated and cleaned with warm saline. If there is marked chemosis, orbital oedema or haemorrhage difficulty may be experienced in replacing the globe. The upper and lower lids should be opened. Strabismus hooks may be helpful for this purpose in relieving the pressure on the globe as it is replaced. A canthotomy may be necessary. The lids are then sutured together for 10–14 days. Antibiotics, anti-inflammatories and diuretics may be given. Atropine may be helpful. Lagophthalmos, squint, blindness and phthisis bulbi are common sequelae to proptosis.

THE EYELIDS

The eyelids are composed of skin and conjunctiva, and are therefore susceptible to dermatological as well as ocular diseases. They also represent a mucocutaneous junction. In the cat they form a relatively round palpebral fissure and protect the globe. Cilia are apparently present on the upper eyelids of the cat but are less distinct than the dog (Wyman, 1986). Vibrissae and cilia are innervated by the fifth cranial nerve and elicit the blink reflex. Eyelid closure is brought about by the orbicularis oculi eye muscle, which forms a sphincter around the palpebral fissure. This muscle is innervated by the palpebral branch of the seventh cranial nerve.

Agenesis

Eyelid agenesis (absence of lid tissue) (Plate 9.1) is a rare congenital condition in the cat. It may present as an extensive absence of lateral upper lid tissue or as a notch. The condition may be inherited in the Persian cat. The condition may be unilateral or bilateral. If the affected area

is small, probably no problems will result. However, where the defect is large, eyelid skin comes into direct contact with bulbar conjunctiva and this results in corneal irritation and an exposure keratitis. Other ocular defects have been described together with lid colobomas in the domestic cat (Bellhorn *et al.*, 1971). These include persistent pupillary membranes, lenticonus, choroidal hypoplasia, disc coloboma and microphthalmos. The treatment of choice is surgical correction (Dziezyc & Millichamp, 1989).

Lateral canthal defects

Lateral canthal defects have been reported in the Burmese cat in association with dermoid formation (Whiteley, 1987).

Dermoids

Dermoids are congenital choristomas (normal tissue in an abnormal position) (Plate 9.2). They may be located on the conjunctiva, third eyelid, cornea or eyelids. They should be surgically removed.

Ankyloblepharon

The eyelids are normally fused together for the first 10–14 days of life. Delayed opening may be associated with neonatal conjunctivitis. In the presence of infection it may be necessary to forcibly open the lids to provide drainage when this occurs.

Symblepharon

Symblepharon is the adhesion of palpebral or bulbar conjunctiva to the cornea or other parts of the globe (Plate 9.3). If it is extensive it may restrict eye movement. The nasolacrimal puncta may become occluded, resulting in epiphora or chronic conjunctivitis. The condition may be congenital or acquired as the result of neonatal conjunctivitis. Treatment involves the surgical breakdown of the adhesion and the application of a prosthesis to prevent them re-forming.

Entropion

Entropion is an inward rolling of the eyelids that results in corneal irritation and ulceration. It may be inherited in the Persian, the lower lid being usually involved (Peiffer, 1982a).

Acquired entropion may be spastic or cicatricial. Entropion is not a common condition in the cat; however, non-spastic cicatricial entropion may be secondary to extensive symblepharon. Corneal and conjunctival disease may cause a spastic entropion, which is usually unilateral.

Diagnosis relies on a careful examination of the lid margins. If the lid has been in-turned for any length of time there may be a loss of pigmentation from the affected areas. Epiphora, blepharospasm and photophobia may be present along with conjunctival disease and corneal ulceration in severe cases. Whilst the application of local anaesthetic to the cornea and conjunctiva is a means of differentiating between primary and secondary entropion, secondary spastic entropion in the cat is not always abolished by this technique.

Primary entropion can only be treated by surgical correction of the lid deformity. With secondary entropion it is necessary to treat the primary underlying cause. However, in the cat surgical correction may be necessary for chronic spastic entropion.

Ectropion

This is an outward rolling of the lid resulting in an exposure conjunctivitis and keratitis. It is a rare condition in the cat.

Distichiasis

Distichiasis is the presence of accessory cilia on the margo intermarginalis. This is a rare condition in the cat, and many authorities do not believe that cilia are present along the eyelid margins.

However, Wyman (1986) does report the presence of normal cilia.

Trichiasis

Trichiasis is the angulation of normal eyelashes or facial hair onto the cornea (Plate 9.1). It may be seen in breeds such as the Persian where the anteriorly placed globe also comes into contact with facial hair.

Blepharitis

Blepharitis is an inflammatory disease of the eyelids that may be part of a dermatological disorder. Blepharitis may result from bacterial, fungal or parasitic infection, or secondary to an allergic reaction or autoimmune disease.

Bacterial infection of the lids may result in a dermatitis, cellulitis or abscessation. The condition may be acute or chronic. Staphylococci or streptococci are most commonly involved. In acute blepharitis the lids become swollen, inflamed and encrusted. This may progress to ulceration and alopecia in chronic cases. Staphylococcal infections may become chronic resulting in a hypersensitivity. Diagnosis relies on clinical signs and culturing techniques. Treatment involves the use of systemic and topical broad-spectrum antibiotics. Steroids may be indicated in some situations. Drainage should be established where there is abscessation of the lids. Frequent cleaning of the lid margins and the application of warm compresses may be helpful.

Parasitic blepharitis may result due to *Notoedres cati* or *Sarcoptes scabei* infestation. The infestation may be localized or generalized. Pruritus, alopecia and thickening of the lids result. The diagnosis is confirmed from skin scrapings. Treatment involves the use of rotenones or sulpha ointment.

Microsporum canis and *Tricophyton mentagrophytes* can cause a fungal blepharitis. This is usually seen in young cats. The lids become hyperaemic with crusting and scaling. A diagnosis is made on fungal culture. Treatment involves the use of topical and systemic antifungals.

The causes of allergic blepharitis are often difficult to elucidate. It may result from insect bites, exposure or the application of topical drugs, such as neomycin, food allergy and inhalants. Alopecia, pruritus and excoriation result. A diagnosis is made from an accurate history and examination. Skin testing and biopsy may be of value. Corticosteroids, antihistamine and essential fatty acids may be helpful in the treatment of this condition. Where the blepharitis is localized and possibly drug-induced, withdrawal of all medication will result in an immediate improvement.

Blepharitis may also be seen as part of the pemphigus complex (Manning *et al.*, 1982). Erythema, alopecia and scaling of the face, ears and periorbital areas result. A diagnosis is made on skin biopsy. The condition is steroid-responsive.

The third eyelid

The third eyelid (membrana nictitans) consists of a T-shaped elastic cartilage that is covered by conjunctiva. It is situated at the medial canthus and contributes to the conjunctival sac. At its base on the medial aspect is a seromucous gland or nictitans gland that contributes to lacrimal secretion. The third eyelid contains both smooth and striated muscle and lymphoid tissue, which is particularly evident on the medial aspect. Movement of the third eyelid in the cat may be an active or passive process. Active protrusion of the third eyelid is due to striated muscle which is innervated by the sixth cranial nerve. The smooth muscle (Müller's muscle) which arises from the medial and ventral rectus muscles with its sympathetic innervation is responsible for third eyelid retraction. The third eyelid serves a protective function; it contributes to the precorneal tear film; and it is immunologically active.

Protrusion of the third eyelid

Debilitating systemic disease may result in bilateral passive protrusion of the third eyelid. This may be due to dehydration of orbital contents, loss of retrobulbar fat and/or muscle atrophy, all of which result in enophthalmos. Conversely an increase in orbital mass due to

cellulitis, haemorrhage or neoplasia will cause an exophthalmos and a protrusion of the third eyelid. Active globe retraction in tetanus or as the result of ocular pain will result in a prominence of the third eyelid. The neurogenic causes of third eyelid prominence involve sympathetic denervation and include Horner's syndrome (Plate 9.4) and feline dysautonomia (Key–Gaskell syndrome). Horner's syndrome is a paralysis of the sympathetic innervation to the smooth muscle of the eyeball and its adnexa. This loss of sympathetic tone results in enophthalmos, a narrow palpebral fissure, ptosis, a protrusion of the third eyelid and miosis. The condition may be unilateral or bilateral. The causes are numerous, with mediastinal lesions and otitis media being the commonest in the cat. A 1% solution of phenylephrine will reverse the clinical signs, but a 10% solution is used to confirm the diagnosis (Gelatt, 1981). Bilateral protrusion of the third eyelid may also occur in cats that appear to be clinically normal. It may be associated with a transient gastrointestinal upset. No treatment is necessary but 1% phenylephrine will relieve the clinical signs. The condition may persist for 3–8 weeks. In feline dysautonomia there is bilateral prominence of the third eyelid, dilatation of the pupils and signs of systemic disease.

Inversion of the third eyelids

Inversion of the third eyelid due to a scrolling of the cartilage with or without prolapse of the nictitans gland (Plate 9.5) is an uncommon condition in the cat. The aetiology is not known. The condition is unsightly and may cause corneal ulceration. The Burmese cat would appear to be particularly affected. Surgical correction is indicated (Albert *et al.*, 1982).

Lymphoid hyperplasia

Hyperplasia of the lymphoid tissue on the bulbar aspect of the third eyelid is often associated with chronic conjunctival irritation and/or infection. Lymphoid follicles may also develop on the palpebral aspect of the third eyelid. Treatment is symptomatic. Corticosteroid therapy in conjunction with follicle dispersion by rubbing with a dry gauze swab gives a satisfactory result.

See also 'Neoplasia' below.

THE CONJUNCTIVA

The conjunctiva is a mucous membrane lining the upper and the lower eyelids, covering the third eyelid and the sclera, and merging with the cornea at the limbus. This mucous membrane contains blood vessels, pain fibres, lymphatics, goblet cells and lacrimal tissue. It is normally pale pink in colour, although there may be patchy pigmentation. The conjunctiva plays an important defensive role in preventing and controlling ocular infections. It is the only ocular structure to contain lymphatics.

Conjunctivitis

Inflammation of the conjunctiva causes hyperaemia, chemosis and a discharge. However, these signs may not all be present at any one time and the degree to which they are evident will vary. Chemosis can be an outstanding feature in some cases of conjunctivitis in the cat, whilst being absent in others. Most discharges are not pathognomonic, changing with the course of time. Conjunctivitis is usually an uncomfortable condition manifesting as blepharospasm and photophobia. It is not an acutely painful condition as only a few pain fibres are present in the conjunctiva. Many factors, extrinsic and intrinsic, predispose an animal to conjunctival infection. These may be geographical, climatic or seasonal factors. Breed predisposition along with anatomical features can result in recurring ocular disease. The Persian, for instance, with its compressed face and incomplete lid closure, more commonly suffers from epiphora and recurring bouts of conjunctivitis. When conjunctivitis is recurring or intractable then the physical status of the cat should also be considered. Ocular disease is often a manifestation of an underlying systemic disease.

Clinical examination

The following clinical parameters should be noted before arriving at a diagnosis of conjunctivitis. Cleaning the eye and the use of topical agents such as local anaesthetic should only be performed after an initial assessment has been made.

EYELIDS

The lid contour is important as changes in the palpebral orifice may be the primary cause of eye disease, e.g. entropion, or may be secondary to ongoing ocular pathology, e.g. spastic entropion. The lids serve a protective function and are therefore subject to wounds and abrasions, foreign body penetration and parasitic infestation. Lid spasm will be initiated by trigeminal pain affecting the conjunctival sac and can be abolished by the use of local anaesthesia. This is a useful diagnostic procedure, in differentiating superficial conjunctival/corneal discomfort from deep-seated pain, e.g. glaucoma, in which local anaesthesia will have no effect. By reflection of the lids, the conjunctiva can be examined. The degree of hyperaemia, chemosis and the presence and type of discharge, should be noted. Where the palpebral conjunctiva reflects at the fornices to become bulbar conjunctiva, discharge frequently accumulates and is typical of some forms of conjunctivitis, e.g. keratoconjunctivitis sicca. Foreign bodies may lie and penetrate at this point. The palpebral conjunctiva is subject to chemosis in acute cases of conjunctivitis, and in chronic conjunctivitis thickening, adhesion and follicle formation will occur. Meibomian gland infection is often very evident on lid reflection and the individual glands can be seen full of inspissated pus. Deposition of substances may also occur at this site, e.g. lipid in xanthomatosis (Fawcett *et al.*, 1977).

THIRD EYELID

The nictitating membrane can be examined under local anaesthesia and retracted with a pair of fine forceps. It can be the site of chronic inflammatory change, neoplasia or a foreign body. In cases of chronic conjunctivitis lymphoid follicles may be present on the palpebral surface. The bulbar surface may demonstrate a lymphoid hyperplasia. Adhesions from the conjunctival sacs to the third eyelid may also develop.

NASOLACRIMAL SYSTEM

The nasolacrimal puncta and nasolacrimal duct should be examined and flushed in cases of chronic conjunctivitis. Infection and foreign bodies may localize in this system. Congenital anomalies, e.g. micropuncta, will result in chronic conjunctivitis and epiphora.

DISCHARGE

The type of discharge present in cases of conjunctivitis can be of diagnostic value. It may be serous, mucoid, mucopurulent or purulent. In some cases it may be bloody due to the presence of red blood cells. The position of the discharge in relation to the cornea, conjunctiva and lids may be helpful. It is normal to find a mucus thread in the fornices. However, adherence of a thick mucoid to mucopurulent discharge at this site may be indicative of keratoconjunctivitis sicca. As lacrimal secretion is poor to absent this discharge also adheres to the cornea. In cases of bacterial conjunctivitis a purulent discharge tends to collect along the contours of the lid and at the medial canthus. When the discharge is serous this may manifest as excoriation at the medial canthus and staining down the side of the nose due to continual wetness. Viral and mycoplasma infections are more likely to produce a serous discharge in the early stages.

CHEMOSIS

Chemosis is a feature of chlamydial, feline viral rhinotracheitis and mycoplasmal conjunctivitis (Plate 9.6). The cat would seem to be particularly prone to conjunctival oedema. It is also a feature of non-infectious causes of conjunctivitis such as insect bites, stings and allergies.

HYPERAEMIA

Congestion and vasodilatation of conjunctival blood vessels results in the so-called 'red eye'. The vessels involved are freely movable, super-ficial and blanch when pressure is applied from the limbus to fornix or on the application of adrenaline (epinephrine). This distinguishes them from the deeper episcleral blood vessels that become congested in glaucoma, uveitis and episcleritis and also thereby producing a red eye.

Diagnostic procedures

CYTOLOGY

To obtain a cellular sample from the conjunctival surfaces, a cotton swab, or metal spatula in the form of a Bard Parker handle or preferably a Kimura spatula should be used. If a cotton swab is used it should be moistened. The procedure can be performed under local anaesthesia but if bacteriology or a Schirmer tear test are to be conducted they should be carried out first. Material is collected by rubbing the palpebral conjunctival surface and transposed onto a glass slide. Several smears should be made, air-dried and then stained with Wright, Giemsa and/or Gram stains. Cytology will indicate the type of inflammatory response present, and may sometimes provide a definitive diagnosis, e.g. chlamydia.. However, a certain amount of experience and familiarity is necessary in recognizing the cell types, the presence of inclusion bodies and their differentiation from melanin granules and chromatin.

BACTERIOLOGY

A sterile moistened swab or a calcium alginate swab is placed in the conjunctival fornix to collect a sample for bacteriology. To avoid drying the swab is immediately placed into transport media, or inoculated into culture media. Care should be taken to avoid contamination from the cilia or skin. If the presence of viruses, chlamydia or mycoplasmas is suspected, special transport media are necessary. Appropriate media can be obtained from the respective laboratory. Time is of the essence and ideally these samples should be examined the same day, or certainly within 24 hours.

BIOPSY

A conjunctival biopsy can easily be obtained under general anaesthesia and in some cases it may be possible under local anaesthesia. The tissue sample should be spread out and flattened onto a piece of cardboard to avoid distortion and fixed in formalin, and/or Michelle's media if immunofluorescent studies are to be performed.

FLUORESCENT ANTIBODY TECHNIQUES

These are reliable diagnostic techniques and can be useful in certain infections such as chlamydia and feline herpesvirus. Slides are prepared from a conjunctival scraping as for cytology. They are air-dried and fixed in acetone (5–10 minutes) before being despatched to the laboratory.

SEROLOGY

Serology is a technique of limited value in cases of conjunctivitis. It may be helpful in cases of acute herpesvirus infection. However, it is the recurring infections that require maximum investigation and these may not have a rising or significant titre.

SCHIRMER TEAR TEST

A Schirmer tear test should always be performed in cases of recurring conjunctivitis. The test paper should be placed with one end in the conjunctival sac and the degree of wetness measured over a period of 1 minute. Tear secretion will vary on a diurnal basis and several readings should be taken before a diagnosis is made. The test should be performed before the eye is cleansed or topical agents applied. Readings of less than 10 mm wetting/min are reported to be indicative of an aqueous deficiency in the tear film; however, the normal value for the cat is lower than that for the dog.

Causes of conjunctivitis

Conjunctivitis may be primary or secondary to another ocular problem or to systemic disease. The possible causes of each type are listed in Table 9.1. In onset it may be acute or chronic. The aetiology is not always apparent as the signs

Table 9.1 Possible causes of primary and secondary conjunctivitis.

Primary conjunctivitis	Secondary conjunctivitis
Infections:	Lid abnormalities
viral,	e.g. entropion/ectropion
bacterial,	Poor lacrimal secretion
chlamydial,	Foreign bodies
mycoplasmal	Trauma, insect bites, burns
Parasitic	Dacrocystitis
Allergic	

of chemosis and hyperaemia and the presence of discharge are often non-specific. Bacterial infection is a common secondary complication.

VIRAL CONJUNCTIVITIS

Feline herpesvirus

Ocular disease in the cat may be associated with feline herpesvirus I (feline rhinotracheitis virus) infection. The presenting signs are variable depending on the age and the immune status of the cat. Characteristically the clinical signs of feline herpesvirus infection are of an upper respiratory tract infection in conjunction with ocular signs (see Chapter 14).

The ocular manifestation of feline herpesvirus have been classified into three groups by Bistner *et al.* (1971), depending upon the age of the cat. Neonatal ophthalmia may develop in association with generalized herpesvirus infection in young kittens up to 4 weeks of age. Acute conjunctivitis, accompanied by upper respiratory signs, may occur between 4 weeks and 6 months of age. In older cats, keratitis has also occasionally been seen in association with the more classic signs of feline herpesvirus infection. Corneal involvement is not usually a feature of herpetic conjunctivitis in young kittens.

The incubation period is generally 48 to 72 hours. Initial signs include conjunctivitis, sneezing, and oculonasal discharge. In neonatal kittens, there may be gross distension of the eyelids and a serous ocular discharge may seep onto the lids, becoming purulent with time. Delayed opening of the eyelids results.

Infection acquired after the lids have opened results in severe conjunctivitis. This is acute in onset and bilateral, characterized by a serous discharge which rapidly becomes purulent due to secondary bacterial infection. These ocular signs are invariably accompanied by systemic signs of an upper respiratory tract infection which can be severe in the neonate. The disease, if uncomplicated, is self-limiting over a period of 2–3 weeks.

In kittens over 6 months of age and in older cats occasionally keratitis and corneal ulceration may also occur. Feline herpes virus is the only known upper respiratory tract virus in the cat to produce corneal lesions. Herpetic corneal infection is often insidious in nature and the course of the disease chronic. There is generally either a recent history or concurrent signs of conjunctivitis and upper respiratory tract infection. Although keratitis is less common than neonatal ophthalmia or conjunctivitis, it is a more serious condition (see 'Cornea' below). Feline herpesvirus may also cause keratoconjunctivitis sicca. Where the ocular infection becomes intractable the cat should be tested for immunosuppression, e.g. feline leukaemia virus.

Diagnosis. The classical presentation of bilateral ocular disease in conjunction with upper respiratory tract infection is highly suggestive of feline herpes virus infection. The following laboratory techniques may help to provide a more definitive diagnosis:

1 Culture – a sterile moistened swab obtained from the conjunctival sac or oropharynx over the first 7–10 days of infection should yield virus on culturing. The swab should be placed in virus transport medium and sent by first class post to an appropriate laboratory for testing. The sample should be frozen if posting is delayed. Feline herpesvirus grows rapidly in feline cell cultures producing a typical cytopathic effect. Cats with stromal disease may yield negative cultures.

2 Immunofluorescence – a sample is collected from the conjunctival sac under local anaesthesia. A smear is made onto a glass slide and fixed in acetone and despatched to an appropriate labora-

tory for detection of feline herpesvirus antigen by fluorescent antibody tests. Not all laboratories routinely carry out this test.

3 Cytology – feline herpesvirus infection is characterized by a lymphocytic inflammatory response that becomes neutrophilic with a concurrent secondary bacterial infection. Large mononuclear cells and epithelial syncytial formation may be seen, although the characteristic intranuclear inclusion bodies are rarely present.

4 Serology – this is only helpful in making a diagnosis if two successive (i.e. acute and convalescent, 3–4 weeks later) sera can be obtained. This is usually not practical, however, as the animals are not presented early enough in the course of infection for a rising titre to be demonstrated.

Treatment. Treatment of neonatal ophthalmia should be directed towards opening the swollen lids to allow for drainage and flushing of the conjunctival sacs. Broad-spectrum antibiotics should be applied six times daily. Systemic antibiotics are indicated in the presence of an upper respiratory tract infection. Supportive therapy is often necessary. Corticosteroids are contraindicated. Where there is corneal involvement antiviral drugs may be helpful although their efficacy remains undetermined (see 'Cornea' below). Treatment should be vigorous to avoid secondary complications. Vaccination is available against feline herpesvirus infection but disease may still sometimes occur (see Chapter 14).

Feline calicivirus
In contrast to feline herpesvirus type I infection (see above) signs of feline calicivirus infection are generally less severe. The disease is characterized by mild conjunctivitis, upper respiratory signs, and characteristic oral ulceration. Ulcers generally occur on the tongue, but lesions may also be present elsewhere in the mouth and on the external nares (see Chapter 14). Treatment is symptomatic as there are no specific antivirals available.

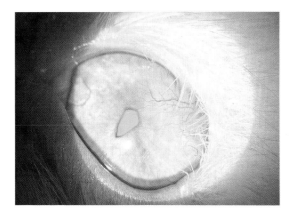

Plate 9.1 Lateral canthal upper lid coloboma resulting in trichiasis and a secondary keratitis.

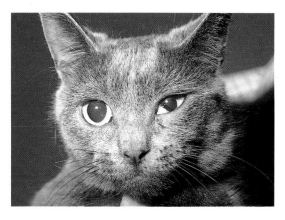

Plate 9.4 Horner's syndrome (left eye).

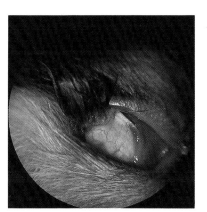

Plate 9.2 Epibulbar dermoid in a Birman cat.

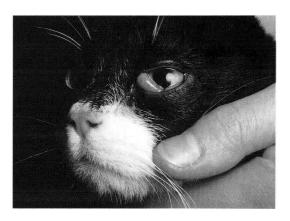

Plate 9.5 Prolapse of the nictitans glands.

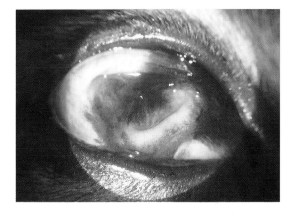

Plate 9.3 Symblepharon.

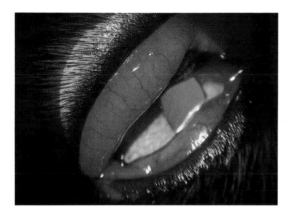

Plate 9.6 Conjunctival chemosis.

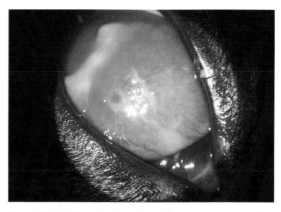

Plate 9.8 Proliferative keratitis. Note the creamy white surface deposit.

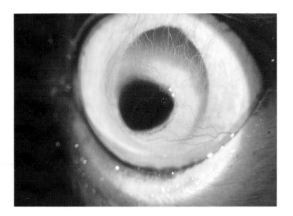

Plate 9.7 Corneal sequestrum in association with extensive corneal vascularization.

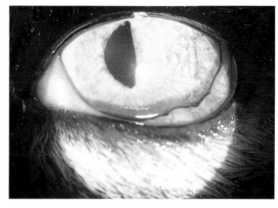

Plate 9.9 'D'-shaped pupil (in association with uveitis; this cat was FIV positive).

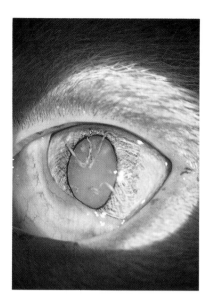

Plate 9.10 Persistent pupillary membranes and cataract.

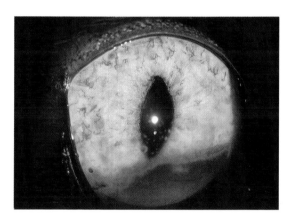

Plate 9.11 Anterior uveitis (*Toxoplasma gondii*). Note keratic precipitates and hyphaema.

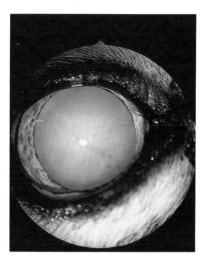

Plate 9.12 Cataract (total).

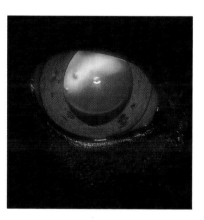

Plate 9.13 Lens luxation (posterior). Note patchy iris pigmentation.

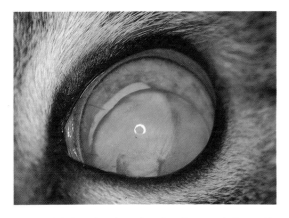

Plate 9.14 Anterior lens luxation in association with uveitis.

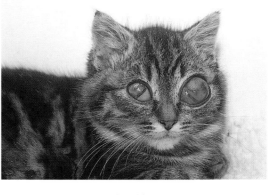

Plate 9.16 Buphthalmos in a kitten.

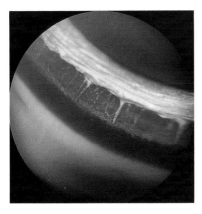

Plate 9.15 Goniophotograph of a normal irido-corneal angle.

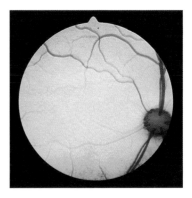

Plate 9.17 Normal ocular fundus (yellow-green) of the cat.

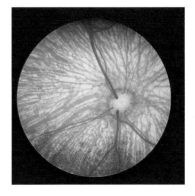

Plate 9.18 Subalbinotic fundus of a blue-eyed white cat.

Feline reovirus
This virus has been shown experimentally to cause a mild serous or mucopurulent conjunctivitis but its significance in the cat population is not known.

BACTERIAL CONJUNCTIVITIS
The conjunctiva of the cat under normal circumstances would appear to be relatively sterile (Shewen *et al.*, 1980). However, *Staphylococcus albus*, *S. aureus*, mycoplasmas, β-haemolytic streptococci and corynebacteria have been isolated from the normal conjunctiva (Campbell *et al.*, 1973). Although their role in conjunctival disease is not clear, they are probably mainly important only as secondary invaders. *Salmonella typhimurium* has been reported to cause conjunctivitis in an adult cat that showed no other signs of clinical disease (Fox, 1977). Acute bacterial conjunctivitis will present with a profuse purulent discharge that may help distinguish it from other causes of conjunctivitis. There will also be hyperaemia, chemosis and blepharospasm. Acute infection in the cat is frequently associated with orbital trauma, or abscessation associated with bite wounds.

MYCOPLASMAS
Several species of mycoplasma have been isolated from the conjunctivae of both normal cats and cats with conjunctivitis (see also Chapter 23). The role of mycoplasmas in causing disease, however, is still not clear, although there are reports that *Mycoplasma felis* may be involved in conjunctivitis (Tan & Miles, 1974; Haesebrouck *et al.*, 1991). The disease is manifest by a localized bilateral serous conjunctivitis (Tan, 1974). The serous discharge becomes purulent with time. Chemosis of the conjunctiva may be marked. Mild sneezing and nasal discharges may also occur. The picture may be confused by the presence of the respiratory viruses or *Chlamydia psittaci*.

Diagnosis

Cytology. The conjunctival inflammatory response is polymorphonuclear.

Culture. Mycoplasmas can be cultured using specific media (Haesebrouck *et al.*, 1991).

Treatment
Tetracycline is the drug of choice in either systemic or topical treatment of ocular mycoplasmosis. Systemic erythromycin, spectinomycin and tylosin may be indicated if there is no response to tetracycline. Mycoplasmas are sensitive to most antibiotics except penicillin and neomycin.

CHLAMYDIA
Chlamydia psittaci is an established cause of conjunctivitis in the cat (see Chapter 21). Respiratory signs may also sometimes be seen. *C. psittaci* is found in many animal species and man, but cat isolates appear to be relatively species-specific. Infection generally takes place in young cats, especially in litters of kittens over 5 or 6 weeks of age. Generally infection presents as an acute conjunctivitis in conjunction with mild rhinitis and pyrexia. Unlike herpesvirus infection, chlamydial conjunctivitis may present initially as a unilateral condition, becoming bilateral over a period of 1–2 weeks. Chemosis is often marked, accompanied by a serous discharge. As the chemosis subsides the discharge may become purulent and the conjunctiva hyperaemic and thickened with the development of papillae. Follicular hypertrophy has been reported, particularly on the inner side of the nictitating membrane, but the role of other possible pathogens in this is not clear. The course of the disease is anything from 2 to 6 weeks, recovery depending on the development of host immunity. Since the organism tends to persist in infected cats, and as immunity is relatively short-lived, conjunctivitis tends to recur, particularly in infected colonies. In some cases, infection may be asymptomatic.

Corneal disease has only been reported under experimental conditions (Sheikh, 1978), but the cats involved were not specific-pathogen-free, and therefore other agents (e.g. feline herpesvirus) may have been involved.

Diagnosis
The diagnostic feature of chlamydial infection is persistent conjunctivitis, with often marked

conjunctival chemosis coupled with only a mild or inapparent upper respiratory tract infection. Unlike infection with the respiratory viruses, the conjunctivitis may initially only be unilateral.

Cytology. Cytology of conjunctival scrapings will reveal a neutrophilic response up to 7 days post-infection. This changes to a mixture of polymorphonucleocytes, macrophages and lymphocytes. Inclusion (intracytoplasmic) bodies are most numerous in the first 4–7 days of infection but are occasionally seen up to 14 days post-infection. These can be stained with Wright or Giemsa stains. Oil-immersion examination is usually necessary to detect their presence in epithelial cells, although the results can often be difficuilt to interpret (see Chapter 21).

Immunofluorescence. In some laboratories immunofluorescent staining is used to detect chlamydial inclusions. The conjunctival smear is air-dried and fixed in acetone. If the specimen is not tested immediately it should be stored at −20°C.

Culture. Samples from the conjunctiva should be obtained with a fresh, dry swab which is immediately transferred to a special transport medium. The specimen should then be sent to the appropriate laboratory and cultured within 24 hours. Chlamydias are intracellular pathogens and for this reason the swab should be taken in an abrasive manner.

Swabs transferred to an appropriate transport medium may also be tested for the presence of the organism by ELISA (see Chapter 21), although this is not quite as sensitive as cell culture, particularly in the later stages of the disease.

Treatment
Treatment is designed to control the infection until host immunity develops over a period of 6 weeks (see Chapter 21). Topical oxytetracycline should be applied three or four times daily for at least 3 weeks and longer if necessary. Systemic therapy may also be indicated since systemic infection in the cat has been demonstrated (see

Chapter 21). Tetracyclines should be used with caution in kittens, although there is little evidence that adverse effects on teeth are a problem. All cats in an infected colony should be treated simultaneously, or reinfection will occur. Stress situations should be avoided and management should be directed towards good husbandry. Unfortunately, immunity is short-lived and recurrence is common, but shedding of organisms probably remains low except when animals are stressed or with the use of immunosuppressive drugs, e.g. corticosteroids.

THE CORNEA

Structure and function

The feline cornea contributes to the outer fibrous tunic of the globe. It merges with the sclera at the limbus where it is at its thickest. The rearrangement of collagen fibres at this junction is said to be responsible for ocular transparency and the ability of the cornea to serve a refractory purpose. The cornea consists of four layers. The outer stratified non-keratinized epithelium may be up to 15 cells thick; the entire corneal epithelium is replaced every 7 days. The stroma makes up 90% of the corneal thickness and consists of collagen lamellae, acid mucopolysaccharides and fibroblasts. Underneath is Descemet's membrane, which is a lipid-rich basement membrane and a very elastic structure in the cat. It is not stained by fluorescein. Lying on this basement membrane are the endothelial cells which have an ability to migrate but limited ability to replicate. In the absence of corneal disease the cornea is avascular, transparent, lacking in pigment and contains non-myelinated sensory nerve fibres.

Corneal disease

The presentation of corneal disease is variable depending on the layers involved. A loss of corneal transparency is a notable feature. This may be due to corneal oedema and/or cellular infiltration. Corneal vascularization may be superficial or deep. The superficial blood vessels are derived from the bulbar conjunctiva. These are large and branching and can be seen crossing the limbus. The smaller deeper vessels have a brush border, are derived from the anterior ciliary vessels and as they cross the limbus are interrupted. Products of metabolism such as lipid and calcium may also be deposited in the cornea. The only time the normal cornea is not transparent is in the neonate, where corneal oedema is present as the eyes open at 10–14 days.

Diagnostic procedures

To examine the cornea some form of magnification is desirable. This can best be achieved with a slit-lamp. The following procedures may be helpful in arriving at a diagnosis:

SCHIRMER TEAR TEST

The Schirmer tear test should be performed prior to cleansing of the eye or the application of local anaesthetic or fluorescein (see 'Conjunctiva' above). The degree of wetting is measured over a period of 1 minute and this should be in the region of 10–15 mm, although normal values for the cat may be lower than the dog.

FLUORESCEIN DYE-IMPREGNATED STRIPS

Fluorescein-impregnated strips are moistened and placed in the conjunctival fornix to demonstrate defects in the corneal epithelium. The use of a cobalt blue filter on an ophthalmoscope or a Wood's lamp may be helpful in demonstrating areas of staining. The dye should be washed out of the eye once the test has been performed. Other stains are available for diagnosing corneal pathology but they are often irritant and of limited value.

CORNEAL SENSITIVITY

Corneal sensitivity can be assessed by drawing a wisp of cotton wool across the cornea. This test will assess the integrity of both sensory (trigeminal nerve) and motor (facial nerve) components of the blink reflex. To assess the motor component alone the blink reflex can be elicited through the menace response or by gently tapping the side of the face.

LOCAL ANAESTHESIA

Local anaesthesia will alleviate corneal pain and make examination of the eye easier. It also differentiates between pain arising from the corneal epithelium or conjunctiva and intraocular pain associated with glaucoma or uveitis. Local anaesthesia will have no effect on the latter. However, it should be remembered that corneal disease may coexist with conjunctivitis, uveitis or glaucoma.

Corneal oedema

The corneal endothelium of the cat has very little capacity to regenerate; when it is compromised oedema will result. Damage to the epithelium will have the same effect. Corneal oedema can be distinguished from other corneal opacities such as fibrosis and lipidosis by applying pressure to the globe. In the presence of corneal oedema there is an immediate increase in corneal opacity, whereas in the presence of other opacities there will be no change.

Corneal dermoids

Corneal dermoids are hereditary in the Birman (Hendy-Ibbs, 1985). They should be more correctly termed epibulbar dermoids.

Corneal lipidosis

Corneal lipidosis is rare in the cat. Lipid deposits are found in the corneal stroma.

Stromal dystrophy

Stromal dystrophy is a non-inflammatory hereditary corneal condition. It occurs in the Manx cat usually at around 4 months of age. The condition presents as one of anterior stromal corneal oedema, the central cornea being most affected. Progression to a bullous keratopathy and epithelial degeneration occurs. Treatment can only be palliative. Affected animals should not be used for breeding as the condition is thought to be inherited as an autosomal recessive trait.

Mucopolysaccharidosis

This condition has been reported in the Siamese and the domestic short-hair (Haskins, 1979). Although the clinical presentation is the same as in gangliosidosis the conditions are biochemically different. Both are lysosomal storage diseases. With mucopolysaccharidosis there is gross skeletal deformity, the flat and long bones being dysplastic. There may be dwarfism, lameness and flattened facial features. Neurological signs may also be present. The corneas are diffusely opaque throughout all layers. A diagnosis can be made on urinalysis.

GM1 gangliosidosis

Gangliosidosis has been reported in the domestic short-hair (Murray *et al.*, 1977). Clinically the condition presents as a neurological disorder, the affected kittens become ataxic with marked head tremors and spasticity. The corneas become progressively opaque due to granular deposition of polysaccharides in corneal fibroblasts and endothelial cells. This condition is progressive and the kittens are blind by 5–6 months of age. Deposits of glycolipid develop in retinal ganglion cells which appear as punctate grey areas. However, the retina is difficult to examine because of the hazy cornea. There is no treatment for this condition and it is probably inherited in an autosomal recessive fashion.

Corneal ulceration

Superficial corneal ulcers, or erosions, arise due to loss of corneal epithelium, which may be the result of trauma, drying of the cornea due to exposure or lack of a tear film, or infection. The position of the ulcer may be of diagnostic value. Lagophthalmos will produce a central exposure keratitis and subsequent ulceration. Entropion will produce ulceration adjacent to the in-turned lid (usually the inferior lateral cornea). The extent of the ulcer can be delineated by the application of fluorescein. Superficial ulcers should heal by epithelialization within 24–72 hours. If this fails to happen the diagnosis should be reviewed and the eye thoroughly examined under local anaesthesia. Herpetic ulcers in cats may present as dendritic or linear epithelial defects which are pathognomonic for herpesvirus infection. In cases with involvement of corneal stroma a deep ulcer develops – a situation which must be regarded as

a serious problem. A descematocele may rapidly lead to perforation and loss of the globe. These ulcers do not stain green with fluorescein, they are not painful, and they have a clear base composed of a bulging Descemet's membrane. They may be accompanied by uveitis.

TREATMENT
Superficial ulcers should be treated by frequent application of a broad-spectrum antibiotic ointment or solution. Contact time and wetting of the cornea can be improved by the use of preparations containing artificial tears. Debridement or chemical cautery is indicated in the presence of dead corneal epithelium or regenerating epithelium that has failed to adhere to the stroma.

Deep ulcers should be regarded as an emergency. The animal should be hospitalized and topical antibiotics applied every 2 hours. If iris spasm is present topical atropine should be given to effect (pupillary dilatation). False tear preparations are also palliative. Surgical intervention is indicated in the presence of a descematocele. Care should be taken in anaesthetizing the patient as a sudden increase in intraocular pressure due to excitement or head shaking can lead to perforation. A conjunctival flap or third eyelid flap should be applied over the affected area. If an ulcer fails to respond to treatment samples should be taken for bacterial and fungal cultures. The eye should be thoroughly examined for the presence of a foreign body, supernumerary eyelashes or the presence of a tumour or other mass that might result in chronic recurrent ulceration.

Keratitis

Keratitis is an inflammation of the cornea and theoretically can be classified as superficial or deep, acute or chronic. However, both superficial and deep keratitis may be present together as in feline herpes keratitis. Accompanying corneal vascularization and a loss of corneal transparency due to oedema and/or cellular infiltration will occur. The signs of keratitis are invariably nonspecific due to a wide variety of insults. The superficial condition is painful, resulting in blepharospasm, photophobia and epiphora.

The principal causes of keratitis are:

1 Infection – viral, mycotic, bacterial.

2 Trauma.

3 Exposure – lagophthalmos, reduced tear film.

4 Extension from other ocular diseases, e.g. scleritis, uveitis, neoplasia.

5 Idiopathic – eosinophilic keratitis, corneal sequestrum.

HERPETIC KERATITIS

Herpetic keratitis is less common than herpes conjunctivitis or neonatal ophthalmia and is most likely to develop in kittens over 6 months of age. Virus replication occurs in the basal cells or the superficial corneal epithelium, resulting in a bullous degeneration. Ulceration occurs in conjunction with a superficial keratitis. The ulcers may be of three types:

1 small and punctate

2 linear

3 dendritic

The dendritic ulcer (branching) is pathognomonic of feline herpesviral infection. A linear or dendritic ulcer may coalesce to form a large geographic ulcer, or deepen to form a descematocele. Secondary bacterial infection may complicate the clinical picture.

Involvement of the corneal stroma may be due to virus replication and/or an immune-mediated reaction resulting in an interstitial (disciform) keratitis. Corneal oedema is said to develop in a typical circular pattern hence the term 'disciform' (Nasisse, 1982). It can progress to a bullous keratopathy, neovascularization and cellular infiltration with polymorphonucleocytes and lymphocytes. The presentation of herpetic keratitis and the course and severity of the infection, depend on the immune status of the cat. Where the condition becomes intractable the possibility of immunosuppression should be considered. The patient should be tested for the presence of feline leukaemia virus or feline immunodeficiency virus.

Diagnosis

See 'Feline infectious conjunctivitis' above.

Treatment

Antivirals. Treatment with antiviral drugs is usually reserved for chronic superficial keratitis. These drugs are said to have little effect on the deep stromal keratitis; however, they may be used on a prophylactic basis to stop epithelial ulceration developing. Virostatic drugs may be used together, or consecutively, if treatment with either one alone fails. They should be applied for a minimum of 2 weeks to avoid the rebound effect if treatment is inadequate.

1 Idoxuridine (IDU) – IDU is a virostatic and relatively insoluble drug and to have any effect on the corneal tissue must have prolonged contact. It is available in ointment form and should be applied four to six times daily for the first week, decreasing to three to four times daily for the second week. Local adverse allergic reactions may occur resulting in chemosis and follicular conjunctivitis.

2 Vidarabine – this drug is less soluble than IDU but may be effective where the latter has failed. It is less likely to cause a local reaction.

3 Trifluoridine – probably the drug of choice as it is very effective and the least toxic. However, it is only available in solution (1%). One drop should be applied every 2 hours until the corneal ulcers have healed. The dose rate is then reduced to one drop every 4 hours for a further week. There may be some initial conjunctival and corneal irritation with this drug.

4 Acyclovir – this preparation is used to treat herpes simplex in man. It has not been evaluated in the cat.

Cautery. Chemical cautery of superficial corneal ulcers may be of value in stimulating epithelialization, particularly where the ulcers are chronic and recurring. However, debridement is probably a better and safer technique in the cat.

Corticosteroids. If corticosteroids are used in the treatment of herpetic keratitis they must be used in combination with antiviral drugs. If used alone they may exacerbate the situation.

MYCOTIC KERATITIS

This is not a common condition but should be considered as a possible cause of chronic ulcerative keratitis. *Aspergillus* spp. and *Candida albicans* are possible causes (Peiffer, 1981). A diagnosis is made on the basis of corneal scrapings and culture. Topical antifungals are the treatment of choice.

CORNEAL SEQUESTRUM

Corneal sequestrum is a degenerative corneal condition probably unique to the cat (Plate 9.7). It has been described under many different terms – corneal mummification, corneal necrosis, corneal nigrum and keratitis nigrum. The condition has been reviewed by Startup (1988). The aetiology is obscure but there would appear to be a breed predisposition in the Himalayan, Persian, Siamese and domestic short-haired cats. There would appear to be neither an age nor sex incidence. The condition is frequently bilateral although both eyes may be affected at different times. The earliest sign is of pigmentation within the corneal stroma. The area affected becomes progressively larger resulting in corneal ulceration and an interstitial vascular keratitis. The sequestrum will eventually slough, sometimes resulting in corneal perforation. Although the aetiology is obscure and there is probably a genetic basis for many cases the eye should be checked for any signs of trauma or chronic irritation, e.g. entropion.

Treatment

In the early stages of the disease medical treatment in the form of topical corticosteroids with antibiotic cover may be successful in controlling the condition. In the presence of corneal ulceration surgical intervention should be considered. Although the sequestrum may slough given time, there is always a danger of corneal perforation. A carefully performed keratectomy and the application of a conjunctival flap will frequently give good results.

PROLIFERATIVE KERATITIS
(EOSINOPHILIC KERATITIS)

Proliferative keratitis (Plate 9.8) as observed in the UK (Bedford & Cotchin, 1983) is a chronic corneal condition that may involve the palpebral, bulbar and membrana conjunctiva. A creamy white surface deposit may be present. Middle-aged cats would appear to be most commonly affected. The presentation is variable. The condition may be unilateral or bilateral. Treatment involves the use of topical corticosteroids (prednisolone 0.5%) applied six times daily, possibly in conjunction with systemic steroids. Alternatively, megestrol acetate may be administered daily (2.5 mg) for a period of 2 weeks; the dose is then tailed off over a period of a further 2 weeks. A combination of both topical corticosteroids and daily megestrol acetate is the third line of treatment. If there is extensive corneal involvement a keratectomy may be appropriate.

Proliferative keratitis in the UK has been distinguished from the eosinophilic keratitis reported in the USA (Brightman *et al.*, 1975). In eosinophilic keratitis the presenting lesion is one of granulation tissue which on biopsy or scraping reveals an abundance of eosinophils. There is no conjunctival involvement and there is an absence of a surface deposit. The lesion in the UK would appear to consist of connective tissue with an infiltration of lymphocytes, histiocytes and plasma cells but an absence of eosinophils. It has been suggested that eosinophilic keratitis is a manifestation of the eosinophilic granuloma complex.

KERATOCONJUNCTIVITIS SICCA

Keratoconjunctivitis sicca is by no means as common in the cat as it is in the dog. The presenting signs are often subtle in the form of a mild conjunctival injection, blepharospasm and secondary bacterial infection. In chronic cases there may be corneal ulceration and vascularization with the accumulation of a mucoid to mucopurulent discharge in the fornices. The age of presentation is variable. There would appear to be a breed predisposition in the Siamese and more particularly the Burmese. The aetiology is often obscure; the condition may be congenital or secondary to feline herpesvirus infection and/or severe symblepharon. Transient keratoconjunctivitis sicca has been reported in conjunction with eosinophilic keratitis (Collins, 1986). A diagnosis is made on the basis of Schirmer tear test readings. A reading below 10 mm of wetting per minute is suggestive of a deficiency in lacrimal secretion, although normal values for the cat are probably lower than those for the dog.

Treatment relies on the frequent (six to ten times daily) application of false tear preparations. In cases where there is secondary corneal change topical steroids are of value. Topical cyclosporin A is probably indicated for treating keratoconjunctivitis sicca in the cat but its efficacy has yet to be proven. If medical treatment, for whatever reason, is unsuccessful, parotid duct transposition may be necessary. However, this should not be considered immediately as in some cases lacrimal secretion may return to normal levels.

THE UVEA

Structure and function

The uvea is the vascular tunic of the eye. It lies between the outer fibrous sclera and the inner neurosensory retina. It can be divided into the iris, the ciliary body and the choroid.

The iris is the most anterior component of the uvea. It acts as a diaphragm separating the anterior and posterior chambers of the anterior segment of the eye. The iris can be divided into a central pupillary and an outer ciliary zone. The pupillary zone is thinner and often darker in colour than the ciliary zone. The vascular supply to the iris is in the form of a lateral and medial ciliary artery that can be seen to enter at 3 and 9 o'clock to form an incomplete arterial circle. The pupillary component rests on a 'cushion' of aqueous humour overlying the lens. Any changes in lens position will result in a loss of support and trembling of the iris (iridodonesis). The pupil in the cat is slit-like and vertically orientated because of the vertical arrangement of the sphincter muscle fibres. The sphincter is supplied by parasympathetic fibres (cranial nerve III) which cause constriction (miosis) of the pupil. Dilatation (mydriasis) of the pupil is brought about by the dilator muscle which is supplied by sympathetic ciliary nerves (cranial nerve V) of which there are two in the cat (lateral and medial). This situation is in contrast to the dog which has five to eight nerve fibres. Localized damage to either one of these sympathetic fibres can result in a D- or inverted D-shaped pupil (Plate 9.9). The anterior layer of the iris, often described as an endothelium, consists mainly of fibroblasts (Gelatt, 1981). The iris stroma is highly vascularized, containing sphincter and dilator muscles, collagen fibres, nerves and pigment. The posterior border of the iris has a double epithelium which is pigmented and forms the pupillary rough. The anterior layer is partially pigmented and contributes to the smooth dilator muscle. This layer continues over the ciliary body to join the retinal pigment epithelium. The posterior layer becomes non-pigmented over the ciliary body and is continuous with the neuroepithelium of the retina.

The ciliary body is triangular in structure and positioned adjacent to the sclera. It can be subdivided into the ciliary processes (pars plicata) and the flat posterior ciliary body (pars plana). The ciliary processes are responsible for the production of aqueous humour and contribute to the blood–aqueous barrier. The pars plana lies adjacent to the vitreous and contains the muscles responsible for accommodation. The lens zonules attach between the ciliary processes and to the pars plana.

The choroid is the most posterior component of the uvea. It consists of an outer lamina fusca, a choroidal vessel layer, the cellular tapetum and the choriocapillaris. The choriocapillaris provides the nourishment for the outer retinal layer. The tapetum occupies the dorsal fundus and is variable in size but roughly triangular in shape. It is slightly more rounded in the cat than the dog. Although the tapetum appears brightly coloured on ophthalmoscopic examination it contains no pigment. It is up to 15 cells thick and these cells are responsible for absorbing and scattering light within its matrix. This action is thought to improve vision in the dorsal fundus which is the ventral visual field. The choroid may contain melanin pigment which contributes to the pigment in the non-tapetal fundus.

Diagnostic techniques

To examine the iris in any depth and detail a slit-lamp biomicroscope is desirable. However, a +20 lens on an ophthalmoscope will give good results. The signs of uveal disease are often subtle, and the good eye should always be used for comparison. The gross relationship of the iris to other intraocular structures may be of importance. Therefore the depth and clarity of the anterior chamber, and the position of the iris in relation to the lens and cornea, should be noted. The following procedures may be helpful in arriving at a diagnosis.

Local anaesthesia
Local anaesthesia will abolish corneal and conjunctival discomfort but will have no effect on intraocular pain. It is a useful diagnostic procedure in differentiating superficial and deep-seated pain and may make an ocular examination easier where corneal lesions are present in conjunction with uveitis.

Tonometry
Measurement of intraocular pressure is a useful diagnostic aid, as intraocular pressure falls when inflammation of the ciliary body occurs. Where a tonometer is not available digital palpation on the globe with the index finger through a closed eyelid, will give a rough guide as to the degree of 'softness' or 'hardness' of the globe. Where uveitis is severe and unilateral it is possible to appreciate a difference in intraocular pressure between affected and unaffected eyes. The important differential diagnosis for uveitis is glaucoma, in which there is a rise in intraocular pressure. The normal intraocular pressure in the cat is 15–30 mmHg.

Tyndall phenomenon
The Tyndall phenomenon occurs with aqueous flare and can be appreciated by shining a light beam (slit beam, focal beam) through the anterior chamber. Suspended particles (inflammatory cells) in the aqueous can be seen to scatter the light.

Aqueocentesis/vitreocentesis
This procedure is regarded by some authorities as being of diagnostic value in anterior and posterior segment disease. However, it is not a recommended diagnostic technique for routine use as it can contribute to intraocular inflammation. It may, however, be of use in evaluating local antibody production. Lappin (1989) has correlated aqueous antibody levels with serum antibody levels in toxoplasma infection. The technique of aqueocentesis has been described (Gelatt, 1981); a 25 gauge needle enters the anterior chamber through the limbus or cornea and the required amount of aqueous is aspirated.

Mydriasis
Dilatation of the pupil using Mydriacil 1% (Alcon) allows for visualization of the fundus, vitreous and lens which is important in cases of posterior uveitis. In the presence of severe anterior uveitis or congenital iridal defects the response to mydriasis is often poor. Its use is contraindicated in glaucoma.

Pupillary light reflex
An inflamed eye may have a slow pupillary light reflex or a miotic pupil. Anisocoria (differing pupil size) is often present in cases of anterior uveitis and is a helpful diagnostic aid.

Congenital conditions

Coloboma
Iris colobomata are usually V-shaped defects involving the inferonasal area. They may be associated with choroidal coloboma (Bellhorn *et al.*, 1971).

Iris cysts
Iris cysts arise from the pigmented iris epithelium. They remain attached to the iris, or they may be free-floating in the anterior chamber.

They should not be confused with iris melanoma (see 'Neoplasia' below). The aetiology of iris cysts is obscure. They can be acquired as a result of uveal inflammation.

Persistent pupillary membrane

The tunica vasculosus lentis, which represents the prenatal blood supply to the lens, regresses post-natally and this should be complete by 2 weeks of age in the kitten. If this fails to occur the pupillary membranes may remain into adult life (Plate 9.10). They may be seen as small strands of iris tissue attached at the iris collarette (mid iris position). They may be free or attached to the cornea or lens causing focal opacities and pigmentation. They should be differentiated from adhesions (synechiae) which are not usually attached at the iris collarette.

Heterochromia

Heterochromia is an incomplete development or absence of pigment in the iris stroma resulting in a blue or a light-coloured iris, or patches of blue coloration within a dark iris. The iris in these cases is quite normal and may be associated with an albinotic or sub-albinotic fundus. In cats and dogs there is a syndrome analogous to Waardenburg's syndrome in man. This condition manifests as a white coat with blue irises and deafness. Vision may be impaired. It is an inherited defect.

Acquired conditions

Uveitis

Uveitis is an inflammation of the uveal tract. It may affect the whole of the tract or it may be localized to the anterior uvea, affecting iris and ciliary body (iridocyclitis), or the posterior uvea, affecting the choroid (choroiditis). This classification is purely anatomical. However, uveitis may also be classified on a histological basis as granulomatous or non-granulomatous. In granulomatous inflammation the reaction is chronic with a mononuclear cell infiltration, e.g. toxoplasma and mycotic infections. Non-granulomatous inflammation is acute and polymorphonuclear cells predominate. Another more satisfactory way of classifying uveitis is on an aetiological basis (see 'Causes of uveitis' below) but in the majority of cases of uveitis the cause remains obscure.

The mediators of uveal inflammation are thought to be prostaglandins. Prostaglandins may be synthesized in the corneal endothelium, conjunctiva and iris, and have a profound effect within the eye. They act directly on the iris sphincter muscle causing miosis. Also they disrupt the tight junctions of the ciliary body non-pigmented epithelium causing a breakdown in the blood–ocular barriers. This action, in conjunction with increased vascular permeability and vasodilatation, results in aqueous flare. Removal of prostaglandins from the eye relies on active transport across the ciliary body. This process may be impaired in inflammation. In the cat prostaglandins have a potent hypotensive effect thought to be due to an increase in outflow facility (Wilkie, 1989).

CLINICAL SIGNS

Anterior uveitis

The clinical presentation of anterior uveitis is classically a red and soft eye with a constricted pupil. The condition is painful and therefore accompanied by epiphora, blepharospasm and particularly photophobia. Both eyes may be affected but usually to differing degrees. Redness is due to deep episcleral and superficial conjunctival blood vessel congestion. The fall in intraocular pressure is related to inflammation of the ciliary body. This is accompanied by breakdown in the blood–aqueous barrier leading to an exudation of inflammatory cells and fibrin resulting in aqueous turbidity or flare. The cell content of the aqueous will vary from a preponderance of polymorphs known as hypopyon to smaller mononuclear precipitates known as keratic precipitates (KPs) (Plate 9.11). The latter can best be seen attached to the corneal endothelium or lens capsule as focal opacities. Bleeding may occur into the anterior chamber (hyphaema) in severe cases.

During an acute attack of uveitis, iris tissue becomes swollen due to vascular engorgement (particularly evident in the cat) leading to a change in iris colour. With time there may be a darkening in iris colour as a result of hyperpigmentation. This darkening of the iris is a useful diagnostic tool. The cornea may become oedematous with severe intraocular inflammation making ophthalmoscopic examination difficult; however, the accompanying fall in intraocular pressure should allow one to make a correct diagnosis.

An acute attack of uveitis renders the iris more susceptible to subsequent attacks which may be immune-mediated due to autosensitivity. Features of chronic uveitis are corneal opacity and neovascularization of both cornea and uvea (rubeosis). Adhesions may develop from iris to lens resulting in pigment deposition on the anterior lens capsule and cataract formation. Extensive posterior synechiae can impede the flow of aqueous from the posterior to the anterior chamber resulting in an iris bomb, a shallow anterior chamber and secondary glaucoma. Glaucoma can also result from an accumulation of inflammatory products and adhesions developing at the angle of filtration. With obstruction of the drainage angle a deep anterior chamber results. In uncontrolled uveitis the sequelae may be secondary glaucoma, lens luxation, cataract and phthisis bulbi.

Posterior uveitis
Posterior uveitis (choroiditis) may present alone or in conjunction with an anterior uveitis. The choroidal involvement frequently affects the retina resulting in a retinochoroiditis. Exudation may occur into the vitreous resulting in vitreal flare. If the retinochoroiditis is extensive then retinal detachment, vitreal haemorrhage and blindness may ensue (see retinal detachment).

The prognosis for cases of uveitis depends on the severity and the duration of the intraocular inflammation. However, it must be guarded in view of the likelihood of recurrence, particularly when the aetiology remains obscure. Of the infectious forms of uveitis, *Toxoplasma* infection

Table 9.2 Classification of uveitis.

Traumatic uveitis
Infectious uveitis
Neoplastic uveitis
Immune-mediated disease
Idiopathic

carries the best prognosis, although regular treatment is necessary.

CAUSES OF UVEITIS
The causes of uveitis are numerous and can be classified on pathogenesis (Table 9.2). The condition may occur in isolation or in conjunction with ocular or systemic disease. Uveitis will frequently accompany scleritis, keratitis, ocular neoplasia and trauma. Uveitis may be one of the signs of systemic disease in the presence or absence of other symptoms. The immune system does appear to play an increasingly important role in uveitis and autosensitivity may be the reason for the chronicity and frequent recurrence of this disease.

Traumatic uveitis
Painful stimuli to the cornea and conjunctiva will cause a local axonal reflex (cranial nerve V) resulting in a transient uveitis. Severe trauma to the eye will cause severe intraocular inflammation involving the uvea. The latter requires aggressive symptomatic treatment to avoid serious sequelae such as secondary glaucoma and phthisis bulbi.

Infectious uveitis
Severe systemic infection may manifest as unilateral or bilateral uveitis. These infections may be viral (feline leukaemia virus, feline infectious peritonitis, feline immunodeficiency virus), protozoal (*Toxoplasma*) or mycotic (blastomycosis, cryptococcosis, histoplasmosis). The latter occur in North America. Presentation of infectious uveitis tends to be similar in all cases irrespective of the aetiology. In the cat FeLV, FIP, FIV and

Toxoplasma should be suspected when a case of uveitis presents.

Neoplastic uveitis
See 'Neoplasia' below.

Toxoplasma gondii
Ocular toxoplasmosis may occur in the absence of systemic disease. The pathogenesis may be due to:
1 Intracellular replication of the organism.
2 Intraocular cyst formation.
3 Delayed hypersensitivity reaction.
4 Immune complex deposition.
5 Toxin production by the organism.
However, it is very difficult to find any evidence of this organism in the eye. The ocular lesions are of an iridocyclitis accompanied by retinochoroiditis. Mutton-fat keratic precipitates are said to be characteristic of the infection.

Diagnosis
1 Serology – this should demonstrate a high titre. If the titre is inconclusive then a further sample should be taken 4 weeks later to demonstrate a rising titre.
2 Aqueocentesis – local antibody production can be measured and correlated with serum antibody levels, which can be diagnostic (Lappin, 1989). It should be remembered that a titre represents exposure to *Toxoplasma* but not necessarily clinical disease.
3 Faecal examination – this may be carried out for the presence of oocysts, which are only shed intermittently.

Treatment. In the absence of systemic disease treatment should be symptomatic. If systemic disease is confirmed then the following drugs may be used: sulphadiazine with pyrimethamine or trimethoprim, clindamycin, chloramphenicol or tetracyclines. In the cat systemic treatment with sulphonamides and pyrimethanine can cause anorexia, depression and bone marrow depression. Clindamycin is reported to control the retinochoroiditis.

Feline infectious peritonitis
Feline infectious peritonitis (FIP) is caused by a coronavirus, and a granulomatous uveitis may be seen with either the effusive or non-effusive forms of the disease. It rarely occurs in the absence of systemic clinical signs, though the ocular signs may precede the systemic signs. The uveitis is the result of a widespread vasculitis that may result in a cyclitis, choroiditis and optic neuritis. Retinal haemorrhage and exudation may occur.

Diagnosis
1 Blood biochemistry – this will usually demonstrate a hyperglobulinaemia resulting from an increase in serum fibrinogen and a polyclonal gammopathy.
2 Serology – high serum anti-coronavirus antibody titres may be suggestive of FIP, but interpretation may be difficult (see Chapter 17).

Treatment. FIP carries a poor prognosis. There is no specific ocular therapy for FIP uveitis therefore any treatment must be symptomatic. It may include the use of ampicillin, prednisolone and cyclophosphamide.

Feline leukaemia virus
Uveitis as a result of feline leukaemia virus (FeLV) infection is usually, but not always, accompanied by systemic signs. The uveitis is severe, relentless and poorly responsive to treatment. The iris may become diffusely or locally infiltrated with neoplastic cells (see 'Neoplasia' below).

Diagnosis. A positive diagnosis may be based on the detection of FeLV antigens in serum, but not all cases are viraemic/antigenaemic. Biopsy of other sites may be helpful.

Treatment. Treatment can be only symptomatic and will give at best a temporary remission (see Chapter 15).

Feline immunodeficiency virus
Infection with feline immunodeficiency virus (FIV) has been reported as a possible cause of uveitis in the cat (English *et al.*, 1990).

Idiopathic uveitis

The majority of cases of uveitis, with or without systemic signs, remain undiagnosed. A recent survey of 53 cats suggested a higher incidence in adult (3–9 years) male cats. FIV may account for some of these cases (Davidson *et al.*, 1989).

Symptomatic treatment. In most cases of uveitis treatment can only be symptomatic thereby attempting to reduce the intraocular inflammation and pain. The following agents may be given alone or in combination.

Mydriatics. The use of mydriatics is often overlooked in the treatment of uveitis; however, they are extremely useful drugs, giving good results when used alone or in combination with anti-inflammatories. Atropine sulphate is both a mydriatic and a cycloplegic (paralyses ciliary muscles). It dilates the pupil thereby preventing synechiae formation and abolishing iris spasm, giving a less painful eye. This drug, by causing mydriasis, also helps to prevent vascular engorgement and therefore reduces cellular infiltration and the formation of a plasmoid aqueous. It also has a stabilizing effect on vascular permeability. The drug should be administered to effect, i.e. pupillary dilatation, and then continued as necessary. Initially one drop may have to be applied two or three times daily to achieve a dilated pupil. It may then only need to be applied at 48–76-hour intervals. Care must be taken in its instillation to avoid atropinizing the cat. The head should be tilted upwards and the nasolacrimal puncta occluded as the atropine is instilled into the eye. The use of ointment instead of drops should be considered. This drug is contraindicated in glaucoma and keratoconjunctivitis sicca.

Phenylephrine (2.5–10%) may be given with atropine if mydriasis is inadequate. The two together have a synergistic effect.

Corticosteroids. These may be administered topically, subconjunctivally or systemically. The latter route should be approached with caution as mycotic and toxoplasma infections will be exacer-

bated by the use of systemic steroids. Where inflammation is mild, hydrocortisone may be adequate. However, in severe cases of uveitis steroids such as dexamethasone or prednisolone acetate are required. All topical steroids should be given frequently in the acute stages of uveitis (four to six times daily) and then the dose decreased with time. Adrenal suppression may occur with topical application.

Non-steroidal anti-inflammatories. Whilst these drugs are of value in the dog their benefit in the treatment of uveitis in the cat has yet to be proven. Topical flubiprofen is the most promising in this field, although not yet available in the UK.

THE LENS

Structure and function

The lens is a transparent, avascular, biconvex structure, situated behind the iris and suspended by the ciliary processes. It consists of a lens capsule, lens epithelium and lens fibres. The lens epithelium gives rise to the collagenous lens fibres that continue to form throughout life. This fact allows the clinician to age lesions that appear within the lens. A nuclear cataract, for instance, is likely to be congenital in origin, whereas a peripheral cataract has probably been recently acquired. Where the lens fibres meet the suture lines result. These suture lines can be seen to form a Y pattern under the anterior lens capsule and an inverted Y under the posterior lens capsule. The lens can be divided into a central nucleus which is a more lucent area than the outer cortex. A nuclear ring may separate the two. The transparency of the lens depends on its lack of blood supply and the solubility of the lens proteins. Aqueous humour supplies the metabolic requirements. The function of the lens, like that of the cornea, is to refract incident light. The cat has limited powers of accommodation (1.75–3.5 dioptres).

Diagnostic techniques

Examination of the lens is facilitated by pupillary dilatation. Tropicamide 1% (Mydriacyl; Alcon)

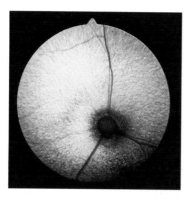

Plate 9.19 Hereditary and progressive retinal atrophy in Abyssinian cat. (Note increased tapetal reflectivity and narrowed blood vessels.)

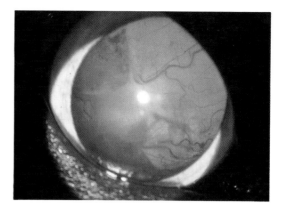

Plate 9.22 Retinal detachment.

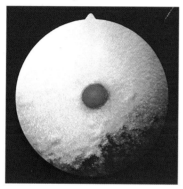

Plate 9.20 Advanced generalized retinopathy in siamese cat. (Note ghost vessels and very reflective tapetal region.) region.)

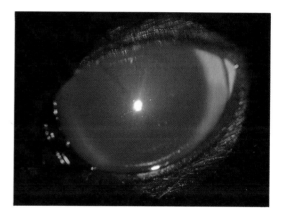

Plate 9.23 Hyphaema in association with retinal detachment.

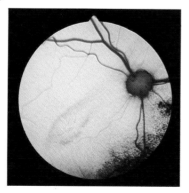

Plate 9.21 Taurine deficiency retinopathy.

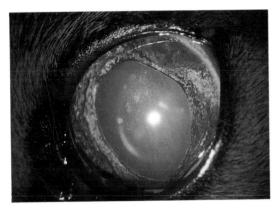

Plate 9.24 Diffuse iris melanoma and secondary glaucoma.

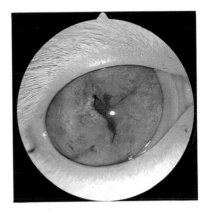

Plate 9.26 Lymphosarcoma (diffuse).

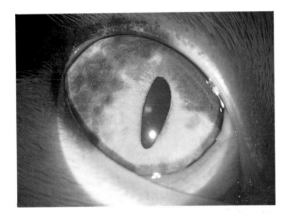

Plate 9.25 Iris pigmentation (normal).

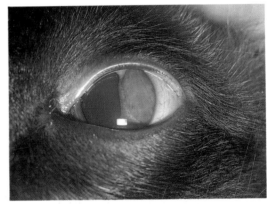

Plate 9.27 Lymphosarcoma (anterior chamber mass).

may cause some salivation. The feline pupil is not very sensitive to phenylephrine. Examination of the lens can be carried out with a direct ophthalmoscope (+20 lens) or a slit-lamp biomicroscope.

Congenital conditions

Aphakia
Aphakia (absence of lens) is a rare condition in the cat. It may occur in association with multiple ocular defects but has been reported in the domestic short-haired cat as a bilateral condition in the absence of other anomalies (Peiffer, 1982b). The clinical signs are of iridodonesis and a direct non-magnified view of the fundus.

Lens deformity
Congenital lens and corneal deformity has been reported in the Persian kitten (Peiffer & Belkin, 1983).

Cataract

A cataract (Plate 9.12) is an opacity of the lens and must be distinguished from lenticular sclerosis, which is age related. On cursory examination the sclerotic lens may appear opaque; however, ophthalmoscopic examination reveals the lens to be clear but with altered refractive properties. A small (or partial) cataract, when viewed by distant direct ophthalmoscopy, will be retro-illuminated and appear as a dark silhouette against the tapetal reflex. Direct illumination with a +10 to +15 lens will show the opacity to be grey or white. The position, size and shape of the cataract may be of diagnostic value. The position of the lens, i.e. whether luxated or not, should also be noted. When a cataract becomes total it is, of course, impossible to examine the posterior segment. However, the pupillary light reflex will give an indication of retinal function but an electroretinogram may be useful if surgery is to be undertaken.

Cataracts may be classified on the basis of their aetiology, their position within the lens, or the age of onset. Cataract in the cat is much less common than in the dog.

Congenital cataract
Congenital cataracts are usually nuclear and non-progressive. They may be associated with a variety of ocular malformations. Persistent pupillary membranes (Plate 9.10) will cause a focal anterior capsular cataract, whilst a persistent hyaloid vessel may cause an axial posterior polar cataract. Congenital cataracts have also been reported in cats with the Chediak–Higashi syndrome (Collier 1979). This is an autosomal recessive disease characterized by partial oculocutaneous albinism, bleeding tendencies and a susceptibility to infection.

Metabolic cataract
Diabetes mellitus is a well-recognized cause of cataract. In the cat it is not a common finding but when present is slowly progressive. This type of cataract indicates undiagnosed or poorly controlled diabetes.

Uveitis
Cataracts may occur secondary to uveitis, which is probably the commonest cause of cataracts in the cat. The cataract usually forms rapidly and may involve the whole of the lens. Adhesions (posterior synechiae) may develop between the iris and the lens. Whilst cataract may develop secondary to iritis the converse is also possible.

Senile cataract
Senile cataracts may develop in the cat and must be differentiated from nuclear sclerosis. However, the two may be present together. Senile cataracts are slowly progressive.

Lens luxation

Displacement of the lens (Plate 9.13) results from breakdown of the zonular attachments and may be due to a variety of causes. Primary lens luxation does occur in the cat but little is known about the aetiology although most cases occur in aged cats; there does not seem to be any breed predisposition. Secondary lens luxation is frequently associated with cataract development and uveitis in the cat. When the zonular attachments rupture, the lens becomes free floating and may move backwards into the vitreous or forwards into the anterior chamber. A posterior lens luxation is usually well tolerated; however, if there is vitreal displacement, secondary glaucoma may result. Retinal degeneration occurs if glaucoma persists. Migration of the lens into the anterior chamber (Plate 9.14) may be accompanied by a rise in intraocular pressure, which will occur due to physical obstruction of the drainage angle by the lens and/or vitreous resulting in an acute congestive glaucoma. Treatment is surgical removal of the lens. When presented with a glaucomatous eye and lens luxation, it is important to try to differentiate between primary glaucoma with secondary lens luxation or primary lens luxation with secondary glaucoma. Surgical removal of the lens in primary glaucoma, although advocated by some authorities, will do little to improve the situation as chronic irreversible ocular damage will have occurred by this stage.

One of the diagnostic features of lens luxation is iridodenesis (trembling of the iris), which occurs because the iris has lost its support from the lens. Iridodenesis is only obvious with ocular movement. The subluxated lens will present with iridodenesis, an aphakic crescent, and possibly small wisps of vitreous at the pupillary edge. The position of the aphakic crescent is variable and if dorsally situated may indicate a primary lens luxation. Location of a luxated lens is not always easy even when anterior. If the lens lies in the anterior chamber it should be possible to see its periphery lying in front of the iris. Secondary corneal oedema can make visualization difficult. If the lens has luxated posteriorly, mydriasis may be helpful. With time a luxated lens will become cataractous. When presented with a case of lens luxation of unknown aetiology the other eye should always be examined. If the condition is primary the second eye will become affected at some time in the future.

GLAUCOMA

Glaucoma refers to an increase in intraocular pressure associated with ocular pathology and results from a decrease in the outflow facility for aqueous humour. Glaucoma may be described as primary or secondary. Primary glaucoma is due to a defective outflow pathway in the absence of obvious ocular disease. The commonest form of glaucoma in the cat is secondary glaucoma, which is usually a sequel to uveitis. The drainage angle may be open, narrow or closed, the latter resulting from deposition of inflammatory products or neoplastic cells. The normal intraocular pressure in the cat is 15–30 mmHg. Feline glaucoma is a comparatively rare condition.

Diagnostic techniques

Gonioscopy
The filtration angle in the cat can be observed using a focal light source. This is possible because of the position of the scleral limbus in relation to the irido-corneal angle. However, for a more detailed examination gonioscopy should be performed (Plate 9.15).

Tonometry
Tonometry is the measurement of intraocular pressure and can be achieved by digital palpation, manometry, indentation tonometry or applanation tonometry. Digital palpation is an inaccurate technique but will give an indication of the changes in intraocular pressure when one eye can be compared with the another. The index or second finger is used to palpate the globe through a closed upper lid.

The Schiotz tonometer has been widely used in small animals. It is a portable instrument and relatively easy to use. The cornea is indented with a corneal footplate and the indentation measured on a recording scale which is then converted using a table (Pickett *et al.*, 1988). More accurate but more expensive tonometers are the applanation models, e.g. the Mackay–Marg. The Tono-Pen is a hand-held, battery-powered instrument that is easy to use. It uses the principle of the MacKay–Marg.

Intraocular pressure should be measured at the same time every day and several readings should be taken at any one time. Diurnal fluctuations do occur in both the normal and glaucomatous eye, which are significant. Higher readings are obtained in the morning in contrast to those taken at night. Other factors such as, drugs, age, arterial and venous pressure and blood osmolarity are just a few of the factors that influence aqueous production and drainage.

Primary glaucoma

Primary glaucoma is uncommon in the cat; it has been described in the Persian, Siamese and domestic short-hair. Congenital glaucoma has also been reported (Wyman, 1986).

The clinical signs of glaucoma in the cat, unlike the dog, are usually more subtle and insidious in onset. However, one survey (Ridgway, 1989) of 29 cats suggests that the signs of glaucoma are perhaps more similar to those of the dog than might be expected, as 57% of the cases presented with corneal oedema, 31% had a dilated pupil and 17% showed episcleral congestion. The cornea, however, may often appear clear and the eye apparently comfortable, and for this reason the cat may not be presented until the signs of glaucoma have become chronic. At this stage the eye may appear buphthalmic (Plate 9.16) and the intraocular pressure may have dropped to within normal limits. In addition the pupil may be fixed and dilated and secondary lens luxation may have occurred. In chronic cases there may be retinal and optic atrophy; the latter is not easy to assess as the cat's optic disc is poorly myelinated. In the early stages of open angle glaucoma tonometry is essential at arriving at a diagnosis. In the later stages, where the intraocular pressure may have dropped to within normal limits, a diagnosis can only be made on the presenting signs.

Secondary glaucoma

Secondary glaucoma in the cat is diagnosed more frequently than primary glaucoma. It may occur as a sequel to uveitis, trauma or neoplasia. In cases of severe uveitis inflammatory cells, fibrin, synechiae and hyphaema are all responsible for preventing aqueous outflow at the irido-corneal angle. In cases of intraocular neoplasia the angle may become infiltrated with tumour tissue. With gonioscopy it is possible to see these changes at the filtration angle.

Treatment

Treatment is aimed at reducing intraocular pressure and can be achieved medically by reducing aqueous humour production and increasing the facility for outflow. The following drugs can be used in combination, although they would appear to be less effective in the cat than the dog.

CARBONIC ANHYDRASE INHIBITORS
Carbonic anhydrase inhibitors reduce the active production of aqueous humour at the ciliary body. The cat is less tolerant than the dog to these drugs and is therefore more likely to show the side-effects of vomiting, acidosis and lethargy. Care should be taken when administring these drugs to the cat. Dichlorophenamide (Daranide*) is probably the drug of choice and may be given at 2–5 mg/kg bodyweight, twice daily, by mouth. However, it is advisable to use the lower dose rate.

MIOTICS
Miotics are used in combination with the carbonic anhydrase inhibitors in the long-term medical treatment of glaucoma. They are contraindicated in secondary glaucoma associated with anterior uveitis. They should be used with caution in the presence of an anterior lens luxation as pupillary block can result. Pilocarpine is a directly acting miotic that may be used alone or in combination with adrenaline (epinephrine) to lower intraocular pressure. Pilocarpine produces an increase in aqueous outflow whilst adrenaline decreases aqueous production. This combination is said to be well tolerated in cats (Manski & Latimer in Sherding, 1989). Pilocarpine is contraindicated in uveitis as it may promote iridal inflammation. Indirectly acting miotics and anticholinesterases increase the outflow of aqueous humour by causing constriction of the ciliary musculature. Demecarium

* Daranide; Merck, Sharpe and Dohme, Hoddesdon, Hants, UK.

bromide (0.125%; Humorsol*) and echothio-
phate (0.125%; Phospholine iodide) can be administered once or twice daily. However, both
may have ocular and systemic side-effects associated with excessive cholinergic stimulation or
local irritation.

OSMOTIC DIURETICS
Osmotic diuretics act by dehydrating the vitreous
and deepening the anterior chamber thereby
opening a compromised angle. Their use is indicated in acute glaucoma. Mannitol (1 g/kg bodyweight as a 20% solution i.v.) will rapidly reduce
ocular hypertension. Water uptake should be
restricted for 2–4 hours after its administration.
Its use may be contraindicated in the presence of
uveitis as an intact blood barrier is required for
effectiveness.

BETA-ADRENERGIC AGENTS
Timolol is a beta-blocker that effectively lowers
intraocular pressure in man but has yet to be
shown to have any therapeutic value in small
animals. It may be used as a 0.25–0.5% solution,
and has been evaluated in the cat under experimental conditions, where it has been shown to
produce a marked decrease in aqueous production
(Colasanti, 1981). There is some indication that it
may be more effective when used at night. Bradycardia and respiratory distress are possible side-
effects.

SURGERY
Surgical treatment of glaucoma is usually reserved
for those cases which fail to respond to medical
treatment. However, in cases of acute glaucoma
rapid improvement is necessary and surgery may
be indicated early in the course of the disease if
any degree of vision is to be retained. A wide
range of surgical techniques are available but
none is entirely satisfactory for the long-term
relief of this serious problem.

* Humorsol, Merck & Co. Westpoint, PA19488, USA.

THE VITREOUS

The vitreous occupies two-thirds of the globe. It
contains 99% water and a framework of collagen
fibrils with hyaluronic acid containing mucopolysaccharides. The vitreous occupies the posterior
segment of the eye and has attachments to the
edge of the optic disc, posterior lens capsule and
the pars plana ciliaris/ora ciliaris retinae. The
hyaloid vasculature may be present for up to 8
weeks in kittens.

Examination
To examine the vitreous, pupillary dilatation is
necessary. Focal illumination, a direct ophthalmoscope (0 to +10 lenses) and a slit-lamp biomicroscope are useful. The latter allows visualization
of the anterior two-thirds of the vitreous. Ultrasonography and vitreous paracentesis (Gelatt,
1981) may be helpful diagnostic techniques.

Congenital anomalies

Persistent hyaloid
Hyaloid remnants are rare in the cat; they are
non-progressive but may be accompanied by a
posterior polar cataract.

Acquired conditions

Hyalitis
Hyalitis occurs due to a breakdown in the blood–
vitreous barrier, a vitreous haze resulting from
protein and cellular deposits. With severe inflammation liquefaction of the vitreous (syneresis)
may occur. The term hyalitis is misleading as the
vitreous is an acellular and avascular structure. In
the cat vitreal involvement may occur with feline
leukaemia virus, toxoplasmosis, feline infectious
peritonitis, cryptococcosis, blastomycosis and histoplasmosis infections.

Vitreous haemorrhage
The cat would appear to be predisposed to intra-
vitreal or preretinal haemorrhage. The cause is
often systemic and may be associated with a
hypertensive retinopathy (diabetes, renal failure).

Local factors such as trauma, chorioretinitis, uveitis, intraocular neoplasia, glaucoma or retinal detachment may also cause haemorrhage into the vitreous.

Herniation of vitreous
The vitreous may herniate into the anterior and posterior chambers following lens luxation, cataract extraction or trauma. Adhesions may form to the iris or the cornea leading to iris bombé, corneal opacity and glaucoma.

THE RETINA

The retina consists of an outer retinal pigment epithelium and an inner neurosensory layer. The retinal pigment epithelium is loosely attached to the rest of the retina and when retinal detachment occurs the separation is between the retinal pigment epithelium and the photoreceptors.

The neurosensory retina consists of nine layers. These are:
1 The receptors (rods and cones).
2 The external limiting membrane (cell membrane connection of the rods, cones and Müller's cells).
3 The outer nuclear layer (receptor nuclei).
4 The outer plexiform layer (axons of receptor nuclei).
5 The inner nuclear layer (nuclei of amacrine, horizontal, bipolar and Müller's cells).
6 The inner plexiform layer (axons of the inner nuclear layer).
7 The ganglion cell layer.
8 The nerve fibre layer.
9 The internal limiting membrane.

The receptors consists of rods and cones which are highly complex structures. The outer segments of the rods are embedded in the retinal pigment epithelium. The rods are sensitive to low-level illumination but have low visual discrimination. In contrast, the cones allow for visual discrimination and possibly colour vision but are less sensitive to light. There is a high cone concentration temporal to the optic disc; this area is devoid of blood vessels and is known as the area centralis, analogous to the macula in man. The feline retina is a rod-rich retina and will function better in dim light and detect movement better than detail or colour. The photoreceptors converge on ganglion cells at the ratio of approximately 130:1 in the cat. The axons of the ganglion cells form the nerve fibre layer. In the cat, unlike the dog, these nerve fibres are unmyelinated until they have passed through the lamina cribrosa. The blood vessels supplying the retina (cilioretinal vessels) lie in this nerve fibre layer. In the cat they can be seen arising in three pairs from the edge of the optic disc. The optic disc has a pitted or mesh-like appearance due to the visible presence of the lamina cribrosa. It is non-myelinated, grey in colour and about 1 mm in diameter.

The tapetum is located within the dorsal choroid and below the choriocapillaris (Plate 9.17). The retinal pigment epithelium overlying the tapetum is usually devoid of pigment or only sparsely pigmented. However, in the ventral non-tapetal fundus the presence of pigment within the retinal pigment epithelium gives a dark-brown appearance. The exception to this appearance is seen in animals that are subalbinotic or albinotic, e.g. Siamese (Plate 9.18). They may lack a tapetum and the retinal pigment epithelium is devoid of pigment thereby producing a fundus where only choroidal vessels are apparent against a white scleral background. Where some pigment is present the fundus will appear uniformly red. The internal limiting membrane may sometimes be visible as a glassy membrane giving a shimmering reflection to the fundus on ophthalmoscopic examination. It covers the entire retina except the optic disc. This appearance is more obvious in the non-tapetal fundus. The normal retina is not visible ophthalmoscopically as it is a transparent structure. However, when retinal detachment occurs it can be seen as a white 'veil' occupying the posterior segment.

Examination techniques

Having examined the eye in diffuse illumination, and assessed the pupillary light reflex, the pupil should be dilated in order to examine the fundus. Ophthalmoscopic examination reveals two distinct areas, a dorsal tapetal fundus (tapetum lucidum) and a ventral non-tapetal fundus (tapetum nigrum). The dorsal tapetal fundus is characterized by a large highly reflective coloured tapetum. It can be divided into two sections transected by the cilioretinal blood vessels giving a dorsolateral and dorsomedial tapetal fundus and a ventral non-tapetal fundus. It is often helpful to follow the three vascular pathways in the tapetal fundus thereby ensuring that the whole of the retina is examined. The optic disc lies in the tapetal fundus near the junction between the tapetum lucidum and tapetum nigrum and provides a good point of reference from which to start an ophthalmoscopic examination. The following parameters should be noted:

1 Optic disc size and colour.
2 Retinal blood vessels. Their presence or absence, tortuosity, degree of vascular filling and the presence of neovascularization.
3 Tapetum. The degree of reflectivity, the presence of abnormal pigment.
4 Retina. The presence of haemorrhages, folds, detachment, tears or exudates.

Fluorescein angiography

This technique allows for the evaluation of retinal vascular defects, the integrity of the blood–retinal barrier and retinal pigment epithelium, as evidenced by the leakage of dye.

Electroretinography

Electroretinography is a recording of the electrical potentials produced by the retina in a characteristic wave form. In the presence of retinal disease this wave form may be modified or absent. It is a useful diagnostic technique in early cases of progressive retinal atrophy or conditions such as sudden acquired retinal degeneration where the retina appears clinically normal. Electroretinography may also be carried out preoperatively in cases of cataract extraction in order to assess retinal function.

Retinal dysplasia

Retinal dysplasia is a congenital condition and implies impaired retinal differentiation. Multifocal retinal dysplasia has been reported in kittens infected prenatally or early in postnatal development with panleucopenia virus. The retinal lesions result in retinal atrophy and pigmentary changes in the non-tapetal fundus but are unassociated with any clinical signs of defective vision (Martin, 1982). Feline leukaemia virus has also been shown to cause retinal dysplasia in experimentally infected cats (Wyman, 1986).

Retinal degeneration

Retinal degeneration may be inherited or acquired. There are certain important features which sometimes allow the clinician to distinguish between the two. Inherited retinal degeneration has a definite breed and age incidence. The condition is always progressive, resulting in blindness. Both eyes are affected simultaneously and, most important of all, the lesions are symmetrical. The inherited retinal degenerations in the cat are generalized, involving both rods and cones, and the whole of the fundus becomes progressively affected. The term 'generalized progressive retinal atrophy' is usually reserved for those retinal degenerations which are inherited. However, the nomenclature is confusing as some generalized progressive retinal atrophies are not inherited, e.g. secondary to trauma. The history, breed and age are therefore of value in arriving at an accurate diagnosis and where there is no proof of inheritance the condition should be described as a retinal degeneration, as opposed to generalized progressive retinal atrophy. The term 'central progressive retinal atrophy' is reserved for retinal degenerations that primarily affect the cones. The lesions therefore correspond in the early stage to the area centralis. In the cat there is no proven inherited central progressive retinal atrophy although taurine deficiency has been described as such in the past.

Acquired retinal degeneration shows no age or breed incidence. The lesions are frequently asymmetrical, with the exception of taurine deficiency, and they are not necessarily progressive. One or both eyes may be affected. They are often secondary to a choroiditis and there may be signs of concurrent retinal or choroidal inflammation such as haemorrhage, retinal detachment and cellular exudation. Abnormal retinal pigment epithelial pigmentation may develop.

The cardinal sign of retinal degeneration, whether inherited or acquired, is tapetal hyper-reflectivity due to retinal thinning. Where the condition is progressive narrowing and finally loss of retinal blood vessels occurs. Optic disc atrophy also occurs and the non-tapetal fundus becomes paler and depigmented. Clinically a progressive loss of the pupillary light reflex accompanies deterioration in vision.

Inherited retinopathies

GENERALIZED PROGRESSIVE RETINAL ATROPHY

In the cat generalized progressive retinal atrophy (GPRA) has been described in the Abyssinian (Plate 9.19), the Persian and the Siamese. In the Abyssinian there would appear to be two distinct presentations for GPRA. In the UK the condition has been described by Barnett and Curtis (1985). It presents at a few weeks of age with nystagmus, dilated pupils and decreased pupillary light reflex, narrowing of retinal blood vessels and tapetal hyper-reflectivity. The kittens are blind. The condition is a rod-cone dysplasia present at birth and is inherited in a dominant fashion.

In Sweden GPRA in the Abyssinian is an autosomal recessively inherited disorder (Narfstrom, 1983). The age of onset is usually 12 months (range 6 months to 2½ years). Most cats are blind by 3 years of age. The area centralis and the area around the optic disc are the first to be affected. This is followed by the mid-peripheral and peripheral fundus and finally the non-tapetal fundus becomes involved. The signs are of discoloration in the tapetal fundus, hyper-reflectivity, blood vessel attenuation and depigmentation of the non-tapetal fundus. This condition is a rod-cone degeneration.

In the UK a late-onset GPRA has been described in the Abyssinian but evidence of inheritance is lacking (Carlile *et al.*, 1984). The situation in the Siamese breed is the same (Barnett, 1965)

(Plate 9.20). In the Persian, GPRA has been described in the USA in kittens of 12 weeks of age (Rubin & Lipton, 1973) and this may be similar to that described above in the Abyssinian in the UK.

GYRATE ATROPHY

A generalized retinal atrophy has been described in the cat that is analogous to gyrate atrophy in man (Valle *et al.*, 1983). Both retina and choroid are affected due to an increase in plasma ornithine. The condition is blinding. In man it is an inherited disorder.

GM1 GANGLIOSIDOSIS

This is a lysosomal storage disease which results in an accumulation of glycolipid in the retinal ganglion cells (Murray et al., 1977). It is an inherited autosomal trait in the cat. See 'The Cornea' above.

Acquired retinopathies

Acquired retinal degeneration may be secondary to a wide variety of insults such as inflammation, trauma, neoplasia, nutritional deficiency and errors of metabolism.

NUTRITIONAL RETINOPATHY

Taurine deficiency

The best described nutritional retinopathy is that of taurine deficiency (Plate 9.21). The condition has been extensively reviewed by Barnett and Burger (1980). Feline central retinal degeneration was initially thought to be an inherited condition and it was some time before the true aetiology was discovered. Taurine is an essential amino acid in the cat and a relative deficiency in the diet results in retinal degeneration and cardiomyopathy although the two do not appear to be present together. Most ocular lesions develop after 6 – 7 months on a taurine-deficient diet. These diets may be semi-purified, vegetable-based diets, dog foods or specialized proprietary diets where taurine has been omitted. All present-day cat foods should contain adequate amounts of taurine.

The retinal lesion presents as a bilateral symmetrical oval or elliptical area originating in the area centralis (temporal and superior to the optic disc). With progression a second lesion may appear on the nasal side. The two coalesce above the optic disc to form one large area of hyper-reflectivity in the tapetal fundus corresponding to the areas of greatest cone density. If the deficiency continues the retinal atrophy becomes generalized. However, if the diet is supplemented with taurine the degeneration is halted.

Thiamine deficiency

Diets high in thiaminase or lacking in thiamine have been reported to result in lesions of the optic disc (peripapillary oedema), neovascularization and a retinopathy (Gelatt, 1981). However, a more recent survey found a total absence of ocular lesions (Davidson, 1992).

INFLAMMATORY RETINOPATHIES

The retina and choroid are often affected simultaneously by inflammatory conditions. The retina becomes secondarily involved in choroiditis and it is often not possible to distinguish clinically between choroidal and retinal inflammation. Active inflammation may result in a cellular infiltration of the fundus. These lesions appear as grey foci with hazy borders. Sheathing may occur around blood vessels and extend into the vitreous (hyalitis). Accumulation of fluid between the retinal pigment epithelium and the neurosensory layers results in an exudative retinal detachment which may be localized or total (Plate 9.22). Exudative detachments are the commonest type of detachment seen in the cat. Detachments may also arise due to tears in the retina, or subsequent to traction as a result of adhesions from the vitreous or through vitreal loss.

Haemorrhage not infrequently occurs in the feline retina. It may be associated with feline leukaemia virus, autoimmune haemolytic anaemia, septicaemia or hypertension. The commonest form of haemorrhage is the intraretinal haemorrhage, which appears as dark-red and punctate in form. However, they may also be pre-retinal (bright-red and large) or haemorrhages in the nerve fibre layer (flat and striated).

Inflammatory retinopathies are usually a manifestation of systemic disease in the cat. Those agents such as feline infectious peritonitis, toxoplasma and feline leukaemia virus that cause uveitis are also possible causes of retinitis.

An association between exudative retinal detachment, haemorrhage and diabetes mellitus induced by megestrol acetate has been recorded (Herrtage & Barnett, 1985). Hypertension is a common cause of retinal problems in man and also a cause of retinal haemorrhage and detachment in the ageing cat. Treatment is difficult as patients are often presented when the condition is advanced and the animal shows signs of complete blindness. However, diuretics and corticosteroids may be helpful in the early stages of exudative chorioretinitis. Small retinal detachments may heal spontaneously.

VASCULAR RETINOPATHIES

Excessive dilatation and tortuosity of retinal vessels, retinal haemorrhage, retinal detachments and papilloedema have been described with congenital heart disease in a 2-year-old cat (Lombard & Twitchell, 1978).

TOXIC RETINAL DEGENERATION

Retinal degeneration of this type has been reported in cats given the potent carcinogen methyl-*N*-nitrosurea (MNU) in combination with ketamine. Bilateral generalized retinal atrophy developed 5 days after injection. When either drug was given alone it did not occur. The lesion is reported as being similar to that of feline central retinal degeneration and may well be the result of a decrease in taurine uptake (Schuller *et al.*, 1981).

HYPERTENSIVE RETINOPATHY

Systemic hypertension in the cat has been recorded with hyperthyroidism, chronic renal disease and idiopathic hypertrophic cardiomyopathy (Lesser, 1990). Systemic hypertension in association with ocular signs, i.e. haemorrhage and retinal detachment, has been recorded in 24 cats, the average age being 15.1 years. There was a sex ratio of 63% males and no breed predisposition. All had some degree of mild renal impairment. Sixteen of the cats had cardiac changes and three were hyperthyroid (Litman, 1990). Another study by Kobayashi *et al.* (1990) demonstrated that hypertension was common in cats with chronic renal failure and hyperthyroidism but none of these cases showed evidence of ocular disease. However, it would appear that where the blood pressures are significantly elevated, particularly for long periods of time, then ocular disease is more likely to develop (Morgan, 1986). Primary or essential hypertension has also been described in the cat in association with a retinopathy. This case had a chronic history of dietary salt supplementation for a lower urinary tract disease (Turner *et al.*, 1990).

The presenting ocular signs in hypertensive cases are of advanced and total retinal detachments (Plate 9.22) in association with haemorrhages into the retina and vitreous and sometimes the anterior chamber (Plate 9.23). Clinically such cases present as acute blindness in one or both eyes. Causes other than hypertension should be considered when presented with such cases and these include clotting deficiencies, systemic disease, neoplasia and hyperproteinaemias.

Treatment is possible and in the acute stages the retina will re-attach and vision is restored. The protocol for treatment is varied depending on the presence or absence of systemic disease. However, good results have been obtained with the use of antihypertensive diuretics, beta-blockers and enzyme inhibitors (captopril). A low salt diet may be helpful.

NEOPLASIA

Tumours affecting the eye, adnexa and orbit may be primary or secondary. These tumours occur less frequently in the cat than the dog, although they are more malignant. Less than 2% of all feline tumours affect the eye.

Orbital neoplasia

Orbital tumours may develop from any of the orbital tissues. They are relatively uncommon but are usually malignant. The prognosis for orbital neoplasia is therefore poor. Primary orbital tumours that have been reported in the cat include osteosarcoma, rhabdomyosarcoma and undifferentiated sarcomas (Peiffer *et al.*, 1988). Secondary orbital tumours are less common. They may arise as direct extension from adjacent tissues, e.g. squamous cell carcinoma (Murphy *et al.*, 1989a). Malignant intraocular tumours such as the melanoma and adnexal tumours, e.g. squamous cell carcinoma, may also infiltrate the orbit. Systemic haematogenous spread may occur with lymphosarcoma and adenocarcinoma (Murphy *et al.*, 1989b).

Clinical signs are related to the development of a space-occupying lesion. The globe becomes exophthalmic, deviated and cannot be retropulsed. Examination of the mouth may reveal oral involvement behind the last molar tooth. The diagnostic techniques are as for exophthalmos. Radiography, tomography and ultrasonography of the orbital area may be helpful. Where metastatic spread is likely, thoracic and abdominal radiographs should be taken. Treatment depends on the nature of the tumour but the prognosis for orbital neoplasia is always poor. If the neoplasm appears to be localized to the orbit then exenteration is the treatment of choice.

The differential diagnoses for orbital neoplasia are orbital abscessation, cellulitis and foreign body penetration. The onset of all these conditions is usually more rapid than with neoplasia.

Eyelid tumours

Tumours of the eyelid are relatively common. A wide variety, including fibromas and fibrosarcomas, neurofibroma and neurofibrosarcoma, haemangiomas and haemangiosarcomas (Williams *et al.*, 1981), and basal cell and mast cell tumours (Peiffer & Gelatt, 1981) have been documented. Many are potentially malignant and a wide surgical excision is the treatment of choice. Papillomas in the cat are rare; the lesion may be sessile or pedunculated and may be self-limiting.

Squamous cell carcinoma

This tumour arises from the epidermis at the eyelid margin and may spread to involve the conjunctiva and limbus. It is a malignant highly invasive and ulcerating neoplasm. It can arise as a primary from the conjunctiva, third eyelid or cornea. Like all squamous cell carcinomas it is more common in white cats and is probably the commonest adnexal tumour in the cat. The diagnosis is made on the histological appearance of the tumour.

Treatment is surgical; cryosurgery and radiotherapy may be of value.

Adenoma/adenocarcinoma

These tumours usually arise from the meibomian glands to involve the eyelids, palpebral conjunctiva or third eyelid. They may present as pigmented or non-pigmented proliferative masses. Surgical excision is the treatment of choice. Metastases are unlikely.

Lymphosarcoma

Lymphosarcomas may arise from the lymphatic tissues in the nictitating membranes. Gross enlargement of the third eyelid results with displacement of the globe. The treatment of choice is wide surgical excision and it is possibly the only indication for the total removal of the third eyelid.

Corneal tumours

Primary tumours of the cornea are very rare. Secondary tumours arise through extension from other tissues. These include the malignant intraocular melanomas, squamous cell carcinoma and lymphosarcoma.

Intraocular tumours

Intraocular tumours may be primary or secondary. The uvea is most commonly involved. Early primary lesions tend not to produce inflammation, whereas secondary metastatic lesions often cause marked inflammation. The most common primary intraocular tumour is the malignant melanoma, whereas lymphosarcoma is the commonest secondary intraocular tumour. Intraocular tumours may also arise as a result of local extension from adjacent tissues.

Diagnosis of intraocular neoplasia is often very difficult. The course of the condition is usually chronic although the patient is frequently presented with an acute history. The eye may be secondarily afflicted with glaucoma, uveitis and cataract formation, which may mask the presence of an intraocular mass. The cornea may be oedematous and bleeding may have occurred in the anterior and/or posterior segments. Diagnosis relies on a thorough intraocular examination. The use of a slit-lamp and gonio lens allows for a detailed examination of the anterior chamber. Mydriasis may reveal the presence of a mass in the posterior segment. Where the ocular media are cloudy, preventing ophthalmoscopic examination, ultrasonography may be helpful. Intraocular biopsy is contraindicated as it may cause seeding of tumour cells, and paracentesis is often hazardous. Treatment should be symptomatic until a diagnosis is reached. The following primary intraocular tumours have been reported in the cat: melanoma, spindle cell sarcoma, adenoma and adenocarcinoma.

Primary intraocular tumours

MELANOMA

Melanoma is a common intraocular tumour with a variable presentation. Diffuse iris melanomas (Plate 9.24) may present as benign looking areas of patchy pigmentation. These proliferate and coalesce over a period of months or years. They are slowly progressive but may involve iris stroma, ciliary body and the drainage angle. It is important to differentiate this type of tumour from normal iris pigmentation (Plate 9.25). A diagnosis of diffuse iris melanoma may depend on frequent examinations at set intervals of time in order to monitor any changes in pigmentation. An added difficulty in diagnosis is the normal change in iris that occurs in age (the irises of older cats are frequently thin with small areas of pigmentation). If treatment is to be undertaken then enucleation should be performed. However, these tumours have been monitored for long periods of time (5 years) without any adverse affects (Wyman, 1986).

Another presentation of the intraocular melanoma is the malignant uveal melanoma arising from the iris and ciliary body. Choroidal involvement is uncommon. This tumour is the most common primary intraocular tumour in the cat and usually occurs in older cats and is unilateral. These tumours are pigmented and present as discrete masses infiltrating the iris and ciliary body. They are highly vascular and may cause necrosis, haemorrhage, intraocular inflammation, secondary glaucoma and cataract. The intraocular melanoma is locally aggressive and may extend to extraocular tissues through the sclera. Metastases to the lung and liver, although they do occur, are not common. No study in the cat has been made to correlate cell type with prognosis or survival time. Enucleation is the only treatment. However, these tumours must be differentiated from iris cysts and benign pigmentary changes.

In addition to the two forms of intraocular melanoma considered above, limbal melanoma has been reported in the cat (Harling *et al.*, 1986). The limbal melanoma usually arises in the superior quadrant as a darkly pigmented mass involving both cornea and sclera. Intraocular examination usually reveals nothing significant and the mass is unassociated with any clinical signs. These tumours are very slow growing and there have been no reports of metastasis.

Treatment in the form of lamellar keratectomy in conjunction either with cryosurgery or preferably beta-irradiation would appear to give extremely good results.

SPINDLE CELL SARCOMA

Primary ocular sarcomas are uncommon but important tumours of the globe. They are thought to arise as a direct result of severe trauma or chronic inflammation within the iris. The latter may be a result of the former. In all reported cases (Dubielzig, 1984; Peiffer *et al.*, 1988) the trauma occurred some time previously, varying from 5 months to 11 years. The affected globes presented as enlarged firm masses, totally disorganized, with the extension of tumour tissue into the optic nerve in some cases. In one series deposits of osteoids were found (Dubielzig, 1984) whereas in another instance the mass was re-

ported to be an osteosarcoma (Miller, 1987). Enucleation of affected eyes and blind phthisical eyes, as a prophylactic measure, is the treatment of choice.

ADENOMA/ADENOCARCINOMA

These tumours do occur in the cat but are rare. They may present as pigmented or non-pigmented masses arising from the ciliary body. The treatment of choice is enucleation. The patient should be given a thorough clinical examination for evidence of metastases before surgery is performed.

Secondary intraocular tumours

LYMPHOSARCOMA

Lymphosarcoma is reported to be the most common secondary intraocular neoplasm in the feline eye. The condition may present as diffuse with severe uveitis (Plate 9.26) or there may be the presence of an anterior chamber mass (Plate 9.27). Systemic disease usually accompanies the ocular signs. An antigen test for FeLV should be carried out. Aqueocentesis may be of value in confirming the diagnosis.

Pupillary abnormalities in the absence of any other ocular signs have been described as the result of systemic FeLV infection. The pupillary light reflex is poor in association with mydriasis. Urinary incontinence may also occur.

ADENOCARCINOMA

Adenocarcinomas may metastasize to the eye from primary sites in the uterus (Bellhorn, 1972), mammary gland (West, 1979) and sweat gland (Moisse, 1982). The presentation may be unilateral or bilateral. The uvea, as in man, appears to be a predilection site for metastases; however, there may also be involvement of extraocular tissue. Tumour tissue may infiltrate iris, choroid and optic nerve, resulting in retinal haemorrhage, detachment and optic neuritis.

Other intraocular tumours that have been reported to occur in the cat are squamous cell carcinoma and haemangiosarcoma (Gelatt, 1991). Metastases usually occur to the anterior uvea and less commonly the posterior uvea. Neoplasia should be suspected in cases of retinal detachment and haemorrhage. Optic nerve involvement may occur with lymphosarcoma, spindle cell sarcoma and adenocarcinoma. Primary tumours at this site have not been reported in the cat.

REFERENCES

Albert R.A., Garrett P.D., Whiteley R.D. *et al.* (1982) Surgical correction of everted third eyelid in two cats. *J. Am. Vet. Med. Ass.* **180**, 763–6.

Barnett K.C. (1965) Retinal atrophy. *Vet. Rec.* **77**, 1543–52.

Barnett K.C. & Burger I.H. (1980) Taurine deficiency retinopathy in the cat. *J. Small Anim. Pract.* **21**, 521–4.

Barnett K.C. & Curtis R. (1985) Autosomal dominant progressive retinal atrophy in Abyssinian cats. *J. Hered.* **76**, 168–70.

Bedford P.G.C. & Cotchin E. (1983) An unusual chronic keratoconjunctivitis in the cat. *J. Small Anim. Pract.* **24**, 85–102.

Bellhorn R.W. (1972) Secondary ocular adenocarcinoma in three dogs and one cat. *J. Am. Vet. Med. Ass.* **160**, 302–7.

Bellhorn R.W., Barnett K.C. & Henkind P. (1971) Ocular coloboma in domestic cats. *J. Am. Vet. Med. Ass.* **159**, 1015–21.

Bistner S.I., Carlson J.H., Shively J.N. *et al.* (1971) Ocular manifestations of Feline Herpes Infection. *J. Am. Vet. Med. Ass.* **159**, 1223.

Blogg J.R. (1980) *The Eye in Veterinary Practice.* Saunders & Co. pp. 247–55.

Brightman A.H., Vestre W.A., Helper L.C. *et al.* (1979) Chronic eosinophilic keratitis in the cat. *Feline Pract.* **9**, 21–4.

Campbell L.H., Fox J.G. & Synders S.B. (1973) Ocular bacteria and mycoplasma of the clinical normal cat. *Feline Pract.* **3**, 10.

Carlile J.L., Carrington S.D. & Bedford P.G.C. (1984) Six cases of Progressive Retinal Atrophy in Abyssinian cats. *J. Small Anim. Pract.* **25**, 415–20.

Cello R.M. (1967) Ocular infections in animals with P.L.I. group organism. *Am. J. Ophthalmol.* **63**, 1270–3.

Colasanti B.K. & Trotter R.R. (1981) Effects of beta, and beta$_2$ adenoreceptor agonists and antagonists on intraocular pressure in the cat. *Invest. Ophthalmol. Visual Sci.* **20**, 69.

Collier L.L. (1979) Ocular manifestations of the Chediak–Higashi syndrome in four species of animals. *J. Am. Vet. Med. Ass.* **175**, 587.

Collins K., Swanson J.F. & MacWilliams P.S. (1986) Eosinophilic keratitis and keratoconjunctivitis in a cat. *Mod. Vet. Pract.* **1**, 32–5.

Curtis R. (1988) Retinal diseases in the dog and cat – an overview and update. *J. Am. Vet. Med. Ass.* **29**, 397–415.

Davidson M.G. (1992) Thiamin deficiency in a colony of cats. *Vet. Rec.* **130**, 94–7.

Davidson M., Nasisse N., Wilcock B. & Jamieson V. (1989) Feline anterior uveitis: 53 cases. *Programme and Transactions of the 20th meeting of the American College of Veterinary Ophthalmologists, New Orleans.*

Dubielzig R.R. (1984) Ocular sarcoma following trauma in three cats. *J. Am. Vet. Med. Ass.* **184**, 578–81.

Dziezyc J. & Millichamp N.J. (1989) Surgical correction of eyelid agenesis in a cat. *J. Am. Anim. Hosp. Ass.* **25**(5), 513–6.

English R.V., Davidson M.G., Nasisse M.P., Jamieson V.E. & Lappin M.R. (1990) Intraocular disease associated with feline immunodeficiency virus and infection in cats. *J. Am. Vet. Med. Ass.* **196**, 7.

Fawcett J., Altman N. & Domray S.Y. (1977) Multiple xanthomatosis in a cat. *Feline Pract.* **7**, 32–3.

Fox J.G. & Galus C.B. (1977) Salmonella-associated conjunctivitis in a cat. *J. Am. Vet. Med. Ass.* **171**, 845.

Gaskell R.M. & Povey R.C. (1979) Feline viral rhinotracheitis: sites of virus replication and persistance in acutely and persistently infected cats. **27**, 167–74.

Gelatt K.N. (1991) *Veterinary Ophthalmology.* Lea & Febiger, Philadelphia.

Haesebrouck F., Devriese L.A., van Rijssen B. & Cox E. (1991) Incidence and significance of isolation of *Mycoplasma felis* from conjunctival swabs of cats. *Vet. Microbiol.* **26**, 95–101.

Harling D.E., Peiffer R.L., Cook C.S. & Belkin P.V. (1986) Feline limbal melanoma: four cases. *J. Am. Anim. Hosp. Ass.* **22**, 595–802.

Haskins M.E. & McDonough S.K. (1979) Mucopolysaccharidosis in a domestic short-haired cat. *J. Am. Vet. Med. Ass.* **175**, 384–87.

Hendy-Ibbs P.M. (1985) Familial feline epibulbar dermoids. *Vet. Rec.* **116**, 13–14.

Herrtage M.E. & Barnett K.C. (1985) Diabetic retinopathy in a cat with megestrol acetate induced diabetes. *J. Small Anim. Pract.* **26**, 595–601.

Kobayashi, Peterson M.E., Graves T.K., Lesser M. & Nichols C.E. (1990) Hypertension in cats with chronic renal failure or hyperthyroidism. *J. Vet. Internal Med.* **4**(2), 58.

Koch S.A. (1979) Congenital ophthalmic abnormalities in Burmese cats. *J. Am. Vet. Med. Ass.* **174**, 90–1.

Lappin M.R., Roberts S.M., Davidson M.G. *et al.* (1989) Detection of *T. gondii*-specific antigens and antibodies in the aqueous humor of cats. In preparation. *Am. J. Vet. Res.*

Leon A. (1988) Diseases of the vitreous in the dog and cat. *J. Small Anim. Pract.* **29**, 448–61.

Lesser M. (1990) Non-invasive blood pressure evaluation in cats with left ventricular hypertrophic disease. *J. Vet. Internal Med.* **4**(2), 117.

Litman M.P. (1990) Spontaneous systemic hypertension in cats. *J. Vet. Internal Med.* **4**(2), 117.

Lombard C.W. & Twitchell M.J. (1978) Tortuosity, sacculations of blood vessels and retinal detachment with the tetrology of fallot. *J. Am. Anim. Hosp. Ass.* **14**, 624–30.

Manning T.O., Scott D.W., Smith C.A. & Lewis R.M. (1982) Pemphigus disease in the feline. *J. Am. Anim. Hosp. Ass.* **18**, 433.

Martin C.L. (1982) Feline ophthalmologic disease. *Mod. Vet. Pract.* **63**, 385.

Miller W.W. & Bousinger T.R. (1987) Intraocular osteosarcoma in a cat. *J. Am. Anim. Hosp. Ass.* **23**, 317.

Moisse N.S., Riis R.C. & Allison N.M. (1982) Ocular manifestation of metastatic sweat gland adenocarcinoma in the cat. *J. Am. Vet. Med. Ass.* **180**, 1100–3.

Morgan G. (1969) Ocular tumors in animals. *J. Small Anim. Pract.* **10**, 563–70.

Morgan G. (1986) Systemic hypertension in four cats. Ocular and medical findings. *J. Am. Anim. Hosp. Assoc.* **22**, 615–21.

Murphy C.J. Koblik P., Bellhorn R.W. *et al.* (1989a) Squamous cell carcinoma causing blindness and ophthalmopegia in a cat. *J. Am. Vet. Med. Ass.* **195**, 7.

Murphy C.J., Canton D.C., Bellhorn R.W. *et al.* (1989b) Disseminated adenocarcinoma with ocular involvement in a cat. *J. Am. Vet. Med. Ass.* **195**, 11.

Murray J.A., Blakemore W.F. & Barnett K.C. (1977) Ocular lesions in cats with GM-gangliosidosis with visceral involvement. *J. Small Anim. Pract.* **18**, 1–10.

Narfstrom K. (1983) Hereditary progressive retinal atrophy in the Abyssinian cat. *J. Hered.* **74**, 273–6.

Nasisse M.P. (1982) Manifestations, diagnosis and treatment of ocular herpes infection in the cat. *Compend. Cont. Educ. Pract. Vet.* **4**, 962–70.

Pedersen N.C. (1988) *Feline Infectious Diseases.* American Veterinary Publications.

Peiffer R.L. (1981) In *Veterinary Ophthalmology* (ed. Gelatt K.N.) Lea & Febiger, Philadelphia.

Peiffer R.L. (1982a) Inherited ocular diseases of the dog and the cat. *Compend. Cont. Educ. Pract. Vet.* **4**(2), 142–66.

Peiffer R.L. (1982b) Bilateral congenital aphakia and retinal detachment in a cat. *J. Am. Anim. Hosp. Ass.* **18**, 128–30.

Peiffer R.L. & Belkin P.V. (1983) Keratolenticular dysgenesis in a kitten. *J. Am. Vet. Med. Ass.* **182**, 124.

Peiffer R.L., Monicello, T. & Bouldin T.W. (1988) Primary ocular sarcomas in the cat. *J. Small Anim. Pract.* **29**, 105–16.

Pentlarge V., Powell-Johnson G., Martin C.L. *et al.* (1989) Orbital neoplasia with enophthalmos in a cat. *J. Am. Vet. Med. Ass.* **195**, 9.

Pickett J.P., Miller P.E. & Majors L.J. (1988) Calibration of the Schiotz tonometer. *Proc. Am. Coll. Vet. Ophthalmologists* **19**, 47–51.

Ridgway M.D. & Brightman A.H. (1989) Feline glaucoma – a retrospective study of 29 clinical cases. *J. Am. Anim. Hosp. Ass.* **25**(5), 485.

Rubin L.F. (1986) Hereditary cataract in Himalayan cats. *Feline Pract.* **16**, 14.

Rubin L.F. & Lipton D.E. (1973) Retinal degeneration in kittens. *J. Am. Vet. Med. Ass.* **162**, 467–9.

Schuller J.P., Wyman M., Weisbrode S.E. *et al.* (1981) Induction of retinal degeneration in cats by methylnitrosurea and ketamine hydrochloride. *Vet. Pathol.* **18**, 239.

Scott F.W., Delahunt A. & Schultz R.D. Teratogenesis in the cat associated with griseofulvin therapy (1974). *Teratology* **11**, 79.

Sheikh H. (1978) Feline chlamydial keratoconjunctivitis – an analogue of trachoma. Thesis. Institute of Ophthalmology, University of London.

Sherding R.G. (1989) *The cat, Diseases and Clinical Management*, vol. 2. Churchill Livingstone, New York.

Shewen P.E., Povey R.C. & Wilson M.R. (1980) A survey of the conjunctival flora of clinically normal cats and cats with conjunctivitis. *Can. Vet. J.* **21**, 231.

Startup F.G. (1988) Corneal necrosis and sequestration in the cat, a review and record of 100 cases. *J. Small Anim. Pract.* **29**, 7.

Tan R.J.S. (1974) Susceptibility of kittens to *Mycoplasma felis* infection. *Jap. J. Exp. Med.* **44**, 235–40.

Tan R.J.S. & Miles J.A.R. (1974) Incidence and significance of mycoplasmas in sick cats. *Res. Vet. Sci.* **16**, 27–34.

Tham K.M. & Studdert M.J. (1987) Clinical and immunological responses of cats to feline herpes type I infection. *Vet. Rec.* **120**, 321–6.

Turner J.L., Brogdon D.J., Lees G.E. & Greco D.S. (1990) Idiopathic hypertension in a cat with secondary hypertensive retinopathy associated with a high salt diet. *J. Am. Anim. Hosp. Ass.* **26**, 647–51.

Valle D., Jezyk P. & Aguirre G. (1983) Gyrate atrophy of choroid and retina. *Comp. Ophthalmol. Bull.* **15**, 2–4.

West C.S., Wolf E.D. & Vainsi S.J. (1979) Intraocular metastases of mammary adenocarcinoma in the cat. *J. Am. Anim. Hosp. Ass.* **15**, 725–7.

Whiteley R.D. (1987) Current concepts in feline ophthalmology. *Canadian Association of Veterinary Ophthalmology and American Society of Vecterinary Ophthalmologists Meeting Quebec, Canada.*

Whiteley R.D. & Moore C.P. (1984) Advances in feline ophthalmology. *Vet. Clin. N. Am. – Small Anim. Pract.* **14**, 1271–88.

Wilkie D.A. (1989) The background of ocular prostaglandins and their role in ophthalmic physiology and pathology. *Programme and Transactions of the Twentieth Annual Meeting of the American College of Veterinary Ophthalmologists, October 26–29, New Orleans.*

Williams L.W., Gelatt K.N. & Gwin R.M. (1981) Ophthalmic neoplasms in the cat. *J. Am. Anim. Hosp. Ass.* **17**, 999.

Wyman M. (1986) *Manual of Small Animal Ophthalmology.* Churchill Livingstone.

Chapter 10 / The Ear

J. G. LANE

INTRODUCTION

In the league table of complaints which cause cat owners to consult veterinary surgeons at first opinion clinics, diseases of the ears rank second equal with such conditions as rhinitis, dermatitis, dental disorders and gingivitis. Subcutaneous abscesses head this chart of discomfort. In primary accession centres otitis externa, most commonly arising through parasitism, predominates whereas in referral hospitals proliferative diseases of the outer and middle ear are more likely to be encountered.

The ears are particularly sensitive structures and therefore disorders which have an inflammatory component are likely to cause considerable distress. The signs of aural diseases which would be obvious to an owner are listed below:

1 Pain and resentment when the ears are touched.
2 Persistent scratching of the ear by the hind-foot. This in turn may cause further trauma to the ear itself and the skin between the base of the ear and the eye may become excoriated.
3 Constant twitching of the ears and head-shaking which produces a characteristic clicking sound.
4 Otorrhoea which may be accompanied by an unpleasant odour.
5 Swelling of the pinna or at the base of the ear.
6 Ulceration and bleeding of the ear flap.
7 Tilting of the head, loss of balance, inco-ordination or a tendency to walk in circles with the head tilted towards the centre of the circle.
8 Pharyngeal obstructive dyspnoea, generally with a nasal discharge.

9 Horner's syndrome: ptosis, anisocoria and prominence of the third eyelid.
10 Deafness.

ANATOMICAL CONSIDERATIONS

It is convenient to divide the ear into three sections to describe the diseases which afflict this region of the cat (Fig. 10.1)

The external ear

The pinna is an erect flap consisting of a thin layer of cartilage providing shape and stability, sandwiched between two layers of skin. On the outside the skin is covered by hair and is similar to the skin covering the remainder of the body. However, on the underside, and at the very edges, the integument is relatively hairless and unprotected.

The feline pinna is highly mobile – well-developed directional hearing is important to domestic and wild cats for the location of prey and predators. The auricular muscles are innervated through the auriculo-palpebral branch of the facial nerve (VII).

The external auditory meatus is a continuation of the pinna; it is cone-shaped to suit its function, which is to condense sound waves towards the tympanic membrane. The tubular canal is angled, with the vertical section supported by the auricular cartilage and the horizontal section by the annular cartilage. The hairless integument becomes thinner in the horizontal canal, and the

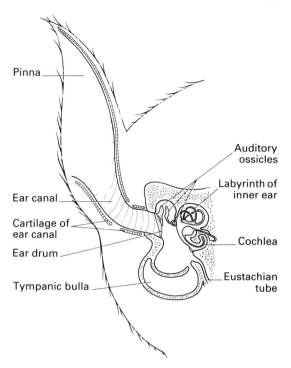

Fig. 10.1 Anatomy of the feline ear (diagrammatic and not to scale).

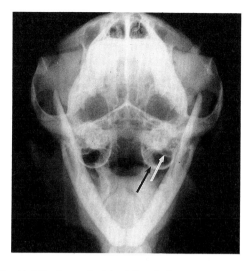

Fig. 10.2 Radiograph of the feline skull, open-mouth projection. The black arrow shows the outer wall of the tympanic bulla. The white arrow shows the wall of the true middle ear cavity.

cerumen and wax-producing glands are most numerous in the vertical segment.

The middle ear

The tympanic membrane forms the lateral limit of the middle ear and divides it from the horizontal canal of the external meatus. The middle ear cavity of the cat differs from that of the dog because the tympanic bulla has a double-shelled configuration with the true middle ear lying within a larger 'false' middle ear. In the past, reports in the North American literature described the feline middle ear as being divided into dorsomedial and ventrolateral compartments and yet it is obvious from radiographs of the feline skull, using the anteroposterior open-mouth projection (Fig. 10.2), that this is incorrect. There are indeed two compartments consisting of a smaller *dorsolateral* cavity, the true middle ear, whose lateral wall is largely formed by the ear-drum and which contains the auditory ossicles dorsally. It is divided by a bony septum, which is incomplete dorsally, from a larger *ventromedial* compartment which also extends somewhat more caudally than the inner shell. The larger compartment, the hypotympanum, corresponds to the fundic portion of the tympanic bulla of the dog.

The tympanic bullae provide the major landmarks on the ventral aspect of the feline skull (Fig. 10.3). Rostrally, these structures are closely related to the temporomandibular joint and, rostromedially, to the nasopharynx, with which they communicate via the eustachian tubes. Ventrally the bullae are thin-walled and have few soft-tissue attachments so that this is the route generally favoured for surgical invasion. The two compartments of the middle ear communicate through a narrow fissure on the caudomedial aspect of the smaller cavity where the dividing bony septum is incomplete. Towards its caudal extremity the fissure widens into a triangular foramen and the round window of the cochlea faces this foramen from the medial wall. The promontory is a rounded bony structure which contains the membranous labyrinth of the inner

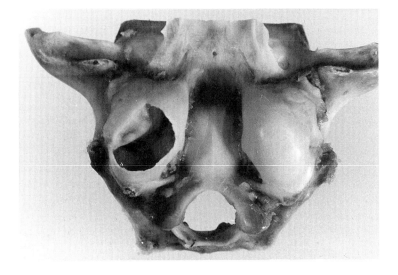

Fig. 10.3 Ventral aspect of the feline skull. Note the prominent tympanic bullae caudomedial to the temporomandibular joints. The left bulla has been opened to show the cavity of the outer shell. The true middle ear can be seen rostrolaterally.

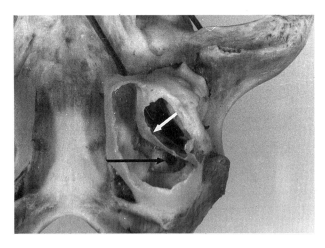

Fig. 10.4 Ventral aspect of right bulla. Both compartments have now been opened. The white arrow shows the broken edge of the septum which divides the cavity. The black arrow points to the position of the round window.

ear and which forms an obvious oval swelling into the dorsomedial wall of the middle ear; as it faces the dividing septum, it is in contact with both compartments (Fig. 10.4). The postganglionic fibres of the cervical sympathetic nerve enter the middle ear at the caudal extremity of the promontory where they fan out across the exposed bony swelling protected only by mucoperiosteum. Thus, they are vulnerable to trauma during middle ear surgery, particularly if the dividing septum is removed. Interruption of the fibres at this level will cause Horner's syndrome.

The middle ear serves two important functions.

First it facilitates the conversion of airborne sound waves at the eardrum into fluid vibrations of the endolymph at the oval window into the inner ear. However, cats, as well as dogs, with damaged eardrums or disrupted ossicular chains retain considerable hearing. Therefore, it is likely that this species relies significantly on sound reverberation through the bones of the skull (osseous conduction) and not exclusively on ossicular transmission. Second, the middle ear acts as a cushion to protect the delicate sensory receptors of the inner ear from the effects of very loud sounds.

Provisions are made for the confined air space

of the middle ear; small pressure changes are accommodated by the slack segment (pars flaccida) of the eardrum. Major pressure adjustments, as well as regular air changes, are made through the eustachian tubes during swallowing. Experimental occlusion of the eustachian tubes has been shown to produce unique effects in cats inasmuch as, in addition to the predictable stagnation of mucus in the middle ear cavity, granulomatous polypoid proliferations develop. It is conjectured that naturally occurring functional tubal occlusion is the cause of middle ear polyps in this species. The auditory os of the eustachian tube occupies the dorsomedial and rostral extremity of each inner compartment. Clearly if polypoid masses are found associated with the eustachian tube openings, the structures of the true middle ear described above are vulnerable to trauma during surgical extirpation.

The inner ear

The organs of hearing and balance are closely related anatomically and physiologically. The cochlea, saccule, utricle and semicircular canals comprise a system of membranous tubes which are bathed in endolymph internally and cushioned from the bony labyrinth by perilymph. The peripheral vestibular apparatus and cochlea have a common embryological origin in the auditory sac. Therefore, it is not surprising that the cochlear and vestibular nerves should unite to form the auditory nerve (VIII). Both systems share a common fluid environment and, hence, diseases which afflict one often afflict both, whether the causes are infectious, toxic, traumatic or more generalized degeneration.

DISEASES OF THE PINNA

Congenital abnormalities

Deformities of the pinnae are rare in the cat although an occasional kitten is born with a crinkled ear or the pinnae may be larger or smaller than is ideal for the breed. Most veterinarians regard cosmetic procedures to rectify congenital abnormalities as totally unethical and, fortunately, requests for such corrections are few and far between.

Trauma to the pinna

Although the pinna may be wounded during fights, the most frequent cause of a split is self-trauma by scratching or headshaking. The underlying cause is invariably otitis externa (see below). Topical treatments to the pinna itself will be futile unless the predisposing otitis is resolved. On the other hand, if therapy is directed towards the otitis, the injury at the ear tip will usually heal spontaneously. Extensive wounds and splits may require debridement of non-vital tissue as well as sutures.

Head shaking secondary to otitis externa may also provoke haematoma formation, but this is not as common in cats as in dogs. The lesion invariably arises between the integument on the underside of the pinna and the supporting cartilage. Although treatment of the underlying otitis is imperative if there is to be any prospect of success, haematomas generally require drainage and compression sutures, for example using discs fashioned from used X-ray film. Other clinicians prefer to drain the haematoma with a stab incision close to the base of the pinna before the insertion of a Penrose drain. Successful and quite rapid results have been claimed in the treatment of feline aural haematomas by the systemic use of dexamethasone after needle aspiration of the contents. The reason for the pursuit of alternative methods is that cicatrization often follows conventional surgery leading to some distortion of the pinna which is particularly obvious in cats.

Scratch and bite wounds frequently occur around the base of the ear and in many instances abscesses form. It is a fundamental surgical principle to establish drainage from the abscess before antibiotic therapy is commenced. Care is essential in the technique and siting of the drainage point. Vertical scalpel incisions should be resisted for fear of transection of the parotid duct. It is safer to puncture the abscess either at its lowest point or at the site of softening using a large-bore needle and then bluntly to enlarge the drainage hole with forceps.

Poor circulation and lack of hair insulation render the tips of the ears susceptible to frostbite injuries. Frostbite should be suspected if a cat that has been outdoors in extreme climatic conditions is found to have cold, pale and painless pinnae.

Other dermatoses

Notoedric mange tends to be most concentrated around the pinnae, but may spread to involve the dorsal surfaces of the head. The infestation causes great irritation and self-mutilation and entire males are particularly susceptible. The diagnosis is confirmed from skin scrapings; treatment with non-toxic acaricides is rapidly effective.

Lesions caused by fleas are much more frequent on the pinnae of cats than on the earflaps of dogs. Dermatophyte infection by *Microsporum canis* also frequently occurs on the ears of cats and produces dry scaly lesions with fragmented hair (see Chapter 1).

Neoplasia

Cats with white hair are vulnerable to solar dermatitis. In the absence of hair and pigment at sites such as the nares, eyelids and ear tips, the ultraviolet component of sunlight produces areas of dermatitis, but in some cases this turns to neoplasia. In the early stages, chronic inflammation of the ear tips is seen with ulceration and the presence of dried blood clots. The lesions may heal during the less sunny winter months, but become progressively more severe with successive summers. The pinna may be deformed by the scar tissue. The development of an ulcerated, bloody and friable surface denotes the onset of squamous cell carcinoma (Fig. 10.5). The natural progress of squamous cell carcinoma at this site is moderately slow metastasis to the adjacent local lymph nodes. Although the progress of the solar dermatitis may be retarded by the frequent application of sun barrier creams, this is tedious and at best only temporarily effective. It is simpler to

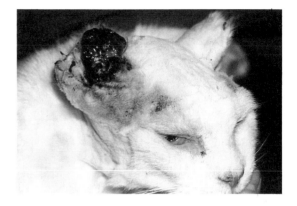

Fig. 10.5 Squamous cell carcinoma on the tips of the pinnae of a white-eared cat.

resect the vulnerable tip of the ear; in cases of true neoplasia, if this partial amputation is performed early, metastasis will be prevented. The cosmetic result of partial amputation can be improved if the skin of the dorsal surface of the pinna can be turned over to the ventral margin of the exposed cartilage. Linear carcinomas at the edge of the pinna are amenable to cryosurgery, but this modality has little value for more rounded lesions because of the poor cosmetic results.

DISEASES OF THE EXTERNAL AUDITORY MEATUS

Otitis externa

The objectives of the management of otitis externa should be to identify and eliminate the factors that initiate the inflammatory reactions in the integument and to reverse any secondary changes that may have arisen. Figure 10.6 illustrates the cycle of events that occurs in the external ear once otitis has been initiated by one of the trigger factors.

Mites

The parasite *Otodectes cynotis* frequently colonizes the feline ear canal. This ubiquitous obligatory parasite has been estimated to be responsible for 50% of otitis in cats. Although most

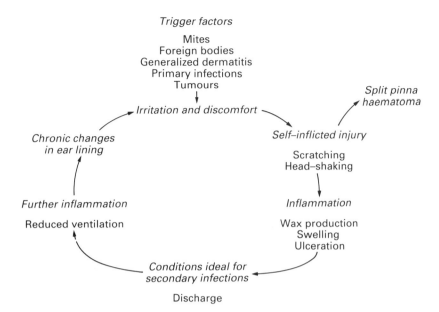

Fig. 10.6 The otitis cycle.

infestations involve the ear canal, ectopic sites may be inhabited in the skin of the neck, head, distal limbs and lumbosacral regions with consequent pruritus. In the ear canal, the mites live on the skin surface protected by debris. They appear to irritate and stimulate the ceruminous glands, and the dark-brown secretions which are produced are thought by many clinicians to be diagnostic of this condition. Otodectic mites feed on the inflammatory products in the ear canal and may sensitize the host to their salivary antigens. In one survey, 87% of a random sample of cats showed immediate wheal and flare reactions to *O. cynotis* antigens; Arthus responses were found in 94% of infested cats and in 54% of those not currently infested. It seems that most cats are exposed early in life to other mite-bearing cats and thus become infected themselves. It has been conjectured that these animals develop an 'immunity' and it would explain why ear mites are most prevalent in young animals. Cats appear to tolerate a significant population of otodectic mites without showing clinical signs, and only when a large colony is present do they show marked evidence of irritation. Even so, mite infestation is easily the most likely explanation

when a cat begins to show signs of aural irritation. Diagnosis by otoscopy is straightforward and treatment with a non-toxic acaricidal agent should be effective. However, the therapy should be sustained for not less than 3 weeks to take account of the life cycle of the mites and all in-contact cats should also be treated if reinfection is to be avoided. Most proprietary drops are oil-based and this helps to soften and break up the cerumen and general debris in the canal, so that pre-cleaning of the ear is not usually necessary. Polypharmaceutical preparations should be used only as directed by the makers; benzyl benzoate suspensions are toxic and should not be used in cats.

Foreign bodies
The relatively open ear canals and the fastidious habits of cats make the incidence of foreign body entrapment much lower in this species than in dogs. Vegetable matter such as grass seeds and barley awns can become lodged in the canal and the shape of grass seeds in particular encourages them to migrate towards the pre-tympanic region. Foreign bodies cause great discomfort, especially when they lie close to the eardrum, and the

clinician's suspicions should be aroused by a history of sudden onset of frenzied head shaking. An aural foreign body should be regarded as an indication for urgent attention because the patient is often in considerable pain. The offending material should be removed without delay but this may require a general anaesthetic if a careful manoeuvre is to be performed on a distressed patient.

Infections

Primary microbial infections of the aural integument of the cat are very unusual. Most organisms that are recovered from the ears of cats with otitis, be they bacteria or yeasts, are commensals which become opportunist pathogens only when the conditions in the ear alter and favour their proliferation, for example in the inflammatory exudates which arise through parasitic otitis. However, secondary infections are important in the exacerbation of otitis and they are a major cause of the otorrhoea and malodour. The purpose of topical medicaments which contain antibiotics is to remove secondary pathogens and thus break the cycle of otitis (see Fig. 10.6). In all cases, it is still correct to attempt to identify and remove the trigger factor before antibiotics are employed.

Generalized dermatitis

A conceptual revolution has taken place in the management of canine otitis in the past decade through the realization that otology is generally a branch of dermatology inasmuch as the changes which occur in the aural integument are frequently localized expressions of generalized dermatoses. The overall predisposition of the cat to otitis is very much lower than the dog, but the same principle applies. Thus, a general assessment of the overall skin health is a necessary part of the examination of cases of otitis externa.

Tumours of the ear canal

Proliferations from the walls of the external meatus compromise natural ventilation and any tendency to ulceration increases the likelihood of opportunist bacterial infections. Malodorous

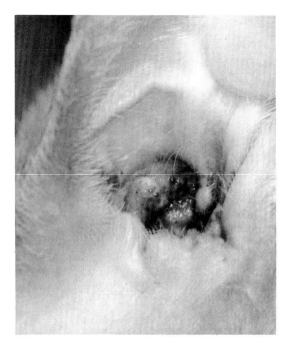

Fig. 10.7 Ceruminous gland adenomas at the opening of the ear canal.

otorrhoea is a frequent presenting sign and cats of any age can be involved. Some tumours will be obvious at the opening to the vertical canal but others may require a deep otoscopic inspection for macroscopic diagnosis and for the retrieval of biopsy samples for confirmation. There is a disparity of opinion regarding the nature and prognosis of the tumours afflicting the feline external ear but this may reflect the difference between the lesions commonly encountered in general practice and those referred to second opinion centres. Ceruminous gland adenomas appear as characteristic blue bubbles (Fig. 10.7) and are rarely solitary. Sometimes the lesions are so numerous that they occlude the lumen of the canal. These lesions rarely metastasize. On the other hand, some authorities hold that at least 50% of ceruminous gland tumours are malignant in the cat. What is not in dispute is that proliferative disorders represent the most common indication for surgery to the ear canal in this species.

This surgery may be aimed at the total extirpation of the tumour(s) or at the provision of improved access to the lower parts of the canal, i.e. by lateral wall resection of the vertical canal. Tumours of the external ear could be confused with polypoid lesions extending through the eardrum into the horizontal canal from the middle ear (see below). Middle ear polyps extending laterally in this way appear as smooth pink fleshy lesions obstructing the horizontal canal. Radiographs of the middle ear will confirm whether or not this is the site of origin of the lesion. It has already been implied that aural carcinomas and adenocarcinomas do occur in cats and all instances of aural integumental neoplasia must be evaluated with this possibility in mind before treatment is commenced. Biopsy sampling is indicated and local lymph nodes should be palpated for evidence of metastasis. Distant metastasis to the mediastinum is highly improbable in the absence of a local lymphadenopathy. Whenever it is established that a malignancy remains confined to the pinna or ear canal appropriate excisional surgery such as amputation of the pinna, vertical canal ablation or total canal ablation with lateral bulla osteotomy can be performed with a good prospect of a favourable long-term outcome. The bubble-like ceruminous gland adenomas can be destroyed by diathermy or cryosurgery if they are accessible and limited in number, otherwise ablation surgery may be indicated.

Secondary changes in the ear canal

The chronic hyperplastic changes which commonly occur in dogs with intractable or neglected canine otitis externa occur in cats but rarely. The appearance is one of keratinized proliferations partly occluding the lumen of the canal with a pale purulent otorrhoea. Initially the hyperplastic changes are likely to be confined to the vertical section of the canal, corresponding to the distribution of glandular elements in the integumental stroma. Thus, surgical removal of the vertical canal can be expected to provide an effective remedy.

Para-aural abscessation (PAA) is occasionally encountered in the cat and this condition arises when the external ear canal is obstructed (i) by a congenital atresia, (ii) by chronic inflammatory changes or, (iii) by neoplasia. The result is that normal secretions which cannot leave the deep parts of the canal eventually break through into the surrounding soft tissues and cause suppuration in the para-aural area. PAA may present either as a swelling in the parotid region and/or as a chronic discharging sinus on the side of the head which might be mistaken for a foreign body abscess. Strictures of the canal following trauma in fights or traffic accidents and post-surgical stenosis of the canal are the most frequent causes of PAA in cats.

Surgery of the external auditory meatus

The indications for ear canal surgery in cats are far less common in cats than in dogs and they have largely been covered above. The technique of lateral wall resection (LWR) is equally applicable to cats although greater attention must be given to the subsequent ear carriage. Vertical canal ablations (VCAs) can be performed using the pull-through technique with excellent cosmetic results. To summarize the indications of the aural resections used in the cat, an LWR is helpful to improve access to the medial wall of the vertical canal and to the horizontal segment and pretympanic region. VCAs are indicated in the removal of chronic inflammatory and neoplastic lesions affecting the upper external meatus. Total canal ablation with lateral bulla osteotomy (TCA/LBO) is used to extirpate lesions involving the whole canal or its horizontal segment and the most frequent indication is neoplasia. The external ear canal is anatomically keyed in to the inner compartment of the middle ear and it is inevitable that integumental elements will be left in the pretympanic area if TCA is attempted without LBO. The result will be a chronic para-aural abscess. TCA/LBO provides limited access to the middle ear itself and is generally not recommended for the treatment of conditions arising from the middle ear, i.e. polyps.

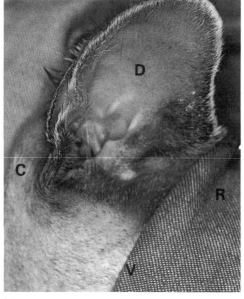

(a)

(c)

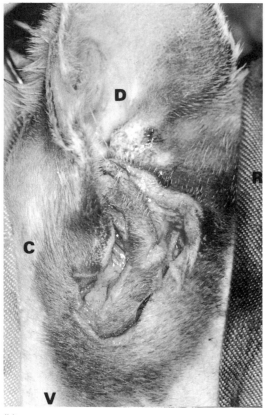

(b)

Fig. 10.8 Lateral wall resection. (a) Ear prepared for
surgery. R = rostral, C = caudal, D = dorsal, V = ventral.
(b) Parallel curved skin incisions. (c) Canal exposed to
show junction between auricular and annular cartilages
(arrowed). (d) After cartilage incisions showing aditus of
horizontal canal. (e) Completion of wound closure.

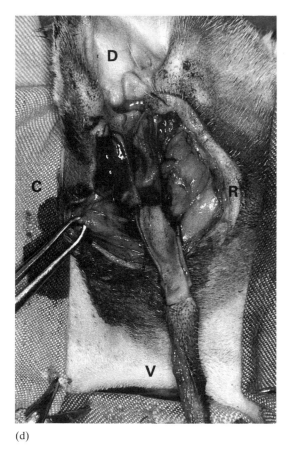

(d)

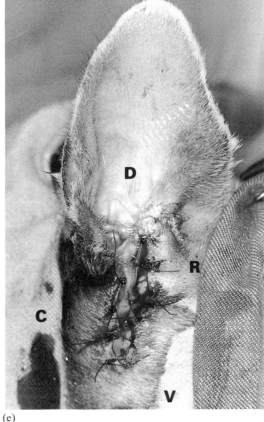

(e)

Lateral wall resection (LWR) (Fig. 10.8)

For LWR, VCA and TCA/LBO surgery the patient is positioned in lateral recumbency with the head extended and supported over a sandbag: this helps to draw loose skin away from the ear. The site is prepared in the usual way for aseptic surgery.

The level of the angle between the horizontal and vertical canals is located by the introduction of a pair of forceps into the meatus. Parallel skin incisions are made 1 cm apart curving forwards and then ventrally to a level 1 cm below that of the horizontal canal. These incisions are rounded to join each other. The skin flap is raised and the soft tissues are cleared to expose the cartilage canal. Care is taken not to traumatize the parotid salivary gland at this stage. The most crucial stage of the LWR is the incision of the cartilage. The spiral shape of the canal easily diverts the anterior

cartilage incision from the lateral aspect of the tube towards its anteromedial surface. Restricted exposure of the additus to the horizontal canal and an inadequate baffle plate will be the results. This technical failure can be avoided if the cartilage incisions are made from the level of the ligamentous attachment between the auricular and annular cartilages. A scalpel is used to puncture the cartilage and integument at this point and the parallel incisions are continued dorsally aiming at the tragal notches. The lateral wall of the ear canal can now be turned downwards and a baffle plate (drainage board) is fashioned with rounded edges to fit the original skin incision. Provided that the incisions have been extended to the level of the annular ligament between the aural cartilages, the ligament itself will act as a hinge so that the baffle plate can lie flush with the side of the face when it is sutured to the skin. The

choice of suture material lies between 3/0 mono-
filament nylon and sheathed multifilament poly-
amide. Any gross cartilaginous projections
should be filleted away before the sutures are
placed, but it may be necessary for the sutures
themselves to penetrate cartilage as well as
integument.

Aftercare consists of a 10-day course of broad-
spectrum antibiotic, and a protective collar is
necessary to prevent self-trauma in some animals.
The patient is re-examined after 5 days so that the
wounds can be cleaned and checked. This may
require a brief anaesthetic to replace any sutures
which have broken down. No attempt should be
made to remove healthy blood clots from the
incisions. The sutures are removed on the 9th day
after surgery – the prolonged presence of non-
absorbable suture material at a site which is inevitably contaminated encourages the possibility
of suture abscessation and wound dehiscence.
Sedatives and bandages are avoided, but a head
collar can provide vital protection against persistent scratching. Owners should be advised that
occasional head shaking is a normal reaction to
the presence of sutures. Head shaking may also
continue during the first month after surgery
whenever the patient is let out into the cold
fresh air.

**Vertical canal ablation (VCA: modified
Tufvesson technique)**
Patient preparation is as for the LWR. In order to
preserve the forward direction of the residual
pinna, the skin incision should take the form of
an inverted L, where the angle lies at the caudal
limit of the natural ear opening. The base of
the inverted L incision is marked with forceps
introduced into the ear canal to the point where
the vertical and horizontal sections meet. The
skin flap is released and the underlying soft tissues
are separated to expose the whole of the vertical
canal. The 'trumpet' of the conchal cartilage is
separated from the residual ear flap by an incision
through the medial wall of the vertical canal at
the level immediately dorsal to the antihelicine
tubercle. The muscular attachments are separated
close to the medial wall of the conchal cartilage so

that the 'trumpet' is mobilized. A baffle plate is
fashioned from the lower vertical canal and lies in
the same position as that described for an LWR.
Again, the ligament between the conchal and
annular cartilages acts as a hinge. The baffle plate
is valuable as it helps to maintain the long-term
patency of the horizontal canal. The choice of
suture materials is as for an LWR, but the soft
tissues deep to the excised canal are included in
the sutures when the L incision is closed so that
the dead space is eliminated. Aftercare of the
patient is similar to that for LWR patients,
although sutures are less inclined to dehisce after
a VCA. Owners should be warned in advance
that the ear carriage will be altered because of the
separation of the muscular attachments from the
medial surface of the vertical canal. Nevertheless
as these rejoin, some improvement in the appearance can be expected in the months following
surgery.

**Vertical canal ablation
(Tigari 'pull-through' technique)**
This modification of the VCA is particularly applicable to cats. It comprises the use of two
circular incisions, one around the opening of the
ear canal, and corresponding to the horizontal
limb of the inverted L described above, and the
other at the level of the additus to the horizontal
canal. The 'trumpet' of the cartilage canal is
mobilized via the upper incision and is then pulled
out through the lower, smaller hole. The pull-
through section is amputated leaving sufficient
tissue to form a baffle plate, and sutured to the
skin around the lower hole using 3/0 monofila-
ment nylon. The advantages of this technique are
that it is simple to perform, leaves little dead
space, gives a superior cosmetic result and closure
needs fewer sutures.

**Total canal ablation (TCA) with lateral bulla
osteotomy** (Fig. 10.9)
The initial stage of the procedure is the same as
for the pull-through technique described above,
but no provision need be made for a horizontal
canal opening and so the entire operation can be
performed through the single larger incision at

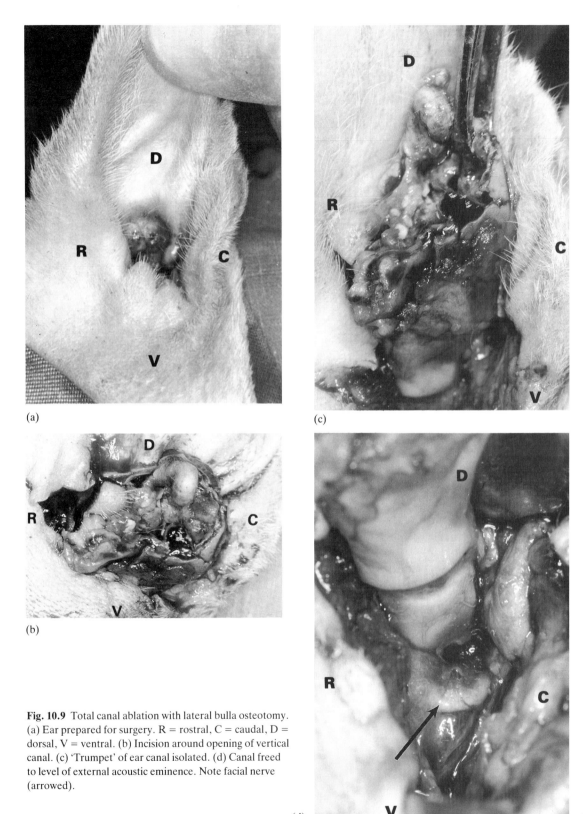

Fig. 10.9 Total canal ablation with lateral bulla osteotomy.
(a) Ear prepared for surgery. R = rostral, C = caudal, D = dorsal, V = ventral. (b) Incision around opening of vertical canal. (c) 'Trumpet' of ear canal isolated. (d) Canal freed to level of external acoustic eminence. Note facial nerve (arrowed).

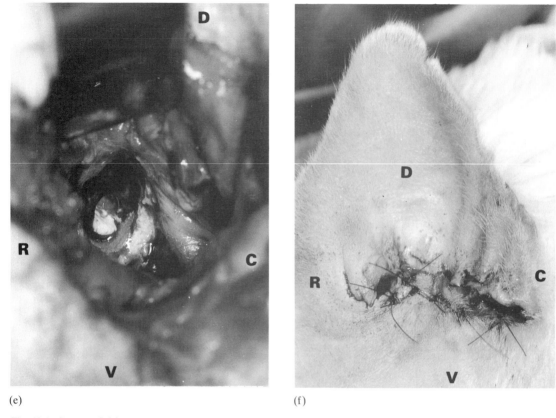

(e)   (f)

Fig. 10.9 *Continued.* (e) Lateral wall of bulla exposed. (f) Closure of linear wound.

the natural opening of the canal. The 'trumpet' of the ear canal is isolated as before and the dissection continues throughout the length of the annular cartilage until the external acoustic eminence is reached. The facial nerve lies adjacent to the horizontal canal passing ventral to the annular cartilage from caudal to rostral. It is carefully drawn away either in a loop of latex rubber drain or by the judicious use of retractors to allow the dissection to proceed. The cartilage canal is then amputated from the bony canal in order to improve visibility at the site and to allow access for the osteotomy. Rongeurs are used to break away the external acoustic eminence and the ventral half of the tympanic ring. The bony resection continues with the piecemeal removal of the lateral wall of the true middle ear as well as that of the hypotympanum. On completion of the lateral osteotomy, the exposed middle ear has a

two-tiered configuration resembling two rings of bone conjoined dorsally. The extent of curettage which follows will depend on the involvement of the middle ear structures in the disease process which the surgery is aiming to ablate. Suffice it to say that great care is required to remove all proliferative tissue and infected material and yet to respect the delicate structures which lie in the area. Facial nerve deficits are not uncommon after this technique but most result from neurapraxia and spontaneous resolution generally takes place within 4–6 weeks of surgery. However, the sympathetic fibres crossing the promontory are possibly more vulnerable to injury when lateral bulla osteotomy is performed than when the ventral route is used (see below). Thus, Horner's syndrome is a frequent iatrogenic sequel which may be permanent. The round window between the middle ear and the membranous labyrinth is a relatively large structure in this species and is vulnerable to trauma if over-zealous debridement is employed. The result of rupture of this structure would be leakage of endolymph leading to peripheral vestibular signs. On completion of the curettage, the site is flushed clear with saline and the wound is closed to eliminate dead space in the soft tissues before the linear skin incision is sutured. A 10–12-day course of prophylactic broad-spectrum antibiotic is advisable.

OTITIS MEDIA

Confusion still exists in the veterinary literature about the terms 'otitis media' and 'otitis interna', with some authors using them synonymously. While these conditions may coexist, a diagnosis of otitis interna should be reserved for those animals in which there is involvement of the peripheral organs of hearing and balance. These cases, which may also be described as 'labyrinthitis', show signs of ataxia, circling, loss of balance, nystagmus and deafness.

Abnormalities of the middle ear

In the dog, where chronic otitis externa is very common, secondary otitis media is often confirmed by radiography or at surgery. The reason why TCA/LBO surgery has become commonplace in dogs is that this technique addresses the objectives of removal of the cause, the diseased ear canal, and the effect, degenerative tissue in the middle ear, all at the same time. The situation in the cat is very different because chronic end-stage otitis externa is rare and secondary otitis media is only likely to arise in association with neoplasia of the external canal and/or para-aural abscessation. Acute ascending otitis media might be suspected when a cat with a short history of head flicking shows no tangible abnormality of the external meatus, but when an otoscopic inspection of the eardrum suggests bulging into the horizontal canal and/or creamy discoloration. Younger cats are likely to be involved and treatment by systemic antibiotics is recommended

in the first instance to eliminate predisposing upper respiratory infections as well as to control infectious agents in the middle ear itself. Sometimes the condition occurs concurrently with labyrinthitis.

By far the commonest cause of chronic otitis in the cat is inflammatory polyps arising in the middle ear cavity. The precise site of origin is the subject of debate but the author's view, based on findings at surgery and histopathology, is that it is at the junctional zone between the middle ear and the eustachian tube Again, young cats are usually afflicted and there are three clinical expressions of the disorder, which may occur singly or in combination:

1 Expansion within the middle ear before passing through the eardrum into the horizontal canal to cause intractable otorrhoea.
2 Extension on a narrow pedicle, by way of the eustachian tube, to the nasopharynx. Here the primary complaint may consist of obstructive dyspnoea and/or a chronic nasal discharge. Some cats with nasopharyngeal polyps are dysphagic.
3 Neurological deficits may be seen as the polyps expand within the middle ear and/or cause compression at the round window with raised pressure in the membranous labyrinth. Horner's syndrome, head tilt, ataxia, circling and nystagmus are possible consequences.

Diagnosis of feline middle ear disorders

The clinical signs outlined above should point to the possibility of a middle ear polyp especially if a young cat is involved. Otherwise the diagnosis of otitis media depends upon a combination of inspection by otoscopy along the horizontal canal, radiology, exploratory surgery and histopathology. The normal feline eardrum consists of two parts: dorsally the pars flaccida, which appears pink and protrudes bubble-like into the horizontal canal, and ventrally the pars tensa, which is stretched between the curved manubrium of the malleus and the tympanic sulcus at the circumference. Fibrous tissue provides the pars tensa with an off-white appearance, much like rice paper. Discharges in the horizontal canal must be

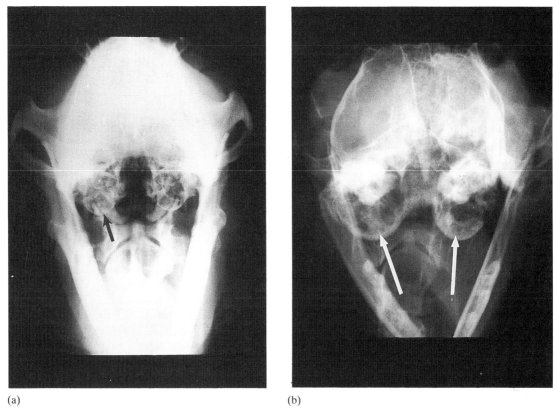

Fig. 10.10 Open-mouth projection of the tympanic bullae of cats with middle ear polyps. (a) Unilateral soft tissue density within bulla (arrowed). (b) Bilateral thickening of outer shell of bullae.

cleared if otoscopy is to be effective. Simple drum ruptures and fleshy polyps may be identified by this means. Palpation for defects with a blunt probe is not recommended as a safe or reliable method. Nasopharyngeal polyps should be sought firstly by transpalatal palpation of the nasopharynx whereby a finger introduced per os compresses the soft palate against the base of the skull and any interposed soft tissue mass is readily detected. This simple technique, while possible in the conscious cat, is more reliable when the patient is anaesthetized. Secondly, polyps at this site are confirmed by drawing the free border of the palatal arch forwards with Alliss forceps to inspect the nasopharynx with an illuminated dental mirror.

The preferred radiographic projections to examine the feline middle ear are the whole skull dorsoventral and open-mouth anteroposterior views. Oblique lateral projections are not satisfactory because it is difficult to obtain consistent results. The normal outline of the tympanic bulla on the open-mouth view shows a thin snail shell-like appearance. Within this, dorsolaterally, will be seen a secondary inner shell (Fig. 10.2). Abnormalities which may be seen on radiographs include loss of normal air contrast within one or both tiers of the bulla, dilation of the middle ear or sclerosis of the bulla walls (Fig. 10.10). The normal contrast in the middle ear cavity may be lost to empyema or to soft tissue proliferations such as polyps. The dorsoventral projection shows the columns of air in the external ear canals which may otherwise show filling defects, and the left and right petrous temporal bones can be compared.

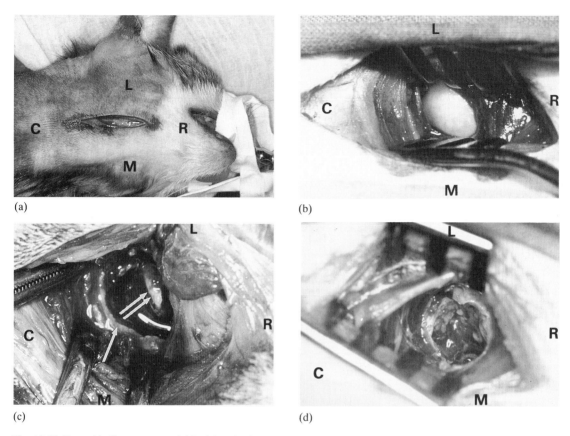

(a)

(b)

(c)

(d)

Fig. 10.11 Ventral bulla osteotomy. (a) Incision site for ventral bulla osteotomy. L = lateral, M = medial, R = rostral, C = caudal. (b) Exposure of the bulla. (c) Outer shell (single white arrow) opened to show inner shell (double white arrows) lying dorsal and lateral. (d) Inner shell opened to show polypoid material within.

Exploratory surgery may become necessary to obtain tissue samples for histological examination and for a definitive diagnosis.

Treatment of otitis media

The medical management of uncomplicated otitis media has been mentioned above. There is little to recommend the former practices of myringotomy and middle ear irrigation, and because of the particular sensitivity of the species to ototoxicity and to neuronal trauma within the middle ear, both techniques should be discontinued.

The presence of radiographic changes within the middle ear is an indication for ventral bulla osteotomy, particularly if soft tissue proliferations can be seen emerging into the horizontal canal, if there is a concurrent nasopharyngeal polyp, or if there are signs of otitis interna. The indications for lateral bulla osteotomy are quite separate and have been presented above. Cats with labyrinthitis, but without evidence of disease in the middle or external sections of the ear, should be managed by systemic medication rather than by topical preparations or middle ear surgery.

Ventral bulla osteotomy (Fig. 10.11)
The pertinent surgical anatomy of the feline middle ear has already been mentioned and in preoperative communications to clients the risks of neuropathies, especially Horner's syndrome, should be outlined although these are most often of a temporary nature. The objective of ventral

bulla osteotomy is usually to remove proliferative tissues, i.e. polyps, or to eliminate infected foci. Invariably this necessitates curettage and herein lies the cause of the trauma to the postganglionic sympathetic nerve fibres. However, an appreciation that these nerves are most vulnerable as they cross the promontory, combined with careful technique both in curettage and during removal of the bony septum dividing the inner and outer compartments, will reduce the incidence of iatrogenic Horner's syndrome. As mentioned already, the round window of the inner ear would be vulnerable to rupture by rough surgery. Although the facial nerve lies within the caudal bony wall of the middle ear, seventh nerve palsy is not a common complication of middle ear disease or ventral bulla osteotomy, but it is a well-recognized risk of the TCA/LBO technique described above.

For ventral bulla osteotomy, the cat is placed in dorsal recumbency with the neck extended over a small roll. Drapes are placed to permit access to the external canal of the affected ear. Some feline candidates for this form of middle ear surgery will already have been subjected to a lateral wall resection which aids access, but otherwise this is not essential as a preparatory measure. A longitudinal skin incision is made anterior and lateral to the larynx and parallel with and medial to the mandible. The skin and a thin layer of muscle, the mylohyoid, are separated to expose the belly of the digastricus muscle laterally and the muscles of the tongue medially. The external maxillary and lingual veins are identified and avoided. Simple blunt dissection between the muscle groups separates the loose connective tissue lateral to the pharynx. During this dissection the hypoglossal nerve and branching internal carotid artery are noted, but again, avoidance presents no difficulties. The bulla lies deep to the fork in the carotid artery and its smooth rounded outline is readily palpable. The incision is held apart with retractors and the soft tissues which overlie the bulla are cleared away. An oval window is fashioned in the ventral wall of the outer shell of the bulla using a chisel or osteotome in the manner of removing the top from a boiled egg.

When this is removed, the contents of the outer compartment can be inspected, but often it is found to be filled with stagnant mucus. This generally proves to be sterile on culture in clinical practice. Once the mucus has been removed by irrigation or suction, the inner shell of the bulla is identified as a smaller rounded structure at the dorsolateral aspect of the outer bulla. This should be entered with care, again by removal of a bony window, but the region where the dividing septum passes towards the promontory requires particular respect if damage to the sympathetic fibres and the promontory itself is to be avoided. Polypoid lesions are likely to arise within the inner shell and these are gently lifted away with forceps. The bony window of the true middle ear should be extended laterally to include the ventral half of the tympanic ring, if only to improve visibility. A blunted probe, curved mosquito forceps or a cotton bud passed down the ear canal from the exterior can be used to displace polyps that have extended laterally through the eardrum back into the middle ear. Indwelling tubes are neither necessary nor desirable for aftercare, and thus wound closure is routine once the cavities of the bulla have been thoroughly cleared and irrigated. Postoperative attention consists of topical application of an appropriate antibiotic preparation via the ear canal and systemic broad-spectrum antibiotic cover.

OTITIS INTERNA AND NEUROLOGICAL DISORDERS RELATING TO THE EAR

The inseparable relationship which exists between the auditory labyrinth (cochlea) and the vestibular system (utricle, saccule and semicircular canals) has been described above and, therefore, it should not be surprising that deafness and disturbances of balance usually occur concurrently in otitis interna (labyrinthitis). The diagnostic challenge, particularly when vestibular disturbances are apparent, is to differentiate between peripheral and central disorders and to identify the causal factors so that specific treatment can be implemented. In general, central vestibular disorders which afflict the vestibular nuclei, cerebellum and midbrain are more persistent, tend to be progressive and are accompanied by additional CNS signs such as deficits of other cranial nerves, behavioural changes and epileptiform seizures.

The signs of unilateral peripheral vestibular disturbances can be dramatic and include head tilt with the affected side down, circling towards the affected side, rolling, falling towards the affected side and horizontal nystagmus in which the fast component is directed away from the affected side. In contrast, the loss of directional hearing which accompanies unilateral deafness may go undetected unless specific audiometric tests are applied.

The damage which is inflicted on the delicate sensory nerve endings, i.e. the hair cells of the organ of Corti in the cochlea, the utricle and saccule, or in the ampullae of the semicircular canals, is likely to be irreparable in many instances regardless of whether the cause is traumatic, toxic or infectious. Fortunately bilateral vestibular dysfunction is most unusual and therefore whenever an animal is afflicted by unilateral labyrinthitis, the contralateral normal side provides a foundation for compensation. Thus, the value of therapy for otitis interna may be difficult to assess because during prolonged treatment simultaneous improvement based on compensation through the normal labyrinth, aided by visual orientation, takes place.

Infection may reach the membranous labyrinth by way of the middle ear or by haematogenous spread. In all cases where there are acquired vestibular signs or deafness, the external ear canal and the middle ear cavity should be investigated by otoscopy and radiography to identify any predisposing lesion. Clearly there can be no virtue in local therapy of the outer or middle segments of the ear without definitive evidence that is the route of infection. In the absence of external or middle ear disease, labyrinthitis should be treated by systemic corticosteroids and a broad-spectrum antibiotic which readily crosses the blood–brain barrier. Prolonged chloramphenicol therapy

should be avoided in cats because of the risk of aplastic anaemia.

Trauma to the head occasionally precipitates peripheral vestibular dysfunction and, provided that there are no central deficiencies, there is a good prospect of resolution with supportive therapy alone.

Congenital deafness

Darwin's statement of 1868 that all blue-eyed white cats are deaf is not absolutely correct because a small number of such animals do have normal hearing. Conversely, not all white cats whose eyes are not blue have normal hearing. The inference is that a genetic factor of high penetrance linked to coat colour, eye colour and ear development is involved. Hereditary deafness is not always complete and there may be residual hearing in the lower frequency ranges. In man more than 70 different syndromes of hereditary hearing deficiency have been characterized, based on the mode of transmission, the characteristics of the deafness itself and associations with other developmental conditions. Thus, to reduce feline hereditary deafness to a single syndrome based on coat and eye colour would be naive. Congenital hearing dysfunction in the cat may not always be inherited. Maternal exposure to ototoxic agents or viral infections may be responsible for a proportion of cases, especially when there is no obvious association with fur or eye colour.

Deafness is a complaint which the new owners of a kitten may not recognize immediately. In fact, several months may pass before the failure to respond to natural sounds is ascribed to anything more than wilfulness. Under current consumer legislation in the UK, the purchasers of a deaf kitten have grounds for redress as it could not be deemed to be 'of merchantable quality' and in support of their claim veterinary evidence may be required. In practice conditions, congenital deafness is assessed by challenging the subject with a variety of natural sounds covering the frequency range of normal hearing and by otoscopic elimination of other causes of deafness.

Brainstem auditory evoked response (BAER) measurement can be applied to cats to add to the specificity of the diagnosis of deafness. This technique depends upon the graphic recording of the electrical activity in the brainstem resulting from the application of pure-tone auditory stimuli; it offers a means to determine the extent of any residual hearing as the frequency of the stimulus which is applied can be controlled.

Congenital vestibular disease

A congenital vestibular disorder has been recognized in Burmese and Siamese cats. Clinical signs begin between 3 and 12 weeks of age and afflicted kittens show the classic signs of vestibular disturbance with the exception that nystagmus is not a feature. No detectable lesions have been recognized at autopsy. Some of the affected kittens may be partly deaf. The signs are not usually progressive; on the contrary, a spontaneous improvement due to compensation is quite likely to occur and, therefore, no specific therapy is indicated.

Ototoxicity

Ototoxicity occurs when the end organs of hearing and/or balance become damaged as a result of a chemical agent administered topically, orally or parenterally. Although it is well known that antibiotics such as streptomycin, dihydrostreptomycin, neomycin and gentamycin can produce irreparable damage to the sensitive structures of the membranous labyrinth when administered parenterally and that cats are particularly susceptible to ototoxicity, a far wider range of medicaments have the potential for similar iatrogenic complications than is generally appreciated. In fact, in veterinary practice the most common route of ototoxicity is the topical application of inappropriate agents in the management of otitis externa.

The list of potentially ototoxic agents and chemicals is formidable and the one given in Table 10.1 simply represents the most common agents incriminated in clinical practice.

Table 10.1 Common ototoxic agents encountered in veterinary practice.

Aminoglycoside antibiotics
 Streptomycin
 Dihydrostreptomycin
 Neomycin
 Gentamycin
 Framycetin

Non-aminoglycoside antibiotics
 Polymyxin B
 Erythromycin
 Chloramphenicol

Antiseptic and cleansing solutions
 Chlorhexidine
 Cetrimide
 Iodine and iodophors
 Ethanol

Miscellaneous chemicals
 Salicylates
 Mercurial compounds
 Arsenicals
 Some detergents

The circumstances of iatrogenic ototoxicity usually consist of the appearance of neurological deficits in a cat recovering from a general anaesthetic administered for the cleansing of the external ear canal of a patient with no previous history of auditory or vestibular dysfunction. Signs such as complete deafness, head tilt, circling, ataxia and nystagmus will be present and it is obvious that such a case is at best professionally highly embarrassing and at worst a potential subject for malpractice litigation. The anaesthetic agent itself can usually be eliminated as the cause of the tragedy and the logical conclusion is that either the irrigation technique was at fault or that the antiseptic/cleansing solution or that topical medicaments were ototoxic. It is implied that the ototoxic solution reached the inner ear by absorption through the round window foramen from the middle ear cavity, which in turn presupposes that the eardrum was ruptured in the first place. Although the changes in the inner ear are irreversible, compensation can be expected in unilateral cases so that the only long-term sign of malfunction is generally slight rotation of the head, which may become more obvious in periods of excitement. The inevitable conclusion is that the only safe medium for lavage of the external ear is sterile saline solution and that particular circumspection in the topical administration of aural medicaments is warranted when there is the possibility of pre-existing eardrum rupture. The practice of myringotomy and middle ear irrigation is contraindicated in the cat and should be discontinued.

Idiopathic feline vestibular syndrome (IFVS)

IFVS consists of a peripheral vestibular disorder of acute onset in mature cats of either sex and any age. The disease is typically, but not exclusively, seen in the months of June–August and, as the name implies, the cause is not known. Clinical examination merely reveals a patient with a severe head tilt (Fig. 10.12), incoordination and apparent discomfort. Nystagmus may be horizontal or rotatory, but there is no evidence of external or middle ear infection. In one survey 75% of affected cats recovered completely within a period ranging from 2 to 6 weeks after onset; the remaining patients had mild residual ataxia and head tilt several months later. The outcome of the condition did not appear to be influenced by treatments with antibiotics, acaricides, tranquillizers or corticosteroids. Nevertheless, it would always be correct to provide therapeutic cover for the possibility of an infectious otitis interna as described above.

Facial paralysis

The signs of facial paralysis comprise loss of motor function of the muscles of facial expression and consist of drooping of the upper lip and muzzle (Fig. 10.13), loss of ear movement and absence of the corneal protection reflex. The axons of the facial nerve pass from the facial nucleus in the medulla, through the internal acoustic meatus into the facial canal within the petrous temporal bone and emerge from the stylomastoid foramen immediately caudal to the external auditory canal. Although the anatomical

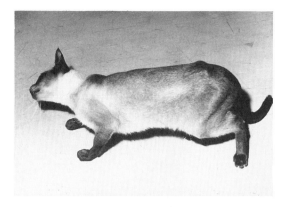

Fig. 10.12 Idiopathic feline vestibular syndrome.

proximity to the ear is as close as in other species, seventh nerve paralysis is rare in cats. However, when it does arise it is often concurrent with vestibular signs and/or Horner's syndrome simply because the cause is likely to be an expansive lesion within the middle ear. Facial paralysis is a recognized potential complication of TCA/LBO surgery.

Horner's syndrome

Horner's syndrome is characterized by retraction of the eyeball (enophthalmos), drooping of the upper eyelid (ptosis) and constriction of the pupil making it smaller than that of the contralateral eye (anisocoria) (Fig. 10.13). It arises through disruption of the sympathetic pathways by lesions in the cervical or anterior thoracic spinal cord, the anterior mediastinum, the carotid sheath, the petrous temporal bone, the floor of the cranium or in the retrobulbar structures. Whenever Horner's syndrome is recognized, the diagnostic procedure aims to identify the site of nerve injury so that appropriate treatment, if applicable, can be instituted. Surveys have shown that the two most common causes of Horner's syndrome in cats are trauma in road accidents and middle ear disease. This is hardly surprising in view of the close anatomical relationship between the post-ganglionic sympathetic fibres and the lining of the middle ear cavity. Horner's syndrome may occur

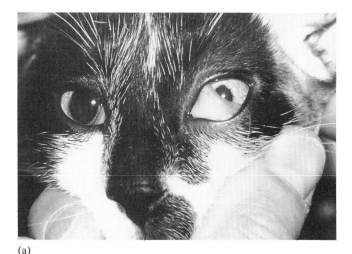

(a)

(b)

Fig. 10.13 Horner's syndrome. (a) Note prominent membrana nictitans and pupillary constriction on affected side. (b) With facial paralysis. Note the pupillary constriction and ptosis on the same side as the saliva drooling from the mouth.

in association with inflammatory polyps or after bulla osteotomy by either ventral or lateral routes.

FURTHER READING

Ader P.L. & Boothe H.W. (1979) Ventral bulla osteotomy in the cat. *J. Am. Anim. Hosp. Assoc.* **15**, 757–62.

August J.R. (1986) Diseases of the ear canal. In: *The Complete Manual of Ear Care*. Veterinary Learning Systems, USA, pp. 37–51.

Bergsma D.R. & Brown K.S. (1971) White fur, blue eyes and deafness in the domestic cat. *J. Hered.* **62**, 171–85.

Burke E.E., Moise N.S., de Lahunta A. & Erb H.N. (1985) Review of idiopathic feline vestibular syndrome in 75 cats. *J. Am. Vet. Med. Assoc.* **187**, 941–3.

Galle H.G. (1985) Ototoxicity. *Proc. Voorjaarsdagenn* 139–41.

Kapatkin A.S., Matthiesen D.T., Noone K.E., Church, E.M., Scavelli T.E. & Patnaik A.K. (1990) Results of surgery and long-term follow-up in 31 cats with nasopharyngeal polyps. *J. Am. Anim. Hosp. Assoc.* **26**, 387–92.

Kern T.J. & Erb H.N. (1987) Facial neuropathy in dogs and cats: 95 cases. *J. Am. Vet. Med. Assoc.* **191**, 1604–9.

Kern T.J., Aromando M.C. & Erb H.N. (1989) Horner's syndrome in dogs and cats: 100 cases. *J. Am. Vet. Med. Assoc.* **195**, 369–73.

Kuwahara J. (1986) Canine and feline aural hematomas: results of treatment with corticosteroids. *J. Am. Anim. Hosp. Assoc.* **22**, 641–7.

Lane J.G. & Watkins P.W. (1986) Para-aural abscesses in the dog and cat. *J. Small Anim. Pract.* **27**, 521–31.

Lane J.G. Orr C.M., Lucke V.M. & Gruffydd-Jones T.J. (1981) Nasopharyngeal polyps arising in the middle ear of the cat. *J. Small Anim. Pract.* **22**, 511–22.

Little C.J.L. & Lane J.G. (1986) The surgical anatomy of the feline bulla tympanica. *J. Small Anim. Pract.* **27**, 371–8.

Rose W.R. (1976) Otitis interna. 1 General considerations. *Vet. Med. Small Anim. Clin.* **71**, 1673–8.

Tigari M. & Pinniger R.S. (1986) Pull-through technique for vertical canal ablation for the treatment of otitis externa in dogs and cats. *J. Small Anim. Pract.* **27**, 123–31.

Tos M., Wiederhold M. & Larsen P. (1984) Experimental long-term tubal occlusion in cats. *Acta Otolaryngol.* **97**, 580–92.

Williams J.M. & White R.A.S. (1992) Total ear canal ablation combined with lateral bulla osteotomy in the cat. *J. Small Anim. Pract.* **33**, 225–7.

Chapter 11 / The Cardiovascular System

P. R. WOTTON AND
T. J. GRUFFYDD-JONES

INTRODUCTION

Recent advances in knowledge have very much improved our understanding of the pathogenesis of cardiac disease in cats. At the same time the increasing use of newer diagnostic techniques such as ultrasonography, alongside more familiar techniques such as radiography and electrocardiography, has increased our ability to assess accurately abnormalities of cardiac function and anatomy, simply and non-invasively. Nevertheless, despite an increasing awareness of the importance of cardiovascular disease, in particular an increasing recognition of both primary and secondary myocardial diseases as major clinical problems, the diagnosis and treatment of cardiovascular disease in cats remain a challenge. This chapter will outline the methods of investigation used before considering the specific congenital and acquired conditions and their management.

CLINICAL HISTORY

A thorough history can provide a first indication of the possible presence of disease of the cardiovascular system, but it is important to realize that the presenting signs of cardiovascular disease and heart failure in cats may differ somewhat from those seen in other species. Signs in cats are often acute in onset, e.g. hindlimb pain and paresis due to aortic thromboembolism, or the sudden development of dyspnoea due to pulmonary oedema. Owners may attribute such signs to the effects of trauma. In other cases, vague and non-specific signs may provide the only evidence of cardiovascular disease. Cats often mask the presence of disease by markedly altering their level of activity. These early subtle signs may easily be overlooked by the owner until more obvious evidence of cardiovascular dysfunction develops.

The usual presenting signs of cardiovascular disease in cats are shown in Table 11.1, in approximate order of frequency of occurrence. Dyspnoea is the most commonly encountered and develops due to the presence of pulmonary oedema or pleural effusion in cases of congestive heart failure, or, much less commonly, due to right-to-left shunting of blood in some congenital cardiac defects (e.g. tetralogy of Fallot). Dyspnoea due to pulmonary oedema can be episodic, and may mimic the clinical presentation of so-called 'feline asthma' (see Chapter 6). Coughing is not common in cats with congestive cardiac failure, nor is ascites, two important differences from the clinical presentation of heart failure in dogs. The accumulation of a significant volume of ascitic fluid in a cat is much more likely to indicate a non-cardiac condition such as feline infectious peritonitis or lymphocytic cholangitis.

Severe congenital cardiac anomalies usually become symptomatic within the first year of life, often within the first few months. Owners may notice stunting of growth, excessive tiring, dyspnoea or, less commonly, syncopal episodes or ascites. It is pertinent to obtain information about the progress of littermates, and any other progeny of the parents, if a hereditary defect is suspected. The breed and sex of the cat may also be relevant in this context as breed and sex predispositions are recognized for certain congenital anomalies

Table 11.1 Presenting signs of cardiovascular disease in cats.

Dyspnoea/tachypnoea/hyperpnoea (may be episodic)
Lethargy and/or weakness/collapse
Anorexia, weight loss
Episodic collapse/syncope
Stunted growth
Paresis, pain, lameness
Coughing
Abdominal enlargement

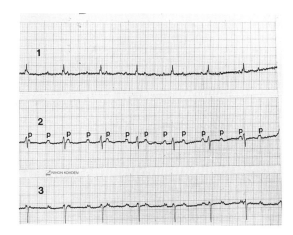

Fig. 11.1 Third degree (complete) atrio-ventricular block. The P waves (marked in lead 2) are unrelated to the QRS complexes. There is also a left axis deviation due to left ventricular hypertrophy and/or left anterior fascicular block. Limb leads 1, 2 and 3 are shown. Paper speed: 50 mm/s; 1 cm = 1 mV.

and acquired diseases. Other important information includes dietary history and any other signs that could indicate the possibility of an underlying primary condition (e.g. an endocrinopathy) to which the cardiovascular disease might be secondary.

CLINICAL EXAMINATION

A careful clinical examination is the most important part of the investigation. It will often provide objective evidence (Table 11.2) for the presence of cardiovascular disease or dysfunction, and can suggest the type of disease involved. Evidence of heart disease (e.g. a murmur caused by a previously unsuspected congenital defect) is sometimes discovered fortuitously, during routine clinical examination or investigation for another unrelated condition. Dyspnoeic cats should be handled carefully during examination and investigation, as their condition can be markedly

Table 11.2 Clinical findings in cats with cardiovascular disease.

Murmur, gallop sounds, dysrhythmia
Altered repiration; abnormal lung sounds
Altered arterial pulse rate, rhythm or character
Altered intensity of apex beat
Paresis, lameness
Pyrexia *or* hypothermia
Jugular distension/abnormal pulsation
Hepatomegaly, ascites
Cyanosis

exacerbated by stressful procedures. In some cases emergency therapy (e.g. thoracentesis of a pleural effusion or management of acute pulmonary oedema with oxygen and intravenous frusemide) is required before diagnostic procedures can be safely carried out.

Particular attention should be paid to the rate and character of the respirations, the colour of the mucous membranes and the rate, rhythm and character of the femoral arterial pulse. Cyanosis may accompany dyspnoea where pulmonary oedema or pleural effusion is severe, or can occur due to a congenital right-to-left shunt. The pulse rate of the normal cat may vary widely from approximately 140 to 240/min. Tachycardia can occur with stress and also in a number of non-cardiac disease states, e.g. pyrexia, anaemia, primary respiratory disorders or hyperthyroidism. The physiological response to heart failure is usually a sinus tachycardia, but sinus bradycardia, sometimes profound, is seen occasionally. Dysrhythmias and conduction deficits are common in primary and secondary myocardial disease and may cause bradycardia (e.g. with complete atrioventricular block; Fig. 11.1), tachycardia or an

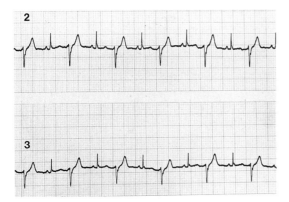

Fig. 11.2 Ventricular bigeminy. Each alternate complex is a ventricular premature complex (negative polarity). Leads 2 and 3. Paper speed: 25 mm/s; 1 cm = 1 mV.

erratic rhythm (Fig. 11.2), the latter often accompanied by a pulse deficit. Careful assessment of the quality of the pulse is also valuable, although the femoral artery may be difficult to palpate in some cats. The pulse becomes hyperkinetic (i.e. strength increased, volume usually reduced) with some congenital cardiac defects (e.g. patent ductus arteriosus) and in diseases characterized by high cardiac output (e.g. anaemia, hyperthyroidism). The pulse will be weak in dilated cardiomyopathy, may be variable in strength with dysrhythmias and is markedly reduced in strength or absent with aortic thromboembolism, accompanied by cold, cyanosed and weak or paretic hindlimbs with pain and contracture of the muscles, particularly the gastrocnemius. Thromboembolism sometimes produces less dramatic signs, as discussed later.

Pyrexia, particularly if chronic or recurrent, might suggest a diagnosis of bacterial endocarditis, but this condition is very rare in cats. Pyrexia of any cause can lead to tachycardia and a functional systolic murmur, which should not be mistaken for evidence of primary cardiac disease. Hypothermia and bradycardia, accompanied by coldness of the extremities due to poor cardiac output (acute forward heart failure or 'cardiogenic shock'), are sometimes seen in cases of dilated cardiomyopathy, and hypothermia may also occur with aortic thromboembolism.

Other important features to note during clinical examination include the presence or absence of a jugular pulse, alteration of thoracic resonance on percussion and the strength of the apex beat on palpation of the thorax. Jugular distension or abnormal jugular pulsation (more than a few centimetres above the thoracic inlet in the standing cat with the head elevated) may be seen in cases where right atrial pressure is elevated (e.g. right atrio-ventricular regurgitation, pericardial effusion). The fur over the jugular furrow must be clipped and/or moistened with surgical spirit in order to be able to see the jugular vein. The apex beat is normally most clearly palpable over the left 5th intercostal space. This may become more prominent if the left ventricle is hypertrophied (e.g. hypertrophic cardiomyopathy, hyperthyroidism) and its intensity is often reduced in dilated cardiomyopathy, or where there is pleural or pericardial effusion or an intrathoracic mass, when the ventral area of dullness on percussion is increased also. Where loud cardiac murmurs are present, palpation of the thorax may reveal a thrill. During the physical examination careful attention should also be paid to the search for thyroid enlargement, the presence of ascites and hepatomegaly and the size and contour of the kidneys. Where ascites is caused by right-sided congestive heart failure, there will usually also be hepatomegaly and jugular distension, and the jugular pulsation may be accentuated by palpation of the liver (the hepatojugular reflex).

Auscultation

Auscultation of the heart and lungs plays a vital part in the investigation of cardiovascular disease, but may be hampered in cats by their purring. The small size of the cat's heart and its rapid rate of contraction also make the localization and characterization of murmurs more difficult. Auscultation should be carried out in a quiet environment. The cat's purring can sometimes be stopped by changing the animal's position, gently blowing on its face or distracting its attention, e.g. by running water. The whole cardiac area should be evaluated methodically, listening on both sides of the thorax at the apex, sternal border and base of the heart; both the bell and diaphragm of the stethoscope should be employed. The positions of the valve areas for auscultation are similar to those in the dog, and are discussed further under 'Congenital heart disease' below. Because of the small physical size of the heart it is much more difficult to define these areas clinically, although the use of a paediatric stethoscope, with a small chest piece, may help. The first and second heart sounds are usually clearly audible, the second often louder than the first, and these are the only heart sounds heard in normal cats. The heart and pulse rates should be compared simultaneously and should be the same; dysrhythmias can produce a pulse deficit. The presence of pleural or peri-cardial effusions or intrathoracic masses often causes muffling of the heart and lung sounds. The heart may become louder on the right side of the thorax if displaced by fluid or a mass. In cats with heart failure of any cause, the third or atrial (fourth) heart sounds often become audible as an extra, usually low-pitched diastolic sound termed a 'gallop sound'. This is generally best heard over the left apex region and may be heard more clearly with the bell of the stethoscope. The pre-sence of gallop sounds is a useful indicator of heart disease, although they are occasionally heard in other situations, e.g. with sedation, or in hypertension due to renal disease.

Murmurs occur frequently in cats with various types of cardiac disease, both congenital and acquired. However, functional or physiological murmurs also occur in non-cardiac diseases, e.g. with anaemia, pyrexia and sometimes with seda-tion. Innocent murmurs (i.e. with no underlying cardiac disease or dysfunction) are encountered in kittens. A murmur can be produced by simply compressing the thoracic wall during auscultation, especially in kittens. Thus the presence of a murmur is not definitive evidence of cardiac dis-ease. If possible, the murmur should be classified according to its timing within the cardiac cycle, loudness, point of maximum intensity, radiation and acoustic profile (character). Auscultation of the thorax should be completed by assessing the loudness and character of the normal respiratory

sounds and noting the presence of any adventitious lung sounds, for instance the crackles (or 'rales') which occur with pulmonary oedema.

DIAGNOSTIC AIDS

While the history and clinical findings may strongly support a diagnosis of cardiovascular disease, further investigation is usually required before a definitive classification of the type of disease and its severity can be made. The most widely used aid to diagnosis is plain radiography, but other tech-niques of imaging, particularly ultrasonography, have become increasingly important. Electrocar-diography is vital for the proper diagnosis and treatment of dysrhythmias. The use and interpre-tation of these techniques can only be discussed briefly here; further details are available in several of the texts and papers cited.

Radiography

The care necessary in handling dyspnoeic cats, particularly for radiography, has already been stressed; in particular a dyspnoeic cat should not be placed in dorsal recumbency, especially if the presence of a pleural effusion is suspected. It may be necessary to remove any significant accumula-tion of thoracic fluid before radiography can safely and usefully be completed, since an effusion obscures the cardiac silhouette as well as compro-mising respiratory function. However, before thoracentesis is attempted it is helpful to take an initial dorsoventral radiograph to confirm the presence and distribution of the effusion.

Radiography allows an assessment to be made of the presence and degree of cardiomegaly and enlargement of specific cardiac chambers. It also allows evaluation of the pulmonary circulation, the great vessels (e.g. Figs. 11.7 & 11.11), the pulmonary parenchyma and pleural space, thus enabling the clinician to detect the common features of heart failure in cats, i.e. pulmonary oedema and pleural effusion. Pulmonary oedema in cats may have a very different radiographic appearance from the 'fluffy' infiltrate typically seen in dogs. It can have a very diffuse distribution in cats or may produce a mottled, patchy or

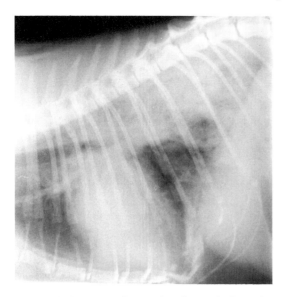

Fig. 11.3 Pulmonary oedema and cardiomegaly. Lateral radiograph from a cat with intermediate cardiomyopathy, aortic thromboembolism and an acute onset of dyspnoea and cyanosis. The pulmonary oedema appears here as an area of intense infiltration.

more uniform infiltrate, sometimes resembling neoplasia (Fig. 11.3).

The usual radiographic projections for the thorax in cases of cardiovascular disease are right lateral and dorsoventral. The conformation and relative shape and size of the thorax and heart are much less variable in cats than in the various breeds of dog, although there is some variation in the alignment of the longitudinal axis of the cat's heart, which may lie almost supine along the sternum in the lateral view in some normal individuals. The heart is more elongated and is smaller relative to the size of the thorax than in dogs. Because the cardiothoracic conformation of cats is relatively uniform, published guidelines and measurements for the detection of cardiomegaly are more useful than in dogs, where thoracic conformation varies widely between breeds. In the lateral projection the width of the normal heart, measured at its widest point and perpendicular to the longitudinal axis, should not exceed the distance between the 5th and 7th ribs at the same level (Van den Broek & Darke, 1987). In the dorsoventral projection the normal heart should not exceed two-thirds of the width of the thorax at its widest point.

The positions of the cardiac chambers within the radiographic cardiac silhouette are shown in Fig. 11.4. Enlargement of the left atrium and ventricle produces elongation of the heart in both projections. In the lateral view this results in elevation of the hilar structures (of which the trachea is most easily seen), which is a useful marker for cardiomegaly even when the heart itself is obscured by pleural effusion. However, intrathoracic masses may also elevate the heart and hilar structures. The apex may remain pointed in shape when the left ventricle is hypertrophied and may appear rounded when there is left ventricular dilatation, but these features do not allow hypertrophy to be reliably distinguished from dilatation. Enlargement of the left atrium may be seen as a caudodorsal bulge in the lateral view or may be more obvious as a left lateral bulge in the dorsoventral view. Enlargement of the right atrium and ventricle is best seen in the dorsoventral projection, producing rounding of the right cardiac border and sometimes craniocaudal widening of the heart in the lateral view. The dorsoventral view is particularly useful in cats, since atrial (especially left atrial) enlargement may produce very obvious widening of the heart and alteration of its shape in this projection, sometimes shifting the apex towards the midline when severe. The term 'valentine-shaped heart' is sometimes used to describe the appearance of a cardiac silhouette with broad 'shoulders' due to marked atrial enlargement, as seen in the dorsoventral view.

A widened aortic arch may be seen cranial to the heart in both projections with congenital defects such as aortic stenosis and patent ductus arteriosus, and may also occur normally in old cats and perhaps secondarily to conditions causing systemic arterial hypertension, e.g. chronic renal failure (Bonagura, 1989). Enlargement of the main pulmonary artery is not readily seen in cats as it is usually hidden within the cardiac silhouette. Inspection of the pulmonary vasculature can show evidence of pulmonary over-circulation in congenital defects with a left-to-right shunt, venous congestion where left atrial pressure is elevated, and wide, sometimes tortuous arteries in cases of pulmonary hypertension. Contrast radiography is sometimes necessary to gain additional information about internal cardiac anatomy in cases of both congenital and acquired cardiac disease. Selective angiography (placing radiographic contrast material into a specific chamber of the heart using an intracardiac catheter) is rarely feasible in practice and has been superseded for many of its applications by ultrasonography. Non-selective angiography (Fig. 11.4) is still of value in some cases (e.g. to distinguish between hypertrophic and dilated cardiomyopathy, to distinguish pericardial distension from cardiomegaly or to show a congenital right-to-left shunt) and is an alternative to ultrasonography where the latter is not available. The procedure is generally well tolerated by cats and may be carried out with the use of sedative cocktails such as ketamine with midazolam, diazepam or acepromazine, following an overnight fast. The dose of ketamine for a healthy cat is 10 mg/kg (maximum 30 mg/cat) mixed in the same syringe with 0.2 mg/kg of midazolam and given intramuscularly. These doses should be reduced by 30–50% for cats with cardiac disease. Midazolam is not approved for use in cats. Atropine should be given if the heart rate is slow. More profound sedation may be obtained using ketamine and xylazine, with caution, at the sedative dose rate. The cat's medical condition (e.g. congestive heart failure, electrolyte imbalance, etc.) must be stabilized first and complications do occur occasionally, ranging from transient bradycardia or vomiting through to cardiac arrest, particularly in cases of dilated cardiomyopathy. An intravenous catheter (20–22G) should be inserted into a cephalic or jugular vein and intravenous radiographic contrast material is injected as quickly as possible, at a dose of approximately 450 mg of iodine/kg bodyweight (less in high-risk cases). A radiograph is taken immediately after injection and then several more as quickly as possible, e.g. 5, 10 and 15 seconds after injection. The construction of a 'cassette tunnel' may help in changing films rapidly (Fox & Bond, 1983).

Ultrasonography (echocardiography)

The use of ultrasonographic imaging has had a tremendous impact on the diagnosis of cardiac disease. In this technique very high frequency sound waves (usually 5–7.5 MHz for echocardiography in cats) are used to generate images of the cross-sectional anatomy of the internal organs. When sound waves, generated by a piezoelectric crystal and transmitted through the soft tissues of the body, meet an interface between tissues of different acoustic impedance (e.g. myocardium and blood), a proportion of the sound is reflected and can be received by the same piezoelectric crystal. This echoed sound deforms the crystal, generating an electrical signal which is used to generate a two-dimensional image. Because this process happens in 'real time', it is possible to show movement and thus gain information on cardiac function as well as anatomy. Information on blood flow may be gained by the use of intravenous echocontrast agents (fluids such as agitated saline or colloids which contain microbubbles and thus strongly reflect ultrasound), for example when looking for an intracardiac shunt. Quantitative information on blood flow patterns and velocities can be derived by the technique of Doppler echocardiography, which makes use of the shift in frequency of sound reflected off moving red blood cells to determine blood flow velocity. These techniques can be carried out safely and non-invasively, without the need for sedation or anaesthesia. It is beyond the scope of this chapter to discuss the theory, techniques or interpretation of echocardiography in any detail, and the reader is referred to the further reading listed (e.g. Moise, 1988; Bonagura, 1989; Barr, 1990; Darke, 1992). Examples of the use of echocardiography are given in the sections on specific cardiac diseases. Figure 11.5 shows cardiac ultrasound images from a normal cat, and some normal values for cardiac measurements determined by M-mode echocardiography are given in Table 11.3.

The most common indication for carrying out echocardiography in cats is to distinguish between the various forms of cardiomyopathy. Echocardiography is also valuable in determining the

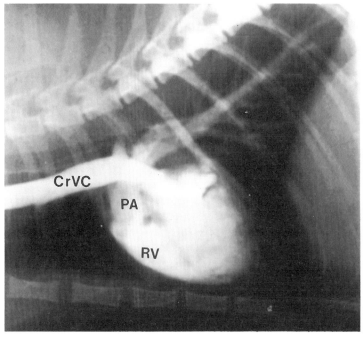

(a)

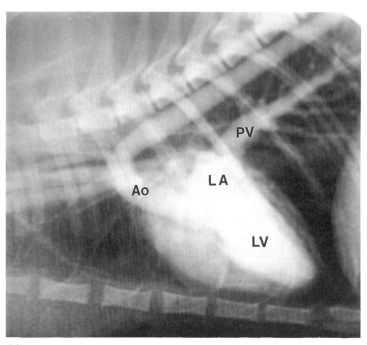

(b)

Fig. 11.4 Non-seletive angiogram from a healthy cat. (a) Initial right ventricular phase outlining the cranial vena cava (CrVC), right ventricle (RV – also partly overlying the left side here) and main pulmonary artery (PA). (b) Left ventricular phase showing the pulmonary veins (PV) emptying into the left artium (LA) then left ventricle (LV) and aorta (Ao).

Table 11.3 Some normal values from M-mode echocardiography.

Diastole	L. ventricular diameter	11.0–16.0 mm
	L. ventricular free wall	2.5–5.5 mm
	Inter-ventricular septum	2.5–5.5 mm
Systole	L. ventricular diameter	6.0–10.0 mm
	L. ventricular free wall	4.0–9.0 mm
	Inter-ventricular septum	5.0–9.0 mm
	L.V. fractional shortening (an indicator of systolic function)	29–55%

Adapted from Bonagura (1989).

Table 11.4 Some normal ECG values (Lead 2).

	Duration (msec)	Amplitude (mV)
P wave	max. 40	max. 0.25
P-R interval	50–100	—
QRS interval	max. 40	max. 1.0
Q-T interval	80–220	—
Heart rate	140–240/min	

nature of congenital anatomical defects, particularly when used with Doppler techniques for detecting abnormal blood flow. Where pleural fluid is present ultrasonography will also help to exclude other causes such as thymic lymphoma and diaphragmatic rupture. Pleural fluid aids ultrasonographic examination whereas it obscures radiographic detail.

Electrocardiography

Disturbances of cardiac electrical activity (impulse formation and conduction) are common in feline cardiovascular disease, especially in both primary and secondary cardiomyopathies. Electrocardiography is essential for defining dysrhythmias, allowing decisions to be made about their significance, and may also give information on cardiac chamber enlargement and metabolic disturbances, but gives no direct indication of the contractile state of the myocardium. Again, it is beyond the scope of this chapter to discuss the theoretical basis, technique and interpretation of electrocardiography, and the reader is referred to the texts cited for a detailed discussion of these areas (e.g. Bonagura, 1989).

Most cats will tolerate the recording of an electrocardiogram (ECG) without the use of sedatives or tranquillizers, and as these may alter the ECG they should be avoided if possible. Whether the patient is placed in right lateral (the position described in standard texts) or sternal recumbency makes little difference to the values recorded; P- and R-wave voltages are in fact slightly greater in sternal recumbency. As most cats tolerate sternal recumbency better, particularly if dyspnoeic, this position is often preferable. Where it is necessary to determine cardiac rhythm only, the cat may be placed in a cage, after attaching the electrodes, and allowed to take up any position which it finds comfortable. Some normal values are given in Table 11.4.

Other diagnostic aids

Thoracentesis
The detection of a significant volume of pleural fluid on thoracic radiographs is an indication for thoracentesis. This technique is described in Chapter 6. Removal of pleural fluid serves to reduce dyspnoea and aids diagnosis by allowing the intrathoracic viscera to be seen more clearly on radiographs. Fluid is also made available for laboratory examination. Both sides of the thorax can generally be drained from one site. The pleural effusion in congestive heart failure is often a transudate, relatively clear in appearance, low in protein (<30 g/l) and containing few cells. However, modified transudates are also found and occasionally the fluid is chylous. Cytological examination of the fluid can help to rule out other causes of pleural effusion, such as thymic lymphoma. In congestive heart failure the fluid contains mainly erythrocytes, mesothelial cells and mature lymphocytes. Pleural effusion is seen most often in the dilated and restrictive forms of cardiomyopathy, although other forms of heart disease cannot be ruled out on that basis.

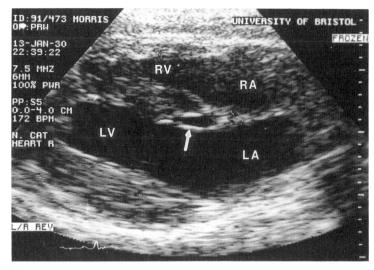

(a)

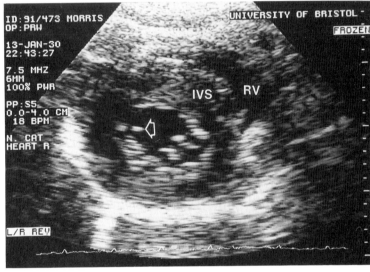

(b)

Fig. 11.5 Cardiac ultrasound images from a healthy cat from the right parasternal position. (a) Long-axis view in diastole; arrow shows open septal cusp of the left A-V valve. (b) Short-axis view at systole; arrowhead shows a chorda.

Laboratory tests

Laboratory investigations are of value in looking for underlying primary causes of cardiac disease and in assessing the effects of heart failure on the function of other organs, as well as any side-effects of therapy.

HAEMATOLOGY

A leucocytosis may be present in cases of endo-carditis or myocarditis, but can be present in other forms of cardiomyopathy. Polycythaemia may occur where a congenital heart defect leads to right-to-left shunting of blood and cyanosis. Moderate/severe anaemia may give rise to a physiological murmur or may lead to signs of secondary cardiac disease.

BIOCHEMISTRY

Assessment of renal function is valuable, as heart failure and the use of diuretics can both cause pre-renal azotaemia; conversely, chronic primary renal failure may give rise to signs of secondary

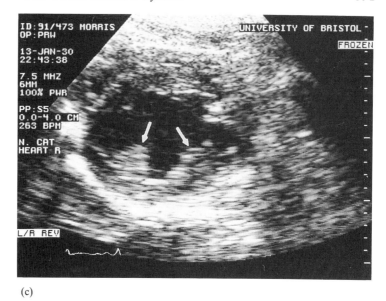

(c)

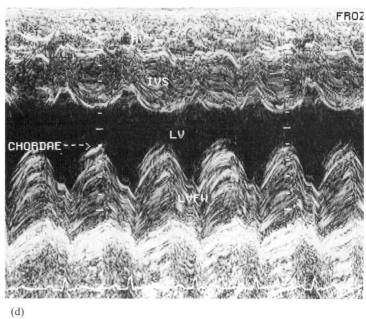

Fig. 11.5 *Continued.* (c) Short-axis view at diastole; arrows show papillary muscles. (d) M-mode display at chordal level – the position used for making measurements of ventricular dimensions and wall thicknesses. (Abbreviations as in Fig. 11.4; also RA = right atrium; IVS = interventricular septum; LVFW = left ventricular free wall.)

(d)

cardiac disease. Renal dysfunction also affects digoxin excretion, and it can be valuable to determine the serum concentration of digoxin in cases where this is of concern. Severe renal failure is seen occasionally due to thromboembolic occlusion of the renal arteries. Electrolyte imbalance, particularly hyperkalaemia, is an important factor in initiating or exacerbating dysrhythmias. Hyperkalaemia and metabolic acidosis occur in cats with thromboembolic disease and renal failure. Hypokalaemia is seen in cats with chronic renal failure and sometimes following the prolonged use of diuretics. Serum alanine-aminotransferase (ALT) is commonly elevated in hyperthyroid cats.

OTHER TESTS

Serum thyroxine levels should always be determined in older cats (>5–6 years) with cardiomyopathy to rule out underlying hyperthyroidism (see Chapter 12). Plasma taurine levels should ideally be measured in cases of dilated cardiomyopathy; a level of less than 20 nM/ml is considered to indicate taurine deficiency. Unfortunately no commercial laboratories currently carry out this assay in the UK. Blood culture is worth while if bacterial endocarditis is suspected.

CONGENITAL HEART DISEASE

The prevalence of congenital heart disease in cats has been estimated to be approximately 2% in post-mortem surveys in the USA (Fox, 1988a). The range of severity is very wide. In many cases (particularly atrio-ventricular valve malformations) the defect is mild and may go unrecognized until the cat reaches maturity or even old age. In others the defect is severe enough to cause death in the first few days or months of life.

The main features of the history and clinical examination associated with congenital heart disease are stunting of growth compared with unaffected littermates, dyspnoea particularly on exertion, poor exercise tolerance, collapse, cyanosis and ascites. Where such signs occur the prognosis is often poor. Sometimes other members of the litter are also affected. Occasionally the presenting signs may appear to be unrelated to the cardiovascular system, e.g. weakness/ataxia or seizures. Auscultation will usually reveal a murmur, which may be loud. However, the finding of a murmur in a kitten is not definitive evidence of the presence of a congenital cardiac anomaly. Innocent murmurs occur, for instance, where no abnormality of the heart can be found; these are usually quiet, occur during systole, and generally disappear by 4–6 months of age. Cardiomyopathy can give rise to a murmur through stretching or distortion of the atrio-ventricular valves, making them incompetent. Cardiomyopathy may occur in kittens as young as 5 or 6 months of age, and even kittens of a few weeks of age may be affected, particularly Burmese and Siamese. Conversely, a

Table 11.5 Relative prevalence of the commoner congenital cardiac anomalies.

Defect	Prevalence (%)
Atrio-ventricular valve dysplasia	19
Ventricular septal defect	17
Patent ductus arteriosus	12
Vascular anomalies	9
Aortic stenosis	7
Tetralogy of Fallot	7
Atrial septal defect	4
Common atrio-ventricular canal	4
Pulmonary stenosis	3

Adapted from Fox (1988a).

severe congenital defect may be present with no audible murmur, although this is uncommon. Further investigations including radiography, ultrasonography, ECG, angiography, cardiac catheterization and post-mortem examination are often required to reach a definitive diagnosis.

Most of the congenital cardiac anomalies recognized in other species have been reported in cats, but many are rare. The relative prevalence of the commoner defects is shown in Table 11.5. It should be noted that this is different from the frequency of occurrence of similar defects encountered in dogs. The commoner defects are considered in more detail below. The medical treatment of congestive heart failure (CHF) of any cause is discussed later in the section on therapy for cardiomyopathy.

Atrio-ventricular valve malformations

Dysplasia of the left (mitral) or right (tricuspid) atrio-ventricular (A-V) valves is the commonest form of congenital cardiac anomaly reported in cats. The range of severity is wide, and the anatomical defects seen include abnormalities of papillary muscle number or position (usually being upwardly displaced), abnormally long or short or fused chordae tendineae, and thickened valve leaflets which may have notches or clefts. The result of these defects is to make the valve incompetent, producing a systolic murmur of A-V valvular insufficiency, although occasionally the valve may also be stenotic. Congenital anomalies may occur in combination; for example, tricuspid dysplasia has been associated with mitral dysplasia and with ventricular septal defects. If the A-V valvular incompetence is severe enough to be haemodynamically significant volume overload occurs, with dilatation of the atrium and ventricle of the affected side.

The clinical effects depend on the severity of the defect. A systolic murmur of A-V valvular insufficiency will usually be audible with maximum intensity over the left or right apex, depending on the side affected; this murmur may radiate widely. In many cases the defect is mild and the cat remains compensated and clinically normal, apart from the presence of a murmur. In more severe cases, volume overload and cardiomegaly of the affected side are detectable radiographically, by ECG and by ultrasonography, the latter being the most sensitive and specific. Ultrasonography shows the atrial and ventricular dilatation and may also demonstrate the anatomical defects of the left or right A-V valves, e.g. thickened or adherent valve leaflets, abnormal chordae and/or papillary muscles (Fig. 11.6). Doppler techniques can be used to show the regurgitant blood flow.

Where congestive heart failure (CHF) does develop, this happens over a variable period. Mitral dysplasia leads to pulmonary oedema, which causes dyspnoea, and in the most severe cases secondary right-sided CHF may follow on from this as a consequence of chronic pulmonary venous congestion and pulmonary hypertension. Tricuspid dysplasia primarily causes right-sided CHF with pleural effusion and/or ascites.

Ventricular and atrial septal defects

Abnormalities of formation of the interventricular and interatrial septa are not uncommon. Ventricular septal defects (VSDs) occur most often, either as isolated lesions or with other defects such as tricuspid dysplasia. Isolated atrial septal defects (ASDs) are infrequently identified, but an ASD may be seen complicating another defect, e.g. with patent ductus arteriosus. The embryology of cardiac septation is complex (the reader is referred to Bishop, 1988, for details) and septal defects are very variable in their size, position, association with other anomalies and haemodynamic effects. A very large sub-aortic VSD is seen as part of the tetralogy of Fallot (see below). A combination of a low (septum primum) ASD with a high VSD can occur forming one large defect, a common atrio-ventricular canal, usually in association with abnormalities of the A-V valves. This complex anomaly results from abnormalities of development of the tissues arising from the embryonic endocardial cushions. It usually causes severe heart failure and carries a very poor prognosis.

The haemodynamic effects of these defects are dependent on the size of the lesion and the nature and severity of any associated anomalies. An ASD allows an abnormal shunting of blood from the left to the right atrium, which, if of sufficient magnitude, results in volume overload and dilatation of the right atrium and ventricle and increased pulmonary blood flow. A quiet systolic murmur of relative pulmonary stenosis is audible at the left heart base due to the larger than normal stroke volume of the right ventricle. A VSD also allows left-to-right shunting and pulmonary overcirculation. The effect here, because of the position of the defect, is predominantly one of increased pulmonary venous return and left-sided volume overload. The effect on the right ventricle is variable; it may be dilated or, if the VSD is large, hypertrophied. A loud holosystolic murmur is typically heard at the right sternal border, and again a murmur of relative pulmonary stenosis may be audible. If pulmonary hypertension develops, perhaps secondary to overperfusion, or if the right ventricle hypertrophies sufficiently, then a right-to-left shunt may occur, leading to cyanosis. This happens if right ventricular systolic pressure increases sufficiently to exceed the pressure on the left side. With a common A-V canal all four cardiac chambers are usually dilated due to the large (usually left-to-right) shunt, A-V valvular incompetence and subsequent severe volume overload.

Clinical signs in cats with septal defects vary

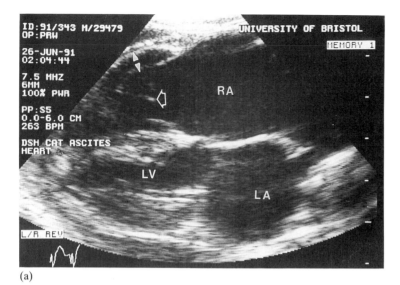

(a)

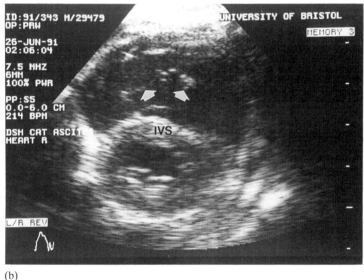

(b)

Fig. 11.6 Cardiac ultrasound images of congenital right A-V valve dysplasia from the right (a–c) and left (d) parasternal positions. (a) Long-axis view; the right atrium is markedly dilated, the right ventricular free wall is hypertrophied (small arrowheads) and an abnormal, thick chorda is visible (open arrowhead). (b, c) Short-axis views at chordal and heart base levels respectively; arrowheads indicate parts of the abnormal A-V valve and chordae. (d) Left apical (4-chamber) view; the right atrium is markedly dilated, the right ventricle less so. (Abbreviations as in Figs 11.4 & 11.5.)

from an asymptomatic murmur through to severe CHF, which may affect the left, right or both ventricles. Severe CHF generally develops in the first year of life with large septal defects. Thoracic radiographs demonstrate cardiomegaly and pulmonary overcirculation, unless a right-to-left shunt has developed, when the lungs appear underperfused. Evidence of CHF, if present, will also be apparent radiographically. Ultrasonography may show the septal defect if it is large enough and will show signs of right ventricular dilatation and volume overload, e.g. septal flattening or paradoxical septal motion. The ECG may show signs of right-sided enlargement, e.g. enlarged P-waves and deep S-waves in leads I, II, III and aVF. Occasionally a conduction deficit is seen due to physical interruption of the conduction system by the septal defect.

Patent ductus arteriosus

Patent ductus arteriosus (PDA) has not been

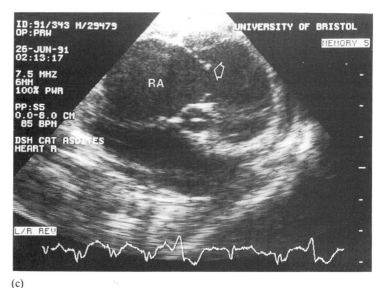

(c)

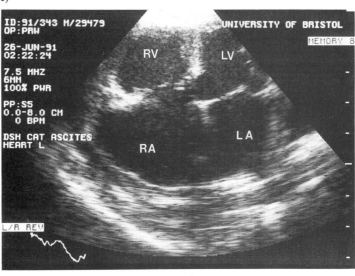

Fig. 11.6 *Continued*

(d)

described commonly in cats (in contrast to dogs where it is the most common congenital cardiac anomaly), but it deserves mention because potentially it can be corrected surgically. There may be a predisposition in the Siamese breed, although it has not been shown to be hereditary. Associations with other congenital anomalies have been reported, including septal defects and tricuspid dysplasia.

Patency of the ductus arteriosus after birth results in a left-to-right shunt and pulmonary over-perfusion with predominantly left-sided volume overload, the severity of which depends on the size of the ductus and pulmonary vascular resistance. A continuous murmur, loudest at the left heart base, and hyperkinetic femoral pulses are the classical clinical findings with PDA. Thoracic radiographs demonstrate varying degrees of left-sided cardiomegaly, pulmonary overperfusion and sometimes enlargement of the great vessels (Fig. 11.7). The ECG may show evidence of left-sided enlargement, e.g. tall R-waves in lead II, wide

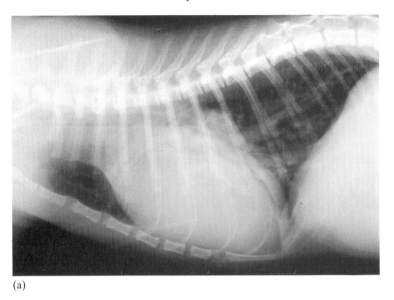

(a)

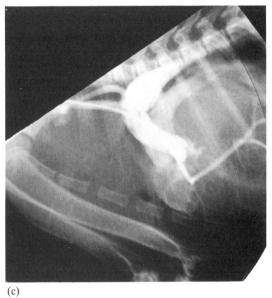

(c)

(b)

Fig. 11.7 Patent ductus arteriosus. Radiographs from a 13-week-old Siamese kitten with a continuous murmur. Lateral (a) and dorsoventral (b) projections show marked generalized cardiomegaly, some patchy pulmonary oedema, a wide aortic arch and wide pulmonary arteries (arrowheads). (c) Injection of contrast material via a catheter in the aortic root outlines both the aorta and the pulmonary artery and a short, wide connection; a coronary artery is also opacified. A small VSD was also found at post-mortem examination.

QRS complexes and wide P-waves. Ultrasonography shows dilatation of the left atrium and ventricle and may also reveal associated defects. If left untreated, PDA will progress to CHF, so surgical closure of the patent vessel is advisable; however, the prognosis should be guarded in cats, particularly if another defect is present. The occurrence of pulmonary hypertension, right ventricular hypertrophy and right-to-left shunting with cyanosis is reported to be rarer in cats than in dogs (Bonagura, 1989).

Aortic stenosis

Aortic stenosis was previously reported to be one of the commonest congenital defects in cats, but more recent surveys have not supported that conclusion. The obstruction to left ventricular outflow may occur at valvular level, or as a supra-valvular or sub-valvular fibrous ring. Associations with other congenital cardiac anomalies are reported. The effect of the obstruction is to produce concentric hypertrophy of the left ventricle with left atrial enlargement and post-stenotic dilatation of the aorta, which is visible in the more severe cases on thoracic radiographs and with ultrasonography. Ultrasound can show the site of obstruction, and a pressure gradient and turbulent blood flow across the aortic valve can be demonstrated using Doppler ultrasound techniques. Clinically a systolic murmur is produced, which is best heard at the left apex or right sternal border (Stepien & Bonagura, 1991). The prognosis for this defect appears to be poor, with most cats developing left-sided CHF, but some cases remain asymptomatic. The clinical and echocardiographic findings in aortic stenosis can be very similar to those of hypertrophic cardiomyopathy, which may lead to some difficulty in diagnosis, particularly if the congenital defect is discovered in an adult cat. This factor may have led to some confusion in previous surveys of prevalence.

Cyanotic congenital heart defects

Cyanosis may arise in cases of congenital heart disease due to right-to-left shunting of desaturated blood into the systemic circulation. This may occur, following the development of pulmonary hypertension and/or right ventricular hypertrophy, with anomalies that normally cause left-to-right shunting, e.g. septal defects or PDA, and also with other severe defects, but the most common in this rare category of conditions is the tetralogy of Fallot. This complex defect arises through abnormalities of development of the embryonic truncus arteriosus into an aorta and a pulmonary artery. This results in: (i) a dextropositioned aorta, overriding the interventricular septum; (ii) a sub-aortic VSD; (iii) pulmonary stenosis (at the level of the valve or outflow tract), which may be severe to the extent of atresia and which causes (iv) secondary right ventricular hypertrophy. The resulting high right ventricular pressures cause a right-to-left shunt of blood through the VSD into the overriding aorta, and thus cyanosis.

Some cats with tetralogy of Fallot may survive to middle-age; others are severely affected in the first year of life. The history, apart from cyanosis, may include dyspnoea, severe exercise intolerance and seizure-like episodes. The latter are thought to be due to hypoxia and to blood hyperviscosity caused by secondary polycythaemia, which occurs as a response to the pulmonary underperfusion. CHF is unlikely to occur, but sudden death is a possible outcome. Clinical examination usually reveals a systolic murmur of pulmonary stenosis at the left heart base, and possibly a murmur from the VSD at the right sternal border; however, the murmurs may be subtle or absent. The cyanosis is often detectable clinically, and severe polycythaemia may produce visible reddening of the mucous membranes. The latter may also produce tortuosity of the retinal vessels. The ECG may show evidence of right ventricular hypertrophy, e.g. a deviation of the mean electrical axis towards the right. Thoracic radiographs show right-sided enlargement and signs of pulmonary underperfusion. Echocardiography shows right ventricular hypertrophy and intravenous echocontrast can be used to show the right-to-left shunt, as can non-selective angiography.

The management of this serious condition is

difficult. Palliative surgical procedures have been described (e.g. subclavian-pulmonary artery anastomosis). Periodic phlebotomy should control the polycythaemia. It has been suggested that β-adrenergic blockers may have some value, in helping to limit the development of ventricular hypertrophy and perhaps also in suppressing dysrhythmias, but there is no information as to their clinical value in this condition.

Other congenital conditions

Endocardial fibroelastosis

This condition has been described previously as a common congenital anomaly with a strong predisposition in the Siamese and Burmese breeds, and was reported as being hereditary in Burmese. The lesions described were dilatation of the left atrium and ventricle with marked fibroelastic thickening of the endocardium. Signs of acute heart failure, with dyspnoea, cyanosis, dysrhythmias and sudden death, were seen in kittens from a few weeks up to a few months of age. However, it is now thought that the marked histological changes of fibroelastosis may merely be a non-specific response to other forms of congenital or acquired cardiac disease. It is thought possible that the original cases were in fact a form of juvenile cardiomyopathy, perhaps due to taurine deficiency.

Vascular ring strictures

This anomaly is reported in kittens, causing regurgitation; it is discussed further in Chapter 8.

Excessive left ventricular moderator bands

Although this probably is a congenital anomaly it is discussed later under 'Restrictive cardiomyopathy'.

Pericardioperitoneal diaphragmatic hernia

This defect is not uncommon and occurs due to incomplete separation of the abdominal and thoracic cavities, allowing abdominal viscera to lie within the pericardial sac. The condition appears to have a predisposition in long-haired cats. The defect may be asymptomatic and re-cognized incidentally, but dyspnoea is more likely and diarrhoea or vomiting are reported. Occasionally affected kittens are simply found dead. There may be associated deformities of the sternebrae (although clinically insignificant deformities of the sternebrae are a common incidental radiographic finding in cats of all ages). Diagnosis is based on radiography, which shows abnormalities of the cardiac silhouette and soft tissue densities within the pericardium. Confirmatory techniques such as barium contrast, non-selective angiography or ultrasonography can be helpful. This condition is treated by surgical reduction of the hernia and closure of the defect.

ACQUIRED HEART DISEASE

Most cardiac disease of clinical significance in cats is acquired, and myocardial disease (cardiomyopathy) accounts for the majority of these cases. The prevalence of cardiomyopathy (of all types) may be as high as 12–15% (Fox, 1988b). Acquired valvular and pericardial diseases are recognized and will be mentioned briefly, but they are not diagnosed commonly.

Cardiomyopathy

Many types of disease involve the myocardium and the term 'cardiomyopathy' may be applied to any pathological process that affects the myocardium primarily and which is not a result of prior congenital heart disease or acquired valvular disease. Myocardial diseases may or may not, depending on their severity, lead to clinically significant impairment of myocardial function. A common effect of myocardial disease is to produce dysrhythmias and/or conduction disturbances that may in themselves affect cardiac function.

Cardiomyopathies are generally classified under one or both of the following headings:
1 Aetiology, either primary/idiopathic (where no aetiology can be identified) or secondary (where there is a known cause); or
2 Effect on cardiac function or anatomy (e.g. dilated, hypertrophic, etc.).

This classification is summarized in Table 11.6.

Table 11.6 Classification of myocardial diseases.

Primary (idiopathic)
   Hypertrophic (obstructive and non-obstructive)
   Dilated
   Restrictive
   Intermediate
   (Excessive left ventricular moderator bands)

Secondary (defined aetiology)
   Metabolic (e.g. endocrine, nutritional)
   Infiltrative (e.g. neoplasia)
   Inflammatory (e.g. FIP, FIV, Lyme disease, ?immune-
     mediated)
   Fibrotic (e.g. post-inflammatory, secondary to other
     cardiac diseases)
   Toxic (e.g. adriamycin/ doxyrubicin)
   Others (e.g. trauma, infarction, chronic renal failure or
     anaemia)

Table 11.7 Secondary cardiomyopathies of potential clinical significance in cats.

Hyperthyroidism
Dietary taurine deficiency
Acromegaly
Chronic renal failure
Chronic severe anaemia
Feline infectious peritonitis
Neoplasia (lymphoma)

As an example of the use of this classification, hyperthyroidism usually causes secondary hypertrophic cardiomyopathy. Secondary cardiomyopathies are of particular importance in cats (Table 11.7) and an attempt should always be made to rule these out before categorizing a case of cardiomyopathy as 'idiopathic', since, if an underlying primary cause can be identified and treated, the prognosis for the cardiomyopathy is much better. Most cases of cardiomyopathy in cats were previously thought to be primary. This situation has been changed by an increasing awareness of the effect of various systemic disease processes on myocardial function, and particularly with the discovery of the role of dietary taurine deficiency as a primary factor in the aetiology of dilated cardiomyopathy. Future research is likely to reduce further the number of cases described as 'idiopathic'.

Three main functional/anatomical classes of cardiomyopathy are recognized in cats. The pathophysiology and relative incidence of these will be described and then the clinical features, diagnosis and treatment of the cardiomyopathies as a whole will be discussed.

Hypertrophic cardiomyopathy (HCM)
In this form of cardiomyopathy there is inappropriate hypertrophy of the left ventricle, papillary muscles and interventricular septum which reduces ventricular compliance (increases 'stiffness') and thus impairs ventricular diastolic function. An increase in left atrial and pulmonary venous pressures is required to fill the 'stiff' ventricle. Contractile (systolic) function is usually unimpaired and the shortening fraction may actually be increased. In some cases (the obstructive form of HCM) asymmetrical hypertrophy of the interventricular septum beneath the aortic valve causes a partial physical obstruction of outflow from the left ventricle during systole. Part of the obstruction to outflow is probably 'dynamic', due to abnormal motion of the septal cusp of the left A-V valve towards the septum during systole ('systolic anterior motion'), which can be demonstrated by M-mode echocardiography. Doppler echocardiography will show a systolic pressure gradient across the outflow tract in hypertrophic obstructive cardiomyopathy (HOCM). The clinical significance of this obstructive component is as yet uncertain.

In the typical form of HCM, massive concentric hypertrophy results in marked reduction of the volume of the left ventricular lumen. In many cases, however, the degree and distribution of hypertrophy of the left ventricle may be quite variable and regional, and the ventricular lumen volume may remain normal (Bright *et al.*, 1992). Because of the elevated filling pressures the left atrium becomes dilated and hypertrophied and left atrial and pulmonary venous pressures may be markedly elevated, resulting in pulmonary oedema. Bouts of acute pulmonary oedema may occur if left ventricular filling is further compromised, e.g. by tachycardia, tachydysrhythmias or anaesthesia, or by further overload of the circulation such as the administration of intravenous fluids. Distortion of the mitral valve apparatus leads to left A-V valvular incompetence and regurgitation, which further increases left atrial pressure and gives rise to a systolic murmur. A systolic murmur may also arise from the area of outflow obstruction. Histological findings are variable, but there may be hypertrophy and cellular disorganization of the myocardiocytes and some interstitial fibrosis. There may also be histological changes in the conduction system, especially the A-V node.

The aetiology of HCM is often unknown. The most notable systemic cause in cats of secondary myocardial hypertrophy and cardiomyopathy is hyperthyroidism, and the possibility of this very treatable condition should always be explored in older cats with signs of cardiomyopathy (see Chapter 12). Other conditions that may lead to mild HCM include chronic anaemia and chronic renal disease with hypertension, although the importance of these conditions as potential causes of overt heart disease or failure is currently unknown. Most cases of HCM are classed as idiopathic. An association between 'primary' HCM and an elevated plasma level of growth hormone has been reported by Kittleson (1991), but the significance of this finding is as yet also unknown. Peterson *et al.* (1990) have also noted cardiomegaly in cats with pituitary adenomas leading to acromegaly. Another suggested aetiology for primary HCM is an abnormal sensitivity of the myocardiocytes to circulating catecholamines, resulting in hypertrophy. Familial forms of HCM are described in humans (Braunwald, 1988).

The clinical and echocardiographic findings in congenital sub-aortic stenosis can be very similar to those in HCM, and as the latter can occur in young cats there is some potential for confusion between these two conditions.

Dilated cardiomyopathy (DCM)
The essential feature of this form of cardiomyopathy (previously termed 'congestive') is systolic failure due to a decrease in the intrinsic inotropic function of the myocardiocytes. The cardiac chambers, especially the left ventricle, are dilated which can be shown readily by echocardiography, and indicators of systolic function (e.g. fractional shortening, ventricular diameter at end-systole, changes in ventricular wall thickness during systole and systolic time intervals) indicate reduced contractility. Ventricular compliance may also be reduced in DCM as in HCM, but the relative haemodynamic significance of this in DCM is not known. A-V valve stretching and valvular incompetence, secondary to ventricular dilatation, gives rise to a systolic murmur. The histological findings in DCM are again variable, including myocardiocyte degeneration and focal fibrosis, and do not reflect the severity of the abnormalities of myocardial function.

The discovery of the role of dietary taurine deficiency as a prime factor in the aetiology of DCM (Pion *et al.*, 1989) can be regarded as a key finding, and has caused considerable interest. DCM is the major form of primary cardiomyopathy in most species, including dogs and humans, and generally carries a poor prognosis. DCM has usually been classed in animals as idiopathic and it has been thought to be the end stage, perhaps after a latent period of months or years, of various possible insults to the myocardium including viral or immune-mediated inflammation or toxins. The aetiopathogenesis of DCM is the subject of a considerable continuing research effort. Cats with naturally occurring DCM were found to have low plasma levels of taurine and the addition of supplementary taurine to their diet, and to the diet of cats with experimentally induced taurine deficiency, resulted in complete reversal of the condition, a unique situation amongst the 'primary' cardiomyopathies. Not all cats on the same diet will develop DCM, so it is likely that other factors (e.g. the bioavailability of the taurine in the food and its absorption or metabolism) are also involved. Taurine depletion has been linked to the feeding of a potassium-depleted acidified diet (Dow *et al.*, 1992). The cat has a particular requirement for taurine, but it is possible that taurine deficiency may also prove to be important in the aetiology of DCM in other species. A form of familial DCM linked to L-carnitine deficiency, described in humans and dogs (boxers), is another example of an apparently diet-related cardiomyopathy (Keene *et al.*, 1991).

Restrictive cardiomyopathy (RCM)

This heterogeneous form of cardiomyopathy is more difficult to define and to diagnose and is probably the least common type seen in cats. It is characterized by varying degrees of focal or diffuse fibrosis of the myocardium or sub-endocardium. This primarily reduces ventricular compliance and restricts filling, thus leading to diastolic failure similar to that caused by HCM. There may also be some myocardial hypertrophy. Depending on the amount of myocardial tissue lost through fibrosis, systolic function may also be reduced. Thus the clinical effects of RCM may encompass aspects of both HCM and DCM, and the term intermediate (or 'intergrade') cardiomyopathy is sometimes applied for this reason. The signs and approach to management are dependent on which aspect (diastolic or systolic failure) predominates.

The aetiology of RCM is unknown, but one possibility is that it may follow a bout or bouts of myocarditis, perhaps after a variable period of latency between the initial 'insult' to the myocardium and the development of clinical signs of diastolic failure (Wynne & Braunwald, 1988). The entity of excessive left ventricular moderator bands is also included within the description of RCM as these structures, which bridge the ventricular lumen, may limit ventricular filling leading to diastolic failure and left atrial enlargement. The excessive moderator bands are probably the result of a congenital abnormality of ventricular development and may occur with other forms of congenital heart disease, but they have also been reported in association with other forms of acquired cardiomyopathy.

Relative prevalence of the cardiomyopathies

Whereas in the majority of species studied DCM is the most frequently encountered form of cardiomyopathy, this does not now appear to be true for the cat. The relative importance of the different

types of cardiomyopathy in cats always seems to have shown some geographical variation. Previously DCM was reported to be the most frequent form in the UK and in some areas of North America, whereas HCM appeared to be more frequent in eastern USA. However, since the discovery of the importance of taurine deficiency in cardiac disease, pet food manufacturers have increased the levels and bioavailability of taurine in commercial cat foods, and the frequency of occurrence of DCM in cats in the UK appears to have markedly decreased; this impression is strongly supported in North America also. DCM due to taurine deficiency is only likely to be seen now in cats eating poorly prepared commercial or home-made diets, although DCM due to causes other than taurine deficiency may still be encountered. A number of other cardiac conditions may, particularly in their end stages, result in a dilated and hypokinetic heart that resembles DCM clinically and echocardiographically. These include acquired valvular disease, severe (and perhaps complex) previously unrecognized congenital heart disease and advanced cases of secondary cardiomyopathy (Table 11.8). Pericardial disease leading to cardiac tamponade can be included here, as this produces a rounded cardiac silhouette on thoracic radiographs that can be difficult to differentiate from the generalized cardiomegaly of DCM if ultrasonography is not available (Fig. 11.8).

With the declining prevalence of DCM, most cases of cardiomyopathy in cats fall into the hypertrophic or restrictive categories. Given the heterogeneous nature of both these forms of cardiomyopathy, however, it may be difficult to make a firm classification in some individuals, even with

Table 11.8 Conditions clinically and radiographically resembling dilated cardiomyopathy.

Acquired valvular heart disease (advanced)
Severe/unrecognized congenital disease
Severe/advanced secondary cardiomyopathies
  (e.g. hyperthyroidism)
Pericardial effusion

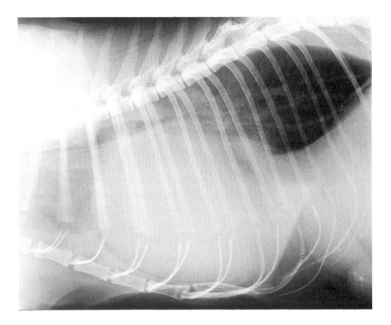

Fig. 11.8 Lateral radiograph from a cat with restrictive cardiomyopathy and marked enlargement of the cardiac silhouette due to pericardial effusion. Some pleural effusion is also present.

the aid of echocardiography. The term 'intermediate cardiomyopathy' (ICM) has been used in cases that show variable hypertrophy, or features of both RCM and HCM, or where there is evidence of both diastolic and systolic dysfunction. Indeed, some authors class the majority of cases of myocardial disease as ICM. However, it is likely that this group will (as mentioned above for DCM) include examples of other forms of cardiac disease, particularly in their more advanced stages, e.g. late recognized congenital disease, acquired valvular disease or secondary cardiomyopathy.

Although it may not be possible to classify an individual case of cardiomyopathy precisely as HCM, RCM or DCM, the most critical decisions to make from the point of view of prognosis and choosing appropriate therapy are:

1 Whether an individual case of cardiomyopathy is primary or secondary; and

2 Whether the disturbance of function is predominantly diastolic or systolic.

This second question is most easily answered by the use of echocardiography. With these questions in mind, the clinical features, diagnosis and treatment of the cardiomyopathies will now be discussed.

Diagnosis of the cardiomyopathies

The reader is referred back to the earlier sections on clinical history, clinical examination and diagnostic aids for a full discussion of these areas, and also to Tables 11.1 and 11.2. This section will concentrate on the features which may help to distinguish the various forms of cardiomyopathy. Harpster (1986) has reviewed the criteria by which a classification may be attempted.

Breed, sex and age

Cardiomyopathy occurs mainly in domestic cats of mixed breeding, but DCM has been associated with pure-bred cats, particularly the oriental breeds (Siamese, Burmese, Abyssinian); whether this is associated with diet or is a true predisposition is not clear. HCM has been associated with long-haired cats. There is a marked male sex predisposition in HCM, with a reported frequency of occurrence of 3–4 times that of females. This predisposition is not reported in DCM and RCM. The age range for HCM and DCM is very wide, with kittens as young as 5 months or less being affected. RCM tends to occur in middle-aged and older cats.

Clinical features

The history and clinical findings are often similar in all three forms of cardiomyopathy. Abnormalities may range from mild to severe; some cases of HCM may remain asymptomatic for long periods of time, whereas signs of acute cardiac output failure ('cardiogenic shock') such as collapse, hypothermia and bradycardia may be seen, especially in DCM. The dietary history may indicate the possibility of taurine deficiency, and in such cases retinal degeneration may also be seen (see Chapter 9).

Dyspnoea is usually the predominant feature in all forms of cardiomyopathy, although this may be episodic, particularly in HCM. Clinical examination may reveal adventitious lung sounds with pulmonary oedema, or muffling of heart and lung sounds and dullness on percussion where there is a pleural effusion. Pulmonary oedema tends to occur more frequently with HCM, pleural effusion with DCM and either may occur with RCM. Other clinical features of cardiomyopathy include lethargy and anorexia, abnormalities on cardiac auscultation (murmurs, gallop sounds and dysrhythmias), signs of thromboembolic disease and abdominal enlargement due to ascites. Ascites may occur more frequently with RCM and murmurs are reported more often in HCM. Unfortunately none of the clinical trends given above are entirely reliable indicators of the form of cardiomyopathy present.

Radiography

Thoracic radiography is used to assess the presence and degree of cardiomegaly and to look for evidence of congestive heart failure, i.e. pulmonary oedema, pleural effusion or venous congestion. Some qualitative differences are reported between the plain radiographic features of the three major forms of cardiomyopathy that may help in distinguishing them. However, it must be stressed that, as with the clinical trends mentioned above, none of these are particularly reliable. Non-selective angiography is much more specific than plain radiography.

In HCM the cardiac silhouette in the dorsoventral projection is often described as 'valentine-shaped' due to the retention of a pointed apex and the broad 'shoulders' caused by atrial and auricular (especially left-sided) enlargement. The apex may be displaced towards the midline (Fig. 11.9). Atrial enlargement is often particularly prominent in HCM and RCM because of the reduced compliance of the ventricle(s). Pulmonary oedema is said to be typical of HCM, although pleural effusions are also seen, especially in long-standing cases. Non-selective angiography shows atrial enlargement and left ventricular hypertrophy, sometimes with very large papillary muscles, and may also indicate the presence of an obstruction in the left ventricular outflow tract. The circulation time from right ventricle to left atrium is generally normal (around 4–6 seconds post-injection). Non-selective angiography may, in any form of cardiomyopathy, demonstrate the presence of an atrial thrombus.

In DCM the typical description is of generalized cardiomegaly with a rounded cardiac apex. There may be pulmonary oedema, pleural effusion or both (Fig. 11.10). Non-selective angiography shows biventricular and bi-atrial dilatation, and sometimes thin ventricular walls are apparent. Pulmonary circulation time is often prolonged and the aorta may appear narrow and poorly opacified.

In RCM the cardiac apex may be rounded and atrial enlargement may be marked. Pulmonary oedema, pleural effusion or ascites may be present (Figs 11.3 & 11.11). Non-selective angiography may be the most reliable means of diagnosing RCM, showing marked atrial enlargement and an irregular outline to the left ventricular endocardium.

Echocardiography

This is the most sensitive and specific means of diagnosing and classifying cardiomyopathy, as it gives information on both the internal anatomy of the heart and its function. The echocardiographic features of the cardiomyopathies have been discussed above, but are summarized here.

In HCM there is hypertrophy of the ventricular (mainly left) free wall and interventricular septum

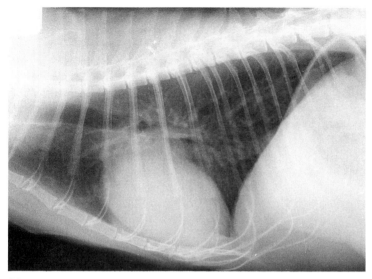

(a)

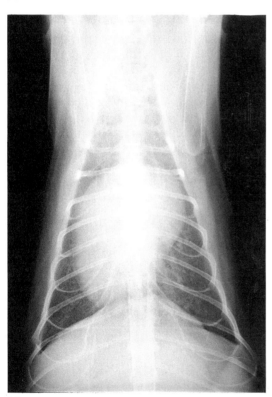

(b)

Fig. 11.9 Lateral (a) and dorsoventral (b) radiographs from a cat with hypertrophic cardiomyopathy. The heart is enlarged and elongated, with an increase in sternal contact in the lateral projection. Left atrial enlargement is seen as a dorsal bulge on the lateral view, elevating the trachea, and a marked lateral bulge on the D-V view; the apex is displaced to the right. Mild pulmonary oedema is seen as a hazy infiltrate.

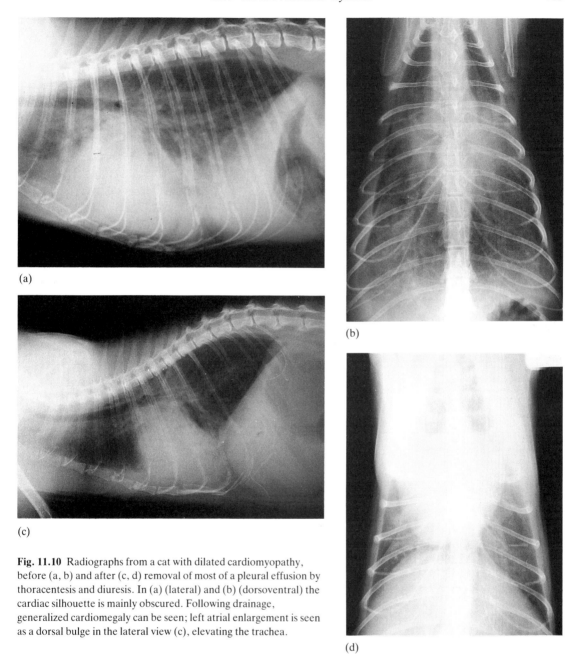

(a)

(b)

(c)

(d)

Fig. 11.10 Radiographs from a cat with dilated cardiomyopathy, before (a, b) and after (c, d) removal of most of a pleural effusion by thoracentesis and diuresis. In (a) (lateral) and (b) (dorsoventral) the cardiac silhouette is mainly obscured. Following drainage, generalized cardiomegaly can be seen; left atrial enlargement is seen as a dorsal bulge in the lateral view (c), elevating the trachea.

(diastolic thickness greater than 5.5 mm). This may be marked and concentric (Fig. 11.12) or variable and regional. There may be asymmetrical hypertrophy of the septum beneath the aortic valve (Fig. 11.13a) leading to partial outflow obstruction, and papillary muscle hypertrophy may be marked. Left ventricular systolic function (as assessed by fractional shortening, for instance) is normal or increased. The left atrium is enlarged. Marked left atrial dilatation is suggestive of the presence of reduced left ventricular diastolic function; the largest left atria are generally seen in cases of HCM and RCM where ventricular compliance is reduced (Fig. 11.14). This finding

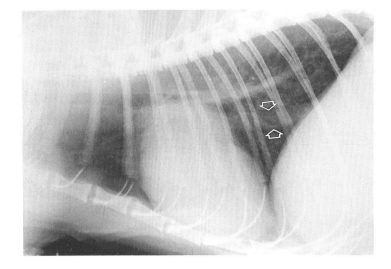

Fig. 11.11 Lateral radiograph from a case of intermediate cardiomyopathy; there is cardiomegaly, widening of the caudal vena cava (arrowheads) and mild pulmonary oedema.

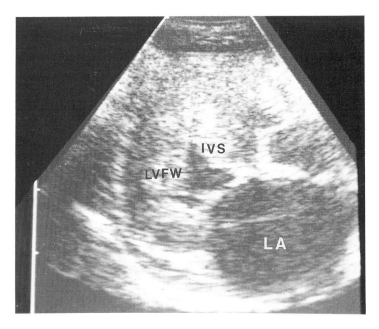

IVS

LVFW

LA

Fig. 11.12 Cardiac ultrasound image of hypertrophic cardiomyopathy. The left atrium is markedly dilated and the left ventricle markedly hypertrophied. (Abbreviations as in Figs 11.4 & 11.5.)

can be a helpful pointer in cases where the degree of hypertrophy is marginal. The echocardiographic assessment of diastolic function is more difficult than that of systolic function. Values such as the rate of ventricular free wall thinning, or the rate of change in ventricular volume during diastole (e.g. relaxation half-time) are used in humans and may prove to be useful in cats (Bright *et al.*, 1992). Left ventricular volume is normal or decreased. A pericardial effusion is seen in some cases. Ultrasonography may, in any form of cardiomyopathy, demonstrate an atrial thrombus.

In DCM the major feature on ultrasonography is a reduction in systolic function (shortening fraction usually less than 30%, Fig. 11.13b). The diameter of the left ventricular lumen at diastole

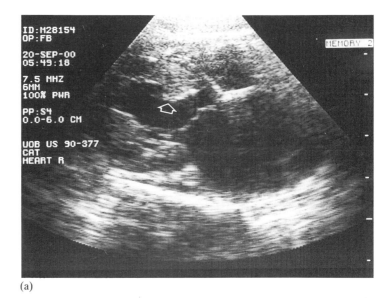

(a)

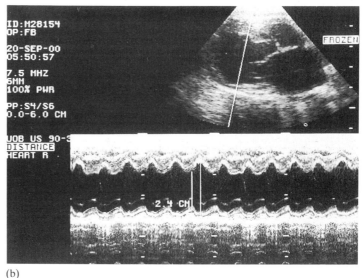

Fig. 11.13 Intermediate
cardiomyopathy. (a) Asymmetrical
hypertrophy of the interventricular
septum (arrowhead) beneath the
aortic valve and marked left atrial
dilatation. (b) An M-mode display
shows poor free wall motion and left
ventricular dilatation; the fractional
shortening is 29% (same case as
shown in Fig. 11.11).

(b)

usually exceeds 16 mm, although this may be less marked or even normal in more acute cases or following diuresis or other therapy. Left ventricular wall thickness may be normal or reduced. The left atrium is usually dilated and the right atrium and ventricle may be dilated also. A small pericardial effusion may be present.

The ultrasonographic features of RCM are reported to be quite variable, with normal, dilated or hypertrophied ventricles, a normal or decreased shortening fraction, left atrial dilatation and a pericardial effusion in some cases (Fig. 11.15).

Electrocardiography

Abnormalities of the ECG, both of rhythm and impulse conduction, are common in cardiomyopathy, but the changes seen are non-specific for the form of cardiomyopathy involved. Abnormalities seen (see Table 11.4 for normal ECG values) include tall or wide P-waves indicating atrial en-

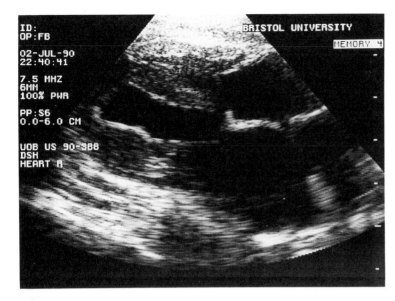

Fig. 11.14 Marked bi-atrial enlargement in a case of intermediate cardiomyopathy; left ventricular hypertrophy was patchy and systolic function was below normal (same case as shown in Fig. 11.3).

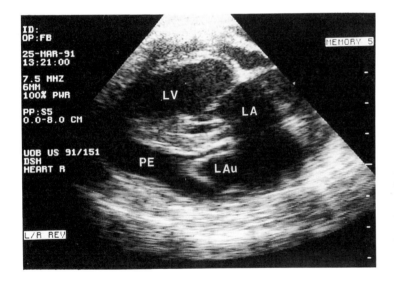

Fig. 11.15 Pericardial effusion in a case of restrictive cardiomyopathy (same case as shown in Fig. 11.8). A grossly dilated left auricular appendage (LAu) is seen within the distended, fluid-filled pericardial sac (PE); the outline of the left ventricle appears somewhat irregular.

largement, widening or, in particular, increased voltages of the QRS complex indicating ventricular enlargement (Fig. 11.16), various supraventricular and ventricular tachydysrhythmias (Fig. 11.2), occasionally sinus bradycardia (e.g. in DCM), and conduction disturbances (Fig. 11.17). Conduction disturbances are reported more frequently in HCM, particularly the abnormality described as left anterior fascicular block, but the latter is also seen in other forms of congenital and acquired cardiac disease (Fig. 11.18).

Prognosis for cardiomyopathy

The prognosis in cases of cardiomyopathy is dependent on factors such as the form of cardiomyopathy involved, its severity, whether any underlying aetiology can be identified and treated,

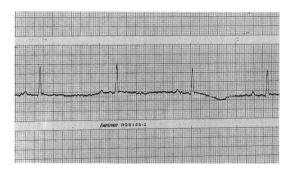

Fig. 11.16 Lead 2 ECG from a cat with hyperthyroidism; R wave voltage increased to 1.5 mV. Paper speed: 100 mm/s; 1 cm = 1 mV.

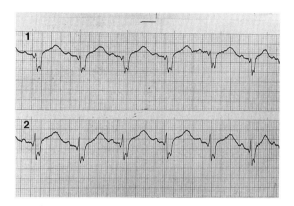

Fig. 11.17 Right bundle branch block in a cat with hypertrophic cardiomyopathy; right axis deviation; QRS interval 60 msec. Leads 1 and 2. Paper speed: 100 mm/s; 1 cm = 1 mV.

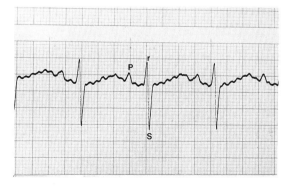

Fig. 11.18 Left anterior fascicular block in a cat with hyperthyroidism; left axis deviation; QRS interval normal. Lead 2. Paper speed: 100 mm/s; 1 cm = 1 mV.

the existence of other complicating related or unrelated conditions (e.g. renal failure, thromboembolic disease) and the response to treatment. The prognosis for HCM is generally better than for other forms of cardiomyopathy, and the occurrence of clinical signs may be very intermittent in HCM. The prognosis for taurine-responsive DCM is good, but poor for cases of DCM where taurine levels are normal. The prognosis is worse in any form of cardiomyopathy where there is a reduction in systolic function.

As mentioned above in the section on relative prevalence, it is very difficult, from clinical and plain radiographic findings alone, to determine the form of cardiomyopathy present in any individual case. If facilities for ultrasonography are not available, and if referral for ultrasonography is not possible, then in view of the apparent decline in the prevalence of DCM in the UK it is probably safest to assume that the case is one of diastolic failure when choosing a therapeutic regime. However, caution should be exercised, particularly in the use of negative inotropic agents, if the functional status of the ventricles has not been determined.

MANAGEMENT OF CARDIOMYOPATHY AND CARDIAC FAILURE

Key considerations in planning a therapeutic regime are the major presenting clinical signs and the prognostic factors mentioned above, i.e. the pathophysiological form of cardiac disease and any underlying cause if identified. Treatment of a primary or predisposing disease improves the prognosis, and it is possible that cardiac function may return to normal. The functional state of the ventricles determines whether inotropic support is indicated. The therapeutic principles covered in this section apply to the treatment of cardiac failure due to any form of cardiac disease, congenital or acquired. Options for treating cardiac failure, and the dose rates of many of the drugs used, are listed in Table 11.9. Table 11.10 summarizes the therapeutic approaches used in specific forms of cardiac disease.

Table 11.9 Therapeutic options in treating cardiac disease.

Diuretics (e.g. frusemide 0.5–2.0 mg/kg *p.o.*/IV q8–12–24 h)
Vasodilators (e.g. glyceryl trinitrate 2% ointment ⅛–¼ inch p.c. q6–8 h;
  ACE inhibitors e.g.
    enalapril 0.5 mg/kg *p.o.* q24 h;
    captopril 3.125–6.25 mg *p.o.* q8–12 h
  hydralazine 0.5–1.0 mg/kg q12 h)
β-adrenergic blockade (e.g. propranolol 2.5–5.0 mg *p.o.* q8–12 h)
Calcium channel blockade (e.g. diltiazem 0.5–1.25 mg/kg *p.o.* q8–12 h)
Positive inotropes (e.g. digoxin 0.005 mg/kg *p.o.* q12–48 h; dobutamine/dopamine 1–5 μg/kg/min IV CRI)
Taurine supplementation 250–500 mg *p.o.* q12 h
Diet change – adequate taurine, low sodium
Aspirin (20–25 mg/kg *p.o.* 2–3 times weekly)
Thoracentesis
Oxygen; bronchodilation (e.g. aminophylline 5–10 mg/kg *p.o.* q8–12 h)
Cage rest/sedation (e.g. acepromazine 0.1 mg/kg s.c.)
Nursing/warmth/intravenous fluids
Treatment of primary cause (e.g. hyperthyroidism)
Surgery for congenital defects (e.g. PDA)

p.o. = *per os*; s.c. = subcutaneously; p.c. = percutaneously; IV = intravenously; CRI = constant rate infusion; ACE = angiotensin convering enzyme.
The doses of captopril and propranolol are not related to bodyweight, but are convenient divisions of standard tablet sizes.
See text for further details of dose rates, indications, etc.
N.B. none of these drugs are approved for use in cats.

Table 11.10 Summary of therapeutic approaches in specific forms of cardiac disease.

Acute pulmonary oedema
  Frusemide (i.v. initially)
  Glyceryl trinitrate
  Cage rest; ? oxyen
  + specific therapy (for type of disease)

Acute cardiac output failure (cardiogenic shock)
  Cage rest and intravenous fluids
  Dobutamine infusion
  Digoxin
  ? diuresis later

Hypertrophic cardiomyopathy
  Frusemide
  Propranolol/diltiazem
  Aspirin
  ? ACE inhibitor

Dilated cardiomyopathy
  Frusemide
  Taurine
  Digoxin
  Aspirin
  ACE inhibitor

Restrictive cardiomyopathy
  Frusemide
  Aspirin
  ? ACE inhibitor
  ? propranolol/diltiazem *or* digoxin (depends on contractile function)

Thromboembolism
  Cage rest, fluids, analgesics, warmth
  ? Frusemide
  Heparin
  Aspirin
  Acepromazine

? = Optional, depending on requirements/severity of the case.

Before discussing therapy for heart failure it is helpful to describe the ways in which the heart and circulation adapt to the presence of cardiac disease. If cardiac output is inadequate to meet the needs of the body, the circulatory system compensates through a series of neuroendocrine mechanisms, which include sympathetically mediated increases in heart rate, contractility and vascular tone, and sodium and water retention mainly brought about by activation of the renin-angiotensin-aldosterone system (for a fuller discussion of this subject see Bonagura, 1989). These adaptive responses (which result in selective vasoconstriction, increased cardiac work, eccentric ventricular myocardial hypertrophy and circulatory volume overload) support circulatory function and allow the cardiovascular system to compensate for the effects of cardiac disease for a variable period, but eventually progress to congestive heart failure in most cases. The clinical signs of heart failure (described earlier in the sections on clinical history and clinical examination) are due to a reduction in cardiac output ('forward heart failure', or 'cardiogenic shock' if severe and acute) and venous hypertension ('backward heart failure'). The latter is produced by a combination of circulatory volume overload, venoconstriction and impaired cardiac diastolic function. The clinical signs of heart failure are often described as being predominantly left- or right-sided, reflecting which valve or chamber is primarily affected. This distinction is useful clinically, although in general the whole circulation is involved.

Management of underlying disease

In view of the relative frequency of occurrence of secondary cardiomyopathies in cats it is vital to search for and, if possible, treat any underlying primary disease. The most important of these are hyperthyroidism (see Chapter 12) and taurine deficiency.

Hyperthyroidism

In many cases of hyperthyroidism the cardiac effects are mild, causing only varying degrees of cardiomegaly (which can be detected radiographically) and tachycardia, without overt heart failure. In such cases it is not necessary to treat for cardiac disease *per se*, except to control excessive tachycardia (>240/min), if present, with propranolol (or other β-blockers, e.g. atenolol) to reduce the heart rate to 150–200/min before surgical or radioiodine thyroid ablation. Some of the clinical signs of hyperthyroidism are due in part to excessive adrenergic stimulation; thus β-blockers are particularly useful in their control. As serum thyroxine levels fall, it may be possible to reduce or stop the propranolol. Where there is overt cardiac failure, treatment for congestive heart failure (as described below) is required alongside anti-thyroid drugs, and surgery should be delayed until circulatory function is stabilized. The prognosis for cats with hyperthyroidism and congestive heart failure is guarded, and is poor where systolic function is reduced. However, in many cases it may be possible to reduce or withdraw cardiac medication following thyroid ablation.

Taurine deficiency

Taurine deficiency should be suspected in all cases of dilated cardiomyopathy, particularly if the diet is poorly balanced or if there are lesions of central retinal degeneration (see Chapter 9). As it is not currently possible to obtain commercial taurine assays in the UK it is prudent to assume that taurine deficiency is present in such cases. Taurine does also have non-specific beneficial effects on myocardial function, and a clinical improvement may occur even when initial plasma taurine concentrations are in the normal range (Sisson *et al.*, 1991). The cat should be placed on a diet containing adequate levels of taurine, and extra taurine (which the owner may be able to obtain in capsule form from a health food shop) is added at the rate of 250–500 mg twice daily. The response to taurine may take several weeks, and treatment for dilated cardiomyopathy is required until cardiac function has returned to normal.

Management of volume overload, oedema and effusions

In all types of cardiac disease, diuretics are the major form of therapy employed to control the effects of circulatory volume overload and venous hypertension, i.e. in treating the pulmonary oedema and the pleural and pericardial effusions (and occasionally ascites) seen in congestive heart failure.

The most frequently used diuretic is frusemide, which can achieve significant diuresis and naturesis in cats. Other less potent diuretics, e.g. hydrochlorothiazide (0.5–2.0 mg/kg bodyweight every 12–24 h), or potassium-sparing diuretics, e.g. spironolactone or amiloride, are also used occasionally, usually in combination with frusemide. These can be useful if effusions prove refractory to frusemide alone or if hypokalaemia is a problem. Frusemide may be administered by various routes and at a wide range of dose rates, depending on the severity of the condition. In cases of acute pulmonary oedema it is best to give it intravenously initially (1–2 mg/kg, 2 or 3 times daily, although up to 4 mg/kg may be used for short periods), along with a venodilator (see below), cage rest, oxygen supplementation if required and, if necessary, where the cat is markedly distressed, sedation (see below under section on thromboembolism). For maintenance therapy, once the oedema or effusion is controlled, then frusemide may be administered orally at about 1 mg/kg once or twice daily. Dosing as infrequently as once every 2–3 days may be sufficient, e.g. in HCM. Conversely, in cases with refractory effusions, higher doses may be needed two or three times daily, or other diuretics or vasodilators (see below) may be used in combination with the frusemide. With pleural effusions, initial thoracentesis is worth while to clear the chest of fluid quickly and thus ease respiration. Periodic drainage of pleural and abdominal effusions may occasionally be necessary as an adjunct to diuresis. A low-sodium diet may be of value in the long-term management of volume overload.

Care must be taken not to cause excessive diuresis, as dehydration, reduced cardiac output and pre-renal azotaemia will result. This is a particular problem with cats as they often do not drink adequately to rehydrate themselves. Electrolyte depletion, particularly hypokalaemia, is a possible danger with high-dose or chronic diuretic therapy, especially where the cat is inappetent, and routine monitoring of plasma sodium and potassium concentrations is advisable in such cases. Where hypokalaemia is identified, oral potassium supplements such as potassium chloride, gluconate or citrate solutions can be used, although these have a low palatability. Tablets and capsules are also available, which may be more palatable. A potassium-sparing diuretic or an angiotensin-converting enzyme (ACE) inhibitor (e.g. enalapril) would be a better alternative (these should not be used in combination with each other).

Vasodilation and reduction of cardiac workload

Vasodilators are used increasingly to treat severe or refractory heart failure in cats and dogs. These agents act directly or indirectly to dilate arterioles and/or veins. The most frequently used vasodilators are glyceryl trinitrate (nitroglycerine), the ACE inhibitors captopril and enalapril, and hydralazine.

Glyceryl trinitrate is a direct-acting venodilator, administered percutaneously as a 2% ointment applied to an area of hairless skin such as inside the pinnae. Gloves should be worn when applying this preparation. By reducing venous pressure and increasing systemic venous pooling of blood, the tendency to form oedema is reduced, thus assisting the action of diuretics. This is of particular value in the management of acute pulmonary oedema, usually in the first 24–48 hours of treatment. More prolonged use results in the development of tolerance to the drug, unless it is used intermittently.

Hydralazine is a direct-acting arteriodilator, and has been advocated for use in refractory DCM and for mitral regurgitaton. Hydralazine can produce hypotension and tachycardia, and the ACE inhibitors are probably easier to use in most circumstances in cats.

Inhibitors of angiotensin-converting enzyme produce arteriolar and venous vasodilation indirectly, predominantly by inhibiting the formation of angiotensin II, which is a potent vasoconstrictor. In addition to causing vasoconstriction, angiotensin II stimulates aldosterone release from the adrenal cortex; thus ACE inhibition will also reduce sodium and water retention. Because ACE inhibitors interfere at a number of levels with the development of congestive heart failure, they are perhaps the most promising of the vasodilators for the treatment of chronic and refractory heart failure, and as experience of their use increases they may be employed even earlier in the course of disease. This group of drugs is among the few to have been shown to prolong survival in human patients with chronic heart failure. Captopril has been widely employed in cats; enalapril seems to be equally effective and may prove easier to use as it need only be given once daily (although the dose can be increased to 0.5 mg/kg *per os* every 12 hours if required), and it seems to have fewer side-effects, such as inappetence. ACE inhibitors may be used as an adjunct to frusemide in any case of refractory heart failure, except in the presence of hypotension, where vasodilators should be used with care or not at all. Hypotension may occur in some cases of DCM, in the obstructive form of severe HCM and in congenital outflow obstruction, such as aortic stenosis.

Vasodilators reduce cardiac workload by reducing afterload and/or preload. Another way of reducing the demands made on the heart, which is simple and effective, is to enforce rest by restricting the cat to a cage. This is particularly valuable in cases of acute pulmonary oedema or thromboembolism, where the cat may be markedly distressed. Drugs that reduce cardiac systolic function (negative inotropic agents) such as β-blockers and calcium channel blockers also serve to reduce myocardial work and oxygen demand. These are discussed further in the next section.

Improving diastolic function

Poor diastolic function of the ventricles is the hallmark of HCM and RCM, and may be important in DCM. Ventricular compliance is also reduced when marked ventricular hypertrophy occurs with congenital defects such as aortic stenosis. β-adrenergic blockers (e.g. propranolol) and calcium channel blockers (e.g. diltiazem) have been used in these situations to reduce contractility and heart rate, thus increasing cardiac output by improving compliance and allowing more time for diastole. Lowering contractility may also reduce any dynamic component of outflow tract obstruction (conversely, arteriodilators may worsen dynamic outflow obstruction).

The negative inotropic agent which has been used most widely in cats is the β-blocker propranolol. This drug also has useful anti-dysrhythmic properties; in fact it is one of the few safe, oral anti-dysrhythmic agents for cats, and is the drug of choice for ventricular tachydysrhythmias. Propranolol should be introduced gradually and the dose titrated slowly upwards, using the minimum effective dose to achieve the desired control of heart rate (its negative inotropic activity is more difficult to quantify) whilst avoiding side-effects such as lethargy and excessive bradycardia. As propranolol is a non-selective β-blocker (i.e. it also blocks the β$_2$-receptors) its use may, in theory, lead to bronchospasm and vasoconstriction, although these potential side-effects do not seem to be a common problem. However, propranolol should be used with care, if at all, in the presence of uncontrolled pulmonary oedema or thromboembolism. Cardio-selective β-blockers are available, but there is little clinical experience of their use in animals. More recently, the calcium channel blocker diltiazem has found favour, although there is as yet little published evidence that this class of drugs is any safer or more effective than the β-blockers for this application (and they may further activate the neuroendocrine mechanisms of congestive heart failure). The calcium antagonists also have anti-dysrhythmic actions, especially against supraventricular tachydysrhythmias, and additionally some vasodilator properties (particularly of the coronary arteries).

A negative inotrope is generally recommended for routine use in HCM. However, they should be used with caution, if at all, in cases where there is systolic dysfunction, hypotension, bradycardia or atrio-ventricular block. Their use in DCM is controversial. There is evidence that β-blockers prolong survival in humans with DCM, and that diastolic function is impaired in DCM. However, most clinicians avoid using negative inotropes, especially β-blockers, in cats with DCM.

Improving systolic function

Where systolic function is impaired, in DCM or any other form of cardiac disease where contractility is reduced, attempts may be made to stimulate myocardial contractility using positive inotropic agents. The most familiar, and the only currently available positive inotrope for oral use of any potency, is digoxin (or other digitalis glycosides). Digoxin acts on the myocardiocyte membrane sodium-potassium pump to increase the strength of contraction, and also, by direct (central vagomimetic) and indirect actions, slows the heart rate, giving more time for diastole. Digoxin is thus also of value in treating supraventricular tachydysrhythmias by suppressing the rate of ventricular response. The digitalis glycosides have many systemic and cardiac toxic side-effects, particularly the induction of dysrhythmias. Digitalis glycosides should be used with great caution in cats. Cats seem especially sensitive to the toxic effects of the glycosides, and there is also much individual variation in susceptibility. It may be of value to monitor the serum concentration of digoxin in some cases (Atkins *et al.*, 1990). Changes in formulation or type of digoxin should be avoided, as this can lead to significant alterations in blood levels, sufficient to cause toxicity. Digitalis glycosides are not indicated in HCM, and may worsen any outflow obstruction.

In advanced cases of DCM and in acute cardiac output failure ('cardiogenic shock'), systolic function may be supported more effectively and immediately by the use of one of the sympathomimetic amines, dopamine or dobutamine. Dobutamine has less of a tendency to produce tachycardia and vasoconstriction; dopamine may be more effective in cardiogenic shock. Both must be given by careful constant rate intravenous infusion, preferably by means of an infusion pump or microdrip set. Excessive infusion rates can result in seizures, although these stop if the infusion rate is reduced. Particular care must be taken not to overuse diuretics in such cases, and circulatory function may even have to be supported by the cautious use of intravenous fluids.

Considerable research effort has been invested in a search for non-glycoside, non-catecholamine positive inotropic agents that are active orally. None are currently available commercially, although some, e.g. milrinone, have shown promise in some veterinary clinical trials. As mentioned above, taurine often improves systolic function, even where plasma taurine concentrations are in the normal range.

Management of dysrhythmias

Most dysrhythmias in cats are associated with primary or secondary cardiomyopathy, and management of the underlying myocardial disease and congestive heart failure, as discussed above, is often adequate for their control. Dysrhythmias

also occur secondarily to systemic disorders such as hyperthyroidism, renal failure, hyperkalaemia, shock, trauma, sepsis, etc. Again, management is generally aimed at the underlying problem, and many such dysrhythmias are transient. Where specific therapy is required, the choice of drugs is limited. Many of the familiar antidysrhythmics, particularly the Class I agents such as lignocaine and procainamide, produce toxic side-effects in cats, and must be used very cautiously if at all. The drug of choice for ventricular tachydysrhythmias is propranolol. Supraventricular tachydysrhythmias may be managed with propranolol, diltiazem or digoxin, depending on the underlying problem and the contractile function of the ventricles. Fortunately cats seem to tolerate dysrhythmias well, without the need for specific therapy in many cases.

Symptomatic bradycardia (<100 beats/min), due to sino-atrial or atrio-ventricular block, is encountered uncommonly in cats without evidence of underlying progressive myocardial disease. The treatment of choice in such cases would be the use of an artificial pacemaker, as anticholinergics and sympathomimetics are generally ineffective in increasing heart rate.

Management and/or prevention of thromboembolism

Thromboembolism is one of the most dramatic and potentially serious consequences of cardiomyopathy, and in a significant proportion of cases is the first sign of disease. Most if not all cases of thromboembolism are associated with underlying cardiomyopathy, where the enlarged left atrium or ventricle allows blood stasis to occur, leading to platelet aggregation and thrombus formation. The exact pathogenesis is not known, and changes in the surface of the endocardium may be involved in activating coagulation. Thromboembolism has been particularly associated with HCM (where a post-mortem prevalence, but not a clinical prevalence, of approaching 50% has been recorded) and with RCM. Atrial enlargement is often greatest in these forms. The incidence in DCM is, however, only slightly less than that in

RCM. Thromboembolism is occasionally seen in cats with cardiomyopathy that have only mild cardiomegaly. A rare cause of thromboembolism is bacterial endocarditis. The clinical signs of thromboembolism arise due to ischaemic neuromyopathy distal to the thrombus, and vary in severity depending on the degree of obstruction and the vessels involved. The ischaemia is caused partly by physical obstruction and partly by vasoconstriction of collateral vessels due to the release of vasoactive substances from the thrombus (see Pion & Kittleson, 1989, for a review of the pathogenesis and treatment of thromboembolism).

The most common form (>90%) in cats is aortic thromboembolism (also called 'saddle embolus'), where an embolus blocks the terminal aorta and iliac trifurcation. The clinial signs are characteristic and distressing, with paresis and painful contracture of the muscles of the hindlimbs, especially the gastrocnemius muscles, marked reduction or absence of the femoral pulse, coldness and pallor. Occasionally only one limb is affected. Thromboembolism to other sites, including the forelimbs (causing lameness, sometimes intermittent and often of a single limb), renal arteries (causing severe azotaemia), mesenteric, coronary, cerebral and other arteries is seen. Potentially fatal complications of thromboembolism include the development of gangrene, renal failure, disseminated intravascular coagulation, metabolic acidosis and hyperkalaemia.

Aspirin has been widely used prophylactically in cats for its ability to reduce platelet aggregation and thus prevent or make less likely the development of thromboembolism. The dose given in Table 11.9 appears to be safe, and there is evidence that it is effective in reducing the risk of thromboembolism.

The prognosis for thromboembolism depends largely on the extent of ischaemic necrosis and the severity of the underlying cardiac disease, in particular whether systolic function is impaired, when the prognosis is much worse. The prognosis may be reasonably good with HCM. Surgical embolectomy has largely been abandoned, in view of the high anaesthetic risk in these cases and the fact that recurrent thromboembolism may occur.

If circulatory function can be supported then the pulse volume and limb function will often improve within a few days, although it may take 6 to 8 weeks for more complete recovery and sometimes permanent abnormalities of gait remain. If no improvement is seen after 2–3 days, then the prognosis becomes very poor. Congestive heart failure should be managed by cage rest and diuresis, with a slow intravenous fluid (dextrose saline plus bicarbonate) infusion if required for hypotension, warmth to combat hypothermia, analgesics (e.g. buprenorphine, morphine) and gentle physiotherapy. Metabolic acidosis and hyperkalaemia may be marked. The use of sodium heparin (200 IU/kg subcutaneously every 8 hours for 2–3 days) has been recommended to try to prevent further extension of the thrombus, and aspirin should be started and continued indefinitely. The coumarin anticoagulant warfarin has also been used prophylactically. Careful monitoring of clotting function is required when anticoagulants are used. Acepromazine (approximately 0.1 mg/kg subcutaneously, or more, to produce visible sedation and nictitating membrane prolapse) provides sedation for the distressed cat and vasodilation of the collateral arterial supply to the limbs. Hydralazine has also been employed as an arteriodilator in this situation. Propranolol should be avoided at this stage as it may lead to vasoconstriction. It has also been suggested that propranolol may interfere with the anti-platelet effects of aspirin. Attempts have been made to produce clot lysis medically. Streptokinase appears to be of little benefit. Genetically engineered tissue plasminogen activator has been reported to be more effective. However, this is extremely expensive and has been associated with a high rate of mortality.

OTHER ACQUIRED CARDIAC DISEASES

Acquired valvular disease
Degenerative valvular heart disease appears to be of little clinical importance in cats, although it is an area that is poorly characterized and

may be overlooked. The most frequent causes of A-V valvular incompetence in cats are ventricular dilatation secondary to cardiomyopathy, and congenital valvular dysplasias. Pulmonary hypertension secondary to chronic left-sided heart failure of any cause is reported to be a significant cause of tricuspid regurgitation (Bonagura, 1989). The murmurs produced by acquired A-V valvular incompetence and their clinical effects are similar to those already described for congenital disease.

Bacterial endocarditis

This has been described in the cat, but appears to be rare. It may follow bacteraemia from an infected focus elsewhere, such as a subcutaneous abscess or a dental infection, or may occur in an immunosuppressed cat. The clinical signs of bacterial endocarditis are those of an infected focus, and resemble an immune-mediated disease such as polyarthropathy – chronic recurrent pyrexia and shifting lameness. A leucocytosis may be present on haematology and blood culture may be positive, allowing antibiotic sensitivity to be determined. Endocarditis affects the mitral valve, producing incompetence and a systolic murmur if of sufficient severity, and/or the aortic valve, again producing incompetence and a diastolic murmur. Vegetations may be seen with ultrasonography. Endocarditis may also lead to myocardial damage, thromboembolism and sepsis in other organs. The response to antibiotic combinations, such as ampicillin or a cephalosporin plus an aminoglycoside (e.g. gentamycin), appears to be poor, and most affected cats die. Antibiotic therapy should ideally be based on blood culture and antibiotic sensitivity testing.

Pericardial disease

This occurs infrequently as a specific entity in cats. Fluid may accumulate in the pericardial sac secondary to cardiomyopathy (this is not uncommon) and in conditions such as feline infectious peritonitis, congenital pericardioperitoneal diaphragmatic hernia and cardiac neoplasia. This can be readily detected by ultrasonography, and may be seen on thoracic radiographs as a rounded 'cardiomegaly'. However, it is uncommon for this

accumulation to have any clinical significance for cardiac function (Rush *et al.*, 1990).

Neoplasia

Neoplasia of the heart is rare in cats. The most commonly encountered cardiac tumour is lymphoma, either as an isolated lesion or as part of more widespread neoplasia.

Cor pulmonale

Infection by the heartworm *Dirofilaria immitis* is seen in cats in those parts of the world where this parasite is endemic, and is reported to have an increasing prevalence (Calvert, 1989). Mild right ventricular enlargement is reported in cats with chronic pulmonary disease (Bonagura, 1989), but in general the importance of chronic thoracic disease for cardiac function in cats is unknown.

Medial hyperplasia/hypertrophy of the pulmonary arteries

This is a common incidental finding at post-mortem examination. It is thought to be associated with pulmonary nematode migration and is not considered to be of any clinical significance.

Acknowledgements

The authors are grateful to colleagues in the Departments of Veterinary Medicine and Surgery, University of Bristol, School of Veterinary Science, for permission to use some of the illustrative material from clinical cases include in this chapter; also to John Conibear for photography.

REFERENCES AND FURTHER READING

Atkins C.E., Snyder P.S., Keene B.W. *et al.* (1990) Efficacy of digoxin for treatment of cats with dilated cardiomyopathy. *J. Am. Vet. Med. Ass.* **196**, 1463–9.

Barr F. (1990) *Diagnostic Ultrasound in the Dog and Cat.* Blackwell Scientific Publications, Oxford.

Bishop S.P. (1988) Developmental anatomy of the heart and great vessels. In Fox P.R. (ed) *Canine and Feline Cardiology.* Churchill Livingstone, New York, pp. 3–14.

Bonagura J.D. (1989) Cardiovascular diseases. In Sherding R.G. (ed) *The Cat: Diseases and Clinical Management.*

Churchill Livingstone, New York, pp. 649–753.

Bright J.M., Golden A.L. & Daniel G.B. (1992) Feline hypertrophic cardiomyopathy: variations on a theme. *J. Small Anim. Pract.* **33**, 266–74.

Calvert C.A. (1989) Feline heartworm disease. In Sherding R.G. (ed) *The Cat: Diseases and Clinical Management.* Churchill Livingstone, New York, pp. 495–510.

Darke P.G.G. (1992) Doppler echocardiography. *J. Small Anim. Pract.* **33**, 104–12.

Dow S.W., Fettman M.J., Smith K.R. *et al.* (1992) Taurine depletion and cardiovascular disease in adult cats fed a potassium-depleted acidified diet. *Am. J. Vet. Res.* **53**, 402–5.

Fox P.R. (1988a) Congenital feline heart disease. In Fox P.R. (ed) *Canine and Feline Cardiology.* Churchill Livingstone, New York, pp. 391–408.

Fox P.R. (1988b) Feline myocardial disease. In Fox P.R. (ed) *Canine and Feline Cardiology.* Churchill Livingstone, New York, pp. 435–66.

Fox P.R. & Bond B.R. (1983) Non-selective and selective angiography. *Vet. Clin. N. Am.: Small Anim. Pract.* **13**, 259–72.

Harpster N.K. (1986) Feline myocardial disease. In Kirk R.W. (ed) *Current Veterinary Therapy IX.* W.B. Saunders, Philadelphia, pp. 380–98.

Keene B.W., Panciera D.P., Atkins C.E. *et al.* (1991) Myocardial L-carnitine deficiency in a family of dogs with dilated cardiomyopathy. *J. Am. Vet. Med. Ass.* **198**, 647–50.

Kittleson M.D. (1991) The changing face of feline cardiomyopathy (abstract). *Paper Synopses of the British Small Animal Veterinary Association Congress.* p. 24.

Moise N.S. (1988) Echocardiography. In Fox P.R. (ed) *Canine and Feline Cardiology.* Churchill Livingstone, New York, pp. 113–56.

Peterson M.E., Taylor R.S., Greco D.S. *et al.* (1990) Acromegaly in 14 cats. *J. Vet. Int. Med.* **4**, 192–201.

Pion P.D. & Kittleson M.D. (1989) Therapy for feline aortic thromboembolism. In Kirk R.W. (ed) *Current Veterinary Therapy X.* W.B. Saunders, Philadelphia, pp. 295–302.

Pion P.D., Kittleson M.D. & Rogers Q.R. (1989) Cardiomyopathy in the cat and its relation to taurine deficiency. In Kirk R.W. (ed) *Current Veterinary Therapy X.* W.B. Saunders, Philadelphia, pp. 251–62.

Rush J.E., Keene B.W. & Fox P.R. (1990) Pericardial disease in the cat: a retrospective evaluation of 66 cases. *J. Am. Anim. Hosp. Ass.* **26**, 39–46.

Sisson D.D., Knight D.H., Helinski C. *et al.* (1991) Plasma taurine concentrations and M-mode echocardiographic measures in healthy cats and in cats with dilated cardiomyopathy. *J. Vet. Int. Med.* **5**, 232–8.

Stepien R.L. & Bonagura J.D. (1991) Aortic stenosis: clinical findings in six cats. *J. Small Anim. Pract.* **32**, 341–50.

Van den Broek A.H.M. & Darke P.G.G. (1987) Cardiac measurements on thoracic radiographs of cats. *J. Small Anim. Pract.* **28**, 125–35.

Wynne J. & Braunwald E. (1988) The cardiomyopathies and myocarditides. In Braunwald E. (ed) *Heart Disease: A Textbook of Cardiovascular Medicine*, 3rd edn. W.B. Saunders, Philadelphia, pp. 1410–69.

Chapter 12 / The Endocrine System

A. C. BLAXTER AND
T. J. GRUFFYDD-JONES

INTRODUCTION

Disorders of the endocrine glands are relatively uncommon in cats but there have been many recent advances in our knowledge concerning the endocrine system and its dysfunction in this species. Although some of the disorders affecting the feline endocrine system are similar to those in the dog, it is important to recognize that for others, such as hyperadrenocorticism and hyperthyroidism, there are very distinct and important differences. The diseases encountered most frequently are diabetes mellitus and hyperthyroidism.

PITUITARY GLAND

The pituitary gland or hypophysis consists of the adenohypophysis (anterior lobe) and the neurohypophysis (posterior lobe). The adenohypophysis contains chromophobe and chromophil cells, the latter being subdivided into acidophils and basophils. The basophil cells secrete thyroid-stimulating hormone (TSH), adrenocorticotrophic hormone (ACTH), melanocyte-stimulating hormone (MSH), follicle-stimulating hormone (FSH), which in the male is interstitial cell-stimulating hormone (ICSH), and luteinizing hormone (LH). Acidophil cells are responsible for the secretion of growth hormone (GH) and prolactin.

The hormones released from the anterior lobe of the pituitary are controlled by the hypothalamus by means of substances referred to as 'factors'. In the case of GH, TSH, ACTH, FSH and LH there is a releasing factor stimulating release of the appropriate hormone, and in the case of GH, MSH and prolactin, there is an inhibiting factor which regulates the release of these hormones. Production and release of these factors in the hypothalamus is controlled by a negative feedback mechanism. Increased levels of a particular target organ hormone inhibit the production and release of that particular target organ hormone. The neurohypophysis acts as a storage depot for vasopressin or antidiuretic hormone (ADH) and oxytocin. These hormones are produced in the nuclei of the hypothalamus (ADH from the supraoptic nucleus and oxytocin from the paraventricular nucleus) and pass along axons to the neurohypophysis. The target organs of these hormones are the kidney (ADH) or mammary gland and uterus (oxytocin).

Pituitary disorders

Neoplasia
Pituitary tumours are generally considered to be uncommon in cats. Some are endocrinologically inactive and any associated clinical signs result from tumour expansion leading to neurological signs or signs associated with failure of pituitary hormone secretion (Smith & Jones, 1966; Martin & Capen, 1975). The major neurological signs are lethargy, depression, weakness, incoordination, pupillary abnormalities and behavioural changes. Rapid, severe weight loss may also be a feature.

In recent years there has been increased recognition of endocrinologically active pituitary tumours in cats. The most prominent feature of these cases is usually an insulin-resistant diabetes mellitus with associated polyuria and polydipsia. These tumours are adenomas and can be of two different types – acidophilic, producing excessive concentrations of growth hormone (GH), or chromophobe adenomas causing excessive ACTH production and hence hyperadrenocorticism. This latter form is considered under adrenal disorders.

Acromegaly

This recently recognized endocrine disease of cats is caused by GH-secreting pituitary tumours. It occurs in older cats and the majority of affected cats reported to date have been males (Peterson *et al.*, 1990).

CLINICAL SIGNS

The signs in acromegaly are related to the excessive secretion of GH. The most prominent of these are polyuria and polydipsia related to diabetes mellitus, which results from the antagonistic effect of GH on the action of insulin. The diabetes is associated with insulin resistance and can be difficult to stabilize, requiring dosages in excess of 20 units of insulin daily. Acromegaly should be considered in any diabetic cat with apparent insulin resistance. Excessive soft tissue development is another prominent feature causing a general weight gain, distended abdomen, development of skin folds, prominent lower jaw and protruding tongue. Articular cartilage may proliferate causing severe arthritis and there may be an increase in interdental tissue leading to separation of the teeth. General organomegaly may occur, particularly involving the heart leading to cardiomegaly. This can be assessed radiographically and congestive heart failure may develop with pulmonary oedema and accumulation of clear thoracic fluid.

DIAGNOSIS

The most important diagnostic feature which will lead to a suspicion of acromegaly is insulin-resistant diabetes mellitus. In such cases it is important initially to eliminate the other major cause of insulin-resistant diabetes mellitus in cats, hyperadrenocorticism, for which confirmatory endocrine tests are more readily available. If this has been eliminated and there is evidence of organomegaly and other soft tissue enlargement, GH estimations are indicated to confirm the diagnosis. A single estimation may be adequate but in some cases a dynamic test is required. This is achieved by assessing the GH response to a glucose load, which should markedly reduce GH concentrations in normal cats. Care should be taken in conducting this test in cats with marked hyperglycaemia to avoid the hyperosmolar syndrome (see 'Diabetes mellitus' below). GH assays suitable for cats are not available in the UK but samples can be sent to the University of Utrecht by prior arrangement. In other species GH secretion has been assessed indirectly by determining counter-regulatory action to insulin-induced hypoglycaemia but the validity of this test in cats is questionable.

If available, brain scans may enable identification of a pituitary tumour but will not differentiate between acidophilic and chromophobe adenomas.

TREATMENT

Irradiation has been shown to be of some valve in managing the pituitary tumour but this technique is unlikely to be available. Somatostatin analogues have proved useful in lowering GH concentrations in humans with acromegaly, but the limited experience to date suggests that either they may be ineffective in cats or that higher dosages are required. Dopaminergic agents have also been used in man and these inhibit GH release. There have been no reports of the use of bromocriptine, a potent dopaminergic drug, in acromegalic cats but the authors have experience of the use of this drug in cats for other conditions. This would currently appear to be the most attractive proposition for treatment. Side-effects (most notably vomiting in other species) have not been a problem in our limited experience and can be minimized by starting at a low dosage of 0.2 mg and gradually increasing.

PROGNOSIS

Although no specific treatments have as yet been demonstrated to be effective in attacking the underlying cause of acromegaly, i.e. the GH-producing pituitary tumour, the major complication of the disease, diabetes mellitus, can be controlled with insulin although exceptionally high dosages may be required. The short-term prognosis is therefore reasonable and cases may be managed successfully in this way for 1 or 2 years or more before severe signs associated with expansion of the pituitary tumour develop.

Pituitary dwarfism

Suspected dwarfism associated with failure of pituitary production of GH has been reported in kittens but appears to be rare. This produces a severe but proportional dwarfism, with the affected individuals appearing as perfect diminutives of their normal littermates. There may be delayed closure of ossification centres and prolonged retention of the deciduous teeth. In the one suspected case seen at our clinic the coat appeared normal although this cat was mature when first presented. The GH deficiency may occur as an isolated phenomenon or part of a panhypopituitarism. In the latter case, evidence of hypofunction of other endocrine organs, such as hypothyroidism, hypoadrenocorticism and hypogonadism, may occur although the GH deficiency appears to be the most prominent feature in early life. Interestingly our suspected case of pituitary dwarfism appeared to have normal thyroid and adrenal function and subsequently bred normally suggesting an isolated GH defect.

Demonstration of low GH concentrations (or somatomedin) with failure to respond to provocative testing with xylazine or clonidine would be required to confirm this diagnosis. However, GH asssays are not readily available (see 'Acromegaly' above). Treatment would entail replacement with GH. The most readily available treatments in man are recombinant human GH and GHRF. However, these drugs are expensive and it is not known whether they are effective in cats.

Diabetes insipidus

Diabetes insipidus (DI) is a rare condition in cats involving an inability to concentrate urine, with subsequent polyuria and polydipsia. It occurs in two forms – cranial or pituitary origin due to failure of production of arginine vasopressin (AVP), and nephrogenic or renal origin due to an inability of the nephrons to respond to AVP. Both forms can be either congenital or acquired. Congenital nephrogenic DI has not been reported in cats although it is recognized in other species. Acquired nephrogenic DI is extremely rare in cats but has been seen in cats with nephrocalcinosis secondary to malignancy-associated hypercalcaemia resulting from lymphosarcoma. Congenital cranial DI is seen in young cats (Winterbotham & Mason, 1983). The acquired cranial form has been reported secondary to trauma and pituitary tumours.

Clinical signs

The predominant clinical sign reported by owners of affected cats is polydipsia. Normal water consumption varies between 40 and 70 ml/kg/day depending on diet (Burger *et al.*, 1980) but may exceed 1 l daily in DI. The polydipsia is secondary to polyuria, although this sign may pass unnoticed by owners unless the cat uses a litter tray or it urinates in the house due to prolonged confinement indoors. Affected cats generally show no other clinical abnormalities.

Diagnosis

The first step in diagnosis of DI is the elimination of other possible causes of polyuria/polydipsia, necessitating assessment of renal function, elimination of hyperthyroidism, diabetes mellitus, etc. Confirmation of diagnosis depends on demonstration of persistently dilute urine with an inability to concentrate. This is most conveniently assessed by performing a water deprivation test. It is imperative that this test is not peformed in cats with renal dysfunction or with prior dehydration as the water restriction may precipitate acute renal failure in such cases. The procedure

Table 12.1 Procedure for water deprivation test.

Time	Procedure
Start of test	Empty bladder Weigh cat Withhold fluids and food Measure plasma urea and osmolality and urine osmolality and SG
4 h and 6 h	Empty bladder Weigh cat Measure plasma urea and osmolality and urine osmolality and SG End test if more than 5% reduction in bodyweight or urea concentrations significantly raised
8 h	Empty bladder Weigh cat Measure plasma urea and osmolality and urine osmolality and SG End test unless results equivocal Test can be continued providing weight loss does not exceed 5% and urea concentrations are not significantly raised, repeating the 4/6 h procedure at 2-h intervals

for the water deprivation test is summarized in Table 12.1. In affected cats the starting urine specific gravity (SG) is likely to be below 1.012, usually below 1.008, and will fail to increase above 1.015 after water restriction. A more prolonged water deprivation test involving partial water restriction has been advocated but is no more sensitive and less convenient to perform. Following demonstration of an inability to concentrate urine it is necessary to repeat the water deprivation test immediately following administration of 1 μg of desmopressin* (DDAVP), a synthetic analogue of AVP. If the cat is still unable to concentrate urine nephrogenic DI is present, but if urine SG increases above 1.015 cranial DI is confirmed. It is claimed that 'psy-

* Desmopressin, 'DDAVP'; Ferning Pharmaceuticals Ltd., Middlesex, UK.

chogenic' polydipsia (primary polydipsia) may be difficult to differentiate from nephrogenic DI, if this has been severe and prolonged leading to medullary wash-out syndrome. However, 'psychogenic' polydipsia has not been reliably reported in cats.

Treatment

Replacement of AVP with DDAVP is the treatment of choice for cranial DI. We prefer to administer the drug by daily injections but it can also be administered conjunctivally or intranasally in a spray form by owners who are unwilling to consider subcutaneous injections. Water consumption should be monitored carefully and the daily dosage of DDAVP progressively decreased until the minimum effective dosage is determined. This may be as low as 0.1 μg daily. The dosage should begin at around 0.4 μg and should not be changed for the first 3 or 4 days as there may be a delay before the nephrons become fully responsive. The duration of action of DDAVP may provide an acceptable degree of control of urine output and it may prove most convenient to administer the drug late in the day to achieve satisfactory overnight control of urination. In congenital cranial DI, lifelong treatment will be required. If the DI was caused by trauma the cat may subsequently regain some ability to secrete AVP. A diagnosis of DI in older cats should raise the suspicion of a pituitary tumour, which will have implications for the long-term prognosis.

Treatment of nephrogenic DI is possible but may not be an important consideration if the underlying cause is malignancy-associated hypercalcaemia. Hydrochlorthiazide can be used at a low dose of 2.5 mg/kg. Although a diuretic, this drug has a paradoxical beneficial effect in DI by creating a mild negative salt balance reducing glomerular filtration rate through decreasing extracellular volume, which results in enhanced fluid resorption in the proximal tubule. Restriction of salt intake potentiates this effect. Treatment with hydrochlorthiazide may lead to hypokalaemia (Court & Watson, 1983) and it is therefore important to monitor potassium levels and, if necessary, provide supplementation. The maximum reduction in water intake that can be expected with this treatment is 50%. Chlorpropamide has been used to treat nephrogenic DI in other species but is not recommended in cats in view of its potential toxicity.

Some owners may not find the polydipsia and polyuria associated with DI unacceptable and in such cases treatment is not necessary although it is important that continual free access to water is available.

PARATHYROID GLANDS

These glands lie next to the thyroid glands and produce parathyroid hormone or parathormone (PTH), which is involved in the regulation of calcium metabolism. The other major hormones involved in this essential process are calcitonin or thyrocalcitonin (CT) and vitamin D_3 or chol-ecalciferol, which is now regarded as a hormone.

Parathyroid hormone (parathormone; PTH)

This hormone is produced in response to low blood calcium concentrations. It has the following effects.

1 To elevate blood calcium and decrease calcium excretion in the urine.
2 To decrease blood phosphate and increase urinary excretion of phosphate.
3 To increase the rate of bone resorption by increasing the activity of osteocytes and osteo-clasts in bone, so mobilizing calcium from bones.
4 To promote absorption of calcium from the gut. This last effect is a much slower process than the mobilization of calcium from the skeleton.

Calcitonin (thyrocalcitonin; CT)

Calcitonin is produced in response to elevated blood calcium and is produced in the C-cells of the thyroid gland as distinct from the follicular cells, which secrete thyroxine (T_4) and triiodothy-ronine (T_3). Calcitonin is secreted continuously while normal blood calcium levels are maintained, but the rate is increased in response to elevation of blood calcium. It functions by interacting with target cells primarily in bone and, to a lesser

extent, in the kidneys and intestine. Calcitonin appears, however, to function as an emergency hormone (in contrast to PTH) to: (i) prevent development of hypercalcaemia during rapid absorption of calcium after food ingestion; and (ii) protect against excessive loss of calcium and phosphate from the maternal skeleton during pregnancy.

Cholecalciferol (vitamin D_3)

This must be activated before it can produce its physiological effects. Control of the final step of this activation is complex and appears to be exerted indirectly with plasma calcium concen-tration influencing the secretion rates of PTH and CT, which in turn influence the activation of cholecalciferol. The function of vitamin D and its metabolites is to increase the absorption of calcium and phosphate from the intestine. It is required, therefore, in young animals for normal bone growth and is also needed for osteoclastic resorption and calcium mobilization in bones.

Parathyroid disorders

Primary hyperparathyroidism

This is a rare condition in cats but has been reported in association with functional para-thyroid tumours (Blunden *et al.*, 1986; Richter *et al.*, 1990). In other species hyperplastic para-thyroidism may occur with involvement of all four parathyroid glands, and hyperplasia or adenomas may also occur as a feature of multiple endocrine gland dysfunction. The resulting in-crease in parathyroid hormone (PTH) concen-trations leads to hypercalcaemia which is respons-ible for the clinical signs.

CLINICAL SIGNS
Hypercalcaemia leads to extreme depression with inappetence, weight loss and vomiting. There may also be muscle weakness, muscle tremors and constipation. Polyuria and polydipsia are seen in other species, associated with nephrocalcinosis leading to nephrogenic DI, but these do not appear to be a consistent feature in cats with

primary hyperparathyroidism, nor does development of calcium uroliths appear to be a feature.

DIAGNOSIS

The major feature is a marked and persistent hypercalcaemia with hypophosphataemia. This must be differentiated from the hypercalcaemia associated with malignancy (see below). It may be possible to demonstrate raised plasma concentrations of PTH but this is a specialized assay which is not readily available. PTH is relatively labile and there may be difficulties in interpretation of results depending on the antiserum used (whether it cross-reacts with cat PTH and the portion of the PTH molecule it recognizes). Recently a double site radioimmunoassay has been described for use in dogs and this appears to offer considerable advantages in this species.

Radiography may show osteoporosis and occasionally metastatic calcification.

TREATMENT

Ideally the abnormal parathyroid should be identified and removed surgically although this may be difficult, particularly if one of the internal parathyroid glands is affected. In the limited number of reported cases a single adenoma has been found and the response to surgical excision has been good. Blood calcium can be lowered in the short term by administration of normal saline, corticosteroids and small doses of frusemide.

Malignancy-associated hypercalcaemia

This is the most common cause of hypercalcaemia in cats but is nevertheless a rare phenomenon and is seen less commonly than in dogs. Recent studies in other species indicate that certain tumours elaborate a polypeptide with PTH-like activity which leads to the hypercalcaemia. Lymphosarcoma is the tumour most often associated with this phenomenon in cats (McMillan, 1985) but it can also be seen with myeloproliferative disorders. The clinical signs are similar to those described for primary hyperparathyroidism. Diagnosis depends on demonstration of the tumour. Although the serum calcium may be lowered using the medical measures suggested for

primary hyperparathyroidism the prognosis is usually poor in view of the underlying neoplasia.

Hypoparathyroidism

Iatrogenic hypoparathyroidism following inadvertent parathyroid removal or damage to their blood supply during thyroidectomy is the most common form of hypoparathyroidism in cats. Hypoparathyroidism has been reported as a rare spontaneous condition (Peterson *et al.*, 1990) and in one case a lymphocytic infiltration of the parathyroids was described (Forbes *et al.*, 1990). Persistent idiopathic hypocalcaemia has been seen rarely in cats at our clinic.

The major clinical manifestations of chronic hypocalcaemia are depression, weakness, restlessness, disorientation, agitation, diarrhoea, ataxia, hyperaesthesia and aggressive behaviour. In more acute cases muscle tremors and tonic muscle spasm leading to opisthotonus and seizures may be seen. Ptyalism was noted in one of the reported cases, and this, together with the various neurological and behavioural signs occurring in a young cat could lead to confusion with the hepatic encephalopathy associated with porto-systemic shunts. Blood examination shows a hypocalcaemia and hyperphosphataemia. This must be differentiated from other causes of hypocalcaemia, most notably eclampsia associated with pregnancy or lactation and the hypocalcaemia associated with hypoalbuminaemia.

The hypocalcaemia can be rectified by supplementing the intake of calcium together with synthetic vitamin D as outlined under postoperative management following thyroidectomy (see below). Blood calcium should be monitored periodically and the supplementation adjusted to maintain levels in the low normal range. Oversupplementation may lead to hypercalcaemia.

ADRENAL GLANDS

There are two endocrine organs in each adrenal gland. The inner adrenal medulla secretes adrenaline and noradrenaline (epinephrine and norepinephrine) and the surrounding outer adrenal cortex secretes steroid hormones. Adrenal medullary hormones are not essential for life, but they help to prepare the individual to deal with emergencies (fight or flight) and their effect on the body organs is identical to those produced by the stimulation of the sympathetic nervous system. The adrenal cortex secretes glucocorticoids such as cortisol and corticosterone (the cat secretes predominantly cortisol) and have widespread effects on the metabolism of carbohydrates, proteins and fats; they also suppress inflammatory and immunological responses in the body. The mineralocorticoids, the main one being aldosterone, are concerned with electrolyte balance of sodium and potassium in the kidney. Adrenocortical secretion is controlled primarily by ACTH from the pituitary, but mineralocorticoid secretion is also subject to control by circulating factors, the most important of which appears to be angiotensin II, a polypeptide formed in the bloodstream under the influence of renin secreted from the kidney.

There are three layers in the adrenal cortex: the outer zona glomerulosa, the middle zona fasciculata and the inner zona reticularis. The zona glomerulosa is responsible for the secretion of mineralocorticoid hormones; the zona fasciculata secretes glucocorticoid hormones; and the zona reticularis secretes sex steroids.

Adrenal disorders

Hyperadrenocorticism (Cushing's syndrome)
Although an uncommon problem hyperadrenocorticism is now being diagnosed with increasing frequency in cats (Nelson *et al.*, 1988). This is largely due to a greater awareness of the presenting features of the condition, which are very different from the classical clinical presentation of Cushing's syndrome in dogs. Most naturally occurring cases result from pituitary chromophobe adenomas but adrenal tumours, both adenomas and carcinomas, have been described. Cats are relatively resistant to side-effects associated with corticosteroid administration but iatrogenic Cushingoid changes can occur following long-term usage of both corticosteroids (Scott

et al., 1982) and progestagens (Watson *et al.*, 1989).

CLINICAL SIGNS
The disease affects middle-aged to older cats. There has been a preponderance of females in the reported cases but it is uncertain whether any true sex predisposition can be inferred from this relatively small number of cases.

The most important clinical features of hyperadrenocorticism in cats are polyuria and polydipsia. These signs do not result directly from the high corticosteroid concentrations (and indeed polyuria and polydipsia are not seen as side-effects of corticosteroid therapy in normal cats) but from the development of secondary diabetes mellitus. Although other clinical signs may be present these are not usually prominent and the disease is therefore not usually recognized until there has been progression to development of diabetes mellitus. Some cases are probably misdiagnosed as idiopathic diabetes mellitus and this may prove to be relatively insulin resistant. Obesity or weight loss and polyphagia may be noted. Alopecia, skin thinning, skin fragility and recurrent infections may also be features but are more likely to be seen in iatrogenic cases in our experience. Disturbances of calcium metabolism occur in Cushing's syndrome and in one of our naturally occurring cases, severe osteoporosis was present which led to the development of pathological fractures and ultimately vertebral collapse.

DIAGNOSIS
Hyperadrenocorticism should be considered in any diabetic cat, particularly if there is insulin resistance. Hyperglycaemia and glycosuria are frequently the only abnormalities detected on routine laboratory testing. Changes consistently seen in Cushingoid dogs, such as lymphopenia, eosinopenia and raised liver enzymes, occur only in a minority of cases.

Assessment of adrenal function is required to confirm hyperadrenocorticism although protocols for this and their interpretation in Cushingoid individuals are less well established than in dogs. We recommend using an ACTH stimulation test administering 0.125 mg synthetic adrenocorticotrophin (tetracosactrin; Synacthen*) intravenously and taking the second sample at 3 hours (Sparkes *et al.*, 1990). This is somewhat later than recommended in applying this test in dogs and in some studies of cats, but will ensure peak concentrations of cortisol are achieved. Mean baseline cortisol concentrations are around 80 nmol/l (range 25–250) rising to 250–640 nmol/l following stimulation. The response of cortisol concentrations to exogenous dexamethasone appears to be rather unpredictable and we do not, therefore, currently routinely recommend a dexamethasone screening test for diagnosis.

Differentiation between pituitary and adrenal tumours in confirmed Cushingoid cats depends on attempts to identify adrenal masses by radiography and ultrasonography. In practice this may be difficult to achieve and may be of less importance in subsequent management than in dogs with Cushing's syndrome (see below). Particular care is necessary in radiographic interpretation since adrenal calcification is a common incidental finding of no clinical significance in old cats, whereas adrenal calcification in cats with hyperadrenocorticism appears to be uncommon. High-dose dexamethasone suppression tests have not been adequately evaluated for differentiation of the underlying cause.

TREATMENT
The optimum treatment for hyperadrenocorticism in cats has not yet been established but current experience suggests that surgery may be preferable to medical management.

Although Lysodren (Mitotane†), the major drug used in medical management of Cushingoid dogs, is a chlorinated hydrocarbon it appears to be well tolerated by cats. However, in our experience, and that of others, it does not appear to induce adrenal suppresssion in Cushingoid cats, at least at the dosages used in dogs, even over prolonged periods. Other drugs such as ketocon

*Synacthen; Ciba Geigy Laboratories, Whittlesford, Cambridge, UK.
†Mitotane; Bristol-Myers, Langley, Slough, Berks, UK.

azole, metyrapone, bromocriptine and cyproheptadine, have been used for medical management in man and dogs with hyperadrenocorticism but all have disadvantages and are not recommended for use in cats with the possible exception of ketoconazole and bromocriptine.

Currently the preferred treatment for Cushing's syndrome in cats is surgical adrenalectomy, both for pituitary dependent cases and adrenal tumours. If a unilateral adrenal tumour is present the unaffected contralateral gland (which may be difficult to recognize due to atrophy induced by negative feedback suppression) should be left. In pituitary dependent cases a bilateral adrenalectomy should be performed. This surgical procedure appears to be relatively well tolerated in cats, certainly in comparison to dogs. Following adrenalectomy replacement glucocorticoid and mineralocorticoid therapy should be instituted with prednisolone (0.1–0.2 mg/kg) and fludrocortisone (initially 0.1 mg). This may be gradually withdrawn in cats undergoing unilateral adrenalectomy but must be continued lifelong in bilateral cases.

Concurrent insulin therapy should be given with both medical and surgical management, to control hyperglycaemia. The requirement for insulin will decrease and subsequently disappear following successful resolution in most cats with hyperadrenocorticism, but must be continued in others.

Hypoadrenocorticism (Addison's disease)
Hypoadrenocorticism is rare in cats. The clinical signs are similar to those seen in dogs but are less likely to be noticed by owners because of their cat's normal lifestyle.

Spontaneous primary idiopathic hypoadrenocorticism has been reported in addition to an iatrogenic form induced by sudden withdrawal of corticosteroids after prolonged corticosteroid treatment (Peterson *et al.*, 1989). Progestagens have also been shown to induce adrenal suppression in experimental trials (Chastain *et al.*, 1981), the potency of this effect depending upon the particular progestagen used (Watson *et al.*, 1989), and we have observed signs suggestive of acute adrenal insufficiency in some cats at our clinic following sudden withdrawal after prolonged usage.

CLINICAL SIGNS

The major signs of hypoadrenocorticism are depression, lethargy, inappetence, weight loss and muscle weakness, which may be so severe that the cat is unable to rise. Less consistent findings are vomiting and bradycardia. There may also be polydipsia and polyuria. The cause of these latter signs is not clear, but they may be related to hyponatraemia leading to an inadequate tubular concentration gradient.

DIAGNOSIS

Most affected cats will show profound electrolyte disturbances with marked hyperkalaemia and hyponatraemia. There may also be a marked uraemia with raised creatinine, which may lead to the misdiagnosis of primary renal failure. Microcardia may be evident on thoracic radiographs.

Confirmation of diagnosis is made by demonstrating a subnormal basal serum cortisol concentration which fails to increase significantly following stimulation with synthetic ACTH (the protocol for this test is described under diagnosis of hyperadrenocorticism).

TREATMENT

Prompt intensive fluid therapy with normal saline and bicarbonate to combat associated acidosis are priorities in the treatment of an acute Addisonian crisis. Corticosteroid should be administered intravenously either as hydrocortisone or dexamethasone (0.5–1.0 mg/kg). The latter has the advantage of not interfering with interpretation of an ACTH stimulation test if this is performed concurrently. Once the acute crisis has been resolved and in chronic cases, supplementation with corticosteroid, in the form of prednisolone (0.1–0.2 mg/kg daily) and mineralocorticoid in the form of fludrocortisone (0.1 mg daily) are required. An increased salt intake may also be beneficial. The electrolytes should be assessed periodically and the dosage of fludrocortisone

adjusted as necessary. If vomiting persists treatment must be given in the short term by injection.

In iatrogenic cases of Addison's disease the corticosteroid or progestagen treatment must be withdrawn very gradually over a long period of time (up to 3 or 4 months).

Hyperaldosteronism (Conn's syndrome)

Conn's syndrome is a rare condition in cats for which there is a single well-documented case report (Eger *et al.*, 1983). We believe that we have seen several cases in our clinic based on the clinical picture and demonstration of striking increases in plasma aldosterone concentrations, but these cats have not subsequently been available for post-mortem examination and confirmation of the suspected diagnosis.

Conn's syndrome results from excessive production of aldosterone associated with a functional adrenal tumour. This leads to excessive urinary potassium loss and consequently hypokalaemia.

CLINICAL SIGNS

The one documented cat with hyperaldosteronism and those suspected cases seen at our clinic have all been elderly cats. The most striking sign is muscle weakness associated with the hypokalaemia. This may appear as ataxia, poor exercise tolerance with episodic collapse or polymyopathy with hyperflexion of the neck. Affected cats are in poor condition with weight loss and an unkempt coat. There may be polydipsia and polyuria.

DIAGNOSIS

The major findings on blood examination are a persistent but variable hypokalaemia with marked increases in creatinine phosphokinase. The condition must be differentiated from other causes of hypokalaemia such as vomiting, diarrhoea, diuretic usage, periodic hypokalaemic paralysis of Burmese cats and, most notably, renal failure. Excessive urinary potassium loss is a peculiar feature of renal failure in cats and if exacerbated by a marginally low potassium intake may lead to clinical signs of polymyopathy. This is the most common cause of hypokalaemia and polymyopathy in elderly cats but differentiation from hyperaldosteronism is important. Dehydration in cats with hyperaldosteronism may cause some increase in blood urea and creatinine but determination of plasma aldosterone concentrations* will readily differentiate the two conditions, markedly elevated levels occurring in Conn's syndrome. Adrenal enlargement may be detectable on radiography or ultrasonography.

TREATMENT

The adrenal cortical adenocarcinoma in the documented case of primary aldosteronism was found to be locally invasive at post-mortem examination and surgical removal would not have been possible. This cat and the suspected cases seen at our clinic improved following potassium supplementation (500 mg of potassium chloride daily) and the administration of spironolactone, an aldosterone antagonist, at a dosage of up to 50 mg/kg. Signs of muscle weakness resolved temporarily but the prognosis is poor.

Phaeochromocytoma

Phaeochromocytomas have been reported in cats but were not endocrinologically active (Carpenter *et al.*, 1987).

ENDOCRINE PANCREAS

The pancreas consists of two parts: the exocrine acinar cells which secrete enzymes involved with digestion of food; and the endocrine cells in the islets of Langerhans. These islets are scattered throughout the pancreas and contain α-cells, which secrete glucagon, and β-cells, which secrete insulin. Glucagon increases glycogenolysis, gluconeogenesis and lipolysis, thereby elevating the blood concentration of glucose. Insulin acts principally in the cells of liver, muscle and adipose tissues. It increases the transfer of glucose in these cells, enhances glucose oxidation and glycogenesis and stimulates lipogenesis and proteo-

genesis. It also decreases the rate of lipolysis, proteolysis, ketogenesis and gluconeogenesis.

The secretion of insulin is increased and that of glucagon reduced by an elevated blood glucose level, whereas hypoglycaemia depresses insulin secretion and stimulates glucagon secretion. In this way, the endocrine part of the pancreas provides a consistent blood glucose level and maintains the flow of glucose into the cells. Insulin secretion can be decreased by adrenaline and noradrenaline and increased by ACTH and corticosteroids.

Diabetes mellitus

In its untreated state diabetes mellitus is characterized by persistent hyperglycaemia. It can be defined as a chronic endocrine disorder with an abnormal response to a glucose load and with disturbances of carbohydrate, lipid and protein metabolism. The underlying pathogenesis is related to deficiency of insulin action, either as an absolute insulin deficiency or relative insulin deficiency associated with resistance to insulin at the peripheral tissues.

The incidence of diabetes mellitus in the feline population is unknown but it is considered to be less common in comparison to the dog and to man. However, it is an important condition to recognize as it is readily confused clinically with other causes of weight loss in old cats, such as chronic renal disease, and unlike such conditions is potentially treatable.

Aetiology

The pathogenesis of feline diabetes mellitus is not well understood, and although comparisons have been made with the condition in dogs and man, it is clear that research is required in this area. An insulin-dependent type of diabetes is well documented, cats requiring lifelong insulin therapy to maintain life, and a causal relationship with pancreatic amyloid deposition and subsequent β-cell degeneration has been demonstrated (Yano *et al.*, 1981a,b). More recently a novel polypeptide hormone has been identified in islet amyloid in cats and it is thought that this

---

* Plasma aldosterone determination; currently available by prior arrangement with the Department of Chemical Pathology, St Mary's Hospital.

may regulate endocrine function in some way (Westermark *et al.*, 1987).

Peripheral tissue resistance to insulin leading to deficiency of insulin action and diabetes mellitus may be more common than previously acknowledged, usually associated with insulin antagonism by other hormones. The most common concurrent conditions reported as inducing insulin resistance in the cat are hyperadrenocorticism and acromegaly (Fox & Beatty, 1975; Feldman & Nelson, 1987). The authors have also seen a single case of hyperthyroidism inducing insulin-resistant diabetes mellitus in an elderly cat that became normoglycaemic after thyroidectomy. Obesity is acknowledged as inducing insulin resistance in man, but the role of this in feline diabetes is unknown.

Administration of drugs with an anti-insulin action may also induce insulin resistance, which stimulates endogenous hyperinsulinaemia and hyperglycaemia. If such stimulation is prolonged irreversible pancreatic β-cell depletion occurs and permanent diabetes results. The most common association made is with progestagen therapy, and in particular with megestrol acetate (Ovarid*), used widely in the treatment of feline skin disease (Moise & Reimers, 1983; Herrtage *et al.*, 1985).

History, clinical signs and clinical examination

Diabetes has been recognized in all breeds of cats, but is most common in middle-aged to elderly animals of at least 6 years of age or older. An early report of 30 cases from the USA suggested that the Siamese breed may be predisposed to diabetes but this has not been substantiated (Schaer, 1977). Unlike the condition in the dog the disease appears to be more common in males.

The classical signs of diabetes occur when fasting blood glucose concentrations rise from the normal range (3.5–5.0 mmol/l) to the renal threshold (10–12 mmol/l). The osmotic effects of glycosuria result in polyuria, and then to a compensatory polydipsia. If gross hyperglycaemia persists pronounced polyphagia occurs because of

---

* Ovarid; Glaxovet.

the lack of insulin action on the satiety centre of the hypothalamus, and weight loss can be profound, with the animal's inability to utilize any calorific intake. As the condition progresses other signs can predominate, possibly associated with the development of ketoacidosis, but the incidence and severity of these is very variable. Depression, anorexia, lethargy or weakness, diarrhoea, a poor hair coat, tachypnoea and dyspnoea, and a distinctive plantigrade stance (hocks touching the ground) have been recorded. Blindness associated with cataract is comparatively rare in cats in comparison to the dog and ocular haemorrhage induced by retinopathy may be a more common ocular abnormality.

Clinical examination is often unremarkable but palpable hepatomegaly associated with hepatic lipidosis is common; jaundice has been recorded, ketones may be discernible on the breath and dehydration may be pronounced.

Differential diagnosis

Elderly cats with weight loss are a common occurrence and it is important to recognize that diabetes shares such a presentation with chronic renal failure, hyperthyroidism and alimentary lymphosarcoma. Other features of these conditions can mimic those of diabetes. For example, polyphagia is also pronounced in hyperthyroidism; polydipsia/polyuria is a cardinal sign of compensated renal disease; and diarrhoea may occur in association with gastrointestinal neoplasia.

Hyperadrenocorticism and acromegaly are rare conditions in the cat but present primarily with induced insulin-resistant diabetes. This suggests that diabetic cats with a poor response to insulin therapy and necessary replacement insulin dosages over 2 IU/kg bodyweight/24 hours may have diabetes as a result of a concurrent condition.

Diagnosis

Diagnosis is based on demonstrating the presence of a fasting hyperglycaemia over the renal threshold and glycosuria, in an animal with appropriate clinical signs. Glycosuria without hyperglycaemia can occur in renal tubular disease (also termed the acquired Fanconi syndrome), and is classically associated with the acute toxic tubular necrosis of ethylene glycol poisoning. However, the major problem associated with the diagnosis of feline diabetes that frightened, 'stressed' or ill animals commonly have acute and transient elevations in blood glucose, often over the renal threshold for glucose. It is vital to interpret blood glucose results in this light and to be prepared to hospitalize hyperglycaemic animals to allow them to adjust to a frightening environment, or to check urine samples for persistence of glycosuria at home. It is important also to recognize that hyperglycaemia can occur as a result of intravenous fluid therapy containing dextrose, and that most anaesthetics and sedatives, particularly xylazine, can induce hyperglycaemia (Hsu & Hembrough, 1982).

Cats appear to be relatively resistant to the development of ketosis or ketoacidosis, but the presence of serum ketones or ketonuria is strongly suggestive of diabetes in an animal without extreme starvation.

Other serum biochemical abnormalities occur with frequency in diabetic cases but are not diagnostic. These include mild to moderate elevations in alanine amino transferase, serum alkaline phosphatase and gamma glutamyl transferase associated with hepatic lipidosis, mild elevations in serum cholesterol and occasionally elevations in serum bilirubin concentrations. Severely ill animals with pronounced anorexia may also be dehydrated and have abnormalities in serum electrolytes.

Glucose tolerance testing is rarely necessary in aiding a diagnosis of diabetes but may prove useful in identifying 'latent' diabetics, or perhaps in categorizing the type of diabetes. Intravenous tolerance tests give more consistent results in comparison to oral tolerance testing but the same problems arise in the interpretation of results in 'stressed' or chemically restrained cases as outlined above. The protocol involves administering 600 mg/kg dextrose 40% intravenously over 60 seconds and evaluating blood glucose before and 10, 30, 45, 60 and 90 minutes after loading. Blood glucose in normal animals should return to baseline within 60 minutes.

Treatment

ORAL HYPOGLYCAEMIA AGENTS

These are used widely in the treatment of human non-insulin-dependent diabetes mellitus but there is no documented evidence of their efficacy in the cat, and they are acknowledged as being potentially hepatotoxic in cats (Feldman & Nelson, 1987).

INSULIN REPLACEMENT THERAPY

This remains the treatment of choice in most cases, accompanied by therapy of concurrent disorders if insulin antagonism is suspected (e.g. withdrawal of progestagen therapy, treatment of hyperthyroidism). There are obvious management problems associated with the restriction in lifestyle of a free-ranging animal and these should be discussed with owners prior to starting replacement therapy. Owners should be aware of the potential success of treatment, but also of the financial and practical limitations involved in maintaining a diabetic animal.

Maintenance insulin therapy — management goals
Although cases differ widely in their response to therapy, and in the acceptability of a strict lifestyle, a reasonable initial goal is to give a 24-hour-acting insulin preparation subcutaneously once daily at the same time each day with one-third of the total daily food intake. The remainder of the food is given at the time of maximal insulin action, usually 7–8 hours after insulin administration, as illustrated in Fig. 12.1.

Table 12.2 Sliding scale of insulin dosages. The aim of therapy is to maintain glycosuria below 1%. The daily insulin dose is calculated on the basis of that morning's glycosuria as measured by the five drop Clinitest method and the insulin dose of the previous day.

Glycosuria	Action
0%	Go down one unit from the previous day's dose
0.5–0.75%	Give the same dose as the previous day
≥1%	Go up one unit from the previous day's dose

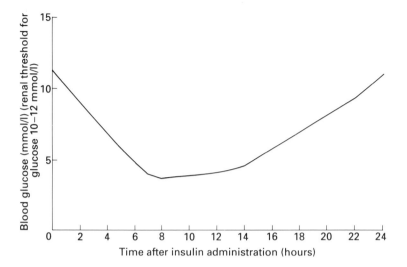

Fig. 12.1 Expected blood glucose response following a '24 hour' insulin preparation in a stabilized diabetic cat.

The diet should be based on weighed canned food to ensure a constant daily calorific intake. Many diabetic cats remain severely polyphagic and the most suitable way to decide on the level of calorie intake is to monitor bodyweight and adjust intake accordingly. Calculation of the insulin dose is best made daily on the basis of morning urinary glucose measurements, although well-stabilized animals usually require once-weekly assessments. The most accurate way to quantify urinary glucose is to use the Clinitest system*, and the instructions in Table 12.2 suggest a sliding scale system to maintain the morning urine glycosuria under 1%, equivalent to a blood glucose measurement around 12 mmol/l. Urine sampling can be problematic in cats, both at home and when hospitalized, and the use of washable litter in sieve type trays is recommended (Mikki trays and litter†).

The choice of insulin for replacement therapy can be difficult as it is acknowledged that individuals respond very differently to particular insulin preparations. In general, cats appear to metabolize insulin far more rapidly than dogs or man,

and to avoid the complications of twice-daily insulin administration it is preferable to use a protamine zinc insulin suspension (PZI). Isophane (NPH) preparations often last well below 12 hours and insulin zinc suspensions (IZS) tend to give between 12 and 18 hours of control (Moise, 1982). Feline insulin is very close to human insulin in structure and it may also be preferable to attempt to use a human monocomponent insulin rather than a purified porcine or bovine one if these become available. The PZI used preferentially in our clinic is Hypurin PZI*, although some cases do appear to achieve 24-hour control with some of the IZS preparations (Insulatard†). It is vital that syringes accurately measure 1 unit (0.01 ml) increments and that a fine-gauge needle is used ('Lo-dose' 0.5 ml U-100 diabetic syringes‡). Insulin can be diluted to give accurate increment changes of less than 1 unit, and diluents are often available on application to the manufacturers of the particular preparation. Although it is recommended that dilutions in sterile saline should be replenished once weekly our experience suggests that once monthly may be adequate.

---

*Clinitest system; Ames Division, Miles Laboratories, UK.
† Mikki urine specimen collection kit for cats; MD Components, Bedfordshire, UK.

* Hypurin; CP Pharmaceuticals Ltd., Wrexham, UK.
† Insulatard; Novo Pharmaceuticals Ltd., Crawley, UK.
‡ Lo-dose syringes, Micro Fine IV; Becton Dickinson Co., New Jersey, USA.

Stabilization on insulin replacement therapy

Cases may be divided into one of three groups: those that are bright, without obvious complications and are non-ketotic; those that are keto-acidotic and are clinically depressed, anorexic and dehydrated; and those with non-ketotic hyperosmolar syndrome characterized by severe hyperglycaemia over 30 mmol/l, hyperosmolarity, severe dehydration and collapse in the absence of ketoacidosis. Most cases belong to the non-complicated group as ketosis is rare in the cat and hyperosmolar non-ketotic syndrome has only been well documented in a single case in the cat (Schaer, 1975).

Stabilization is best achieved by hospitalizing the animal although it can be performed on an out-patient basis, keeping in touch with the owner in the morning after home assessment of urinary glycosuria, and taking blood samples for glucose estimation in the afternoon when the insulin preparation is at it most active (see Fig. 12.1). It is essential that the clinic is able to measure blood glucose accurately and quickly in animals undergoing stabilization and the authors strongly recommend the use of the inexpensive portable blood glucose analysers which require only a drop of blood (e.g. Glucometer*).

Suggested protocols for the stabilization of each category of case are given in Tables 12.3, 12.4 and 12.5.

COMPLICATIONS OF INSULIN THERAPY

It is important to recognize that continuing clinical signs suggest that blood glucose control is inadequate. Diabetic animals are prone to bacterial infections, particularly cystitis, and these should be treated promptly. The microangiopathies involving the kidney and peripheral nerves, and the deterioration in peripheral vascular control common in human diabetics have not been well documented in the cat. Complications usually fall into one of two categories, insulin resistance and hypoglycaemia.

* Glucometer; Ames, Slough, UK.

Table 12.3 Stabilization procedure in non-complicated diabetics.

---

1 Once the diagnosis has been confirmed establish a blood glucose baseline after an overnight fast. Weigh the cat and decide on the exact size of meals

2 Decide on a routine the owner can follow at home, e.g. test urine at 8.30 a.m., insulin and breakfast at 9.00 a.m., supper 8 hours later at 5.00 p.m. and follow this while hospitalized

3 Monitor water intake accurately and obtain clean urine samples first thing each morning

4 Start the insulin dose at 0.5 IU/kg bodyweight

5 Monitor the blood glucose at the time of peak insulin action (with PZI 7–8 hours after insulin injection) to ensure the cat is responding to insulin

6 Make daily adjustments to the insulin dose on the basis of morning glycosurias, afternoon blood glucose estimations and daily water intake. It is preferable to change the insulin dose slowly (i.e. 1 unit daily)

7 Stabilization is complete when urine glucose is between 0.25 and 1%, afternoon blood samples show that blood glucose is reaching the normal range and water intake approaches normal

---

Insulin resistance

This is defined as occurring when hyperglycaemia persists despite insulin dosages exceeding 2 IU/kg bodyweight/24 hours, far in excess of the normal physiological rate of endogenous insulin secretion. Improper storage of insulin or usage of insulin preparations by owners, including frequent incorrect injection technique, will result in an apparent, but spurious, insulin resistance. The most commonly identified causes of true insulin resistance involve insulin antagonism and are strongly associated with hyperadrenocorticism and acromegaly in the cat (Eigenmann *et al.*, 1984; Nelson *et al.*, 1988). As indicated elsewhere in this chapter the main presentation of both these rare conditions is as insulin-resistant diabetics. Other situations that may induce insulin resistance include concurrent hyperthyroidism, severe obesity, severe bacterial infections and prolonged ketosis.

To investigate such cases it is wise first to hospitalize the animal and ensure that the routine reported by the owner has induced true insulin

Table 12.4 Stabilization procedure in ketoacidotic diabetics.

1 Animals have to be hospitalized and an indwelling intravenous catheter inserted. If possible assess extent of dehydration, metabolic and electrolyte imbalances as well as degree of hyperglycaemia
2 Fluid therapy – suggested empirical doses: 0.9% NaCl (approx. 500 ml plus losses in vomiting), then 0.45% NaCl (approx. 2 ml/kg/h)
3 Soluble insulin therapy (e.g. Actrapid*) – 1 unit/kg bodyweight as an intravenous bolus repeated 3 to 4 hourly until blood glucose begins to fall. Ketones have a half-life of well over 48 hours in blood so will persist despite resolution of hyperglycaemia
4 Correct acidosis if present – ideally this should be based on an assessment of blood gases, but in the absence of this an empirical dose of 2.5 ml/kg bodyweight of 4.2% sodium bicarbonate solution should be added to the intravenous infusion over 6–8 hours. Repeat 12-hourly
5 Potassium therapy – intensive insulin therapy may result in hypokalaemia and serum potassium should be monitored. Supplementation is best given orally with either 'Slow K' or an effervescent potassium preparation
6 Supportive care – antiemetics, antibiotics, etc.
7 The aim of therapy is to switch to a 24-hour-acting insulin preparation as soon as the animal is non-ketotic, is willing to eat, and no longer requires fluid replacement. This may take several days. At this point switch to the procedure for the non-complicated group.

* Actrapid; Novo Pharmaceuticals Ltd., Crawley, UK.

Table 12.5 Stabilization procedure in non-ketotic hyperosmolar diabetes mellitus.

1 Animals have to be hospitalized and assessed as in Table 12.4. Hyperosmolar coma occurs at blood glucose levels over 33 mmol/l
2 Fluid therapy – slow intravenous administration of 0.45% NaCl
3 Soluble insulin therapy – 0.5 unit/kg bodyweight intravenously and 0.5 unit/kg bodyweight intramuscularly. Assess response and repeat 3–6-hourly
4 Revert to Table 12.4 once blood glucose has reduced

resistance. It may be advisable to use a previously unopened bottle of the cat's usual insulin preparation to check the potency of the bottle used at home. If insulin resistance is confirmed then the case should be evaluated for the presence of concurrent endocrine disease.

Hypoglycaemia
The clinical signs of hypoglycaemia in the cat are similar to those in other species and early features include disorientation, agitation, vocalization and extreme hunger. These progress quickly to ataxia or weakness, apparent blindness, convulsions and collapse. Treatment should be prompt and involves oral administration of dextrose to effect. The easiest way for owners to do this is to crush dextrose tablets (e.g. Dextrosol) and rub them on the gums, or to dissolve dextrose in water and administer orally by syringe. Administration should be continued until the animal's condition starts to improve, but if no response is gained within 5 minutes veterinary intervention is required. Intravenous 5% dextrose saline is an appropriate strength of solution for reversal of hypoglycaemia and care should be taken not to overadminister glucose intravenously as this can induce hyperosmolar coma with cerebral damage. Obviously the insulin dose and the management routine should be reviewed prior to insulin administration the next day.

Hypoglycaemia occurs as a result of a relative insulin overdose and can occur for a number of obvious management reasons. Owners may miscalculate the insulin dose, the cat may fail to eat despite having been given insulin, or there may be an inadvertent change in insulin preparation – all may result in hypoglycaemia. Clinical signs are most likely to appear at the time of the insulin preparation's peak activity, in the case of PZI being 7–8 hours after administration. However, in cats an important phenomenon is recognized as inducing hypoglycaemia. Administering an overdose of insulin to a patient results in subclinical or overt hypoglycaemia that inevitably initiates secretion of counter-regulatory hormones such as adrenaline, cortisol and glucagon, resulting in rapid 'rebound' hyperglycaemia. This will induce gross glycosuria the following morning and owners may increase the insulin dose in an attempt to reduce this. This leads to an increase in severity of the hypoglycaemia attacks and increasing signs of glycaemic instability such as polydipsia/polyuria. This 'Somogyi' phenomenon has been well documented as a common complication in cats (McMillan & Feldman, 1986), and may be related to their ability to metabolize many insulin preparations rapidly. Diagnosis requires assessment of serial blood glucose estimations to demonstrate hypoglycaemia followed by hyperglycaemia in one 24-hour period (Feldman & Nelson, 1987) as urine glucose and single afternoon blood glucose determinations are often potentially misleading. It is confirmed when drastically reducing the insulin dose by 50–75% reduces glycosuria and improves blood glucose control.

Insulinoma

Functional tumours of the islet cells are a well-recognized cause of hypoglycaemia and episodic neurological signs in dogs but are very rare in cats. There have been a few reports of this tumour affecting older cats. The major signs are episodic ataxia, weakness and seizures. Frequent feeding may protect against clinical signs. Diagnosis depends on demonstration of a persistent hypoglycaemia associated with hyperinsulinaemaia. Surgical excision or medical management with diazoxide can be considered but there is little information about their value and the prognosis must be considered to be guarded.

Gastrinoma

There is a single report of a pancreatic tumour in a cat causing gastrin release leading to duodenal ulceration and vomiting (Middleton & Watson, 1983).

THYROID DISEASE

Hyperthyroidism

Hyperthyroidism was not recognized as a clinical problem in cats until around 1979. However, there were several earlier reports of pathological abnormalities of the thyroid glands of cats although their relevance to clinical disease was not appreciated at that time. Hyperthyroidism is now considered to be the most common endocrine condition of cats and one of the major causes of disease in older cats. It is of importance not only because of its frequency but also because it is eminently treatable, in contrast to many other feline conditions of the older patient. Greater familiarity with the clinical presentation and ready availability of thyroid hormone estimations has led to increasing frequency of diagnosis of feline hyperthyroidism but it has also been suggested that there has been a genuine increase in the incidence of the condition in recent years (Taylor *et al.*, 1989).

Causes

Thyroid adenomas or adenomatous hyperplasia account for the vast majority of cases. Carcinomas of the thyroid are often endocrinologically active in cats and are responsible for around 1–3% of all cases of feline hyperthyroidism. This form is of particular importance in view of its implications for treatment and prognosis (see below). In large series of hyperthyroid cats reported from the USA the adenomas have been bilateral in over 70% of cases and unilateral in under 30%. At our clinic the proportion of bilateral cases has been larger. Radioactive thyroid scans have shown that although only one gland may appear abnormal on gross examination both glands may be affected. Furthermore, in a high proportion of cats which have been unilaterally thyroidectomized in the belief that only one gland is affected there is a recurrence of hyperthyroidism resulting from abnormalities of the remaining gland. This suggests that the ratio of bilateral to unilateral cases may be underestimated and this is an important factor to consider in the management of hyperthyroid cats (see below).

Thyroid adenomas are considered to be analogous to toxic nodular goitre in man and the underlying cause is not clear. A number of epidemiological associations have been recognized with hyperthyroidism in the USA – with regular flea treatment, exposure to agrochemicals, confinement indoors, living in multicat households and a diet of predominantly canned food (Scarlett *et al.*, 1988) – but the significance, if any, of these associations is not understood. Thyroid-stimulating immunoglobulins, as found in human patients with Graves's disease, have not been found in affected cats although thyroid growth-stimulating antibodies have been identified (Peterson *et al.*, 1987b). A lymphocytic infiltration of the thyroid glands has also been reported in some hyperthyroid cats (Kennedy & Thoday, 1988). The relevance, if any, of these findings to the pathogenesis of feline hyperthyroidism is not clear and it is possible that they may result from, rather than be a cause of the disease.

History and clinical signs

Hyperthyroidism is primarily a disease of older cats. It has been reported in cats as young as 6 years of age but is seen mainly in cats over 10 years old with a mean age of around 12 years. There is no sex or breed predisposition although a relatively low prevalence in pedigree cats has been noted in the USA and at our clinic. It is possible that this reflects differences in the life expectancy of pedigree compared to mixed breed cats.

Thyroid hormones influence the function of many body systems and therefore in hyperthyroidism the clinical signs are very varied. These are summarized in Table 12.6. The major sign is progressive weight loss frequently accompanied by polyphagia. Increased appetite is an uncommon clinical sign in feline medicine apart from lymphocytic cholangitis and inflammatory bowel disease and perhaps diabetes mellitus. Affected cats are frequently hyperactive and irritable, resenting clinical examination. In view of its insidious development this sign is frequently overlooked by owners and dismissed as part of the normal ageing process. Cardiac abnormalities are

Table 12.6 Clinical features of hyperthyroidism.

Weight loss
Polyphagia
Hyperactivity
Polydipsia
Steatorrhoea
Palpable thyroid nodule
Tachycardia
Poor coat
Depression
Vomiting

common and there is usually a tachycardia with a heart rate in excess of 240/minute. In addition there may be a gallop rhythm with an extra heart sound, a murmur and/or dysrhythmia. The heart sounds may be louder than usual and audible over a wide area. In severe cases there may be development of heart failure with dyspnoea resulting from either pulmonary oedema or (more rarely) accumulation of thoracic fluid. Diarrhoea with voluminous fatty faeces is a common feature. Although no specific skin changes will usually be present, the coat frequently becomes matted and unkempt giving the cat a dishevelled appearance. Polydipsia and polyuria are common but are signs which may pass unnoticed by owners. Although most hyperthyroid cats are polyphagic and hyperactive a small proportion (accounting for about 10%) of advanced cases are presented with severe depression, muscle weakness and anorexia. This is described as the 'apathetic' clinical presentation. There may be muscle weakness, most often seen as a peculiar ventral neck flexion. Heat intolerance with panting, vomiting and dysphonia may also be noted. In most cases there will be palpable enlargement of one or both thyroids, which may have a nodular feel. Thyroid palpation requires both care and practise. Glands are usually located just below the larynx but in hyperthyroid cats may descend down the neck and occasionally pass through the thoracic inlet.

Differential diagnosis

Although the clinical signs are both variable and diverse the combination of signs is usually very suggestive of hyperthyroidism. A frequent comment from practitioners is that once the first case of hyperthyroidism has been diagnosed subsequent cases are recognized readily. The most important differentials for hyperthyroidism are other causes of progressive weight loss – mainly alimentary lymphosarcoma, chronic renal disease, diabetes mellitus and simple ageing. Polydipsia with polyuria may have been noted in cats with renal disease and there may also be muscle weakness and ventral flexion of the neck associated with hypokalaemic-induced polymyopathy. Diabetes mellitus may also result in polyphagia. Since hyperthyroidism is a disease of older cats other coincidental diseases are not uncommon, including diabetes mellitus and particularly chronic renal disease.

Diagnosis

There are frequent abnormalities of a number of routine blood tests but the diagnosis is most readily confirmed by estimation of thyroid hormone concentrations.

HAEMATOLOGY

The most frequent haematological change is a relative polycythaemia with increases in all the red cell parameters and a macrocytosis with increased mean corpuscular volume (MCV). Less common is a mild non-regenerative anaemia.

CLINICAL CHEMISTRY

An increase in liver enzymes including ALT, SAP and gamma GT is a consistent feature although the reason for this is not clear. There may be other biochemical changes, particularly an increase in urea, creatinine and phosphate in cats with concomitant renal disease. These features may have implications for the prognosis of the condition.

ELECTROCARDIOGRAPHY

Apart from tachycardia the most consistent electrocardiographic change is the presence of tall R waves particularly on lead II which results from left ventricular hypertrophy. Various dys-

rhythmias may be present such as ventricular ectopics and conduction disturbances.

RADIOGRAPHY AND ULTRASONOGRAPHY

Hyperthyroid cats with secondary cardiac disease usually show a marked cardiomegaly which is evident on both radiography and ultrasound examination. In the early stages this is predominantly left-sided although in time it may also affect the right side. The features are usually typical of hypertrophic cardiomyopathy – an elongated, lemon-shaped heart with increased sternal contact and marked atrial dilatation. Ultrasound examination shows that the ventricular enlargement is primarily the result of hypertrophy with a greatly reduced intra-ventricular volume. Occasionally the cardiac changes are more typical of dilated cardiomyopathy with generalized dilatation of all cardiac chambers and a hypomotile heart.

THYROID HORMONE ASSAY

The most reliable test for confirming hyperthyroidism is demonstration of an elevated basal T_4 or free T_4 concentration (generally considered to be over 65 nmol of T_4 or free T_4 >15 pmol/l). There is usually no advantage in determining T_3 concentrations (which occasionally remain within a normal range) or in performing a TSH or TRH (thyrotrophin-releasing hormone) stimulation test. However, significant daily variations have been shown to occur in T_4 concentrations in hyperthyroid cats and in occasional cases the level may at times fall within the normal range (Peterson *et al.*, 1987a; Broome *et al.*, 1988). If hyperthyroidism is suspected on clinical grounds but cannot be confirmed by repeated basal T_4 estimations, a T_3 suppression test can be performed. A morning blood sample is collected for T_4 estimation and 25 µg of T_3 is given followed by the same dosage every 8 hours for the next 2 days. Four hours after the seventh dosage of T_3 a second blood sample is collected for T_4 estimation. In a normal cat this treatment will usually result in a greater than 30–50% suppression of the basal T_4 but not in hyperthyroid cats.

THYROID IMAGING

Administration of radioactive technetium or iodine can be used to perform thyroid scans for diagnosing hyperthyroidism if a gamma camera is available. There is some salivary gland uptake of technetium but the thyroids can generally be clearly identified, abnormal glands showing increased uptake. This technique can show whether both glands are involved (which is valuable if surgical thyroidectomy is subsequently to be performed) and has the advantage of identifying glands which have descended into the thorax through the thoracic inlet or the rare cases of abnormal ectopic thyroid tissue within the thorax. It is also particularly useful in assessing cats which are showing a recurrence of signs following previous thyroidectomy and it may help in the identification of thyroid carcinomas.

Treatment

There are three options for treatment of hyperthyroidism in cats. The optimum method for treatment depends on a number of factors including whether the underlying lesion is an adenoma or a less common carcinoma, although this may not be established until the thyroid glands have been examined.

RADIOACTIVE IODINE

Administration of ^{131}I has proved to be an effective method for treating hyperthyroid cats. It is possible to attempt to determine the optimal dosage by assessing uptake of labelled iodine but some workers report that a standard dose is equally effective (Meric & Rubin, 1990). The major disadvantage of this method of treatment is the need for specialized facilities to house the cats whilst treatment is carried out and to dispose of urine, faeces, etc. Handling of the patient should be avoided for the first week after treatment and the minimum amount of time should be used for feeding and clearing of the cage. The cat can be returned home after 1–2 weeks but handling and close contact should be minimized for a further week. For those reasons, this method of treatment has not been widely used in the UK. One potential disadvantage is that should any problems arise during the early stage of treatment, the need to avoid close contact during this period may cause difficulties particularly if the cat should require additional medication such as treatment for an associated cardiomyopathy. Radioactive iodine treatment may be particularly indicated in cats with thyroid carcinomas when local invasion or metastasis can complicate surgical removal. In such cases higher dosages of ^{131}I of up to 30 m G may be required (Turrel *et al.*, 1988).

SURGERY

Surgical thyroidectomy is the method of treatment most frequently used in the UK. It is a relatively simple and straightforward procedure although the degree of surgical skill is a critical factor in determining whether postoperative complications arise both in terms of hypoparathyroidism and recurrence of hyperthyroidism. Prior medical treatment (discussed below) for 2–4 weeks or more is indicated to improve the cat's condition and minimize the potential complications arising from the hyperthyroidism, such as catecholamine-induced cardiac irregularities. Special consideration is necessary in the choice of premedicants and atropine should be avoided as this increases the risk of tachycardia and arrhythmias. Ketamine and xylazine should also be avoided for this reason. Acetylpromazine premedication protects against arrhythmias and also against autonomic signs associated with hyperthyroidism.

The surgical approach to the thyroid glands is straightforward and involves blunt separation of the sternohyoid muscles. Prior thyroid scans will not usually be available but these do enable both differentiation between bilateral and unilateral cases and localization of the thyroid glands. A number of different surgical techniques for thyroidectomy have been described and these have certain advantages and disadvantages (Flanders *et al.*, 1987; Welches *et al.*, 1989). An extracapsular technique minimizes the risk of leaving abnormal thyroid tissue but increases the risk of compromising parathyroid function. The intracapsular technique is less likely to interfere with parathyroid function but leaves an increased risk of recurrence due to some affected tissue remaining. Both these techniques have been modified and improved. The modified intracapsular technique involves removal of all the capsule with the exception of the part immediately adjacent to the external parathyroid gland. This appears to reduce the risk of recurrence seen with the unmodified technique considerably to a comparable level of risk of recurrence with the extracapsular technique. However, hypocalcaemia does occur in about one-third to a half of cases as opposed to only around 15–20% for the unmodified intracapsular technique. This is presumed to be due to increased traction on the capsule interfering with the vascular supply to the parathyroid glands. In the modified extracapsular technique the caudal vessels supplying the thyroid gland are ligated, but instead of ligating the cranial vessels as for the unmodified technique the thyroid capsule is cauterized around the parathyroid at least 2 mm away from its outer edge. This reduces the risk of compromising the blood supply to the retained external parathyroid glands and hypocalcaemia occurs in around 20% of cases as compared to about 80% with the unmodified extracapsular technique. Since hypoparathyroidism and hypocalcaemia are the major complications of thyroidectomy the modified extracapsular technique is the preferred choice as it minimizes both this risk and recurrence of hyperthyroidism.

Even if the thyroid abnormality is clearly unilateral, as in the minority of cases, every effort should be made to conserve parathyroid tissue in case a further thyroidectomy is required should the remaining gland subsequently become affected. Two pairs of parathyroids are present in cats. The external glands are located close to the proximal pole of the thyroid glands and should be identifiable at surgery; the internal glands are located within the thyroid parenchyma and are inevitably removed at thyroidectomy. A transient hypocalcaemia occurs following unilateral thyroidectomy but this is not associated with any clinical signs.

In most cases of hyperthyroidism both glands are quite obviously grossly abnormal but as discussed above, occasionally one gland may appear normal in bilateral cases and these can be recognized only by prior thyroid scanning without resort to histological examination. The major potential complication of bilateral thyroidectomy is hypocalcaemia associated with hypoparathyroidism. This risk can be minimized by careful surgical technique as described above, but nevertheless is present to some degree following all bilateral thyroidectomies. This complication most often arises 1–3 days after thyroidectomy but clinical signs of hypocalcaemia may develop in some cats within 8 hours of surgery, or not until 5 days following surgery in others. A mild hypocalcaemia (<2.2 mmol/l) is a consistent postoperative feature but clinical signs develop in only a minority of these cases. Signs are more likely to develop with severe hypocalcaemia (<1.8 mmol/l) but the degree of hypocalcaemia is not an entirely reliable predictor of development of clinical signs. In our clinic, blood calcium is measured twice daily for 4 days following thyroidectomy and then at intervals determined by the degree of hypocalcaemia. If blood calcium drops below 2.0 mmol/l or if clinical signs develop, treatment is begun immediately. Undoubtedly this policy leads to treatment of some cats which would not have developed clinical signs. The first signs of hypocalcaemia are general agitation and hyperaesthesia. This rapidly progresses to tonic muscular spasms with opisthotonus. Signs of hypocalcaemia develop very quickly and death may follow rapidly without treatment. The approach we adopt therefore avoids the risk of a hypocalcaemic crisis arising when the cat is not being observed.

If blood calcium falls below 2.0 mmol/l but no clinical signs are evident, 1 g of calcium carbonate and 0.2 mg dihydrotachysterol are administered orally daily. This treatment is adjusted according to subsequent blood calcium estimations, the objective being to maintain concentrations within the normal range. In some cases considerably higher dosages of calcium (up to 3 g daily) and dihydrotachysterol are required in the short term (for the first week or so). If severe clinical signs of hypocalcaemia develop with muscular tetany, up to 2 ml of 2.5% calcium gluconate is given slowly intravenously. Further calcium may be given intravenously to effect (to control muscular spasms but avoiding bradycardia) but with great care. 10–20 ml of the same solution is then administered subcutaneously and oral supplementation begun. Severely affected cats should be monitored carefully after resolution of signs following intravenous calcium as signs may recur quickly. Excessive supplementation should be avoided since hypercalcaemia may result in various complications such as metastatic calcification, particularly of the renal tubules leading to nephrogenic diabetes insipidus. In most cases supplementation can be reduced to approximately 0.3 g calcium daily and 0.05 mg dihydrotachysterol daily. Lack of access to rapid calcium estimations is a severe limiting factor in the short-term management of cats undergoing thyroidectomy. Prophylactic treatment is unsatisfactory since the dosage requirements and length of treatment needed are so variable and oversupplementation is dangerous. Previous attempts to provide prophylactic treatment have proved unsuccessful (Flanders *et al.*, 1987). Although the risk of hypocalcaemia associated with clinical signs may be relatively small with careful surgical technique, we consider that where feasible bilateral thyroidectomies should be performed only in centres with access to calcium estimations.

Two-stage thyroidectomies have been performed in bilaterally affected cats in an attempt to minimize the risk of hypoparathyroidism (Flanders *et al.*, 1987). The thyroidectomy of the remaining gland was performed 1 month after the first thyroidectomy on the basis that the blood supply to the retained parathyroid would have returned to normal by this stage. Some slight reduction in the frequency of hypocalcaemia was noted but it was concluded that this approach did not provide any substantial advantage in surgical management and that surgical expertise is the factor most critical to success.

Our experience concurs with reports of a large series of cases (Welches *et al.*, 1989) that calcium and vitamin D supplementation can be withdrawn in all cats that have shown hypoparathyroidism following thyroidectomy. Even if the parathyroids are inadvertently removed ectopic

parathyroid tissue has been reported to be present in up to 50% of cats, located in the mediastinum, pericardium or peritracheal area, and it is presumed that this undergoes compensatory hypertrophy. Revascularization of damaged or remnant parathyroid tissue may also account for the re-establishment of calcium homeostasis.

Horner's syndrome and voice loss associated with damage to the recurrent laryngeal nerve are other possible postoperative complications but may resolve with time. Interestingly in the report of two-stage thyroidectomies five of the nine cats became euthyroid and one became hypothyroid, as judged by the estimations, shortly after the first thyroidectomy. The owners of the other three cats did not return their pets until signs of hyperthyroidism recurred, which was not until 9–19 months after the first thyroidectomy.

The need for thyroid hormone replacement therapy following thyroidectomy is questionable; 0.1–0.2 mg of thyroxine (T_4) daily within one or two days of surgery has been recommended (Welches *et al.*, 1989). However, another approach is to assess T_4 concentrations 4–6 weeks after surgery. No signs of hypothyroidism generally become evident in this period, and in most cases T_4 concentrations are within the normal range implying that there has been compensatory hypertrophy of either residual or ectopic thyroid tissue. Thyroid replacement has not been found necessary in cats undergoing bilateral thyroidectomy at our clinic.

Early recurrence (within 6–12 months) of hyperthyroidism is rare in cats in which unilateral disease is demonstrated by thyroid scans. Recurrence will occasionally occur in 2–3 years. In some bilateral cases only one of the affected glands may appear grossly normal as described above and this is the most likely explanation for early recurrence in most apparently unilateral cases.

Up to 10% of bilateral cases show recurrence, usually 2–3 years after initial surgery. Thyroid scans have shown that this results from regeneration of residual affected tissue and the risk of recurrence depends on the surgical technique used. There is considerably increased risk of hypoparathyroidism in attempting further surgical treatment and such cases are most satisfactorily managed by either radioactive iodine or long-term medical treatment.

MEDICAL TREATMENT

The major indication for medical treatment is to prepare hyperthyroid cats for surgical thyroidectomy – to improve their general condition and to reduce the risk of complications arising during surgery. Medical treatment based on antithyroid drugs may also be used for long-term management as an alternative to radioactive iodine or surgical treatment. This is less satisfactory since these drugs block thyroid hormone synthesis rather than having a cytotoxic effect on the neoplastic thyroid tissue and therefore do not influence the underlying cause. In addition their use may be associated with adverse side-effects (see below). Nevertheless, medical treatment may be the only treatment option that some owners will consider and it may be indicated in cats with other concurrent diseases. The most important complicating concurrent disease is renal dysfunction, which is relatively common in old cats. Our experience indicates that thyroidectomy carries a poor prognosis in such cases and we recommend medical management.

Carbimazole is the antithyroid drug now most widely used in the UK. It is closely related to methimazole, which has been extensively used in the USA for management of hyperthyroid cats (Peterson *et al.*, 1988). It reduces thyroid hormone synthesis by interfering with the organification of iodine in the thyroid.

The objective of carbimazole treatment is to return the cat to a euthyroid state and reduce the serum T_4 concentration to the normal range. The dosage required to achieve this is very variable. We begin treatment at a dosage of 5 mg three times daily although this may be adjusted according to our assessment of the severity of the disease. The cat is checked every 1–2 weeks for clinical response and the serum concentration of T_4 is determined. It may be necessary to increase the dosage up to 15 mg three times daily to achieve this objective. In most cases 2–4 weeks of medical

treatment are required to prepare cats for subsequent surgical thyroidectomy. The major side-effects of carbimazole treatment in cats are vomiting and marrow suppression leading to leucopenia and less commonly thrombocytopenia. Although the marrow suppression is reported to occur in the early stages (within 1 month) of treatment with methimazole, for which extensive data have been published from the USA (Peterson *et al.*, 1988), our more limited experience with carbimazole suggests that this occurs after more prolonged treatment. The blood picture should be monitored periodically to check for this side-effect, initially every 1–2 weeks, and every 2–4 weeks with prolonged treatment. It will resolve shortly after cessation of treatment. If long-term medical management is to be used as an alternative to thyroidectomy the aim of monitoring should be to use the minimum dosage to maintain T_4 within the normal range to reduce the risk of side-effects developing. The use of propylthiouracil as an antithyroid drug is no longer recommended as it carries an unacceptably high risk of side-effects, particularly autoimmune haemolytic anaemia.

Propranolol is indicated in cats with severe tachycardia and dysrhythmias although it should be used with care if clear evidence of heart failure is present. It may also help to protect against stress-induced tachycardia. We continue propranolol treatment in cats undergoing surgical thyroidectomy until the tachycardia resolves although treatment is withheld during the immediate postoperative period if the cat is stressed by administration of tablets. In most cats the secondary cardiomyopathy appears to resolve after thyroidectomy.

Hypothyroidism

Hypothyroidism may be seen following thyroidectomy (see above) but has not been convincingly documented as a spontaneous acquired condition. Recently, however, congenital hypothyroidism has been recognized with increasing frequency as a cause of stunting in young kittens. Several reported cases have been associated with thyroid dysgenesis. There have also been two reported cases in which a defect in organification has been demonstrated (Arnold *et al.*, 1984) and a number of such cases have been identified at our clinic. We have studied one particular family of cats with an organification defect and have strong evidence to suggest that this particular defect is inherited as an autosomal recessive trait. However, in man organification defects represent a hetereogeneous group of congenital errors of metabolism which involve different abnormalities of normal organification.

Clinical signs

The most striking feature of this disorder is stunting, although this may not become apparent until affected kittens reach 1 month of age or more. In contrast to growth hormone (GH) deficiency, which leads to proportional stunting, affected individuals have a disproportionate appearance with short, rounded body, rounded, squat heads and abnormally short limbs. Some affected kittens develop severe constipation which may prove refractory to treatment. A goitre develops but this may not become evident until the kittens are several months of age. Mental impairment was noted in both one of the reported cases and one of our affected cats, but was not evident in any of the other individuals. In man there are a number of different organification defects which result in variable clinical signs and the same may apply to this disorder in cats.

Diagnosis

A thyroid function test will enable confirmation of diagnosis. Either thyroid-stimulating hormone (TSH) or thyrotrophin-releasing hormone (TRH) can be used for provocative testing at a dosage of 1 unit and $100\,\mu g$ intravenously respectively with the post-stimulation samples being taken 7 or 4 hours later. In affected individuals basal T_4 levels are low ($<20\,$nmol/l) and these fail to increase after thyroid stimulation. Primary congenital hypothyroidism must be differentiated from the multiple endocrine abnormalities including GH deficiency seen in panhypopituitarism (see 'Pituitary dwarfism' above).

Determination of the precise underlying nature of the defect is of limited practical importance and requires specialized facilities for assessing thyroidal uptake of radioactive iodine and subsequent discharge following administration of perchlorate, a potent oxidizing agent.

Treatment

Supplementation with thyroxine can be considered but most of our affected individuals appear to have compensated to some extent for the defect by developing thyroid hypertrophy and treatment may not be necessary.

REFERENCES

General

Feldman E.C. & Nelson R.W. (1987) *Canine and Feline Endocrinology and Reproduction.* W.B. Saunders.

Peterson M.E. & Randolph J.F. (1989) The endocrine system. In Sherding R.G. (ed) *The Cat.* Churchill Livingstone, p. 1095.

Both provide an extensive review of feline endocrine disorders.

Pituitary disorders

Pituitary tumours

Martin S.L. & Capen C.C. (1975) *Feline Medicine.* American Veterinary Publications Inc., Santa Barbara.

Smith M.A. & Jones T.C. (1966) *Veterinary Pathology*, 2nd edn. Lea & Febiger.

Acromegaly

Peterson M.E. *et al.* (1990) Acromegaly in 14 cats. *J. Vet. Intern. Med.* **4**, 192.

Diabetes insipidus

Burger I.H., Anderson R.S. & Holme D.W. (1980) In Anderson R.S. (ed) *Nutrition of the Dog and Cat.* Pergamon Press.

Court M.H. & Watson A.D.T. (1983) Idiopathic neurogenic diabetes insipidus in a cat. *Aust. Vet. J.* **60**, 245.

Gradual water deprivation over 8 days was used to determine the cat's ability to concentrate urine. Hypokalaemia developed following treatment with hydrochlorthiazide, but this was controlled with spironolactone.

Winterbotham J. & Mason K.V. (1983) Congenital diabetes insipidus in a kitten. *J. Small Anim. Pract.* **24**, 569.

Parathyroid disorders

Hyperparathyroidism

Blunden A.S., Wheeler S.J. & Davies J.V. (1986) Hyperparathyroidism in the cat of probable primary origin. *J. Small Anim. Pract.* **27**, 791.

Richter K.P., Kallet A.J., Feldman E.C. & Brum D. (1990) Primary hyperparathyroidism in seven cats. *J. Vet. Intern. Med.* **4**, 115.

Malignancy-associated hypercalcaemia

McMillan F.D. (1985) Hypercalcemia associated with lymphoid neoplasia in two cats. *Feline Pract.* **15**(3), 31.

Hypoparathyroidism

Forbes S., Nelson R.W. & Guptil L. (1990) Primary hypoparathyroidism in a cat. *J. Am. Vet. Med. Assoc.* **196**, 1285.

Peterson M.E. *et al.* (1990) Naturally occurring hypoparathyroidism in the cat. *J. Vet. Intern. Med.* **4**, 41.

Adrenal disorders

Testing

Sparkes A.H., Adams D.T., Douthwaite J.A. & Gruffydd-Jones T.J. (1990) Assessment of adrenal function in cats: Response to intravenous synthetic ACTH. *J. Small Anim. Pract.* **31**, 2.

Hyperadrenocorticism

Nelson R.W., Feldman E.C. & Smith M.C. (1988) Hyperadrenocorticism in cats: seven cases (1978–1987). *J. Am. Vet. Med. Ass.* **193**, 245.

Scott D.W., Manning T.O. & Reimes T.J. (1982) Iatrogenic Cushing's syndrome in the cat. *Feline Pract.* **12**(2), 20.

Iatrogenic Cushing's syndrome was induced only after prolonged, high-dosage administration of corticosteroids. A marked hyperglycaemia developed but no other blood biochemical changes. Clinical signs were minimal and included curling of the ear tips.

Watson A.D.J., Church D.B., Emslie D.R. & Middleton D.J. (1989) Comparative effects of proligesterone and megestrol acetate on basal plasma glucose concentrations and cortisol responses to exogenous adrenocorticotrophic hormone in cats. *Res. Vet. Sci.* **47**, 374.

Hypoadrenocorticism

Chastain C.B., Graham C.L. & Nichols C.E. (1981) Adrenocortical suppression in cats given megestrol acetate. *Am. J. Vet. Res.* **42**, 1029.

Peterson M.E., Greco D.S. & Ortho D.N. (1989) Primary hypoadrenocorticism in ten cats. *J. Vet. Intern. Med.* **3**, 55.

Watson A.D.J., Church D.B., Emslie D.R. & Middleton D.J. (1989) Comparative effects of proligesterone and megestrol acetate on basal plasma glucose concentrations and cortisol responses to exogenous adrenocorticotrophic hormone in cats. *Res. Vet. Sci.* **47**, 374.

Conn's syndrome

Eger C.E., Robinson W.F. & Huxtable C.R.R. (1983) Primary aldosteronism (Conn's syndrome) in a cat: a case report and review of comparative aspects. *J. Small Anim. Pract.* **24**, 293.

Phaeochromocytoma

Carpenter J.L., Andrews L.K. & Holzworth J. (1987) Tumours and tumour like lesions. In Holzworth J. (ed) *Diseases of the Cat*. W.B. Saunders, p. 549.

Endocrine pancreatic disorders

Diabetes mellitus

Eigenmann J.E., Wortman J.A. & Haskins M.E. (1984) Elevated growth hormone levels and diabetes mellitus in a cat with acromegalic features. *J. Am. Anim. Hosp. Assoc.* **20**, 747.

Feldman E.C. & Nelson R.W. (1987) *Canine and Feline Endocrinology and Reproduction*. W.B. Saunders, Philadelphia, USA.

Fox J.G. & Beatty J.O. (1975) A case report of complicated diabetes mellitus in a cat. *J. Am. Anim. Hosp. Assoc.* **11**, 129.

Herrtage M.E., Barnett K.C. & MacDougall D.F. (1985) Diabetic retinopathy in a cat with megeostrol acetate induced diabetes. *J. Small Anim. Pract.* **26**, 595.

Hsu W.H. & Hembrough F.B. (1982) Intravenous glucose tolerance test in cats: influenced by acetylpromazine, ketamine, morphine, thiopental and xylazine. *Am. J. Vet. Res.* **43**, 2060.

McMillan F.D. & Feldman E.C. (1986) Rebound hyperglycaemia following overdosing of insulin in cats with diabetes mellitus. *J. Am. Vet. Med. Assoc.* **188**, 1426.

Moise N.S. (1982) Insulin therapy in diabetic cats. *American College of Veterinary Internal Medicine Scientific Proceedings, Salt Lake City*, 80.

Moise N.S. & Reimers T.J. (1983) Insulin therapy in cats with diabetes mellitus. *J. Am. Vet. Med. Assoc.* **182**, 158.

Nelson R.W., Feldman E.C. & Smith M.C. (1988) Hyperadrenocorticism in cats: seven cases (1978–1987). *J. Am. Vet. Med. Ass.* **193**, 245.

Schaer M. (1975) Diabetic hyperosmolar nonketotic syndrome in a cat. *J. Am. Anim. Hosp. Assoc.* **11**, 42.

Schaer M. (1977) A clinical survey of thirty cats with diabetes mellitus. *Am. Anim. Hosp. Assoc.* **13**, 23.

Westermark P., Wernstedt C., O'Brien T.D., Hayden D.W. & Johnson K.H. (1987) Islet amyloid in Type 2 human diabetes mellitus and adult diabetic cats contains a novel putative polypeptide hormone. *Am. J. Pathol.* **127**, 414.

Yano B.L., Hayden D.W. & Johnson K.H. (1981a) Feline insular amyloid: incidence in adult cats with no clinicopathological evidence of overt diabetes mellitus. *Vet. Pathol.* **18**, 310.

Yano B.L., Hayden D.W. & Johnson K.H. (1981b) Feline insular amyloid associated with diabetes mellitus. *Vet. Pathol.* **18**, 621.

Insulinoma

McMillan F.D., Barr B. & Feldman E.C. (1985) Functional pancreatic islet cell tumour in a cat. *J. Am. Anim. Hosp. Assoc.* **21**, 741.

Gastrinoma

Middleton D.J. & Watson A.D. (1983) Duodenal ulceration associated with gastrin-secreting pancreatic tumour in a cat. *J. Am. Vet. Med. Ass.* **183**, 461.

Thyroid disorders

Hyperthyroidism

DIAGNOSIS

Broome M.R., Feldman E.C. & Turrel J.M. (1988) Serial determination of thyroxine concentrations in hyperthyroid cats. *J. Am. Vet. Med. Assoc.* **192**, 49.

Peterson M.E. & Becker D.V. (1984) Radionucleotide thyroid imaging in 135 cats with hyperthyroidism. *Vet. Radiology* **25**, 23.

Peterson M.E. & Graves T.K. (1988) Triiodothyronine (T_3) suppression test: an aid in the diagnosis of mild hyperthyroidism in cats. In: *Proc. 5th American College of Veterinary Internal Medicine Conference.*

Peterson M.E., Graves T.K. & Cavanagh I. (1987a) Serum thyroid hormone concentrations fluctuations in cats with hyperthyroidism. *J. Vet. Int. Med.* **1**, 142.

TREATMENT

Broome M.R., Turrel J.M. & Hays M.T. (1988) Predictive value of tracer studies for ^{131}I treatment in hyperthyroid cats. *Am. J. Vet. Res.* **49**, 193.

Flanders J.A., Harvey H.J. & Erb H.N. (1987) Feline thyroidectomy. A comparison of postoperative hypocalcemia associated with three different surgical techniques. *Vet. Surgery* **16**, 362.

Meric S.M. & Rubin S.I. (1990) Serum thyroxine concentrations following fixed-dose radioactive iodine treatment in hyperthyroid cats: 62 cases (1986–1989). *J. Am. Vet. Med. Ass.* **197**, 621.

Peterson M.E., Kintzer P.P. & Hurvitz A.I. (1988) Methimazole treatment of 262 cats with hyperthyroidism. *J. Vet. Internal Med.* **2**, 150.

Swalec K.M. & Birchard S.J. (1990) Recurrence of hyperthyroidism after thyroidectomy in cats. *J. Am. Anim. Hosp. Ass.* **26**, 433.

Turrel J.M., Feldman E.C., Nelson R.W. & Cain G.R. (1988) Thyroid carcinoma causing hyperthyroidism in cats: 14 cases (1981–1986). *J. Am. Vet. Med. Ass.* **193**, 359.

Welches C.D., Scavelli T.D., Matthiesen D.T. & Peterson M.E. (1989) Occurrence of problems after three techniques of bilateral thyroidectomy in cats. *Vet. Surgery* **18**, 392.

OTHER ASPECTS

Bond B.R., Fox P.R., Peterson M.E. & Skavaril R.V. (1988) Echocardiographic findings in 103 cats with hyperthyroidism. *J. Am. Vet. Med. Ass.* **192**, 1546.

Kennedy R.L. & Thoday K.L. (1988) Autoantibodies in feline hyperthyroidism. *Res. Vet. Sci.* **45**, 300.

Labuc R.H. & Jones B.R. (1988) Feline hyperthyroidism – a review. *N.Z. Vet. J.* **36**, 77.

Peterson M.E., Kintzer P.P., Cavanagh P.G., Fox P.R., Ferguson D.C., Johnson G.F. & Becker D.V. (1983) Feline hyperthyroidism: Pretreatment clinical and laboratory evaluation of 131 cases. *J. Am. Vet. Med. Ass.* **183**, 103.

Peterson M.E., Livingston P. & Brown R.S. (1987b) Lack of circulating thyroid stimulating immunoglobulins in cats with hyperthyroidism. *Vet. Immunol. Immunopathol.* **16**, 277.

Scarlett J.M., Moise N.S. & Rayl J. (1988) Feline hyperthyroidism: a descriptive and case-control study. *Preventive Vet. Med.* **6**, 295.

Taylor J.A., Jacobs R.M., Lumsden J.H. & Bennett B.N. (1989) Perspectives on the diagnosis of feline hyperthyroidism. *Canad. Vet. J.* **30**, 477.

Hypothyroidism

Arnold U., Opitz M. & Grosser I. (1984) Goitrous hypothyroidism and dwarfism in a kitten. *J. Am. Anim. Hosp. Assoc.* **20**, 753.

Peterson M.E. & Randolph J.F. (1989) The endocrine system. In Sherding R.G. (ed) *The Cat*. Churchill Livingstone, p. 1128.

PART 2
INFECTIOUS DISEASES

Chapter 13 / Feline Panleucopenia

R. M. GASKELL

Feline panleucopenia (FP) is a highly infectious and ubiquitous disease affecting not only the domestic cat but also other members of the Felidae (for example tigers, lions and leopards), the Mustellidae (e.g. mink and ferret), Procyonidae (e.g. coatimundi, racoon) and Viverridae (e.g. civet cat) (Scott, 1987). The disease is characterized by a marked decrease in circulating white blood cells (i.e. a panleucopenia) and destruction of the intestinal mucosa leading to enteritis.

THE AGENT

Feline panleucopenia was the first disease of the cat that was shown to be viral in origin, but it was not until 1964 that Johnson achieved the breakthrough of being able to grow the virus in tissue culture (Johnson, 1964). Subsequently it was shown to be a parvovirus, a small (20 nm diameter), unenveloped, single-stranded DNA virus, with only one serotype of the virus known, and which is also indistinguishable serologically from mink enteritis virus. The recently emerged canine parvovirus (CPV) is also closely related but minor differences do exist, both antigenically and in the viral DNA, which mean that a possible origin of CPV from FP virus remains speculative (Tratschin et al., 1982; Parrish et al., 1982). Interestingly, the original CPV that emerged in the 1970s has now been replaced globally by very closely related, but antigenically and genetically slightly different variant, possibly because they replicates more efficiently in dogs (Parrish et al., 1985). Although undoubtedly a rare event, the ability of parvoviruses to mutate, and on occasion to cross

species, should be noted because presumably the potential is there for it to happen again.

Parvoviruses are an interesting group of viruses, one characteristic of which is an affinity and requirement of the virus for actively dividing cells (Pollock, 1984). Indeed it is this feature that determines the pathogenicity of the agent in the cat.

FP virus is a remarkably stable virus, resistant to heat and many disinfectants, and may persist in infected premises for up to a year (Johnson, 1966, 1969). Scott (1980), reporting on 27 products tested at the manufacturers' recommended concentrations, found that only three solutions — hypochlorite (household bleach, diluted 1 in 32), formaldehyde, or gluteraldehyde — had sufficient virucidal activity against FP virus. Hypochlorite is best used with another antiseptic such as a quaternary ammonium compound (e.g. washing-up liquid) to improve its cleaning properties. Although formalin has good activity against the virus it is highly irritant and toxic to both cats and their owners; with care, however, it may be useful for disinfecting empty buildings and equipment as described by Povey (1976).

PATHOGENESIS AND PATHOLOGY

The pathogenesis of the disease may be predicted from the requirement of the virus for rapidly dividing cells (Fig. 13.1). Virus enters the body mainly through the nose or mouth, and probably multiplies initially in the oropharyngeal tissues (Csiza et al., 1971a,b). It then spreads via the bloodstream to its main target organs, i.e. the

445

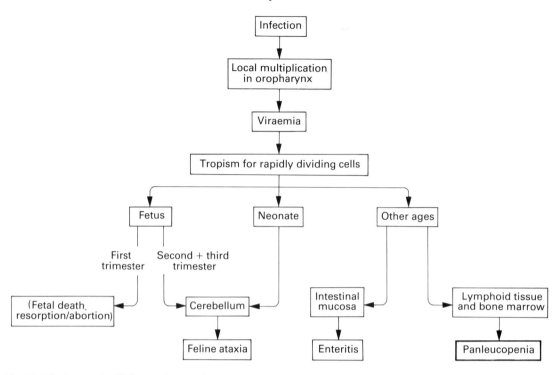

Fig. 13.1 Pathogenesis of feline panleucopenia.

rapidly dividing cells of lymphoid tissue and the bone marrow, leading to panleucopenia; and the crypt epithelium of the intestinal mucosa, leading to enteritis (Fig. 13.1). Virus localizes in the intestinal crypt cells because these are the most mitotically active; the cells are destroyed by the virus and no new cells are then available to migrate from the crypts to replace the absorptive cells at the villus tips. This results in malabsorption and increased permeability leading to diarrhoea. Thus, factors that may determine the mitotic rate in intestinal crypt cells, such as the presence of bacterial flora and whether or not the animal is fasting, may also be important in the pathogenesis of FP (Kahn, 1978). Therefore in experimental germfree and specific pathogen-free (SPF) cats, the disease is usually mild (Rohovsky & Griesemer, 1967; Hosokawa *et al.*, 1987), and even in conventional cats held under laboratory conditions, intestinal lesions may be only minimal (Larsen *et al.*, 1976).

On post-mortem examination, changes may be slight and not detected by casual examination. The cat will appear dehydrated and there may be evidence of vomiting and a fetid diarrhoea. The jejunum and ileum may appear dilated and oedematous and there is usually hyperaemia or petechial haemorrhages producing a 'rose-red' appearance on the serosal and mucosal surfaces (Johnson, 1969). The mesenteric lymph nodes may also be oedematous and haemorrhagic.

Microscopically, lesions are usually present in the mucosa of the jejunum and ileum, but necrosis may also occur in the duodenum and colon. Lesions vary from mild to nearly total destruction of the epithelial lining, with dilatation of the crypts. These are often filled with cellular debris and in early cases, transient intranuclear inclusion bodies may be seen (Gillespie & Scott, 1973).

Lymphocyte depletion and reticuloendothelial cell hyperplasia are regularly seen in lymphoid tissues, particularly in mesenteric lymph nodes,

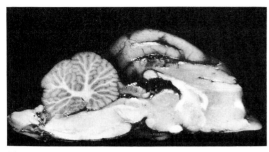

(a)

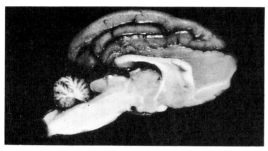

(b)

Fig. 13.2 Sagittal sections of brain from (a) normal kitten; (b) kitten with cerebellar hypoplasia.

Peyer's patches and spleen. In younger animals, the thymus may be similarly depleted. In the bone marrow, there is a general depression in myeloid activity with a marked reduction in neutrophils; the reticulum cell meshwork is also depleted (Langheinrich & Nielsen, 1971).

Feline ataxia

Transplacental infection in pregnant queens may also occur with FP virus, and indeed this is not surprising in view of its predilection for actively dividing cells. The virus infects and replicates in placental cells, and can then infect the fetus (Fig. 13.1) (Kilham *et al.*, 1967). It has been postulated that infection early in pregnancy may lead to early fetal death and resorption (Gillespie & Scott, 1973), but later on (from the middle third of gestation to immediately postnatally) it has been shown that it will lead to cerebellar hypoplasia (Fig. 13.2). Histologically there is a marked reduction in the numbers of granular cells and Purkinje cells. The retina may also be affected but this is usually of no clinical significance.

Hydrocephalus and hydranencephaly may also be seen (Greene & Scott, 1990).

Although present at birth, clinical signs are not usually observed in these kittens until they attempt to walk at 2–3 weeks of age and not all the litter are necessarily affected (Csiza *et al.*, 1972). Affected cats show symmetrical ataxia, a characteristic hypermetria, incoordination and often intention tremors. These signs persist for life. Nevertheless, the kittens may learn to compensate and continue to thrive in other respects.

CLINICAL SIGNS

The severity of the disease varies considerably in susceptible individuals, ranging from either a subclinical infection or a mild transient fever and leucopenia to a severe syndrome where the animal may be found dead. In general, the disease tends to be more severe in young kittens.

In the typical case, however, the incubation period is approximately 2–10 days, and the first signs of illness are lethargy, fever and anorexia with apparent thirst, but refusal to drink. Affected cats generally vomit, but diarrhoea is less common, particularly in the early stages (Carpenter, 1971; Greene & Scott, 1990). Abdominal palpation reveals gas and fluid-filled intestines, and may elicit pain. After 2–3 days, if death has not already occurred, signs are variable. There may be fever or a subnormal temperature, the latter carrying a grave prognosis. Profuse watery diarrhoea or dysentery may occur and there is severe dehydration and electrolyte imbalance.

The mortality rate in the natural disease varies from 25 to 75% (Gillespie & Scott, 1973). Most fatalities occur within 3–5 days of the first signs of illness, and are probably due to overwhelming bacterial infection, dehydration and electrolyte imbalance. Animals that recover generally take several weeks to regain condition, and in the meantime may be prone to a variety of secondary infections as a result of their panleucopenia. Erythrocytopoiesis appears to remain unaltered during FP (Larsen *et al.*, 1976). In any case the longer surviving red blood cell makes its numbers less susceptible than the white cell series to the effects of the bone marrow suppression: nevertheless, anaemia may develop in cats ill for longer than 10 days, especially if there is serious intestinal bleeding.

DIAGNOSIS

A presumptive diagnosis may be made on the basis of the clinical and vaccination history, and presenting clinical signs; often the cat has had some recent exposure to a possible source of infection, for example a visit to a boarding cattery, but this is not necessarily so. Diagnosis can usually be confirmed in the acute stages of the disease by a blood smear, which can easily be obtained by an ear prick, stained with Giemsa or methylene blue, and is nearly devoid of leucocytes. Laboratory haematology usually shows a white blood count of below $7 \times 10^9/l$ and often below $2 \times 10^9/l$, although if the cat survives for over a week or so after the onset of clinical signs, it may start to show a neutrophilia with a left shift.

In fatal cases, the characteristic gross pathological findings may be used to aid diagnosis: samples of small intestine (jejunum and ileum), mesenteric lymph node and spleen may also be sent in formal saline for histopathology. Specialist diagnostic virology laboratories can also be used to confirm the diagnosis, although, depending on the technique used by the laboratory, a negative result does not necessarily rule out the disease. From the live animal, an oropharyngeal swab in transport media, a faeces sample, and acute and convalescent sera should be sent, and from a freshly dead cat, samples of spleen, mesenteric lymph node, ileum and faeces should suffice.

A number of other syndromes may be confused with feline panleucopenia (Carpenter, 1971; Cotter, 1979). These include the presence of intestinal foreign bodies, especially if associated with obstruction or with infection; acute bacterial septicaemia, not necessarily secondary to FP; toxoplasmosis; poisoning; and occasionally lymphosarcoma. A similar condition but associated with feline leukaemia virus infection has also been described.

TREATMENT

Treatment should be supportive whilst the cat's own natural defence mechanisms overcome the virus, and should be aimed specifically at combating the propensity for secondary bacterial infection, dehydration and electrolyte imbalance. Because of vomiting, and impairment of both gut absorption and the animal's immune response, a parenteral, bactericidal, broad-spectrum antibiotic should be given (Cotter, 1980), such as ampicillin or cephalosporin.

Fluid therapy is also essential; in some cases subcutaneous fluids may be adequate, but where the animal is severely depressed and dehydrated and the circulation collapsed, an intravenous drip may be necessary. Suitable fluids include 5% dextrose saline, lactated Ringer's solution and other more complex balanced electrolyte solutions. The use of whole blood has been advocated, although its use is equivocal since patients are rarely anaemic or thrombocytopenic. Nevertheless, it may be useful in the very early stages of the disease (less than 5 days), as a means of giving hyperimmune serum, i.e. antibody from a recovered cat, or one that has been vaccinated several times, particularly with a live vaccine. Care should be taken, however, since, rarely, disseminated intravascular coagulation may occur with FP (Greene & Scott, 1990).

Antiemetics (e.g. metoclopromide, Chapter 8) may be useful in reducing fluid loss, but the use of anticholinergic drugs (e.g. atropine) is not advisable because they may cause sustained ileus of the bowel (Greene & Scott, 1990). Oral fluids and liquidized foods may be given in the later stages of the disease when gastrointestinal signs have diminished. Low doses of oral or parenteral diazepam can be used just before feeding to stimulate appetite. Vitamin supplements may also be beneficial, particularly the B vitamin complex.

Good nursing care and attention is also essential, and unless the cat requires hospital intensive care, this is best done at home by the owner in a warm, clean, quiet environment. Many cats respond favourably to such attention and so sustain the will to live. Hospital intensive care requires isolation facilities and scrupulous attention to hygiene, bearing in mind the marked resistance of the virus to the environment and to many common disinfectants.

‹EPIDEMIOLOGY

FP is a highly infectious disease and in cat populations which are predominantly unvaccinated, it will almost certainly be endemic. Although most ages may be affected, it is primarily a disease of young kittens who succumb when their maternal antibody has waned. Natural exposure then results in most cases in a lifelong immunity to the disease. Although the morbidity of the disease in a susceptible population will often approach 100%, not all affected cats will necessarily show severe clinical signs; in many cases the disease will only be mild or subclinical. In some areas in the USA, the disease appears to have a seasonal incidence with peaks occurring in the summer and autumn coincident with the appearance of large numbers of susceptible kittens as a result of a seasonal pattern to the birth rate (Gillespie & Scott, 1973; Reif, 1976).

FP virus is perpetuated in the cat population in three main ways. First, it is perpetuated in the cat by contact spread from acutely infected clinical cases to susceptible cats, but only if there is a sufficient number of susceptible animals in the population and sufficient opportunity for contact between them. Virus is shed in large quantities in infected animals, mainly in faeces, but it is also present in saliva, urine, vomitus and blood. It should also be remembered that in pregnant queens transplacental infection may occur.

Secondly, the virus can persist in the recovered cat because of the existence of immune carriers. The recovered clinical case may harbour virus in its tissues for several months, and in the tissues of ataxic kittens and in the faeces of mink, the virus has been shown to persist for up to a year (Bouillant & Hanson, 1965; Csiza *et al.*, 1971c). However, persistence of virus in these immune carriers is probably not particularly important — far more significant in the epidemiology of the disease

is the remarkable ability of the virus to survive in the environment (see above).

Thus once one clinical case has occurred, the environment — e.g. cages, food dishes, litter trays and the clothing of personnel — will be heavily contaminated from the infected discharges, and unless adequate disinfection procedures are carried out (see above), any cat or kitten with inadequate immunity is a good target for infection.

Finally, biting and flying insects such as fleas have also been suspected of mechanically transmitting the agent, but it seems unlikely that this plays a significant role in the epidemiology of the disease. Similarly, although FP may occur in other species, it seems highly unlikely that this will have a significant impact on the epidemiology of the disease in the domestic cat.

VACCINATION AND CONTROL

Vaccination against feline panleucopenia has been extremely successful, where it has been carried out. There is only one serotype of the virus, the virus is highly immunogenic and both natural and vaccine-induced immunity is high and long-lived.

Both modified live (attenuated) and inactivated (killed) systemic vaccines are available, and although antibody titres are generally lower with inactivated vaccines, both types confer entirely adequate immunity. Modified live vaccines probably induce a more rapid onset of protection, and are perhaps more likely to be able to overcome low levels of maternally derived antibody (MDA), although some inactivated products may also be capable of this, depending for example on their antigenic mass and the nature of the adjuvant. Inactivated vaccines have the advantage that they may be administered safely to pregnant queens; modified live vaccines are contraindicated in this situation since FP virus can cross the placenta and induce cerebellar hypoplasia in kittens. In addition inactivated vaccines are free from the, albeit small, risk of contamination by extraneous agents or of reversion to virulence. Recently, problems with one modified live vaccine have been reported in particular breeds of cats under certain conditions (Carwardine, 1990), but in general such vaccines appear to be perfectly safe, having been used widely for many years.

Most cats of breeding age have acquired either a natural or vaccine-induced immunity to the disease, and this immunity is passed on via the colostrum from queens to their kittens. This maternally derived immunity in kittens subsequently declines at a uniform rate (with a half-life of 9.5 days), but whilst present, is capable of interfering with the kitten's vaccination programme. The optimum age for initial vaccination of kittens, therefore, should be as soon as possible after their passive antibody has waned. Unfortunately, as with canine parvovirus infection, low levels of MDA may interfere with vaccination, but may not protect against infection. Such a potential immunity gap is not usually such a problem in the cat disease, however, possibly because of lower levels of challenge virus in the environment.

As there is a high degree of correlation between antibody titres in the queens and MDA levels in kittens, normographs have been used to predict the optimum age of vaccination of an individual litter (Scott *et al.*, 1970). However, not all kittens will suckle to the sane extent, and therefore the amount of colostrum-derived antibody in an individual kitten may vary. More important, in feline panleucopenia it has been found that such an approach is not usually necessary. In most breeding colonies, where this might be applied, the balance between the virus and host immunity is in a reasonably steady state because of a long tradition of vaccination coupled with an absence of clinical disease.

In most kittens born to mothers with moderate titres acquired through vaccination, MDA has declined to non-interfering levels by 8–12 weeks of age. Thus from 12 weeks of age onwards, for most vaccines one dose of vaccine is usually sufficient. Where MDA is likely to be unusually high (for example, if the queen was known to have had the disease or was vaccinated with live virus just before or during pregnancy) an extra dose should be give at 16 weeks. In kittens less than 12 weeks of age, additional doses at 2–4-week intervals are

required, ensuring the last dose is at 12 weeks of age or over. In rare circumstances where MDA is thought to be inadequate (i.e. queen never vaccinated or exposed, or kittens deprived of colostrum) and there is the likelihood of exposure, vaccination may be carried out from the age of 6 weeks onwards, or exceptionally, 4 weeks, with additional doses given as above. In this age of kitten, an inactivated vaccine should be used.

The duration of immunity following either the natural disease or vaccination is thought to be very long. In the natural disease, Scott *et al.* (1970) have shown that recovered animals possess very high serum neutralizing antibody titres, whereas those vaccinated with attenuated vaccines have more moderate titres which, nevertheless, in cats kept in strict isolation, have been shown to persist for at least 4 years (O'Reilly & Hitchcock, 1976). Titres in cats vaccinated with inactivated vaccines are slightly lower, but have similarly been shown to persist for over 1 year (Bittle *et al.*, 1970; Davis *et al.*, 1970). Undoubtedly too, in the natural situation there is much natural boosting of immunity, although this should not be relied upon to confer adequate long-term protection, particularly in isolated household pets. On balance, it is probably sensible to advocate an initial booster at 1 year of age, followed by further doses at 1–2-yearly intervals, depending on the type of vaccine used and the likelihood of exposure, for example, entry into a boarding cattery.

A regular vaccination programme in adults and kittens, as outlined above, should ensure a good level of protection in most animals. Nevertheless, in open colonies and even in well-controlled colony situations, breakdowns may occur. For example, there may be lapses in vaccination schedules, intercurrent disease, immunological incompetence or overwhelming infection. Kittens may be unprotected because they have just lost their passive immunity, or because they were vaccinated whilst passive antibody was still present at interfering levels.

Once one clinical case has occurred, the environment will be heavily contaminated, and this may then lead to further cases. Adequate disinfection (see earlier) of all contaminated pens,

bedding, feeding and cleaning utensils, and the hands and clothing of personnel is essential. Booster vaccinations should be given to all cats, and killed vaccine given to any pregnant queens. Following adequate disinfection, a cat vaccinated 2 weeks previously may safely be introduced onto the premises almost immediately. If disinfection is difficult, or the replacement kitten is too young for the vaccination course to be completed, it is advisable to wait for several months or to confine the cat to different quarters.

With new entrants to a cattery, vaccination should have been completed at least 2 weeks before entry, and the cat quarantined for at least 2 weeks on arrival. In boarding catteries, all cats should be housed individually, with their own equipment and utensils, and any animals with suspect clinical signs kept in strict isolation and fed last. Other measures designed to minimize the spread of disease in such situations are described in Chapter 14.

REFERENCES

Bittle J.L., Emrich S.A. & Gauker F.B. (1970) Safety and efficacy of an inactivated tissue culture vaccine for feline panleucopenia. *J. Am. Vet. Med. Ass.* **157**, 2052.

Bouillant A. & Hanson R.P. (1965) Epizootiology of mink enteritis: III. carrier state in mink. *Can. J. Comp. Med. Vet. Sci.* **29**, 183.

Carpenter J.L. (1971) Feline panleucopenia: clinical signs and differential diagnosis. *J. Am. Vet. Med. Ass.* **158**, 857.

Carwardine P.C. (1990) Adverse reactions to vaccine. *Vet. Rec.* **127**, 243.

Cotter S.M. (1979) Some uncommon diseases in the cat. *Proc. Am. Anim. Hosp. Ass.*, pp. 115–7.

Cotter S.M. (1980) Feline panleucopenia. In Kirk R.W. (ed) *Current Veterinary Therapy VII. Small animal practice.* W.B. Saunders, Philadelphia, pp. 1286–8.

Csiza C.K., Scott F.W., De Lahunta A. & Gillespie J.H. (1971a) Pathogenesis of feline panleucopenia virus in susceptible newborn kittens, I. Clinical signs, haematology, serology, and virology. *Infect. Immun.* **3**, 833.

Csiza C.K., Scott F.W., De Lahunta A. & Gillespie J.H. (1971b) Pathogenesis of feline panleucopenia virus in susceptible newborn kittens. II. Pathology and immunofluorescence. *Infect. Immun.* **3**, 838.

Csiza C.K., Scott F.W., De Lahunta A. & Gillespie J.H. (1971c) Immune carrier state of feline panleucopenia virus-infected cats. *Am. J. Vet. Res.* **32**, 419.

Csiza C.K., De Lahunta A., Scott F.W. & Gillespie J.H. (1972) Spontaneous feline 'ataxia'. *Cornell Vet.* **62**, 300.

Davis E.V., Gregory G.G. & Beckenhauer W.H. (1970) Infectious feline panleucopenia – a tissue culture origin formalin-inactivated vaccine. *Vet. Med. Small Anim. Clin.* **65**, 237.

Gillespie J.H. & Scott F.W. (1973) Feline viral infections II. Feline panleucopenia (FPL) infection. *Adv. Vet. Sci. Comp. Med.* **17**, 164.

Greene C.E. & Scott F.W. (1990) Feline panleucopenia. In Greene C.E. (ed) *Infectious Diseases of the Dog and Cat.* W.B. Saunders, Philadelphia, pp. 291–9.

Hosokawa S., Ichijo S. & Goto H. (1987) Clinical, hematological and pathological findings in specific pathogen-free cats experimentally infected with feline panleucopenia virus. *Jap. J. Vet. Sci.* **49**, 43–50.

Johnson R.H. (1964) Isolation of a virus from a condition simulating feline panleucopenia in a leopard. *Vet. Rec.* **76**, 1008.

Johnson R.H. (1966) Feline panleucopenia virus III. Some properties compared to a feline herpes virus. *Res. Vet. Sci.* **7**, 112.

Johnson R.H. (1969) Feline panleucopenia. *Vet. Rec.* **84**, 338.

Kahn D.E. (1978) Pathogenesis of feline panleucopenia. *J. Am. Vet. Med. Ass.* **173**, 628.

Kilham L., Margolis G. & Colby E.D. (1967) Congenital infections of cats and ferrets by feline panleucopenia virus manifested by cerebellar hypoplasia. *Lab. Invest.* **17**, 465.

Langheinrich K.A. & Nielsen S.W. (1971) Histopathology of feline panleucopenia: a report of 65 cases. *J. Am. Vet. Med. Ass.* **158**, 863.

Larsen S., Flagstad A. & Aalback B. (1976) Experimental feline panleucopenia in the conventional cat. *Vet. Pathol.* **13**, 216.

O'Reilly K.J. & Hitchcock L.M. (1976) Persistence of antibody to feline panleucopenia induced by a modified live virus vaccine. *J. Small Anim. Pract.* **17**, 549.

Parrish C.R., Carmichael L.E. & Antczak D.F. (1982) Antigenic relationships between canine parvovirus type 2, feline panleucopenia virus and mink enteritis virus using conventional antisera and monoclonal antibodies. *Arch. Virol.* **72**, 267–78.

Parrish C.R., O'Connell P.H., Evermann J.F. & Carmichael L.E. (1985) Natural variation of canine parvovirus. *Science* **230**, 1046–8.

Pollock R.V.H. (1984) The parvoviruses. Part 1. Feline panleucopenia virus and mink enteritis virus. *Compend. Cont. Educ. Pract. Vet.* **6**, 227–41.

Povey R.C. (1973) Feline panleucopenia – which vaccine? *J. Small Anim. Pract.* **14**, 399.

Povey R.C. (1976) Viral diseases of cats: current concepts. *Vet. Rec.* **98**, 293.

Reif J.S. (1976) Seasonality, natality and herd immunity in feline panleucopenia. *Am. J. Epid.* **103**, 81.

Rohovsky M.W. & Griesemer R.A. (1967) Experimental feline infectious enteritis in the germ-free cat. *Path. Vet.* **4**, 391.

Scott F.W. (1971) Comments on feline panleucopenia biologics. *J. Am. J. Vet. Med. Ass.* **158**, 910.

Scott F.W. (1980) Virucidal disinfectants and feline viruses. *Am. Vet. Res.* **41**, 410.

Scott F.W. (1987) Viral diseases. Panleucopenia. In Holzworth J. (ed) *Diseases of the Cat: Medicine and Surgery*. W.B. Saunders, Philadelphia, pp. 182–93.

Scott F.W., Csiza C.K., & Gillespie J.H. (1970) Maternally derived immunity to feline panleucopenia. *J. Am. Vet. Med. Ass.* **156**, 439.

Tratschin J-D., McMaster G.K., Kronauer G. & Siegl G. (1982) Canine parvo virus: relationship to wild-type and vaccine strains of feline panleucopenia virus and mink enteritis virus. *J. Gen. Virol.* **61**, 33.

Chapter 14 / Viral-Induced
Upper Respiratory Tract Disease

R. M. GASKELL AND S. DAWSON

INTRODUCTION

Respiratory disease has always been a major problem in feline medicine. This chapter deals with feline viral upper respiratory tract (URT) disease, the syndrome which is also commonly known as 'cat flu'. Despite the advent of vaccination in the mid-1970s, viral-induced respiratory disease in cats still commonly occurs, although vaccination has reduced the overall severity of the condition seen.

AETIOLOGY

The majority of cases of infectious respiratory disease in cats are caused by one of two viruses: feline viral rhinotracheitis virus (feline herpesvirus 1 (FHV1)) and feline calicivirus (FCV) (Table 14.1). Both viruses occur worldwide and have traditionally been isolated in approximately equal frequency from cases of the disease. Recently, however, FCV has been isolated more frequently than FHV 1 (Knowles *et al.*, 1989; Harbour *et al.*, 1991). This may be explained in part by the antigenic diversity amongst FCV isolates compared to the one serotype of feline herpesvirus, and the consequent relative efficacy of the two vaccines. FHV 1 is probably a more significant pathogen to the cat when it occurs, however, as the disease it induces is generally more severe.

Other agents implicated in the syndrome include a feline strain of *Chlamydia psittaci*, feline reovirus, cowpox virus and possibly feline infectious peritonitis virus (feline coronavirus), and bacteria and mycoplasmas (Table 14.1).

Feline *C. psittaci* has been identified as a significant cause of disease problems where the predominant clinical sign is a persistent conjunctivitis; mild respiratory signs may also sometimes be present. Feline reovirus has long been cited as a possible cause of mild conjunctival and respiratory disease in cats, on the basis of some experimental work done in the USA a number of years ago. Its importance in the field has never been established, however, and in recent virological studies we have found no evidence of infection in over 150 conjunctival samples from cats with conjunctivitis.

Other agents, such as cowpox virus and feline coronavirus, have only peripheral or suspected involvement with feline respiratory disease. Cowpox virus infection is cats primarily causes skin lesions, but occasional respiratory or ocular signs may also be seen. Feline infectious peritonitis virus is probably mainly initially an enteric pathogen, but primary respiratory signs have also been suggested by some.

Bacteria, such as staphylococci, β-haemolytic streptococci, *Pasteurella* spp. and coliforms, and mycoplasmas, have been implicated in feline respiratory disease, although their main importance is probably as secondary invaders following damage to the respiratory mucosa by a primary viral agent. Nevertheless, a more primary role for mycoplasmas has been suggested by some, particularly for conjunctivitis. The importance of *Bordetella bronchiseptica*, which has been isolated from cats with respiratory disease in laboratory colonies, has yet to be determined (Fisk & Soave, 1973). Recently, it has also been associated with

Table 14.1 Causes and significance of infectious respiratory disease in the cat.

Agents	Significance
Feline viral rhinotracheitis virus (feline herpesvirus 1)	Approximately 40% of cases. Tends to be more severe
Feline calicivirus	Approximately 40% of cases, possibly more. Usually mild
Feline *Chlamydia psittaci*	Approximately 30% of cases of persistent conjunctivitis
Feline reovirus	Mild disease experimentally
Cowpox virus	Occasional respiratory/ocular signs but other, skin signs also present
Feline infectious peritonitis virus (feline coronavirus)	Most likely a primary, enteric pathogen, but respiratory signs also suggested by some
Bordetella bronchiseptica	Some laboratory and field colonies. Clinical significance?
Other bacteria e.g. *Staphylococcus*, *Streptococcus* and *Pasteurella* spp.; coliforms, mycoplasmas	Mainly secondary invaders

Possibly primary, mainly secondary infection |

severe respiratory signs and deaths in kittens in the field (Willoughby *et al.*, 1991). Whether or not it is a common primary or secondary pathogen in cats is still unclear.

In addition to the above agents, concurrent infection with known immunosuppressive agents such as feline leukaemia virus and feline immunodeficiency virus (Chapters 15 and 16) should be considered (see below). Not only might the primary viral infection be exacerbated by such agents, but the effects of secondary bacterial infection may also be enhanced.

It should also be remembered that many of these pathogens are likely to coexist. In general, they are highly infectious and thrive in situations where cats are brought together, for example for breeding, boarding and showing. Moreover, relatively little work has been done on respiratory diseases of cats compared to some other species, and it is quite possible that other pathogens may be discovered.

This chapter deals primarily with the two major viral respiratory diseases of cats, feline viral rhinotracheitis (FHV 1 infection) and feline calicivirus infection. Subsequent chapters give more detailed information on feline coronavirus (Chapter 17), feline poxvirus (Chapter 18), feline reovirus (Chapter 20), feline *C. psittaci* (Chapter 21) and feline mycoplasmal infections (Chapter 23).

Feline herpesvirus 1 (FHV 1)

FHV 1 is a typical herpesvirus, containing double-stranded DNA, and with a glycoprotein-lipid envelope. Its morphological, physicochemical, cultural and other properties have beeen reviewed elsewhere (Crandell, 1973; Povey, 1979; Gaskell, 1988).

As with many herpesviruses, FHV 1 is comparatively labile. In the external environment, it will probably survive in secretions for only up to 18 hours in a damp environment and up to 12 hours in a dry environment (Povey & Johnson, 1970) and it is also relatively unstable as an aerosol (Donaldson & Ferris, 1976). Because of its lipoprotein envelope, it is highly susceptible to the effects of heat, acids and to all common disinfectants (Scott, 1980). A useful disinfectant, also recommended for other feline viruses, is bleach diluted 1 in 32 in water with washing-up liquid.

All isolates of the virus examined so far appear to constitute one serotype on the basis of conventional serological cross-neutralization tests. Isolates also appear to be very similar when examined by restriction enzyme analysis of the viral DNA, although some minor differences may be detected with this technique (Herrmann *et al.*, 1984; Rota *et al.*, 1986). This high degree of similarity between strains is in general reflected in the relatively uniform pathogenicity of isolates. Nevertheless, strains of modified virulence do exist, having been produced in recent years for vaccines. In addition, although no controlled comparisons with different isolates have been done, some isolates do appear to be associated with more severe disease.

FHV 1 appears to be unrelated antigenically to several herpesviruses tested from other species, and infection appears to be confined to members of the cat family. However, one group of investigators has isolated herpesviruses indistinguishable from FHV 1 from dogs with diarrhoea (Evermann *et al.*, 1982), although the clinical and epidemiological significance of the finding is unclear.

Feline calicivirus (FCV)

FCV is a small, unenveloped single-stranded RNA virus, a member of the calicivirus family. These viruses show characteristic cup-like depressions on their surfaces from which the name 'calicivirus' is derived. As far as is known, FCV only infects members of the Felidae, although caliciviruses antigenically similar to FCV have been recovered from dogs (Evermann *et al.*, 1981). Properties of the virus have been reviewed by Gillespie and Scott (1973) and of caliciviruses in general by Studdert (1978).

Although they are both relatively short-lived in the external environment, the survival time of FCV is slightly longer than that of FHV 1. It may survive for up to 1 week, or possibly slightly longer if the environment is damp (Povey & Johnson, 1970). The virus is generally more resistant to low pH than FHV 1, and is not as susceptible to so many disinfectants (Scott, 1980); nevertheless, the bleach/detergent solution recommended for use with FHV 1 should also be effective for FCV.

A number of different strains of feline calicivirus exist, which may differ both in antigenicity and pathogenicity. However, most strains so far examined are quite closely related and probably constitute one serotype (Povey, 1974; Kalunda *et al.*, 1975). Nevertheless, there is still antigenic variation within the group, and although clinically there is a reasonable level of cross-protection between the majority of these variants, cats may still be sequentially infected with some of the strains (Povey & Ingersoll, 1975; Pedersen et al., 1983; Knowles *et al.*, 1990).

Strains selected for use in vaccines are those whose antigenic specificity is considered broad enough to encompass most of the antigenic variations seen in the remainder of the group. Thus F9, which was shown to be broadly cross-reactive in the mid-1970s has been widely used as a vaccine virus. It still appears to be similarly cross-reactive, neutralizing at least 50% of more recent field isolates (Kalunda *et al.*, 1975; Knowles *et al.*, 1990).

Nevertheless, some strains of FCV occur which current vaccines do not appear to protect against (Pedersen *et al.*, 1983) and widespread use of vaccines based predominantly on one strain may encourage selection for these. Indeed, the apparent recent increase in isolation rate of FCV compared to FHV 1 may be a reflection of this. Thus future vaccines may need to incorporate several complementary, cross-protective isolates in order to ensure more complete protection against disease, and it may also be necessary to monitor the predominant antigenic types of feline calicivirus which, at any one time, are occurring in the field. There is already some evidence that there has been a change in the antigenic spectrum of feline caliciviruses isolated recently in the UK, compared to 15 or more years ago (Knowles *et al.*, 1990).

PATHOGENESIS AND PATHOLOGY

Feline herpesvirus infection

The natural route of infection by FHV 1 is almost certainly intranasal, oral or conjunctival, though experimentally other routes have been investigated. In pregnant queens, for example, intravaginal instillation of virus has led to vaginitis and congenitally infected kittens (Bittle & Peckham, 1971) and intravenous inoculation has led to transplacental infection and abortion (Hoover & Griesemer, 1971a).

In the typical respiratory infection, however, virus replication takes place predominantly in the mucosae of the nasal septum, turbinates, nasopharynx and tonsils; other tissues including conjunctivae, mandibular lymph nodes and upper trachea are also often involved (Gaskell & Povey, 1979b; Nasisse *et al.*, 1989). Virus shedding may be detected in nasal and oropharyngeal secretions as early as 24 hours after inoculation, and generally persists for 1–3 weeks. A viraemia, and other evidence of virus generalization, for example the presence of virus in visceral tissues, has only occasionally been reported. FHV 1 viraemia appears to be associated with peripheral blood leucocytes (Tham & Studdert, 1987a).

Pathological findings have been reviewed in detail elsewhere (Crandell, 1973; Povey, 1979). Briefly, replication of the virus in the epithelium, as shown by the presence of intranuclear inclusion bodies, leads to areas of multifocal epithelial necrosis with neutrophilic infiltration and exudation with fibrin. Resolution is generally slow, but by 2–3 weeks, epithelial regeneration with some squamous cell metaplasia, and sometimes hypertrophy, may be seen. The disease is apparently not dependent upon the presence of microbial flora, for it has been reproduced experimentally in germ-free cats (Hoover *et al.*, 1970). Nevertheless, it is likely that the effects of the disease may be enhanced by secondary invasion by bacteria.

Feline calicivirus infection

The natural routes of infection are similar to those described for FHV 1 infection. The various strains of FCV differ in their tissue tropisms and pathogenicity, however. Virus replication occurs mainly in the oral cavity and upper respiratory tract tissues (Wardley & Povey, 1977a), but some strains have an apparent predilection for the lung (Kahn & Gillespie, 1971). Virus may also sometimes be found in visceral tissues and faeces, and also occasionally in urine. In addition, viral antigen has been detected within macrophages in joints (Bennett *et al.*, 1989; Dawson, 1991), but the significance of this in the pathogenesis of the lameness syndrome sometimes seen following FCV infection is unknown.

Lingual and palatine ulcers are usually a prominent pathological feature of FCV infection. They begin as vesicles which subsequently rupture, with necrosis of the overlying epithelium and infiltration by neutrophils at the periphery and base. Pulmonary lesions appear to result from an initial focal alveolitis, which leads to areas of acute exudative pneumonia, and then to the development of a proliferative, interstitial pneumonia (Love, 1975; Ormerod *et al.*, 1979). These workers have also suggested that although primary interstitial pneumonia can occur in FCV infection, it may have been overemphasized in the past as a result of experimental studies using aerosols, rather than the more natural intranasal route of infection.

CLINICAL SIGNS

Feline herpesvirus infection

FHV 1 infection is generally a severe upper respiratory disease particularly in young, susceptible animals (Crandell *et al.*, 1961). The incubation period is usually 2–6 days, but may be longer. Experimentally, it has been shown that increasing virus dosage is significantly correlated with a shortening of the incubation period and to some extent with the severity of clinical signs (Gaskell & Povey, 1979a), but in general the syndrome is reasonably uniform.

Early signs of the disease include depression, marked sneezing, inappetence and pyrexia, followed rapidly by serous ocular and nasal discharges; sometimes in the early stages there is excessive salivation and drooling. Conjunctivitis usually develops, and as the disease progresses, the ocular and nasal discharges gradually turn mucopurulent (Plate 14.1). Dyspnoea and coughing may develop and sometimes there may be a recurrence of the pyrexia. A leucocytosis with a left shift is present throughout the course of the disease.

Other signs seen less commonly include tongue ulcers (Karpas & Routledge, 1968), ulcerative and interstitial keratitis (Bistner *et al.*, 1971) and a primary viral pneumonia (Love, 1971); generalized disease may also occasionally occur, particularly in younger or immunosuppressed animals (Spradbrow *et al.*, 1971; Shields & Gaskin, 1977; Van Pelt & Crandell, 1987). These and other, rarer, manifestations such as skin ulcers and nervous signs have been reviewed by Gaskell and Wardley (1978). It is probable that abortions, sometimes associated with the respiratory form of FHV 1 infection, are secondary to the severe debilitating respiratory infection rather than to a direct effect of the virus itself (Hoover & Griesemer, 1971a).

Although it may be a distressing disease, the mortality rate is not usually high, except sometimes in very young kittens or immunosuppressed animals. Fatalities most often result from dehydration, and also secondary bacterial infection, which may lead to bronchopneumonia. Signs generally resolve within 10–20 days, but in some cats the severe necrosis and ulceration of the mucous membranes seen in the acute phase of the disease may lead to permanently damaged areas of mucosae, prone to recurrent microbial infection. In the turbinate region there may be necrosis and resorption of the underlying bone itself. A predilection of the virus for the growth regions of the skeleton, including the turbinates, has also been shown experimentally following intravenous inoculation of young kittens (Hoover & Griesemer, 1971b). Thus cats may be left with chronic rhinitis or sinusitis, and some may show chronic conjunctivitis. In some cases, persistent or recurrent signs may follow recrudescence of viral shedding in carrier cats.

Feline calicivirus infection

FCV infection is typically milder than FHV 1 infection, although the large number of strains of feline calicivirus can cause a spectrum of disease, ranging from a more severe syndrome similar to that seen with FHV 1 infection to a subclinical infection (Povey & Hale, 1974; Hoover & Kahn, 1975). However, in general, there are certain features of FCV infection which may be used to differentiate it from FHV 1 infection (Table 14.2). Mouth ulceration is a frequent and characteristic feature of the disease and indeed in some cases it may be the only clinical sign (Plate 14.2). Ulcers may occur on the tongue, hard palate, lips and on the nostrils, particularly in the median cleft. Lingual ulcers usually begin as vesicles, which subsequently rupture.

General malaise is usually less marked than in FHV 1 infection and sneezing, conjunctivitis, and ocular and nasal secretions are not as prominent. Keratitis does not occur. Excessive drooling of saliva is not a feature of the disease, although some cats with severe ulcers may show slight wetness around the mouth. There may be dyspnoea and other signs associated with pneumonia in cats infected with more virulent strains of FCV.

Some strains of FCV cause pyrexia, joint and muscle pain and lameness with or without associated signs of oral/respiratory disease (Studdert *et al.*, 1970; Pedersen *et al.*, 1983; Dawson, 1991). In some cases, the syndrome has been reported to occur after vaccination, though the significance of this is as yet unclear (see below). The pathogenesis of the lameness is not understood, though recently some evidence of viral localization to the joints and immune complex formation has been found in experimentally infected cats (Bennett *et al.*, 1989; Dawson, 1991). Most cases resolve spontaneously, although possible long-term effects on the joints (e.g. with respect to chronic polyarthritis) are unknown (Chapter 3). Another possible pathogenic role for FCV is in

Table 14.2 Comparison of the relative importance of individual clinical signs seen in the major respiratory infections of cats.

Clinical signs	FHV infection	FCV infection*	Feline *Chlamydia psittaci* infection
General malaise	+++	+	+
Sneezing	+++	+	+
Hypersalivation	++	−	−
Conjunctivitis	++	++	+++†
Ocular discharge	+++	++	+++
Nasal discharge	+++	++	+
Oral ulceration	+	+++	−
Keratitis	+	−	−
Primary pneumonia	(+)	+	+/−
Limping	−	+	−

* Strain variation occurs.
† Often persistent.
(+) Rare, but has been reported.
+/− Lesions may be present, but not usually seen clinically.

chronic gingivitis/stomatitis. Approximately 85% of affected cats are shedding FCV from the oropharynx, compared to 20% or less of controls (Thompson *et al.*, 1984; Knowles *et al.*, 1989). Whether this is causal in the disease is not yet known. Other factors, for example FIV (Chapter 16), may also be involved; approximately 80% of affected cats in the more recent UK study also had antibody to FIV.

Recently, in experimental co-infection studies with FIV and FCV we have observed that cats previously infected with FIV tended to experience more widespread acute disease following FCV challenge, compared to FCV alone, though chronic stomatitis was not induced (Dawson *et al.*, 1991). Significantly more of the FIV-infected cats remained as FCV carriers (see below), and for longer, compared to FCV alone. This may in part explain the apparent association of these two viruses in the field in cases of chronic stomatitis, but the pathogenesis of the syndrome is still unclear.

DIAGNOSIS

To a large extent FHV 1 infection and FCV infection may be distinguished on presenting clinical signs. Table 14.2 summarizes the essential fea-

tures of each condition and includes feline *Chlamydia psittaci* infection as a differential. In general, a more severe syndrome, with marked sneezing and copious ocular and nasal discharges, might suggest FHV 1 infection. If milder upper respiratory and ocular signs are present, however, and especially if there is also oral or nasal ulceration, then it is more likely to be FCV infection. Feline *C. psittaci* infection should always be suspected if the major presenting sign is persistent or recurrent conjunctivitis, particularly in colonies that have been fully vaccinated against the respiratory viruses.

Apart from differences between virus strains and infecting dosages, other factors may also influence the host's response to infection, making differentiation on clinical grounds alone problematical. Factors such as age, genotype, general health and nutritional status, may account for some individual variation in response. Intercurrent disease, particularly with feline leukaemia virus or feline immunodeficiency virus, may predispose the cat to a more severe syndrome. Differences in microbial flora may also affect the course of the disease, as discussed previously: the more severe cases seem to be associated with upper respiratory populations of *Bordetella bronchiseptica* (Willoughby *et al.*, 1991), β-haemolytic streptococci, haemolytic staphylococci and *Pasteurella multocida* (Povey & Johnson, 1970). Finally, of course, clinical signs will be reduced or absent in cats that are wholly or partially immune, either from vaccination, previous exposure or from the presence of maternally derived antibody.

In most circumstances accurate diagnosis is not essential unless specific advice on control in a colony situation is required, or unless antiviral drugs become widely used. Diagnosis may be confirmed by isolation of the agent in feline cell cultures. Oropharyngeal swabs should be taken, placed in appropriate transport media, and sent by first-class post to a specialist laboratory. Ideally, samples should be taken within 1 week of the onset of clinical signs. In cases where persistent or recurrent conjunctivitis is the predominant sign, swabs should also be taken for chlamydia isolation (see Chapter 21). In unvaccinated cats serology may be helpful in establishing a diagnosis of chlamydia infection, but it is generally not helpful for the respiratory viruses becaue of the more widespread immunity from vaccination.

When virus is successfully isolated from a case of acute URT infection, it is reasonable to assume that in the majority of cats it is the actual cause of the disease. However, particularly for FCV, the results may sometimes be equivocal, because of the large percentage of apparently healthy cats that also appear to carry the virus (see below).

Bacterial culture and sensitivity testing is important in cases which fail to respond to an initial course of antibiotics, and in some cases of chronic rhinitis. The most valuable material is obtained from the nasal chambers, after the nares have been cleaned with antiseptic solution. Chronic rhinitis classically improves, albeit temporarily, after a prolonged course of antibiotics; failure to do so might suggest concurrent FIV or FeLV infection or other, much rarer diagnoses such as nasal mycoses or neoplasia (see Chapter 6).

TREATMENT

At present no antiviral drugs are in widespread use to control FHV 1 infection and FCV infection. However, 5-iododeoxyuridine (IUdR) has been used in cases of ulcerative keratitis associated with FHV 1 infection, and there are anti-herpesvirus drugs that have been used successfully in other species that may prove useful in FHV 1 infection. IUdR therapy should be given in the form of 0.1% ophthalmic solution 4–6 times daily for 3–5 days.

The main emphasis in treatment is the use of broad-spectrum antibiotics (such as ampicillin, potentiated sulphonamide and oxytetracycline) to help control secondary bacterial infection and to try and prevent chronic sequelae. Since swallowing may be painful, antibiotics may be given by paediatric syrups or long-acting injections. Animals should be re-examined after 4–5 days, and antibiotics continued if necessary. If there is no improvement after a week of treatment, bacterial culture and sensitivity testing should be performed.

Multivitamin supportive therapy (vitamins A, B, C, as oral drops, and vitamin B_{12}) may also be helpful, but corticosteroids are contraindicated because they retard the healing process and may potentiate the virus infection.

Good nursing care is essential and is best given at home if the owner is conscientious – the will to live seems to be a significant factor in recovery in some cats. Hospital intensive care requires an isolation unit and scrupulous hygiene to prevent cross-infection. Affected cats should be kept in a clean, warm and well-ventilated environment and kept groomed. Discharges from around the eyes and nose should be frequently wiped away and a bland ointment applied to prevent excoriation. Nebulizers and steam inhalation (e.g. sitting the cat in a steamy bathroom) to clear airways are tolerated better by cats than nasal decongestants.

The cat should be encouraged to eat by offering strongly flavoured, aromatic foods because affected cats may lose their sense of smell. Baby food or liquidized food may be helpful when mouth or throat ulceration makes eating painful. If dehydration is a problem, food may be diluted with water. In severe cases, subcutaneous or intravenous fluids may be indicated for dehydration, and where anorexia is prolonged, the use of a gastrotomy tube may be indicated (Tennant & Willoughby, 1993).

The treatment of chronic sinusitis and rhinitis is

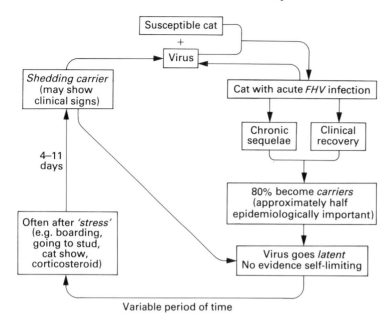

Fig. 14.1 FHV 1 carrier state: epidemiology.

discussed in Chapter 6. However, it should be emphasized that the best treatment for this condition is prevention, i.e. adequate therapy in the acute phase of the disease. Once the intranasal structures are irreversibly damaged, the long-term prognosis is relatively poor.

EPIDEMIOLOGY

Both FCV and FHV 1 are highly successful pathogens of the cat, and most animals tested prior to vaccination were shown to have antibodies to both viruses. However, infection is generally more widespread in colony animals compared to isolated household pets. Thus, the disease appears mainly in boarding catteries, breeding colonies, stray-cat homes or other situations where a large number of cats have been brought together.

The feline respiratory viruses persist in such populations in three main ways.

1 By passing directly from acutely infected to susceptible animals. This depends on the presence of a sufficient number of susceptible animals in the population and sufficient opportunities for contact between them.

2 By persisting in the environment. Although this is for only relatively short periods of time, it is long enough for indirect transmission to occur, particularly within the close confines of a cattery where secretions may contaminate cages, feeding or cleaning utensils, or personnel.

3 By persisting in the recovered cat as a carrier state. In the acute stages, most of the clinical signs and virus shedding cease by 2 to 3 weeks after infection. However, for both viruses, the carrier state is a common sequel to infection. Despite vaccination, carriers are widespread in the population and are therefore an important factor to consider in relation to the epidemiology and control of feline URT disease.

The FHV 1 carrier state
(Fig. 14.1)

FHV 1 is a typical alphaherpesvirus, the carrier state being virtually the normal sequel to infection and characterized by periods of latency interspersed with intermittent episodes of virus shedding, particularly after a stress. In the latent phase, virus is undetectable by normal sampling techniques, but during shedding episodes, virus is present in oronasal and conjunctival secretions and the cats are infectious to other cats (Gaskell & Povey, 1982).

Although over 80% of FHV 1-recovered cats remain as virus carriers, approximately only half of these are likely to be of epidemiological importance, i.e. likely to shed virus under natural conditions. Shedding may occur spontaneously (approximately 1% of a group of carriers on any one day), but is most likely following stress (Gaskell & Povey, 1973, 1977; Ellis, 1981; Goddard, 1984). Experimentally, corticosteroid treatment may induce shedding in approximately two-thirds of a group of carrier cats, and it has also been shown that a change of housing may induce shedding in approximately one in five carrier animals. This has also been confirmed in the field situation where FHV 1 re-excretion was recorded in three out of 75 cats 9–12 days after entering a boarding cattery (Gaskell & Wardley, 1978).

There is some evidence that the stress of lactation may also precipitate a shedding episode in queens, but the clinical outcome in the kittens will depend on their levels of maternally derived antibody (MDA) at that time. It is also possible for kittens to become infected subclinically under cover of MDA and become latent carriers without ever having shown clinical signs (Gaskell & Povey, 1982). Shedding in the post-partum period is obviously an ideal mechanism for the virus to perpetuate itself in the next generation, particularly if it can occur without the hazards associated with the development of clinical disease.

Virus shedding episodes do not occur immediately after the stress; there is a lag period of about a week, followed by a shedding episode lasting for up to two weeks. In some cases carriers may show mild clinical signs when shedding. Occasionally though, clinical signs may be seen in carriers unassociated with detectable episodes of virus re-excretion.

The mechanism of stress-induced re-excretion is not clear. Whatever the event that leads to the presence of detectable virus, however, it is probable that the immune response plays a role in determining the duration of the shedding episode.

Interestingly, in studies on cats re-excreting virus after the natural stress of re-housing, Goddard (1984) found (i) that the cats that shed had experienced significantly more severe primary disease than those that did not; (ii) that they had a significantly greater 'stress' response (i.e. loss of appetite and nervous withdrawal) to re-housing than the non-shedder cats; and (iii) that they tended to have lower mean antibody levels (as assessed by antibody/complement lytic capacity) prior to re-housing compared to the non-shedders.

The duration of the carrier state has not been determined, but there is no evidence to suggest that it may be self-limiting. Nevertheless, there is some evidence that animals are less likely to shed in the immediate few months after an episode (Gaskell & Goddard, 1984). The site or sites of latency of the virus are not known for certain, but it is probable that the trigeminal ganglia or other nervous tissue is involved (Gaskell & Povey, 1979b; Gaskell *et al.*, 1985).

The practical implications of these findings are as follows.

1 FHV 1 carriers are difficult to identify because of their intermittent shedding pattern, though the chances of detecting virus shedding might be increased either following a stress or when clinical signs are present. However, it is inadvisable to use corticosteroid to induce detectable virus shedding in carriers because occasionally severe disease may result. If FHV 1 is isolated from a cat then it is almost certainly virulent virus, unless an intranasal vaccine has recently been used. Systemic vaccine virus does not normally generalize (see below). In unvaccinated cats, serology may be helpful in detecting possible carriers.

2 Any animal with a known history of respiratory disease, or with persistent or recurrent signs of respiratory disease, should be suspected of being a carrier. Similarly any queen who repeatedly produces litters that develop respiratory disease is probably a carrier and it may be advisable to use other queens for breeding.

3 Although FHV 1 carriers should always be regarded as potentially infectious as they may shed virus spontaneously at any time, they are much more likely to be so in the 3-week period

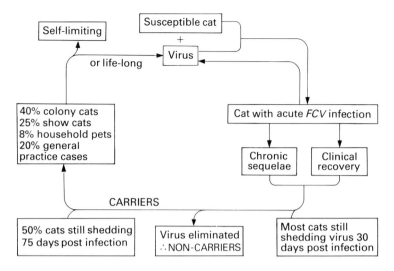

Fig. 14.2 FCV carrier state: epidemiology.

after a stress. In the field such stresses may include any change of housing, such as going to a cat show, to stud or into a boarding cattery; or the stress of kittening and lactation. Mild clinical signs may also indicate that the cat is actually shedding infectious virus.

4 Animals may become field virus carriers without ever having shown clinical signs, under protection from either maternally derived immunity (Gaskell & Povey, 1982), or from systemic vaccination (Orr *et al.*, 1978). Thus, there is always the possibility that a cat obtained from a colony that has endemic respiratory disease might be a carrier, even though it may never have shown clinical signs itself and it may be fully vaccinated.

5 There is no evidence that vaccination will 'cure' pre-existing carriers, though it is possible it may reduce episodes of virulent virus shedding.

The FCV carrier state
(Fig. 14.2)

Unlike FHV 1, the FCV carrier state is characterized by more-or-less continuous virus shedding. Such animals are therefore a constant hazard to susceptible cats. Although in some cats the carrier state appears to be lifelong, most animals at some point spontaneously recover and suddenly eliminate the virus. Experimentally it has been shown that with some strains of

virus, most animals will still be shedding FCV in oropharyngeal secretions 30 days after infection. Generally there is then an exponential decline in the proportion of animals that remain as carriers, with approximately 50% of the animals still shedding virus 75 days after infection, and a small proportion probably continuing to shed for the rest of the animal's life (Wardley & Povey, 1977b; Gaskell *et al.*, 1982). There is some recent evidence that pre-existing FIV infection may increase both the proportion of cats that remain FCV carriers after infection and the length of time that they shed (Dawson *et al.*, 1991).

FCV carriers may be arbitrarily divided into high-, medium- or low-level shedders, each shedding a fairly constant amount of virus which fluctuates around a mean for that individual cat (Wardley, 1976). High-level excreters appear to have more epidemiological importance in that they may more easily, with only brief contact, infect susceptible individuals. Low-level excreters are probably not so infectious and may be more difficult to detect: a series of swabs over several weeks may be needed, since sometimes the amount of virus shed falls below the level of sensitivity of the test.

Feline calicivirus carriers are very common, despite vaccination. Before vaccines were introduced, in the 1970s, surveys showed that approximately 8% of household pets, 25% of cats attending cat shows, and 40% of colony cats were shedding the virus (Wardley *et al.*, 1974). Younger cats had a higher isolation rate than older animals, which probably reflects their high susceptibility to infection once passive immunity has waned. Recently, it has been found that approximately 20% of veterinary hospital cases and general practice cases, referred for reasons other than that of respiratory disease, were shedding FCV (Knowles *et al.*, 1989; Harbour *et al.*, 1991), thus confirming that despite vaccination, the virus is still very widespread. Experimentally vaccination does not protect against virus shedding (Gaskell *et al.*, 1982; Dawson *et al.*, 1991).

Virus persists in tonsil and other oropharyngeal tissues (Wardley & Povey, 1977a; Dick & Johnson, 1989). Unfortunately, tonsillectomy does not terminate the carrier state.

The practical implications of these findings are as follows.

1 In general, FCV carriers may be identified by isolation of virus from a single oropharyngeal swab, but ideally several samples should be taken over a 4- to 6-week period. Although a positive isolation probably indicates that the cat is a field virus carrier, many carriers do manage to eliminate the virus in the months following infection, and so it is worth re-testing. In addition, a small proportion of isolates may represent transient reinfection or infection with a non-pathogenic strain. Animals vaccinated intranasally may also become carriers of vaccine virus (Orr *et al.*, 1980). Thus, results should be interpreted in conjunction with the clinical and vaccination history of the colony.

2 Where virus isolation facilities are not available, carriers may have to be identified, as for FHV 1, on the basis of their clinical history and circumstantial evidence.

3 Systemically vaccinated cats may become carriers following subclinical infection with field virus (Gaskell *et al.*, 1982), and the same may occur in kittens with maternally-derived antibody (Johnson & Povey, 1984). There is no evidence that vaccination will 'cure' a pre-existing carrier state.

In summary, then, URT disease tends to appear wherever cats are congregrated together, and in-

fection is often introduced by the often clinically normal carrier. Once enzootic, the disease is generally seen in the acute form in young kittens at the stage during which passive immunity is lost and they are exposed to shedding carriers. In older cats the presence of infection may be noted by the existence of chronically affected cats with persistent or recurrent rhinitis, sinusitis or conjunctivitis.

TRANSMISSION

Transmission occurs mainly by direct cat-to-cat contact via infectious discharges. Both viruses are shed primarily in ocular, nasal and oral secretions. Feline calicivirus may also be shed in urine and faeces, but this is probably not of great epidemiological significance.

Indirect transmission via contaminated secretions on cages, feedbowls, cleaning utensils, personnel, etc. may also occur, particularly within the close confines of a cattery. Since the viruses are relatively short-lived outside the cat, however, the environment is not usually a long-term source of virus. Factors which will reduce external virus survival include an optimal environmental temperature, low relative humidity and adequate ventilation (i.e. 15–20 air changes per hour).

Aerosol transmission is not thought to be of major significance, as there is some evidence that the cat does not produce an infectious aerosol of the respiratory viruses during normal respiratory movements (Wardley & Povey, 1976; Gaskell & Povey, 1982). However, sneezing may propel macrodroplets over a distance of 1–2 metres (Povey & Johnson, 1970).

The efficacy of transmission also depends on the amount of virus shed by the infecting animal, and the duration and intimacy of contact (Wardley, 1976; Gaskell & Povey, 1982). Although amounts of virus shed may be similar, transmission is in general more easily achieved by animals in the acute stages of the disease, rather than by carriers, because the discharges are usually more copious. However, carriers are undoubtedly of importance, particularly where close contact occurs, for example in colonies.

IMMUNITY

Although a number of conventional serological tests have been developed for use with the feline respiratory viruses, most studies have concentrated on the detection of serum virus neutralizing (VN) antibody. Following primary infection in FHV 1 infection, VN antibody is slow to rise and even by 40 days may only be present in about 70% of cats (Gaskell & Povey, 1979a). Titres are often low, and in some cases absent, but VN titres are not necessarily indicative of resistance to infection. In herpesvirus infections particularly, because the viruses tend to be cell-associated and there is cell-to-cell spread, other mechanisms, especially cell-mediated immunity (CMI), are also considered important because virus-infected cells can be lysed by various cytotoxic mechanisms. Some of these have been described for FHV (Wardley *et al.*, 1976; Goddard & Gaskell, 1984; Tham & Studdert, 1987a,b).

In FCV infection, serum VN antibody titres are also usually used as an indicator of resistance to infection. However, even in calicivirus infections, where an early response and high levels of VN antibody generally occur, it is probable that other immune mechanisms also play a role. Indeed, partial heterologous cross-protection with FCV strains has been observed even in the absence of detectable VN antibody to the cross-infecting strain (Knowles *et al.*, 1991). Tham and Studdert (1987c) have demonstrated several types of CMI responses in FCV infected and vaccinated cats, including an apparently MHC-restricted cytotoxic T (Tc) cell response. Knowles (1988) observed in *in vitro* studies that FCV remained cell-associated for a prolonged period after maximal cell-associated titres were obtained, and infected cells were also shown to release cytoplasmic buds containing FCV antigen: this could suggest a possibly greater importance for CMI responses in FCV infection than previously thought. Such findings may also be relevant to the *in vivo* carrier state.

Local immunoglobulin responses have been examined by several groups. In studies on early protection with an intranasal FHV 1 vaccine,

although apparently specific protection was operating by 6 days after vaccination, no detectable neutralizing antibody was present in nasal washings or serum although there were low levels of IgA and IgM (Cocker *et al.*, 1986). In studies on FCV infection, Johnson (1981) found that although IgA and IgG were present in nasal and oropharyngeal secretions IgG appeared to mediate virus neutralizing activity. In more recent work on FCV, Knowles *et al.* (1991) have found all three immunoglobulin classes present in saliva over the course of the infection.

There is little information on the duration of immunity to the two viruses as determined by resitance to reinfection. Walton and Gillespie (1970) demonstrated resistance to challenge with FHV 1 21 days after infection, and partial protection after 5 months. For FCV, there appears to be some variation depending upon the virus strain involved, and whether or not homotypic or heterotypic protection is being considered (Bartholomew & Gillespie, 1968; Povey & Ingersoll, 1975). Homotypic antibody appears sooner than heterotypic antibody and is present in higher titres (Kahn *et al.*, 1975; Gaskell *et al.*, 1982).

The duration of immunity following vaccination is not known. Most challenge experiments have been done within 3 months of initial vaccination, but equivalent protection has been reported after 1 year for FHV 1 infection, and 10–12 months for FCV infection (Bittle & Rubic, 1975). Most manufacturers recommend yearly revaccination or 6-monthly revaccination in some circumstances (e.g. stud cats).

Available data for FHV 1 infection suggest that maternally derived (essentially colostral) antibody in kittens may persist for 2–10 weeks with mean levels falling below detectable levels by 6–9 weeks of age (Edwards *et al.*, 1977; Gaskell & Povey, 1982). For FCV infection, Johnson and Povey (1983) found that titres may be more persistent than for FHV 1 infection, antibody declining to undetectable levels by 10–14 weeks of age. However, with FCV infection low levels of maternally derived antibody in kittens do not necessarily give protection against infection or disease (Kahn & Gillespie, 1971; Johnson & Povey, 1984). This latter group showed that kittens born to carrier queens became infected between 3 and 9 weeks old when they still had some maternal antibody; the kittens showed varying degrees of clinical signs, with some infections subclinical. In contrast, in FHV1 infection some kittens with no detectable antibody were protected against the disease, though not necessarily against infection (Gaskell & Povey, 1982).

It is perhaps interesting that colostrally-derived immunoglobulin appears to be able to protect kittens against challenge by the respiratory route, since it is taken up by the gut into the systemic circulation. It is probable that, as with immunity derived from systemic vaccination, limited local replication of virus takes place, allowing some leakage of systemic immunoglobulin onto the mucosal surface.

PREVENTION AND CONTROL

The prevention and control of viral respiratory disease in different types of cat populations is described below. Vaccination has been available for a number of years, and in general, where it has been carried out, it has been relatively successful in controlling the disease. However, milder forms still sometimes occur, and problems can arise, for example in stray cat homes, or in young kittens in catteries as they lose their maternally derived antibody. Both respiratory viruses are extremely widespread in the cat population and clinically healthy carriers are common, thus ensuring that there is plenty of exposure. Essentially, therefore, control is best attempted through a combination of vaccination and management.

Vaccination

Three types of vaccine are available in the UK for the protection of cats against viral respiratory disease: modified live systemic vaccines, modified live intranasal, or inactivated adjuvanted systemic. The FHV 1 virus component of the current inactivated vaccine available in the UK is a sub-unit glycoprotein fraction, designed to avoid an apparent hypersensitivity reaction noted with whole virus preparations by that particular manufacturer. Elsewhere in the world inactivated whole virus preparations are marketed. Recently a genetically engineered feline herpesvirus has been described with a deleted thymidine kinase gene, and this may prove useful as a vaccine (Nunberg *et al.*, 1989).

In previously healthy, unexposed cats, all types of vaccines induce reasonable protection against disease, though not necessarily against infection, and all may be used with reasonable confidence in routine vaccination programmes. Ideally, vaccination of the whole cat population should be the aim. Whilst stressing the advantage of a vaccination programme, however, the client should also be made aware of its possible limitations. To a large extent, such limitations are due to the ubiquity of the viruses and the nature of the epidemiology of feline respiratory disease, but the vaccines themselves also have some limitations.

Most vaccines marketed are modified live systemic, and in most situations these are quite satisfactory. However, they should be administered carefully since there are occasional reports that if they are inadvertently given via the respiratory route (e.g. if a cat licks the injection site or an aerosol is made with the syringe) then respiratory signs can develop (Povey, 1977). Although when given correctly such vaccines are not normally considered to generalize, recently, under experimental conditions, we have observed the apparent localization to the oropharynx of a modified live FCV vaccine when given to previously immune cats (Bennett *et al.*, 1989). The epidemiological implications of this are not clear, but presumably if significant levels of such virus were shed, then transmission to in-contact animals could theoretically occur. In completely virus-free colonies or where in-contact animals are totally susceptible, therefore, an inactivated vaccine might be preferable.

Intranasal vaccines probably induce marginally better protection than systemic vaccines but at the expense of often greater side-effects. Generally, these take the form of mild sneezing some

5–9 days later in up to 60% of cats, although some ocular and nasal discharges and oral and nasal ulceration have been reported (Orr *et al.*, 1980; Gaskell, 1981). The intranasal route is useful, however, where rapid onset of protection is important, for example in a stray cat home, or during an outbreak of disease. Only one dose of intranasal vaccine is required to induce immunity in a primary vaccination course, and specific immunity appears very rapidly. Complete protection against challenge has been shown 4 days after intranasal vaccination and partial protection after 2 days (Cocker *et al.*, 1984).

The optimum age for vaccination of young kittens can be difficult to determine. In general, kittens should be vaccinated with systemic vaccines initially at 9 weeks of age, when in most cases maternally derived antibody has declined to non-interfering levels, with the second dose 3–4 weeks later.

Because of the variable and sometimes short duration of MDA in kittens (see above), and because of the high prevalence of carriers in the cat population, respiratory disease often occurs in young kittens before they have been successfully vaccinated. Vaccination of queens during pregnancy with an inactivated vaccine can help protect such kittens by prolonging the duration of MDA (Iglauer *et al.*, 1989). In addition, earlier vaccination schedules can be used in kittens in an attempt to reduce the immunity gap, but management measures are often also necessary (see below) to ensure kittens are not already incubating the disease at the time of vaccination, or perhaps are already carriers.

Thus it has been suggested that systemic vaccines may be used from 3 or 4 weeks of age, vaccinating at 3–4-week intervals until 12 weeks old. However, although Johnson and Povey (1985) have shown that an inactivated adjuvanted systemic vaccine can provide protection against FHV1 infection when given to kittens at 5 and 7 weeks of age with residual MDA, others have found that a modified live virus systemic vaccine did not provide protection in similar circumstances (Slater & York, 1976). It is difficult to extrapolate from such work for other vaccines,

for they may differ in factors such as strain of virus, antigenic mass or adjuvant which could well affect the efficacy of particular vaccines in particular situations.

An alternative approach is the use of intranasal vaccination. Although this should normally be initiated at 12 weeks of age and is not licensed in the UK for earlier use, in some circumstances it can be useful for preventing disease in very young kittens, particularly in colonies where the disease is endemic, because it is not interfered with by maternally derived antibody (Slater & York, 1976; Wilson, 1978; Pickering, 1981). Since intranasal vaccine itself can sometimes induce mild clinical signs, vaccination of very young kittens should only be attempted where there is a high and unavoidable risk of exposure. The age at which the vaccine should be given depends to some extent on when clinical signs in young kittens have been occurring; for example, if disease has been occurring at 4–5 weeks of age, then vaccination should be performed at 3 weeks of age, and then probably at 8 and 12 weeks (Morris, 1990). However, there is evidence that multiple doses of intranasal vaccine may not be necessary and a single dose may suffice (Johnson & Povey, 1985). Additional vaccination of the queen via the intranasal route on the day of parturition has also been advocated (Wilson, 1978).

In general, immunity in feline viral respiratory disease is not particularly high or long-lived. Annual boosters are usually recommended for vaccines, but in some circumstances (for example, a stud cat, or an old cat going for the first time into a boarding cattery) then 6-monthly boosting is probably advisable.

Vaccine reactions and breakdowns
Probably the most common reason why apparent vaccine reactions occur (i.e. clinical disease which appears within a week or so of vaccination) is because the cat is already incubating the disease at the time of vaccination. This is particularly true in young kittens, which are generally vaccinated just as their maternally derived antibody wanes and therefore when they are also susceptible to field virus infections. The incubation period of

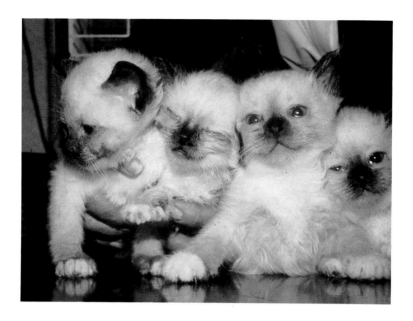

Plate 14.1 A litter of kittens with early FHV infection. The kitten second from the left is more severely affected than the others with marked conjunctivitis, ocular discharge and nasal discharge.

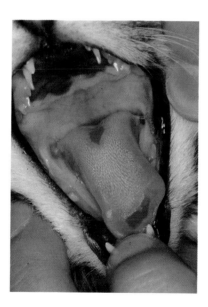

Plate 14.2 Two lingual ulcers on the tongue of a cat infected with feline calicivirus.

the feline respiratory viruses is generally 2–10 days, but just occasionally it may be longer, up to 2–3 weeks.

The second point is that the cat might already be a field virus carrier. Such animals may have a history of having had respiratory disease, but they may not if they were infected subclinically under cover of vaccine-induced immunity or maternally derived antibody. Both FHV 1 infection and feline calicivirus carriers are very widespread in the population, and both may show persistent or recurrent signs related to damage from the original infection. In addition, FHV 1 infection carriers may shed and show signs as a result of 'stress', and it has been suggested that vaccination and the attendant disruption of routine may sometimes initiate this. It is unlikely that vaccination will 'cure' carriers, though it is just possible that in FHV 1 infection it may reduce the severity of the shedding episodes.

Modified live systemic vaccines should not induce disease if administered correctly, although as already discussed, they may still induce signs if they are inadvertently given oronasally, and perhaps in some circumstances virus may generalize following vaccination of previously immune animals. Clinical signs that may occur following intranasal vaccination have already been discussed.

Clinical signs that are commonly reported as vaccine reactions include upper respiratory and ocular signs and mouth ulceration (Dawson *et al.*, 1993). More recently, lameness and fever have also been reported. Typically such reactions occur approximately 6–7 days after vaccination, often after primary vaccination, and it has been suggested that this syndrome may be associated with the calicivirus component of particular vaccines. Whilst some of the isolates appear to be similar to vaccine virus, in cases examined so far the majority of isolates appear to be field viruses (Dawson *et al.*, 1993).

In general, vaccine reactions attributable to live virus vaccines are uncommon, though it should be remembered that differences in microbial flora and any intercurrent disease, especially with the immunosuppressive cat diseases such as feline leukaemia virus infection or feline immunodeficiency virus infection, may lead to signs that might not otherwise be seen.

Apparent vaccine breakdowns may also be explained in a number of ways. Assuming the vaccine was potent and had been stored and given correctly, even under ideal conditions, protection is not necessarily complete in all animals. In the field, there may be intercurrent disease (especially with the immunodeficiency viruses) or overwhelming infection, or maternally derived antibody may have interfered with the original vaccination programme. Recently we have observed that previous infection with FIV renders subsequent vaccination with an inactivated FCV vaccine significantly less effective in protecting against FCV challenge (Dawson *et al.*, 1991).

In colonies, respiratory disease may occur in young kittens as previously discussed, because of the 'immunity gap' and because of high risk of exposure from carriers. Furthermore, vaccination does not eliminate infection from cats that are already carriers, and in addition, a previously unexposed systemically vaccinated cat can subsequently become infected subclinically and become a field virus carrier under cover of vaccine immunity (Orr *et al.*, 1978; Gaskell *et al.*, 1982). Intranasally vaccinated cats may become carriers of the, albeit attenuated, calicivirus vaccine component, but there is some evidence that intranasal vaccination may protect against the development of the FHV 1 carrier state, at least in the short term (Orr *et al.*, 1980).

It is also becoming increasingly apparent that the vaccines currently widely used in the UK probably do not protect against all isolates of calicivirus, and future vaccines may need to incorporate several complementary, cross-protective isolates. Finally it should be emphasized that apparent breakdowns may be due to another agent, such as *C. psittaci* or *Bordetella bronchiseptica*, not included in the viral vaccines.

Disease control in different situations

Household pets

All household pets should be regularly vaccinated with any of the available vaccines. They are most likely to be exposed to the respiratory viruses when entering a boarding cattery or a veterinary hospital. Exposure is less likely to occur between neighbouring household pets, except in an urban environment with a high-density cat population. Cats are mainly territorial animals and with neutered animals, once their territory is established, any contact with other cats is usually too brief to encourage extensive transmission of virus. In addition, the respiratory viruses are relatively fragile outside the cat, and therefore indirect transmission will be a rare event. Thus, the individual cat should, if possible, be routinely vaccinated and should avoid stress and social contact as far as possible. From the point of view of infectious disease, ideally a friend or neighbour should feed the cat whilst the owner is on holiday, but if it does go into a boarding cattery, then it should be given a booster vaccination before entry unless it has been very recently vaccinated (within the previous 6 months).

Boarding catteries
All cats admitted to the cattery should have an up-to-date vaccination record. This means that young kittens should have completed the full vaccination course, i.e. two vaccines 3–4 weeks apart at least 7 days before admission, and adult cats should have had their annual booster preferably at least 7 days before. Where vaccination has lapsed for longer than 18 months it might be advisable to give a full course. In exceptional circumstances, where there is no alternative and rapid protection is required, intranasal vaccine may be used. However, it must be remembered that such vaccines may themselves induce mild clinical signs.

However, cattery owners should not rely solely on adequate vaccination for disease control, for virus will inevitably be present in the cattery either from the occasional animal incubating the disease, or, more likely, from carriers. Thus, precautions should still be taken to prevent any possible cross-infection and reduce the concentration of virus in the environment. Such measures are outlined in Table 14.3. Although at first sight they may appear complicated, in practice they are

Table 14.3 Recommendations to prevent spread of the respiratory viruses in a boarding cattery.

1 Make sure all incoming cats are fully vaccinated
2 House cats individually, unless from same household
3 Build cattery with solid partitions between pens. Ensure frontages are at least 1 m apart, and the surface of the pen is easily washable
4 Arrange pen so food bowl and litter tray may be removed routinely without entering the pen, i.e. do not handle cats more than necessary
5 Either wash hands in disinfectant bucket between visiting each pen; or have an individual pair of rubber gloves on a peg by each pen for use only with that pen. Disinfect thoroughly before use with a new boarder
6 Wear rubber boots and, if it is necessary to enter the pen, step into a disinfectant bath
7 Either: use disposable food trays; or have two sets of feed bowls used on alternate days. Soak used set in 1 in 32 bleach/detergent solution (see earlier) for several hours, and then leave thoroughly rinsed and dried until re-use 24 hours later
8 Prepare food in central area
9 Replace badly soiled litter trays with another previously disinfected and pre-filled in a central area, i.e. a similar system to the feed bowls
10 When cat goes home, thoroughly disinfect cage, allow to dry, and preferably leave empty for 2 days before re-using
11 Put cats with any signs of a previous respiratory infection (e.g. ocular discharge, chronic rhinitis), cats known to have had respiratory disease, and any suspect carrier cats from past experience in one section, or at one end of the cattery, and feed last
12 Feed cats in same order every day and attend to each pen completely before moving onto the next
13 Reduce concentration of virus in environment by adequate ventilation, low relative humidity, and optimum environmental temperature

not difficult to implement, and in our experience, can actually increase efficiency within a cattery. In addition they will also generally inhibit the spread of other pathogens.

Stray cat homes
In general, the same measures apply as with boarding catteries, but it is often impossible to separate animals to the same extent. However,

animals should be segregated or batched and quarantined as far as possible, and those with clinical signs kept apart. Unless animals can be isolated on arrival for 3–4 weeks, systemic vaccines may not have time to become effective. In these circumstances, it may be advisable to use the intranasal route.

Breeding catteries
In disease-free colonies cats should be vaccinated routinely if there is any contact at all, directly or indirectly, with other cats. Inactivated vaccines are preferable, though if administered carefully, modified live vaccines should be satisfactory. Great care should be taken to avoid bringing virus into the colony: *any* cat with a history of respiratory disease or from a household with a history of respiratory disease may be a carrier. It should be remembered that cats can become infected subclinically under cover of maternal or vaccine-induced immunity. Thus stud cats and new breeding stock should be from a respiratory disease-free colony. There is a possible risk of infection from cat shows, but the greatest risk of infection to a disease-free household is from stud cats and new breeding stock where exposure is more prolonged.

Cats entering the colony should be quarantined for 3 weeks to avoid animals incubating the disease, and screened virologically at least twice a week during this time. This increases the probability of detecting FHV 1 re-excretion and low-level FCV carriers. Even so there is still a risk of importing a latent FHV 1 carrier or a very low-level FCV carrier which may be a source of infection. With unvaccinated cats, this risk can be minimized by not accepting cats that have seroconverted to FHV 1 or FCV. Since FIV infection seems to potentiate FCV infection, it is probably wise to test for FIV, and indeed FeLV, as well.

In breeding colonies where the disease is endemic, in some circumstances it may be feasible to re-stock the colony with virus-free cats and to employ a barrier system to keep the viruses out. A commercial or institutional colony could achieve this using specific-pathogen-free stock; a

pedigree cat breeding unit could hand-rear kittens of existing stock in isolation, bearing in mind that the viruses are very widespread and it might be difficult to ensure that even with vaccination, the colony would then remain virus-free. However, in many situations, the only reasonable course is to attempt disease control. This may be done by:
1 Regular vaccination programmes.
2 Giving booster vaccinations to queens either prior to mating or during pregnancy (if the latter, by using a killed vaccine only).
3 Keeping cats as stress-free as possible and employing good management practices to reduce spread of viruses within the colony.
4 Avoiding the use of particular queens with a history of respiratory disease in their kittens.
5 Moving queens into isolation to kitten at least 3 weeks before term, so that the kittens are not exposed to carriers in the colony, and any shedding episode from the queen as a result of the move will be over before kittening.
6 Early-weaning kittens into isolation away from their mother as soon as it is feasible (ideally at 4–5 weeks) if it is likely she is a carrier.
7 Vaccinating all kittens as soon as maternally derived antibodies are at a non-interfering level (normally 9+ weeks) and keeping them in strict isolation until a week after the second dose.
8 Earlier vaccination schedules, the starting age depending on the age in that particular colony that kittens first become affected. Both intranasal and systemic vaccines have been suggested in such circumstances, and the advantages and disadvantages of each have been discussed above.

REFERENCES

Review articles or those of general interest

Crandell R.A. (1973) Feline viral rhinotracheitis (FVR). *Adv. Vet. Sci. Comp. Med.* **17**, 201.
Donaldson A.I. & Ferris N.P. (1976) The survival of some air-borne animal viruses in relation to relative humidity. *Vet. Microbiol.* **1**, 413.
Fisk S.K. & Soave O.A. (1973) *Bordetella bronchiseptica* in laboratory cats from central California. *Lab. Anim. Sci.* **23**, 33.
Gaskell R.M. (1981) An assessment of the use of feline

respiratory virus vaccines. In Grunsell C.S.G. & Hill F.W.G. (eds) *The Veterinary Annual, 21st Issue*. Wright-Scientechnica, Bristol, p. 267.

Gaskell R.M. (1988) Herpesviruses of cats. In Darai G. (ed) *Virus Diseases in Laboratory and Captive Animals*. Martinus Nijhoff Publishers, Boston.

Gaskell R.M. & Gaskell C.J. (1988) Infectious causes of reproductive failure in dogs and cats. In Laing J.A., Brinley-Morgan W.J. & Wagner W.C. (eds) *Fertility and Infertility in Veterinary Practice*, 4th edn. Balliere Tindall, London, p. 262.

Gaskell R.M. & Wardley R.C. (1978) Feline viral respiratory disease: a review with particular reference to its epizootiology and control. *J. Small Anim. Pract.* **19**, 1.

Gillespie J.H. & Scott F.W. (1973) Feline viral infections. *Adv. Vet. Sci. Comp. Med.* **17**, 163.

Iglauer F., Gartner K. & Morstedt R. (1989) Maternal protection against feline respiratory disease by means of booster vaccinations during pregnancy – a retrospective clinical study. *Kleintierpraxis* **34**, 235.

Morris T.H. (1990) Vaccination during URT disease in kittens. *Vet. Rec.* **126**, 250.

Pickering J.G. (1981) A vaccination technique to break the transmission cycle of chronic respiratory disease in breeding catteries. *New Zeal. Vet. J.* **29**, 63.

Povey R.C. (1977) Feline respiratory disease – which vaccine? *Feline Pract.* **7**(5), 12.

Povey R.C. (1979) A review of feline viral rhinotracheitis (feline herpesvirus 1 infection). *Comp. Immun. Microbiol. Infect. Dis.* **2**, 373.

Povey R.C. & Johnson R.H. (1970) Observations on the epidemiology and control of viral respiratory disease in cats. *J. Small Anim. Pract.* **11**, 485.

Scott F.W. (1980) Viricidal disinfectants and feline viruses. *Am. J. Vet. Res.* **41**, 410.

Studdert M.J. (1978) Caliciviruses: Brief review. *Arch. Virol.* **58**, 157.

Tennant B. & Willoughby K. (1993) The use of enteral nutrition in small animal medicine. *Comp. Cont. Educ.* **15**, 1054.

Wardley R.C., Gaskell R.M. & Povey R.C. (1974) Feline respiratory viruses; their prevalence in clinically healthy cats. *J. Small Anim. Pract.* **15**, 579.

Willoughby K., Dawson S., Jones R.C., Symons M., Daykin J., Payne-Johnson C., Gaskell R.M., Bennett M. & Gaskell C.J. (1991) Isolation of *B. bronchiseptica* from kittens with pneumonia in a breeding cattery. *Vet. Rec.* **129**, 407–8.

Wilson J.H.G. (1978) Intranasal vaccination against upper respiratory tract disease (URD) in the cat. 11. Results of field studies under enzootic conditions in the Netherlands with a combined vaccine containing live attenuated calici- and herpesvirus. *Comp. Immunol. Microbiol. Infect. Dis.* **1**, 43.

Feline viral rhinotracheitis

Bistner S.I., Carlson J.H., Shiveley N.J. & Scott F.W. (1971) Ocular manifestations of feline herpesvirus infection. *J. Am. Vet. Med. Ass.* **159**, 1223.

Bittle J.L. & Peckam J.C. (1971) Comments: genital infections induced by feline rhinotracheitis virus and effects on newborn kittens. *J. Am. Vet. Med. Ass.* **158**, 927.

Cocker F.M., Gaskell R.M., Newby T.J., Gaskell C.J., Stokes C.R. & Bourne F.J. (1984) Efficacy of early (48 and 96 hour) protection aganist feline viral rhinotracheitis following intranasal vaccination with a live temperature-sensitive mutant. *Vet. Rec.* **114**, 353.

Cocker F.M., Newby T.J., Gaskell R.M., Evans P.A., Gaskell C.J., Stokes C.R., Harbour D.A. & Bourne J.F. (1986) Responses of cats to nasal vaccination with a live, modified feline herpesvirus type 1. *Res. Vet. Sci.* **41**, 323.

Crandell R.A., Rehkemper J.A., Niemann, W.H., Ganaway, J.R. & Maurer F.D. (1961) Experimental feline viral rhinotracheitis. *J. Am. Vet. Med. Ass.* **138**, 191.

Edwards B.J., Buell D.J. & Acree W.M. (1977) Evaluation of a new feline rhinotracheitis vaccine. *Vet. Med. Small Anim. Clin.* **72**, 205.

Ellis T.M. (1981) Feline respiratory virus carriers in clinically healthy cats. *Austr. Vet. J.* **57**, 115.

Evermann J.F., McKiernan A.J., Ott R.L. & Reed L.A. (1982) Diarrhoeal condition in dogs associated with viruses antigenically related to feline herpesvirus. *Cornell Vet.* **72**, 285.

Gaskell R.M. & Goddard L.E. (1984). The epizootiology of feline viral rhinotracheitis with particular reference of the nature and role of the carrier state. In *Current Topics in Veterinary Medicine and Animal Science EEC Symposium. Latent Herpesvirus Infections in Veterinary Medicine* Martinus Nijhoff, Boston, p. 337.

Gaskell R.M. & Povey R.C. (1973) Re-excretion of feline viral rhinotracheitis virus following corticosteroid treatment. *Vet. Rec.* **93**, 204.

Gaskell R.M. & Povey R.C. (1977) Experimental induction of feline viral rhinotracheitis virus re-excretion in FVR-recovered cats. *Vet. Rec.* **100**, 128.

Gaskell R.M. & Povey R.C. (1979a) The dose response of cats to experimental infection with feline viral rhinotracheitis virus. *J. Comp. Rath.* **89**, 179.

Gaskell R.M. & Povey R.C. (1979b) Feline viral rhinotracheitis: sites of virus replication and persistence in acutely and persistently infected cats. *Res. Vet. Sci.* **27**, 167.

Gaskell R.M. & Povey R.C. (1982) Transmission of feline viral rhinotracheitis. *Vet. Rec.* **111**, 359.

Gaskell R.M., Dennis P.E., Goddard L.E., Cocker F.M. & Wills, J.M. (1985) Isolation of felid herpesvirus 1 from the trigeminal ganglia of latently infected cats. *J. Gen. Virol.* **66**, 391.

Goddard L.E. (1984) Immunological studies during acute and latent felid herpesvirus 1 infection. PhD thesis, University of Bristol.

Goddard L.E. & Gaskell R.M. (1984) Immunity to felid herpesvirus 1. In *Current Topics in Veterinary Medicine and Animal Science EEC Symposium. Latent Herpesvirus Infections in Veterinary Medicine.* Martinus Nijhoff, Boston, p. 351.

Herrmann S., Gaskell R.M., Ehlers B. & Ludwig H. (1984) Characterisation of the feline herpesvirus genome and molecular epidemiology of isolates from natural outbreaks and latent infections. In *Current Topics in Veterinary Medicine and Animal Science EEC Symposium. Latent Herpesvirus Infections in Veterinary Medicine.* Martinus Nijhoff, Boston, p. 321.

Hoover E.A. & Griesemer R.A. (1971a) Experimental feline herpesvirus infection in the pregnant cat. *Am. J. Path.* **65**, 173.

Hoover E.A. & Griesemer R.A. (1971b) Bone lesions produced by feline herpesvirus. *Lab. Invest.* **25**, 457.

Hoover E.A., Rohovsky M.W. & Griesemer R.A. (1970) Experimental feline viral rhinotracheitis in the germ-free cat. *Am. J. Path.* **58**, 269.

Johnson R.P. & Povey R.C. (1985) Vaccination against feline viral rhinotracheitis in kittens with maternally derived feline viral rhinotracheitis antibodies. *J. Am. Vet. Med. Ass.* **186**(2), 149.

Karpas A. & Routledge J.K. (1968) Feline herpesvirus: isolation and experimental studies. *Zbl. Vet. Med.* **15**, 599.

Love D.N. (1971) Feline herpesvirus associated with pneumonia in a kitten. *Vet. Rec.* **89**, 178.

Nasisse M.P., Guy J.S., Davidson M.G., Sussman W.A. & Fairley N.M. (1989) Experimental ocular herpesvirus infection in the cat. Sites of virus replication, clinical features and effects of corticosteroid administration. *Invest. Ophthalmol. Vis. Sci.* **30**(8), 1758.

Nunberg J.H., Wright D.K., Cole G.E., Petrovskis E.A., Post L.E., Compton T. & Gilbert J.H. (1989) Identification of the thymidine kinase gene of feline herpesvirus: use of degenerate oligonucleotides in the polymerase chain reaction to isolate herpesvirus gene homologs. *J. Virol.* **63**(8), 3240.

Orr C.M., Gaskell C.J. & Gaskell R.M. (1978) Interaction of a combined feline viral rhinotracheitis, feline calicivirus vaccine and the FVR carrier state. *Vet. Rec.* **103**, 200.

Orr C.M., Gaskell C.J. and Gaskell R.M. (1980). Interaction of an intra-nasal combined feline viral rhinotracheitis, feline calicivirus vaccine and the FVR carrier state. *Vet. Rec.* **106**, 164.

Rota P.A., Maes R.K. & Ruyechan W.T. (1986) Physical characterisation of the genome of feline herpesvirus-1. *Virol.* **154**, 168.

Shields R.P. & Gaskin J.M. (1977) Fatal generalised feline viral rhinotracheitis in a young adult cat. *J. Am. Vet. Med. Ass.* **170**, 439.

Slater E. & York C. (1976) Comparative studies on parenteral and intra-nasal inoculation of an attenuated feline herpesvirus. *Develop. Biol. Standards.* **33**, 410.

Spradbrow P.B., Carlisle C. & Watt D.A. (1971) The association of a herpesvirus with generalised disease in a young kitten. *Vet. Rec.* **89**, 542.

Tham K.M. & Studdert M.J. (1987a) Clinical and immunological responses of cats to feline herpesvirus type 1 infection. *Vet. Rec.* **120**, 321.

Tham K.M. & Studdert M.J. (1987b) Antibody and cell-mediated immune responses to feline herpesvirus 1 following inactivated vaccine and challenge. *J. Vet. Med. B.* **34**, 585.

Van Pelt C.S. & Crandell R.A. (1987) Pancreatitis associated with a feline herpesvirus infection. *Comp. Anim. Prac.* **1**, 7.

Walton D.E. & Gillespie J.H. (1970) Feline viruses VII. Immunity to the feline herpesvirus in kittens inoculated experimentally by the aerosol method. *Cornell Vet.* **60**, 232.

Wardley R.C., Rouse B.T. & Babiuk L.A. (1976) Observations on recovery mechanisms from feline viral rhinotracheitis. *Can. J. Comp. Med.* **40**, 257.

Feline calicivirus infection

Bartholomew P.T. & Gillespie J.H. (1968) Feline viruses. 1. Characterisation of four isolates and their effect on young kittens. *Cornell Vet.* **58**, 248.

Bennett D., Gaskell R.M., Mills A., Knowles J.O., Carter S. & McArdle F. (1989) Detection of feline calicivirus antigens in the joints of infected cats. *Vet. Rec.* **124**, 329.

Bittle J.L. & Rubic W.J. (1975) A feline calicivirus vaccine combined with feline viral rhinotracheitis and feline panleucopenia vaccine. *Feline Parct.* **5**(6), 13.

Dawson S. (1991) Studies on feline calicivirus and its role in feline disease. PhD thesis, University of Liverpool.

Dawson S., Smyth N.R., Bennett M., Gaskell R.M., McCracken C.M., Brown A. & Gaskell C.J. (1991) Effect of primary stage feline immunodeficiency virus infection on subsequent feline calicivirus vaccination and challenge in cats. *AIDS* **5**, 747–50.

Dawson S., McArdle F., Bennett D., Carter S.D., Bennett M., Ryvar R. & Gaskell R.M. (1993) Investigation of vaccine reactions and breakdowns after feline calicivirus vaccinations. *Vet. Rec.* **132**, 346.

Dick C.P. & Johnson R.P. (1989) Sites of persistence of feline calicivirus. *Res. Vet. Sci.* **47**, 367.

Evermann J.F., Bryan C.M. & McKeirnan A.J. (1981) Isolation of a calicivirus from a case of canine glossitis. *Canine Pract.* **8**, 36.

Gaskell C.J., Gaskell R.M., Dennis P.E. & Wooldridge M.J.A. (1982) Efficacy of an inactivated feline calicivirus (FCV) vaccine against challenge with United Kingdom field strains and its interaction with the FCV carrier state. *Res. Vet. Sci.* **32**, 23.

Hoover E.A. & Kahn D.E. (1975) Experimentally induced feline calicivirus infection: clinical signs and lesions. *J. Am. Vet. Med. Ass.* **166**, 463.

Johnson R.P. (1981) Immunity to feline calicivirus in kittens. *Dissertation Abstracts International* **41B**, 2922.

Johnson R.P. & Povey R.C. (1983) Transfer and decline of maternal antibody to feline calicivirus. *Can. Vet. J.* **24**, 6.

Johnson R.P. & Povey R.C. (1984) Feline calicivirus infection in kittens borne by cats persistently infected with the virus. *Res. Vet. Sci.* **37**, 114.

Kahn, D.E. & Gillespie J.H. (1971) Feline viruses: pathogenesis of picornavirus infection in the cat. *Am. J. Vet. Res.* **32**, 521.

Kahn D.E., Hoover E.A. & Bittle J.L. (1975) Induction of immunity to feline caliciviral disease. *Infect. Immun.* **11**, 1003.

Kalunda M., Lee K.M., Holmes D.F. & Gillespie J.H. (1975) Serologic classification of feline calicivirus by plaque reduction neutralisation and immunodiffusion. *Am. J. Vet. Res.* **36**, 353.

Knowles J.O. (1988) Studies on feline calicivirus with particular reference to chronic stomatitis in the cat. PhD thesis, University of Liverpool.

Knowles J.O., Gaskell R.M., Gaskell C.J., Harvey C.E. & Lutz H. (1989) Prevalence of feline calicivirus, feline leukaemia virus and antibodies to FIV in cats with chronic stomatitis. *Vet. Rec.* **124**, 336.

Knowles J.O., Dawson S., Gaskell R.M., Gaskell C.J. & Harvey C.E. (1990) Neutralisation patterns amongst recent British and North American feline calicivirus isolates from different clinical origins. *Vet. Rec.* **127**, 125.

Knowles J.O., McArdle F., Dawson S., Carter S., Gaskell C.J. & Gaskell R.M. (1991) Studies on the role of feline calicivirus in chronic stomatitis in cats. *Vet. Microbiol.* **27**, 205.

Love D.N. (1975) Pathogenicity of a strain of feline calicivirus for domestic kittens. *Austr. Vet. J.* **51**, 541.

Ormerod E., McCandlish I.A.P. & Jarrett O. (1979) Diseases produced by feline caliciviruses when administered to cats by aerosol or intranasal instillation. *Vet. Rec.* **104**, 65.

Pedersen N.C., Laliberte L. & Ekman S. (1983) A transient febrile limping syndrome of kittens caused by two different strains of feline calicivirus. *Fel. Pract.* **13**, 26.

Povey R.C. (1974) Serologic relationships among feline caliciviruses. *Infect. Immun.* **10**, 1307.

Povey R.C. & Hale C.J. (1974) Experimental infections with feline caliciviruses (picornaviruses) in specific-pathogen-free kittens. *J. Comp. Path.* **84**, 245.

Povey R.C. & Ingersoll J. (1975) Cross-protection among feline caliciviruses. *Infect. Immun.* **11**, 877.

Studdert M.J., Martin M.C. & Peterson J.E. (1970) Viral diseases of the respiratory tract of cats: isolation and properties of viruses tentatively classified as picornaviruses. *Am. J. Vet. Res.* **31**, 1723.

Tham K.M. & Studdery M.J. (1987c) Antibody and cell-mediated immune responses to feline calicivirus following inactivated vaccine and challenge. *J. Vet. Med. B.* **34**, 640.

Thompson R.R., Wilcox G.E., Clark W.T. & Jansen K.L. (1984) Association of calicivirus infection with chronic gingivitis and pharyngitis in cats. *J. Small Anim. Pract.* **25**, 207.

Wardley R.C. (1976) Feline calicivirus carrier state. A study of the host/virus relationship. *Arch. Virol.* **52**, 243.

Wardley R.C. & Povey R.C. (1976) Aerosol transmission of feline caliciviruses. An assessment of its epidemiological importance. *Br. Vet. J.* **133**, 504.

Wardley R.C. & Povey R.C. (1977a) The pathology and sites of persistence associated with three different strains of feline calicivirus. *Res. Vet. Sci.* **23**, 15.

Wardley R.C. & Povey R.C. (1977b) The clinical disease and patterns of excretion associated with three different strains of feline calicivirus. *Res. Vet. Sci.* **23**, 7.

Chapter 15 / Feline Leukaemia Virus

O. JARRETT

INTRODUCTION

Feline leukaemia virus (FeLV) is an important cause of death in young adult cats. The virus was recognized originally as the cause of lymphosarcoma (Jarrett *et al.*, 1964) and other haemopoietic tumours, but it is now clear that it is also associated with many non-malignant conditions that may be more common than cases of neoplasia. FeLV-related diseases occur in cats that have a permanent infection characterized by a persistent viraemia. In these cats the latent period between infection and the development of clinical disease is often long and although cats may remain quite healthy during this time, they excrete virus and may transmit the infection to other susceptible cats. The control of FeLV infections depends partly on the isolation of viraemic carrier cats from susceptible animals, and partly on vaccination.

Many diseases associated with FeLV involve the haemopoietic and lymphoid systems. Thus, diseases are encountered which are characterized by proliferation, including lymphosarcoma and myeloid leukaemia, as well as those in which cell populations are depleted, as in anaemia, marrow aplasia and immunodeficiency.

This chapter presents an outline of the characteristics of FeLV which are relevant to the pathogenesis and epidemiology of the virus, a description of the clinicopathological features of the major diseases associated with FeLV infection, and a discussion of the measures which have been evolved to control FeLV infections.

STRUCTURE AND REPLICATION OF FeLV

FeLV is a retrovirus with a genome of RNA, surrounded by a protein core and an external envelope. The most abundant of the core proteins has a molecular weight of 27 000 and consequently is called p27. Surrounding the core and comprising the external surface of the particle is an envelope in which are inserted glycoprotein spikes. The antigens which induce the production of virus-neutralizing (VN) antibodies reside in these spikes.

The basis of FeLV persistence in cats may be found in the life cycle of retroviruses within infected cells, a crucial stage of which is the integration of a DNA copy of the viral genome into the cellular chromosomes. This FeLV provirus remains indefinitely in infected cells and directs the synthesis of new viral particles. Infected cells are not harmed in this process and may continue to divide. As a result of virus synthesis, the major core protein, p27, is produced in large quantities in the cytoplasm of infected cells and is also released from the cells. The detection of p27 in the blood is important in the diagnosis of FeLV infections in cats.

Another important characteristic of retroviruses is that virus is released by infected cells only during mitosis. This feature is important in pathogenesis by FeLV since the virus grows mainly in those tissues which contain rapidly dividing cells, as in the bone marrow and in the stem cells of epithelial surfaces.

PATHOGENESIS OF
FeLV INFECTION

Source of infection

The source of FeLV is the persistently viraemic cat that may be suffering from FeLV-related disease or, more likely, is a healthy carrier. Transmission occurs in two main ways. First, FeLV is transmitted by contact (Hardy *et al.*, 1973; Jarrett *et al.*, 1973). The virus is excreted from the mouth of infected cats and licking is likely to be the means of transfer of virus. FeLV is also excreted in the urine, faeces and milk. A second important method of transmission is congenital, probably by passage of virus through the uterus of infected queens to her developing embryos.

The importance of indirect transmission of virus is not clear. It is generally considered that owing to the lability of FeLV and the relatively large quantity of virus that must be transmitted to achieve a successful infection, indirect spread of virus occurs rarely, if at all.

Consequences of infection

Most cats that are exposed to FeLV recover, develop an immunity and do not become excreting carriers. The proportion of cats that recover varies greatly according to the circumstances of exposure to the virus. The alternative and less favourable outcome is that a permanent infection is established.

Persistent FeLV infection

Following infection by transfer of FeLV-containing saliva into the mouth, the virus grows in cells in the oropharynx and is transported in blood mononuclear cells to tissues in which extensive viral replication can occur (Rojko *et al.*, 1979), notably the bone marrow which consists of a large population of dividing cells. The virus grows in the marrow, eventually infecting essentially all of the dividing cells and consequently is produced in very large amounts. Free virus and p27 antigen are released into the plasma. The blood also contains neutrophils which have p27 antigen in their cytoplasm.

The virus produced in the bone marrow reaches many other organs by haematogenous spread and multiplies in many tissues where there are dividing cells, such as the epithelial cells of the oropharynx, the upper respiratory tract and the salivary glands from which the virus is excreted into the mouth.

The incubation period between infection and the first appearance of virus in the blood is approximately 2 weeks following experimental administration of virus into the oropharynx, but in natural conditions this period can be extremely variable ranging from 4 to 30 weeks. When an FeLV carrier cat is introduced into a household of susceptible animals, a considerable period is required before a state of socializing is achieved which permits sufficient contact for the transfer of virus (Madewell & Jarrett, 1983).

Transient FeLV infections

Most cats exposed to FeLV undergo a temporary infection from which they ostensibly recover (Jarrett *et al.*, 1982a). Following infection of the oropharynx, the extent of spread of virus in the body varies. In some animals the virus may not reach the bone marrow before the infection ends, exposure to virus being inferred from the subsequent appearance of antibodies in the serum. In other cats, infection goes a stage further so that transient viraemia is apparent before the virus is eliminated. The duration of the transient viraemia is variable and may last from 1 or 2 days up to 8 weeks. During the period of transient viraemia the cat usually excretes virus from the mouth.

Latent FeLV infections

Of the cats which appear to recover from FeLV infection, over half do not eliminate the virus immediately but maintain it for a time in bone marrow, and perhaps other, cells in a latent form. However, these cells do not usually release virus in sufficient quantities to either establish a viraemia or be excreted from the mouth. Latent infections are most effectively uncovered by detection of virus in cell cultures established from bone marrow biopsies (Rojko *et al.*, 1982).

Latency is generally short-lived, but around 10% of cats retain their latent infection for over 3 years (Pacitti *et al.*, 1986).

The significance of healthy latent carriers in the spread of FeLV is not clear. Based on experience of the control of FcLV infections, it is assumed that such cats do not act as a major source of infectious FeLV (McClelland *et al.*, 1980). However, transmission of FeLV in the milk from a latently infected queen to her kittens has been recorded (Pacitti *et al.*, 1986). It is not established if cats with latent infections are at risk of developing FeLV-related diseases.

Determinants of the outcome of FeLV infections

The two most important factors which determine whether a cat becomes permanently infected or recovers from FeLV are the age at which it is infected and the dose of virus to which it is exposed. The most susceptible animal is the developing fetus and all kittens born of persistently viraemic queens have a permanent infection. Young kittens less than 8 weeks old are also very susceptible, but after that age the proportion which resist infection increases rapidly so that only a minority of cats over the age of 16 weeks develop a persistent infection following exposure (Hoover *et al.*, 1976).

Another important factor is virus dose, which is related in large measure to the circumstances in which the cat is maintained. Among free-range cats the degree of contact between excreting and susceptible cats, and hence the amount of virus which is transmitted, is limited. Although FeLV exposure is common among these cats, very few become permanently infected (Hosie *et al.*, 1989). By contrast in closed, multi-cat households into which the virus is introduced, the dose of virus transmitted is large and approximately 30–40% of susceptible cats become persistently viraemic.

Prognosis for persistently viraemic cats

Cats with persistent FeLV infections have a very high risk of developing an FeLV-related disease.

In one study 85% of viraemic cats died within 3.5 years of natural exposure compared to 15% of recovered or uninfected cats (McClelland *et al.*, 1980). Another important demonstration of the effect of FeLV viraemia is that approximately half of cats die within 6 months of the time of diagnosis of FeLV viraemia. Such cats, of course, may have had the infection for a long period before diagnosis.

Immunity to FeLV

Fortunately, most cats that are exposed to FeLV recover and do not continue to excrete virus. Resolution of a transient FeLV infection is due to an immune response. Virus-neutralizing (VN) antibody is found in the serum of recovered (and latently infected) cats but very rarely in viraemic cats. Cats with VN antibodies are resistant to infection with FeLV. VN antibodies are transferred to kittens in the colostrum and protect them from early FeLV infection for about the first 4 weeks of life (Hoover *et al.*, 1977; Jarrett *et al.*, 1977).

EPIDEMIOLOGICAL SITUATIONS

The consequences of FeLV infections for cat populations depend to a large extent on how the animals are maintained. Two reasonably distinct epidemiological patterns may be discerned, the major characteristics of which are shown in Table 15.1.

Free-range cats

The first pattern involves free-range cats. Most probably the cycle of transmission of FeLV in these cats involves the excretion of small amounts of virus for short periods by transiently viraemic animals. In this way, there is widespread dissemination of virus throughout the community with the majority of cats being exposed. However, the dose of virus is small and most cats recover. A second factor which alleviates the consequences of infection is that most cats in this community are more than 16 weeks of age before they en-

Table 15.1 Epidemiological patterns in FeLV infections.

Free-range cats	
High exposure rate	
Low prevalence of immunity	4% of cats have virus-neutralizing antibodies [VNA]
Low viraemia rate	5% of cats viraemic
Low incidence of FeLV-related disease	
FeLV-infected multi-cat households	
High exposure rate	
High prevalence of immunity	70% of FeLV-negative cats have VNA
High rate of viraemia	30–40% of cats viraemic
High incidence of FeLV-related diseases	

counter the virus and consequently are relatively resistant. Few of these cats develop VN antibodies (the hallmark of the resistant cat), suggesting that they may be susceptible to subsequent re-infection. In a survey in the UK about 5% of healthy cats were found to be viraemic (Hosie *et al.*, 1989).

Multi-cat households

In marked contrast to the free-range cat, the cat in a multi-cat household into which FeLV is introduced has a very high risk of developing a persistent infection and an FeLV-related disease (Hardy *et al.*, 1973). Close association of cats leads to the continuous transmission of large doses of virus and often very young cats are exposed. Approximately 30–40% of cats in houses in which FeLV is enzootic are found to be persistently viraemic. The non-viraemic cats usually have VN antibodies and are resistant to the infection. A great deal of the FeLV-related disease which is encountered is in multi-cat households, and consequently often in the pedigree breeds. There is no real evidence, however, that any one breed is more or less susceptible to FeLV than any other.

FeLV-RELATED DISEASES

Diseases associated with FeLV infection tend to occur in young adult cats between 2 and 4 years of age (Hosie *et al.*, 1989) although there are notable exceptions such as alimentary lymphosarcoma, as discussed below. The major diseases associated with FeLV infection are summarized in Table 15.2.

Diseases of the haemopoietic system

As described in Chapter 4, the haemopoietic system consists of two main components, myeloid and lymphoid. In the bone marrow reside the pluripotential stem cells, from which committed myeloid and lymphoid stem cells are derived. The myeloid stem cell then gives rise to blast cells, which differentiate along separate lineages to provide the erythrocytes, granulocytes, monocytes or platelets of the blood. In the other component, precursor lymphoid cells differentiate into T- or B-lymphocytes which migrate from the marrow to populate the peripheral lymphatic tissues and take part in immune responses to infectious agents. FeLV can exert profound effects on the differentiation of each of these cell types, producing the proliferation of cells which is recognized as lymphoid or myeloid neoplasia, or extinction of cells leading to conditions such as anaemia or immunodeficiency.

Haemopoietic tumours

Approximately 90% of the malignancies of the haemopoietic system in cats involve lymphoid

Table 15.2 FeLV-related diseases.

Malignant haemopoietic diseases

Lymphosarcoma   thymic lymphosarcoma, multicentric lymphosarcoma, alimentary lymphosarcoma, lymphatic leukaemia

Myeloid leukaemias   mycloid leukaemia, erythroleukaemia, acute erythraemia

Non-malignant haemopoietic diseases

Anaemias   haemolytic anaemia, erythroid hypoplasia,
Immunodeficiency
Marrow aplasia

Other diseases

Infertility
Enteritis

---

cells. Tumours of the other elements of the haemopoietic system, myeloid and erythroid cells, are less frequently diagnosed, but are almost certainly more common than is generally realized.

LYMPHOSARCOMA

In lymphosarcoma, malignant lymphoid cells infiltrate into compartments of the lymphoid tissues throughout the body. Lymphosarcoma is by far the most common malignant tumour of the cat, representing about one-third of all tumours. Lymphosarcoma is more commonly diagnosed in cats than in any other species of domestic animal or man, occurring with an annual incidence of around 200 per 100 000 cats at risk. Since it is uniformly fatal, the disease is a major cause of death in adult cats.

There are several quite distinct forms of lymphosarcoma which are defined by the distribution of the tumour cells within the lymphatic system. This localization almost certainly reflects the localization of the normal counterparts of the malignant lymphoid cells.

Four major types of lymphoid neoplasms are recognized. These are thymic lymphosarcoma, multicentric lymphosarcoma, alimentary lymphosarcoma and lymphatic leukemia. In addition, several other types of lymphosarcoma, involving individual organs, are encountered. The major clinical and diagnostic features of lymphosarcoma are summarized in Table 15.3.

Thymic lymphosarcoma

In this form there is a large mass in the anterior mediastinum as shown in Fig. 15.1. All thymic lymphosarcomas consist of T-cells. Lymph node involvement varies. The thoracic lymph nodes are always enlarged but further dissemination of the tumour cells to other nodes is unusual. Likewise, tumour cells are seldom found in the blood. There is often some degree of pleural effusion.

The clinical signs are due mainly to the space-occupying effects of the tumour and pleural fluid on the thoracic organs (see Chapter 6). The tumour may develop over a period of weeks or months and weight loss is common, but the tumour is often remarkably large before any specific clinical signs become apparent. Pressure on the lungs and trachea produces tachypnoea, dyspnoea and exercise intolerance. There is muffling of heart sounds and decreased thoracic resonance. The anterior thorax is often incompressible. If the oesophagus is restricted, there may be difficulty in swallowing.

Diagnosis is based mainly on the clinical signs. Thymic lymphosarcoma is more common in young cats (average 2.5 years). Radiographic examination of the thorax will demonstrate the space-occupying mass, dorsal displacement of the trachea and the presence of pleural fluid (Fig. 15.2). Cytology of the pleural fluid obtained by thoracentesis will reveal malignant lymphoid

Table 15.3 Diagnostic features in lymphosarcoma (LSA).

Type of LSA	Diagnostic features
Thymic LSA	Weight loss Tachypnoea, dyspnoea, exercise intolerance Regurgitation Young animal (average 2.5 years) Radiography: mass in anterior mediastinum; displacement of trachea Cytology on pleural fluid: malignant lymphoblasts FeLV test positive in 80%
Multicentric LSA	Bilateral enlargement of peripheral lymph nodes Splenomegaly Histology of lymph node biopsy: malignant cells FeLV test positive in 60%
Alimentary LSA	Tumour masses palpable in abdomen Weight loss, inappetence/anorexia Wasting, vomiting or diarrhoea Pallor of mucous membrances Anaemia FeLV test positive in only 30%
Lymphatic leukaemia	Intermittent pyrexia Weakness, inappetence/anorexia Pallor of mucous membranes Petechial haemorrhages in mucous membranes and skin Haematology: raised WBC count and malignant cells, anaemia FeLV test positive in 60%

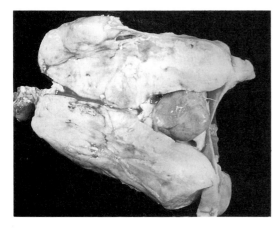

Fig. 15.1 Thymic lymphosarcoma. A huge tumour mass is present in the mediastinum anterior to the heart.

cells. Haematology may be helpful although tumour cells are not always found in the blood. Tests for FeLV are useful since about 80% of cats with thymic lymphosarcoma are FeLV-positive.

Multicentric lymphosarcoma
As the name suggests, the multicentric form of lymphosarcoma involves lymphatic tissues throughout the body. As shown in Fig. 15.3, the lymph nodes are grossly enlarged due to infiltration of malignant lymphoid cells, and on examination at biopsy or post-mortem examination they are pale with loss of cortico-medullary differentiation. The white pulp of the spleen is infiltrated and protrudes when the surface is cut. The liver may also be involved.

Clinically, there is bilateral enlargement of the

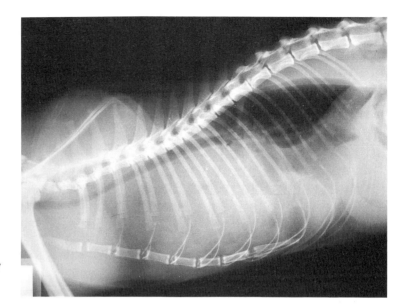

Fig. 15.2 Thymic lymphosarcoma. The radiograph shows a tumour mass in the anterior thorax with displacement of the trachea dorsally and the presence of pleural fluid. (Courtesy of Prof. Robin Lee.)

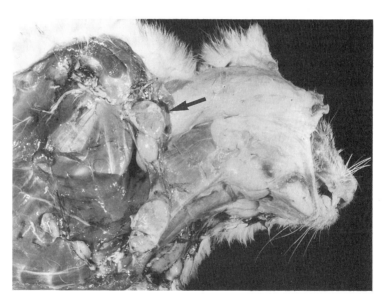

Fig. 15.3 Multicentric lymphosarcoma. Grossly enlarged cervical (arrowed) and retropharyngeal lymph nodes are evident.

peripheral lymph nodes. Splenomegaly is usual but hepatomegaly is less common. A moderate anaemia is apparent in about half of cases but obvious tumour cells are found in the blood in less than 20% of cases. The average age of cats with multicentric lymphosarcoma is about 4 years. Definitive confirmation of the diagnosis is by histological examination of a lymph node biopsy. Approximately 60% of cases of multicentric lymphosarcoma are FeLV-positive.

Alimentary lymphosarcoma
The tumour mass in alimentary lymphosarcoma consists of malignant B-lymphocytes and occurs

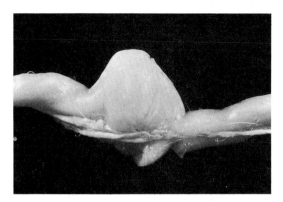

Fig. 15.4 Alimentary lymphosarcoma: tumour mass in wall of ileum.

in the gastrointestinal wall at some point in the tract (Fig. 15.4), commonly spreading to the associated mesenteric lymph nodes. The usual sites are the small intestine, caecum or colon and, less frequently, the stomach or rectum. Occasionally a diffuse infiltration of a large part of the bowel is found. The kidneys may also be involved. Erosion of the tumour into the lumen may occur.

Clinically, weight loss and anorexia are common. The particular signs are associated with intestinal obstruction, for example vomiting if the upper small intestine is occluded. Diarrhoea and wasting are found when there is diffuse involvement of the small intestine or lower bowel. The tumour mass is often palpable in the abdomen although the clinical effects may be due to quite small tumours. Anaemia is common. In general, alimentary lymphosarcoma occurs in older cats (average age 8 years) and the majority are free of FeLV, only about 30% of cases being FeLV-positive.

Lymphatic leukaemia
Lymphatic leukaemia primarily involves the bone marrow. The growth of tumour cells in the marrow has a harmful effect on haemopoiesis. The leukaemic cells spread haematogenously to other organs rather than by the lymphatic system and are found in the blood, spleen and liver. There may be a greatly increased white blood cell count due to the circulating leukaemic cells.

Haematology also usually reveals anaemia and thrombocytopenia.

The first clinical sign may be intermittent pyrexia over a period of a few weeks. Weakness and loss of appetite are noticed as anaemia develops. Thrombocytopenia may lead to petechial haemorrhages in the skin and mucous membranes. There is splenomegaly and usually hepatomegaly, but lymph node enlargement is not common.

Confirmation of the diagnosis relies on haematology. An increased white cell count together with the presence of large numbers of malignant cells on a blood smear are pathognomonic. Bone marrow biopsy will demonstrate the replacement of the marrow by malignant cells. The FeLV test is positive in 60% of cases.

Other forms of lymphosarcoma
The four forms described above are the most commonly diagnosed types of lymphosarcoma. However, other forms occur more rarely in which essentially a single organ or tissue is involved. These are found mainly in the kidney, skin, eye or central nervous system. Kidney tumours may be relatively small but are commonly large, invading the cortex. In the skin, the tumour masses are discrete and raised, up to 2 cm in diameter. In the eye, lymphosarcoma is the most common intraocular tumour and may involve any of the ophthalmic structures, with one or both eyes being affected. The growth of tumour in the central nervous system produces clinical effects depending on the part involved.

FeLV-negative lymphosarcoma
Many cases of lymphosarcoma in cats are free of FeLV by all established criteria and as described above, many are of the alimentary type. An important question is whether or not FeLV is implicated in the pathogenesis of these tumours, perhaps by initiating the leukaemogenic process before being eliminated from the cat. Evidence in favour of this interpretation is that an epidemiological association in multi-cat households has been described between FeLV infection and the occurrence of cases of virus-negative lympho-

sarcoma as well as virus-positive cases (Hardy *et al.*, 1980). On the other hand, virus-free lymphosarcoma has been observed in cats that were never exposed to FeLV, and there is no evidence that FeLV DNA is present in the virus-negative tumour cells, as one might expect if the cells had been infected by FeLV at some time.

In view of the finding that virus-negative lymphosarcoma cases occur more frequently than expected in households in which FeLV is enzootic, it is wise to check the FeLV status of other cats in a house in which this type of lymphosarcoma occurs. Since tumours of B-lymphocytes, including alimentary lymphosarcomas, are quite commonly associated with feline immunodeficiency virus infection (Callanan *et al.*, 1992), diagnostic tests for that virus must also be considered.

MYELOID LEUKAEMIA

Neoplastic diseases of cells in the myeloid compartment of the haemopoietic system are less commonly diagnosed than lymphoid tumours. Myeloid tumour cells arise in the bone marrow and spread haematogenously to other organs, notably the spleen, liver and lymph nodes. It is likely that the primary defect occurs in a haemopoietic stem cell committed to the myeloid lineages. Subsequently, a clone of malignant cells becomes dominant, producing a large proportion of abnormal cells in the bone marrow and blood. There is considerable variety in the extent of the defect, so that in some cases the leukaemic cells are poorly differentiated blast cells, while in others there may be a degree of differentiation, with granulocytes which appear almost normal present in the blood. Variety also occurs in the cell lineage that is involved, so that malignant cells of more than one series may be apparent. The main characteristics of the myeloid leukaemias are summarized in Table 15.4. In addition, a few cases of monocytic, megakaryocytic and eosinophilic leukaemias have been recorded in the cat.

While the conditions summarized in Table 15.4 are considered here separately, it should be appreciated that in many cases strict categor-

Table 15.4 Diagnostic features in myeloid leukaemias.

Myeloid leukaemia
Bone marrow. The tumour cells may be poorly differentiated with very few mature neutrophils, or well differentiated with late members of the neutrophil or (rarely) eosinophil series in the blood. WBC count varies considerably
Anaemia is macrocytic and normochromic with reticulocytosis
Extramedullary haemopoiesis invariably occurs

Erythroleukaemia
Proliferation of malignant cells of both the erythroid and granulocytic series. In the blood, granulocytic cells are usually well differentiated, while cells of the erythroid series are often primitive with many aberrant blast forms

Acute erythraemia
Malignant cells are erythroid
The blood contains large numbers of malignant erythroblasts and normoblasts

ization is extremely difficult. The clinical and pathological features of myeloproliferative diseases, however, tend to be similar. The signs are a reflection of grossly abnormal haemopoiesis and dissemination of malignant cells in the blood, although there is not necessarily an increased white blood cell (WBC) count. The major clinical feature is a progressive anaemia. Intermittent pyrexia and weight loss is common. There is usually splenomegaly, hepatomegaly and a variable degree of lymphadenopathy. Thrombocytopenia may lead to haemorrhages in the skin and mucous membranes while leucopenia renders the cat very susceptible to bacterial infections.

A precise diagnosis of the type of myeloproliferative disease relies upon cytology, and blood and bone marrow smears.

FeLV is found in the majority of cases of myeloid leukaemia and the disease has been induced experimentally by the virus. However, all cases of eosinophilic leukaemia have been FeLV-negative.

Non-malignant haemopoietic diseases

PRIMARY FeLV-ASSOCIATED ANAEMIA

Severe anaemia is diagnosed more commonly in cats than in other domestic animals. There are several causes, the most important being FeLV. FeLV-associated anaemia may be consequent upon lymphoid or myeloid leukaemia with their harmful effects on haemopoiesis, or it may be a primary effect of the virus.

Erythroid hypoplasia

The main type of primary FeLV-related anaemia is erythroid hypoplasia, a condition similar to pure red cell aplasia in man, in which only cells of the erythroid series are affected (Hoover *et al.*, 1974; Mackey *et al.*, 1975). A complete block in erythropoiesis occurs so that the numbers of erythroblasts, normoblasts and reticulocytes in the bone marrow, and erythrocytes in the blood, decline rapidly (Onions *et al.*, 1982). Granulocytes and platelets are produced in normal amounts. This condition is often referred to as 'non-regenerative' anaemia.

Cats are usually presented in the later stages of the disease when the signs are of a severe, progressive anaemia. The haematocrit is very low, often below 10%, but the WBC count is usually within the normal range. The red blood cells (RBCs) are normocytic and normochromic. Nucleated RBCs may be present in the blood, but reticulocytes are absent. Extramedullary haemopoiesis is not usually apparent at this late stage.

Haemolytic anaemia

Haemolytic anaemia associated with FeLV infection may be common, but often remains undiagnosed until the condition becomes severe. Of cats with a haematocrit of less than 20%, approximately one-sixth will have a haemolytic anaemia (Hardy, 1981). The anaemia is macrocytic and normochromic with evidence of reticulocytosis and extramedullary haemopoiesis.

Experience of the treatment of anaemias in FeLV-positive cats is not encouraging.

FeLV-ASSOCIATED IMMUNODEFICIENCY

General immunodeficiency is reflected clinically in the susceptibility of viraemic cats to infections by microbial agents which would normally be insignificant in the uncompromised individual.

The mechanism by which FeLV causes immunodeficiency is complex and is not fully understood. The strain of virus may be important and some strongly immunosuppressive isolates which kill T-lymphocytes *in vitro* have been described (Hoover *et al.*, 1987). In young kittens with FeLV infections, the thymus atrophies very rapidly and the maturation of T-lymphocytes may be adversely affected (Anderson *et al.*, 1971). Another suggested mechanism is that a viral protein, p15(E) is directly cytotoxic to lymphocytes (Mathes *et al.*, 1979). Whatever the mechanism, viraemic cats are often very susceptible to respiratory tract infections, enteritis, gingivitis, abscesses and septicaemia, and may show prolonged wound healing times. Any cat with a chronic inflammatory condition should be suspected of being infected with FeLV. Such cats should also be tested for the presence of the lentivirus, feline immunodeficiency virus.

MARROW APLASIA

In marrow aplasia there is hypoplasia of the myeloid cells in the bone marrow with a consequent severe leucopenia. The pathogenesis of this condition is uncertain. Possibly FeLV-induced immunodeficiency may allow colonization of the gut with bacteria which produce toxins responsible for the severe depression of myelopoiesis. Alternatively, FeLV may exert a direct aplastic effect on the bone marrow.

The major clinical signs are weight loss, anorexia, pyrexia, depression and dehydration. Frequently, bacterial involvement causes dysentery and on post-mortem examination there is a severe haemorrhagic enteritis throughout the intestine with haemorrhagic mesenteric lymph nodes.

ENTERITIS

Two types of FeLV-associated 'panleucopenia-like' syndromes have been reported. In the first, lesions in the intestine are distinct from those of panleucopenia, occurring at the tips of the villi rather than in the crypts (Hardy, 1981). There is depletion of lymphoid tissue in the intestinal wall and of granulocytes in the bone marrow. By contrast, in the second type the lesions in the intestine are identical to those of panleucopenia with degeneration of epithelial cells of the crypts of the villi and villous atrophy (Reinacher, 1987). However, there is no degeneration of lymphoid follicles in the gut or other lymphoid organs. A further distinction is that this syndrome is subacute or chronic compared to the generally acute clinical course of panleucopenia. Severe enteritis has also been described in association with infection by the immunodeficiency-causing strain of FeLV (Hoover *et al.*, 1987).

FeLV-related reproductive disease

FeLV is the single most common cause of infertility in queens. This is not to say that all queens persistently viraemic with FeLV have reproductive problems. Indeed, it is quite usual for queens with a recent history of infertility to have had one or two normal pregnancies.

FeLV is much more frequently associated with fetal resorption than abortion. A common history is that a queen has had at least one previous unsuccessful pregnancy. In the present pregnancy mating was normal and 3–4 weeks later conceptual swellings were palpable and the queen showed other signs of early pregnancy. However, at 5–7 weeks there was a sudden reduction in abdominal size, which might or might not have been associated with a slight, bloody vaginal discharge.

The mechanism by which FeLV causes fetal resorption is not known. Egg transfer experiments indicate that the virus is transmitted across the placenta to the post-implantation embryo, but whether the pathogenesis involves an effect on the embryo or the placenta is not clear, although the latter is suggested by the occurrence of an endometritis in a large proportion of cases.

TREATMENT OF LYMPHOSARCOMA

Treatment is by administration of a combination of cytotoxic drugs. In a report of 103 cases, complete remission was achieved in 62% with a median survival time of 7 months, and about 20% survived for over 12 months (Mooney *et al.*, 1989). A protocol suggested by Squires and Gorman (1990) is reproduced in Table 15.5. On recurrence of the tumour, the treatment for weeks 2–8 should be repeated but with an increased prednisolone dose of $40 \, mg/m^2$. An effective, but expensive, treatment for subsequent tumour recurrences is L-asparaginase $(10\,000 \, IU/m^2)$ subcutaneously every 3 weeks until the tumour becomes resistant, then doxorubicin $(30 \, mg/m^2)$ intravenously every 3 weeks until the cumulative dose is $240 \, mg/m^2$.

Continuous monitoring of possible harmful effects of therapy such as leucopenia and thrombocytopenia is essential. The success of treatment may be assessed by radiography for thymic lymphosarcoma, or the reduction in lymph node size combined with histology of lymph node biopsies in the case of multicentric lymphosarcoma. Little success has been achieved in the treatment of lymphatic or myeloid leukaemia.

DIAGNOSIS OF FeLV INFECTION

The methods used for FeLV diagnosis are outlined in Table 15.6. The most commonly used screening test is the enzyme-linked immunosorbent assay (ELISA) which detects FeLV p27 antigen in the blood. This test is available in kit form for use by veterinary practitioners and is sensitive, specific and rapid.

Other diagnostic methods are virus isolation (VI) and immunofluorescence (IF). VI is considered to be the definitive diagnostic test but has the disadvantages that it is relatively expensive and time-consuming.

It is essential that if control programmes may result in euthanasia of an apparently healthy cat,

Table 15.5 Chemotherapy of lymphosarcoma.

Stage	Timing	Drug	Dose/m^2	Route
Induction	Day 1	L-asparaginase	10 000 IU	s.c.
		Vincristine	0.5 mg	i.v.
	Day 1–7	Prednisolone	40 mg	oral
	Day 3–6	Cyclophosphamide	50 mg	oral
	Weeks 2–8:			
	Daily	Prednisolone	20 mg	oral
	Every 2 days	Cyclophosphamide	50 mg	oral
	Weekly	Vincristine	0.5 mg	i.v.
Maintenance	Every 2 days	Cyclophosphamide	50 mg	oral
	Every 2 days	Prednisolone	20 mg	oral
	Every 2 weeks	Vincristine	0.5 mg	i.v.
[Alternative]	Every 2 days	Chlorambucil	2 mg	oral
	Every 2 days	Prednisolone	20 mg	oral
	2–3 times/week	Methotrexate	2.5 mg	oral

Adapted from Squires and Gorman (1989) with permission.

Table 15.6 Diagnostic methods for FeLV.

Method	FeLV component detected	Sample
ELISA	p27 antigen	Plasma
Virus isolation	Infectious virus	Plasma
Immunofluorescence	Antigen in neutrophils	Blood smear

the diagnostic methods used to detect viraemic cats must be very reliable. From comparisons of these tests in routine diagnosis, it is clear that a negative result in any test indicates that the cat is FeLV-free (Jarrett *et al.*, 1982b). However, about 10% of healthy cats which are positive by ELISA are found to be negative when tested by VI or IF. The basis of this 'discordant' state is not known. The cat may be at the beginning or, more likely, at the end of a transient infection when there is antigen but no virus in the blood. Alternatively the cat may have a latent infection or a focal productive infection, in which antigen, but not virus, gains access to the blood.

The important questions which arise are whether or not 'discordant' cats excrete virus and are a danger to susceptible cats and whether they are at a higher risk than uninfected cats of developing an FeLV-related disease. Present evidence suggests that they are not an important source of infectious virus. However, it is not yet known whether such cats have a higher than normal risk of developing FeLV-related disease.

In the present state of knowledge discordant cats should be isolated and retested after 12 weeks. If they have been undergoing transient infection or were at the start of an infection, the situation may be resolved during this interval and the cat will be either negative or positive on both tests. There is a tendency for discordant cats to become negative on both tests even though they may have been positive by ELISA on two occasions, 4 weeks apart (Jarrett *et al.*, 1991). However, some of these cats will continue in the discordant state indefinitely and should be treated with suspicion. While they are unlikely to spread virus by contact, such queens may transmit the infection in the milk (Pacitti *et al.*, 1986). Therefore, discordant cats should not be used for breeding.

VACCINATION

At present two vaccines are available in the UK. One (*Leucocell 2**) consists of inactivated viral products while the second (*Leucogen†*) is a genetically engineered subunit vaccine containing the protein part of the surface glycoprotein of FeLV. Both claim to provide 80–100% protection against challenge. Two doses of vaccine are given with an interval of 3 weeks between doses, and kittens can be vaccinated from 9 weeks of age. An annual booster vaccination should be given. It is strongly recommended that cats should be tested for FeLV before vaccination otherwise if a vaccinated cat is subsequently found to be FeLV positive, there is no way of knowing whether the infection was acquired before or after vaccination. Vaccination of viraemic cats is apparently safe, but has no useful effect on the infection. The diagnostic tests for FeLV are not affected by vaccination.

CONTROL OF
FeLV INFECTIONS

A programme of control

There is considerable demand for the control of FeLV infections, especially from the owners of pedigree cats in multi-cat households. The method of control is the detection and isolation or elimination of the source of infection – the persistently viraemic cat. A typical control programme is illustrated in Table 15.7. The reasons for re-testing after 12 weeks are, first, to establish whether or not a positive cat is still positive and therefore likely to have a permanent infection,

* Leucocell 2; SmithKline Beecham, Animal Health, Tadworth, Survey, UK.
† Leucogen; Virbac Ltd.

Table 15.7 A programme for the control of FeLV infections.

1 Test all cats for FeLV
2 Separate FeLV-positive and FeLV-negative cats Quarantine the house: no removals or additions. Wash and disinfect all bowls, litter trays, baskets, etc.
3 Re-test cats after 12 weeks
4 FeLV-positive cats are considered permanently viraemic and should be euthanased or kept in permanent isolation. FeLV-negative cats are considered free of infectious FeLV. If any negative cats are now positive, return to step 2
5 Re-test all cats at 6–12-month invervals. Test all cats before entry to house. Isolate introductions for 12 weeks and re-test to ensure FeLV-negative before mixing with existing cats

and second, to ensure that a negative cat is still negative and was not incubating an infection at the time of the first test.

Household bleach diluted to concentrations used for normal domestic use can be used to disinfect objects contaminated with FeLV.

Once FeLV has been eliminated from a household, the possible future sources of infection for a cat are new introductions into the house, and contact with other cats at cat shows or at stud. Present evidence suggests that cat shows are not a major source of infection. A re-test at intervals of 6–12 months is strongly recommended for breeding cats which come into contact with queens or toms from other households. It is common practice for owners of stud cats to demand a very recent certificate of freedom from FeLV before allowing a queen to visit. The success of control programmes is well established (Hardy *et al.*, 1976; Weijer *et al.*, 1986).

The decision about the disposal of healthy FeLV-positive cats depends on individual circumstances and will be reached after discussion between the owner and the veterinarian. Many factors have to be considered when making a decision. Many owners will not consider euthanasia of their pet under any circumstances and will elect to retain it in the house. If there is no other cat in the house, this is a reasonable decision since the cat may enjoy many months or years of good health, although the long-term prognosis is not good. However, when it is known that a cat is FeLV-positive, an ethical problem arises since the cat excretes virus and is a potential hazard to other animals, both in the same household or in the local community, if the cat is free-ranging. Owners should be strongly advised to keep such animals away from susceptible cats. This may not be a problem if there are only FeLV-positive cats in the household or the in-contact FeLV-negative cats have been in the house for a sufficient period to assume that they are immune. Susceptible cats can be vaccinated and consequently ought to be resistant to infection. Some owners who wish to remove positive cats from a multi-cat household give them to friends in another house with the instructions that they should not meet other cats.

Owners must be discouraged from breeding from an FeLV-positive queen since all of her kittens will be born with a persistent infection. Infected tom cats should not be used for breeding.

REFERENCES

Anderson L.J., Jarrett W.F.H., Jarrett O. & Laird H.M. (1971) Feline leukemia virus infection of kittens: mortality associated with atrophy of the thymus and lymphoid depletion. *J. Nat. Cancer Inst.* **47**, 807.

Callanan J.J., McCandlish I.A.P., O'Neil B., Lawrence C.E., Rigby M., Pacitti A.M. & Jarrett O. (1992) Lymphosarcoma in experimentally induced feline immunodeficiency virus infection. *Vet. Rec.* **130**, 293.

Hardy W.D. Jr (1981) Feline leukemia virus non-neoplastic diseases. *J. Amer. Anim. Hosp. Assoc.* **17**, 941.

Hardy W.D. Jr, Old L.J., Hess P.W., Essex M. & Cotter S.M. (1973) Horizontal transmission of feline leukaemia virus. *Nature* **244**, 266.

Hardy W.D. Jr, McClelland A.J., Zuckermann E.E., Hess P.W., Essex M., Cotter S.M., MacEwan E.G. & Hayes A. (1976) Prevention of contagious spread of FeLV and the development of leukaemia in pet cats. *Nature* **263**, 326.

Hardy W.D. Jr, McClelland A.J. & Zuckerman E.E. (1980) Development of virus non-producer lymphosarcomas in pet cats exposed to FeLV. *Nature* **288**, 90.

Hoover E.A., Kociba G.J., Hardy W.D. Jr & Yohn D.S. (1974) Erythroid hypoplasia in cats inoculated with feline leukemia virus. *J. Nat. Cancer Inst.* **53**, 1271.

Hoover E.A., Olsen R.G., Hardy W.D. Jr, Schaller J.P. & Mathes L.E. (1976) Feline leukemia virus infection: age-related variation in response of cats to experimental infection. *J. Nat. Cancer Inst.* **57**, 365.

Hoover E.A., Schaller J.P., Mathes L.E. & Olsen R.G. (1977) Passive immunity to feline leukemia: evaluation of immunity from dams naturally infected and experimentally vaccinated. *Inf. Imm.* **16**, 54.

Hoover E.A., Mullins J.I., Quackenbush S.L. & Gasper P.W. (1987) Experimental transmission and pathogenesis of immunodeficiency syndrome in cats. *Blood* **70**, 1880.

Hosie M.J., Robertson C. & Jarrett O. (1989) Prevalence of feline leukaemia virus and antibodies to feline immunodeficiency virus in cats in the United Kingdom. *Vet. Rec.* **128**, 293.

Jarrett O., Russell P.H. & Stewart M.F. (1977) Protection of kittens from feline leukaemia virus infection by maternally-derived antibody. *Vet. Rec.* **101**, 304.

Jarrett O., Golder M.C. & Stewart M.F. (1982a) Detection of transient and persistent feline leukaemia virus infections. *Vet. Rec.* **110**, 225.

Jarrett O., Golder M.C. & Weijer K. (1982b) A comparison of three methods of feline leukaemia virus diagnosis. *Vet. Rec.* **110**, 325.

Jarrett O., Pacitti A.M., Hosie M.J. & Reid G. (1991) Comparison of diagnostic methods for feline leukemia virus and feline immunodeficiency virus. *J. Amer. Vet. Med. Assoc.* **199**, 1362.

Jarrett W., Jarrett O., Mackey L., Laird H., Hardy W. & Essex M. (1973) Horizontal transmission of leukemia virus and leukemia in the cat. *J. Nat. Cancer Inst.* **51**, 833.

Jarrett W.F.H., Martin W.B., Crighton G.W., Dalton R.G. & Stewart M.F. (1964) Leukaemia in the cat. A virus-like particle associated with leukaemia (lymposarcoma). *Nature* **202**, 566.

McClelland A.J., Hardy W.D. Jr & Zuckerman E.E. (1980) Prognosis of healthy feline leukemia virus infected cats. In Hardy W.D. Jr., Essex M. & McClelland A.J. (eds) *Feline Leukemia Virus*. Elsevier-North Holland, New York, pp. 121–6.

Mackey L., Jarrett W., Jarrett O. & Laird H. (1975) Anemia associated with feline leukemia infection in cats. *J. Nat. Cancer Inst.* **54**, 209.

Madewell B.R. & Jarrett O. (1983) Recovery of feline leukaemia virus from non-viraemic cats. *Vet. Rec.* **112**, 339.

Marciani D.J., Kensil C.R., Beltz G.A., Hung C., Cronier J. & Aubert A. (1991) Genetically engineered subunit vaccine against feline leukaemia virus: protective immune response in cats. *Vaccine* **9**, 89.

Mathes L.E., Olsen R.G., Heberbrand L.C., Hoover E.A., Schaller J.P., Adams P.W. & Nichols W.S. (1979) Immunosuppressive properties of a 15000-dalton virion polypeptide protein from feline leukemia virus. *Cancer Res.* **39**, 950.

Mooney S.C., Hayes A.A., MacEwen E.G., Matus R.E., Geary A. & Shurgot B.A. (1989) Treatment and prognostic factors in lymphoma in cats: 103 cases (1977–1981). *J. Amer. Vet. Med. Assoc.* **194**, 696.

Onions D., Jarrett O., Testa N., Frassoni F. & Toth S. (1982) Selective effect of feline leukaemia virus on early erythroid precursors. *Nature* **296**, 156.

Pacitti A.M., Jarrett O. & Hay D. (1986) Transmission of feline leukaemia virus in the milk of a non-viraemic cat. *Vet. Rec.* **118**, 381.

Reinacher M. (1987) Feline leukemia virus-associated enteritis: a condition with features of felines panleukopenia. *Vet. Pathol.* **24**, 1.

Rojko J.L., Hoover E.A., Mathes L.E., Olsen R.G. & Schaller J.P. (1979) Pathogenesis of experimental feline leukemia virus infection. *J. Nat. Cancer Inst.* **63**, 759.

Rojko J.L., Hoover E.A., Quackenbush S.L. & Olsen R.G. (1982) Reactivation of latent feline leukaemia virus infection. *Nature* **298**, 385.

Squires R.A. & Gorman N.T. (1990) Antineoplastic chemotherapy in cats. *In Practice* **12**, 101.

Weijer K., Uytdehaag F. & Osterhaus A. (1986) Control of feline leukaemia virus infection by a removal programme. *Vet. Rec.* **119**, 555.

Chapter 16 / Feline Immunodeficiency Virus

C. D. HOPPER, A. H. SPARKES
AND D. A. HARBOUR

INTRODUCTION

In 1986, investigation of an outbreak of disease in a previously healthy colony of rescued cats in Northern California by workers at the University of California (Davis) Veterinary School resulted in the isolation of a new retrovirus from the affected cats (Pedersen *et al.*, 1987). These cats exhibited a variety of clinical signs suggestive of an immunodeficiency disorder, but the colony was, and had been, kept free of feline leukaemia virus (FeLV) infection by a rigorously applied screening programme. The new virus was shown to belong to the lentivirus subfamily of retroviruses and was tentatively named the feline T-lymphotropic lentivirus (FTLV). By international agreement, and to bring the nomenclature into line with that of other T-lymphotropic lentiviruses (including human immunodeficiency virus (HIV), the cause of AIDS in man) the name was changed to feline immunodeficiency virus (FIV). FIV has been shown to be a significant cause of disease in cats worldwide.

THE AGENT

FIV virions are similar to other lentiviruses, but are slightly smaller at 100–110 nm in diameter. They consist of a cylindrical core, containing a helical ribonucleoprotein strand, surrounded by a membrane which is derived from the outer membrane of the infected cell as the virus particle is externalized by budding. Into the membrane are inserted molecules of a viral glycoprotein of about 130 kDa molecular weight, against which

neutralizing antibodies are directed. This protein appears as short spikes projecting from the membrane. Like other lentiviruses, FIV possesses a Mg^{2+}-dependent reverse transcriptase which distinguishes it from the Mn^{2+}-dependent reverse transcriptase of FeLV. When the virus enters a cell, following uncoating, the reverse transcriptase (which is an integral component of the virion structure) makes a double-stranded DNA copy of the virion RNA genome. The double-stranded DNA copy is integrated into the chromosomal DNA of the host cell. The integrated DNA is known as a provirus, and is essential for further replication of the virus; replication can only take place once the provirus is integrated. Transcription of the provirus leads to the manufacture of virus proteins. Apart from the reverse transcriptase and membrane glycoprotein, there is a transmembrane protein of about 40 kDa and core proteins of 28, 18 and 10 kDa molecular weight.

EPIDEMIOLOGY

Testing of stored serum has shown that antibodies to FIV were present in samples collected in the UK in 1975 (Gruffydd-Jones *et al.*, 1988), and in the USA in 1968 (Shelton *et al.*, 1990a). The worldwide distribution of FIV indicates that the virus has almost certainly existed for many years prior to 1968, and therefore this is a newly recognized (rather than a newly evolved) virus which is likely to be endemic in the general cat population. A survey of exotic cats (Barr, 1989) showed evidence of FIV infection in several zoo

Table 16.1 Results of epidemiological surveys for FIV.

Country	No. of cats tested	% FIV antibody positive	Reference
UK	1007 (healthy)	6	Hosie *et al.* (1989)
	1204 (sick)	19	Hosie *et al.* (1989)
UK	224 (healthy)	6	Hopper *et al.* (1991)
	1450 (sick)	17	Hopper *et al.* (1991)
France	208 (sick)	22	Lutz *et al.* (1988)
Netherlands	123 (healthy)	1	Lutz *et al.* (1988)
	98 (sick)	3	Lutz *et al.* (1988)
Switzerland	178 (healthy)	3	Lutz *et al.* (1988)
	775 (sick)	4	Lutz *et al.* (1988)
Japan	1584 (healthy)	12	Ishida *et al.* (1989)
	1739 (sick)	44	Ishida *et al.* (1989)
USA	361 (healthy)	1	Shelton *et al.* (1989)
	226 (sick)	10	Shelton *et al.* (1989)
USA	585 (various)	2	Witt *et al.* (1989)
USA	83 (healthy)	4	Grindem *et al.* (1989)
	40 (sick)	15	Grindem *et al.* (1989)
USA	511 (low risk*)	1	Yamamoto *et al.* (1989)
	2212 (high risk*)	14	Yamamoto *et al.* (1989)
Canada	42 (high risk*)	19	Yamamoto *et al.* (1989)
Australia	72 (healthy)	29	Robertson *et al.* (1990)
	211 (sick)	28	Robertson *et al.* (1990)

* Low risk indicates healthy cats; high risk indicates cats with chronic problems and those in contact with them.

populations, including snow leopards, lions, tigers and jaguars, and also in free-roaming populations of Florida panthers and bobcats.

Serological surveys have been conducted in several countries to determine the current prevalence of FIV infection in various cat populations. The findings are summarized in Table 16.1. The particularly high prevalence of FIV infection in Japanese cats is thought to be linked to the high density of free-roaming cats found in the Japanese cities from which the samples were obtained. Most surveys show that the prevalence of FIV infection is much greater amongst sick cats, i.e. those with clinical problems, than healthy cats. However, in Switzerland, The Netherlands and Australia there was little difference between sick and healthy cats. It is possible that these latter findings may alter once greater numbers of cats are studied. Alternatively, if pathogenicity does vary between strains of FIV, it may be that the strains occurring in these three countries are less pathogenic than those found elsewhere.

Detailed information is available from the UK (Hosie *et al.*, 1989), American (Yamamoto *et al.*, 1989) and Japanese (Ishida *et al.*, 1989) surveys. A breakdown of the cats tested, according to age, breed, sex and management, is shown in Table 16.2. In cats less than one year of age FIV infection was rare, but the prevalence increased

Table 16.2 Details of UK,[a] American/Canadian[b] and Japanese[c] surveys.

Detail	UK		USA		Japan	
	Total tested	% FIV seropositive	Total tested	% FIV seropositive	Total tested	% FIV seropositive
Sex distribution						
F	819	6	663	8	1330	22
NF	286	16				
M	663	15	855	20	1993	34
NM	443	19				
Age distribution (yrs)						
<1	509	3	198	4	690	4
1–5	987	9	678	10	1871	29
6–10	518	27	390	24	612	54
11–15			205	24	135	33
>15	197	18	19	16	15	47
Breed distribution						
Domestic	1609	15	577	16	2627	34
Siamese			71	6	171	18
Persian	602*	5	40	0	193	8
Abyssinian			9	0	36	11
Environmental status						
Indoor (owned)			61	8	236	7
Outdoor (owned)			33	33	165	39
Indoor/outdoor (owned)			90	20	437	36
Outdoor (unowned)			28	25	55	40

[a] Hosie *et al.* (1989); [b] Yamamoto *et al.* (1989) (only details of high risk cats given); [c] Ishida *et al.* (1989).
* All pedigree cats.

steadily with age, being highest in middle-aged and older cats. This is in contrast to FeLV infection since cats usually become infected with FeLV at an early age. All surveys demonstrate a clear male predisposition to FIV infection. Non-pedigree cats were more frequently infected than pedigrees and infection was much more common amongst free-ranging cats than those which were totally confined.

These epidemiological trends can be interpreted by considering the effect of each factor on the frequency with which a cat will encounter other cats outside its own household. In almost all cases the highest prevalence of infection occurs in those cats which most often meet and have contact with other cats. For example, older cats venture further, and have better developed social and aggressive behaviour than young cats; males tend to roam further and fight more frequently than females; non-pedigree cats are usually allowed to roam freely, whilst pedigree cats are often kept partially or totally confined. The one exceptional finding was that in the UK survey the prevalence of infection was lower in the entire males than the neutered males, even though entire tom cats would be expected to encounter other cats outdoors more frequently than neutered toms. However, in another UK survey (Hopper *et al.*, 1991) the prevalence was highest in both entire males and entire females, when compared with their neutered counterparts.

Additional serological findings in specific popu-

Table 16.3 Prevalence of FIV in various cat populations.

Population	No. tested	No. FIV seropositive (%)	Reference
Feral cats	90	24 (27)	Bennett *et al.* (1989a)
	77	29 (38)	Hopper, unpublished
Farm cats	50	12 (24)	Hopper, unpublished
Pedigree show cats	77	0	Hopper, unpublished

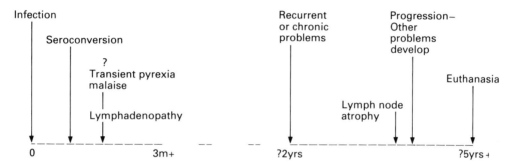

Fig. 16.1 Possible time course of FIV infection.

lations of cats in the UK such as pedigree show cats, farm and feral cats (see Table 16.3) highlight the strong association of FIV infection with free access to the outdoor environment. Although these results should be interpreted with caution, since the numbers studied were small, the high prevalence of infection amongst the feral and farm cats (the majority of which were semi-wild) indicates that such cats may form a reservoir of FIV infection in the general cat population.

PATHOGENESIS

The pathogenesis of FIV is as yet poorly understood since the virus appears to have a long incubation period, perhaps several years, before the characteristic signs of immunodeficiency manifest themselves in clinical disease. A postulated time course of FIV infection in an infected cat is shown in Fig. 16.1.

A distinct primary phase of FIV infection has been observed in cats experimentally infected with the virus (Yamamoto *et al.*, 1988; Hopper, unpublished observations) and it is probable that naturally infected cats also undergo a similar phase subsequent to initial infection. Following inoculation of cats with FIV, after about 2 weeks virus can be isolated from peripheral blood lymphocytes, and seroconversion is seen at around the same time. Pyrexia (usually mild, but lasting several days) may occur in some cats around 5 weeks post-inoculation. Almost all cats develop generalized lymphadenopathy at 4–6 weeks post-inoculation, and this usually persists for several months. In addition, during the primary phase of infection, many cats develop haematological abnormalities including absolute and relative neutropenia, and leucopenia.

Under natural conditions, following the primary phase of infection, there is probably a prolonged period (perhaps months to years) of asymptomatic infection in most, if not all, infected cats. It is uncertain precisely how long this period lasts, but it probably varies greatly between individuals. Eventually, however, as the FIV-induced immune dysfunction progresses, the majority of infected cats are thought to develop clinical signs in association with this (see also 'Clinical signs'). As with HIV infection in man, cats with naturally occurring FIV infection become progressively depleted of CD4+ T-lymphocytes (T-helper cells) and develop an inverted CD4+/CD8+ T-cell ratio (Novotney *et al.*, 1990). These findings are confirmed by experimental studies (Torten *et al.*, 1991), where cats developed CD4+ depletion within 6 months of infection and T-cell-dependent immune dysfunction became evident at 25–44 months post-infection. T-independent B-cell function was not affected during this period.

The typical acquired immunodeficiency syndrome, which appears to be characteristic of cats naturally infected with FIV, has yet to be observed under experimental conditions in cats infected with FIV alone. There are probably two main reasons for this. First the immunodeficiency syndrome is thought to represent an advanced stage of infection, and there may not have been sufficient time for this to occur in the experimental studies; secondly, the development of this stage of infection may depend in part on exposure to additional pathogens. Experimental studies have demonstrated that chronic clinical signs can be induced when cats with FIV are co-infected with chlamydia (O'Dair, personal communication) and calicivirus (Hopper, unpublished observations). Additionally, Pedersen *et al.* (1990) were able to show that pre-existing FeLV infection in experimentally infected cats enhanced the severity of both the acute and chronic stages of subsequent FIV infection.

Other factors may also be relevant to the development of disease, such as the age of the cat at the time of infection, exposure dose, route of infection and potential variation in viral pathogenicity.

TRANSMISSION

Experimental work has shown that FIV can be readily transmitted by intravenous, subcutaneous or intraperitoneal inoculation. Subcutaneous inoculation is successful even in cats with high levels of maternal antibody. Infection by the oral route is not successful unless extremely high doses of virus are used (N. Pedersen, personal communication).

Less is known about the natural modes of FIV transmission. Current knowledge suggests that biting, often as a result of territorial fighting, is the *primary* route of transmission. Virus is shed in the saliva of infected cats (Yamamoto *et al.*, 1988) and efficient transmission was shown to occur under experimental conditions when the skin of an uninfected cat was punctured by the canine teeth of an infected cat (Yamamoto *et al.*, 1989). Epidemiological studies consistently demonstrate that FIV infection is most common amongst free-roaming, mature male cats, i.e. those which are most likely to fight and bite. Clinically ill cats, particularly those with mouth lesions, will probably be most infective as much greater quantities of virus are shed in the saliva of these cats (Yamamoto *et al.*, 1988).

Other possible routes of transmission must be considered since, on rare occasions, in closed colonies of cats where there is no evidence of biting or scratching, FIV has been transmitted to in-contact cats (Pedersen *et al.*, 1987; Hopper, unpublished observations). A potential route of indirect FIV transmission is through salivary contamination of food and food bowls. If it does occur this would probably be an inefficient means of transmission, since FIV appears to be relatively labile in the environment and cats would only be exposed to very low levels of virus. Therefore a considerable period of contact would be necessary before infection occurred. Urine and faeces are highly unlikely to be major sources of FIV and hence the shared use of litter trays is probably not significant in transmission. Prolonged periods of intimate contact may facilitate direct transmission through mutual grooming and the licking of scratches and wounds. However, studies in which infected and uninfected cats were housed together for up to 14 months (Yamamoto *et al.*, 1988) and over (Hopper, unpublished observations) showed little or no evidence of transmission, so direct and indirect contact were considered unimportant.

Recently the use of the highly sensitive polymerase chain reaction (PCR) technique (see also 'Diagnosis'), to test blood from cats which had been in prolonged close contact with infected cats, has shown that in some cases very low levels of virus are present even though infection cannot be demonstrated by virus isolation or serology (N. Pedersen, personal communication). Therefore transmission through direct or indirect contact may arise more frequently than was first suggested, but it is still likely to be uncommon. The possibility of variation in the transmissibility between different strains of FIV is under investigation.

There has been no success to date in demonstrating sexual transmission, either from infected male to uninfected female, or from infected female to uninfected male. Epidemiological evidence indicates that sexual activity bears little or no relationship to the prevalence of FIV. Vertical transmission has been studied by breeding from infected queens. It is known that FIV can be spread from queens to their kittens but the route of infection and factors influencing transmission have not been established (Barr, 1988; Callanan *et al.*, 1991; Hopper, unpublished observations). As yet FIV has not been isolated from colostrum or milk, or from the kittens at birth. However, virus was recovered from the thymus of an aborted fetus from a queen in the acute phase of infection (Harbour, unpublished observation). Further studies are necessary in this area. The spread of FIV by blood-sucking insects such as fleas remains to be investigated, but epidemiological evidence suggests that vector transmission is not significant. Iatrogenic infection resulting from the use of surgical instruments contaminated with infected blood is a possibility.

CLINICAL SIGNS

Clinical signs associated with FIV infection may arise either as a direct result of the viral infection, or as a consequence of the immunodeficiency syndrome that is associated with infection.

Information regarding these signs has come largely through the observation of clinical cases,

and a substantial amount of data has now been collected. In addition, some information is also available from experimental studies of FIV infection.

There may be a distinct primary phase of FIV infection occurring shortly after inoculation of the virus, and in some or all infected cats this is followed by the development of a progressive immunodeficiency syndrome.

Primary phase of infection

A primary phase of FIV infection is recognized in cats experimentally infected with FIV (see under 'Pathogenesis'), and naturally infected cats probably also undergo a similar distinct phase following initial infection. The main clinical signs associated with this phase are pyrexia and generalized lymphadenopathy. Opportunistic infections (e.g. pyodermas) have also been observed in some cats, probably arising as a result of the neutropenia and leucopenia that are frequently seen during the primary phase.

Following the primary phase of infection most cats are thought to undergo a prolonged period when they are free of clinical signs attributable to FIV infection. Nevertheless, experimentally infected cats have been shown to develop a progressive deterioration in immune function, and probably in the majority of naturally infected cats this eventually leads to the development of clinical signs.

Immunodeficiency phase of infection

The later stages of FIV infection are characterized by the development of clinical signs related to a progressive immunodeficiency syndrome. The signs that develop have frequently been likened to the non-neoplastic findings that occur in association with FeLV infection (FeLV is also known to cause immunosuppression in cats – see Chapter 15). Clinical signs during this stage of the disease are frequently associated with secondary opportunistic infections, or inappropriate immune responses to antigens. The course of infec-

Table 16.4 Clinical signs associated with FIV infection.

Common signs	Other reported signs
Malaise/lethargy/depression	Otitis externa
Chronic gingivitis/stomatitis	Chronic abscessation
Inappetence/anorexia	Vomiting
Weight loss/emaciation	Recurrent cystitis
Chronic upper respiratory tract infection	Renal disease/failure
Pyrexia	Neurological disorders
Chronic diarrhoea	Behavioural abnormalities
Lymphadenopathy	Reproductive failure/abortion
Chronic dermatoses, including	Neoplasia, including
Demodicosis	Lymphoma
Notoedric mange	Myeloproliferative disorders
Pustular dermatitis	
Miliary dermatitis	
Alopecia	
Chronic ocular signs, including	
Conjunctivitis	
Keratitis	
Uveitis	
Ocular discharge/epiphora	

tion, and range of clinical signs shown in any individual case, appear to be very variable but, from the information available, certain common trends can be seen.

A picture of the range of clinical signs found in FIV-infected cats has been compiled from surveys of cats seropositive to FIV (Hopper *et al.*, 1989; Ishida *et al.*, 1989; Yamamoto *et al.*, 1989). Table 16.4 lists both the common, and some of the less common, signs that have been observed.

The most frequent findings are diseases of the oral cavity, respiratory tract and gastrointestinal tract. Non-specific signs such as lethargy, malaise, weight loss, lymphadenopathy and pyrexia are also very common. Oral cavity diseases are encountered most frequently and include chronic gingivitis, stomatitis and periodontitis of varying severity. In some cases extremely severe purulent and necrotizing gingivitis has been seen.

In addition, specific concurrent or opportunistic infections have often been identified in FIV-infected cats. These have included conditions such as cowpox, demodicosis, notoedric mange, bacterial cystitis, toxoplasmosis, haemobartonel-losis, feline calicivirus infection, feline herpesvirus infection, bacterial pneumonia, systemic candidiasis, coccidiosis, pyothorax and feline infectious peritonitis. Some of these infections are unusual and would immediately suggest the possibility of an underlying immunosuppression, whereas the role of FIV infection in others is uncertain.

Some workers have noted an unexpectedly high incidence of neoplasia in FIV-infected cats, and a retrospective study has demonstrated a significant correlation between FIV infection and lymphoid malignancies independent of FeLV infection (Shelton *et al.*, 1990a). Since FIV is not thought to be an oncogenic virus, it is possible that the high incidence of neoplasia is related to the immunosuppressive properties of the virus. A high incidence of certain tumours is also seen in humans infected with HIV.

Neurological abnormalities have been observed in a small proportion of infected cats (see also 'Pathology'). The signs seen are very variable, but are sometimes dramatic and have included psychomotor abnormalities, aggression, anisocoria and convulsions. These signs are likely to be directly related to the FIV infection since FIV, like HIV, is known to be neurotropic (Dow *et al.*, 1990).

Many clinical cases have a history of chronic illness. Often this appears to start as episodes of sporadic or recurrent illness, which are frequently interspersed with (sometimes prolonged) periods of clinical normality. Some cats have shown a rapid advancement of clinical signs, whilst others have shown little indication of deterioration in clinical condition, even over prolonged periods of time. In most cats, however, as the disease progresses, the clinical signs become more persistent and more severe. Characteristically, and especially in advanced cases, the clinical signs may be multiple, and cats may become severely ill such that death occurs, or euthanasia is required on humane grounds. Because the clinical signs arise largely from secondary diseases, or opportunistic infections, none is in any way diagnostic of FIV infection. However, underlying FIV infection should be suspected in cats with a history of chronic illness; in cats with severe, unexplained clinical signs; in individuals which do not respond as expected to normal therapeutic measures; and in those cats which have a combination of several clinical signs. Clinicopathological abnormalities may also arouse suspicion.

Although a gradual clinical deterioration is clearly evident in many cats infected with FIV, there can often be problems in assessing the significance of FIV infection in certain individuals. This is especially true if a cat is presented with clinical signs that are not immediately suggestive of an immunodeficiency state, and where there is no history of chronic illness. In the future, as knowledge of FIV and of feline immunology expands, it should be possible to develop laboratory and clinical guidelines to establish the degree or stage of immunosuppression in infected cats. This should enable a clearer understanding of the clinical significance of FIV infection in an individual, and of the likely prognosis.

LABORATORY FINDINGS

Clinicopathological abnormalities occur in most cats infected with FIV. However, the number and severity of these abnormalities will vary greatly between individuals, and will depend on a number of factors, including the stage of disease.

Haematological abnormalities are common and the changes seen are often both diverse and multiple. The abnormalities seen during the investigation of FIV infection in a series of cats referred to our clinic are shown in Table 16.5.

In some cases there are obvious explanations for the observed changes, for example hypersensitivity disorders (e.g. flea bite hypersensitivity) in cats with eosinophilia and/or basophilia, and concurrent infections or stress in some cats showing neutrophilia and leucocytosis. However, the reasons for many of these abnormalities remain unclear, and are probably multifactorial. The factors involved are likely to include direct effects of FIV on circulating cells or bone marrow, concurrent or opportunistic diseases, immune-mediated mechanisms, and effects of drug therapy. FIV is known to be T-lymphotropic and lymphopenia is a common finding in infected

Table 16.5 Common haematological and serum biochemical abnormalities in a series of FIV-infected cats.

Abnormality	% Affected
Leucocytosis	13
Neutrophilia	27
Lymphocytosis	4
Monocytosis	23
Eosinophilia	11
Basophilia	16
Leucopenia	13
Neutropenia	11
Lymphopenia	29
Anaemia	18
Hyperproteinaemia	38
Hyperglobulinaemia	25
Hypergammaglobulinaemia	67
Hyperalpha-2-globulinaemia	91
Hypoalbuminaemia	12

Reproduced from Sparkes *et al.* (1993).

cats. Direct viral destruction of lymphocytes probably contributes to many cases of lymphopenia, whilst the stress of FIV, and other concurrent infections, is likely to be another important cause. As in HIV infection, a reduction in the CD4+ subset of lymphocytes is seen in FIV-infected cats. Neutropenia is not commonly seen in feline diseases, but has been observed in a substantial proportion of FIV cases. An inhibitory substance present in the serum and directed at the granulocyte/macrophage lineage of cells in the bone marrow has been shown to occur in at least one infected cat (Shelton *et al.*, 1989b), and may be an important cause of neutropenia.

It appears that generally the cytopenias (anaemia, neutropenia, lymphopenia and leucopenia) are both more common and more severe in cats with clinically advanced immunosuppression (Shelton *et al.*, 1990b; Sparkes *et al.*, 1992). Progressive anaemia has been observed in several cats which were terminally ill. A similar pattern of cytopenias is also seen in HIV-infected humans, where again the cytopenias are more common in advanced immunosuppression (particularly AIDS). Where the haematology of infected cats has been monitored over a prolonged period of time, abnormalities have become more frequent, and often more profound as the disease progresses.

In addition to the haematological changes, serum biochemical abnormalities may also be seen in infected cats. In the cases of FIV infection seen at our clinic, the most commonly observed changes appear to be elevations in serum proteins (see Table 16.5). The hyperproteinaemia and hyperglobulinaemia may be profound on occasions, and it appears that elevated levels of IgG may be partly responsible for this in many cases. Serum protein electrophoresis shows that a high proportion of infected cats have mild to moderate elevations of alpha-2-globulin and/or gammaglobulin levels. Interestingly, hypergammaglobulinaemia is a frequent finding in HIV-infected humans and appears to arise from polyclonal activation of B-lymphocytes. Other serum biochemical abnormalities have been seen

with FIV infection, but generally appear to reflect involvement of disease with specific organs.

PATHOLOGY

There is still much to be learned about the pathology of FIV infection. Experimental studies have helped to provide information on the early phase of infection. Less is known about the pathology of the intermediate phase of infection, when cats are usually asymptomatic. Since the full-blown immunodeficiency stage of infection has not yet been demonstrated experimentally, the pathology in the advanced phase can only be studied in cats with naturally acquired FIV infection. The progression of the pathological changes throughout infection has not yet been investigated in any detail.

The principal pathological finding in the early or acute phase of FIV infection, which may last 10–40 weeks, is peripheral generalized lymphadenopathy (Yamamoto *et al.*, 1988). Microscopically there is enlargement of the cortical zone of the lymph node as a result of follicular hyperplasia (Fig. 16.2a). Disruption of the mantle zone of the follicles occurs. The germinal centres are increased in size, as well as number, and are often irregularly shaped; as a result they may extend into the pericortex and also the medulla. In addition there is widespread erythrophagocytosis in the medullary sinuses. Other lesions which have been found at this stage of infection in experimental cats include the expansion of lymphoid tissue in the lung and intestine, and expansion of the B-cell compartment of the splenic white pulp (W. Jarrett, personal communication). The splenic red pulp may also be hypercellular. Multiple pyogranulomatous lesions were found in the colon of an experimentally infected kitten which developed progressive pancytopenia and anaemia 8 weeks after inoculation (Yamamoto *et al.*, 1988).

During the intermediate stage of infection the lymph nodes may show either hyperplasia or involution. Some nodes have both lesions concurrently (known as a mixed pattern). There is evidence that chronic inflammatory lesions may

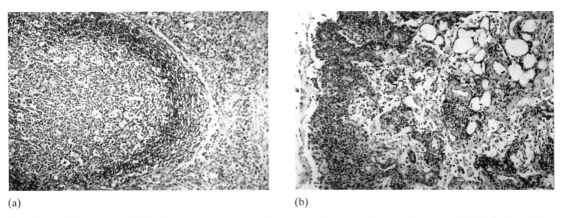

(a)   (b)

Fig. 16.2 (a) Hyperplastic follicle in the cortical zone of a lymph node from a cat in the initial stages of FIV infection. (b) An atrophic lymph node from a cat with chronic FIV infection. The follicles are indistinct and have been replaced by aggregates of hyaline material.

be present in the intestine of some cats at this stage.

In the terminal stages of FIV infection, gross pathological findings are often unspectacular, which is surprising, considering that cats have usually become severely ill. Those changes which do occur tend to be directly related to the presenting clinical signs, and because of the wide range of clinical problems associated with FIV, the pathological findings in chronic infection are very variable and none is pathognomonic. Microscopic lesions are more consistent but again are not specific for FIV. Generally there are inflammatory lesions in a variety of tissues and organs, together with abnormalities in the lymph nodes.

The alimentary tract is most commonly affected. The lesions accompanying gingivitis, stomatitis and periodontitis usually involve diffuse infiltration by lymphocytes and plasma cells. In the small intestine and colon, foci of chronic inflammation are not uncommon, even in cats which have not shown signs of enteritis. In some cases mucosal ulceration occurs at these sites with additional infiltration by inflammatory cells through the thickness of the gut wall. Irregularity and dilation of the crypts has been seen in the small intestine of some cats. There are no reports of specific aetiological agents associated with any of these lesions.

Perivascular mononuclear infiltration of the brain has been seen in a cat with mild neurological signs. Other cats have been found to have meningoencephalitis involving lymphocytic-plasmacytic infiltration even though neurological signs had not been observed (Brown *et al.*, 1991). Lymphocytic infiltration of the liver and, more commonly, the lung are also known to occur.

Changes in the lymph nodes seen in the chronic stages of infection usually involve generalized atrophy or a mixed pattern. In the atrophic nodes the follicles appear either small and indistinct or have a 'burned-out' appearance because of the loss of cells and the aggregation of hyaline material (Fig. 16.2b). The medullary cords are generally hypocellular. In severely involuted nodes the connective tissue and vascular skeleton are very prominent.

DIAGNOSIS

Diagnostic methods

Routine testing for FIV infection is currently performed by the use of commercial kits to detect antibodies to the virus in serum or plasma. More complex techniques of antibody detection may be employed by research laboratories. The various types of antibody tests are described below. It is important to note that the presence of antibody indicates persistent FIV infection since, in contrast to most viral infections, the immune response to FIV does not eliminate the virus.

Other methods of diagnosis include virus isolation, detection of the retroviral enzyme reverse transcriptase and detection of the viral genome in infected cells by either *in situ* hybridization or polymerase chain reaction (PCR). These latter diagnostic methods as yet have their principal use as research tools; the major methods are briefly described below. The development of serological tests to detect viral antigen (the routine method of FeLV diagnosis) has been hampered by the fact that there appears to be very little free FIV antigen present in the blood.

Serology

Indirect immunofluorescence was first used for the detection of FIV antibodies. However, this technique is time-consuming and is complicated by the cross-reaction with antibodies to another retrovirus, feline syncytium-forming virus (FeSFV). An enzyme-linked immunosorbent assay (ELISA) was developed, and in April 1988 the introduction of commercially available ELISA kits into the UK enabled large-scale FIV testing to begin.

The ELISA kit (Petchek FIV*) is used by most diagnostic laboratories. It consists of 96-well microtitre plates, each well coated with partially purified FIV as the capture antigen. A serum sample and FIV antigen conjugated with the enzyme horse-radish peroxidase are added to each well and FIV antibodies present will bind to the viral proteins to form the ELISA 'sandwich'. After unbound components are washed away, substrate for the peroxidase is added and the test result is read spectrophotometrically. The test is simple and rapid and is reported to have an acceptable sensitivity, specificity and reproducibility. Cross-reaction with antibodies to FeSFV is minimal and should not be confused with a genuine positive result.

The introduction of a combination concentration immunoassay technology kit (CITE FeLV/FIV COMBO; Idexx), which tests for

*Petchek FIV; Idexx, High Wycombe, Bucks, UK.

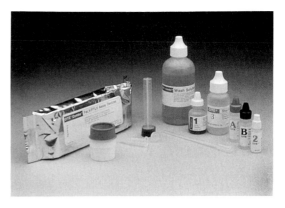

Fig. 16.3 An individual CITE combo device, with reagents, which is suitable for testing for FIV/FeLV in the practice laboratory.

FeLV and FIV simultaneously, has further improved the availability of FIV diagnosis. The CITE test requires no sophisticated equipment and is designed for use in the practice laboratory. An individual CITE device (Fig. 16.3) is used for each sample. The principle of the procedure is exactly the same as that for the Petchek ELISA with the exception that the FIV capture antigen is bound to a membrane rather than a plastic microwell. The incorporation of a separate membrane filter means that whole blood can be tested as well as serum or plasma. The test is very rapid, and reliable providing the manufacturer's instructions are followed carefully.

The above methods cannot distinguish antibody responses to *individual* viral proteins. Reasearch laboratories are able to use the more complicated and demanding techniques of Western blotting (immunoblotting – Fig. 16.4) and radioimmunoprecipitation assay (RIPA) to detect antibodies, present in serum or plasma, which are directed against specific viral proteins. It is hoped that further study will demonstrate that the presence and/or absence of antibodies to particular viral proteins may be useful as prognostic indicators.

Virus isolation

The isolation of FIV, and other related immunodeficiency viruses, has been made possible by the

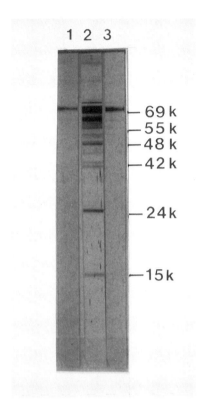

Fig. 16.4 Immunoblotting can be used to show the presence of specific antibodies to individual viral proteins. A positive sample (track 2) has antibodies to several protein bands (molecular weights shown on right).

information and technological advances gained from the study of HIV. Thus the procedure for isolation of FIV from peripheral blood lymphocytes closely resembles that used for the isolation of HIV and is given in detail elsewhere (Harbour *et al.*, 1988). If the lymphocytes are infected then cytopathic effects, including ballooning degeneration, syncytium formation and increased cell death occur, usually after 5–14 days of culturing. The presence of virus in the culture can be confirmed by immunofluorescence, electron microscopy and reverse transcriptase assay (see below) or with a commercial antigen ELISA test. Virus isolation is not suitable for large-scale testing because it is expensive, labour-intensive and does not give a rapid result.

Reverse transcriptase (RT) assay

The presence of a Mg^{2+}-dependent reverse transcriptase in lymphocyte culture fluid indicates the active replication of a lentivirus. Although this test is not specific for FIV, it distinguishes a lentivirus from FeLV (an oncovirus) and FeSFV (a spumavirus).

FIV antigen ELISA

This commercial kit has been developed primarily for use by research laboratories. An antigen capture technique, using microtitre wells coated with monoclonal antibody to FIV p26 antigen, binds viral antigen which is present in a sample of lymphocyte culture supernatant. Enzyme-labelled FIV monoclonal antibody, plus substrate, are added to detect the antibody/antigen complexes. As mentioned previously this assay cannot be used to detect viral antigens in the blood.

In situ hybridization and polymerase chain reaction (PCR)

These techniques, already established in HIV diagnosis, are being adapted and developed for FIV. Almost certainly their use will be limited to research laboratories but it is possible that in future these tests will be important in the detection of infected cats which have no antibody to FIV. *In situ* hybridization involves the use of a radiolabelled FIV RNA probe. It can detect viral RNA when less than 1 in 10^4 cells is infected. PCR is likely to be even more effective in detecting very low levels of virus – it should be possible to detect one infected cell in a million. PCR is a method for amplification of specific sequences of DNA in the FIV provirus. The amplified FIV sequences are then detected by hybridization with radiolabelled. virus-specific oligonucleotide probes.

Problems in diagnosis

Generally speaking, diagnosis of FIV is reliable. However, it is possible for equivocal, false negative and false positive results to occur. Most of the difficulties arise from antibody testing.

Some tests, notably the antibody ELISA and immunoblotting, occasionally give equivocal results which are impossible to interpret. In such cases it may be necessary to repeat the test successively over a period of time until a definitive result is obtained. An alternative method of testing should also be used if possible. However, further problems may arise because there is not always good correlation between results obtained by different antibody tests. One study showed that both CITE and ELISA gave *more* positive results than immunoblotting (Hosie & Jarrett, 1990) whilst another study demonstrated *fewer* positive samples with ELISA than immunoblotting (Bennett *et al.*, 1989b). The CITE has been found to give fewer positives than ELISA (Hosie & Jarrett, 1990). Unfortunately virus isolation was not performed in these studies so at present it is not possible to determine which test is most accurate. However, these discrepancies indicate that in some instances (as yet undetermined) all three test methods may occasionally give false positive or negative results.

There is another important reason why a seronegative result should not exclude the possibility of FIV infection. By virus isolation, a number of cats were shown to be infected with FIV despite being seronegative by several serological methods (Hopper *et al.*, 1989; P. Anderson, personal communication). Some of these cats were monitored for up to 18 months, and remained seronegative throughout. Further investigation is necessary to determine the proportion of infected cats which are not detected by antibody testing alone, but preliminary studies show that the figure may be as high as 20% (Hopper, 1990). Experimental studies show that the majority of cats seroconvert between 3 and 4 weeks after inoculation, but Yamamoto *et al.* (1988) reported that one cat did not develop significant levels of antibody until 14 months after inoculation. The late development of antibodies is seen in some humans infected with HIV. In addition some HIV-infected patients have reduced levels of antibody in the later stages of infection because increased levels of viral antigen in the blood bind antibody to form immune complexes. There is evidence that a decline in antibody levels also occurs in some cats (Alexander *et al.*, 1989).

Unfortunately there is currently no routinely available test to detect virus itself. Opportunities for virus isolation are very limited, and even this technique is not infallible since the interpretation of viral cytopathic effect is rather subjective and the confirmatory tests cannot guarantee to detect very low levels of virus in lymphocyte cultures. Further work is necessary to develop a more accurate test suitable for large-scale screening.

TREATMENT AND PROGNOSIS

Specific therapy

Currently there are no specific antiviral agents effective against FIV that can be recommended for use in cats. However, because of the importance of FIV as a comparative model for HIV studies, there has been considerable attention devoted to the efficacy of chemotherapeutic agents against FIV. Many of the drugs known to inhibit HIV replication are also effective against FIV, at least *in vitro*. One such drug, 9-(2-phosphonomethoxyethyl)adenine (PMEA), has been shown to be effective *in vivo*, producing clinical improvement in field cases of FIV infection in which secondary infections were apparent (Egberink *et al.*, 1990). Future clinical trials will determine the safety of other antiviral agents for use in FIV-infected cats. Unfortunately, in the immediate future, even if agents are shown to be safe and effective *in vivo*, it is unlikely that treatment with these drugs will be economically viable for most cats. As with HIV, these agents may slow down the progression of disease, but are unlikely to be able to eliminate infection. Vaccination will probably be the most successful method of preventing FIV infection.

Although anti-viral therapy may play an important role in the treatment of HIV-infected humans, treatment of specific or concurrent infections is also considered to be of great importance, and it is this aspect of therapy that we must focus on for cats.

As has already been shown, numerous specific

concurrent infectious and non-infectious diseases have been identified in FIV-infected cats, and establishing a diagnosis of FIV should not preclude further investigation of a sick cat. It is important to try to establish what, if any, other disease processes are ongoing, and to institute appropriate treatment for these. It is perhaps also relevant to consider ways of reducing exposure of an infected cat to potential pathogens, perhaps by attempting to minimize contact with other cats, especially free-roaming cats (see also 'Control').

Symptomatic therapy

Despite further investigations, it is not always possible to find specific concurrent diseases, and in these cases symptomatic therapy based on clinical signs is always justified. Many such cases have shown a favourable response to the use of antibiotics (presumably indicating that secondary bacterial infections are common in FIV-infected cats, although not always immediately apparent). If antibiotics are to be used empirically it is probably sensible to use a broad-spectrum bactericidal agent.

We have also found a (perhaps surprising) value in the use of corticosteroids in some infected cats. In a number of cases, particularly of pyrexia, inappetence or stomatitis/gingivitis that have failed to show response to conventional therapy, we have often seen a dramatic response to the use of corticosteroids. In most cases a good response has been achieved by the use of daily or alternate-day prednisolone, often at quite low doses (0.5–1 mg/kg), though higher doses may be necessary. Part of the benefit of corticosteroids would appear to be derived from their potent anti-inflammatory activity; however, these agents are known to be immunosuppressive and therefore the long-term consequences of their use may be deleterious. This does not preclude their use, although caution should be exercised and, before embarking on corticosteroid therapy, other lines of treatment should be attempted (where appropriate). If there is any suspicion of involvement of bacterial pathogens, it is clearly essential to use antibiotics.

Other supportive and symptomatic measures may be of value in certain cases, including fluid therapy, anabolic steroids in cases of severe weight loss, and possibly blood transfusions. Attention should also be paid to the diet, to ensure that cats are consuming a balanced food meeting their nutritional requirements, and again where weight loss is a problem, provision of a palatable high-calorie food may be valuable. The supplementation of the diet with essential fatty acids (EfaVet Regular [EfaMol Vet Ltd.], one 550 mg capsule once daily) has been shown to produce clinical improvements in most infected cats, though the improvements are usually less marked in cats which have advanced clinical signs (Hopper, unpublished data). Vitamin supplementation may also be helpful.

Prognosis

The prognosis for FIV-infected cats must be guarded. If the diagnosis of FIV infection is made early in the course of the disease, there may be a long period during which the cat is free of clinical signs related to FIV and so the outlook may be less bleak. Although it is not certain that all infected cats go on to develop an immunodeficiency syndrome, the evidence available suggests that the majority do, and in all cats the infection appears to be permanent (in common with other lentivirus infections in other species). The prognosis for a cat infected with FIV and showing clinical signs suggestive of an immunodeficiency syndrome is poor. It is difficult to give any reliable estimate of the mortality rate amongst FIV-infected cats. Surveys have given different results, ranging from around 15% (Ishida *et al.*, 1989) to over 45% (Hopper *et al.*, 1989) during a 6–12-month follow-up period. The mortality rate will vary according to which population of cats is studied (e.g. referral cases or first opinion cases), and the picture is further complicated by the fact that in some cases owners choose to have cats euthanased for reasons other than the severity of clinical signs. Nevertheless, FIV infection is undoubtedly a major cause of disease in cats, and is frequently associated with mortality. Owners should be made aware of these facts, and whilst many cats initially show a good response to supportive and symptomatic therapy, in most cases deterioration will eventually occur, necessitating euthanasia on humane grounds.

In humans with HIV infection, a careful and precise system has been developed to stage the progress of the infection. At present there is no established system of staging FIV infection, but the future development of a reliable system should enable a more accurate prognosis to be given in individual cases.

CONTROL

At present control measures relating to FIV are restricted to details of management since the development of a vaccine is unlikely in the near future. Conventional methods of vaccination appear to be inappropriate for FIV for the following reasons. The lentiviruses as a group show antigenic variation of the envelope proteins and therefore the immune system remains one step behind as it has to respond to a succession of viral proteins. In addition, lentiviruses are able to remain latent within target cells and therefore avoid host immune surveillance mechanisms. The principal target cells of FIV are lymphocytes and the monocyte/macrophage cell lines, all of which play an important role in the immune response, so FIV can actively disrupt the immune response mounted against it. To overcome these problems, new methods of vaccine design are being investigated, but progress is likely to be slow. To date the most effective results have been achieved using a formaldehyde-inactivated whole cell vaccine (Yamamoto *et al.*, 1991).

Management of uninfected cats

In order to achieve minimal risk of FIV infection, there should be as little contact with cats outside the house as possible, and in particular it is important to avoid contact with stray and feral cats. However, once a cat has begun to venture away from home, and establishes its territory, it is then very difficult to prevent wandering without taking drastic measures. Often a cat must be left to live with the risk, and the best compromise is to keep it in at night. Owners of new kittens should be advised to consider either keeping their cat as an indoor cat, or attempting to discourage it from leaving the garden. It is also possible to reduce the tendency for a cat to roam (and therefore to socialize and fight with other cats) by ensuring that it is neutered. This is best done at the earliest opportunity but is likely to be beneficial at any age.

Management of infected cats

Decisions regarding the management of an infected cat depend largely on individual circumstances and the views and conscience of the owner. At present the uncertainties about modes of transmission, outcome of infection, and the reliability of serodiagnosis make it unwise to recommend a definite policy.

Infected cats within the household

If there are infected and uninfected cats within a household then the owner will face a dilemma: should the infected cats be kept separately or should they remain in contact with the other cats? Separation of cats is often very difficult, and totally impractical in some cases. In addition, since FIV does not appear to be readily transmitted by close contact between cats, the risk avoided by keeping infected cats separately may not justify the difficulty and stress that can arise from such measures. The problem of ensuring that all infected cats are detected must also be considered (see 'Diagnosis'). Finally it is worthwhile remembering that if the uninfected cats have outdoor access then there is probably a greater risk of infection from neighbouring cats than from those within the household, provided that there is no fighting amongst the cats in the household. Given these considerations, most owners decide to keep their cats together. Another alternative is to re-home the infected or uninfected cat(s), whichever proves easier. If all cats within a household are infected, then considerations are limited to the confinement of the cats. At the present time the euthanasia of an FIV-infected cat is recommended only on humane grounds when the cat is severely ill, and not purely because of the FIV infection.

Outdoor management of infected cats

Ideally, infected cats should be isolated from neighbouring cats. However, in practice this often proves extremely difficult since it is usually adult cats which are diagnosed with FIV infection and at this stage it is hard to change their behaviour patterns. A compromise may be necessary, and confinement at night, at least, is suggested. If a cat is aggressive and is known to bite then enforced confinement to house and garden is strongly recommended. If this is not practical, euthanasia may be considered regardless of the health status of the cat. Generally, the neutering of entire infected cats is suggested, providing they are well enough to receive an anaesthetic. This measure should help to reduce the tendency for wandering and aggressive behaviour in both male and female cats.

Advice for breeding colonies

In order to minimize the risk of introducing FIV into the colony, breeders are advised to prevent their breeding cats having free access outdoors, or having contact with any cats that are allowed outdoors. Regular testing of breeding cats, e.g. annually, and of new cats prior to introduction, is sensible. If an infected cat is identified then appropriate measures must be taken. These are summarized in Table 16.6.

It is very important that there is no breeding

Table 16.6 Suggested procedure following the identification of an FIV-infected cat in a breeding colony.

1 Stop breeding
2 Test all other cats
3 Remove/separate infected cats
4 Retest all cats in 3–6 months
5 Resume breeding if all negative
6 Avoid overcrowding, and isolate each queen before and after kittening
7 Retest all cats in a further 6 months

from FIV-infected queens since transmission of FIV to kittens can occur (see also 'Transmission'). In fact there should be no breeding whilst *any* infected cat remains in the colony. If the breeder wishes to continue breeding then it will be necessary to test all cats and remove, or completely separate, those which are infected. This procedure is complicated by the fact that not all infected cats may be identified by routine antibody testing. At present the most satisfactory answer to this problem is to retest all cats at 6-monthly intervals and resume breeding once no further infected cats are identified. Retesting again 6 months after resumption of breeding is strongly advised.

Although current knowledge suggests that sexual transmission rarely occurs, if ever, it is nevertheless strongly recommended that FIV-infected toms are not used at stud.

Advice for cat rescue centres and organizations

Special consideration must be given to rescue cats and in some instances the advice will differ from that given to owners of pet cats infected with FIV.

Testing for FIV

Financial constraints are likely to prevent the routine screening for FIV in all cats. If this is not possible, it is suggested that testing is reserved for those cats which are showing clinical signs. In addition it would be wise to test cats which are obviously aggressive and bite other cats – often the adult entire males. If financial provisions allow, the testing of stray and feral cats would also be sensible since these are the cats most likely to be infected with FIV.

Dealing with infected cats

Careful consideration is necessary before a cat rescue society knowingly re-homes a cat with FIV since an infected cat (particularly if ill when the diagnosis of FIV infection was made) has a poor prognosis and is likely to need regular veterinary attention. Infected cats should not remain for a lengthy period in the foster home or shelter so the most realistic and responsible option may be euthanasia, even if the cat is relatively healthy.

Prevention of the spread of FIV within a rescue centre

It is recommended that aggressive cats are housed alone whilst at the centre, and tested for FIV if possible. Secondly, it is advisable to keep cats in the smallest groups possible; this is an important measure in preventing spread of any infectious agent. A policy of neutering cats before re-homing should also be effective in reducing transmission of FIV since neutered cats are less likely to fight and bite.

PUBLIC HEALTH SIGNIFICANCE

At present there is no evidence that FIV can be transmitted to humans or other animals. As a family, the lentiviruses are highly adapted to the species of animal which they infect and they do not readily cross-infect other species. FIV is antigenically distinct from other lentiviruses, including HIV (Olmsted *et al.*, 1989; Talbott *et al.*, 1989) and genetic sequencing has shown that FIV has not recently evolved from any of the known lentiviruses. Although more extensive work is necessary, attempts to grow FIV in a number of cell lines from humans, mice, dogs and sheep have been unsuccessful.

Serum samples from 18 people who had close contact with FIV-infected cats did not contain antibody to FIV (Yamamoto *et al.*, 1989). This survey included two people who had been bitten by infected cats and three who had accidentally been injected with infected material.

REFERENCES

Alexander R., Robinson W.F., Mills J.N., Sherry C.R., Sherard E., Paterson A.J., Shaw S.E., Clarke W.T. & Hollingsworth T. (1989) Isolation of feline immunodeficiency virus from three cats with lymphoma. *Austral. Vet. Practitioner* **19**, 93–7.

Barr M. (1988) Feline immunodeficiency virus. *Feline Health Topics for Veterinarians* (Cornell Feline Health Centre) **3**(3), 1–8.

Barr M.C., Calle P.P., Roelke M.E. & Scott F.W. (1989)

Feline immunodeficiency virus infection in non-domestic felids. *J. Zoo Wildlife Med.* **20**, 265–72.

Bennett M., McCracken C., Lutz H., Gaskell C.J., Gaskell R.M., Brown A. & Knowles J.O. (1989a) Prevalence of antibody to feline immunodeficiency virus in some cat populations. *Vet. Rec.* **124**, 397–8.

Bennett M., Knowles J.O., McCracken C., Gaskell R.M. & Gaskell C.J. (1989b) Diagnosis of FIV infection. *Vet. Rec.* **124**, 520–1.

Brown P.J., Hopper C.D. & Harbour D.A. (1991) Pathological features of lymphoid tissues in cats with natural feline immunodeficiency virus (FIV) infection. *J. Comp. Pathol.* **104**, 345–55.

Callanan J.J., Hosie M.J. & Jarrett O. (1991) Transmission of feline immunodeficiency virus from mother to kitten. *Vet. Rec.* **128**, 332–3.

Dow S.W., Poss M.L. & Hoover E.A. (1990) Feline immunodeficiency virus: a neurotropic lentivirus. *J. Acquired Immune Deficiency Syndromes* **3**, 658–68.

Egberink H., Borst M., Niphuis H., Balzarini J., Schellekens H., DeClercq E., Horzinek M. & Koolen M. (1990) Suppression of feline immunodeficiency virus infection in vivo by 9-(2-phosphonomethoxyethyl)adenine. *Proc. Natl. Acad. Sci. USA* **87**, 3087–91.

Grindem C.B., Corbett W.T., Ammerman B.E. & Tomkins M.T. (1989) Seroepidemiologic survey of feline immunodeficiency virus infection in cats of Wake County, North Carolina. *J. Am. Vet. Med. Ass.* **194**, 226–8.

Gruffydd-Jones T.J., Hopper C.D., Harbour D.A. & Lutz H. (1988) Serological evidence of feline immunodeficiency virus infection in UK cats from 1975–76. *Vet. Rec.* **123**, 569–70.

Harbour D.A., Williams P.D., Gruffydd-Jones T.J., Burbridge J. & Pearson G.R. (1988) Isolation of a T-lymphotropic lentivirus from a persistently leucopenic domestic cat. *Vet. Rec.* **122**, 84–6.

Hopper C.D. (1990) Comparison of antibody testing and virus isolation for the diagnosis of feline immunodeficiency virus. *British Small Animal Veterinary Association Congress, 19–22 April 1990, Paper Synopses and Free Communications*, p. 195.

Hopper C.D., Sparkes A.H., Gruffydd-Jones T.J., Crispin S.M., Muir P., Harbour D.A. & Stokes C.R. (1989) Clinical and laboratory findings in cats infected with feline immunodeficiency virus. *Vet. Rec.* **125**, 341–6.

Hopper C.D., Cripps P.J., Howard P.E., Harbour D.A. & Gruffydd-Jones T.J. (1991) The epidemiology of feline immunodeficiency virus infection in cats in the United Kingdom. *Proceedings of the Society for Veterinary Epidemiology and Preventative Medicine, 17–19 April 1991*, pp. 67–74.

Hosie M.J. & Jarrett O. (1990) Serological responses of cats to feline immunodeficiency virus. *AIDS* **4**, 215–20.

Hosie M.J., Robertson C. & Jarrett O. (1989) Prevalence of feline leukaemia virus and antibodies to feline immunodeficiency virus in cats in the United Kingdom. *Vet. Rec.* **125**, 293–7.

Ishida T., Washizu T., Toriyabe K., Motoyoshi S., Tomoda I. & Pedersen N.C. (1989) Feline immunodeficiency virus infection in cats of Japan. *J. Am. Vet. Med. Ass.* **194**, 221–5.

Lutz H., Egberink H., Arnold P., Winkler G., Wolfensberger C., Jarrett O., Parodi A.L., Pedersen N.C. & Horzinek M.C. (1988) Felines T-lymphotropes lentivirus (FTLV): Experimentelle infektion und vorkommen in einigen Landern Europas. *Kleintierpraxis* **33**, 455–9.

Novotney C., English R.V., Housman J., Davidson M.G., Nasisse M.P., Jeng C., Davis W.C. & Tompkins M.B. (1990) Lymphocyte population changes in cats naturally infected with feline immunodeficiency virus. *AIDS* **4**, 1213–8.

Olmsted R.A., Hirsch V.M., Purcell R.H. & Johnson P.R. (1989) Nucleotide sequence analysis of feline immunodeficiency virus: genome organisation and relation to other lentiviruses. *Proc. Natl. Acad. Sci. USA* **86**, 8088–92.

Pedersen N.C., Torten M., Rideout B., Sparger E., Tonachini T., Luciw P.A., Ackley C., Levy N. & Yamamoto J. (1990) Feline leukemia virus as a potentiating cofactor for the primary and secondary stages of experimentally induced feline immunodeficiency virus infection. *J. Virol.* **64**, 598–606.

Robertson I.D., Robinson W.F., Alexander R., Shaw S.E. & Sutherland R.J. (1990) Feline immunodeficiency virus and feline leukaemia virus in cats. *Austral. Vet. Pract.* **20**, 66–9.

Shelton G.H., Waltier R.M., Conor S.C. & Grant C.K. (1989a) Prevalence of feline immunodeficiency virus and feline leukemia virus infections in pet cats. *J. Am. Anim. Hosp. Ass.* **25**, 7–12.

Shelton G.H., Abkowitz J.L., Linenberger M.L., Russell R.G. & Grant C.K. (1989b) Chronic leukopenia associated with feline immunodeficiency virus in a cat. *J. Am. Vet. Med. Ass.* **194**, 253–5.

Shelton G.H., Grant C.K., Cotter S.M., Gardner M.B.,

Hardy W.D. & DiGiacomo R.F. (1990a) Feline immunodeficiency virus and feline leukemia virus infections and their relationships to lymphoid malignancies in cats: a retrospective study (1968–1988). *J. Acquired Immune Deficiency Syndromes* **3**, 623–30.

Shelton G.H., Linenberger M.L., Grant C.K. & Abkowitz J.L. (1990b) Hematologic manifestations of feline immunodeficiency virus infection. *Blood* **76**, 1104–9.

Sparkes A.H., Hopper C.D., Millard W., Gruffydd-Jones T.J. & Harbour D.A. (1993) Feline immunodeficiency virus infection: clinicopathologic findings in 90 naturally occurring cases. *J. Vet. Intern. Med.* **7**, 85–90.

Talbott R.L., Sparger E.E., Lovelace K.M., Fitch W.M., Pedersen N.C., Luciw P.A. & Elder J.H. (1989) Nucleotide sequence and genomic organisation of feline immunodeficiency virus. *Proc. Natl. Acad. Sci. USA* **86**, 5743–7.

Torten M., Franchini M., Barlough J.E., George J.W., Mozes E., Lutz H. & Pedersen N.C. (1991) Progressive immune dysfunction in cats experimentally infected with feline immunodeficiency virus. *J. Virol.* **65**, 2225–30.

Witt C.J., Moench T.R., Gittelsohn A.M., Bishop B.D. & Childs J.E. (1989) Epidemiological observations on feline immunodeficiency virus and *Toxoplasma gondii* coinfection in cats in Baltimore, Md. *J. Am. Vet. Med. Ass.* **194**, 229–33.

Yamamoto J.K., Sparger E., Ho E.W., Andersen P.R., O'Connor T.P., Mandell C.P., Lowenstine L., Munn R. & Pedersen N.C. (1988) Pathogenesis of experimentally induced feline immunodeficiency virus infection in cats. *Am. J. Vet. Res.* **49**, 1246–58.

Yamamoto J.K., Hansen H., Ho E.W., Morishita T.Y., Okuda T., Sawa T.R., Nakamura R.M. & Pedersen N.C. (1989) Epidemiologic and clinical aspects of feline immunodeficiency virus infection in cats from the continental United States and Canada and possible modes of transmission. *J. Am. Vet. Med. Ass.* **194**, 213–20.

Yamamoto J.K., Takiko O., Ackley C.D., Louie H., Zochlinski H., Pembroke E. & Gardner M.B. (1991) Experimental vaccine protection against FIV. *Proceedings of the First International Feline Immunology and Immunodeficiency Workshop, 28–31 May 1991*, p. 49.

Chapter 17 / Feline Coronavirus Infections

M. E. STODDART AND M. BENNETT

INTRODUCTION

Coronavirus infection of cats can have a variety of clinical sequelae including wet and dry feline infectious peritonitis (FIP), enteritis or no obvious clinical signs at all. Classical or wet FIP is characterized by the development of tacky straw-coloured fluid in the peritoneal and pleural cavities. Dry FIP, however, is characterized by the development of chronic granulomatous lesions in a wide variety of organs resulting in a correspondingly large range of clinical signs. Both wet and dry FIP are almost invariably fatal. The first published account of wet FIP is probably that of Holzworth (1963), but it was not until over 20 years later that the causative virus was first isolated (Horzinek & Osterhaus, 1977). Mild feline enteritis associated with coronavirus infection was first reported in 1981 (Pedersen et al., 1981), although previous serological surveys, in which up to 20% of household cats and 95% of colony cats were found to have antibody (Pedersen, 1976; Osterhaus et al., 1977), had indicated that feline coronavirus infection was not always fatal. In addition to the strains of feline coronaviruses causing FIP (the FIP viruses; FIPV) and enteritis (the feline enteric coronaviruses; FECV), some canine coronavirus strains can also infect and cause disease in cats, at least experimentally (Stoddart et al., 1988a; Barlough et al., 1984; McArdle et al., 1992).

AETIOLOGY

The coronaviruses are a family of pleomorphic enveloped RNA viruses, approximately 100 nm in diameter and surrounded by a characteristic corona (or crown) of large petal-like projections (the peplomers or spikes). The peplomers are involved in attachment of virus to cells, and also seem to be the main target for virus-neutralizing and, in the case of FIPV, virus-enhancing antibody (Vennema et al., 1990).

Coronaviruses are relatively labile, the feline viruses generally being inactivated within one day in both dry and moist conditions. They are readily inactivated by heat and most disinfectants, but are relatively resistant to phenols, low temperature and low pH.

The classification of the coronaviruses which infect cats is confusing and will probably only be clarified by study of their molecular biology. FIPV and FECV, although originally regarded as separate species, are now often looked upon as extremes of a spectrum of feline coronaviruses of varying infectivity and pathogenicity (Pedersen, 1987a). Indeed, it has been suggested that FIPV strains are mutants of FECV (Pedersen et al., 1981). Certainly they are very closely related and difficult to distinguish in the laboratory. However, some workers have found what appear to be consistent differences between FIPV and FECV strains using monoclonal antibodies (Fiscus & Teramoto, 1987).

FIPV and FECV are members of a larger group of antigenically related coronaviruses which also includes transmissible gastroenteritis virus (TGEV) of swine and canine coronavirus (CCV). Consistent differences in antigenicity and the genomes of TGEV and FIPV have been found which clearly distinguish these two viruses, but

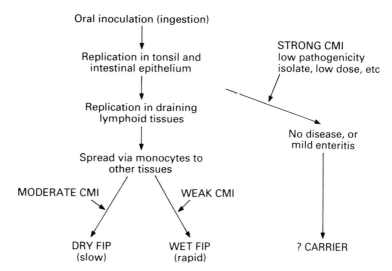

Fig. 17.1 Possible pathogenesis of feline coronavirus infection in cats. (Modified from Pedersen, 1987b, with permission.)

little work appears to have been done on distinguishing FIPV from CCV. Given that several recent publications have shown that CCV cannot only infect cats but sometimes produce clinical disease (Barlough *et al.*, 1984; Stoddart *et al.*, 1988a; McArdle *et al.*, 1992), more work in this area is obviously needed.

PATHOGENESIS

The clinical outcome of coronavirus infection in cats depends on several factors including species, strain and dose of virus, and the age, immune status and other innate characteristics of the cat. In particular the strain of virus and the ability of the cat to mount a strong cell-mediated immune response to it appear to be important in determining the outcome of infection (Pedersen & Black, 1983; Stoddart *et al.*, 1988b; Weiss & Cox, 1989). The role of antibody in FIP is complex, as circulating IgG can even cause enhancement of the disease (Pedersen & Boyle, 1980; Weiss & Scott, 1981). Figure 17.1 and the following text describe the possible course of events following infection, although it should be stressed that what follows is largely hypothetical.

The usual route of infection is now generally agreed to be oral, although some authorities believe that inhalation and respiratory infection

may also be important. Transplacental transmission can also occur although its relevance in the field is not known (Pedersen, 1987b). Following oral inoculation with FIPV, FECV or CCV, virus can be isolated from both the saliva and faeces of experimentally infected cats. The initial sites of virus replication are in tonsil and small intestine (Hyashi *et al.*, 1982; Stoddart *et al.*, 1988a,b,c; McArdle *et al.*, 1990), although some virus can also be found in the mesenteric lymph nodes draining the gut, probably having been carried there by macrophages. Enteric infection is sometimes associated with mild, or occasionally more severe, diarrhoea, although it is usually asymptomatic.

According to the model in Fig. 17.1, if the virus is of low pathogenicity or if the cat produces a strong cell-mediated immune response, virus is eliminated (or at least its spread is controlled) and no further clinical signs develop. This appears to be what happens after infection with FECV or most CCV strains, and probably accounts for those cats (approximately one in five in the authors' experience) which recover from experimental infection with even very pathogenic FIP-inducing strains. Even cats which do not eliminate virus usually stop shedding virus in saliva and faeces within several weeks of inoculation, although shedding may recommence later with the appearance of clinical signs (Stoddart *et al.*, 1988b).

After infection with more pathogenic, FIP-inducing virus strains, and in the absence of a strong cell-mediated immune response, a viraemia develops and virus is disseminated to a variety of tissues and organs (Weiss & Scott, 1981). Macrophages appear to play an important role in the dissemination of virus, and one recent study showed that FIP-inducing strains are better able to replicate in macrophages than are FECV strains (Stoddart & Scott, 1989). Whether a cat develops wet FIP or dry FIP after generalization of the virus is thought to depend on the strength of the cat's cell-mediated immune response. It seems likely that cats which produce a weak cell-mediated response rapidly develop acute wet FIP, whereas those producing a moderate cell-mediated response gradually develop the more chronic granulomatous lesions characteristic of dry FIP (Pedersen, 1987b). Some experimental evidence exists in support of an important role for the cell-mediated immune response in determining whether or not a cat recovers (Stoddart *et al.*, 1988b; Weiss & Cox, 1989), but as yet there is little direct evidence for its role in determining between wet and dry FIP. Clinical signs of wet FIP often first appear 3 weeks after experimental inoculation. The time taken to develop signs of dry FIP is rather greater.

The role of antibody in the pathogenesis of FIP is complex. Although infected cats produce large amounts of circulating antibody which can neutralize virus in cell culture, pre-existing IgG can often cause accelerated and enhanced wet FIP in cats (Pedersen & Boyle, 1980; Weiss & Scott, 1981; Pedersen, 1987a,b; Vennema *et al.*, 1990). The mechanism of this enhancement is not known, although it has been suggested that it may result from opsonization of the virus by bound antibody, thus increasing virus uptake by macrophages, in which it replicates (Weiss & Scott, 1981; Hohdatsu *et al.*, 1991; Olsen *et al.*, 1992). Alternatively, enhancement may result from immune-complex deposition and complement activation in vascular endothelium (Jacobse-Geels *et al.*, 1982). The phenomenon of antibody enhancement obviously must be borne in mind when considering vaccination, but its role in the pathogenesis of most field cases of FIP is not known.

CLINICAL SIGNS

There are several clinical syndromes associated with feline coronavirus infection in the field, although in most cases no clinical signs are observed. Enteritis associated with low virulence coronavirus (e.g. FECV) infection is generally mild and of short duration. It is most common in kittens, particularly just after weaning (Pedersen, 1987c). Diarrhoea generally develops 2–7 days after experimental inoculation and lasts 2–3 days (Pedersen *et al.*, 1981). Sometimes the diarrhoea is preceded by transient vomiting. More severe diarrhoea may be associated with secondary bacterial infection, but the fatal haemorrhagic diarrhoea reported by McKeirnan *et al.* (1981) is rare.

The initial signs of both wet and dry FIP are similar, rather non-specific and often missed in field cases. They include pyrexia (39.5°C), anorexia and lethargy. Occasionally some cats may also develop mild upper respiratory signs or diarrhoea. In wet FIP these vague signs are rapidly followed by the development of ascites (Fig. 17.2) with weight loss, depression, anaemia and death. As well as ascites, pleural effusion occurs in about 20% of cases and in these cats dyspnoea is a prominent clinical sign. Jaundice is also sometimes seen, especially in the later stages.

In dry FIP granulomatous lesions develop in a variety of organs and the clinical signs reflect the organs involved. Most frequently affected are organs in the abdominal cavity (particularly the liver and kidney), the CNS and eyes (Pedersen, 1987b). The most common presenting signs are therefore chronic pyrexia, weight loss and depression. Involvement of the central nervous system may lead to a variety of neurological signs including ataxia, paresis, paralysis, disorientation, nystagmus, fits, hyperaesthesia and peripheral nerve palsies. In some cases of FIP

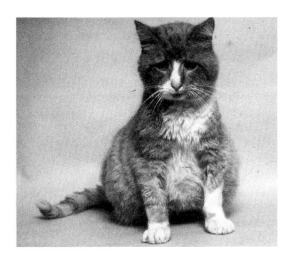

Fig. 17.2 A cat with wet or effusive FIP, showing gross abdominal distension.

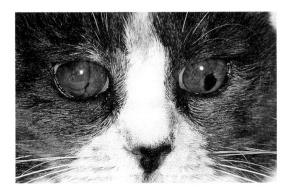

Fig. 17.3 Iritis associated with dry FIP.

involvement of the eye, e.g. hyphaemia, iridocyclitis and retinitis of varying severity, may be the only clinical manifestation of FIP (Fig. 17.3).

Although FIP is usually described as two discrete syndromes, as might be predicted from the model in Fig. 17.1, wet and dry FIP are not mutually exclusive descriptions. Eye or CNS lesions may be clinically apparent in up to 10% of cases of wet FIP and many cats with wet FIP have some lesions of dry FIP at necropsy. There are also occasional accounts of cats with wet FIP apparently recovering but then developing dry FIP.

DIAGNOSIS

Making a diagnosis of FIP, especially dry FIP, can be difficult, and should be based on a combination of clinical signs and laboratory findings. In particular, microscopic examination of tissue sections is often necessary if a definitive diagnosis is to be reached (Barlough, 1985; Addie, 1989).

Because of the non-specific nature of the clinical syndromes associated with, in particular, the dry form of the disease, FIP should be considered in any cat with weight loss, inappetence or persistent pyrexia. Other infectious diseases which need to be considered in such cases include FeLV or FIV infection and toxoplasmosis. Careful ophthalmic examination should be carried out on these cats as the eyes may contain the only readily detectable lesion. When ascites or pleural effusion occurs, FIP is one of the major differential diagnoses. FIP should also be considered in neurological conditions in which the cause is not immediately obvious.

Wet FIP has to be differentiated from other causes of ascitic and/or pleural effusion such as lymphocytic cholangitis, tumours, pyothorax, bacterial peritonitis, heart failure and liver cirrhosis. Aspiration and analysis of fluid will distinguish it from most other diseases, although cats with lymphocytic cholangitis may produce ascitic fluid with similar biochemical properties (Lucke *et al.*, 1974). In wet FIP the fluid is often yellow or grey and is very tacky and viscous. It has a high protein concentration (32–118 g/l) – largely gammaglobulin – and froths easily when shaken. If left to stand it may clot. Microscopic examination of the fluid often reveals neutrophils, lymphocytes, macrophages and mesothelial cells. In cats with ocular or CNS disease increased amounts of proteins and cells are also sometimes found in the aqueous humour and cerebrospinal fluid (Pedersen, 1987b).

Haematological changes in wet and dry FIP are similar. There is usually a leucocytosis with neutrophilia but lymphopenia. A mild non-regenerative anaemia is present in about half of all cases. Co-infection with FeLV causes more profound anaemia and is often accompanied by panleucopenia.

Serum protein levels are one of the more useful routine biochemical tests for FIP. In both wet and dry FIP there is often a hyperproteinaemia (>80 g/l) with raised globulin fraction largely due to large amounts of circulating anti-coronavirus antibody. Early in the development of clinical signs, blood clotting times may be markedly reduced, but later in the course of the disease they often increase. Other biochemical parameters, such as liver enzymes, bilirubin and urea, may be elevated owing to granulomatous lesions in the relevant organs.

Isolation of coronavirus from clinical cases of FIP is not usually possible, partly owing to the relatively small amounts of virus excreted during the clinical stages of the disease, but largely owing to the general difficulty of growing field strains of feline coronaviruses in cell culture. In the future techniques such as assays for circulating immune complexes, antigen-capture ELISA or the use of nucleic acid probes and the polymerase chain reaction may make virus detection routine, but at present virus detection is rarely even attempted. Serological tests, including ELISA, immunofluorescence and virus neutralization assays, are commonly used as indicators of coronavirus infection. The main disadvantages of serological tests are the difficulties of distinguishing between infection with FIP-inducing and enteric strains, and between past and present infection. In general, very high titres are more indicative of generalized infection, and, if accompanied by clinical signs, are often taken as diagnostic of FIP. Lower antibody titres are usually interpreted as indicating local, enteric infection. However, serum from some cats with acute wet FIP may contain low concentrations or even no detectable antibody. Conversely high antibody titres are sometimes detected in cats with no clinical signs, possibly reflecting past infection and recovery from an FIP-inducing strain. This illustrates the need for caution in interpreting the results of serological tests for FIP and the dangers of relying on serology alone for making a diagnosis. Certainly euthanasia should never be performed purely on the basis of a serological test.

A definitive diagnosis of FIP is often only possible by histological examination of biopsy or post-mortem material. Therefore if a colony is at risk from the disease necropsy should always be performed on any suspected cases of FIP and fixed tissues examined for characteristic histopathological changes.

Pathology

Gross findings

The most striking feature on opening the abdomen of a cat with wet FIP is usually the large amount of ascitic fluid. Although it may amount to as little as a few millilitres, the total volume of abdominal fluid is more often several hundred millilitres. The fluid is generally yellowish or grey and may be clear or contain flakes of fibrin. Pleural effusions have a similar appearance. Many serosal surfaces are covered by a greyish-white fibrinous exudate, and the omentum is often opaque, thickened and granular. Granulomatous lesions within organs appear as white foci on cut surfaces. In the thorax, pleural lesions often extend into the lung.

In dry FIP, abdominal fluid and fibrinous exudates are rare, and variably sized granulomatous lesions are often more prominent. Although many of the granulomatous lesions found in cats with dry FIP are small and very similar to those found in cats with wet FIP, in some organs, particularly the liver, kidney and lymph nodes, the lesions may be several centimetres in diameter. Gross lesions are rarely seen, however, in the CNS. Gross lesions in the eye have been described earlier.

Histopathology

In wet FIP there is a fibrinous or fibrinocellular exudate on the serosal surface of most abdominal organs. The omentum and serosa contain numerous small pyogranulomas, some of which are visible with the naked eye, and foci of mesothelial hyperplasia, especially on the spleen. The granulomas usually consist of a necrotic centre and neutrophils, surrounded by lymphocytes, plasma cells and many large, active macrophages. Perivascular cuffing both within the serosa and extending along venules into the underlying tissue is frequently reported (Pedersen, 1987b). Granulomatous infiltrations in the liver may involve the biliary tree, and a necrotic, thrombic vasculitis of the wall of the gall bladder has also been described. The lymphoid organs of the abdomen and thorax are frequently affected; marked follicular hyperplasia, necrotic foci and pyogranulomatous lesions are common findings in abdominal lymph nodes and the spleen.

The histopathological changes associated with dry FIP are similar to those of wet FIP although there is far less exudation, and the granulomatous lesions are usually much larger, surrounded by more fibrosis and are often found outside the abdomen and thorax. In the CNS, phlebitis of the meninges and choroid plexus is common, but thrombosis does not usually occur. In the eye inflammation may be focal or diffuse. The uvea and retina are affected as are the meninges of the optic nerves. Fibrinocellular exudates are seen within the eye giving the aqueous humour a cloudy appearance. Excess melanin may accumulate in the uvea. Lesions in skeletal muscle, testes, peripheral nerves and the bladder are rare.

TREATMENT

Once clinical signs of wet or dry FIP have developed the prognosis is very poor. Aspiration of fluid generally provides only temporary relief as fresh fluid soon accumulates. An early report suggesting that tylosin and prednisolone might be effective (Colgrove & Parker, 1971) has not been confirmed, although some cats may improve with large doses of corticosteroids or other immunosuppressants (Pedersen, 1987b; Weiss, 1991). Such improvement is, however, usually only temporary, and in the longer term corticosteroids may even worsen the condition by suppression of cellular immunity. Although ribavirin and interferon inhibit feline coronavirus replication *in vitro* (Weiss & Oostram-Ram, 1989; Weiss & Toivio-Kinnucan, 1989; Barlough & Scott, 1990), they do not appear to be effective in diseased cats. Some clinical success has, however, recently been described for the immunomodulator promodulin (Weiss, 1991).

Rarely, some cats do recover from FIP, although the role played in their recovery by any treatment regime is usually unclear. Probably symptomatic treatment and dedicated nursing are most effective, especially if started early in the development of the disease.

EPIDEMIOLOGY AND CONTROL

Feline coronavirus infection has been reported in domestic cats from throughout the world (Horzinek & Osterhaus, 1979) and also in a range of wild cat species, mainly kept in zoos (Pedersen, 1987b). Serological surveys of cats suggest that infection is common; up to 25% in household cats and up to 95% in some colonies (Pedersen, 1976; Osterhaus *et al.*, 1977). Such surveys cannot, of course, differentiate between infection with FIP-inducing strains, FECV or CCV. On the other hand, if FIP-inducing strains are simply variants or mutants of FECV, differentiation may be deceptive in terms of disease potential. Clinical FIP is certainly nothing like so common as coronavirus infection; in household pets it occurs only sporadically, and even outbreaks among cats living in colonies usually only affect 5–10% of the population (Pedersen, 1988) although up to 50% may be affected sometimes (Potkay *et al.*, 1974).

Clinical FIP can occur in cats of any age, although it is most frequently seen in young animals (less than 2 years of age) and in older cats (greater than 11). In Britain FIP seems to be more common in certain breeds of cat, for example Burmese and Persian (Addie, 1992). While pedigree cats might be expected to show an increased incidence associated with a colony environment, it is possible that genetic factors may also be involved. Neither infection nor disease appear to be sex-linked.

Most cats in colonies probably become infected either from their dam or from other adults or kittens during the first few weeks of life (Addie & Jarrett, 1990, 1991), although horizontal spread among susceptible adults can also occur. Spread among adults is probably more important in household pets than in closed colonies, although it can also be a means of introducing virus into a colony. Some canine coronaviruses can also infect cats, although their role in the epidemiology of field disease is not known (McArdle *et al.*, 1992).

Feline (and canine) coronaviruses have been shown experimentally to be excreted in the faeces and saliva of cats for several days to weeks prior to the onset of clinical FIP (Stoddart *et al.*, 1988b). Therefore infected cats are likely to be a source of infection for other cats long before disease is suspected, and this obviously makes it difficult to control spread through a colony. Furthermore, epidemiological and experimental studies suggest that cats can become persistently infected with coronaviruses, and that these carrier cats may be a source of infection to others. However, the mechanism and sites of persistent infection, the amounts of virus shed and how long cats can remain persistently infected are not at all clear (Pedersen, 1987a).

Although no commercial vaccine is available in the UK at the time of writing, an attenuated live FIP vaccine which appears to provoke protective mucosal immunity (Christianson *et al.*, 1989; Gerber *et al.*, 1990; Reeves *et al.*, 1992), is currently licensed in the USA and is undergoing both laboratory and field trials in Europe. Other experimental approaches to vaccination include the development of subunit vaccines, i.e. vaccines which contain only part of the FIP virus. These subunit vaccines can either be dead or, by inserting the genes for specific FIPV proteins into another virus (e.g. vaccinia virus), live. Current research using these approaches is concentrated on finding those parts of the virus which might induce a protective rather than enhancing immune response (Vennema *et al.*, 1990, 1991).

It can therefore be appreciated that control of coronavirus infection can be difficult; serology cannot reliably differentiate between infection with pathogenic and non-pathogenic strains, nor can it give any indication of protective immunity. Furthermore, some cats with antibody may be recovered and immune, whereas others might be asymptomatic carriers. Virus isolation is rarely possible, and even if it were, laboratory differentiation of pathogenic and non-pathogenic isolates is not yet feasible. No vaccine is available in the UK at present. There are therefore two main approaches to control: total eradication of all coronavirus infection or pragmatic tolerance. The former approach is usually only practicable in limited situations, for example in breeding colonies of experimental cats. In many colonies control depends largely on strict hygienic precautions combined with tolerance of some infection. Diseased and in-contact cats should be isolated and their housing thoroughly cleaned and disinfected. Quarantine and serological testing will help keep out new infection. In seropositive colonies, kittens separated from their mothers and the rest of the colony at 2–6 weeks old rarely seroconvert (Addie & Jarrett, 1991); such early weaning and rearing in isolation may enable eradication of the virus from a colony. As FeLV is known to cause more severe disease, FeLV should be tested for and eradicated.

REFERENCES

Addie D.D. (1989) Interpretation of feline coronavirus serology. *In Practice* **11**, 232–5.

Addie D.D. (1992) Studies on the humoral immune response to feline coronavirus. PhD Thesis, University of Glasgow.

Addie D.D. & Jarrett O. (1990) Control of feline coronavirus infection in kittens. *Vet. Rec.* **126**, 164.

Addie D.D. & Jarrett O. (1991) A study of naturally occurring feline coronavirus infections in kittens. *Vet. Rec.* **126**, 164.

Barlough J.E. (1985) Cats, coronaviruses and coronavirus antibody tests. *J. Small Anim. Pract.* **26**, 353–63.

Barlough J.E. & Scott F.W. (1990) Effectiveness of three antiviral agents against FIP virus *in vitro*. *Vet. Rec.* **126**, 556–8.

Barlough J.E., Stoddart C.A., Sorresso G.P., Jacobson P.H. & Scott F.W. (1984) Experimental inoculation of cats with CCV and subsequent challenge with FIPV. *Lab. Anim. Sci.* **34**, 592–7.

Christianson K.K., Ingersoll J.D., Landon R.M., Pfeiffer N.E. & Gerber J.D. (1989) Characterisation of a temperature sensitive feline infectious peritonitis coronavirus. *Arch. Virol.* **109**, 185–96.

Colgrove D.J. & Parker A.J. (1971) Feline infectious peritonitis. *J. Small Anim. Pract.* **12**, 225–32.

Fiscus S.A. & Teramoto Y.A. (1987) Antigenic comparison of feline coronavirus isolates: evidence for markedly different peplomer glycoproteins. *J. Virol.* **61**, 2607–13.

Fiscus S.A., Rivoire B.L. & Teramoto Y.A. (1987) Epitope specific antibody responses to virulent and avirulent feline infectious peritonitis isolates. *J. Clin. Microbiol.* **25**, 1529–34.

Gerber J.D., Pfeiffer N.E., Ingersoll J.D., Christianson K.K., Landon R.M., Selzer N.L. & Beckenhauer W.H. (1990) Characterisation of an attenuated temperature sensitive feline infectious peritonitis (FIP) virus vaccine that protects cats against FIP. In Cavanagh D. & Brown D. (eds) *Coronaviruses.* Plenum Press, New York & London, pp. 481–9.

Hohdatsu T., Nakamura M., Ishizuka Y., Yamada H. & Koyama H. (1991) A study on the mechanism of antibody dependent enhancement of FIPV infection in feline macrophages by monoclonal antibodies. *Arch. Virol.* **120**, 207–17.

Holzworth J. (1963) Some important disorders in cats. *Cornell Vet.* **53**, 157–60.

Hyashi T., Watabe Y., Nakayama H. & Fujiwarak K. (1982) Enteritis due to FIPV. *Jpn. J. Vet. Sci.* **44**, 97–106.

Horzinek M.C. & Osterhaus A.D.M.E. (1977) Feline infectious peritonitis virus. *Zbl. Vet. Med. B* **24**, 398–405.

Horzinek M.C. & Osterhaus A.D.M.E. (1979) Feline infectious peritonitis; a worldwide survey. *Am. J. Vet. Res.* **40**, 1487–92.

Jacobse-Geels H.E., Dala M.R. & Horzinek M.C. (1982) Antibody, immune complexes and complement activity fluctuations in kittens with experimentally induced feline infectious peritonitis. *Am. J. Vet. Res.* **43**, 666–70.

Lucke V.M. & Davies J.D. (1984) Progressive lymphocytic cholangitis in the cat. *J. Small Anim. Pract.* **25**, 249–60.

McArdle F., Bennett M., Gaskell R.M., Tennant B., Kelly D.F. & Gaskell C.J. (1992) Induction and enhancement of feline infectious peritonitis by canine coronavirus: a preliminary study. *Am. J. Vet. Res.* **53**, 1500–6.

McKeirnan A.J., Evermann J.F., Hargis A., Miller L.M. & Ott R.L. (1981) Isolation of feline coronaviruses from two cats with diverse disease manifestations. *Feline Pract.* **11**, 16–20.

Olsen C.W., Corapi W.V., Ngichabe C.K., Baines J.D. & Scott F.W. (1992) Monoclonal antibody to the spike protein of feline infectious peritonitis virus mediates antibody dependent enhancement of infection of feline macrophages. *J. Virol.* **66**, 956–65.

Osterhaus A.D.M.E., Horzinek M.C. & Reynolds D.J. (1997) Seroepidemiology of feline infectious peritonitis virus using transmissible gastroenteritis virus as an antigen. *Zbl. Vet. Med. B* **24**, 835–41.

Pedersen N.C. (1976) Serologic studies of naturally occurring feline infectious peritonitis. *Am. J. Vet. Res.* **37**, 1449–53.

Pedersen N.C. (1987a) Virologic and immunologic aspects of feline infectious peritonitis virus infection.

In Lai M.M.C. & Stohlman S.A. (eds) *Coronaviruses.* Plenum Press, New York and London, pp. 529–50.

Pedersen N.C. (1987b) Feline infectious peritonitis virus. In Appel M. (ed) *Virus Infections of Carnivores.* Elsevier Science Publishers BV, Amsterdam, Oxford, New York & Tokyo, pp. 267–86.

Pedersen N.C. (1987c) Feline enteric coronavirus. In Appel M. (ed) *Virus Infections of Carnivores.* Elsevier Science Publishers BV, Amsterdam, Oxford, New York & Tokyo, pp. 261–5.

Pedersen N.C. & Black J.W. (1983) Attempted immunisation of cats against FIP using avirulent live virus or sublethal amounts of virulent virus. *Am. J. Vet. Res.* **44**, 229–34.

Pedersen N.C. & Boyle J.F. (1980) Immunologic phenomena in the effusive form of feline infectious peritonitis. *Am. J. Vet. Res.* **41**, 868–76.

Pedersen N.C., Boyle J.F., Floyd K., Fudge A. & Barker J. (1981) An enteric coronavirus infection of cats and its relationship to feline infectious peritonitis. *Am. J. Vet. Res.* **42**, 368–77.

Potkay B.A., Bacher J.D. & Pitts T.W. (1974) Feline infectious peritonitis in a closed breeding colony. *Lab. Anim. Sci.* **24**, 279–89.

Reeves N.C.P., Pollock R.V.H. & Thurber E.T. (1992) Long-term follow-up study of cats vaccinated with a temperature sensitive feline infectious peritonitis vaccine. *Cornell Vet.* **82**, 117–23.

Stoddart C.A. & Scott F.W. (1989) Intrinsic resistance of feline peritoneal macrophages to coronavirus infection correlates with *in vivo* virulence. *J. Virol.* **63**, 436–40.

Stoddart C.A., Barlough J.E., Baldwin C.A. & Scott F.W. (1988a) Attempted immunisation of cats against feline infectious peritonitis using canine coronavirus. *Res. Vet. Sci.* **45**, 383–8.

Stoddart M.E., Gaskell R.M., Harbour D.A. & Gaskell C.J. (1988b) Virus shedding and immune responses in cats inoculated with cell culture adapted FIPV. *Vet. Microbiol.* **16**, 145–58.

Stoddart M.E., Gaskell R.M., Harbour D.A. & Pearson G.R. (1988c) The sites of early viral replication in feline infectious peritonitis. *Vet. Microbiol.* **18**, 259–71.

Vennema H., De Groot R.J., Harbour D.A., Dalderup M., Gruffydd-Jones T., Horzinek M.C. & Spaan W.J.M. (1990) Early death after feline infectious peritonitis virus challenge due to recombinant vaccinia virus immunisation. *J. Virol.* **64**, 1407–9.

Vennema H., De Groot R.J., Harbour D.A., Horzinek M.C. & Spaan W.J.M. (1991) Primary structure of the membrane and nucleocapsid genes of feline infectious peritonitis virus and immunogenicity of recombinant vaccinia viruses in kittens. *Virol.* **181**, 327–35.

Weiss R.C. (1991) The diagnosis and clinical management of feline infectious peritonitis. *Vet. Med.* **86**, 308–19.

Weiss R.C. & Cox N.R. (1989) Evaluation of immunity to feline infectious peritonitis in cats with cutaneous viral-induced delayed hypersensitivity. *Vet. Immunol. Immunopath.* **21**, 293–309.

Weiss R.C. & Oostram-Ram T. (1989) Inhibitory effects of ribavirin alone or combined with human alpha interferon on feline infectious peritonitis virus replication *in vitro. Vet. Microbiol.* **20**, 255–65.

Weiss R.C. & Scott F.W. (1981) Pathogenesis of feline infectious peritonitis; nature and development of viremia. *Am. J. Vet. Res.* **42**, 382–90.

Weiss R.C. & Toivio-Kinnucan M. (1989) Inhibition of feline infectious peritonitis virus replication by recombinant human leukocyte (α) interferon and feline fibroblastic (β) interferon. *Am. J. Vet. Res.* **49**, 1329–35.

Chapter 18 / Feline Poxvirus Infection

R. M. GASKELL AND M. BENNETT

INTRODUCTION

The first case of cowpox in a domestic cat was seen in 1978 (Thomsett *et al.*, 1978; Baxby *et al.*, 1979), although an outbreak of cowpox in cheetahs at a British zoo had been recorded the previous year (Baxby *et al.*, 1979, 1982). Since then many further cases have been reported (e.g. Gaskell *et al.*, 1983; Hoare *et al.*, 1984; Martland *et al.*, 1985; Bennett *et al.*, 1986, 1990), and more cases of cowpox are now seen each year in domestic cats than in any other species. However, cowpox virus is not endemic in cats, and the reservoir host is believed to be a small wild rodent.

Cowpox virus is infectious to man, and cat-to-man transmission has been recorded on several occasions (Willemse & Egberink, 1985; Pether *et al.*, 1986; Casemore *et al.*, 1987). Veterinary surgeons and owners should therefore take care when handling infected cats.

In addition to cowpox virus, occasional accounts of feline orf exist (Hamblet, 1993). The clinical signs of feline orf appear generally similar to those of cowpox, but the source of infection is probably farm animals. Little is known about feline orf, but it may be transmissible to man. The rest of this chapter refers only to cowpox virus.

AETIOLOGY

Cowpox virus is a poxvirus in the genus *Orthopoxvirus*, which also includes smallpox virus (now eradicated) and the virus of smallpox vaccine, vaccinia. The orthopoxviruses are all closely related and are antigenically very similar, but each species can be identified by a combination of biological tests, minor serological differences and by genome analysis (Thomsett *et al.*, 1978; Bennett *et al.*, 1985; Naidoo *et al.*, 1992). Although Jenner apparently used cowpox material for the original smallpox vaccine, the modern day vaccine, vaccinia virus, is clearly different from cowpox virus and its origins are not known (Baxby, 1981).

Like many poxviruses, cowpox virus is very resistant and may remain viable for several years at room temperature if kept dry. It is susceptible, however, to many disinfectants, particularly hypochlorites.

PATHOGENESIS

Clinical surveys suggest that the usual route of infection is by skin inoculation, although oronasal infection can also occur, at least experimentally (Bennett *et al.*, 1986, 1989). Virus replication at the site of entry may cause the development of a primary skin lesion or mild coryza. Virus is transported from the inoculation site to draining lymph nodes, where further virus replication causes viraemia and the subsequent development of widespread secondary skin lesions. During the viraemia much virus can be isolated from a variety of lymphoid organs and from the respiratory tract, including the lungs (Gaskell *et al.*, 1983; Bennett *et al.*, 1989), although clinical signs of respiratory disease are uncommon. Inoculation of low doses of virus, or oronasal inocu-

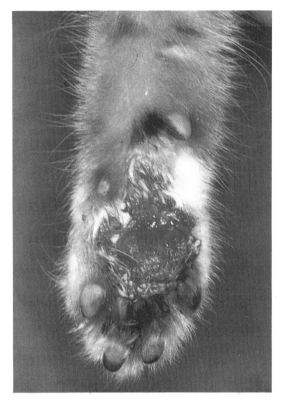

Fig. 18.1 Ulcerated cowpox virus lesion on paw.

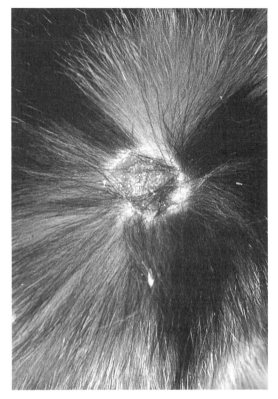

Fig. 18.2 Hairless scabbed lesion on dorsum.

lation may cause less severe disease (Bennett *et al.*, 1989), whereas immunosuppression, for example after treatment with corticosteroids or infection with feline immunodeficiency virus, may result in severe disease and death.

CLINICAL SIGNS

Most cats with cowpox are first presented for veterinary attention with widespread skin lesions, although closer examination of the cat and questioning of the owner will often reveal a history of an original, single skin lesion on the head, neck or a forelimb. This primary lesion can vary in character from a large abscess to small, scabbed papules or ulcers, but will often be described as having originated as a small, bite-like wound (Bennett *et al.*, 1986, 1990).

Secondary skin lesions develop a few days to a few weeks after the primary lesion is first noticed. They first appear as small, randomly distributed dermal nodules, which over 3–5 days develop into ulcerated papules up to 1 cm in diameter (Figs. 18.1 and 18.2). Occasionally, vesicles may be seen, particularly on the tongue or inner aspect of the pinna. The secondary lesions quickly become scabbed, and, over the following 2–3 weeks, the scabs dry and separate to leave small bald patches of healing skin. New hair soon grows, and most cats are completely recovered in 6–8 weeks. The lesions are sometimes pruritic, especially the primary lesion and healing secondary lesions.

In addition to the skin lesions, some cats may be mildly pyrexic during the viraemic stage of the disease, i.e. just before and during the early development of secondary lesions. Some cats, up to about 20%, may also develop a mild, serous nasal discharge, conjunctivitis or transient diarrhoea, and occasionally cats may be depressed and anorexic. More severe or long-standing systemic signs, or delayed healing of skin lesions may result from heavy secondary bacterial infection, especially of the primary lesion, or immunodeficiency either resulting from corticosteroid treatment or due to severe concurrent disease or infection with feline leukaemia virus (FeLV) or feline immunodeficiency virus (FIV) (Hoare *et al.*, 1984; Webster & Jefferies, 1984; Bennett *et al.*, 1986; Brown *et al.*, 1989). Severe systemic signs indicate a poor prognosis, and euthanasia might be considered in these cases.

DIAGNOSIS

A history of a primary skin lesion followed by the development of widespread secondary skin lesions enables a clinical diagnosis of cowpox to be made in many instances, but a laboratory diagnosis is required for confirmation (Bennett *et al.*, 1985, 1986). The more common differential diagnoses include cat bite abscesses, neoplasia, eosinophilic granuloma and miliary eczema.

Dry, unfixed scab material can be sent through the post without need for special transport medium. Examination of scab homogenate by electron microscopy enables a diagnosis to be made in three-quarters of cases, often on the day of receipt, while virus isolation in cell culture is more sensitive but may take up to 10 days. Tissue fixed in 5% formol-saline can be sent for histological examination. The histopathological changes associated with cowpox include epidermal hyperplasia and hypertrophy, multilocular vesicle formation and the presence of large, eosinophilic, intracytoplasmic inclusion bodies. However, healing lesions or those with extensive secondary bacterial infection may not always contain such diagnostic features. Immunostaining may be useful in these cases (Bennett *et al.*, 1990).

Serological tests including immunofluorescence (IF), virus neutralization (VN) and haemagglutination inhibition (HAI) tests can help in reaching a diagnosis, especially retrospectively, although since cowpox virus is not endemic in cats, a fairly certain diagnosis of cowpox can usually be made based on serology alone. HAI and IF antibodies are detectable before VN antibody, and are therefore useful for diagnosis early in disease. Both VN and IF antibodies can persist for several years and may be more useful when making a retrospective diagnosis.

EPIDEMIOLOGY

Cowpox virus, unlike pseudocowpox virus, is only found in Eurasia and is rarely isolated from cattle (Baxby, 1977). The virus is believed to be endemic in a small wild mammal reservoir (Fig. 18.3) (Baxby, 1977; Bennett *et al.*, 1986; Fenner *et al.*, 1988) from which it can be spread to a variety of 'incidental' hosts. In addition to domestic cats, cattle and man, cowpox virus has been isolated from exotic cats in British and European zoos (Baxby *et al.*, 1979, 1982), from elephants, rhinoceroses, okapi, big cats and anteaters in zoos in mainland Europe and from wild susliks and gerbils in Turkmenistan (Marennikova *et al.*, 1984; Pilaski & Woolf, 1988).

Most cases of cowpox recognized in Britain nowadays are in domestic cats, and the epidemiology of the disease in cats fits well with the theory of infection through contact with small wild mammals. Affected cats are usually adult and come from rural environments; almost all are known by their owners to hunt small mammals; and the primary skin lesion often first appears as a bite-like wound on the head or a forelimb. Most cases occur in the autumn (Bennett *et al.*, 1986), possibly because many small wild mammals are at their maximum population size and are most active at that time of year.

There is circumstantial field evidence and good experimental evidence that cat-to-cat transmission does occur, but generally causes only subclinical infection in the recipient cat (Bennett *et al.*, 1986, 1989). Further cat-to-cat transmission has not been reported, and serological surveys confirm that cowpox virus is not endemic in cats. Cat-to-human transmission can also occur, and

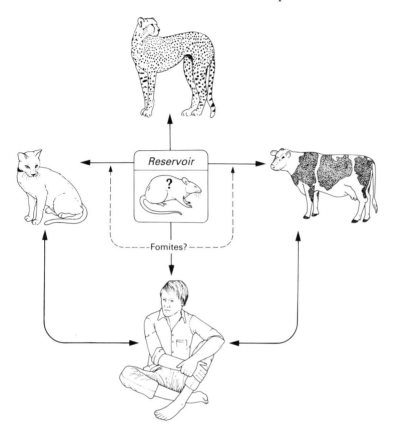

Fig. 18.3 Probable epidemiology of cowpox.

several recent cases in man have been traced to contact with an infected cat.

TREATMENT AND PREVENTION

There is no specific treatment for cowpox virus infection, so it is fortunate that most cats recover uneventfully. Treatment usually consists of broad-spectrum antibiotics to control secondary and concurrent bacterial infection, bathing of large lesions in a mild antiseptic solution, and, if necessary, use of an Elizabethan collar or bandaging to prevent scratching. Severely ill cats, especially if immunosuppressed, have a poor prognosis and euthanasia might be considered in these cases. Corticosteroids should be avoided as they may exacerbate the condition.

No vaccine is available, and feline cowpox is probably not common enough to warrant the development of one. As the source of infection for cats is not known, prevention is therefore difficult unless the cats are housed entirely indoors in rodent-proof accommodation. Among pet cats, cat-to-cat transmission is uncommon and usually causes only seroconversion without clinical signs in the recipient cat, so unless the in-contact cats are thought to be at extra risk of severe disease, isolation is probably not necessary. In big cat collections thought to be at risk, vaccination with vaccinia virus might be considered, although little is known about the immunizing value of vaccinia virus in big cat species (Baxby *et al.*, 1982). Control of disease in big cat collections relies largely on prompt diagnosis and isolation of affected individuals.

Public health aspects

Approximately half of recent cases of human cowpox have been traced to contact with infected cats (Willemse & Egberink, 1985; Lancet, 1987), and the possibility of such contact should always be considered when investigating cases of human cowpox. Human infection usually causes a single lesion on the hand or face, although spread to other sites around the body may occur through direct contact, for example hand to face, or locally in immunosuppressed individuals or those with a pre-existing skin disease (Baxby, 1977, 1988). In addition to the skin lesion(s), cowpox may also cause systemic illness including nausea, pyrexia and headaches, and many patients require bed rest, sometimes in hospital. Very rarely, cowpox can be fatal in man (Eis-Hubinger *et al.*, 1990). It should be noted that smallpox vaccination, even recent, may not provide complete protection against primary cowpox virus infection, although it might help prevent more severe disease.

Although cats do appear to be one of the more frequent sources of human cowpox, cat-to-man transmission is uncommon, and transmission to humans is unlikely if basic hygienic precautions are taken. Veterinary surgeons and others handling infected cats should wear gloves and take care not to allow infected material into wounds or the eyes. Young children, the elderly, those with a pre-existing skin condition or debilitative or immunosuppressive disease should avoid contact with the cat while it remains infective (i.e. until the scabs have gone). If these elementary procedures are followed then the risk of human infection should be small, and it is rarely necessary to kill an affected cat on public health grounds.

REFERENCES

Baxby D. (1977) Is cowpox misnamed? A review of 10 human cases. *Br. Med. J.* **i**, 1379–81.

Baxby D. (1981) *Jenner's Smallpox Vaccine. The Riddle of Vaccinia Virus and its Origin.* Heinemann Educational Books, London.

Baxby D. (1988) Human poxvirus infection after the eradication of smallpox. *Epidem. Inf.* **100**, 321–34.

Baxby D., Ashton D.G., Jones D.M., Thomsett L.R. &

Denham E.M. (1979) Cowpox virus infection in unusual hosts. *Vet. Rec.* **104**, 175.

Baxby D., Ashton D.G., Jones D.M. & Thomsett L.R. (1982) An outbreak of cowpox in captive cheetahs; virological and epidemiological studies. *J. Hyg.* [Camb.] **89**, 365–72.

Bennett M., Baxby D., Gaskell R.M., Gaskell C.J. & Kelly D.F. (1985) The laboratory diagnosis of *Orthopoxvirus* infection in the domestic cat. *J. Small Anim. Pract.* **26**, 653–61.

Bennett M., Gaskell C.J., Gaskell R.M., Baxby D. & Gruffydd-Jones T.J. (1986) Poxvirus infection in the domestic cat; some clinical and epidemiological observations. *Vet. Rec.* **118**, 387–90.

Bennett M., Gaskell R.M., Gaskell C.J., Baxby D. & Kelly D.F. (1989) Studies on poxvirus infection in cats. *Arch. Virol.* **104**, 19–33.

Bennett M., Gaskell C.J., Baxby D., Gaskell R.M., Kelly D.F. & Naidoo J. (1990) Feline cowpox virus infection; a review. *J. Small Anim. Pract.* **31**, 167–73.

Brown A., Bennett M. & Gaskell C.J. (1989) Fatal poxvirus infection in a cat associated with FIV infection. *Vet. Rec.* **124**, 19–20.

Casemore D.P., Emslie E.S., Whyler D.K., Baxby D., Bennett M. & Davies A.B. (1987) Cowpox in a child, acquired from a cat. *Clin. Exp. Derm.* **12**, 286–7.

Eis-Hubinger A.M., Gerritzen A., Schneweis K.E., Pfeiff B., Pullman H., Mayr A. & Czerny C.-P. (1990) Fatal cowpox-like virus infection transmitted by a cat. *Lancet* **ii**, 880.

Fenner F., Henderson D.A., Arita I., Jezek Z. & Ladnyi I.D. (1988) *Smallpox and its Eradication.* WHO, Geneva.

Gaskell R.M., Gaskell C.J., Evans R.J., Dennis P.E., Bennett A.M., Udall N.D., Voyle C. & Hill T.J. (1983) Natural and experimental poxvirus infection in the domestic cat. *Vet. Rec.* **112**, 164–70.

Hamblet C.N. (1993) Parapoxvirus infection in a cat. *Vet. Rec.* **132**, 144.

Hoare C.M., Gruffydd-Jones T.J., Bennett M., Gaskell R.M. & Baxby D. (1984) Cowpox in cats. *Vet. Rec.* **114**, 22.

Lancet (1987) What's new pussy-cat? Cowpox. *Lancet* **ii**, 668.

Marennikova S.S., Shelukhina E.M. & Efremova E.V. (1984) New outlook on the biology of cowpox. *Acta. Virol.* **28**, 437–44.

Martland M.F., Poulton G.J. & Done R.A. (1985) Three cases of cowpox infection in the domestic cat. *Vet. Rec.* **117**, 231–3.

Naidoo J., Baxby D., Bennett M., Gaskell R.M. & Gaskell C.J. (1992) Characterisation of orthopoxviruses isolated from feline infections in Britain. *Arch. Virol.* **125**, 261–72.

Pether J.V.S., Trevains P.H., Harrison S.R.B., Baxby D.,
Bennett M. & Gibb A.P.R. (1976) Cowpox from cat to
man. *Lancet* **i**, 38–9.

Pilaski J. & Wolff A.R. (1988) Poxvirus infections in zoo-
kept animals. In Darai G. (ed) *Virus Diseases in Laboratory and Captive Animals*. Martinus Nijhoff, The Hague,
pp. 55–100.

Thomsett L.R, Baxby D. & Denham E.M.M. (1978)
Cowpox in the domestic cat. *Vet. Rec.* **16**, 567.

Webster J. & Jefferies A.R. (1984) Cowpox in cats. *Vet.
Rec.* **114**, 151.

Willemse A. & Egberink H.F. (1985) Transmission of
cowpox virus infection from domestic cat to man. *Lancet*
i, 1515.

Chapter 19 / Rabies

P.-P. PASTORET, B. BROCHIER
AND R. M. GASKELL

INTRODUCTION AND HISTORY

Rabies is a neurotropic disease of virtually all mammals. It exists worldwide, except in places such as Australia and New Zealand, and it has been eradicated from the British Isles by quarantine and other measures.

The disease has been recognized since antiquity. The Latin word *rabies* comes from an old Sanskrit word *Rabhas*, which means 'to do violence' (Steele, 1975). In Britain, the earliest mention of the disease was in 1026, but it was not until the late 18th and 19th centuries that it became frequent. Dogs were recognized as the major source of infection (urban rabies) and the first attempt to deal with it on a national basis was made in 1831 when a Bill was drafted to 'prevent the spreading of canine madness' (Waterhouse, 1971). The Bill did not become law but local authorities were later given the power to require muzzling, to restrict the movement of dogs, and to destroy strays. These methods were only partly successful when left to local authorities, but when the Board of Agriculture assumed overall responsibility, and introduced quarantine amongst other measures, there was a marked decline in the number of rabies cases each year. The disease appeared to have been eradicated in 1903, was reintroduced in 1918, but was finally eliminated by 1922.

The absence of records of rabies in wildlife in Britain, and the success of the straightforward measures by which the disease was eventually eliminated through the control of dogs, suggest that it was never established in British wildlife in a permanent and widespread form. Between 1886 and 1903 in the whole of Great Britain, 3056 animals are known to have died of rabies, but of these, the only wild animals affected were a herd of deer, and it is presumed that this outbreak originated from attacks by a stray, rabid dog (Waterhouse, 1971).

Since the final eradication of rabies from Great Britain in 1922, although a number of cases have occurred in animals whilst in quarantine, only two cases have occurred in dogs which had passed through the specified 6-month quarantine period (Morgan-Jones, 1969; Peace & Hopes, 1970). Fortunately, in both these cases, the disease was contained, but as a result of this, quarantine procedures were changed and animals entering quarantine are now required to be vaccinated (see below). Only two deaths from rabies have since occurred in quarantine (King *et al.*, 1985; P. Thomas, personal communication, 1993). Rabies control measures in the UK may change, however, as a result of EC regulations currently under review (see below).

THE CAUSATIVE AGENT

Rabies virus is a bullet-shaped virus, a member of the Rhabdoviridae. The Rhabdoviridae are enveloped RNA viruses characterized by their shape (Greek *rhabdos*, rod), and by the presence of helical ribonucleocapsids enclosed in a lipid envelope bearing surface projections. The genome is a single molecule of negative sense single-stranded RNA which is non-infectious and is transcribed into five mRNAs, each of which codes for a single protein. The gene order is 3′-N-NS-M-G-L-5′, representing respectively the nucleocapsid protein (N), the non-structural protein (NS), the matrix protein (M), the envelope glycoprotein (G), and a large protein (L), the RNA-dependent RNA polymerase (Tordo *et al.*, 1988; Wunner *et al.*, 1988; Pastoret & Brochier, 1990).

Rabies virus belongs to the genus *Lyssavirus*, named after rabies in Greek (Greek *Lyssa*, madness). For many years rabies virus was thought to be unique. It is now clear that antigenic variation exists within rabies virus itself (Schneider, 1982) and the existence of several distinct rabies-related viruses is now recognized (Bourhy *et al.*, 1993). Five rabies-related viruses described so far (Lagos bat, kontonkan, Mokola, Obodhiang and Duvenhage viruses) are all African viruses (King *et al.*, 1990; Pastoret & Brochier, 1990). A virus closely related to the African Duvenhage virus has also been isolated from European insectivorous bats. These viruses can be distinguished from rabies virus by using conventional sera or monoclonal antibodies. The exact significance of rabies-related viruses in the epidemiology of classical rabies is not well understood but some rabies-related viruses may infect cats (Foggin, 1982; King & Crick, 1988).

The biological behaviour of conventional isolates of rabies virus also varies in that there are differences in pathogenicity between strains, depending on their species of origin or on their passage history in the laboratory; the dose and route of exposure also influence the outcome of infection (Charlton, 1988). There is also an intrinsic difference in species susceptibility to rabies virus infection in that the amount of infectious virus needed to induce the disease experimentally differs markedly between species (Sikes, 1962; Parker & Wilsnack, 1966; Smith & Baer, 1988). The level of virus excretion and the percentage of virus excretors within an infected group also vary according to the species and the infecting virus strain (Blancou & Barrat, 1988). In some species a paradox has been observed when a high dose of virus has been used for infecting animals: such animals seem to be more resistant to challenge than animals given a lower infecting dose (Blancou *et al.*, 1983).

Rabies virus is sensitive to lipid solvents and emulsifying agents and thus is quickly inactivated by a number of disinfectants, including formalin, soap and quaternary ammonium compounds (Waterhouse, 1971; Dean, 1975). The virus is easily inactivated by heat and sunlight, but stable at low temperatures. Under normal environmental conditions, therefore, it does not remain infective for long outside the host in contamined secretions.

PATHOGENESIS AND PATHOLOGY

Rabies virus is excreted in the saliva of infected animals and is mainly transmitted by biting, or less frequently, by contamination of mucosa or a superficial wound (Afshar, 1979). In the USA, airborne transmission has also been recorded in man, coyotes and foxes following exposure to caves heavily populated by infected bats (Constantine, 1962; Winkler, 1975). However, several dogs and cats exposed in the same way did not become infected. Experimentally, rabies has been transmitted by the oral route to various laboratory animals, foxes, skunks and cats, and infection of dogs from eating rabid fox carcases has been reported from the Arctic (Soave, 1966; Bell & Moore, 1971; Charlton, 1988). An important sequel to the demonstration of oral infection is the development of oral rabies vaccines for wildlife.

On gaining entry to the body, the virus multiplies locally within myocytes at the site of exposure before moving up the axon of the associated nerve to the central nervous system to produce an encephalitis: there is also evidence that in some cases virus may enter peripheral nerves directly, without preliminary replication in non-nervous tissue (Murphy *et al.*, 1973a,b; Baer, 1975a; Charlton, 1988). During the spread of virus through the CNS, virus moves centrifugally into the peripheral nerves, viral antigens appearing in nerve endings in salivary glands, skin, mucosal surfaces, gut and most other organs. Thus saliva may be infective for a few days before clinical signs appear.

As in other species, infection of the salivary glands is important in the spread of the disease: at least 70% of rabid cats have virus in their saliva and are able to transmit infection (Vaughn *et al.*, 1963; Chantal & Blancou, 1985; Blancou & Pastoret, 1990).

Gross pathological findings are minimal in rabies. The carcase may be emaciated and there may be evidence of self-trauma. Although in dogs there may be foreign bodies in the alimentary tract as a result of pica, this is less common in cats. Histologically, there is a diffuse encephalitis with mononuclear cell perivascular cuffing and focal gliosis, constituting an inflammatory response typical of any non-suppurative infection of the brain (Jubb & Kennedy, 1985). Spongiform lesions in the brains of rabid animals have also been reported (Charlton, 1988).

There may also be a ganglioneuritis in the paravertebral ganglia and degenerative changes in the salivary gland. Neuronal degeneration in rabies is usually relatively severe compared to some other viral infections of the CNS, and in carnivores particularly it is often quite extensive. In addition, the neurons may contain characteristic intracytoplasmic inclusions containing viral antigen, called Negri bodies. These can occur in several areas of the brain but are usually most prominent in the hippocampus: they are pathognomonic for rabies in most species (Atanasiu, 1975). In cats, however, some confusion may arise, in that even in normal cats, inclusions which resemble Negri bodies may be found in the cytoplasm of some nerve cells (Szlachta & Habel, 1953).

Although Negri bodies are found in the majority of cases of rabies (McQueen, 1960; Tustin & Smit, 1962) and have in the past been used extensively in diagnosis, their absence does not exclude the disease. In addition, when identification of Negri bodies was used as the predominant method of rabies diagnosis, it was usually considered necessary to keep the animal alive until it died naturally, to increase the sensitivity of the test (Tierkel, 1959). The technique has therefore now been superseded in most countries by more reliable techniques in terms of specificity, sensitivity and speed of diagnosis (see below).

As already mentioned, the susceptibility of animals to rabies virus varies a great deal, depending on the animal species, the virus dose and the virus strain (biotype). For example, foxes are highly susceptible to their own virus, but humans seem to be fairly resistant to this biotype. In general, cats are probably of intermediate susceptibility (Jaeger & Barth, 1979; Soulebot *et al.*, 1981). Cats appear to be more susceptible than dogs to certain vaccine strains of virus (Dean & Guevin, 1963; Vaughn, 1975; Pastoret *et al.*, 1985). Other factors significant in determining an individual's susceptibility to the disease include the age of the animal, and the nature and site of the wound. Thus, a young cat suffering a deep wound in the head region, heavily contaminated with saliva, is more likely to develop the disease, with a shorter incubation period, than an older animal with a superficial wound on the extremities. In mice, resistance to rabies virus infection has been shown to be under genetic control (Lodmell, 1988). This resistance is a dominant trait, controlled by one or two genes and not linked to the H-2 locus. The mechanisms involved in genetic variability have not been elucidated.

Experimentally in cats the incubation period has been shown to range from 9 to 51 days (median 18 days), while the periods of clinical illness until death ranged from 1 to 8 days (median 5 days) (Vaughn *et al.*, 1963). Virus was first detected in the saliva of these cats, by conventional virological techniques, one day before the appearance of clinical signs, and virus shedding usually then continued until the cat died. Under natural conditions, the incubation period is generally similar, though in occasional cases it may be much longer, probably up to 6 months or more. In dogs, for example, cases have occasionally been recorded beyond this time (Waterhouse, 1971).

CLINICAL SIGNS

The clinical course of rabies is classically described as three, often overlapping, phases: the prodromal period, the excitative phase ('furious' rabies; Fig. 19.1), and the paralytic stage ('dumb' rabies; Fig. 19.2). In cats, the prodromal phase

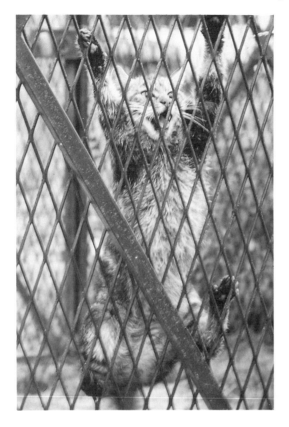

Fig. 19.1 Furious form of rabies in a cat.
(Acknowledgement: CNEVA-EID, Nancy, France.)

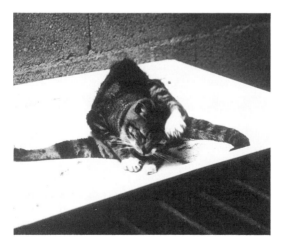

Fig. 19.2 Paralytic form of rabies in a cat.
(Acknowledgement: CNEVA-EID, Nancy, France.)

usually lasts 1 day only and is manifested by a marked change in behaviour (Vaughn, 1975). Sullen cats may become more alert, restless and friendly, whereas amicable cats may scratch or bite without provocation, or become depressed and withdrawn, hiding in dark places. Aggression is more commonly observed in the cat than the dog (Tierkel, 1959). During this initial period, there may be slight pyrexia, and some dilatation of the pupils with an impaired corneal reflex.

Gradually, the excitement phase predominates, and it is in this form that rabies is most easily recognized, and the animals are at their most hazardous to others. The cat becomes increasingly nervous, irritable and vicious, and may show muscle tremors, flaccidity or incoordination. As in humans, there is difficulty in swallowing due to spasm, and eventual paralysis of the muscles of deglutition. This in turn leads to the accumulation of saliva, and drooling or frothing. As the cat enters the paralytic stage, muscular incoordination and convulsions gradually lead to generalized paralysis, coma and death. The excitement phase may last up to 7 days, but sometimes it is virtually non-existent and cats progress directly from the prodromal phase to the paralytic stage.

Although in classical rabies there is undelayed progression of the characteristic clinical signs, through to death, in some cases infection may lead to a more variable outcome. Thus in dogs in Ethiopia, a carrier state has been reported, which may or may not be associated with a period of clinical signs (Andral & Serie, 1965; Fekadu, 1975; Carey & McLean, 1983; Charlton, 1988). Chronic recrudescent rabies has also been observed experimentally in a cat (Perl *et al.*, 1977).

Recovery from CNS infection in both animals and humans has also been reported, albeit rarely (Bell, 1975; Fekadu *et al.*, 1981; Charlton, 1988). A serological survey in South America has shown that 1% of the cats included in the study had antirabies neutralizing antibodies (Diaz *et al.*, 1975). However, this may have been only as a result of peripheral infection, and its significance is not clear.

IMMUNITY

Since most animals die from rabies, and no serological response can be detected before the onset of clinical signs, most information on protective immune mechanisms in rabies has been obtained from vaccination studies. There is a good correlation between antibody titres obtained after vaccination and protection (Blancou *et al.*, 1986) and protection against rabies can be obtained through passive transfer of specific antibodies. However, vaccinated animals without detectable neutralizing antibodies can still resist challenge, and undoubtedly other immunological mechanisms are involved in protection. Although the importance of cell-mediated immunity has not been fully evaluated, in humans it has been suggested that the protective mechanisms following post-exposure treatment with rabies vaccine involve T-cells and interferon induction (Macfarlan, 1988).

DIAGNOSIS AND ACTION IN SUSPECT CASES

In Britain, where rabies is not endemic, most veterinary surgeons are inexperienced in dealing with the disease. Nevertheless, because of the public health risk, and the great danger that the disease may become established in the wildlife of the country, a diagnosis of rabies should always be considered when certain clinical signs are present. The furious form of rabies, where the cat shows unprovoked aggression, is probably most easily recognizable but should be distinguished from pseudorabies (Aujeszky's disease – see Chapter 20). However, it is when an incoordinate, paralytic or moribund animal is presented that there may be most difficulty. The differential diagnosis includes toxoplasmosis, CNS infection, neoplasia or trauma, thiamin deficiency, oral and pharyngeal foreign bodies, and poisoning with substances such as lead, organochlorine compounds, benzoic acid and strychnine. The very rare syndrome of spongiform encephalopathy should also be considered (Wyatt *et al.*, 1990). The severe weakness seen in animals moribund from infectious diseases such as panleucopenia and feline leukaemia virus infection may also on occasion simulate paralytic or terminal rabies.

A detailed account of the action to be taken in Britain in a case of suspected rabies has been given by members of the State Veterinary Service (Anon, 1976a,b, 1982). Briefly, a suspect case should be detained in isolation of the premises on which it has been examined and the local divisional veterinary officer of the Ministry of Agriculture must be notified immediately. The veterinary surgeon and any other handler should carry out a thorough personal disinfection in soap or detergent and water and any contaminated clothing should be changed. If anyone is bitten or scratched, it is imperative to wash and flush the wound immediately with soap or detergent (not both, as soap inhibits quaternary ammonium compounds) and water, then water alone, followed by the application of 40–70% alcohol, tincture or aqueous solutions of iodine, or 0.1% quaternary ammonium compounds (e.g. cetrimide B.P.). No further animals should enter the consulting room until the case is diagnosed as negative, or the premises satisfactorily cleansed and disinfected under the supervision of the Ministry veterinary officer. The names and addresses of any contacts (e.g. those in the waiting room) should be recorded. The veterinary officer will inform the medical officer for environmental health of any necessary further action.

If the animal dies or is killed, the head and neck should be removed by an MAFF veterinary officer and transported fresh and intact to an appropriate diagnostic laboratory (in the UK, the Central Veterinary Laboratory, Weybridge). It should be packed in a sealed container, held at a low temperature, but not frozen.

A combination of several laboratory techniques is generally used to diagnose rabies.
1 Fluorescent antibody test on brain smears to demonstrate viral antigen. Results within 2–3 hours, high degree of accuracy – correlates well with mouse inoculation.
2 Histological examination of brain material, usually from the hippocampus, for the specific Negri body inclusions. Results within 2 days, but

only 40–50% accuracy, especially if the animal is killed (Kissling, 1975). Formalin-fixed brain tissue may also be examined by the fluorescent antibody test, if the tissues are trypsin treated (Webster & Casey, 1988). Immunochemical techniques have also been developed.

3 Mouse inoculation. Mice are inoculated intracerebrally with a suspension of brain tissue, and observed for up to 28 days for mortality: if sufficient mice are inoculated the observation time may be reduced by sacrificing mice at intervals and examining their brains by the fluorescent antibody test (Koprowski, 1973; Webster & Casey, 1988).

4 Cell culture isolation – recently it has been found that some cell cultures (such as BHK-21 cells and a murine neuroblastoma (NA) cell line) appear to be equally if not more sensitive than mouse inoculation for isolation of virus, and this has replaced the mouse inoculation test in several laboratories (Crick & King, 1988; Webster & Casey, 1988).

5 Panels of monoclonal antibodies may be used in fluorescent antibody tests on brain smears or infected cell cultures, in order to determine the origin of the rabies virus, e.g. vaccine or field virus (Esh *et al.*, 1982; Bellinger *et al.*, 1983; Whetstone *et al.*, 1984); or rabies or rabies-related virus (Webster & Casey, 1988); or for epidemiological typing, e.g. skunk versus fox rabies (Smith & Baer, 1988).

6 More recently detection of rabies virus nucleic acid after gene amplification has been described (Bourhy & Sureau, 1990).

EPIDEMIOLOGY

Although virtually every mammal is susceptible to rabies, the natural disease occurs predominantly in carnivores. Thus, in Europe, the red fox is the most important species affected, whereas in Asia it is the domestic dog (Blancou, 1988). In the USA and Canada, rabies is enzootic in several species of animals, such as skunks, foxes and racoons (Smith & Baer, 1988). Monoclonal antibody studies have shown that although each strain of rabies virus has the potential to infect many species, in different geographical areas usually only one or two vectors predominate.

In many parts of the world, including Europe and the Americas, bats also harbour rabies. However, bat rabies exists largely as an independent cycle, and is not generally linked to terrestrial rabies although spill-over can and does occur (Smith & Baer, 1988). In contrast, in Latin America, vampire bats are a frequent source of infection for cattle, although the dog is the major vector for humans. In Latin America, therefore, sylvatic rabies (i.e. in wildlife) and urban rabies (i.e. in dogs) coexist. Sylvatic and urban rabies also coexist in parts of Eastern Europe, Africa, and Asia, but here a number of wildlife species, including wolves, jackals and mongooses, also act as reservoir hosts – animals which fill the same ecological niche as foxes in other countries (Winkler, 1975; Pastoret *et al.*, 1988b).

Fox rabies in Europe

In continental Europe, epizootics of fox rabies have occurred several times in the past, but the disease then appeared to terminate without specific control measures around the end of the 19th century (Winkler, 1975; Blancou, 1988). In 1939, however, a new, stable, epizootic began, numerous cases of rabies being reported in foxes and badgers in Poland and since then it has become an increasing and important problem (Pastoret *et al.*, 1989).

The present European epizootic of rabies has spread some 1400 kilometres westward from Poland since 1939. For several years the front of the epizootic advanced 20–60 kilometres per year (Toma & Andral, 1977; Macdonald, 1988) (Fig. 19.3). This epizootic is sylvatic: the reservoir of infection is in wildlife. While it involves all susceptible species, both wild and domestic, the red fox (*Vulpes vulpes*) is involved in more than 75% of cases. The red fox is both the vector of the disease and its reservoir. It plays a key role in the maintenance of the disease but usually it does not transmit it directly to man. Man is mainly at risk from affected domestic animals such as cattle and

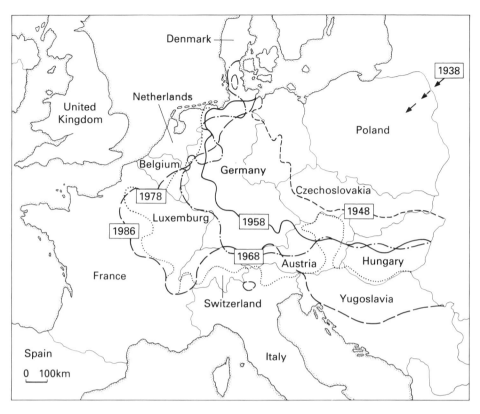

Fig. 19.3 Progress of fox rabies through Europe from 1938 to 1986. (Acknowledgement: CNEVA-EID, Nancy, France.)

cats, although human deaths in Europe from rabies are now very rare (Blancou, 1988).

The percentage of rabid foxes is almost certainly underestimated for several reasons (Braunschweig, 1982). For example, the occurrence of the disease in cubs in the den is always neglected but may, in fact, be relatively frequent (Thiriart *et al.*, 1985). The fox seems to be the only species to play a role in the maintenance of the present epizootic; it has been shown that where rabies has been eliminated from the fox population in certain areas of Europe, the disease then disappears from all other species (except bats) (Wandeler, 1988).

The prevailing hypothesis is that the virus originated in dogs and became adapted, by successive passages, for foxes (Winkler, 1975). This virus is classified as lyssavirus serotype 1. The virus is highly pathogenic for the fox: a dose of 0.3 mouse

intracerebral LD-50 is sufficient to kill one fox out of every two, whereas domestic carnivores require a dose 100 000 times greater to produce the same effect (Blancou, 1985). When the disease front penetrates a new area the foxes within the area suffer an epizootic of rabies. When the fox population is heavily decimated, the incidence of the disease decreases and remains low for a 'silent' period of some 2–3 years. After the initial epizootic, secondary enzootic outbreaks recur, often at intervals of 3–5 years (Aguilar-Setién *et al.*, 1985; Macdonald & Voigt, 1985).

Superimposed upon the annual variation in the incidence of reported cases of vulpine rabies is a seasonal pattern. Cases tend to peak in late winter and reach a trough in mid-summer. The late-winter/early-spring peak of rabies seems to be linked to the mating season of foxes. In recent years the advance of the rabies epizootic seemed to have stopped, but has now started again. This is exemplified by the situation in France (Blancou *et al.*, 1988a).

In Europe, the fox is the animal which is most susceptible to rabies. The proportion of rabid foxes that excrete the virus is very high: 93–100% of rabid foxes harbour the virus in the salivary glands and excrete it in large quantities in saliva. Furthermore, virus may be excreted for 5 days or more before the onset of the disease (Blancou *et al.*, 1979a,b; Aubert *et al.*, 1991). The incubation period of the disease in foxes depends mainly on the dose of virus with which the animal has been infected and varies from 10 to 41 days. The clinical disease lasts 3–5 days. The symptoms are variable (George *et al.*, 1980). The furious form is relatively rare; instead, most animals become apathetic and develop paralysis (Steck & Wandeler, 1980).

Rabies virus is transmitted by biting. Since the dumb or apathetic form of the disease predominates in the fox, rabid foxes usually do not wander far from their original territory (Artois & Aubert, 1985). This may explain why the front of a fox rabies epizootic progresses slowly.

In continental Europe, rabies in domestic animals tends to follow the pattern of disease seen in wildlife (Blancou & Barrat, 1988). Thus when the incidence of rabies increases in foxes, it also increases in domestic species such as cattle, sheep, cats and dogs. Human exposure occurs through contact with infected domestic species. Cats become infected relatively often, possibly because they tend to have regular contact with wildlife and vaccines are used less frequently in this species (Wachendörfer, 1962; Diesch *et al.*, 1982). There is no evidence, however, that rabies persists among cats in areas where canine (urban) and wildlife (sylvatic) rabies have been eliminated.

In other areas of the world where urban rabies occurs, stray dogs are common and these animals are one of the reservoirs of infection. Human exposure tends to reflect human–animal contact and the control of the disease in the dog population by vaccination leads to a marked drop in human exposure rates (Larghi *et al.*, 1988).

PREVENTION AND CONTROL

Introduction

There are two aspects to be considered with respect to rabies vaccination, i.e. preventive vaccination and post-exposure treatment. The first human vaccination by Louis Pasteur in 1885 was for post-exposure treatment. Nowadays human post-exposure treatment requires several vaccinations, together with an injection of specific immunoglobulin if the exposure was severe. Veterinarians and others exposed to an increased risk of infection should be protected by preventive vaccination. In animals only preventive vaccination is generally carried out. In some countries, post-exposure vaccination of domestic animals may be allowed but only if the animal has previously been vaccinated.

Whether current vaccines based on serotype 1 (classical rabies virus) confer adequate protection against the rabies-related viruses is still not clear; some studies have demonstrated adequate protection whereas others have not, and it has been suggested there may be a case for producing polyvalent vaccines in some parts of the world (King & Crick, 1988).

Conventional vaccines for human use

Only inactivated vaccines have been licensed for human use. Inactivated vaccines prepared in the nervous systems of adult animals have been used for protection against rabies. However, their use can lead to problems because of post-vaccinal nervous system reactions. Such reactions are due to the myelin content of nervous tissues; foreign myelin may be responsible for the induction of hypersensitivity reactions in the recipient, leading to paralysis. Because myelination is delayed in neonatal mice, the use of suckling mouse brain reduces this risk, but some reactions may still occur and thus such vaccines are best avoided.

Since rabies virus can nowadays be grown in cell culture, most current vaccines are derived from cell cultures and are perfectly safe. They can be used both for preventive vaccination or for post-exposure treatment in conjunction with specific immunoglobulin therapy. In some parts of the world, however, cost precludes the use of such improved vaccines. New cell culture vaccines (Vero cells) or new vaccination procedures (intradermal) may reduce the cost. Vectored vaccines (canaripox) are presently being developed for human use (Pastoret *et al.*, 1991).

Vaccines for domestic animals

Attenuated virus vaccines have been widely used in the past for immunization of domestic animals. However, all of them still had some residual pathogenicity for some species, and cases of vaccine-induced rabies occasionally occurred, often in cats (Dean & Guevin, 1963; Esh *et al.*, 1982; Bellinger *et al.*, 1983; Whetstone *et al.*, 1984; Pastoret *et al.*, 1985). The use of monoclonal antibodies has made it much easier to distinguish such cases from infection with wild-type virus. Humans exposed to attenuated vaccine strain for veterinary use are treated in the same way as after wild-type virus exposure.

In the last few years, safe and potent inactivated vaccines have been developed for veterinary use, and these have now largely superseded attenuated vaccines. Rabies virus strains have been adapted to cell cultures so that large amounts of virus can be produced without the hazards associated with vaccines prepared in nervous tissue, and newer adjuvants have increased the immunogenicity of such vaccines. More recently, a recombinant vaccinia-rabies glycoprotein vaccine has been developed, and it has been shown to be both safe and efficacious for the cat (Kieny *et al.*, 1984; Blancou *et al.*, 1989).

Control measures for rabies in Britain

The presence of rabies in continental Europe poses a considerable threat to Britain (Wright, 1977). At present, control measures for rabies in Britain rely on a rigorously enforced 6-month quarantine period for all mammals, except farmstock and some other herbivores which are subject to other controls (Anon, 1976b). All quarantine kennels are under veterinary supervision and regularly inspected by Ministry veterinary officers.

The 1971 Committee of Inquiry on Rabies (Waterhouse, 1971) (initiated after two cases of the disease occurred in dogs which had passed through the specified 6-month period) made a number of recommendations that were then implemented concerning quarantine kennels. Basically, these were designed to prevent the possible spread of infection within kennels, for the inquiry had concluded that although nonbite transmission in the dog had not previously been recorded, they could not exclude the possibility that in one of these cases it might have occurred. In addition, all animals entering quarantine are required to be vaccinated, with an approved vaccine. Vaccination of other animals, other than in quarantine or for export, is not allowed in Britain at present.

At the time of writing (1993), EC regulations with respect to rabies and the importation of dogs and cats are under review, and from July 1994, under certain conditions, commercially traded animals will be able to move more freely between member states and the UK.

Control measures in countries where rabies is endemic

In countries where rabies is endemic, apart from measures aimed at wildlife control, the incidence of the disease in cats and dogs may be reduced by the elimination of stray animals, by licensing, by restricting movement and by vaccination. A number of vaccines are available for use in dogs and cats (e.g. for the USA, see vaccines listed under the Compendium of Animal Rabies Control, 1990). Since the use of any live vaccine carries an inherent risk and since potent inactivated vaccines are now available, the latter are now generally preferred.

In cats and dogs, primary vaccination is generally not recommended before 3 months of age, followed by a booster 1 year later; thereafter annual or triennial boosters are recommended, depending on the vaccine. At least 1 month should be allowed for the development of immunity. It should be remembered, however, that although

available vaccines do confer reasonable protection, fully vaccinated cats may in some cases still
develop rabies.

Veterinarians and others exposed to an increased risk of infection should also be protected
by prophylactic vaccination. Vaccination of
animals, other than in quarantine or for export, is
not allowed in the UK.

Control of rabies in wildlife

Fox rabies is still present in most of continental
Western Europe (Blancou et al., 1988a) despite
the prophylactic measures taken in the past (Taylor, 1976; Bögel et al., 1981). The destruction
of foxes has not prevented the spread of the
epizootic, for although such measures may be
temporarily effective the fox population rapidly
recovers and rabies then recurs.

In Western Europe, rabies is considered a significant source of economic loss and, above all,
hampers the movement of animals between the
different member states of the European Community. This has serious implications for the 'open
market' since some member states (e.g. Great
Britain, Ireland and Spain) are currently rabies-
free and wish to maintain their disease-free status.
Therefore, the control of rabies requires a common strategy established by the European
Community.

During recent years, most of the research on
the control of fox rabies has concentrated on the
development of methods of vaccination of the fox
by the oral route (Mayr et al., 1972; Baer, 1975b;
Steck et al., 1982a,b) After an initial trial,
this method has now been used extensively in
some European countries (Kappeler et al., 1988;
Schneider & Cox, 1988; Brochier et al., 1988c)
under the control of the World Health Organ-
ization (Blancou et al., 1988b).

One of the vaccines used (SADB19 attenuated
strain of rabies virus) consists of 1.8 ml of virus
suspension in a hermetically sealed capsule contained in a bait (Schneider & Cox, 1988). Initially
chicken head baits were used, but baits now
consist of a machine-made mixture of fat, bone
and fish meal. When a fox chews the bait, the
vaccine capsule bursts and the virus suspension

spreads over the oral mucosa. Each bait contains
150 mg of tetracycline which is used as a marker
of bait uptake.

Attempts to control rabies by vaccinating wild
carnivores seem very promising, and many areas
of Europe are now free from rabies as a result
of this (Wandeler, 1988). However, the use of
attenuated rabies virus remains controversial as
far as safety and stability are concerned (Leblois
& Flamand, 1988) since these vaccine strains are
pathogenic for some non-target species, such as
rodents. There is no evidence, though, that they
can become established in the small mammals in
the wild (Wandeler, 1988).

In order to improve both the safety and the
stability of the vaccine, a recombinant vaccinia
virus (VVTGgRAB 187 XP-26D3 strain) expressing the immunizing glycoprotein of rabies virus
has been developed (Kieny et al., 1984; Wiktor et
al., 1984). The potential of this VVTGgRAB
strain to protect foxes against rabies has been
demonstrated (Blancou et al., 1986; Brochier et
al., 1988a).

The safety of this recombinant virus for non-
target species has been tested in many laboratory
animals, domestic animals and wild animals. In
addition, horizontal transmission of the recombinant virus did not occur in foxes, badgers, wild
boars, cattle, dogs and ferrets (Brochier et al.,
1988b, 1989b). However, the long-term interaction of this recombinant virus with naturally
occurring orthopoxviruses in the field should be
investigated. The site as well as the degree of
multiplication of the recombinant virus in the
fox was also studied: the virus multiplied for a
short time only in the same organs as the vector
vaccinia strain without any modification of its
tissue specificity (Thomas et al., 1990). Under
experimental conditions, vaccination of rabid
foxes during the incubation period with the recombinant virus did not produce asymptomatic
carriers of the virus (Brochier et al., 1989a).

An initial, restricted trial was carried out with
this recombinant vaccine in foxes in October 1987
in Belgium (Pastoret et al., 1988a). Larger trials
were then carried out in 1988, 1989 and 1990, and
the vaccine is currently used in all rabies-infected
areas of Belgium (Newmark, 1988; Brochier et

al., 1990, 1991). The recombinant vaccinia-rabies glycoprotein vaccine has also been shown to be efficacious and safe for the oral immunization of the main vectors in North America (Rupprecht *et al.*, 1986; Tolson *et al.*, 1987). Because of its high thermostability it should also be tested for the control of wildlife rabies in Africa.

ACKNOWLEDGEMENTS

The authors are most grateful to A. King, J.W. Wilesmith and P. Thomas, (MAFF) for their help in the preparation of the manuscript. We also want to thank Jean Blancou for the figures and his help and Marinette Muys for her skilful secretarial work.

REFERENCES

Afshar A. (1979) A review of non-bite transmission of rabies virus infection. *Brit. Vet. J.* **135**, 142.

Aguilar-Setien A., Thomas I., Brochier B., Thiriart C., Schwers A. & Pastoret P.P. (1985) La rage vulpine. *Cahiers d'Ethologie Appliquée* **5**, 51–70.

Andral L. & Serie C. (1965) Etudes experimentales sur la rage en Ethiopie. *Ann. Inst. Pasteur* **108**, 442–50.

Anon (1976a) Action in a case of suspected rabies: notes for guidance. *Vet. Rec.* **99**, 168.

Anon (1976b) Dealing with the rabies risk: official policy. *Vet. Rec.* **99**, 169–72.

Anon (1982) *Rabies Guidance Notes for Practising Veterinary Surgeons*. Ministry of Agriculture, Fisheries & Food, UK.

Artois M. & Aubert M.F.A. (1985) Behaviour of rabid foxes. In Artois M., Blancou J. & Kempf C. (eds) *Ecology and Epidemiology of Wild and Feral Canids in the Pal<u>e</u>artic Zone*. Revue d'Ecologie (La Terre et la Vie) vol. 40, pp. 171–6.

Atanasiu P. (1975) Animal inoculation and the Negri body. In Baer G.M. (ed) *The Natural History of Rabies*, vol. I. Academic Press, New York, pp. 374–400.

Aubert M.F.A., Blancou J., Barrat J., Artois M. & Barrat M.J. (1991) Transmission et pathagénic de la renard roux de deux isolats á dix ans d'intervalle du virus de la rage vulpine. *Ann. Rech. Vet.* **22**, 77–93.

Baer G.M. (1975a) Pathogenesis to the central nervous system. In Baer G.M. (ed) *The Natural History of Rabies*, vol. I. Academic Press, New York, pp. 181–98.

Baer G.M. (1975b) Wildlife vaccination. In Baer G.M. (ed) *The Natural History of Rabies*, vol. II. Academic Press, New York, pp. 261–6.

Bell J.F. (1975) Latency and abortive rabies. In Baer G.M. (ed) *The Natural History of Rabies*, vol. II. Academic Press, New York, pp. 331–55.

Bell J.F. & Moore G.J. (1971) Susceptibility of carnivora to rabies virus administered orally. *Am. J. Epidem.* **93**, 176.

Bellinger D.A., Chang J., Bunn T.O., Dick J.R., Murphy M. & Rahija R. (1983) Rabies induced in cats by high-egg-passage Flury strain vaccine. *J. Am. Vet. Med. Ass.* **183**, 997–8.

Blancou J. (1985) La rage du renard. *Ann. Med. Vet.* **129**, 293–307.

Blancou J. (1988) Epizootiology of rabies: Eurasia and Africa. In Campbell J.B. & Charlton K.M. (eds) *Rabies, Developments in Veterinary Virology*. Kluwer Academic Publishers.

Blancou J. & Barrat J. (1988) Rôle épidémiologique des diverses espèces animales dans la contamination rabique de l'homme en Europe. *Bull. Acad. Vét. de France* **61**, 497–512.

Blancou J. & Pastoret P.P. (1990) La rage du chat et sa prophylaxie. *Ann. Méd. Vét.* **134**, 315–24.

Blancou J., Aubert M.F.A., Andral L. & Artois M. (1979a) Rage expérimentale du renard roux (*Vulpes vulpes*). I. Sensibilité selon la voie d'infection et la dose infectante. *Revue de Médecine Vétérinaire* **130**, 1001–15.

Blancou J., Andral L., Samudio & Silva-Crispin L.S. (1979b) Rage expérimentale du renard roux (*Vulpes vulpes*). II. Excrétion du virus rabique après infection. *Revue de Médecine Vétérinaire* **130**, 1473–82.

Blancou J., Aubert M.F.A. & Soulebot J.P. (1983) Differences dans le pouvoir pathogenes des souches de virus rabique adaptées au renard ou au chien. *Ann. Virol.* [Inst. Pasteur] **134E**, 523–31.

Blancou J., Artois M., Barrat J. & Prave M. (1986a) Vaccination du chat contre la rage; taux d'anticorps et resistance a l'epreuve un an apres la vaccination. *Revue de Médicine Vétérinaire* **137**, 29–36.

Blancou J., Kieny M.P., Lathe R., Lecocq J.P., Pastoret P.P., Soulebot J.P. & Desmettre P. (1986b) Oral vaccination of the fox against rabies using a live recombinant vaccinia virus. *Nature* **322**, 373–5.

Blancou J., Aubert M.F.A. & Artois M. (1988a) La rage sylvatique en Europe. In Pastoret P.P., Brochier B., Thomas I. & Blancou J. (eds) *Vaccination to control rabies in foxes. La vaccination antirabique du renard.* Commission of the European Communities, EUR 11439 EN-FR, pp. 14–21.

Blancou J., Pastoret P.P., Brochier B., Thomas I. & Bögel K. (1988b) Vaccinating wild animals against rabies. *Rev. Sci. tech. Off. int. Epiz.* **7**, 1005–13.

Blancou J., Artois M., Brochier B., Thomas I., Pastoret P.P., Desmettre P., Languet B. & Kieny M.P. (1989) Innocuité et efficacité d'un vaccin antirabique recombinant des virus de la vaccine et de la rage administré par voie orale au renard, au chien et au chat. *Ann. Rech. Vét.* **20**, 195–204.

Bögel K., Moegle H., Steck F., Krocza W. & Andral L. (1981) Assessment of control in areas of wildlife rabies. *Bulletin of the World Health Organization* **59**, 269–79.

Bourhy H., Kissi B. & Tordo N. (1993) Molecular diversity of the *Lyssavirus* genus. *Virology*, **194**, 70–81.

Bourhy H. & Sureau P. (1990) *Laboratory Methods for Rabies Diagnosis*. Institut Pasteur, Paris.

Braunschweig A. (1982) Ein modell für die Fuchspopulationsdynamik in der Bundesrepublik Deutschland. In *The Red Fox: Behaviour and Ecology*. Zimen Junk, The Hague, pp. 97–106.

Brochier B., Languet B., Blancou J., Kieny M.P., Lecocq J.P., Costy F., Desmettre P. & Pastoret P.P. (1988a) Use of recombinant vaccinia-rabies virus for oral vaccination of fox cubs (*Vulpes vulpes*) against rabies. *Vet. Microbiol.* **18**, 103–8.

Brochier B., Languet B., Blancou J., Thomas I., Kieny M.P., Lecocq J.P., Desmettre P. & Pastoret P.P. (1988b) Innocuité du virus recombinant vaccine-rage chez quelques espèces non-cibles. In Pastoret P.P., Brochier B., Thomas I. & Blancou J. (eds) *Vaccination to Control Rabies in Foxes. La vaccination antirabique du renard*. Commission of the European Communities, EUR 11439 EN-FR, pp. 118–23.

Brochier B., Thomas I., Iokem A., Ginter A., Kalpers J., Paquot A., Costy F. & Pastoret P.P. (1988c) A field trial in Belgium to control fox rabies by oral immunization. *Vet. Rec.* **123**, 618–21.

Brochier B., Blancou J., Aubert M.F.A., Kieny M.P., Desmettre P. & Pastoret P.P. (1989a) Interaction between rabies infection and oral administration of vaccinia-rabies recombinant virus to foxes (*Vulpes vulpes*). *J. Gen. Virol.* **70**, 1601–4.

Brochier B., Blancou J., Thomas I., Languet B., Artois M., Kieny M.P., Lecocq J.P., Costy F., Desmettre P. & Pastoret P.P. (1989b) Use of recombinant vaccinia-rabies glycoprotein virus for oral vaccination of wildlife against rabies: innocuity to several non-target bait consuming species. *J. Wildl. Dis.* **25**, 540–7.

Brochier B., Thomas I., Bauduin B., Leveau T., Pastoret P.P., Languet B., Chappuis G., Desmettre P., Blancou J. & Artois M. (1990) Use of a vaccinia-rabies recombinant virus for the oral vaccination of foxes against rabies. *Vaccine* **8**, 101–4.

Brochier B., Kieny M.P., Costy F., Coppens P., Bauduin B., Lecocq J.P., Languet B., Chappuis G., Desmettre P., Afiademanyo K., Libois R. & Pastoret P.P. (1991) Large scale eradication of rabies using recombinant vaccinia-rabies vaccine. *Nature* **354**, 520–2.

Carey A.B. & McLean R.G. (1983) The ecology of rabies: evidence of co-adaptation. *J. Appl. Ecol.* **20**, 777–800.

Chantal J. & Blancou J. (1985) Le virus rabique. In *Pasteur et la Rage*. Inf. Tech. Serv. Vét., No. 92–95, pp. 281–92.

Charlton K.M. (1988) The pathogenesis of rabies. In Campbell J.B. & Charlton K.M. (eds) *Rabies, Developments in Veterinary Virology*. Kluwer Academic Publishers, Boston, pp. 101–50.

Compendium of Animal Rabies Control (1990) *J. Am. Vet. Med. Ass.* **196**, 36.

Constantine D.G. (1962) Rabies transmission by non-bite route. *Publ. Hlth. Report. Wash.* **77**, 287.

Crick J. & King A. (1988) Culture of rabies virus *in vitro*. In Campbell J.B. & Charlton K.M. (eds) *Rabies, Developments in Veterinary Virology*. Kluwer Academic Publishers, Boston, pp. 47–66.

Dean D.J. (1975) Local wound treatment. In Baer G.M. (ed) *The Natural History of Rabies*, vol. II. Academic Press, New York, pp. 305–17.

Dean D.J. & Guevin V.H. (1963) Rabies vaccination of cats. *J. Am. Vet. Med. Ass.* **142**, 367.

Diaz A.M.O. de, Fuenzalida E. & Bell J.F. (1975) Non-fatal rabies in dogs and cats. *Ann. Microbiol.* [Inst. Pasteur] **126B**, 503–9.

Diesch S.L., Hendrickx S.L. & Currier R.W. (1982) The role of cats in human rabies exposures. *J. Am. Vet. Med. Ass.* **181**, 1510.

Esh J.B., Cunningham J.G. & Wiktor T.J. (1982) Vaccine-induced rabies in four cats. *J. Am. Vet. Med. Ass.* **180**, 1336.

Fekadu M. (1975) Asymptomatic non-fatal canine rabies. *Lancet* i, 569.

Fekadu M., Shaddock J.H. & Baer G.M. (1981) Intermittent excretion of rabies virus in the saliva of a dog two and six months after it had recovered from experimental rabies. *Am. J. Trop. Med. Hyg.* **30**, 1113.

Foggin C.M. (1982) Atypical rabies in cats and a dog in Zimbabwe. *Vet. Rec.* **110**, 338.

George J.P., George J., Blancou J. & Aubert M.F.A. (1980) Description clinique de la rage du renard. Etude expérimentale. *Revue de Médecine Vétérinaire* **131**, 153–60.

Jaeger D. & Barth R. (1979) Experimental infection of cats with rabies street virus strain NYC. *Berliner und Münchener Tierärzliche Wochenschrift* **92**, 27.

Jubb K.V.F., Kennedy P.C. & Palmer N. (1985) Viral infections of the nervous system. In *Pathology of Domestic Animals*, 3rd edn. vol. 1. Academic Press, Orlando, pp. 293–96.

Kappeler A., Wandeler A.I. & Capt S. (1988) Ten years of rabies control by oral vaccination of foxes in Switzerland. In Pastoret P.P., Brochier B., Thomas I. & Blancou J. (eds) *Vaccination to Control Rabies in Foxes. La vaccination antirabique du renard*. Commission of the European Communities, EUR 11439 EN-FR, pp. 55–60.

Kieny M.P., Lathe R., Drillien R., Spehner D., Skory S., Schmitt D., Wiktor T., Koprowski H. & Lecocq J.P. (1984) Expression of rabies virus glycoprotein from a recombinant vaccinia virus. *Nature* **312**, 163–6.

King A. & Crick J. (1988) Rabies-related viruses. In Campbell J.B. & Charlton K.M. (eds) *Rabies, Developments in Veterinary Virology*. Kluwer Academic Publishers, Boston, pp. 177–99.

King A.A., Davies P. & Crick J. (1985) Rabies in a quarantine kennel in the U.K.: the Irish wolfhound from Florida. *State Vet. Journal* **39**, 42–4.

King A., Davies P. & Lawrie A. (1990) The rabies viruses of bats. *Vet. Microbiol.* **23**, 165–74.

Kissling R.E. (1975) The fluorescent antibody test in rabies. In Baer G.M. (ed) *The Natural History of Rabies*, vol. l. Academic Press, New York, pp. 401–16.

Koprowski H. (1973) The mouse inoculation test. In Campbell J.B. & Koprowski H. (eds) *Laboratory Techniques in Rabies*. World Health Organization, Geneva, pp. 85–93.

Larghi O.P., Arrosi J.C., Nakajata-A.J. & Villa-Nova A. (1988) Control of urban rabies. In Campbell J.B. & Charlton K.M. (eds) *Rabies, Developments in Veterinary Virology*. Kluwer Academic Publishers, Boston, pp. 407–22.

Leblois H. & Flamand A. (1988) Studies on pathogenicity in mice of rabies virus strains used for oral vaccination of foxes in Europe. In Pastoret P.P., Brochier B., Thomas I. & Blancou J. (eds) *Vaccination to Control Rabies in foxes. La vaccination antirabique du renard*. Commission of the European Communities, EUR 11439 EN-FR, pp. 101–4.

Lodmell P.L. (1988) Genetic control of resistance to rabies. In Campbell J.B. & Charlton K.M. (eds) *Rabies, Developments in Veterinary Virology*. Kluwer Academic Publishers, Boston, pp. 151–61.

Macdonald D.W. (1988) Rabies and foxes: the social life of a solitary carnivore. In Pastoret P.P., Brochier B., Thomas I. & Blancou J. (eds) *Vaccination to Control Rabies in Foxes. La vaccination antirabique du renard*. Commission of the European Communities, EUR 11439 EN-FR, pp. 5–13.

Macdonald D.W. & Voigt D.R. (1985) The biological basis of rabies models. In *Population Dynamics of Rabies in Wildlife*, pp. 71–108.

Macfarlan R.I. (1988) Immune responses to rabies virus: vaccines and natural infection. In Campbell J.B. & Charlton K.M. (eds) *Rabies, Developments in Veterinary Virology*. Kluwer Academic Publishers, Boston, pp. 163–76.

McQueen J.L. (1960) Rabies diagnosis. Special application of fluorescent antibody techniques. *Proc. 63rd meeting U.S. Livestock Sanit. Ass. San Francisco, 1959*, pp. 356–63.

Mayr A., Kraft H., Jaeger O. & Haacke H. (1972) Orale immunisierung von fuchsen gegen tollwut. *Zentbl. Vet. Med. B* **19**, 615–25.

Morgan-Jones K.R. (1969). The case of rabies in Surrey. *Vet. Rec.* **85**, 476.

Murphy F.A., Bauer S.P., Harrison A.K. & Winn W.C. Jr (1973a) Comparative pathogenesis of rabies and rabies-like viruses. Viral infection and transit from inoculation site to the central nervous system. *Lab. Invest.* **28**, 361.

Murphy F.A., Harrison A.K., Winn W.C. & Bauer S.P. (1973b) Comparative pathogenesis of rabies and rabies-like viruses. Infection of the central nervous system and centrifugal spread of virus to peripheral tissues. *Lab. Invest.* **29**, 1.

Newmark P. (1988) New vaccine and initiative mean end of rabies in sight for Europe? *Nature* **336**, 416.

Parker R.L. & Wilsnack R.E. (1966) Pathogenesis of skunk rabies virus: quantitation in skunks and foxes. *Am. J. Vet. Res.* **27**, 33.

Pastoret P.P. & Brochier B. (1992) Rhabdovirus, infection and immunity. In Roitt I.M. & Delves P.J. (eds) *Encyclopedia of Immunology*. Saunders, Orlando, Florida Academic Press, 1329–32.

Pastoret P.P., Thomas I., Brochier B. & Schwers A. (1985) Les problèmes associés à la vaccination antirabique des animaux domestiques. *Ann. Méd. Vét.* **129**, 361–74.

Pastoret P.P., Brochier B., Languet B., Thomas I., Paquot A., Bauduin B., Kieny M.P., Lecocq J.P., De Bruyn J., Costy F., Antoine H. & Desmettre P. (1988a) First field trial of fox vaccination against rabies using a vaccinia-rabies recombinant virus. *Vet. Rec.* **123**, 481–3.

Pastoret P.P., Thiry E., Brochier B., Schwers A., Thomas I. & Dubuisson J. (1988b) Diseases of wild animals transmissible to domestic animals. *Rev. Sci. tech. Off. int. Epiz.* **7**, 705–36.

Pastoret P.P., Brochier B., Thomas I., Leveau T., Bauduin B. & Costy F. (1989) Fox rabies in Europe. *Ir. Vet. J.* **42**, 93–5.

Pastoret P.P., Brochier B., Chappuis G. & Desmettre P. (1993) Vaccines against rabies virus. In Hoglund S. & Pausley R. (eds) *Progress in Vaccinology, vol. 4. Veterinary Vaccines*. SpringerVerlag, pp. 139–62.

Peace C.K. & Hopes R. (1970) The case of rabies at Newmarket. *Vet. Rec.* **86**, 299.

Perl D.P., Bell J.F., Moore G.J. & Stewart S.J. (1977) Chronic recrudescent rabies in a cat. *Proc. Soc. Exp. Biol. Med.* **155**, 540–8.

Rupprecht C.E., Wiktor T.J., Johnston D.H., Hamir A.N., Dietzschold B., Wunner W.H., Glickman L.T. & Koprowski H. (1986) Oral immunization and protection of raccoons (*Procyon lotor*) with a vaccinia-rabies glycoprotein recombinant virus. *Proc. Natl. Acad. Sci. USA* **83**, 7947–50.

Schneider L.G. (1982) Antigenic variants of rabies virus. *Comp. Immunol. Microbiol. Infect. Dis.* **5**, 101.

Schneider L.G. & Cox J.H. (1988) Eradication of rabies through oral vaccination: the German field trial. In Pastoret P.P., Brochier B., Thomas I. & Blancou J. (eds) *Vaccination to Control Rabies in Foxes. La vaccination antirabique du renard.* Commission of the European Communities, EUR 11439, EN-FR, pp. 22–38.

Sikes R.K. (1962) Pathogenesis of rabies in wildlife 1. Comparative effect of varying doses of rabies virus inoculated into fox and skunks. *Am. J. Vet. Res.* **23**, 1041–7.

Smith J.S. & Baer G.M. (1988) Epizootiology of rabies: The Americas. In Campbell J.B. & Charlton K.M. (eds) *Rabies, Developments in Veterinary Virology.* Kluwer Academic Publishers, Boston, pp. 267–99.

Soave O.A. (1966) Transmission of rabies to mice by ingestion of infected tissue. *Am. J. Vet. Res.* **27**, 44.

Soulebot J.P., Brun A., Chappuis G., Guillemin F., Petermann H.G., Precausta P. & Terre J. (1981) Experimental rabies in cats: immune response and persistence of immunity. *Cornell Vet.* **71**, 311.

Steck F. & Wandeler A.I. (1980) The epidemiology of fox rabies in Europe. *Epidemiologic Reviews* **2**, 71–96.

Steck F., Wandeler A.I., Bichsel P., Capt S. & Schneider L.G. (1982a) Oral immunisation of foxes against rabies. A field study. *Zentralbl. für Veterinärmed.* **29**, 372.

Steck F., Wandeler A.I., Bichsel P., Capt S., Hafliger V. & Schneider L.G. (1982b) Oral immunisation of foxes against rabies: laboratory and field studies. *Comp. Immun. Microbiol. Infect. Dis.* **5**, 165–71.

Steele J.H. (1975) History of rabies. In Baer G.M. (ed) *The Natural History of Rabies*, vol. I. Academic Press, New York, pp. 1–29.

Szlachta H.L. & Habel R.E. (1953) Inclusions resembling Negri bodies in the brains of non-rabid cats. *Cornell Vet.* **43**, 207.

Taylor D. (1976) Rabies: epizootic aspects. *Vet. Rec.* **99**, 157.

Thiriart C., Iokem A., Costy F., Schwers A., Brochier B., De Meurichy A., Peharpe D. & Pastoret P.P. (1985) Immunization of young foxes against rabies: interaction between vaccination and natural infection. *Ann. Vet. Res.* **16**, 289–92.

Thomas I., Brochier B., Languet B., Blancou J., Peharpre D., Kieny M.P., Desmettre P., Chappuis G. & Pastoret P.P. (1990) Primary multiplication site of the vaccinia-rabies glycoprotein recombinant virus administered to foxed by the oral route. *J. Gen. Virol.* **72**, 37–42.

Tierkel E.S. (1959) Rabies. *Adv. Vet. Sci.* **v**, 183.

Tolson N.D., Charlton K.M., Stewart R.B., Campbell J.B. & Wiktor T.J. (1987) Immune response in skunks to a vaccinia virus recombinant expressing the rabies virus glycoprotein. *Can. J. Vet. Res.* **51**, 363–6.

Toma B. & Andral L. (1977) Epidemiology of fox rabies. In Lauffer M.A., Bang F.B., Maramorosch K. & Smith K.M. (eds) *Advances in Virus Research.* vol. 21. Academic Press, New York, pp. 1–36.

Tordo N., Poch O., Ermine A., Keith G. & Rougeon F. (1988) Génétique moléculaire du virus de la rage, un siècle après Pasteur. *Molecular Biology and Infectious Diseases.* Elsevier, Paris, pp. 31–40.

Tustin R.C. & Smit J.D. (1962) Rabies in South Africa. An analysis of histological examinations. *J. S. Afri. Vet. Med. Ass.* **33**, 295.

Vaughn J.B. (1975) Cat Rabies. In Baer G.M. (ed) *The Natural History of Rabies*, vol. II. Academic Press, New York, pp. 139–54.

Vaughn J.B., Gerhardt P. & Paterson J.C.S. (1963) Excretion of street rabies virus in saliva of cats. *J. Am. Med. Ass.* **184**, 705.

Wachendörfer G. (1962) Role of cats in the present rabies epidemic in Germany. *Dtsch. Tierärz. Wschr.* **69**, 555.

Wandeler A.I. (1988) Control of wildlife rabies: Europe. In Campbell J.B. & Charlton K.M. (eds) *Rabies, Developments in Veterinary Virology.* Kluwer Academic Publishers, Boston, pp. 365–80.

Waterhouse R. (Chairman) (1971) *Rabies in Europe with particular reference to Great Britain. Report of the Committee of Inquiry on Rabies. Final Report.* HMSO London, Cmnd. 4696.

Webster W.A. & Casey G.A. (1988) Diagnosis of rabies infection. In Campbell J.B. & Charlton K.M. (eds) *Rabies, Developments in Veterinary Virology.* Kluwer Academic Publishers, Boston, pp. 201–22.

Whetstone C.A., Bunn T.O., Emmons R.W. & Wiktor T.J. (1984) Use of monoclonal antibodies to confirm rabies in ten dogs, two cats, and one fox. *J. Am. Vet. Med. Ass.* **185**, 285–8.

Wiktor T.J., McFarlan R.J., Reagan K.J., Dietzschold B., Curtis P.J., Wunner W.H., Kieny M.P., Lathe R., Lecocq J.P., Mackett M., Moss B. & Koprowski H. (1984) Protection from rabies by a vaccinia virus recombinant containing the rabies virus glycoprotein gene. *Proc. Natl. Acad. Sci. USA* **81**, 7194–8.

Winkler W.G. (1975) Fox rabies. In Baer G.M. (ed) *The Natural History of Rabies*, vol. II. Academic Press, New York, pp. 3–22.

Wright A.I. (1977) Waiting for rabies. In Bodley-Scott R. & Fraser J. (eds) *The Medical Annual.* John Wright & Sons, Bristol, pp. 347–53.

Wunner W.H., Larson J.K., Dietzschold B. & Smith C.L. (1988) The molecular biology of rabies viruses. *Rev. Infect. Dis.* **10**, S771–S784.

Wyatt J.M., Pearson G.R, Smerdon T., Gruffydd-Jones T.J. & Wells G.A.H. (1990) Spongiform encephalopathy in a cat. *Vet. Rec.* **126**, 513.

Chapter 20 / Other Feline Virus Infections

R. M. GASKELL AND M. BENNETT

An undoubtedly incomplete list of reported virus infections of cats is shown in Table 20.1. Most of the more important and better understood viruses have already been discussed, and this chapter aims to discuss briefly a few of the others.

FELINE REOVIRUS

Reoviruses are double-stranded RNA viruses, 75 nm in diameter, and are found in many mammalian and avian species. Mammalian reoviruses can be divided into three serotypes (types 1, 2 or 3), regardless of their species of origin (Rosen, 1960). They are very stable viruses, and can resist heat, ether, acid phenol, hydrogen peroxide, formalin and lysol: they can be inactivated, however, by 70% ethanol (Stanley et al., 1953).

The clinical importance of feline reovirus infection in the cat population is unknown, though there is some evidence that infection itself may be widespread. Limited serological surveys have shown that in the USA approximately 70% of cats had antibodies to reovirus type 1 and 50% to type 3 (Scott et al., 1970; Hong, 1970), whereas in Europe approximately 12% of cats had antibodies to type 1, 17% to type 2, and 70% to type 3 (Lazarowicz, 1977).

It is not known how commonly reovirus causes disease in the field. It has been isolated from cats with a variety of clinical conditions, but in many of these cases it was probably not the cause of disease. Experimental inoculation of kittens with feline reovirus type 3 induced a mild syndrome, mainly consisting of conjunctivitis, photophobia and serous ocular discharges, and transmission of clinical disease to in-contact kittens (Scott et al., 1970). Animals were depressed but showed no pyrexia, anorexia or leucocytosis. Some cats developed mucopurulent ocular discharges and one or two animals also showed gingivitis or nasal discharge. Kittens inoculated with feline reovirus type 2 developed mild diarrhoea (Muir et al., 1992). Newborn kittens inoculated with feline reovirus type 1 nursed poorly and died 2 days later (Hong, 1970). At post-mortem examination, cytoplasmic reovirus inclusions were seen in their bronchiolar epithelium.

Thus it is possible that reoviruses may contribute to the upper respiratory tract syndrome in the field, particularly cases of mild conjunctivitis. However, in a recent survey we found no evidence of reovirus infection among 150 cases of conjunctivitis.

Virus in faeces may be detected by direct electron microscopy, or it can be isolated from rectal and pharyngeal swabs using special cell culture techniques (Gillespie & Scott, 1973a).

Although infection is widespread, control measures are probably not indicated because infection is thought to be subclinical or at most mild. As the virus appears to be shed mainly in faeces, however, any attempt to eliminate it from the environment will require thorough cleansing and disinfection.

In summary, feline reovirus infection appears to be widespread, but clinically does not appear to be of major significance. However, this may merely reflect a paucity of information on the subject, and more studies are necessary to de-

Chapter 20

Table 20.1 Some virus infections of domestic cats.

Virus	Comments
Feline herpesvirus type 1 Feline calicivirus Reovirus	Mainly respiratory infections
Feline parvovirus Feline coronavirus Canine coronavirus Rotavirus Astrovirus Torovirus	Mainly enteric infections
Feline leukaemia virus Endogenous retroviruses Feline immunodeficiency virus Feline syncytium-forming virus	Retroviruses
Cowpox virus Hantavirus Rabies virus Aujeszky's disease virus Feline herpesvirus type 2 Influenza virus Canine distemper virus Paramyxoviruses	Miscellaneous and generally not endemic in cats
Venezuelan equine encephalitis virus Flaviviruses Tenshaw virus Rift valley fever virus	Arthropod-borne; not endemic in cats

termine the true clinical significance of feline reovirus infections.

FELINE ROTAVIRUS

Rotaviruses are double-stranded RNA viruses, approximately 70 nm in diameter. They have been isolated from many mammalian species and in a number of these, for example humans, cattle, sheep and pigs, they are a well-established cause of acute diarrhoea (reviewed by McNulty, 1978). Typically, rotavirus infection occurs initially in neonatal animals, although further, usually milder or subclinical, infections may occur at intervals throughout life. Rotaviruses from different species share a group-specific antigen, and

it has also been shown that viruses may be transmitted between species. Nevertheless, other antigens do vary, and it appears likely that specific serotypes are mostly pathogenic for only certain species.

There are very few reports of rotavirus infection in cats, and in general it is probably not a disease of any major significance. Nevertheless, serological evidence of past infection has been found in five out of six cats sampled in Northern Ireland (McNulty *et al.*, 1978), in 28–99% of cats in Great Britain (Snodgrass *et al.*, 1979, Muir *et al.*, 1990), in 10 out of 15 cats in Belgium (Dagenais *et al.*, 1980), and in 33% of cats in New York State, USA (Hoshino *et al.*, 1981a). In Britain rotavirus particles have been detected in association with two separate cases of mild diarrhoea, one in an adult cat and one in a 6-week-old kitten, and the disease was also reproduced in two kittens experimentally (Snodgrass *et al.*, 1979; Chrystie *et al.*, 1979). However, in the USA, attempts to produce clinical disease experimentally with one of five isolates made from hospitalized cats with no gastroenteric signs were unsuccessful (Hoshino *et al.*, 1981a). Both Hoshino *et al.* (1981a) and Chrystie *et al.* (1979) showed their isolates to be antigenically distinct from human rotavirus.

Rotavirus infections in general do not cause systemic disease and virus replication appears to be confined to the sides and tips of villi in the small intestine. The limited experimental work reported suggests this may also be true for the cat (Flewett & Woode, 1978; Snodgrass *et al.*, 1979). In the cat, the available evidence suggests that subclinical infection is probably most common, and diarrhoea, if it occurs, is only mild and transient. Nevertheless, it is always possible that more severe disease may occur if the situation is complicated by other pathogens or predisposing factors, and in some cases, therefore, the disease might not be recognized. Diagnosis is usually by detection of particles in faeces by electron microscopy. Other methods might include virus isolation on specially treated cell cultures (expensive), the use of antigen capture ELISA kits (although these are presently designed to detect human serotypes and may miss animal strains; Scott, 1988; Scott *et al.*, 1988) or electrophoresis of genomic RNA through polyacrylamide gels (Herring *et al.*, 1982; Birch *et al.*, 1985). Treatment, other than 24-hour fasting, is unlikely to be necessary, but in any cases of prolonged diarrhoea parenterally administered fluid therapy may be indicated.

Rotaviruses are highly infectious, and in species living in colonies or herds spread occurs mainly through faecal-oral contamination at an early age, the source of infection being either other neonates or adult carriers. In species living in smaller groups, however, infection may be delayed until later in life. For example, recent evidence suggests that most dogs do not become infected until over 6 months old (Tennant *et al.*, 1990). Thus the risk of infection in cats probably depends on the environment in which they live, cats living in colonies being more likely to meet infection earlier in life than most household pets. Virus particles are shed in the faeces of infected cats for 10–14 days, although in some cats periodic shedding has been reported to occur (Hoshino *et al.*, 1981a), and bovine rotavirus can survive in dried faeces for up to 9 months (Woode, 1978). The environment in a colony can therefore be heavily contaminated, and if the disease is thought to be a problem, suitable disinfection should be carried out. Hypochlorite, widely used in cat virus disease as a disinfectant, does not appear to be effective against rotaviruses, and 4% iodophore, 5% lysol or 10% formol saline are recommended following removal of organic matter on surfaces (Snodgrass & Herring, 1977), although care should be taken as phenolics such as lysol can be toxic to cats.

FELINE ASTROVIRUS

Astroviruses are small (29 nm diameter) RNA viruses with a characteristic five- or six-pointed star-shaped morphology by electron microscopy. Little has been published on the epidemiology or clinical significance of feline astrovirus infection, although one report suggests that less than 10% of cats in the UK have antibody to the virus (Harbour, 1990).

Most isolations have been made from cats with diarrhoea (Hoshino *et al.*, 1981b; Harbour *et al.*, 1987; Harbour, 1990). The diarrhoea has been described as persistent (4–14 days), green and watery, and may be accompanied by vomiting, pyrexia and depression. Mild diarrhoea, with an 11–12-day incubation period, has been reproduced experimentally in kittens (Harbour *et al.*, 1987). Although kittens seem most affected, adults may also be infected and develop clinical signs (Harbour, 1990).

Diagnosis is by submission of faeces to a laboratory for electron microscopic examination. Treatment is symptomatic.

FELINE TOROVIRUS

The toroviruses are a group of viruses similar to the coronaviruses, but with a characteristic rod or doughnut-shaped core. They include Berne virus, isolated from a horse (Weiss *et al.*, 1983), Breda virus, isolated from cattle (Woode *et al.*, 1982), and several torovirus-like isolates from humans (Beards *et al.*, 1984). The human and bovine isolates have been associated with diarrhoea, but the equine isolate appears to cause only asymptomatic infections.

Recently, torovirus-like particles and antibody reacting with Breda virus types 1 and 2 have been also detected in cats (Muir *et al.*, 1990). Although not reproduced experimentally, there is some evidence to link this virus in cats to a clinical syndrome involving diarrhoea and protrusion of the nictitating membrane (Muir *et al.*, 1990). This syndrome is a common presentation of persistent diarrhoea in cats, and is frustrating to treat, although often eventually self-limiting. An infectious cause has been postulated in the past (Gruffydd-Jones *et al.*, 1977), and if a torovirus is shown to be the responsible agent then the development of measures for control and prevention may be possible.

FELINE SYNCYTIUM-FORMING VIRUS

Feline syncytium-forming virus (FeSFV) is a member of the foamy virus group (the Spumavirinae) in the family Retroviridae. Spumaviruses have been isolated from many species but, unlike the oncoviruses and lentiviruses, they generally do not appear to be pathogenic, and their main importance at present lies not in clinical medicine but as potential contaminants in research and vaccine production.

In the USA, FeSFV is ubiquitous in the cat population, the prevalence of infection ranging from 30 to 90% depending on the population tested (Hackett *et al.*, 1970; Gaskin & Gillespie, 1973). In limited studies in Britain it appears to be present in approximately 20–30% of cats (Jarrett *et al.*, 1974; Gaskell *et al.*, 1979), whereas in some other parts of the world the prevalence appears to be very low (Sabine & Love, 1973; Mochizuki & Konishi, 1979; Ellis, 1981). The virus has been isolated both from clinically healthy cats (Hackett *et al.*, 1970; Jarrett *et al.*, 1974) and from cats with a variety of diseases (reviewed by Gillespie & Scott, 1973b), but no signs of disease have been produced when the agent has been inoculated into cats experimentally, even in the long-term (Kasza *et al.*, 1969; Gaskell *et al.*, 1979). Nevertheless, the possibility still exists that FeSFV may induce or predispose animals to disease, perhaps in conjunction with other agents or in cats of a particular histocompatibility type. Such an association has been suggested for FeSFV and possibly FeLV in the feline chronic progressive polyarthritis syndrome (Pedersen *et al.*, 1980).

Infected cats appear to harbour virus indefinitely. Virus may be isolated in cell culture from throat swabs, buffy coat cells, urine and tissues (Shroyer & Shalaby, 1978; Gaskell *et al.*, 1979). Carrier cats may also be reliably detected by screening for antibody to the virus using immunofluorescent or immunodiffusion techniques (Gaskin, 1973; Gaskin & Gillespie, 1973).

FeSFV may be transmitted vertically or horizontally. Thus it has been detected in fetuses and in embryo cultures obtained during hysterectomy of pregnant queens (Hackett *et al.*, 1970; Jarrett *et al.*, 1974). However, this is probably not a frequent occurrence, for other workers have been unable to demonstrate *in utero* transmission of the virus in several litters of kittens born to carrier queens (Gaskin, 1973). Since infection is widespread in the cat population, and the virus is shed in oropharyngeal secretions and in urine, it would seem likely that horizontal transmission via the oronasal route would be the predominant mode of spread. However, even with the close contact that occurs between queens and their kittens, infection does not under normal circumstances appear to spread very readily between cats. Thus, in order to account for the high incidence of infection in some cat populations, it has been suggested that transmission may occur more readily during outbreaks of respiratory disease because of the copious oronasal discharges that occur (Gaskin, 1973). Bite wounds are another possible means of cross-infection.

In conclusion, infection with this agent would appear to be of little consequence for the clinician and therefore at present no control measures are necessary. When initiating a specific-pathogen-free cat colony, however, it would be wise to consider testing parent stock for the presence of FeSFV because of the possibility of vertical transmission.

HANTAVIRUS

Hantavirus is a genus in the family Bunyaviridae. Hantaviruses are enzootic worldwide in wild and laboratory rodent populations, and are often zoonotic, causing haemorrhagic fever and renal syndrome in man (Schmaljohn, 1988). Different areas of the world appear to have their own local strains, which can be distinguished serologically and which circulate in the local rodent species. The various strains also vary in their pathogenicity to man; in general strains from Eastern Europe and Asia seem to be more pathogenic than strains from Western Europe and North America, which usually cause only mild or no clinical signs.

Hantavirus antibody in cats was first detected in laboratory-housed cats in Belgium (Desmyter *et al.*, 1983), and a recent survey in Britain (Bennett *et al.*, 1990) found serum antibody to *Hantavirus* in around 10% of cats from a variety of disease and environmental backgrounds. The clinical significance of *Hantavirus* infection in cats is not known, although the same British survey did suggest a possible association between *Hantavirus* antibody and chronic disease. *Hantavirus* has not yet been isolated from a domestic cat, and it is not known if cat-to-cat or cat-to-human transmission can occur. However, there is no evidence to suggest that cats are a frequent source of human infection; the overall prevalence of antibody in man in the UK is only 0.5%, with higher prevalences found in those whose work or recreation exposes them to rodents (Lloyd, 1985).

AUJESZKY'S DISEASE

Aujeszky's disease (pseudorabies, mad itch) is primarily a disease of pigs. It is caused by a herpesvirus, *Herpesvirus suis*. Although infection is often subclinical, in older pigs it can produce dullness and anorexia, and in breeding sows and gilts reproductive failure. In young piglets nervous signs predominate, and mortality can be very high (Baskerville *et al.*, 1973). Sometimes respiratory signs are seen and indeed the virus is mainly spread between pigs by direct or aerosol contact with infected oral and nasal secretions. The virus may persist in the environment for several weeks, and thus indirect transmission is also thought to be possible (Wittman, 1982). Recovered pigs remain as latent carriers of the virus, which may be reactivated by stress (Wittman *et al.*, 1982).

Although pigs are the reservoir host for Aujeszky's disease virus (ADV), other animals, including cattle, sheep, dogs, cats and rats, can also be infected. These species are thought to be 'dead end' hosts, however, and are not thought to transmit the disease themselves, although cats may shed virus in their oral and nasal secretions (Maes & Pensaert, 1987). There are several reports of Aujeszky's disease in cats, all of whom had either close contact with pigs or who had eaten uncooked, infected pig meat (Dow & McFerran, 1963; Horvath & Papp, 1967; Cartwright, 1982).

Aujeszky's disease in dogs and cats is almost always fatal, and often rapidly so. The first clinical signs seen in Aujeszky's disease in cats and dogs are usually behavioural changes and include restlessness, anorexia and hypersalivation. Often no clinical signs will be seen in free-roaming cats as they will run off to hide early in disease development (Maes & Pensaert, 1987). Intense pruritus, commonly localized around the face or mouth (Galloway, 1938; Dow & McFerran, 1963; Metianu *et al.*, 1971; Hagemoser *et al.*, 1980) is often described as a characteristic sign of Aujeszky's disease, but many infected cats are not pruritic (Horvarth & Papp, 1967; Hagemoser *et al.*, 1980; Maes & Pensaert, 1987). Those that are pruritic may become frenzied in an attempt to alleviate the intolerable itching, and gross self-mutilation can often result. It is in this form that the disease may be mistaken for rabies; but unlike rabid cats, cats with Aujeszky's disease are rarely aggressive. Terminal signs, which develop usually within 48 hours of the onset of clinical signs, include paralysis, and coma. Some cats may die suddenly without showing any prior clinical signs (Howard, 1986).

At gross post-mortem examination, few lesions are usually visible apart from evidence of local trauma and self-mutilation. Histological examination reveals cutaneous areas of non-specific inflammation associated with characteristic viral lesions in the ganglia of the related spinal or cranial nerves (Dow & McFerran, 1963).

There is no treatment for the disease, no vaccine available for use in cats and all cases are rapidly fatal once signs have appeared. A definitive diagnosis can be made by isolation of ADV from nervous tissue related to the site of pruritus such as the brainstem region, or by immunostaining fixed or frozen tissues, particularly brain and tonsil. Distribution of virus and lesions is usually localized to a small area in the brain or spinal cord, so that selection of CNS tissue is critical. Antibody tests are not generally useful as cats normally die before circulating antibody appears.

In Britain, an eradication programme for Aujeszky's disease in pigs has proved very successful, so it seems highly unlikely that the disease in cats will occur in Britain to any significant extent in the near future. Aujeszky's disease is, however, prevalent in pigs in most of Europe and North and South America, and thus the disease may continue to occur in cats in these places.

FELINE HERPESVIRUS 2

A second, cell-associated feline herpesvirus has been described, serologically distinct from feline herpesvirus 1, the virus of feline viral rhinotracheitis (Fabricant & Gillespie, 1974) (see Chapter 14). This virus, tentatively named feline herpesvirus 2 (FHV-2), has been found to induce chemical crystal formations in infected cell cultures, and has also been implicated as a possible aetiological agent in the feline urological syndrome (FUS) (Fabricant, 1977). Other workers, however, have so far been unable to confirm the transmissibility of FUS, and have failed to isolate a similar agent (Jackson, 1975; Gaskell *et al.*, 1979; Kruger *et al.*, 1990).

Recently, antigenic and molecular studies on FHV-2 have shown it to be very closely related to bovid herpesvirus 4 (BHV-4) (Kruger *et al.*, 1989). BHV-4 has been isolated from cattle with respiratory and reproductive disease in continental Europe, and has been associated with abortion in Great Britain (Fitton *et al.*, 1990). The European type strain of BHV-4 (Movar) does not appear to be infectious to cats (Thiry *et al.*, 1991). Further studies are needed to determine the origin of FHV-2 and whether it is a true feline virus or if it originated in cattle.

OTHER VIRUSES

Influenza virus can infect cats following experimental inoculation, and there is some serological evidence of infection in the field. However, there is no evidence that cat-to-human transmission might occur, the reverse being more likely during human influenza pandemics.

Several reports also exist of paramyxovirus infection of the CNS in cats; these infections have been associated with demyelinating encephalitis and with clinical neurological signs (Cook & Wilcox, 1981; Wilcox *et al.*, 1984). In addition avian Newcastle disease virus can cause disseminated meningoencephalitis in kittens inoculated intranasally (Luttrell & Bang, 1958). The relevance of these reports to the field is not known.

Canine distemper virus (CDV) can infect domestic cats both experimentally and in the field but generally causes no clinical signs (Appel *et al.*, 1974). In big cats, however, natural CDV infection has been associated with encephalitis (Blythe *et al.*, 1983).

Cats in some parts of the world may also become infected with several arthropod-borne viruses. Infection is usually asymptomatic but occasionally causes encephalitis (Greene, 1990).

ACKNOWLEDGEMENTS

The authors are grateful to Dr M.S. McNulty, the Veterinary Research Centre, Stormont, for critically reviewing the rotavirus and Aujeszky's disease sections.

REFERENCES

Appel M., Sheffy B.E., Percy D.H. & Gaskin J.M. (1974) Canine distemper virus in domesticated cats and pigs. *Am. J. Vet. Res.* **35**, 803.

Baskerville A., McFerran J.B. & Dow C. (1973) Aujeszky's disease in pigs. *Vet. Bull.* **43**, 465.

Beards G.M., Hall C., Green J., Flewett T.H., Lamouliatte F. & Du Pasquier P. (1984) An enveloped virus in the stools of children and adults with gastroenteritis that resembles the Breda virus of calves. *Lancet* **i**, 1050.

Bennett M., Lloyd G., Jones N., Brown A., Trees A.J., McCracken C., Smyth N.R., Gaskell C.J. & Gaskell R.M. (1990) The prevalence of antibody to Hantavirus in some cat populations in Britain. *Vet. Rec.* **127**, 548–9.

Birch C.J., Heath R.L., Marshall J.A., Lui S. & Gust I.D. (1985) Isolation of feline rotaviruses and their relationship to human and simian isolates by electropherotype and serotype. *J. Gen. Virol.* **66**, 2731.

Blythe L.L., Schmitz J.A., Roelke M. & Skinner S. (1983) Chronic encephalomyelitis caused by canine distemper virus in a Bengal tiger. *J. Am. Vet. Med. Assoc.* **183**, 1159.

Cartwright S. (1982) Epidemiology and control of Aujeszky's disease in Great Britain. In Wittman G. & Hall S.A. (eds) *Aujeszky's Disease.* Martinus Nijhoff, The Hague, pp. 237–44.

Chrystie I.L., Goldwater P.N. & Banatvala J.E. (1979) Rotavirus infection in a domestic cat. *Vet. Rec.* **105**, 404.

Cook R.D. & Wilcox G.E. (1981) A paramyxovirus-like agent associated with demyelinating lesions in the CNS of cats. *J. Neuropathol. Exp. Neurol.* **40**, 328.

Dagenais L., Schwers A., Lansival B. & Pastoret P.-P. (1980) Survey of antibodies against bovine rotavirus in the serum of dogs, cats and horses in Belgium. *Annales de Med. Vet.* **124**, 423.

Desmyter J., Leduc J.W., Johnson K.M., Brasseur F., Deckers C. & Van Ypersele de Strihou C. (1983) Laboratory rat-associated outbreaks of haemorrhagic fever with renal syndrome due to Hantaan-like virus in Belgium. *Lancet* **ii**, 1445.

Dow C. & McFerran J.B. (1963) Aujeszky's disease in the dog and cat. *Vet. Rec.* **75**, 1099.

Ellis T.M. (1981) Feline respiratory virus carriers in clinically healthy cats. *Austr. Vet. J.* **57**, 115.

Fabricant C.G. (1977) Herpesvirus-induced urolithiasis in specific pathogen-free male cats. *Am. J. Vet. Res.* **38**, 1837.

Fabricant C.G. & Gillespie J.H. (1974) Identification and characterisation of a second feline herpesvirus. *Infect. Immun.* **9**, 460.

Fitton J., Beenham J. & Edwards S. (1990) Bovid herpesvirus-4 antibody in cattle in Great Britain. *Vet. Rec.* **126**, 173.

Flewett T.H. & Woode G.N. (1978) The rotaviruses. Brief review. *Arch. Virol.* **57**, 1.

Galloway I.A. (1938) Aujeszky's disease. *Vet. Rec.* **50**, 745.

Gaskell R.M., Gaskell C.J., Page W., Dennis P. & Voyle C.A. (1979) Studies on a possible viral aetiology for the feline urological syndrome. *Vet. Rec.* **105**, 243.

Gaskin J.M. (1973) Feline syncytia-forming virus: an occult virus and its host. PhD Thesis, Cornell University, New York.

Gaskin J.M. & Gillespie J.H. (1973) Detection of feline syncytia-forming virus carrier state with a microimmunodiffusion test. *Am. J. Vet. Res.* **34**, 245.

Gillespie J.H. & Scott F.W. (1973a) Feline viral infections. IV Feline reovirus (FRV) infection. *Adv. Vet. Sci. Comp. Med.* **17**, 188.

Gillespie J.H. & Scott F.W. (1973b) Feline viral infections. V Feline syncytium-forming virus (FSV) infection. *Adv. Vet. Sci. Comp. Med.* **17**, 192.

Greene C.E. (1990) Arboviral infections. In Greene C.E. (ed) *Infectious Diseases of the Dog and Cat.* W.B. Saunders, Philadelphia, pp. 393–6.

Gruffydd-Jones T.J., Orr C.M. & Flecknell P.A. (1977) A new syndrome in cats. *Vet. Rec.* **101**, 413.

Hackett A.J., Pfiester A. & Arnstein P. (1970) Biological properties of a syncitia-forming agent isolated from domestic cats (feline syncitia-forming virus). *Proc. Soc. Exp. Biol. Med.* **135**, 899.

Hagemoser W.A., Kluge J.P. & Hill H.T. (1980) Studies on the pathogenesis of pseudorabies in domestic cats following oral inoculation. *Can. J. Comp. Med.* **44**, 192.

Harbour D.A. (1990) Feline astroviral infections. In Greene C.E. (ed) *Infectious Diseases of the Dog and Cat.* W.B. Saunders, Philadelphia, pp. 313–4.

Harbour D.A., Ashley C.R., Williams P.D. & Gruffydd-Jones T.J. (1987) Natural and experimental astrovirus infection of cats. *Vet. Rec.* **120**, 555.

Herring A.J., Inglis N.F., Ojeh C.K., Snodgrass D.R. & Menzies J.D. (1982) Rapid diagnosis of rotavirus infection by direct detection of viral nucleic acid in silver stained polyacrylamide gels. *J. Clin. Microbiol.* **16**, 473.

Hong C. (1970) Studies on a strain of reovirus type 1 isolated from a feline leukemia cell culture. MS Thesis, Cornell University, New York.

Horvath Z. & Papp L. (1967) Clinical manifestations of Aujeszky's disease in the cat. *Acta. Vet. Hung.* **17**, 49.

Hoshino Y., Baldwin C.A. & Scott F.W. (1981a) Isolation and characterisation of feline rotavirus. *J. Gen. Virol.* **54**, 313.

Hoshino Y., Zimmer J.F., Moise N.S. & Scott F.W. (1981b) Detection of astrovirus in faeces of a cat with diarrhoea. *Arch. Virol.* **70**, 373.

Howard D.R. (1986) Pseudorabies in dogs and cats. In Kirk R.W. (ed) *Current Veterinary Therapy IX*. W.B. Saunders, Philadelphia, pp. 1071–2.

Jackson O.F. (1975) The case against a viral aetiology in feline urolithiasis. *Vet. Rec.* **97**, 70.

Jarrett O., Hay D. & Laird H.M. (1974) Infection by feline syncytium-forming virus in Britain. *Vet. Rec.* **94**, 201.

Kasza L., Hayward A.H.S. & Betts A.O. (1969) Isolation of a virus from a cat sarcoma in an established canine melanoma cell line. *Res. Vet. Sci.* **10**, 216.

Kruger J.M., Osborne C.A., Whetstone C.A., Goyal S.M. & Semlak R.A. (1989) Genetic and serologic analysis of feline cell-associated herpesvirus-induced infection of the urinary tract in conventionally reared cats. *Am. J. Vet. Res.* **50**, 2023.

Kruger J.M., Osborne C.A., Goyal S.M., O'Brien T.D., Pomeroy K. & Semlak R.A. (1990) Clinicopathologic analysis of herpesvirus-induced urinary tract infection in specific pathogen-free cats given methylprednisolone. *Am. J. Vet. Res.* **51**, 878.

Lazarowicz M. (1977) A serological survey in cats for antibodies to respiratory viruses and Chlamydia. *Zeitschrift fur Veruchstierkunde* **19**, 325.

Lloyd G. (1985) Hantavirus: cause for concern in the United Kingdom? *PHLS Microbiol. Dig.* **2**, 37.

Luttrell C.N. & Bang F.B. (1958) Newcastle disease encephalomyelitis in cats. 1. Clinical and pathological features. *AMA Arch. Neurol. Psychiatr.* **79**, 647.

McNulty M.S. (1978) Rotaviruses. *J. Gen. Virol.* **40**, 1.

McNulty M.S., Allan G.M., Thompson D.J. & O'Boyle J.D. (1978) Antibody to rotavirus in dogs and cats. *Vet. Rec.* **101**, 81.

Maes L. & Pensaert M. (1987) Pseudorabies virus (Aujeszky's disease). In Appel M.J. (ed) *Virus Infections of Carnivores*. Elsevier Science Publishers BV, Amsterdam, pp. 241–6.

Metianu T., Lucas A., Vallee A. & Laurent R. (1971) Contribution a l'étude de la maladie d'Aujeszky en France: isolement du virus chez deux chats. *Bull. Acad. Vet. Fr.* **44**, 221.

Mochizuki M. & Konishi S. (1979) Feline syncytial virus spontaneously detected in feline cell cultures. *Jap. J. Vet. Sci.* **41**, 351.

Muir P., Harbour D.A., Gruffydd-Jones T.J., Howard P.E., Hopper C.D., Gruffydd-Jones E.A.D., Broadhead H.M., Clarke C.M. & Jones M.E. (1990) A clinical and microbiological study of cats with nictitating membrane protrusion and diarrhoea; isolation of a novel virus. *Vet. Rec.* **127**, 324.

Muir P., Harbour D.A. & Gruffydd-Jones T.J. (1992) Reovirus type 2 in domestic cats. Isolation and experimental transmission. *Vet. Microbiol.* **30**, 309–16.

Pedersen N.C., Pool R.R. & O'Brien T. (1980) Feline chronic progressive polyarthritis. *Am. J. Vet. Res.* **41**, 522.

Rosen L. (1960) Serologic grouping of reoviruses by haemagglutination inhibition. *Am. J. Hyg.* **71**, 242.

Sabine M. & Love D.A. (1973) Feline foamy virus incidence in Australia. Brief report. *Arch. Virol.* **43**, 397.

Schmaljohn C.S. (1988) Hantavirus. In Darai G. (ed) *Virus Diseases in Laboratory and Captive Animals*. Martinus Nijhoff, Boston, p. 535.

Scott F.M.M. (1988) Rotavirus diagnostic kits. *Vet. Rec.* **123**, 39.

Scott F.M.M., Snodgrass D.R., Molyneux P. & Winter G. (1988) Rotavirus diagnostic kits. *Vet. Rec.* **122**, 262.

Scott F.W., Kahn D.E. & Gillespie J.H. (1970) Feline viruses; isolation, characterisation and pathogenicity of a feline reovirus. *Am. J. Vet. Res.* **31**, 11.

Shroyer E.L. & Shalaby M.R. (1978) Isolation of feline sincytia-forming virus from oropharyngeal swab samples and buffy coat cells. *Am. J. Vet. Res.* **39**, 555.

Snodgrass D.R. & Herring J.A. (1977) The action of disinfectants on lamb rotavirus. *Vet. Rec.* **101**, 81.

Snodgrass D.R., Angus K.W. & Gray E.W. (1979) A rotavirus from kittens. *Vet. Rec.* **104**, 222.

Stanley N.F., Dorman D.C. & Ponsford J. (1953) Studies on the pathogenesis of a hitherto undescribed virus (hepato-encephalomyelitis) producing unusual symptoms in suckling mice. *Austr. J. Exp. Med. Sci.* **31**, 147.

Tennant B.J., Gaskell R.M., Jones R.C. & Gaskell C.J. (1991) Prevalence of antibodies to some major canine viral diseases in a U.K. hospital population. *J. Small Anim. Pract.* **32**, 175–9.

Thiry E., Chappuis G., Bublot M., Vanbressem M.F., Dubuisson J. & Pastoret P.-P. (1991) Failure to infect cats with bovine herpesvirus type 4 strain Movar 33/63. *Vet. Rec.* **128**, 614–5.

Weiss M., Steck F. & Horzinek M.C. (1983) Purification and partial characterisation of a new enveloped RNA virus (Berne virus). *J. Gen. Virol.* **64**, 1849.

Wilcox G.E., Flower R.L.P. & Cook R.D. (1984) Recovery of viral agents from the central nervous system of cats. *Vet. Microbiol.* **9**, 355.

Wittmann G. (1982) Introduction: Aujeszky's disease. In Wittmann G. & Hall S.A. (eds) *Aujeszky's Disease*. Martinus Nijhoff, The Hague, pp. xi–xiii.

Wittmann G., Rziha H.-J. & Doller P.C. (1982) Occurrence of clinical Aujeszky's disease in immunosuppressed latently infected pigs. In Wittmann G. & Hall S.A. (eds)

Aujeszky's Disease. Martinus Nijhoff, The Hague, pp. 211–4.

Woode G.N. (1978) Epizootiology of bovine rotavirus infection. *Vet. Rec.* **103**, 32.

Woode G.N., Reede D.E., Runnels P.L., Herrig M.A. & Hill H.T. (1982) Studies with an unclassified virus isolated from diarrhoeic calves. *Vet. Microbiol.* **7**, 221.

Chapter 21 / Feline Chlamydial Infection

J. M. WILLS AND R. M. GASKELL

INTRODUCTION

Infection of cats with *Chlamydia psittaci* was first described by Baker (1942), when the organism was isolated from the lungs of naturally infected cats. At that time the organism was considered to be the major cause of feline upper respiratory tract disease, and all respiratory infections were called 'feline pneumonitis', apparently caused by *C. psittaci*. Since the recognition of feline herpesvirus (FHV) and feline calicivirus (FCV) as significant causes of respiratory disease in cats (Povey & Johnson, 1971; Gaskell & Wardley, 1978) (see Chapter 14), further investigation into the importance of *C. psittaci* in the cat has shown that it is primarily a conjunctival rather than a pulmonary pathogen, and pneumonia is not a common clinical feature (Hoover *et al.*, 1978; Wills *et al.*, 1984). Therefore, the disease is perhaps better described as feline chlamydial infection, or feline chlamydiosis (FC), rather than feline pneumonitis.

THE AGENT

The aetiological agent is a feline strain of *Chlamydia psittaci*. This organism is in the genus *Chlamydia*, family Chlamydiaceae, order Chlamydiales. The genus contains two species: *C. trachomatis* and *C. psittaci*. Strains of *C. trachomatis* generally only infect man, causing ocular and genital tract infections, whereas strains of *C. psittaci* can cause respiratory disease, conjunctivitis, abortion and arthritis in many animal species.

Chlamydiae form an unusual group of organisms and initially, because of the small size of the infectious particle (approximately 300 nm) and their dependence on the host cell for energy (adenosine triphosphate) and replication, they were regarded as viruses. However, they have a rigid cell wall similar in structure and content to that of Gram-negative bacteria, contain both DNA and RNA, divide by binary fission without an initial eclipse phase, and are susceptible to certain antibiotics. Chlamydiae are therefore generally regarded as highly specialized obligate intracytoplasmic bacteria.

Chlamydiae are relatively unstable outside their host; *C. psittaci* in conjunctival discharges will become inactivated within 3 days at room temperature. Even at 0°C considerable inactivation occurs after several days and long-term storage is best achieved at −70°C (Cello, 1971a) or by lyophilization. Their lipid-containing cell wall is rapidly inactivated by a number of lipid solvents and detergents, although they resist acids and alkalis (Gillespie & Timoney, 1981). A 1 in 1000 dilution of a quaternary ammonium compound is recommended for hospital use.

PATHOGENESIS AND CLINICAL SIGNS

Conjunctival epithelium would appear to be the chief target for feline *C. psittaci*. The organism replicates within an inclusion, in the cytoplasm of epithelial cells. The life cycle of *C. psittaci* in the cat takes approximately 48 hours, after which time the parasitized epithelial cell usually disintegrates, releasing further infectious organisms. In experimentally induced infection, clinical signs of conjunctivitis appear after 3–5 days in cats challenged by the conjunctival route (Wills *et al.*, 1987). In a more natural situation, new introductions to an infected colony can take 14 days or longer to become infected, depending on how social the cats are.

In the initial stage of disease, there is marked serous ocular discharge, blepharospasm, chemosis and hyperaemia of the palpebral conjunctivae (Plates 21.1 and 21.2). Initially only one eye may be affected, but the other eye is usually involved 5–21 days later. As the disease progresses, the conjunctivae become more hyperaemic, and discharges become mucopurulent. Secondary invaders such as streptococci, staphylococci, pasteurellae, pseudomonas and mycoplasmas may become involved (Plate 21.3). Giemsastained conjunctival smears from affected cats show neutrophils in large numbers in the first 7 days of ocular discharge, after which mononuclear cells are the predominant inflammatory cell. In most untreated cases, severe clinical signs generally resolve in 3–4 weeks, but conjunctival hyperaemia and intermittent mucopurulent ocular discharge may persist for months (Plate 21.4). Chlamydiae can be shed from the conjunctiva for long periods of time, and up to 18 months has been reported experimentally (Woodland & Darougar, 1986).

Follicular hyperplasia of the conjunctival lymphoid tissue of the inner surface of the nictitating membrane has been described (El Sheikh, 1978). Corneal ulceration, punctate keratitis and pannus have also been described (El Sheikh, 1978) but in these cases the presence of other feline infectious agents known to infect the eye itself was not investigated. Eye involvement has not been observed in specific pathogen-free (SPF) cats challenged with feline *C. psittaci* by the conjunctival route (Wills, 1986a).

Mild nasal discharge and sneezing may also occur, and there may be mild pyrexia for several days during the initial stages of the disease. However, affected cats usually continue to eat and are generally well, apart from the initial conjunctival discomfort, particularly if chemosis is present.

Despite the original name 'feline pneumonitis', pneumonia is not usually clinically apparent, but mild pulmonary lesions may be found at postmortem examination (Hoover *et al.*, 1978).

The respiratory viruses (see Chapter 14) have been isolated in conjunction with chlamydiae (Newberne *et al.*, 1959; Studdert *et al.*, 1981). Feline calicivirus has been isolated from oropharyngeal swabs taken from chlamydia-infected cats (Wills *et al.*, 1988a). It is likely that chlamydial conjunctivitis is aggravated by infection with FCV or FHV, and co-infection may account for the more serious clinical signs of pneumonitis reported previously for chlamydial infection (Baker, 1944).

Chlamydiae can also infect the cat's genital tract (Darougar *et al.*, 1977; Wills *et al.*, 1987) and gastrointestinal tract (Hargis *et al.*, 1983). Isolation of chlamydiae from vaginal swabs can occur 8–25 days after initial conjunctival challenge, and excretion from this route may persist for months. Infection is not usually associated with vaginal discharge. The female genital tract may become infected before the conjunctivae, in the natural situation (Wills, 1986a). Other workers have shown that salpingitis and adhesion formation can occur after a feline strain of *C. psittaci* was inoculated directly into the oviducts of cats (Kane *et al.*, 1985) but it is unlikely that this would be the consequence of a vaginal chlamydial infection, due to the presence of 'valve' systems in the feline uterus and oviduct that would inhibit ascending infection. The effect of persistent vaginal excretion on both pathology and clinical disease in the cat, and its significance in the epidemiology of FC, is still unclear. Occasionally, the organism has been associated with neonatal conjunctivitis in kittens (Cello, 1967; Shewen *et al.*, 1978), although there has been little success in isolation of the organism from the queen's vaginal tract in these cases. In some colonies, abortion has been noted in some cats infected with *C. psittaci* (Shewen *et al.*, 1978; Wills *et al.*, 1984), although the role of chlamydiae in reproductive failure in the cat has yet to be established. Indeed, queens that have experienced an earlier conjunctival and vaginal infection have produced healthy litters, as have queens that have been infected conjunctivally prior to mating and during pregnancy (Wills *et al.*, 1988b).

Chlamydiae have been isolated from rectal swabs of cats naturally infected with FC (Gethings *et al.*, 1987) and cats experimentally challenged by the conjunctival route (Wills *et al.*, 1987). In these cases, there was no association with diarrhoea. Hargis *et al.* (1983) identified *Chlamydia* post mortem in superficial gastric mucosal cells of cats; there was no consistent association with clinical disease, as infection was present in apparently healthy cats as well as those with a variety of clinical disease, including weight loss. These cats had no conjunctival or respiratory disease, but aerosol and oral inoculation of SPF kittens with gastric chlamydiae grown in cell culture produced conjunctivitis and rhinitis (Gaillard *et al.*, 1984). These authors suggested that the stomach may be a site of persistent infection for FC in cats. Undoubtedly, independent infection of genital and gastrointestinal tracts does occur, and excretion from these routes has been recorded for 7 months after initial infection (Wills, 1986a) and from the conjunctiva for 18 months (Woodland & Darougar, 1986).

INCIDENCE AND DISTRIBUTION

In the USA *C. psittaci* is thought to be one of the most common causes of conjunctivitis in cats and is estimated to account for 5–10% of all feline respiratory illnesses (Kahn & Hoover, 1976). Previous attempts to isolate chlamydiae from diseased cats in Britain have mostly been unsuccessful (Prydie, 1969) with only sporadic reports of its existence (Gledhill, 1952; Osborne, 1963). However, several groups of workers have now confirmed the presence of the organism in the domestic cat population in Britain (Darougar *et al.*, 1977; Johnson, 1984; Wills *et al.*, 1984). In a recent survey, chlamydiae were isolated from 226 of 753 (30%) conjunctival swabs from household cats with conjunctivitis and occasionally ad-

ditional signs of upper respiratory disease (Wills *et al.*, 1988a) (Table 21.1). The cats were classified by their age, breed and sex, and the data analysed by multifactorial regression analysis. The prevalence of chlamydial infection was found to be higher in male cats than females, the significance of which is unclear. The prevalence of chlamydial infection was highest in cats of both sexes of the age group 5 weeks to 9 months, and lowest in kittens under 5 weeks old. This confirms a clinical observation that the disease is usually one of litters of kittens, often presenting with 'sticky eyes', and kittens under 5 weeks old seem less likely to become infected with chlamydiae (Plate 21.5).

Feral and farm cat populations were also examined for the presence of chlamydiae, by isolation and serology, and these results are also presented in Table 21.1. Chlamydiae were isolated from 10 of 41 (24.4%) feral cats from three colonies; if present in a feral colony, infection is likely to be endemic. This was reflected in the prevalence of chlamydial antibodies in 69.4% of sera obtained from the feral cats.

DIAGNOSIS

Isolation

A tentative diagnosis may be based on the characteristic, often persistent clinical signs of conjunctivitis, and also indirectly by responses to different antibiotics. Examination of Giemsa-stained conjunctival scrapings or smears in early untreated cases may reveal the presence of intracytoplasmic inclusions. These infected cells are most numerous in the first 4–7 days of clinical disease, and are only occasionally seen from 7 to 14 days. Although their presence is diagnostic, it is an unreliable technique in more chronic cases of chlamydial conjunctivitis. The technique is described in more detail by Cello (1971b), together with possible hazards of interpretation.

A definitive diagnosis of infection must rely on the isolation and identification of the organism. Chlamydiae are obligate intracytoplasmic organisms, and therefore require living tissue culture

Table 21.1 Prevalence of *Chlamydia psittaci* in different cat populations in Britain, by isolation and serology.

Cat type	Chlamydia isolation*	(%)	Serology† titres >32	(%)
Household cats				
No conjunctivitis or URT disease	0/40	(0)	3/40	(7.5)
Conjunctivitis	226/753	(30)	64/116	(55.2)
Active chlamydial conjunctivitis			68/71	(95.8)
Feral cats (three colonies)	10/41	(24.4)	25/36	(69.4)
Farm cats	3/49	(6.1)	23/51	(45.1)

* Isolation in tissue culture and staining by indirect immunofluorescence (Wills *et al.*, 1987).
† Indirect immunofluorescence on *C. psittaci* (cat strain) infected cells (Wills, 1986a).

cells for their replication in a laboratory environment. Some specialist laboratories in Britain will attempt to isolate the organism in tissue culture, from conjunctival swabs. Chlamydiae are relatively unstable outside their host, and special transport medium is required for transportation for cell culture purposes. Some media will enable chlamydiae to survive transit in the post (Wills, 1986a). Either immunofluorescence or conventional histochemical stains can then be used to identify the intracytoplasmic chlamydial inclusions, after a period of incubation in tissue culture (Wills, 1988) (Plate 21.6).

Commercial veterinary laboratories are under increasing pressure to provide a reliable chlamydia diagnostic service, but lack of tissue culture facilities has inhibited its development. As a result, commercial opportunities for noncultural methods have developed in the human field, where either viable or non-viable chlamydiae can be used. Several kits are now available which can be used for the detection of *C. psittaci*. These kits use a genus-specific monoclonal or polyclonal antibody, which has been fluorescein-labelled for use in the direct examination of conjunctival smears or has been incorporated into an ELISA. However, cell culture has been shown to be more sensitive than ELISA for the detection of *C. psittaci* in cat conjunctival swabs, and in those cases where low quantities of organism are suspected, for example, in chronic

chlamydial conjunctivitis, cell culture is more reliable (Wills *et al.*, 1986).

Serology

A positive serological response, or the demonstration of a rising titre to chlamydia may be helpful in diagnosis. Indirect immunofluorescence (IF) and complement fixation tests (CFT) have both been used. However, not all cats known to have been infected with *C. psittaci* will develop positive titres by CFT, although the same cats will have high titres by IF (Shewen *et al.*, 1980; Wills, 1986a).

Chlamydial antibody titres measured by IF on *C. psittaci* (cat strain)-infected cells are significant over 32, whilst titres <16 are considered seronegative. In experimentally induced infection, cats not previously exposed to the organism will produce antibody titres by 2 weeks postchallenge. These titres will rise to ≥512 by 4 weeks post-challenge.

High IF titres to chlamydiae can persist in previously infected cats for over a year (Wills, 1986a). Whether this represents antibodies with a long half-life, or persistent infection with the organism that is stimulating antibody production is not known; therefore, high antibody titres do not necessarily suggest current infection.

Clinical cases of chlamydial conjunctivitis are likely to have high antibody titres. Sera from cats with an active chlamydial conjunctivitis, confirmed by isolation of the organism in tissue culture, had titres of ≥1024 in 62 of 71 samples (87.3%) (Wills *et al.*, 1988a).

Cell-mediated responses (as assessed by lymphocyte transformation) have been recorded by Shewen *et al.* (1980).

IMMUNITY

Persistent infection is characteristic of chlamydial conjunctivitis, and organisms have been isolated 18 months after infection (Woodland & Darougar, 1986). However, there is both clinical and microbiological protection to experimental challenge 3 months after initial challenge, and partial protection after 18 months (J.M. Wills, unpublished observations).

Kittens born to previously infected queens have maternally derived colostral antibodies to chlamydia. In a study of 26 kittens born to seven queens, the estimated half-life of passively derived colostral antibody to chlamydia measured by indirect IF was 13 days (Wills *et al.*, 1988b). In most kittens, antibody persisted until 9 weeks old, and in some cases until 12 weeks old, and the evidence suggests that in many cases this maternally derived antibody may be protective (see below).

TREATMENT

Chlamydia have cell walls that are similar in structure to Gram-negative bacteria, and thus they are susceptible to certain antibiotics. The tetracyclines are the drugs of choice for all *C. psittaci* infections. As systemic infection with the organism has been demonstrated in the cat, it might be advisable to treat both topically and systemically. Ophthalmic preparations that contain tetracycline or oxytetracycline can be applied 3–4 times daily (Achromycin Oil Suspension,*

Terramycin Ophthalmic Ointment†). Oxytetracycline has been shown *in vitro* to be more effective than chlortetracycline, probably because chlortetracycline is unstable at 37°C, at neutral or slightly alkaline pH, or in the presence of protein (Katz, 1956); for this reason, ophthalmic ointments containing chlortetracycline should ideally be applied 12 times daily.

Oxytetracycline or doxycycline (a tetracycline derivative; Ronaxan‡) can be given systemically to cats. Doxycycline has been shown to be effective in the treatment of FC (El Sheikh, 1978). Doxycycline has a longer half-life than oxytetracycline, and therefore only needs to be given once daily. It can also be given mixed in food, with no adverse effect on absorption. The dose rate is 5 mg/kg, once daily. All cats in a household should be treated simultaneously, for 4 weeks, or for at least 2 weeks after clinical signs have disappeared (Shewen *et al.*, 1978). Systemic tetracyclines may be contraindicated in pregnancy or in kittens, where calcification is occurring. However, there is little evidence that long-term administration of oxytetracycline or doxycycline adversely affects kittens' teeth, or causes gastrointestinal upsets.

Other antibiotics that have been used to kill other strains of *C. psittaci* include erythromycin and tylosin. However, no controlled experimental trials have been carried out in the cat. *C. psittaci* is not sensitive to sulphonamides or neomycin, and only slightly sensitive to penicillin and chloramphenicol. The agent can be recovered from the conjunctivae of cats in which chloramphenicol ophthalmic preparations have been used.

EPIDEMIOLOGY AND CONTROL

Chlamydial infection is probably mainly transmitted between cats by direct contact of infectious conjunctival, and occasionally nasal, secretions. Infected individuals may further disseminate the organism by means of soiled paws

---

* Achromycin Oil Suspension; Lederle.

† Terramycin Ophthalmic Ointment; Pfizer.
‡ Ronaxan, Rhône Mérieux.

wiping away infectious discharges. Fomite transmission is probably also important in the short term. Thus, measures designed to stop the spread of the feline respiratory viruses (see Chapter 14) should also help to prevent the spread of chlamydiae.

Once endemic in a cat colony, clinical signs may persist in an individual for some weeks and recurrent episodes can occur. Some of these episodes may be hormonally induced, and stress factors may be involved. Thus chlamydiae were isolated from the conjunctiva of seven out of ten previously infected queens (12 litters) during lactation, for variable periods of time ranging from 1 to 50 days post-partum (Wills *et al.*, 1988b). The stress of parturition and early lactation may be sufficient to reactivate a chlamydial infection, and there is some experimental evidence to suggest that chlamydial growth may be regulated hormonally. Despite close contact between queen and kittens when suckling, transmission of chlamydiae only occurred in one of the litters. Chlamydial conjunctivitis developed in a 16-day-old kitten. However, the rest of the litter did not become infected until 43, 50 (two kittens) and 65 days old, despite large amounts of the organism shed from the infected kitten, and close contact with its siblings. Thus, suckling kittens born to chlamydia-infected queens are usually protected from chlamydial infection from their dam, and this protection may stem from maternally derived colostral antibodies.

Natural immunity to chlamydial infection appears to be relatively inefficient in some individuals. Whether or not the organism persists in an infected colony as a true latent infection that requires activation before further excretion of infectious organisms, or as a slowly replicating, persistent infection where low numbers of organisms are disseminated continuously, is still not clear. The possible role of natural genital and gastrointestinal infection in the epidemiology of the disease is still unclear, but these may be sites of persistent infection. Nevertheless, in practice, infection does appear to be perpetuated in colony situations for some months, if not years.

Apparent breakdowns of recurrent conjunctivitis after long-term systemic treatment of a confirmed active chlamydial case may not be attributable to chlamydia alone; in these cases it is advisable to reassess the infectious agents involved, in particular the feline respiratory viruses FCV and FHV.

Vaccination against FC has been used in the USA for a number of years, either as a monovalent product or in combination with panleucopenia, FCV and FHV. Initially, the vaccine contained live, egg-grown chlamydia, but more recently it has been tissue-culture produced. The vaccine is live, and is administered subcutaneously. There has been some discussion as to the efficacy of the vaccine in the past. Various studies have shown that it can produce good protection (McKercher, 1952; Kolar & Rude, 1977; Mitzel & Strating, 1977), partial protection (Shewen *et al.*, 1980) or no protection (Cello, 1971a). When a live egg-grown, tissue-cultured passaged vaccine was used to protect cats from challenge with a British field isolate of feline *C. psittaci*, clinical signs of conjunctivitis were significantly reduced, but it did not prevent prolonged excretion from the eye, or dissemination of chlamydia to the genital and gastrointestinal tracts (Wills *et al.*, 1987).

ZOONOTIC IMPLICATIONS

Feline-associated *C. psittaci* has been implicated as the source of infection in four separate human cases, although it can be argued that the evidence presented in each case is not conclusive. The first case reported described a 21-year-old man with an acute unilateral follicular conjunctivitis, and conjunctival scrapings were positive for chlamydial agents by fluorescent antibody test (Schachter *et al.*, 1969; Ostler *et al.*, 1969; Ostler & Schachter, 1972). The patient had a 12-week-old kitten which had experienced unilateral ocular discharge for 1–2 weeks prior to the patient's illness. Chlamydial agents were identified in conjunctival scrapings taken from the cat.

The other reports are based on serological evidence, and are reviewed by Wills (1986b). The most recent report is that of a 25-year-old woman with acute follicular keratoconjunctivitis, who had a cat with rhinitis and conjunctivitis (Jahn & Bialasiewicz, 1986). Both patient and cat had IgM antibody titres to *C. psittaci*, but no organism was isolated from either human or cat, possibly because of pretreatment with tetracycline.

In our own studies, conjunctivitis was not a feature noted in owners of cats that had an active chlamydial infection (Wills, 1986a). The role of feline *C. psittaci* as a cause of human disease is therefore still unclear, but nevertheless, where *C. psittaci* has been isolated from a cat, the owner should be advised to maintain hygienic precautions, with washing of hands after petting or treatment of the infected cat, and after cleaning litter trays.

REFERENCES

Baker J.A. (1942) A virus obtained from a pneumonia of cats and its possible relation to the cause of atypical pneumonia in man. *Science* **96**, 475–6.

Baker J.A. (1944) A virus causing pneumonia in cats and producing elementary bodies. *J. Exp. Med.* **79**, 159–72.

Cello R.M. (1967) Ocular infections in animals with PLT (Bedsonia) group agents. *Am. J. Ophthalmol.* **63**, 1270–3.

Cello R.M. (1971a) Microbiological and immunologic aspects of feline pneumonitis. *J. Am. Vet. Med. Assoc.* **158**, 932–8, 943.

Cello R.M. (1971b) Clues to differential diagnosis of feline respiratory infections. *J. Am. Vet. Med. Ass.* **158**, 968.

Darougar S., Monnickendam M.A., El-Sheikh H., Treharne J.D., Woodland R.M. & Jones B.R. (1977) Animal models for the study of chlamydial infections of the eye and genital tract. In *Non-Gonococcal Urethritis and Related Infections*. American Society of Microbiology, Washington D.C., pp. 186–98.

El Sheikh E.H.A. (1978) Feline chlamydial keratoconjunctivitis as an analogue of trachoma. PhD Thesis, University of London.

Gaillard E.T., Hargis A.M., Prieur D.J., Evermann J.F. & Dhillon A.S. (1984) Pathogenesis of feline gastric chlamydial infection. *Am. J. Vet. Res.* **45**, 2314–21.

Gaskell R.M. & Wardley R.C. (1978) Feline viral respiratory disease: a review with particular reference to its epizootiology and control. *J. Small Anim. Pract.* **19**, 1–16.

Gethings P.M., Stephens G.L., Wills J.M., Howard P.E.,

Balfour A.H., Wright A.I. & Morgan K.L. (1987) Prevalence of chlamydia, toxoplasma, toxocara and ringworm in farm cats in South West England. *Vet. Rec.* **121**, 213–6.

Gillespie J.H. & Timoney J.F. (1981) The Chlamydiaceae. In Hagen W.A. & Bruner D.W. (eds) *Infectious Diseases of Domestic Animals*, 7th edn. Cornell University Press, p. 334.

Gledhill A.W. (1952) Feline enteritis: paper presented to BVA Congress, 1952. *Vet. Rec.* **64**, 723–33.

Hargis A.M., Prieur D.J. & Gaillard E.T. (1983) Chlamydial infection of the gastric mucosa in twelve cats. *Vet. Pathol.* **20**, 170–8.

Hoover E.A., Kahn D.E. & Langloss J.M. (1978) Experimentally induced feline chlamydial infection (feline pneumonitis). *Am. J. Vet. Res.* **39**, 541–7.

Jahn G.J. & Bialasiewicz A.A. (1986) Keratokonjunktivitis durch *Chlamydia psittaci*. *Klin. Mbl. Augenheilk.* **188**, 47–9.

Johnson F.W.A. (1984) Isolation of *Chlamydia psittaci* from nasal and conjunctival exudate of a domestic cat. *Vet. Rec.* **114**, 342–4.

Kahn D.E. & Hoover E.A. (1976) Infectious respiratory diseases of cats. *Vet. Clin. North Am.* **6**(3), 399.

Kane J.L., Woodland R.M., Elder M.G. & Darougar S. (1985) Chlamydial pelvic infection in cats: a model for the study of human pelvic inflammatory disease. *Genitourin. Med.* **61**, 311–8.

Katz E. (1956) The activity of tetracycline on feline pneumonitis virus infection of chick embryos. *J. Infect. Dis.* **98**, 177.

Kolar J.R. & Rude T.A. (1977) Clinical evaluation of a commercial feline pneumonitis vaccine. *Feline Practice* **7**, 47–50.

McKercher D.G. (1952) Feline pneumonitis. I. Immunization studies in kittens. *Am. J. Vet. Res.* **13**, 557–61.

Mitzel J.R. & Strating A. (1977) Vaccination against feline pneumonitis. *Am. J. Vet. Res.* **38**, 1361–3.

Newberne J.W., Bittle J.L. & Mayer K. (1959) Clinical differentiation of feline viral diseases. *Allied Vet.* **30**, 50–3.

Osborne A.D. (1963) Conditions of importance in cat practice. Discussion after paper at BVA Congress 1963. *Vet. Rec.* **75**, 1206.

Ostler H.B. & Schachter J. (1972) Bedsonia (chlamydia) of epizootic origin. *Rev. Int. Trach.* **49**, 37–43.

Ostler H.B., Schachter J. & Dawson C.R. (1969) Acute follicular conjunctivitis of epizootic origin. *Arch. Ophthalmol.* **82**, 587–91.

Povey R.C. & Johnson R.H. (1971) A survey of feline viral rhinotracheitis and feline picornavirus infection in Britain. *J. Small. Anim. Pract.* **12**, 233–47.

Prydie J. (1969) Viral diseases of cats. *Vet. Rec.* **79**, 729–38.

Schachter J., Ostler H.B. & Meyer K.F. (1969) Human

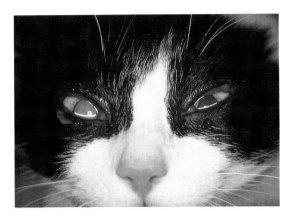

Plate 21.1 Blepharospasm and ocular discharges (serous and mucopurulent) in a domestic short-haired cat, 7 days after infection with *C. psittaci*.

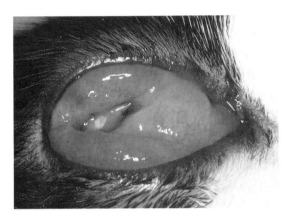

Plate 21.2 Severe case of chemosis, 7 days after infection.

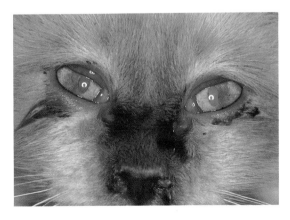

Plate 21.3 Birman cat with chlamydial conjunctivitis and secondary *Haemophilus* infection.

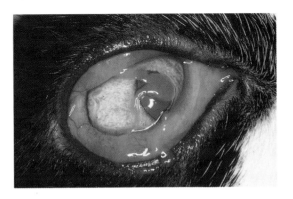

Plate 21.4 Severe hyperaemia with mucopurulent ocular discharge 16 days after infection. Same cat as Plate 21.1.

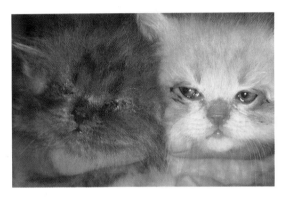

Plate 21.5 Eyelids sealed with mucopurulent ocular discharge in 6-week-old Persian kittens infected with *C. psittaci*.

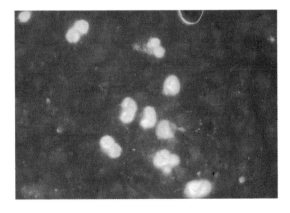

Plate 21.6 Green intracytoplasmic inclusions of *C. psittaci* in McCoy cells stained by indirect IF (or immunofluorescence) after 40 hours incubation.

infection with the agent of feline pneumonitis. *Lancet* **i**, 1063–5.

Shewen P.E., Povey R.C. & Wilson M.R. (1978) Feline chlamydial infection. *Can. Vet. J.* **19**, 289–92.

Shewen P.E., Povey R.C. & Wilson M.R. (1980) A comparison of the efficacy of a live and four inactivated vaccine preparations for the protection of cats against experimental challenge with *Chlamydia psittaci. Can J. Comp. Med.* **44**, 244–51.

Studdert M.J., Studdert V.P. & Wirth H.J. (1981) Isolation of *Chlamydia psittaci* from cats with conjunctivitis. *Aust. Vet. J.* **57**, 515–7.

Wills J.M. (1986a) Chlamydial infection in the cat. PhD Thesis, University of Bristol.

Wills J.M. (1986b) Chlamydial zoonoses. *J. Small Anim. Pract.* **27**, 717–31.

Wills J.M. (1988) Feline chlamydial infection (feline pneumonitis). In Chandler E.A. (ed) *Advances in Small Animal Practice 1*. Blackwell Scientific Publications, Oxford.

Wills J.M., Gruffydd-Jones T.J., Richmond S.J. & Paul I.D. (1984) Isolation of *Chlamydia psittaci* from cases of conjunctivitis in a colony of cats. *Vet. Rec.* **114**, 344–6.

Wills J.M., Millard W.G. & Howard P.E. (1986) Evaluation of a monoclonal antibody based ELISA for detection of feline *Chlamydia psittaci. Vet. Rec.* **119**, 418–20.

Wills J.M., Gruffydd-Jones T.J., Bourne F.J., Richmond S.J. & Gaskell R.M. (1987) Effect of vaccination on feline *Chlamydia psittaci* infection. *Infect. Immun.* **55**, 2653–7.

Wills J.M., Howard P.E., Gruffydd-Jones T.J. & Wathes C.E. (1988a) Prevalence of *Chlamydia psittaci* in different cat populations in Britain. *J. Small Anim. Pract.* **29**, 327–39.

Wills J.M., Roberts K., Richmond S.J. & Gruffydd-Jones T.J. (1988b) Transmission of feline *Chlamydia psittaci* from dam to kittens. In *Proceedings of the European Society for Chlamydia Research*, p. 61.

Woodland R.M., & Darougar S. (1986) Feline keratoconjunctivitis – an animal model of persistent chlamydial conjunctivitis. In Oriel D., Ridgway G., Schachter J., Taylor-Robinson D. & Ward M. (eds) *Chlamydial Infections*. Cambridge University Press, pp. 412–5.

Chapter 22 / Feline Infectious Anaemia

R. J. EVANS

INTRODUCTION

Parasitic infection of the red blood cells may give rise to haemolytic anaemia. Several such parasitic haemolytic anaemias are known in the cat. That due to *Haemobartonella felis* is known as feline infectious anaemia (FIA). It is the only one encountered in Britain and occurs worldwide. Feline infectious anaemia was first recognized in South Africa by Clark (1942). Although the overall incidence of the condition is probably not high, it is a widespread and troublesome clinical condition and diagnosis may prove difficult. Treatment of the condition may have an unsatisfactory outcome in some cases: relapses and fatalities are not uncommon. Understanding of the pathophysiology and epidemiology of the condition remains rudimentary. It now appears likely that uncomplicated haemobartonellosis causes little problem but that intercurrent conditions, particularly FeLV infection, may lead to the manifestation of clinical anaemia (Bobade *et al.*, 1988).

AETIOLOGY

The disease is associated with parasitism of the red blood cells by the rickettsial organism *Haemobartonella felis*, formerly known as *Eperythrozoon felis*. The organism is stained by Giemsa and other Romanowsky stains, by acridine orange (which is bound to DNA and RNA) and can also be demonstrated by immunofluorescence using specific antibodies. After Giemsa-staining the organisms appear as faintly to strongly purple ring-like or coccoid structures on the surface of the red

cell and as dots or rods around its periphery (Small & Ristic, 1967).

Electron microscopy reveals coccoid, rod and ring forms of the parasite and the coccoid forms may be in chains. The parasites are attached by fine filaments to the red cell membrane; they invaginate the membrane to form shallow pits and folds in which they lie. The parasites do not penetrate the membrane but do erode its surface (Demaree & Nesmith, 1972; Jain and Keeton, 1973).

The parasite has been described as reproducing by binary fission and by budding but its exact mode of replication remains unclear. The disease can be transmitted by infected blood but since the organism has not been cultured, Koch's postulates are not satisfied.

PATHOGENESIS

In experimentally infected cats a period of some 2–20 days elapses before the parasite is detectable on red blood cells (Harvey & Gaskin, 1977). The behaviour of the parasite in this period is not known; however, once parasitaemia is established single or recurrent anaemic crises may occur. After its appearance the parasitaemia increases until a period of rapid clearance, which may precede or accompany a fall in packed cell volume (PCV). The fall in packed cell volume may be due to red cell destruction or may be caused by red cell sequestration in the spleen; in the latter case the PCV may increase rapidly from its trough value after parasite clearance.

Red cell destruction in FIA appears to be primarily extravascular (Maede & Hata, 1975; Maede, 1978; Maede & Murat, 1978), although some would dispute this. The organism damages the erythrocyte membrane without puncturing it and there are alterations in the lipid composition of the membrane. There is a concomitant increase in red cell fragility which might be expected to produce some intravascular haemolysis. The finding of decreased haptoglobin concentrations in some affected animals supports this contention. There is, on the other hand, convincing evidence for splenic, hepatic and pulmonary sequestration of red blood cells and for erythrophagocytosis in the spleen and also the circulation. It also appears that splenic macrophages can pit the organism from the surface of the red cell with survival of the erythrocytes; release of such cells from the spleen probably accounts for the rapid increase in PCV which can sometimes be seen following clearance of the organism from the blood. Autoantibodies may have a role to play in red cell phagocytosis or lysis since it is reported that many cats with FIA become Coombs' positive. It has been reported that cold agglutinins are present in some animals infected with *H. felis* (Zulty & Kociba, 1990) but the validity of this finding has been questioned (Bücheler & Giger, 1991). There is evidence for shortening of red cell life span to around 50% of normal. Red cell destruction may well involve multiple mechanisms (Maede & Hata, 1975; Maede, 1978).

The fate of the parasite after pitting and phagocytosis is not known. Parasites have been visualized in phagocytic vacuoles (Maede & Murat, 1978). If parasites were able to survive and multiply in phagocytes this might explain the common occurrence of relapses.

EPIDEMIOLOGY

The epidemiology of FIA is poorly understood. The disease may occur in cats of any age but is more prevalent in younger animals, around 50% of cases being between 1 and 3 years of age. Males are seemingly at greater risk than females; there is no clear seasonal variation.

The disease can certainly be transmitted to healthy cats by the injection of a small volume of blood from an affected animal, or even by giving infected blood by mouth. There is no convincing evidence as to how the organism is transmitted naturally. Small epizootics are occasionally seen in colonies (Ojeda & Skives, 1978) but it is usually a disease of individual cats. Arthropod ectoparasites, fight wounds and bites have all been proposed as mechanisms of transmission although none can be considered proven (Harbutt, 1963). The higher incidence in male cats may be related to fighting. There is some evidence to support the possibility of transmission from dam to kittens and this may occur *in utero*.

The epidemiology is complicated by the incidence of silent carriers. It is not known whether these cats can spread the organism or whether transmission only occurs in the clinically active phase of infection. It has been assumed that the carrier state is of clinical importance. FIA is considered to be stress-related, with the implication that stress or intercurrent disease could precipitate clinical disease in carriers. In a study (Harvey & Gaskin, 1978) of experimentally infected cats, all the cats developed an acute haemolytic crisis and some cats had repeated episodes. All the cats that survived this acute phase became carriers, some after a single crisis. This study challenges the concept of stress-induced recrudescence of disease in carrier animals. Immunosuppression of carrier animals with cyclophosphamide or 6-mercaptopurine produced no flare-up of parasitaemia. Splenectomy or glucocorticoid administration induced moderate parasitaemia but no clinical signs. None the less, clinically there is a correlation between the occurrence of clinically apparent FIA and feline leukaemia virus (FeLV) infection (Essex *et al.*, 1975; Bobade *et al.*, 1988) or the presence of other intercurrent disease (Bobade *et al.*, 1988). This has been thought to be due to the stress of intercurrent disease or to immunosuppression by FeLV. It seems likely that FeLV and *Haemobartonella* infection have a synergistic effect in the induction of anaemia (Bobade *et al.*, 1988).

Infected animals develop antibodies directed

against *Haemobartonella felis*. It is not known whether these protect the cat against reinfection or what effect they may have on the course of infection.

CLINICAL SIGNS

Infection with *Haemobartonella felis* may be clinically inapparent. Clinical disease is more common when there is also FeLV infection or other intercurrent disease (Bobade *et al.*, 1988). When clinical disease does result from infection, the course may be acute, subacute or chronic. The main features of the disease are those associated with any anaemia, but the balance of signs depends on the severity and rate of onset.

Most commonly the chronic manifestation of the condition is encountered. There is generally a history of lethargy, weakness, anorexia and chronic weight loss. The disease shows an undulant course with cycles of haemolysis giving a progressive decline in PCV and haemoglobin levels. The cat's general condition may fluctuate, with periods of relapse and remission, and the ability of the cat to adapt its life style often results in such animals being severely anaemic on presentation. The mucous membranes show moderate to marked pallor, capillary refill time is prolonged and the pulse collapsing. Tachycardia is often present, sometimes with an accompanying haemic murmur and increased apical impulse. Pyrexia is a less common finding, being noted in about a fifth of cases, and dehydration may occasionally be present. There is slight to moderate lymph node enlargement in about 10–15% of cases, and occasionally splenomegaly. The animal may be tachypnoeic at rest or on slight exertion.

The subacute course results in similar signs but is more rapidly progressive and less obviously undulant.

The acute disease is the rarest form seen clinically and presents with a haemolytic crisis. There is apathy, anorexia, weakness and often collapse. The animal may be markedly dyspnoeic. Icterus and haemoglobinuria may occur but are found only occasionally even in acute disease. Animals may die within hours of signs appearing and moribund animals may be hypothermic. Many animals do, however, survive acute haemolytic crises.

DIAGNOSIS

The clinical signs associated with anaemia are non-specific and the diagnosis of feline infectious anaemia depends upon laboratory investigation. Haematological examination reveals an anaemia. In mild cases the anaemia may be normochromic and normocytic, and this is particularly the case in animals in which FeLV is not also present (Bobade *et al.*, 1988). In more severe cases the features are of a macrocytic regenerative anaemia, often with a haemoglobin of 4 g/dl or less, unless there is some intercurrent disease interfering with the marrow response. There is marked anisocytosis and polychromasia with some poikilocytosis. The mean cell volume is increased and may reach 100–105 fl because of a prominent reticulocytosis. The majority of erythrocytes may be reticulocytes and large numbers of nucleated red cells may be present in the circulation. Intermediate as well as late normoblasts may be found. The MCHC may be reduced. Howell–Jolly bodies are present in a much increased proportion of the red blood cells. Late in the disease marrow aplasia may supervene and the anaemia becomes non-regenerative. Bilirubinaemia may also be detected.

The critical diagnostic criterion is the identification of the causal organism in stained blood films, in association with an appropriate anaemia. This, however, presents biological, technical and interpretative difficulties. First, as already mentioned, the parasitaemia is transient or cyclical. Marked parasitaemia may last a number of days but occurs just prior to the haemolytic episode, which is generally associated with clearance of the organism. By the time the affected animal is presented with clinically obvious disease, very few or no parasites may be detectable on a blood film. Thus a single negative finding does not rule out the condition. It is necessary, therefore, to examine a number of blood films, over a period of 4–10 days, before it may be concluded that the patient has, or is free from, the infection. The parasite may detach from the red cells during storage of anticoagulated samples. Films for examination for the presence of *H. felis* should therefore be prepared immediately after blood is drawn, preferably without the addition of anticoagulant, and gently dried by waving them in the air.

The staining of smears requires attention to detail if they are to be of diagnostic quality (see Butt, 1990, for detailed discussion). Blood smears in which the organism has been stained either by acridine orange or by immunofluorescence are the most sensitive, and are in good agreement. These techniques are, however, beyond the scope of many practice laboratories, and less sensitive Romanowsky staining techniques are normally used: Giemsa is probably the most satisfactory but the organism is also well shown by Wright's stain. Precipitates readily form in solutions of these stains and the resulting deposits can be difficult to differentiate from the parasite. Attention to details in staining technique, in order to avoid such artefacts, is therefore essential. The slides used should be scrupulously clean and grease-free (acid-alcohol washed) and the stain should be filtered before use. Slides are best stained inverted over a shallow trough or dish and the stain solution should not be allowed to dry out. The film should be thoroughly but gently washed with a stream of purified water prior to drying and examination.

The stained film should be searched carefully for the single or multiple, round, rod-shaped or ring-form organisms in the size range 0.8–1.5 μm lying attached to red cell membranes. The parasites are sometimes seen lying free in the intercellular spaces, probably due to detachment of the organism from erythrocytes during sample storage.

The white cell changes in this disease are highly variable. In the early stages a marked neutrophilia may occur but later in the course of the disease neutropenia is not unusual. This may be related to concurrent FeLV infection in many cases. Bizarre monocytoid cells, some of which have phagocytosed red cells, may be encountered.

Since emergence of clinical FIA appears to be associated with stress, with intercurrent disease and particularly with FeLV infection, it is essential that investigation of such cases is not abandoned once the diagnosis of FIA is secure. Underlying disease should be sought diligently and in particular all cases of FIA should be tested for FeLV and FIV.

As with many haematological conditions, a diagnosis of FIA must be made during life because post-mortem examination, although it can provide corroborative evidence, cannot be diagnostic. At necropsy generalized pallor of the carcass is noted whilst jaundice is only occasionally present. There is often emaciation and the lymph nodes are slightly to moderately enlarged. The spleen is usually substantially enlarged with a bulging cut surface and, in some cases, hepatomegaly is also noted. The red marrow is increased in extent in the long bones and is solid in texture.

Histological examination often reveals extramedullary haemopoiesis, erythrophagocytosis and haemosiderin deposition. The lymph nodes show reactive hyperplasia. Many plasma cells are present in the spleen and lymph nodes. In the liver, centrilobular anoxic necrosis is noted. The bone marrow is hypercellular but the cells are present in approximately normal proportions. In chronic cases, less marked changes are often found and, as mentioned, marrow aplasia may occur.

TREATMENT

The treatment of feline infectious anaemia has two main elements. First, every effort should be made to eliminate the causal organism although this is rarely successful. The drug of choice is generally considered to be oxytetracycline (20 mg/kg t.i.d.) but doxycycline (5 mg/kg daily p.o.) can also be used. Therapy should be continued for at least 14 days and further blood films should be examined for the presence of the parasite before and after discontinuing treatment.

Second, supportive measures may be needed of which the most useful is blood transfusion (see Chapter 4 for details) if the PCV is below 0.15 l/l.

Fluid therapy may be considered but it must be appreciated that haemodilution will aggravate the anaemia and its effect on oxygen transport. Other supportive therapy may be helpful; in particular, vitamin supplementation and a high-protein diet can be of some value. The administration of haematinics is not indicated. The administration of immunosuppressive doses of glucocorticoids has been advocated in the belief that autoantibodies contribute significantly to the haemolysis but their value is unsubstantiated.

PROGNOSIS

It is difficult to give an accurate assessment of the prognosis of FIA although a mortality rate of around 25% is often cited. In an experimental study (Harvey & Gaskin, 1977), every cat that recovered became a carrier and this is also probably the case in natural infection. The incidence of development of the carrier state is apparently substantially lower after successful therapy of milder cases. None the less relapses are not uncommon and, after a short period of remission, anaemia may develop again and prove fatal. Careful observation of apparently recovered cats is, therefore, desirable. The carrier state may persist for many months and relapses may be triggered by intercurrent disease.

OTHER INFECTIOUS ANAEMIAS

Other red cell parasites which give rise to infectious haemolytic anaemias are recognized. On the African continent, the protozoon *Babesia felis* is found in the domestic cat. It has also been encountered in a variety of other cat species, both in the wild and in collections. In the southern USA another protozoal species, *Cytauxzoon felis*, produces a rapidly fatal disease for which there is no effective therapy (Keir, 1984).

REFERENCES

Bobade P.A., Nash A.R. & Rogerson P. (1988) Feline haemobartonellosis: clinical, haematological and pathological studies in natural infections and the relationship to infection with feline leukaemia virus. *Vet. Rec.* **122**, 32–6.

Bücheler J. & Giger U. (1991) Cold agglutinins in feline haemobartonellosis. *J. Amer. Vet. Med. Assoc.* **198**, 740.

Butt M.T. (1990) Diagnosing erythrocyte parasitic diseases in cats. *Compend. Contin. Educ. Pract. Vet.* **12**, 628–38.

Clark P. (1942) *Eperythrozoon felis* (sp. nov.) in a cat. *J. S. Afr. Med. Ass.* **13**, 15–6.

Demaree R.S. Jr & Nesmith W.B. (1972) Ultrastructure of *Haemobartonella felis* from a naturally infected cat. *Amer. J. Vet. Res.* **33**, 103.

Essex M., Cotter S.M., Hardy W.D., Hess P., Jarrett W., Jarrett O. *et al.* (1975) Feline oncornavirus-associated cell membrane antigen IV. Antibody titres in cats with naturally occurring lymphoma, leukaemia and other diseases. *J. Natl. Cancer Inst.* **55**, 463–7.

Harbutt P.R. (1963) A clinical appraisal of feline infectious anaemia and its transmission under natural conditions. *Austr. Vet. J.* **39**, 401–4.

Harvey J.W. & Gaskin J.M. (1977) Experimental feline haemobartonellosis. *J. Amer. Anim. Hosp. Assoc.* **13**, 28.

Harvey J.W. & Gaskin J.M. (1978) Feline haemobartonellosis: attempts to induce relapses of clinical disease in chronically infected animals. *J. Amer. Anim. Hosp. Assoc.* **14**, 453.

Jain N.C. & Keeton K.S. (1973) Scanning electron-microscopic features of *Haemobartonella felis*. *Amer. J. Vet. Res.* **34**, 697–700.

Kier A.B. (1984) Cytauxzoonosis. In Greene C.E. (ed) *Clinical Microbiology and Infectious Diseases of the Dog and Cat*. W.B. Saunders, Philadelphia, pp. 791–5.

Maede Y. (1978) Studies on feline haemobartonellosis V. Role of spleen in cats infected with *H. felis*. *Jap. J. Vet. Sci.* **40**, 141–6.

Maede Y. & Hata R. (1975) Studies on feline haemobartonellosis II. The mechanism of anaemia produced by infection with *Haemobartonella felis*. *Jap. J. Vet. Sci.* **37**, 49–54.

Maede Y. & Murat H. (1978) Ultrastructural observations on the removal of *H. felis* from erythrocytes in the spleen of a cat. *Jap. J. Vet. Sci.* **40**, 203–5.

Ojeda J.H. & Skives H.R. (1967) Haemobartonella infection of cats: report of an outbreak and its treatment. *Vet. Mexico* **9**, 55–60.

Small E. & Ristic M. (1967) Morphological features of *Haemobartonella felis*. *Amer. J. Vet. Res.* **28**, 845–51.

Zulty J.C. & Kociba G.J. (1990) Cold agglutinins in cats with haemobartonellosis. *J. Amer. Vet. Med. Assoc.* **196**, 907–10.

Chapter 23 / Other Feline Infections

M. BENNETT AND K. WILLOUGHBY

The aim of this chapter is to discuss some of the infectious diseases and significant asymptomatic infections of cats not covered elsewhere in this book. A thorough discussion of every type of feline infection reported is obviously not possible, and we have attempted to concentrate on those infections which occur most commonly or which may be zoonotic.

BACTERIAL DISEASES

Feline abscess

Abscesses and cellulitis are probably the most common infections encountered in cats. They are mostly due to bites and scratches received through fighting with other cats, but occasionally with other species, for example rats. Wounds may also be caused by other means and the possibility of foreign bodies, including grass seed-heads and airgun pellets, should be investigated. Infection often involves several bacterial species, anaerobes and facultative anaerobes being most frequently isolated in surveys, e.g. *Pasteurella multocida*, *Bacteroides*, *Streptococcus* and *Fusobacterium* and sometimes *Actinomyces*, *Nocardia* or *Rhodococcus*. Enteric bacteria such as *E. coli* are also commonly found in wound infections.

The clinical signs vary according to site and severity. Abscesses due to bite or scratch wounds are generally found on the head, leg, back or base of tail. They are usually painful, often accompanied by pyrexia, depression, inappetence and enlarged local lymph nodes. Large, mature abscesses can be palpated, but they may be less obvious early in development, and owners often notice only the systemic signs or behavioural changes. Diagnosis is based on clinical signs and history, careful examination, and may be aided by haematology. Possible sequelae depend on the site of the abscess, but may include pyothorax, osteomyelitis, rhinitis, otitis, meningitis or pyaemia with localization at distant sites. Perhaps surprisingly, in view of the frequency with which cat abscesses occur, bacterial endocarditis is rare.

Treatment depends on the extent of infection and stage of development of the abscess. Antibiotics are generally unable to penetrate abscess walls, but may be useful for treating cellulitis and help prevent recurrence after drainage and other complications. The penicillins and their derivatives (ampicillin and amoxycillin) are effective against most abscess-forming bacteria, with cephalosporins, lincomycin, clindamycin and metronidazole as second choice for their particular activity against anaerobes. In addition, a single injection of penicillin G given within 24 hours of being bitten may prevent the development of cellulitis and/or abscess formation. Surgical drainage should only be undertaken once the abscess has matured, a process which can be enhanced by the use of warm saline compresses. Surgically or naturally drained abscesses can be debrided if necessary, cleaned with either a proprietary wound cleaner (e.g. Dermasol*), dilute

* Dermasol; SmithKline Beecham, Animal Health, Tadworth, Surrey, UK.

hydrogen peroxide or cetrimide solutions, there-after being left open for drainage. Partial suturing and drain placement is rarely indicated as even large deficits usually heal rapidly.

If abscesses recur or persist, a more thorough investigation is called for. An undetected foreign body may still be present or complications as listed above may have developed, requiring further surgery as appropriate. Alternatively, a persistent infection with less common agents such as *Mycobacterium*, *Nocardia*, *Actinomyces*, *Dermatophilus*, or fungi may have developed, or the cat may be immunosuppressed by concurrent infection with feline immunodeficiency virus (FIV) or feline leukaemia virus (FeLV). Myco-plasmas have also been isolated from feline abscesses. Squamous cell carcinoma may mimic chronic abscessation.

Castration can be effective at reducing the incidence of cat bite abscesses in males, even in adult cats.

Actinomycosis and nocardiosis

Members of the genera *Actinomyces* and *Nocardia* are Gram-positive, pleomorphic branching rods and filaments which can be dif-ficult to distinguish except by culture. They are both facultative anaerobic bacteria, but whereas *Actinomyces* spp. are part of the normal flora of the oral cavity and respiratory tract, *Nocardia* spp. are common soil saprophytes. Both can cause persistent pyogranulomatous lesions in cats, and are most frequently isolated from abscesses, cellulitis and pyothorax. *Nocardia* spp. are more rarely isolated than *Actinomyces* spp. and may cause more severe disease with marked regional lymph node involvement. Pus from lesions caused by either organism frequently contains 'sulphur granules' consisting of bacterial colonies and dead tissue. Actinomycosis and nocardiosis can be dif-ficult to treat, and, whatever the site of the lesion, drainage and removal of pus is essential if sub-sequent antibiotic therapy is to be effective. *Actinomyces* spp. are usually susceptible to penicillins, but, unlike many other anaerobes, are not sensitive to metronidazole. *Nocardia* spp. are

often sensitive only to sulphonamides with or without potentiation, but an antibacterial sen-sitivity test should be carried out to find the appropriate antibacterial agent.

Chlamydiosis

Chlamydia psittaci var. *felis* is a frequent cause of chronic conjunctivitis and, less commonly, of upper respiratory tract disease in cats (see Chapter 21). It has also been isolated from vaginal swabs of queens both with and without repro-ductive failure or abortion, and the significance of infection of the reproductive tract is therefore currently unknown. The strains responsible for feline infection are readily distinguishable from avian and ovine strains in cell culture and by genetic methods. Although some anecdotal ac-counts of zoonotic spread exist, there is no good evidence that feline chlamydiosis poses any risk to human health.

Bordetellosis

Bordetella bronchiseptica may infect the feline upper respiratory tract secondary to a primary viral infection, and, in some circumstances, *B. bronchiseptica* may be a primary pathogen and a cause of purulent bronchopneumonia in cats (see Chapters 6 and 14).

Streptococcal infections

Beta-haemolytic streptococci of Lancefield group G are part of the normal flora of the upper respiratory tract, oropharynx, lower genital tract and skin of cats. Most cats probably become infected at birth from their mother's genital tract, with infection entering through the umbilicus and then spreading to various sites around the body via the liver. In otherwise healthy kittens born of older queens, maternal antibody protects against clinical disease, but in young kittens born of younger queens, or when the kittens or queen is immunocompromised by FeLV or other infec-tions, septicaemia and severe systemic disease, often culminating in death, may develop. In older kittens, up to about 6 months old, subclinical infection in the tonsils may develop into clinically apparent tonsillitis and cervical lymphadenopathy, but rarely more severe disease unless, again, the cats are immunosuppressed.

Streptococci are also frequently isolated from wounds and abscesses in adult cats and as opportunist pathogens secondary to upper respiratory and other mucosal infections.

Streptococci are susceptible to penicillins, and early treatment with penicillin, together with cleansing of abscesses or wounds, is usually effective. In colonies with a history of neonatal disease, topical application of antiseptic to the navel and treatment at birth with a long-acting penicillin or penicillin derivative may help prevent further disease.

In addition to group G streptococci, cats can also harbour asymptomatic infections of group A streptococci in their oropharynx. These infections are acquired from man, and can be transmitted back to man. Hence a family pet may become a reservoir for human infection and the source of recurrent tonsillitis or pharyngitis in a family. Isolation of group A streptococci from a cat's oropharynx may be difficult, and if a cat is suspected of being a source of human infection it may be advisable to treat the cat anyway with penicillin or a cephalosporin.

Tuberculosis, feline leprosy and other mycobacterial infections

Cats can be infected with *Mycobacterium tuberculosis*, *M. bovis*, *M. avium* or *M. microti*, which cause tuberculosis, or *M. lepraemurium*, the cause of feline leprosy. In addition, various other mycobacteria may be involved in chronic wounds and abscesses.

Tuberculosis

Tuberculosis is a rare disease of cats. *M. tuberculosis* and *M. bovis* infection is generally contracted through contact with infected humans, although cattle and certain wild mammals might be an alternative source of *M. bovis* infection in some areas. *M. avium* is a saprophyte found in soil and water, and only an opportunist pathogen of animals and man, while the main source of *M. microti* is believed to be voles. *M. avium* and *M. microti* infections are extremely rare in cats.

Tuberculosis may be acquired by the respiratory, gastrointestinal or percutaneous routes. Infection is most often subclinical, but, if clinical signs do develop, they generally reflect the location of granulomas. Chronic ulcerative infections of the oropharynx, tonsils and draining lymph nodes or bronchopneumonia may present as retching, a non-productive cough, dysphagia or hypersalivation. Anorexia, wasting, vomiting or diarrhoea may accompany intestinal malabsorption owing to granuloma formation in the alimentary tract. Pleural or peritoneal effusions may also be present, and intestinal infection often causes palpably enlarged mesenteric lymph nodes. Skin and ocular forms can also occur in the cat.

Diagnosis is by history and demonstration of acid-fast organisms in biopsies or smears of exudates. Isolation may be possible on special media, but can be a lengthy process. Radiography may reveal large granulomas in the respiratory tract or abdomen. Skin tests are unreliable work in cats. Very often diagnosis is made at necropsy.

Improvement of clinical signs following treatment of cats with either isoniazid or streptomycin has been reported, but was not considered to have produced bacteriological cure. Successful treatment of dogs experimentally infected with *M. tuberculosis* has been reported with rifampicin, isoniazid and streptomycin for 23 months.

Although zoonotic spread from cats and dogs has not been reported, cats can excrete *M. tuberculosis* and *M. bovis* in exudates and faeces. Elderly or immunosuppressed owners might be particularly at risk, and euthanasia of the cat should therefore be considered on public health grounds. The zoonotic risk of *M. avium* infection has not been reported, but infection from a common source is probably as likely as zoonotic spread.

Feline leprosy

Feline leprosy is caused by *M. lepraemurium* ('rat leprosy'). It is an uncommon condition thought to be contracted from rat bites. The lesions develop between 2 weeks and several months following injury, and generally consist of single or multiple, fleshy, sometimes ulcerated nodules on the head or extremities. Unlike skin tuberculosis, caseation is not a feature of feline leprosy. Spread of the infection up a limb may be accompanied by lymphangitis and regional lymphadenopathy. Diagnosis depends on finding acid-fast organisms in impression smears or biopsies. *M. lepraemurium* is very difficult to grow *in vitro*, so isolation is not usually attempted. Treatment is by surgical removal, but local infiltration with streptomycin, oral rifampicin or dapsone at 50 mg twice a day for 2 weeks may be worth trying when complete surgical excision is not possible. Haemolytic anaemia and neurotoxicity have been reported with the use of dapsone in cats, and the canine dose rate of 1 mg/kg three times daily may be advisable. Even following apparently successful surgical excision, recurrence at the same or other sites may occur.

Other atypical mycobacterial infections

Various saprophytic mycobacteria have been isolated from superficial or, more rarely, deeper, persistent abscesses or ulcerative or granulomatous lesions of cats. Sinus formation is common but lymphatic involvement is unusual. Species isolated from these 'atypical' mycobacterial infections of cats include *M. fortuitum-M. chelonei* complex, *M. smegmatis*, *M. xenopi* and *M. phlei*. It is thought that the organisms obtain entry through a wound into already damaged or concurrently infected tissue. In man, infection is often associated with immunosuppression. Diagnosis depends on the demonstration of acid-fast organisms in impression smears or biopsies. Mycobacterial organisms may be scarce in lesion material and easily missed. Treatment includes surgical removal of as much of the lesion as possible, and at least 6 weeks of antibiotic therapy: gentamicin, amikacin and potentiated sulphonamides have been used with apparent success. Some lesions heal spontaneously, but the prognosis for such infections is guarded as recurrence is common.

Tyzzer's disease

This is an uncommon disease of cats caused by *Bacillus piliformis*, which is part of the normal intestinal flora of many rodent species, but can cause clinical disease if the host animal is stressed or immunosuppressed in some way. Cats are thought to become infected through contact with rodents, and may also be more susceptible to disease if immunosuppressed or under stress. The bacteria originally replicate inside intestinal epithelial cells, may cause ileocolitis and, given the right conditions, spread via the portal vein to cause focal necrotic hepatitis. Clinical signs include rapid onset of anorexia, depression, abdominal pain, hepatomegaly and abdominal distension, jaundice and death within 2 days. A diagnosis is usually made post mortem.

Leptospirosis

Clinical leptospirosis is rare in cats, despite the presence of antibody to leptospires in some cat populations. Surveys from various countries have demonstrated antibody in 5–20% of cats, and in Britain antibody has been demonstrated in 6.8% of cats. Various serovars have been isolated from individual cases, including *icterohaemorrhagiae*, *pomona* and *bratislava*. The pathogenesis of experimental leptospirosis in the cat is similar to the dog, yet clinical signs rarely appear despite development of bacteraemia and histological evidence of renal and hepatic inflammatory responses. Clinical signs, if present, are referable to acute systemic illness or renal and hepatic disease. Cats have been shown to be capable of excreting the organism in urine for up to 3 months following experimental infection.

Salmonellosis

Cats are extremely resistant to experimental infection with *Salmonella* spp., and clinical salmonellosis is uncommon in cats, although epidemics may occur, especially in kittens. When it does occur clinical salmonellosis is often associated with concurrent enteric infections or immunosuppression. Surveys of the prevalence of *Salmonella* spp. in cat faeces vary between 1% and 20%. Salmonellae were isolated from 7% of enteric or faecal samples from cats at Liverpool University in 1991, although this figure is probably an underestimate as selective media were not used in most cases. The serotypes isolated are mostly *S. typhimurium*, but reflect local conditions and include whatever serotypes dominate at the time.

Although most cases of salmonellosis in cats are asymptomatic, clinical syndromes reported associated with infection include acute and chronic gastroenteritis, and pyrexic episodes (up to 106°F, 41°C) lasting several days, sometimes accompanied by vomiting, pneumonia, conjunctivitis, abortion, stillbirths and fading kittens. Severe infection may result in bacteraemia and endotoxaemia, with depression, hypothermia and collapse. Transient bacteraemias sometimes result in abscess formation in internal organs such as the liver, lung, spleen, lymph nodes or bone marrow with subsequent clinical signs appropriate to the affected organ.

Treatment should initially be symptomatic, and may include supportive fluid therapy in severe cases. Antibiotics should be avoided whenever possible as they rarely eliminate the organism, may cause selection of resistant strains and may prolong shedding. When systemic disease occurs and antibacterial treatment is necessary, the choice of antibiotic must be based on the results of a sensitivity test as many salmonellae carry multi-resistance plasmids. Salmonellosis is one of the most common zoonotic infections, and can cause severe illness, and even death, in man. The role played by pet animals in the epidemiology of salmonellosis has not been thoroughly studied, although it seems likely that cats are far less important as a source of human infection than are food animals and other humans. In an outbreak, the possibility of humans having been the source of infection for cats should not be ignored.

Other enteric bacterial infections

Escherichia coli

Although a much studied cause of enteritis and systemic disease in man and animals, little is known about the role played by *E. coli* in feline disease. *E. coli* form part of the normal flora of the alimentary tract, but some recent studies suggest that some cases of acute diarrhoea might be caused by *E. coli* capable of producing a verotoxin (VT) apparently related to the VT1 produced by enteropathogenic *E. coli* of other species. Further work is required to determine fully the role of toxigenic *E. coli* in feline enteritis.

E. coli can often be isolated from the urine of healthy cats, although many such isolations probably reflect faecal contamination of the sample. High numbers ($>10^3$/ml urine), however, may be associated with pyelonephritis or acute cystitis. *E. coli* are also frequently isolated from many sites and the blood of fading kittens, from abscesses, wounds, pyometra and from peritonitis following bowel injuries or rupture.

The antibiotics used to treat *E. coli* infections in cats should be chosen with regard to the site of the infection (for example, urinary tract, enteric or superficial infections) and an antibiotic sensitivity test. As part of the normal flora of the gut, *E. coli* are exposed to almost all the antibiotics ever given to a cat and also have frequent contact with *E. coli* from other animals, including the cat's owners. Although they may not themselves colonize the cat's gut, these exogenous *E. coli* may be a source of resistance factors to the normal flora. *E. coli* are therefore particularly likely to be multi-resistant to antibiotics. Most isolates are resistant to ampicillin and tetracycline, so other agents should be used while awaiting the results of an antibiotic sensitivity test.

Campylobacter infection

Cats can become infected with several species of *Campylobacter* although most reports concern the isolation of *C. jejuni*. Surveys suggest that 5% of cats may be excreting *C. jejuni* in their faeces, and, as in dogs, there is no clear association between infection and disease. It may be that clinical campylobacteriosis is usually secondary to infection with other enteric pathogens such as coronaviruses or *E. coli*. Some *Campylobacter* strains are difficult to isolate, and diagnosis may depend on getting faecal samples in transport medium rapidly to the laboratory.

Campylobacteriosis is a common cause of enteritis in man, especially in young children, and cats and dogs are frequently blamed for human infection. Although owners should be warned of the zoonotic potential of campylobacteriosis if it is diagnosed in a cat, it may be that cats, dogs and their owners are frequently infected from a common source rather than the pet being the main source of human infection. Recently, jackdaws pecking at milk bottles have been incriminated in several outbreaks of human disease in the UK, and many birds, particularly carrion feeders, excrete *Campylobacter* in their faeces.

Yersiniosis and pseudotuberculosis

Yersinia enterocolitica and *Y. pseudotuberculosis* can be isolated from the faeces of many animals, including cats and dogs, and are therefore also frequent soil contaminants. They generally cause no clinical signs in cats, although *Y. pseudotuberculosis* can cause non-ulcerative gastritis and enteritis, abdominal lymphadenitis and multiple caseous abscesses in the liver, kidneys and spleen.

In man, particularly young children, both can cause severe disease. Most often the source of human infection cannot be traced, but there are reports of children becoming infected with *Y. pseudotuberculosis* through direct contact with cat faeces in sand pits. If a cat is shown to be shedding *Y. enterocolitica* or *Y. pseudotuberculosis* in its faeces, then treatment with tetracycline or potentiated sulphonomides may be thought appropriate.

Anaerobiospirillum

Anaerobiospirillum is a genus of motile spiral bacteria some species of which are a normal part of the intestinal flora of cats and dogs; in one survey they were isolated from the faeces of 7/10 cats and 3/10 dogs. They are not, however, part of the normal human intestinal flora, and their

isolation in human faeces is often associated with enteritis and diarrhoea in children. There are several reports providing good evidence of zoonotic spread from puppies to babies, and it is probable that cats can also be a source of human infection.

***Capnocytophaga* (DF-2 and DF-2-like) infection**

Capnocytophaga is a genus of fastidious, non-motile, Gram-negative, pleomorphic bacilli. They are frequently isolated from the oropharynx and faeces of cats and dogs, in which they cause no disease. Human infection occurs through bites and scratches, and is also generally asymptomatic. In immunocompromised individuals, however, *C. canimorsus* (originally called dysgonic fermenter-2, DF-2) can cause septicaemia, severe systemic illness, meningitis, coma and death, and even in immunologically normal children it may cause severe keratitis if inoculated into the eye by, for example, a cat scratch. *C. cynodegmi* (previously known as DF-2-like organism) is usually associated with less severe human disease, in particular with localized wound infections.

Eugonic fermenters

Eugonic fermenter-4 (EF-4), is a Gram-negative bacterium with cultural properties similar to those of *Pasteurella*. It is apparently part of the normal commensal flora of the oral cavity of cats and dogs, and is also isolated from bite wounds of both animals and man. EF-4 has also been associated with fatal pneumonia in cats, causing severe dyspnoea or sudden death. Recent transportation or other stresses may be predisposing factors.

Tetanus

Cats are even less susceptible to tetanus than dogs, and feline tetanus is therefore a very uncommon condition. *Clostridium tetani* replicates in the gut of many animals, and is excreted in their faeces, but toxin produced in the intestine is largely destroyed by digestion. Clinical signs are caused by the production of a toxin, tetanospasmin, by the organism growing anaerobically in a wound. Spastic paralysis first develops in muscles nearest the wound, usually within 2 weeks of trauma. The cat may first develop paralysis in one limb before the toxin's effects spread to involve more of the CNS. Generalized tetanus is characterized by stiffness of all limbs and contracture of facial muscles, making the ears erect and giving the animal a surprised look. Protrusion of the nictitating membrane, trismus and loss of voluntary defecation and urination may occur. Treatment involves thorough debridement and cleansing of the wound, and administration of intravenous penicillin for at least 5 days. Prompt therapy with antitoxin has been recommended either intravenously (100–500 μm/kg) or by local infiltration, but as it does not penetrate the CNS, the efficacy of treatment with antitoxin is debatable. Such treatment also carries some risk of anaphylactic reactions to the antiserum. Animals should be kept in a quiet and darkened room and disturbed as little as possible as they may be hyperaesthetic to touch and noise. Benzodiazepine, barbiturate or phenothiazine group drugs may be helpful to control tetanic spasms. General nursing care is also important to empty the bladder and rectum and to ensure adequate nutrition and hydration. Nutritional support (enteral or parenteral) may be necessary.

Botulism

Botulism is caused not by infection but by ingestion of *Clostridium botulinum* toxin in water or food. Cats are very resistant to botulinum toxin, and the disease is therefore very rare. Experimentally, the clinical signs develop within hours or over a week or more, depending on the amount of toxin ingested, and include muscle weakness, paresis and flaccid paralysis. Paralysis of the iris may cause a decreased pupillary reflex, and paralysis of the tongue and muscles involved in swallowing may result in dysphagia. Urinary retention and constipation may follow autonomic paralysis. Treatment is supportive: antibiotics,

laxatives and enemas may help remove any ingested clostridia and toxins; enteral or parenteral nutrition may be necessary; and the bladder may need to be emptied by manual pressure, catheterization or by cystocentesis.

Plague

In some parts of North America, cats can become infected with the plague organism through contact with wild mammals or their fleas. They may pass the infection on to man, veterinary surgeons being particularly at risk. The prevalence of *Yersinia pestis* infection in European wildlife is not known but is probably low, and the risk of feline infection in Europe is therefore probably small. The most common form of the disease in cats is bubonic plague, clinical signs of which include pyrexia, dehydration and lymphadenopathy. Septicaemic plague is often fatal within several days with few signs other than collapse and shock. Pneumonic plague is rare in cats.

Cat scratch disease

Cat scratch disease is not a disease of cats but of man. It is a usually benign, self-limiting lymphadenopathy, most commonly seen in children. Lymphadenopathy generally develops within about 2 weeks of the appearance of a papule, characteristically at the site of a cat scratch, but often at the site of a wound from another cause. Although around 30% of patients may have suffered no known cat scratch, over 95% of patients have had recent contact with a cat or dog. More severe forms of the disease, including systemic disease, may occur in up to 10% of patients, and are more common in those with HIV infection. The cause appears to be either *Afipia felis* and/or *Rochalimae henselae*. Both the organisms are difficult to grow in the laboratory, and laboratory diagnosis can only be undertaken at a few specialist centres.

Mycoplasma infection

Little is known about the role played by *Myco-plasma felis* in feline disease. *M. felis* can be isolated from many cases of upper respiratory tract disease, but is thought to be mainly a secondary pathogen. Some workers have suggested that *M. felis* may be a primary cause of conjunctivitis, at least in some cases, but other workers have isolated it from the conjunctiva of apparently healthy cats. *M. felis* has also been associated with reproductive disorders in cats, with pneumonia and with abscesses and pyothorax. The other *Mycoplasma* species most frequently isolated from cats is *M. gateae*. This organism appears to be part of the normal flora of the cat's oropharynx, respiratory and reproductive tracts, but has also been associated with polyarthritis. Other *Mycoplasma* species have also been isolated from cats and their role in disease is not known.

Other bacterial infections

Listeria monocytogenes is a rare cause of disease in cats. Following ingestion, septicaemia and widespread microabscess formation can occur causing signs related to the organs most affected. Anthrax (caused by *Bacillus anthracis*) can also infect cats, usually causing severe inflammation and necrosis of the upper alimentary tract, head and neck. Feline anthrax is extremely rare, and is a notifiable disease. *Brucella canis* can infect cats experimentally, but field infection does not occur.

FUNGAL INFECTIONS

Mycetoma

Mycetomas are chronic pyogranulomatous actinomycotic or mycotic infections of the skin and deeper tissues which form firm, often large and multiple masses, possibly with discharging sinuses. Various oral or soil-originating organisms such as *Actinomyces*, *Nocardia* and *Strepto-myces* spp. may be involved in actinomycotic mycetomas. Mycotic mycetomas appear to be

rare in the cat but there are reports of cases involving *Torula* spp. and *Microsporum canis*. Wound inoculation is the most likely route of infection. Therapy includes radical surgical resection and antifungal therapy (ketoconazole or griseofulvin) but is frequently unsuccessful.

Aspergillosis

Aspergillosis is far less common in cats than in dogs. Although it can cause chronic nasal disease (see Chapter 6), feline aspergillosis appears to be more often a systemic infection, causing granu-lomatous pneumonia or infiltrative intestinal lesions. Rarely, other sites may be affected such as the bladder, oral cavity or cornea and con-junctiva. Dermal sensitivity may develop to *As-pergillus* spp. As in other species, aspergillosis in the cat is usually associated with immuno-suppression, for example by FeLV, FIV or pan-leucopenia virus infections, or, less often, as a secondary invader following other upper respir-atory tract infections. Diagnosis depends on cul-ture, although serology may be helpful, but is unfortunately often only made post mortem. Treatment is possible; the use of amphotericin and 5-fluorocytosine has been reported. Thia-bendazole or ketoconazole may also be effective, but, whatever the treatment, the prognosis is poor.

Cryptococcosis

Cryptococcosis occurs worldwide and has been reported, but is rarely diagnosed, in Britain. The causative organism is *Cryptococcus neoformans*, an encapsulated yeast which exhibits fungal dimorphism and is frequently associated with pigeon droppings. In man, infection is associated with immunosuppression and this may also be the case in the domestic cat. Many organ systems can be involved, but the upper respiratory tract is the most common site of infection, causing unilateral or bilateral nasal discharge progressing to the development of polyp-like lesions protruding from one or both nostrils (see Chapter 6). There may also be local lymph node or oral involvement.

Other presentations include firm, nodular facial lesions and neurological disease; more rarely, joint infections, eye lesions and disseminated disease have been reported. Diagnosis is based on demonstration of the organism from lesions or cerebrospinal fluid, and serology may be useful to detect antigen or antibody. A positive antigen titre is probably diagnostic, but a negative result does not exclude the diagnosis. Treatment can be attempted with ketoconazole or a combination of amphotericin B and 5–fluorocytosine, but the prognosis is always guarded.

Although *Cryptococcus* is capable of infecting man, there is no evidence that it can spread directly between animals or from animal to man. However, care may be advisable with children, the elderly or immunosuppressed owners.

Candidiasis

Candida albicans is a rare pathogen of the cat, but may occur in chronic infections of the skin, ears and mucosal surfaces. Lesions are typically greyish mucoid plaques with a foul-smelling odour. Intestinal candidiasis, causing chronic diarrhoea, has also been reported. As in man, clinical candidiasis is often associated with immunosuppression, for example debilitation or infection with feline immunodeficiency virus, or it may be secondary to chronic infection or prolonged antibacterial therapy.

Yeast-like organisms can be seen in smears of lesions and biopsy material, and colonies rapidly grow on Sabouraud's agar. Topical therapy with gentian violet or nystatin has been recommended, and systemic ketoconazole or 5-fluorocytosine may be used. The predisposing cause should, if possible, be treated.

PROTOTHECOSIS

Prototheca is a genus of algae, several species of which can be pathogenic to the dog and cat. It is found mainly in sewage, from which it can contaminate drinking water, soil and food. Animal-to-animal spread does not occur. Infection is usually associated with immunosuppression,

especially of cell-mediated immunity. Cats generally develop cutaneous nodules on the head or feet. Occasionally, however, systemic infection occurs with clinical signs which include intermittent, chronic, bloody diarrhoea, weight loss and signs of CNS and eye infection. Diagnosis depends on demonstration of the organism in biopsies or in smears of vitreous fluid, CSF or, sometimes, urine. *Prototheca* will grow in Sabouraud's medium. Treatment in cats is by surgical excision of skin lesions. There is no known effective treatment for systemic infection.

Q FEVER

Q fever is caused by the rickettsia *Coxiella burnetii*. Although, like other rickettsiae, *C. burnetii* can be transmitted between and from ticks, in Britain at least, *C. burnetii* appears to be maintained in wild and domestic animal populations mainly by ingestion and inhalation of infective material such as placentas, urine and faeces. Apart from occasional abortions in sheep, *C. burnetii* generally causes no disease in most of its hosts. The main exception is man, in which infection can cause general malaise, pyrexia, pneumonia, myalgia, vomiting and diarrhoea. Traditionally, those most at risk have been veterinary surgeons, abattoir workers and farmers, but more recently urban outbreaks have occurred where the source of infection was difficult to determine. There have also been several reports from North America of Q fever contracted from parturient and aborting cats. Antibody to Q fever is apparently quite common in domestic cats; surveys in the USA and UK suggest that up to 40% of cats may have been infected at some time. The role of *C. burnetii* in feline disease, and the role of cats in the epidemiology of human infection are not known and require further investigation.

BACKGROUND
AND FURTHER READING

Abaas S., Franklin A., Kuhn I., Orskov F. & Orskov I. (1989) Cytotoxin activity on Vero cells among *Escherichia coli* strains associated with diarrhea in cats.

Am. J. Vet. Res. **50**, 1294.

August J.R. (1988) Dysgonic fermenter-2 infections. *J. Am. Vet. Med. Ass.* **193**, 1506.

Ball M.R. (1951) Salmonella in cats and dogs of Los Angeles, Honolulu and Bermuda areas. *J. Am. Vet. Med. Ass.* **118**, 164.

Biberstein E.L. & Holzworth J. (1987) Bacterial diseases. In Holzworth J. (ed) *Diseases of the Cat, Medicine and Surgery*, vol. 1. W.B. Saunders, Philadelphia, p. 279.

Bryson D.G. & Ellis W.A. (1976) Leptospirosis in a British domestic cat. *J. Small Anim. Pract.* **17**, 459.

Carithers H.A. (1985) Cat scratch disease. An overview based on a study of 1200 patients. *Am. J. Dis. Childhood* **139**, 1124.

Carpenter P.D., Heppner B.T. & Gnann J.W. (1987) DF-2 bacteraemia following cat bites. Report of two cases. *Am. J. Med.* **82**, 621.

Carro T., Pedersen N.C., Beaman B.L. & Munn R. (1989) Subcutaneous abscesses and arthritis caused by a probable bacterial L-form in cats. *J. Am. Vet. Med. Ass.* **194**, 1583.

Coloe P.J. & Allison J.F. (1982) Protot/thecosis in a cat. *J. Am. Vet. Med. Ass.* **180**, 78.

Cox E.G. (1974) Prototthecosis; a case of disseminated algal infection. *Lancet* **ii**, 379.

Dickie C.W. (1979) Feline pyothorax caused by a Borrelia-like organism and Corynebacterium pyogenes. *J. Am. Vet. Med. Ass.* **174**, 516.

Dillberger J.E. *et al.* (1988) Prototthecosis in two cats. *J. Am. Vet. Med. Ass.* **192**, 1557.

Dow S.W., Jones R.L., Henik R.A. & Husted P.W. (1989) Clinical features of salmonellosis in cats: six cases (1981–1986). *J. Am. Vet. Med. Ass.* **194**, 1464.

Eidson M., Thilsted J.P. & Rollag O.J. (1991) Clinical, clinicopathologic and pathologic features of plague in cats: 119 cases (1977–1988). *J. Am. Vet. Med. Ass.* **199**, 1191.

English C.K., Wear D.J., Margileth A.M., Lissner C.R. & Walsh G.P. (1988) Cat scratch disease: isolation of the bacterial agent. *J. Am. Med. Ass.* **259**, 1347.

Fenner W.R. (1989) Botulism. In Sherding R.G. (ed) *The Cat, Diseases and Clinical Management*. Churchill Livingstone, New York, p. 1195.

Fessler J.F. & Mortimer R.L. (1964) Experimental feline leptospirosis. *Cornell Vet.* **54**, 176.

Fox J.G. & Beaucage C.M. (1979) The incidence of Salmonella from random-source cats purchased for use in research. *J. Infect. Dis.* **139**, 362.

Fox J.G., Ackerman J.I. & Newcomer C.E. (1985) The prevalence of Campylobacter jejuni in random source cats used in biomedical research. *J. Infect. Dis.* **151**, 734.

Fukushima H.K., Nakamura R., Iitsuka S., Ito Y. & Saito K. (1985) Presence of zoonotic pathogens (Yersinia spp., Campylobacter jejuni, Salmonella spp. and leptospira

spp.) simultaneously in dogs and cats. *Zentralblatt für Bakteriologie. Abt 1 Orig B* **181**, 430.

Fukushima H., Gomyoda M., Ishikura S., Nishio T., Moriki S., Endo J., Kaneko S. & Tsubokura M. (1989) Cat contaminated environmental substances lead to Yersinia pseudotuberculosis infection in children. *J. Clin. Microbiol.* **27**, 2706.

Gillespie J.H. & Baker J.A. (1952) Experimental Q fever in cats. *Am. J. Vet. Res.* **13**, 91.

Goodall S.A., Lane J.G. & Warnock D.W. (1984) The diagnosis and treatment of a case of nasal aspergillosis in a cat. *J. Small Anim. Pract.* **25**, 627.

Greene C.E. (1988) Zoonotic aspects of group A streptococcal infections in dogs and cats. *J. Am. Anim. Hosp. Ass.* **24**, 218.

Greene C.E. (1990) Mycobacterial infections. In Greene C.E. (ed) *Infectious Diseases of the Dog and Cat*. W.B. Saunders, Philadelphia, p. 558.

Haesebrouck F., Devriese L.A., van Rijssen B. & Cox E. (1991) Incidence and significance of isolation of Mycoplasma felis from conjunctival swabs of cats. *Vet. Microbiol.* **26**, 95.

Hall A.V., Roberts C.M., Maurice P.D., McLean K.A. & Shousha S. (1988) Cat scratch disease in patient with AIDS: atypical skin manifestation. *Lancet* **ii**, 453.

Hardie E.M. (1990) Actinomycosis and nocardiosis. In Greene C.E. (ed) *Infectious Diseases of the Dog and Cat*. W.B. Saunders, Philadelphia, p. 585.

Herring A.J., McClenaghan M. & Aitken I.D. (1986) Nucleic acid techniques for strain differentiations and detection of Chlamydia psittaci. In Oriel D., Ridgeway G., Schachter J., Taylor-Robinson D. & Ward M. (eds) *Chlamydial Infections*. Cambridge University Press.

Higgins R. & Paradis M. (1980) Abscess caused by *Corynebacterium equi* in a cat. *Can. Vet. J.* **21**, 63.

Holzworth J. (1987) Mycotic diseases. In Holzworth J. (ed) *Diseases of the Cat, Medicine and Surgery*, vol, 1. W.B. Saunders, Philadelphia, p. 320.

Hudson S.J., Sobo A.O., Russel K. & Lightfoot N.F. (1990) Jackdaws as potential source of milk-borne Campylobacter jejuni infection. *Lancet* **i**, 1160.

Kirkpatrick C.E. & Glickman C.E. (1989) Cat scratch disease and the role of the domestic cat: vector, reservoir or victim? *Medical Hypothesis* **28**, 145.

Kosatsky T. (1984) Household outbreak of Q fever pneumonia related to a parturient cat. *Lancet* **ii**, 1447.

Kunkle G.A. (1990) Feline leprosy and atypical mycobacterial infections. In Greene C.E. (ed) *Infectious Diseases of the Dog and Cat*. W.B. Saunders, Philadelphia, p. 567.

Lucas S.B. (1991) Cat scratch disease. *J. Pathol.* **163**, 91.

Lucke, V.M. and Crowther, S.T. (1965) The incidence of leptospiral agglutination titres in the domestic cat. *Veterinary Record*, **77**, 647.

McCarthy M. & Zumla A. (1988) DF-2 infection. *Brit. Med. J.* **297**, 1355.

McCaw D., Franklin R., Fales W., Stockham S. & Lattimer J. (1984) Pyothorax caused by Candida albicans in a cat. *J. Am. Vet. Med. Ass.* **185**, 311.

McParland P.J., O'Hagen J., Pearson G.R. & Neill S.D. (1982) Pathological changes associated with group EF-4 bacteria in the lungs of a dog and a cat. *Vet. Rec.* **111**, 336.

Madewell B.R. & McChesney A.E. (1975) Salmonellosis in a human infant, a cat and two parakeets in the same household. *J. Am. Vet. Med. Ass.* **167**, 1089.

Mair N.S., Harbourne J.F., Greenwood M.T. & White G. (1967) Pasteurella pseudotuberculosis in the cat: two cases. *Vet. Rec.* **81**, 461.

Malik R., Love D.N., Hunt G.B., Canfield P.J. & Taylor V. (1991) Pyothorax associated with a Mycoplasma species in a kitten. *J. Small Anim. Pract.* **32**, 31.

Malnick H., Jones A. & Vickers J.C. (1989) Anaerobiospirillum: cause of a new zoonosis? *Lancet* **i**, 1145.

Margileth A.M., Wear D.J. & English C.K. (1987) Systemic cat scratch disease: report of 23 patients with prolonged or recurrent severe bacterial infection. *J. Infect. Dis.* **155**, 390.

Mayer G. (1983) Recurrent pharyngitis in a family of four. *Postgrad. Med.* **74**, 277.

Medleau L., Marks A., Brown J. & Borges W.L. (1990) Clinical evaluation of a cryptococcal antigen test for diagnosis of cryptococcosis in cats. *J. Am. Vet. Med. Ass.* **196**, 1470.

Millar W.H. & Goldschmidt M.H. (1986) Mycetomas in the cat caused by a dermatophyte. *J. Am. Anim. Hosp. Ass.* **22**, 255.

Paton B.G., Ormerod L.D., Peppe J. & Kenyon K.R. (1988) Evidence for a feline reservoir for dysgonic fermenter 2 keratitis. *J. Clin. Microbiol.* **26**, 2439.

Pedersen N.C. (1987) Mycoplasmal infections. In Holzworth J. (ed) *Diseases of the Cat, Medicine and Surgery*, vol. 1. W.B. Saunders, Philadelphia, p. 308.

Randhawa A.S., Jolley W.B., Dietrich W.H. & Hunter C.C. (1974) Coxiellosis in pound cats. *Feline Pract.* **4**(6), 37.

Roos K., Lind L. & Holm S.E. (1988) Beta-haemolytic streptococci group A in a cat as a possible source of repeated tonsillitis in a family. *Lancet* **ii**, 1072.

Rutgers H.C. (1989) Diarrhoea in the cat. *In Practice* **11**, 139.

Sawyer L.A., Fishbein D.B. & McDade J.E. (1987) Q fever: current concepts. *Rev. Infect. Dis.* **9**, 935.

Schlossberg D., Krouse T.B., Wear D.J. & English C.K. (1989) Culture-proved disseminated cat scratch disease in AIDS. *Arch. Int. Med.* **149**, 1437.

Scott D.W. (1989) Candidiasis. In Sherding R.G. (ed) *The Cat, Diseases and Clinical Management*. Churchill Livingstone, New York, p. 1549.

Sherding R.G. (1989) Diseases of the intestines. In Sherding R.G. (ed) *The Cat, Diseases and Clinical Management*. Churchill Livingstone, New York, p. 955.

Shimi A. & Barin A. (1977) Salmonella in cats. *J. Comp. Pathol.* **87**, 315.

Skirrow M.B. (1990) Campylobacter. *Lancet* **336**, 921.

Skirrow M.B., Turnbull G.L., Walker R.E. *et al.* (1980) Campylobacter jejuni enteritis transmitted from cat to man. *Lancet* **i**, 1188.

Swindle M.M., Narayan O., Luzzarage M. & Bobbie D.L. (1980) Contagious streptococcal lymphadenitis in cats. *J. Am. Vet. Med. Ass.* **177**, 829.

Swindle M.M., Narayan O., Luzarrage M. & Bobbie D.L. (1981) Pathogenesis of contagious streptococcal lymphadenitis in cats. *J. Am. Vet. Med. Ass.* **179**, 1208.

Tan R.J.S. (1974) Susceptibility of kittens to Mycoplasma infection. *Jap. J. Exp. Med.* **44**, 235.

Tilman P.C., Dodson N.D. & Indiveri M. (1982) Group G streptococcal epizootic in a closed cat colony. *J. Clin. Microbiol.* **16**, 1057.

Timony J.F., Neibert H.C. & Scott F.W. (1978) Feline salmonellosis: a nosocomial oubreak and experimental studies. *Cornell Vet.* **68**, 271.

Tyler D.E. (1990) Protothecosis. In Greene C.E. (ed) *Infectious Diseases of the Dog and Cat*. W.B. Saunders, Philadelphia, p. 74.

Van den Broek A.H.M. & Thoday K.L. (1987) Eumycetoma in a British cat. *J. Small Anim. Pract.* **28**, 827.

Warren J.S. & Allan S.D. (1986) Clinical and laboratory features of Capnocytophaga infections. *Am. J. Clin. Pathol.* **86**, 513.

Wilkinson G.T. (1977) Feline leprosy. In Kirk R.W. (ed) *Current Veterinary Therapy VI*. W.B. Saunders, Philadelphia, p. 569.

Wilkinson G.T. (1979) Feline cryptococcosis: a review and seven case reports. *J. Small Anim. Pract.* **20**, 749.

Wilkinson G.T., Bate M.J., Robins G.M. & Croker A. (1983) Successful treatment of four cases of cryptococcosis. *J. Small Anim. Pract.* **24**, 507.

Wilson H.D., McCormick J.B. & Feeley J.C. (1976) Yersinia enterocolitica infection in a 4-month old infant associated with infection in household dogs. *J. Pediatrics* **89**, 767.

Wolff A. (1966) Tuberculosis in a domestic cat. *Vet. Med. Small Animal Clinician* **61**, 553.

Yanagawa Y., Maruyama T. & Sakai S. (1978) Isolation of Yersinia enterocolitica and Yersinia pseudotuberculosis from apparently healthy dogs and cats. *Microbiol. Immunol.* **22**, 634.

Zumla A. (1989) Dysgonic fermenter type 2 infection. *Lancet* **ii**, 627.

PART 3
OTHER ASPECTS

Chapter 24 / Feline Nutrition and Disease

R. S. ANDERSON

INTRODUCTION

With increasing urbanization domestic cats have become more and more reliant on their owners to provide for their nutritional needs. Although a small proportion of house cats are fed fresh food, many receive most, if not all, of their sustenance from prepared foods. The need to establish the safety and reliability of these foods has provided a strong stimulus for research, and over the last 10 or 15 years much that was previously unquantified or even unrecognized has been published on the special nutritional requirements of cats. In many countries there is also a statutory obligation for manufacturers to ensure that products claimed to be complete should supply all the known nutritional needs of cats in a balanced form.

The nutritional profile which has emerged from clinical and research findings on cats is of an animal which, despite centuries of domestication and unlimited opportunity to change, has adhered faithfully to its carnivorous lifestyle and metabolism. Although some of the details of these special characteristics have no direct implications for the clinician and will receive only passing mention, others are important for a better understanding of the cat's susceptibility to some diseases and the logical routes to their prevention or treatment.

Cats have been domesticated for thousands of years. A well-preserved mandible, thought to belong to a domestic cat, was uncovered in 1983 from a neolithic site (c. 6000 B.C.) in Cyprus (Davis, 1987). By 1600 B.C., cats were not only domesticated but were regarded as sacred by the Egyptians, and there are even some early dietary recommendations (bread, milk and slices of Nile fish) from this era (McDonald et al., 1984). These early origins of the domestic cat in the hot, dry lands of the Middle East may well account for some aspects of its behaviour and metabolism, particularly in relation to its sparing use of water.

Despite their prolonged association with man, cats have retained much of their behavioural independence and food-procuring habits from the wild. They are, in general, better equipped to meet their nutritional needs in the feral state than dogs. This ability has advantages and disadvantages. There seems little doubt that the predatory skills of cats have, by supplementing their nutrient intake with the bodies of small mammals and birds, preserved them from dietary deficiencies which might otherwise have arisen had they become wholly dependent on man for their food. Their efficiency in catching their own food has, however, made them more vulnerable than dogs to nutritional mismanagement since they have not had to adapt their metabolism to diets which are not primarily of animal origin. It is interesting to speculate whether the cat's success as a predator and true carnivore prevented or made unnecessary the development of greater metabolic adaptability or whether its inability to make these metabolic adaptations locked it into its carnivorous status.

Metabolic constraints due to a carnivorous lifestyle

Despite the fact that cats do require special consideration of their status as true carnivores, they are not complete metabolic cripples when faced with foods of vegetable origin. They are, for instance, efficient converters to energy of the starches and sugars, which they would rarely encounter in a carnivorous diet (Morris *et al.*, 1977). There are, however, significant constraints to be considered in meeting the nutritional needs of cats.

Vitamin A
In many animals, including dogs, preformed vitamin A in the diet is not essential so long as there is sufficient dietary carotene from which their retinol or vitamin A requirement can be synthesized. The cat, however, is unable to make the necessary conversion of dietary carotenes to vitamin A and, since preformed vitamin A is absent from plant materials, it requires either materials of animal origin or a supplementary source of vitamin A to meet its requirements.

Taurine
Taurine is an amino-sulphonic acid, not present in protein, which, like vitamin A, effectively occurs only in tissues of animal origin. Most animals can meet their dietary requirements from methionine and cystine via conversion to cysteine and thence to taurine. Although cats are able to carry out this metabolic conversion to a limited extent, the activity of the enzymes essential to the latter stages of the pathway is too low to produce enough for their needs from diets which are low or deficient in taurine. The problem is compounded by the continued requirement to conjugate taurine with cholic acid in bile. Thus, even when there is a dietary deficiency of taurine, cats continue to leak their remaining stores into their digestive tracts as taurocholic acid. This is in contrast to the dog and other mammals which, when taurine is in short supply, can substitute glycine for taurine to form glycocholic acid. Insufficient dietary taurine and low levels of dietary cystine and methionine have been shown to cause irreversible degenerative changes in the retina (feline central retinal degeneration, FCRD), a reversible cardiomyopathy (Pion *et al.*, 1987), reproductive failure in queens and developmental abnormalities in kittens.

Taurine is, therefore, another nutrient, absent from plant materials and present only in animal tissues, which is a dietary essential for the cat.

Water
Cats have been said to have a relatively high urinary concentrating capacity inherited, as a means of economizing on water turnover, from their desert-dwelling ancestors. Although several other desert-living species form a much more concentrated urine than most cats (Chew, 1965), some individual cats appear to have a characteristically high concentration (Thrall & Miller, 1976). Cats make less precise and rapid compensatory changes in voluntary water intake than dogs in response to changes in the water content of their food (Anderson, 1983). Similarly, their compensatory drinking response to dehydration due to increased environmental temperature is less effective than dogs (Adolph, 1947).

This apparent weakness of the cat's thirst drive to respond to changes in its state of hydration and the capability of some individuals to form a more concentrated urine than others may contribute to the cat's susceptibility to the feline urological syndrome (FUS).

Essential fatty acids
Provided that there is an adequate dietary supply of the essential fatty acid (EFA), linoleic acid (and possible alpha-linolenic acid), dogs and other mammals are capable of synthesizing enough of the other metabolically active EFAs to meet their needs (McLean & Monger, 1989). Cats, however, are relatively deficient in at least one of the enzymes (Δ6-desaturases) necessary to convert linoleic acid to arachidonic acid, a step which is essential for the formation of the prostaglandins. Unlike other mammals, they thus require a dietary source of the EFA arachidonic acid.

This requirement for the long-chain arachidonic acid, found only in animal tissues, is not unique to cats but occurs in other strict carnivores, such as the lion.

Protein

Cats have a relatively high protein requirement for maintenance – about three times that of dogs (Schaeffer *et al.*, 1989). The reason is not that they have an exceptional requirement for essential amino acids, but that, unlike dogs and rats, for instance, they are unable to adapt to low-protein diets (Rogers *et al.*, 1977); hepatic enzymes in cats fed low-protein diets continue to catabolize nitrogen as if it were plentiful, thus incurring a negative nitrogen balance; dogs and rats, on the other hand, adapt to diminished nitrogen intake by a marked reduction in nitrogen catabolism (Schaeffer *et al.*, 1989).

This inability to adapt to a low intake of dietary protein is another manifestation of the cat's strictly carnivorous lifestyle. There is no evolutionary pressure on a strict carnivore to economize on protein when all of its natural food sources contain protein, in abundance.

Niacin

The niacin requirements of many species can be satisfied by synthesis of the vitamin from tryptophan. In cats, however, because of the active removal of an intermediate compound by the enzyme picolinic carboxylase, tryptophan contributes little to the cat's niacin requirements (MacDonald *et al.*, 1984). The cat's niacin requirements, which are similar in amount to other species, are better supplied by animal tissues, in which the vitamin is more plentiful than in plants.

Other constraints

There are other metabolic characteristics which distinguish cats from dogs, such as their acute sensitivity to a dietary deficiency of the essential amino acid arginine, their relatively high dietary requirement for the sulphur amino acids, and their excretion in the urine of a unique branched-chain sulphur amino acid (felinine). There is little doubt that more are awaiting discovery. However, the foregoing six characteristics have been highlighted either because they illustrate well the characterization of the cat as a strict carnivore or because they are significant in relation to the vulnerability of cats to some diseases associated with nutrition.

FEEDING BEHAVIOUR

Compared to dogs, cats are usually unhurried in their meals. Some seem to examine each particle of food carefully before taking into their mouths; even with semi-homogeneous foods they will discard relatively small particles which displease them, particles which most dogs would be unaware were present. This careful and occasionally selective behaviour has given them the reputation of being fussy or finicky eaters. Although it has been argued that cats' finickiness has been exaggerated by owners who pander to their dietary whims, there is little doubt that they are more discriminating than dogs with respect to some dietary constituents such as textured vegetable protein. This reputation generally earns them higher quality dietary ingredients (in both commercial and home-prepared foods) than their canine companions.

Despite their long history of domestication cats are still effective and enthusiastic predators, killing and eating a wide variety of prey, such as mice, birds, rats and rabbits, even when well fed by their owners. Mice are said to be the commonest prey of domestic cats (Eberhard, 1954; Coman & Brunner, 1972) and the fact that each 'average' mouse contributes about 30 kcal (126 kJ) of the cat's 250–300 kcal/day (1046–1255 kJ) energy requirement has been cited as an explanation for the experimental observation that cats will eat 10–20 times in every 24 hours, eating periods being distributed throughout the periods of light and darkness.

This explanation does not, however, hold good for cats which kill and partially consume half-grown rabbits; this behaviour is more compatible with the experimental observations that the more work a cat does to obtain a meal, the fewer meals and the larger meal size it will take (MacDonald *et al.*, 1984).

Feeding frequency

KITTENS

Ten-week-old kittens (weighing about 1 kg) require an energy intake of about 250 kcal/kg (1046 kJ/kg) bodyweight (NRC, 1986). In order to meet this requirement from a canned food containing 100 kcal/100 g (418 kJ/100 g), they must consume 250 g/day, or 25% of their bodyweight. These figures underline two important points:

1 Young kittens require to be fed frequently (4–5 times per day), or be provided with prolonged or continuous access to food.

2 Kitten food should have a relatively high energy content.

ADULTS

Adults may be meal fed or, particularly with dry foods, given continuous access. Not uncommonly, a combination of these systems is used, giving one or two meals of a fish- or meat-based food and providing access to a dry food or most of the day.

Taste and palatability

Many cats will eat a novel food in preference to one they are accustomed to, provided they are not put in a stressful situation (Mugford & Thorne, 1980); they also prefer warm (35–40°C) to cold food (Edney, 1973), as might be expected of a carnivore which eats its prey soon after it has been killed.

Evidence of the cat's ability to discriminate between solutions of different sweetness is conflicting, depending on whether the solutions are presented in water, milk or saline (Frings, 1951; Pfaffman, 1955; Carpenter, 1956; Bartoshuk *et al.*, 1971). As the picture is further clouded by the fact that pure water has a taste effect on cats, it can be assumed that sweetness is not an important factor in the taste and palatability of foods for cats.

Gustatory sensitivity to a wide variety of other substances, including protein hydrolysates, meat extracts and individual amino acids, is documented by Kane (1989).

Food odour is clearly an important factor in whether or not cats approach and consume or reject a particular food and Mugford (1977) demonstrated the effectiveness of a cooked rabbit odour in re-initiating ingestive behaviour after a meal of dry food.

Other factors which are influential in determining food palatability for cats are texture, moisture, fat content, particle size and hardness. With dry foods, the effectiveness of the high palatability components of the food, such as fat and protein hydrolysates, is increased by spraying these on the outside of the particles rather than incorporating them with other less palatable ingredients in the feed mix.

NUTRIENT REQUIREMENTS

The most recent estimates of the minimum nutrient requirement for growing kittens are given in Appendix 24.1 (NRC, 1986). In interpreting these data, account must be taken of the comments of the NRC subcommittee which drew them up.

1 Although a margin of safety was not incorporated, some of the values, although known to be adequate, are probably greater than minimum requirements.

2 Many of the values, for instance the amino acids, were established using purified diets and therefore in conventional foods an allowance must be made for lower digestibility and/or availability.

3 The values are given for growing kittens, since most have been derived from these rather than adult cats. The minimum requirements for the adult cat for maintenance are not known, though it is likely that all will be lower than those given for the growing kitten.

4 The minimum requirements for reproduction for the adult male or female cat are not known. However, the values shown for growing kittens would probably be adequate for reproduction if the following values are substituted for those in the table of Appendix 24.1: Vitamin A, 6000 IU/kg diet; taurine, 500 mg/kg diet (this value for taurine is only relevant for semipurified diets. Recommended levels in canned and dry foods are given (see p. 581)).

Energy

Control of intake
Dietary energy intake is generally well matched to energy expenditure in cats (although cats confined to individual cages in catteries tend to put on more weight than when kept in communal conditions). They have the ability to make compensatory changes in the intake of foods of differing energy densities (Castonguay, 1981; Kane *et al.*, 1981c) and obesity is, therefore, less common in cats than dogs (Anderson, 1973).

Hunger and satiety centres are located in the hypothalamus and the neuropathways and the glucostatic cues on which they depend appear to be the same for the short-term control of food intake, as in other animals (MacDonald *et al.*, 1984).

Dietary energy
Dietary energy (expressed as kcal or kJ) is provided by the protein, fat and carbohydrate in the food (1 kcal = 4.184 kJ). The actual amount of energy available to the animal from the food, the metabolizable energy (ME), is dependent on the total or gross energy (GE) in the food (determined by combustion in a bomb calorimeter) less the GE excreted in the faeces (F) and urine (U). Digestible energy (DE) is the GE less the faecal energy (F). Thus:

$$ME = GE - (F + U)$$

$$DE = GE - F$$

The simplest way of calculating the metabolizable energy in pet foods is to multiply the protein (CP), fat (AEE) and carbohydrate (NFE) values by energy conversion factors. For human food these factors (the modified Atwater factors, 4.0 (16.7), 9.0 (37.7) and 3.75 (15.7) kcal (kJ) for protein, fat and carbohydrate respectively) provide a satisfactory estimate of the metabolizable energy in kcal/g (kJ/g). For cat food, however, the modified Atwater factors overestimate the

metabolizable energy by 24% on average (Kendall *et al.*, 1985), since the apparent digestibility of protein, fat and carbohydrate assumed by the Atwater factors for human foods is greater than was found for a range of cat foods. For canned foods Kendall *et al.* (1985) found that the factors of 3.9 (16.3), 7.7 (32.2) and 3.0 (12.6) kcal/g (kJ/g) for protein, fat and carbohydrate gave a close approximation to *in vivo* ME values. For dry foods the best estimate of metabolizable energy was to use the gross energy (GE) as determined by calorimetry in the equation

$$ME\ (kcal/g) = 0.84\ GE - 0.6$$

or

$$ME\ (kJ/g) = 3.5\ GE - 2.5$$

The ME values of dry food are particularly affected by the vegetable fibre content (from cereal) which in the above study ranged from 0.2 to 23.1 g/kg.

In summary, therefore, the best estimates of the energy content of cat foods are as follows:

Canned food:

$$ME\ (kcal/g) = 3.9\ CP + 7.7\ AEE + 3.0\ NFE - 0.05$$

or

$$ME\ (kJ/g) = 16.3\ CP + 32.2\ AEE + 12.6\ NFF - 0.21$$

Dry food:

$$ME\ (kcal/g) = 0.84\ GE - 0.6$$
or
$$ME\ (kJ/g) = 3.5\ GE - 2.5$$

For practical purposes, the NRC (1986) uses the ME values given in Table 24.1 in calculating food allowances for cats.

The DE or ME content of the individual ingredients of cat foods has not been determined *in vivo*, but a list of values, determined in swine, is contained in the NRC booklet (NRC, 1986), some of which have been verified in other single-stomached animals.

Table 24.1 Approximate metabolizable energy (ME) content of cat foods.

	Food		
	Dry	Semi-moist	Canned
Dry matter (%)	90	70	25
ME: kcal/g (kJ/g) dry matter	3.5 (14.6)*	4.2 (17.6)*	4.4 (18.4)*
ME: kcal/g (kJ/g) as fed	3.2 (13.4)*	3.0 (12.6)*	1.1 (4.6)*

* From NRC (1986) with permission.

Table 24.2 Apparent digestibility of commercial and other foods for cats and dogs.

	Apparent digestibility (%)	
	Cats	Dogs
Crude protein (CP)	82	87
Fat (AEE)	76	92
Nitrogen-free extract (NFE)	67	70
Energy	79	89

From Kendall *et al.* (1982) with permission.

Digestibility

Comparisons between dogs and cats receiving the same foods have shown that, on average, dogs obtain 11 and 9% more digestible energy per unit of food eaten than cats (Kendall *et al.*, 1982). Table 24.2 shows the mean values of the apparent digestibility of protein (CP), fat (AEE), carbohydrate (NFE) and energy of a range of commercial foods, fresh minced meat and semi-purified diets for both cats and dogs.

Energy requirements

The bodyweights of mature domestic cats (2–6 kg) range less widely than those of dogs and their lifestyle and energy expenditure is also less variable. For practical purposes, therefore, there is little advantage in relating energy requirement

to metabolic bodyweight (e.g. $W^{0.73}$) (Kendall *et al.*, 1983) and values for cats are, in contrast to those for dogs, usually expressed on bodyweight (kg) basis.

ADULT CATS

The values for adult cats range from 60 kcal (251 kJ) ME/kg bodyweight (BW) for inactive animals to 80–90 kcal/kg BW (335–377 kJ) for those with greater scope for exercise. A recommended value for practical purposes is 80 kcal/kg BW (335 kJ) (NRC, 1986).

KITTENS

From birth until they start taking solid food at 3–5 weeks old, kittens are largely dependent on the queen's milk, which has a relatively high energy density (142 kcal/100 g) (594 kJ) compared to cow's milk (65 kcal/100 g) (272 kJ) (Paul & Southgate, 1978). At 5 weeks of age the daily ME requirements are about 250 kcal/kg BW (1046 kJ) (Miller & Allison, 1958) decreasing with age to about 180 kcal/kg BW (753 kJ) at 10 weeks (BW = 0.98 kg) and about 150 kcal/kg BW (628 kJ) at 20 weeks (BW = 2.130 kg) (Loveridge, 1987). After weaning, young kittens clearly require a diet which is sufficiently rich in energy to meet their needs for growth and maintenance; ideally such a diet should provide at least 100 kcal (418 kJ) ME per 100 g of diet as fed. Kittens fed foods of lower energy density tend to become pot-bellied as a result of attempting to consume sufficient food to meet their energy needs.

There are significant differences in bodyweights and energy intakes of male and female kittens from 6 and 9 weeks of age respectively (Fig. 24.1) (Loveridge, 1987). These data, collected from a colony of specific pathogen-free (SPF)-derived cats, showed that by 52 weeks of age males (average weight 4.12 kg) were 45% heavier than females (2.83 kg).

PREGNANT AND LACTATING QUEENS

The weekly bodyweights of queens during gestation and lactation are shown in Fig. 24.2. These values obtained from an SPF-derived colony show that from mating, pregnant queens show a steady

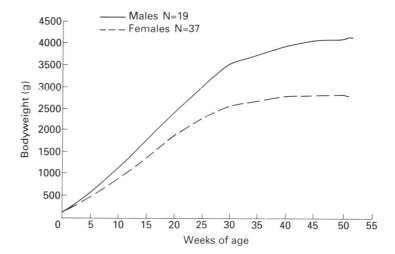

Fig. 24.1 Growth from birth to 52 weeks. (From Loveridge, 1987, with permission.)

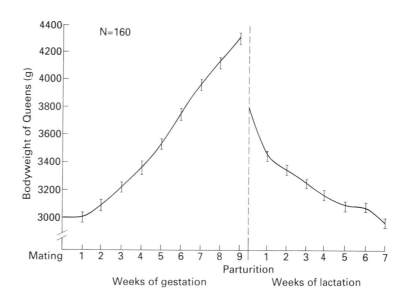

Fig. 24.2 Mean bodyweights of queens during gestation and lactation. (From Loveridge, 1986, with permission.)

increase in bodyweight, accompanied by increased energy intake (until the last week of gestation) (Fig. 24.3). This is in contrast to the pregnant bitch in which there is characteristically relatively little increase in bodyweight or energy intake during the first five of the nine weeks of pregnancy (Rainbird, 1988). The average increase in energy intake per queen during pregnancy was from 270 to 470 kcal (1130 to 1966 kJ), an increase of 74% and, depending on the number of kittens conceived, bodyweight in-

creased from 3.03 kg at mating to 4.32 kg immediately prior to parturition, an increase of 43% (Loveridge, 1986). Weight loss immediately after parturition was only 40% of the weight gained during gestation, so much of the gain shown during pregnancy was due to maternal rather than fetal tissue growth (see Loveridge & Rivers, 1989). (The ingestion of fetal membranes after parturition would, to some extent, offset the initial losses due to these tissues at parturition.) This increase in maternal tissue during pregnancy

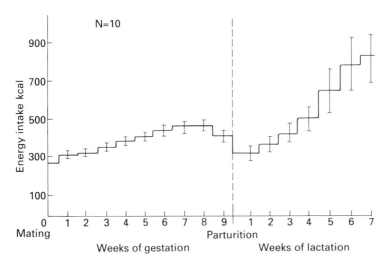

Fig. 24.3 Energy intake of queens during gestation and lactation. Lactation includes intake of kittens from about 3 weeks. (From Loveridge, 1986, with permission.)

does not appear to be such a well-marked feature during pregnancy in bitches, which within a day or so following parturition typically lose much of the weight gained during pregnancy (Holme, 1982). The weight of the dam at mating appears to have a significant effect on the weights of the kittens from about 2 weeks of age until 20 weeks; on the other hand the growth rates of the kittens were, surprisingly, not significantly affected by the numbers of kittens (from three to six) per litter (Loveridge, 1987).

During lactation queens show a decrease in bodyweight (Fig. 24.2), the number of the kittens in the litter in these observations having little or no effect on the weight loss (Fig. 24.4). (Queens with very large litters, i.e. six or seven, are, nevertheless, likely to show substantial decreases in bodyweight during lactation.) The food intake of the queens is, however, markedly affected by the number of kittens in a litter; by week 3 of lactation queens with litters of four kittens consume 80% more than a queen with a single kitten (269 kcal) (1110 kJ). In these circumstances, therefore, queens appear to be able to limit their weight losses regardless of the number of kittens in the litter provided they have ad lib access to good quality food. By week 3 of lactation (before the kittens had started taking solid food) the average energy intake of all the queens was 56%

more than that at mating. Despite the increased food intake, all queens continued to lose weight during lactation so that bodyweight at the time of weaning had returned to approximately that at mating. Later studies (Munday & Earle, 1991) show that the energy intake of queens by week 6 of lactation was two or more times that of pre-pregnancy levels, depending on litter size.

There are several features worth emphasizing in the above studies (Loveridge, 1986, 1987).
1 Although bodyweight of the queens at mating had no effect on birthweight of the kittens, those born from the heavier queens grew faster during lactation and retained this advantage during the subsequent growth period (to 20 weeks). Whether the lighter kittens eventually caught up at maturity is not known.
2 The queens showed a steady weight increase during pregnancy, together with an increased food intake. Much of this weight increase was due to maternal tissue accretion so that bodyweight immediately after parturition was substantially greater than that at mating. This tissue stored during preg enancy acted as a reserve energy source during lactation.
3 Unless queens are provided with sufficient high-quality food to permit this laying down of maternal tissue during pregnancy, it seems likely that the inevitable mobilization of maternal tissue

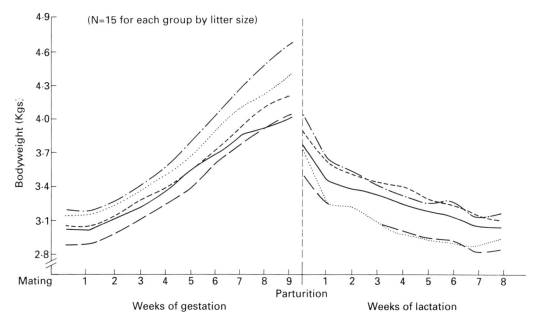

Fig. 24.4 Bodyweight changes of queens during gestation and lactation for litter sizes 1–5. Littersize = 1 ——, 2 -----, 3 — —, 4 ·····, 5 —.—..

during lactation will be a limiting factor on milk production and kitten growth.

4 Provided that feeding and management is good, queens are well able to rear litters of six kittens, and kittens from such large litters appear to suffer little or no disadvantage compared to kittens from smaller litters.

Energy allowances

The approximate amount of food (dry, semi-moist or canned) required to meet the ME allowances for cats is in Table 24.3.

Protein

Under natural conditions, the cat's carnivorous lifestyle ensures that, so long as prey is available, the proportion of protein in its food is likely to be high and therefore sufficient to meet its needs. Although protein deficiency could, in theory, occur in animals fed entirely by their owners, it is unlikely for the following reasons:

1 Cats tend to select high-protein (animal origin) ingredients from mixtures of high- and low-protein foods.

2 Household cats receive a substantial amount of their nutritional needs from commercial canned foods, which are largely dependent on animal protein to achieve the palatability and texture needed to maintain their market position. Although palatability can be achieved with a low-protein dry food, the importance of protein of satisfactory quality and quantity is so well recognized by food manufacturers that the possibility of dietary deficiency is remote.

Amino acids

The amino acids essential for kitten growth are arginine, histidine, lysine, leucine, isoleucine, methionine, phenylalanine, threonine, trypto-phan and valine (Rogers & Morris, 1979).

Arginine is of particular interest in cats (and other carnivores) because of the severe metabolic disturbance which occurs if it is omitted from the

Table 24.3 Estimated daily food allowances for cats.

Cat	Weight[a] of cat (kg)	Dry type[b] (g/kg body wt.)	(g/cat)	Semi-moist (g/kg body wt.)	(g/cat)	Canned[d] (g/kg body wt.)	(g/cat)
Kitten							
10 weeks	0.9–1.1	78	70–86	83	75–91	227	204–250
20 weeks	1.9–2.5	41	78–103	43	82–108	118	224–295
30 weeks	2.5–3.8	31	78–118	33	83–125	91	228–346
40 weeks	2.9–3.8	25	73–95	27	78–103	73	212–277
Adult[e]							
Inactive	2.2–4.5	22	48–90	23	51–99	64	141–288
Active	2.2–4.5	25	55–113	27	59–122	73	160–329
Gestation	2.5–4.0	31	78–124	33	83–132	91	228–364
Lactation	2.2–4.0	78	172–312	83	182–332	227	499–908

[a] Derived from Figure 1 by setting lower limit at mean weight of females minus one standard deviation and the upper limit at mean weight of males plus one standard deviation.
[b] Dry matter, 90%; ME, 3.2 kcal/g (13.4 kJ/g).
[c] Dry matter, 70%; ME, 3.0 kcal/g (12.6 kJ/g).
[d] Dry matter, 25%; ME, 1.1 kcal/g (4.6 kJ/g).
[e] Fifty weeks of age or older.
[f] Queens nursing 4–5 kittens in week 6 of lactation.
From NRC (1986) with permission.

Table 24.4 Taurine content of selected foods.

Item	Uncooked mean (mg/kg)
Beef muscle	362
Beef liver	192
Beef kidney	225
Lamb muscle	473
Lamb kidney	239
Pork muscle	496
Pork liver	169
Chicken muscle	337
Cod	314
Cows' milk (colostrum)	38
Cows' milk	1.3
Cats' milk	359

From NRC (1986) with permission.

diet. Within hours of an arginine-deficient meal, cats show severe signs of ammonia intoxication manifested as lethargy, emesis, vocalization, hypersalivation, hyperactivity, hyperaesthesia, ataxia, emprosthotonus, extended limbs and exposed claws; the most severely affected develop hypothermia, bradypnoea and cyanosis followed in some cases by death (McDonald *et al.*, 1984). These dramatic events, which occur only under experimental conditions are, nevertheless, a further indication of the inability of the cat to cope with diets which do not supply sufficient nitrogen as protein or amino acid.

Cats have a relatively high requirement for the sulphur-containing amino acid methionine or methionine plus cystine. Possible contributory factors are the demands for hair growth and the urinary excretion of the unique branched-chain sulphur amino acid, felinine. Felinine, present in highest concentration in the urine of adult male cats, may have a role in territorial marking or perhaps in the regulation of sterol metabolism.

The amount of methionine or methionine and cystine in the diet affects the cat's requirement for dietary taurine (see below). The sulphur-containing amino acids are usually the most limiting amino acids in the cat's diet and in order to meet their high requirements, cats need about 19% of animal protein in the diet.

Taurine

Mention has already been made of dietary taurine in characterizing the cat as an obligate carnivore. The pathogenesis of feline central retinal degeneration (FCRD) and cardiomyopathy which occur in association with low plasma taurine levels in cats are described elsewhere, but some further elaboration of the relevant nutritional details is given below.

As an amino-sulphonic acid, taurine does not occur in protein in association with other amino acids, being the end-product of sulphur amino-acid metabolism. It is known to be conjugated with bile acids to form bile salts (taurocholates), is involved in nerve function in the central nervous system and is also found in high concentrations in the retina and myocardium (Pion *et al.*, 1987). Its occurrence in various food materials of animal origin is shown in Table 24.4.

The minimum recommended taurine content of food for kitten growth is 400 mg/kg diet, dry basis (NRC, 1986). These values were, however, based on semi-purified diets and there are marked individual differences in the plasma taurine levels of cats receiving the same foods. Furthermore, the same dietary level of taurine in foods of different categories (dry or canned) appears to give different plasma concentrations (Morris *et al.*, 1989). Whole blood taurine levels provide a better indicator of taurine status than plasma levels: higher taurine concentrations are required in canned food (2000–2500 mg/kg dry matter) to supply adequate taurine compared to dry foods (1200 mg/kg dry matter).

The effects of low-taurine diets on the development of FCRD have been observed mainly from experimental work with semi-purified diets in which plasma taurine and the development of retinal degeneration over a period of months was found to be dependent on the sulphur-amino acid content of the diet as well as the taurine content. Naturally occurring FCRD was first reported by Aguirre (1978) in household cats maintained largely on dry commercial dog food containing little or no taurine.

Taurine has also been implicated in myocardial failure in cats (Pion *et al.*, 1987). In 23 cases of cats with echoradiographic evidence of dilated cardiomyopathy (DCM), all but one had low concentrations of plasma taurine and eight had retinal lesions (FCRD) indicating long-term taurine deficiency. Clinical improvement and subsequent echocardiographic evidence of resolution of the DCM were attributed to correction of the taurine deficiency.

Taurine insufficiency has also been implicated in impaired reproductive function typified by fetal resorption, low birthweight of kittens and poor survival rate. Abnormalities in neurological function and skeletal growth also occur. These effects, which are accompanied by reduced tissue levels of taurine in queens, their offspring and in maternal milk, are prevented by supplementation of the diet with taurine.

An adequate supply of dietary taurine is, therefore, important for the maintenance of health and reproduction in cats. Unlike some other nutrients in which deficiency is theoretically possible but rarely occurs in practice, dietary taurine deficiency should clearly be given serious consideration in the investigation of retinal degeneration, cardiomyopathy and reproductive dysfunction in cats. The adequacy of dietary taurine is affected by a number of factors, including the sulphur amino acid content and the method of processing the diet. Cats fed unconventional diets low in ingredients of animal origin, such as dog biscuits, are at risk of taurine depletion – particularly if they are kept inside and thus prevented from supplementing their diets by hunting.

Fat

Animal fat makes an important contribution to both the palatability and the nutritional value of the feline diet. Vegetable oils are in general less palatable than animal fats (Kane *et al.*, 1981a). Cats will willingly consume diets with a high animal fat content (25–30%) but since such diets have a high energy density, total food intake is usually reduced in compensation (Schneck & Cumberland, 1968). Because of this compensatory decrease in intake, the concentration of all other essential nutrients in high-fat diets must be greater than in diets with a lower energy content. The apparent digestibility of fat in a number of commercial dog and cat foods, fresh meat (minced) and semi-purified diets is less for cats (76%) than for dogs (92%) (Kendall *et al.*, 1982). This difference in apparent digestibility is particularly apparent at low levels of fat intake and is due, at least in part, to the relatively high content of metabolic fat in the cats' faeces. Fat digestibility at higher levels of intake may be as high as 99% (NRC, 1986).

Apart from its nutritional value as a rich and palatable energy source, fat has two other major roles – as a carrier of the fat-soluble vitamins and as a source of essential fatty acids. There are, however, no minimum fat levels specified for cats as it would be impossible to provide a diet made up of animal materials which did not contain a significant amount of fat – and certainly sufficient to act as a vehicle for the fat-soluble vitamins.

The levels of fatty acids in the diet are, however, critical. Because of the cat's inability to synthesize arachidonic from linoleic acid (see above) minimum amounts of both these nutrients are specified (Appendix 24.1)

There is an extensive literature on EFA metabolism in cats in which the cat's relative inability to convert the 18C linoleic acid to the longer chain (20C) fatty acids has been investigated. For practical purposes, deficiency of essential fatty acids is, however, unlikely if cats are provided with food containing ingredients of mixed animal tissues.

Dietary EFA supplementation has been widely used in dogs in the treatment of allergic skin disease and claims have been made for its efficacy in cats with intractable skin problems (see Chapter 1).

Carbohydrate

Although the food of cats in the wild contains little carbohydrate, they are, nevertheless, able to utilize a range of carbohydrates (Morris *et al.*, 1977); dry cat foods containing 50% or more of carbohydrate can maintain adult cats indefinitely and also support satisfactory growth in kittens. Carbohydrate appears to be most acceptable in high levels in the dry expanded form found in dry cat foods. In canned foods, although adequate palatability can be achieved, the presence of carbohydrate tends to decrease palatability, possibly by its effect on the texture of the wet food.

The carbohydrate content of the queen's milk (approximately 4%) (Keen *et al.*, 1982) is much the same as that of other animals and remains at a fairly constant level throughout lactation; kittens are, therefore, well able to utilize carbohydrate as a significant (about 17% of total energy) part of the diet. In adult cats lactose, sucrose, glucose, dextrin and starch have apparent digestibilities of 96% or more when fed at 20% of a ground beef and mutton diet (Trudell & Morris, 1975). In commercial, fresh and semi-purified foods, values ranging from an average of 69% (Kendall *et al.*, 1982) to 82–95% (NRC, 1986) are recorded. The relatively low values for apparent digestibility of carbohydrate in canned and dry food found by Kendall *et al.* (1982) are partly attributable to the inclusion of soluble (e.g. carrageenan) and insoluble (e.g. cellulose) dietary fibre in their calculations. The relatively higher fibre component in dry foods makes it more difficult to predict the apparent digestibility of total carbohydrate (or nitrogen-free extract) in these foods.

A dietary source of carbohydrate is not apparently required by cats at any stage of their life cycle, as might be expected in an animal which has a strictly carnivorous lifestyle. Insoluble fibre, though not digested by cats, may, like the undigested connective tissue of their prey, play a useful role in providing sufficient dietary bulk to regulate the passage of digesta through the bowel and reduce the occurrence of constipation.

Minerals

In the wild, cats obtain an adequate and balanced supply of the main minerals and the trace elements by consumption of the whole bodies of their prey, which provide a suitably balanced supply of these essential nutrients in an available form. Even under domesticated conditions many cats may obtain a proportion of their mineral requirements from their hunting activities. Abnormalities of mineral nutrition are, therefore, a feature of the misguided or negligent provision of unbalanced or deficient food materials resulting in an over- or under-supply or the unavailability of one or more minerals. The occurrence of rickets in monkeys, lions, bears and birds in London Zoo and its cure by the addition of bone dust and cod liver oil was recorded over a hundred years ago, but there is still a lack of appreciation among many animal owners that a 'meat only' diet is not equivalent to a carnivorous diet, and is deficient in nutrients present in the whole animals which provide cats with their natural food.

In general, the mineral requirements of cats do not differ substantially from those of dogs (Morris & Rogers, 1989) but there is relatively little quantitative work on the requirements of cats for growth, reproduction and maintenance and much of the existing data are taken from experimental diets which have proved adequate in practice.

Calcium and phosphorus

Like other animals, growing kittens require more calcium and phosphorus than any other minerals in their diets; minimum requirements for maintenance of adults are not known, but they are likely to be substantially less than for growth (NRC, 1986).

The calcium content of queen's milk increases by over 200% during the first 3 weeks of lactation (from 545 to 1725 mg/l) (Keen *et al.*, 1982). This is equivalent to 8.9 g/kg dry matter and approximates to the minimum recommendation (8 g/kg DM) for the growing kitten (NRC, 1986). The calcium content of cow's milk (1200 mg/l) (Paul & Southgate, 1978) is similar to that of the queen. The calcium levels in commercial cat foods for which nutritional data are readily available usually incorporate a generous safety margin, so calcium supplementation is unnecessary and may even contribute to calcium/phosphorus imbalance.

There is little specific information on the phosphorus requirements of kittens. Phosphorus is present in relatively greater amounts than calcium in most muscle and other edible animal material. The calcium:phosphorus ratio in muscle meat is about 1:20 and in liver about 1:50 (Paul & Southgate, 1978). Since the recommended calcium:phosphorus ratio is between 0.9:1 and 1.1:1, it is not surprising that cats fed diets consisting largely of unsupplemented muscle meat or liver encounter disturbances of bone metabolism.

Although various proprietary calcium supplements are available, it is essential, if recommending supplementation of an unbalanced diet, that a rough estimate be made of the calcium and phosphorus status of the diet and of the supplement before making any recommendation, otherwise the imbalance may be exacerbated rather than corrected. Although vitamin D supplementation may prevent or alleviate rachitic or osteomalacic changes due to calcium-deficient diets, it may cause other bone defects if dietary mineral deficiency is severe (Campbell & Douglas, 1965). Sterilized bone flour (approximately 30% calcium and 14% phosphorus) is a useful, cheap and readily available calcium/phosphorus supplement for muscle meat; 15 g will adequately supplement about 1 kg of meat. It is, however, simpler and probably more effective to advise feeding a complete commercial food which the manufacturers, with the benefit of detailed analytical information on their raw materials and finished products, have adjusted to deliver the appropriate 'package' of minerals and vitamins in relation to the energy content of the food.

Absorption of calcium may be impaired by the phytate present in plant materials such as cereal grains and oil seed products; however, so long as the levels present in the diet are not marginal, the presence of cereal phytates is probably of minor importance.

Nutritional secondary hyperparathyroidism in kittens, especially Siamese, was described by Bennett (1976) as the most commonly encountered bone disease in cats, being particularly associated with the feeding of 'owner compiled meat-rich diets'. Although the feeding of such diets is still a potential hazard to the development of kittens, the increasing use of commercial foods, some of which are specifically formulated for kittens, should result in a reduction in the occurrence of such cases.

Although calcium and phosphorus requirements for maintenance of the adult cat are probably quite low, there is an increased requirement during pregnancy and lactation. The increased intake of food during these periods (see above), particularly during lactation, is probably sufficient to meet the increased need, provided that the food is palatable and contains at least the recommended calcium content for growing kittens. Experience with cat colonies in which many hundreds of litters have been bred indicates that hypocalcaemic tetany associated with pregnancy or lactation is very rare under good management and dietary conditions.

Magnesium
Magnesium is present in varying amounts in animal tissues but in sufficient quantities to meet the cat's requirements for growth and maintenance. Clinical deficiency has never been reported in cats. The role of excessive magnesium intake in the feline urological syndrome (FUS) has, however, received considerable attention. Experimentally it was shown that the syndrome could be reproduced by the consumption of diets containing high levels of magnesium (>3.5 g/kg diet) in dry diets (Buffington *et al.*, 1989) and epidemiological studies (Walker *et al.*, 1977); Willeburg (1984) identified a number of predisposing factors including low water intake and dry diets.

While current evidence has established the critical importance of a high urinary pH in predisposing to the formation of the struvite crystals associated with FUS (Buffington *et al.*, 1989), dietary magnesium remains an essential component of the syndrome. The relatively high magnesium content of raw materials such as meat and bone meal (11 g/kg) and dried fish meals (13 g/kg), which are potentially useful as ingredients in dry foods, are potential contributors to increased urinary magnesium levels. While foods may be formulated to provide an acid urinary pH, other physiological or metabolic factors may intervene to elevate urinary pH to levels which allow the precipitation of magnesium ammonium phosphate crystals, and it is therefore essential to use only ingredients which give magnesium levels substantially lower than those known to have been associated with FUS.

Potassium
Potassium is present in all plant and animal materials and it is unlikely that primary deficiency will occur in healthy animals. However, if intake is marginal, intercurrent disease or therapy may precipitate clinical effects due to hypokalaemia. Feline hypokalaemic polymyopathy has been reported as a sporadic disorder in the USA (Dow *et al.*, 1987), in the UK as a possible hereditary condition in young Burmese kittens (Blaxter *et al.*, 1986) and in an adult Siamese cat (Hopkins, 1989). A number of metabolic dysfunctions may account for potassium shifts or excessive renal losses. These respond to parenteral or oral potassium supplementation.

Sodium and chloride
Dietary deficiency of salt is unlikely in healthy cats fed on fresh or commercial diets. Cats, like other animals, respond to increased salt intake by increasing their fluid intake (Anderson, 1982) and, provided that adequate water is available, are able to excrete the additional salt without ill-effect over a prolonged period. There is no evidence for or against a relationship between salt intake and hypertension in cats.

Minimum sodium requirements for cats have not been established. By extrapolation from the requirements of other small mammals, a minimum salt level of 500 mg/kg dry diet has been recommended (NRC, 1986). Since the salt content of lean, uncooked meat is approximately

1500 mg/kg dry weight (Paul & Southgate, 1978) and most other food materials for cats, such as fish and liver, have greater amounts, the likelihood of dietary salt deficiency in healthy cats fed fresh foods is remote. Most commercial foods contain varying amounts of salt added with other minerals in amounts sufficient to ensure a generous safety margin.

Low-salt prescription diets are available for supportive treatment and long-term maintenance in conditions featuring sodium retention, such as chronic cardiac failure. The role of dietary sodium restriction in renal failure in cats is less well defined and individual clinical assessment is necessary before embarking on a low-salt dietary regime. Michell (1989) argues against the need for salt restriction in canine renal disease on the grounds that sodium depletion can cause a rapid impairment of renal function. Very low dietary salt levels affect food palatability with the possible reduction in the intake of other essential nutrients.

Iron and copper
The iron content of queen's milk (4 mg/l) is much higher than that of human (0.2–0.5 mg/l) or cow's milk (0.2–0.3 mg/l) but lower than that reported for dogs (approximately 10 mg/l) (Keen *et al.*, 1982). The iron content of feline milk increases during the first week of lactation but, as in other species, levels decrease during the later stages of lactation.

Iron values in milk substitutes for cats are not readily available in the published literature (Baines, 1981) but in a growth trial with kittens from about 1 to 20 days of age, kittens reared on a milk substitute showed similar weight gains to controls reared by their dam (though overall weight gains were less than those recorded in other growth trials) (Loveridge, 1987).

Iron deficiency in healthy cats fed diets substantially made up from animal tissues is unlikely since the iron in haemoglobin and myoglobin is usually well utilized. The recommended dietary iron level for cats is, however, substantially greater than that for dogs (Morris & Rogers, 1989) and this seems a safe and rational recommendation in view of the cat's characteristically carnivorous diet in which iron would usually be present and available in ample amounts. The availability of dietary iron may be materially reduced by the presence of other nutrients such as zinc or phytic acid.

Copper levels in queen's milk, ranging from about 1.6 mg/l in early lactation to 0.6 mg/l in the late stages (Keen *et al.*, 1982) are higher than human and cow's milk (0.3–0.6 and 0.2–0.3 mg/l respectively) but similar to that of the bitch (2.0 mg/l).

Deficiency of copper is unlikely in growing or adult cats as copper is present in varying amounts in most tissues of animal origin normally fed to cats. Some meat, fish and bone meals have very high copper levels (NRC, 1986) and although excessive dietary levels of copper have not been reported, foods containing these materials could have relatively high copper levels.

Iodine
Iodine deficiency has been reported in zoo felids and domestic cats (NRC, 1986). Clinical signs include thyroid hypertrophy, alopecia, abnormal calcium metabolism and fetal resorption (MacDonald *et al.*, 1984). Iodine administration alleviated clinical signs of deficiency in cats given all-meat or low-calcium diets. Hyperthyroidism, including signs such as polyphagia, increased activity, polydipsia, polyuria and vomiting, with increased circulating levels of thyroxine and tri-iodothyronine has been reported in cats (Peterson *et al.*, 1983), though its relation to dietary iodine levels was not clear. Colouring agents used in commercial products may contain iodine which, though it contributes to iodine levels by analysis, is virtually unavailable for absorption. A source of available iodine is, therefore, incorporated into commercial foods.

Zinc
The concentration of zinc in cats' milk (0.6 mg/l) is about the same as in other species (Keen *et al.*, 1982). Although zinc deficiency has been produced experimentally in kittens (Kane *et al.*, 1981b), its spontaneous occurrence has not been

reported. Like other species, deficient male cats show testicular degeneration and thus appear more sensitive than females to marginal zinc intakes. Deficient kittens showed perioral skin lesions with erythema, scaling and crusting of increasing severity. The coats became thin, lustreless and scaly.

Bone, meat and fish meals are a rich source of zinc, but zinc is present in variable amounts in all animal tissue. Zinc absorption is decreased in the presence of high concentrations of dietary calcium and phytate, so it is not unrealistic to propose that cats kept under the same conditions which caused taurine deficiency (Aguirre, 1978) – i.e. fed on a low-quality, dry dog food with a high calcium content – could also be vulnerable to zinc deficiency.

Manganese, cobalt and selenium

Deficiencies of these elements have not been reported and it appears likely that healthy cats receiving diets primarily of animal origin will receive adequate amounts.

Vitamins

Quantitative information on the vitamin requirements of cats is rather patchy, depending on isolated pieces of research, on experimental diets which had rather arbitrary vitamin levels or on extrapolation from studies on other species.

Vitamin A

The cat's inability effectively to convert the vitamin A precursor, beta-carotene, found in plant materials, to vitamin A makes it dependent on animal sources of the vitamin. Muscle meat and white fish contain only traces of vitamin A, the main sources in animal materials being in liver, kidneys, milk and oily fish such as herring or mackerel. Vitamin A deficiency is associated with conjunctivitis, xerosis and keratinization of the cornea, photophobia, delayed pupillary response to light and possibly retinal degeneration. Squamous metaplasia of the respiratory tract and susceptibility to lung infections are also features of cats experimentally made deficient.

Vitamin A, however, is better known for the toxic effects of hypervitaminosis than for deficiency. Cats fed predominantly on raw liver develop crippling bone disease due to the excessive intake of vitamin A (English & Seawright, 1964). After several months of consuming such a diet, they develop cervical spondylosis associated with dullness, lethargy, unkempt coat, lack of appetite and general disinterest in normal activities. Lameness is usually present in one or both forelegs and movement is slow and cautious. The pain and difficulty in movement is associated with bony exostoses and ankylosis of spinal vertebrae, particularly in the cervical region (Fry, 1989).

Removal of the source of vitamin A results in some clinical improvement, if the signs are recognized early; advanced cases are less likely to respond to treatment.

Liver or other vitamin A-rich foods in modest proportions present no hazard to cats, since the amounts required to produce bony lesions (17–35 mg retinol or 56 000–116 000 IU vitamin A per kg bodyweight) are only achieved by prolonged and virtually exclusive feeding of liver. Calf liver (UK) contains an average retinol content of 14.6 mg/100 g (Paul & Southgate, 1978) thus more than 100 g of liver per day would be required to attain the lower level of toxicity reported by Seawright *et al.* (1967). It is, however, worth noting that the vitamin A content of liver from sheep and cattle is highly variable and it is probably significant that hypervitaminosis in cats was first observed in Australia, where the levels in the livers of grazing cattle and sheep have a higher concentration than in other countries.

Vitamin D

Rickets occurred in vitamin D-deficient diets fed experimentally to growing kittens (Gershoff *et al.*, 1957); however, Rivers *et al.* (1979) found that although plasma levels of vitamin D_3 decreased initially in kittens fed vitamin D-deficient diets and shielded from ultraviolet light, no signs of bone disease occurred. Requirements are, therefore, low for both growing and adult cats and naturally occurring deficiency is unlikely.

Gross and prolonged overdosage with vitamin D is associated with calcification of soft tissues.

Vitamin E

Dietary deficiency of vitamin E in cats is associated with steatitis or yellow fat disease. It was first observed in kittens fed a canned fish-based diet (Cordy & Stillinger, 1953), the yellowness of the fat resulting from the painful deposition of ceroid pigment in fat cells.

Cats or kittens receiving diets with a high level of polyunsaturated fats and inadequate vitamin E supplementation are vulnerable. Such diets, especially those containing fish oil, require a higher level of vitamin E supplementation than normal diets. Clinical steatitis due to the combination of high polyunsaturates and low vitamin E intake occurs occasionally in practice (Gaskell *et al.*, 1975).

Vitamin K

Deficiency of vitamin K has not been produced experimentally nor encountered clinically.

Vitamin B complex

Thiamin

Unlike most of the other B vitamins, clinical dietary deficiency of thiamin in cats may be encountered (Davidson, 1992). Thiamin is readily destroyed by heating, so manufacturers of prepared food take account of its thermolabile nature by incorporating sufficiently high levels in the ingredients prior to cooking. Thiamin may also be destroyed in fresh, uncooked food by the thiaminase present in species of fish such as carp and herring. Thus, while thiamin deficiency is unlikely to occur in cats receiving prepared foods, because of the thiamin added to counteract processing losses, home-prepared foods, particularly if subjected to prolonged cooking, could have a low thiamin content. The onset of thiamin deficiency in cats is characterized by anorexia followed by neurological disorders with postural abnormalities such as ventroflexion of the head, impaired righting reflexes, dilated pupils and slow pupillary light reflex. Terminally there is progressive weakness, prostration and death. Diagnostic tests include measurement of blood thiamin pyrophosphate and measurement of

erythrocyte transketolase stimulation by thiamin pyrophosphate (NRC, 1986).

Niacin

The potential vulnerability of the cat to niacin deficiency because of its inability to synthesize the vitamin from tryptophan has been mentioned above. However, naturally occurring niacin deficiency has not been recorded. Cats are, however, dependent on a dietary source of niacin to meet their requirements.

Riboflavin, pyridoxine, pantothenic acid, biotin, vitamin B_{12} and choline

Although experimental deficiencies of these members of the vitamin B group have in many cases been produced in kittens or cats, and under exceptional conditions could occur, the likelihood is very low.

Vitamin C (ascorbic acid)

Despite repeated trials, there is no evidence that cats have a dietary requirement for vitamin C.

FOODS FOR CATS

In the past the traditional foods for cats were fish, meat, liver, and milk. The animals probably survived a range of nutrient deficiencies on such diets by supplementing their intake with the more complete nutrition offered by the whole bodies of the small mammals and birds which they caught.

These traditional foods have, however, been replaced to a very large extent by commercially prepared complete foods, with the result that the great majority of the cats in Britain and many other countries receive part or all of their nutritional requirements from these prepared foods. The international pet food industry has both carried out and supported substantial research into assessing the nutritional needs of cats and the fact that disease of nutritional origin is rarely reported is a measure of their success in applying current nutritional knowledge to food products on the market. Research, however, continues and it seems not unlikely that the range of present knowledge of the cat's specialized nutrient needs will be extended in the future. Present knowledge does, nevertheless, allow manufacturers to claim with confidence, supported by the evidence of growth, reproduction and maintenance trials, that cats can be maintained in good health when fed solely and exclusively on one or more prepared foods.

These fall into three main categories – canned, semi-moist and dry. As the names suggest, their differing water content is one of their main distinguishing features.

Canned foods

Because of their relatively high water content (75–85%) these foods must be commercially sterilized and maintained sterile in sealed, impervious containers. This method of processing and packaging virtually guarantees their microbiological safety (unless a container is damaged after processing). On the rare occasions when a can is under-processed and thus incompletely sterilized, bacterial multiplication occurs rapidly, often with gas formation, resulting in the 'blown' can, apparent from a domed deformation of the lid and the escape of gas on opening. The feeding of meat from sealed containers after thorough sterilization virtually eliminates the possibility of food poisoning of dietary origin (in contrast to the relative prevalence of food poisoning organisms in uncooked fresh meat for human consumption). The impervious container also renders unnecessary the use of additives for preservation and, although a very slow decrease in vitamin levels occurs with time, such foods have a long shelf-life.

The contents of cans, mainly fresh or frozen meats such as lung, liver, kidney, spleen, tripe, udder, bone, blood, poultry by-products and/or fresh or frozen fish, are mixed with the appropriate additional minerals and vitamins to bring the total nutrient content to exceed that recommended for cats (NRC, 1986). Some products also contain cereal or cereal by-products and possibly soya. The actual nutrient levels in the final product are related to its energy content, so that a food with a relatively high energy content

must also contain a relatively high content of other nutrients, since the quantity of food (and its contained nutrients) ingested for a given energy requirement will be relatively less for the high-energy food than for a lower energy food.

Nutrient content per unit of wet or dry weight

Because of the wide range of moisture content of different categories of prepared foods – from about 8% moisture (dry) to 85% moisture (canned) – comparisons of nutrient contents of foods of different categories on a 'wet weight' basis are not particularly meaningful. Thus although the protein content of a canned food may be shown as, say, 8% on the label, compared to a dry food with a claimed value of 30% protein, the levels expressed on a dry weight basis, assuming the respective moisture contents are 80% and 8% (20% and 92% dry matter) are:

Canned food:

20 g dry matter contains 8 g of protein

$$\therefore 100\,\text{g of dry matter contains } \frac{8 \times 100}{20}\,\text{g}$$

$$= 40\,\text{g}/100\,\text{g dry matter}$$

Dry food:

92 g dry matter contains 32 g of protein

$$\therefore 100\,\text{g of dry matter contains } \frac{32 \times 100}{92}\,\text{g}$$

$$= 38\,\text{g}/100\,\text{g dry matter}$$

As a percentage of the total nutrients, therefore, the canned food contains a slightly greater protein content than the dry food. The same calculation is relevant for the comparison of all nutrients in foods of widely differing water content.

Canned foods have in general the highest palatability and protein digestibility of the three categories of prepared foods. Within the canned category those without added cereal, usually presented as chunks in gravy or jelly, have the highest palatability and cost, and a relatively low energy content. Those with added cereal, sometimes called loaf product, have a slightly lower palatability and cost, with a higher energy content. Sterilized foods in small, rigid aluminium foil packs offer a new and highly palatable option within this category of canned or wet foods. Like all pet foods, canned foods are required to state on the label whether they are complete, i.e. whether they are capable of meeting all the cat's nutritional needs when fed alone according to instructions.

The energy concentrations of canned foods are usually greater, when expressed on a dry weight basis, than dry foods, but on a wet weight basis they are, of course, lower. When energy and other nutrient requirements are particularly high, as in the early stages of growth and during lactation, canned foods with a relatively high energy density are the most appropriate. Some canned foods are specifically formulated for these special physiological requirements.

Semi-moist foods

As their name suggests, semi-moist foods occupy an intermediate position between canned (wet) and dry foods, having a moisture content of 15–30%. As they are not sterile and not packaged in impervious containers, preservation is effected by the incorporation of water-soluble solids such as sugar, sorbates and low molecular weight alcohols such as propylene glycol. These substances stabilize the products by reducing the availability of water for growth of spoilage organisms.

Semi-moist foods have been less successful for cats than dogs but, nevertheless, play a useful role in the range of foods available. Because of the preservative, they do not dry out or spoil when left in the bowl and can be used in the same way as dry foods in ad lib feeding regimes.

Since they are much less dependent on retaining the texture of the raw materials than canned foods, a wide range of ingredients can be used among which are fresh or frozen meats, animal products and fish meals, cereals and cereal by-products, and soya bean meals.

Semi-moist products can be used as complete diets, having a higher energy density than canned foods and much the same as dry foods. It is important to take their possibly high sugar content into account when recommending diets for cats with diabetes mellitus.

Dry foods

The low moisture content of dry foods (8–12%) prevents fungal or bacterial spoilage if stored in dry conditions. Dry foods for cats are usually expanded extruded biscuits and, although cereal-based, contain substantial amounts of meals of animal origin providing a relatively higher protein content (30%) than comparable complete dry dog foods. Dry milk products such as dried whey, dried skimmed milk and sodium caseinate may also be included to contribute protein. Fat levels of 6–8% are achieved partly from the fat levels in the mix and partly by spraying liquefied fat onto the surface of the extruded particles. Most dry cat foods are complete (in contrast, in the UK, to dry dog foods in which most are used as biscuit mixers with canned foods).

Although dry foods of good quality can provide a satisfactory complete diet for maintenance, growth and reproduction, it is necessary to moisten them with water or milk for young kittens and, in some cases, for lactating queens. The digestibility of dry foods is usually lower for cats than for dogs (Kendall *et al.*, 1982) and is also lower than wet or canned foods, particularly if there is much cereal fibre.

Cats require substantially more drinking water when fed dry or semi-moist foods than when fed canned foods. Dry foods provide a substantial proportion of the prepared cat food market worldwide and although generally of lower palatability than canned foods, have a significant place in cat nutrition.

Home-made diets

Unlike dogs, cats are disinclined to accept household scraps and leftovers, unless they happen to be good quality meat or fish. Cats which are not given prepared cat foods usually have meat or fish bought especially for them. There is no doubt that cats can thrive on such diets so long as the owners are sufficiently nutrition conscious to make up for deficiencies in nutrients such as calcium and vitamin A in meat and fish. Milk, which is also a traditional food for cats, makes up for many of the deficiencies which might occur in predominantly meat or fish diets. Cheese and eggs are also useful sources of vitamins and minerals which are acceptable to many cats.

A useful guide to the nutrient content of some meats and meat by-products has been provided by Rainbird (1988) and more detailed tables of the nutrients in a wide range of foodstuffs is provided in *Nutrient Requirements of Cats* (NRC, 1986) and *The Composition of Foodstuffs* (Paul & Southgate, 1978).

WATER

Homeostatic control of water balance in cats differs in some important respects from that of dogs (Anderson, 1982, 1983).

Drinking

Cats will eat and drink at any time of the day and night (in contrast to dogs, which rarely eat or drink during darkness) (Mugford, 1977). Cats, however, appear to exert a less precise control over their state of hydration than dogs and are slower to replenish water losses by drinking (Adolph, 1974).

Water in the food

The water content of the commercial foods commonly fed to cats varies from 8% in dry foods to over 80% in canned foods; thus the amount of drinking water required is affected substantially by the water content of the food. Cats can live for long periods without drinking water when receiving food containing 67–73% water but become dehydrated when the water content of the food is 63% or less (Anderson, 1982). When fed canned food (84% moisture) with access to drinking water, they obtain over 90% of their total water intake from the diet, whereas on dry food, 96% of the total water intake is obtained by drinking. The total free water intake (from food and drinking water) decreases when cats are fed dry food only, so that the water to dry matter intake ratio when fed on commercial dry foods varies from 2.0 to 2.8:1 whereas on canned foods it varies from 3.0 to 5.7:1 (NRC, 1986). Thus for any given dry matter intake cats have a higher water turnover on canned than on dry foods.

Oxidation water

Depending on the diet, water from the oxidation of dietary protein, fat and carbohydrate provides about 10% of the total water intake (Table 24.5).

Although fat provides most water of oxidation per gram, carbohydrate provides the most water per unit of energy. Where water is scarce, a diet of carbohydrate and water is better than water alone, as the carbohydrate spares the oxidation of tissue, protein and fat, thus reducing urinary solutes and volume.

Respiratory water

Respiratory evaporative cooling is an important way of losing heat in most mammals. In cats, however, this method of heat control is relatively ineffective. While dogs show a 12–20-fold increase in respiration rate in response to heat stress (40°C), cats show only a 4–5-fold increase with the consequence that the percentage of their heat output which can be lost by panting is small (10%) compared to that of dogs (57%) (Anderson, 1982). At high environmental temperatures cats, in addition to seeking cool places, will augment their evaporative heat losses by increased salivation and licking and moistening their fur (Robinson & Lee, 1941).

Table 24.5 Water derived from the oxidation of basic nutrients.

Nutrient	Water formed/g (g)	Water formed/kcal (g)
Carbohydrate	0.566	0.133
Fat	1.071	0.113
Protein	0.396	0.092

Table 24.6 Maximum urinary concentrating capacity of various mammals.

Species	Maximum urine concentration (mOsm/l)
Jerboa	6500
White mouse	4300
Cat	3200*
Camel	3170
Dog	2425
Man	1160

* Thrall and Miller (1976) recorded values of 4890 and 3420 mOsm/l in one cat.
From Chew (1965) with permission.

Urinary water loss

In cats fed dry food, 14–30% of total free water intake is excreted via the urine (Anderson, 1983). Their ability to conserve water by excreting a highly concentrated urine is frequently cited as a factor in their predisposition to develop urolithiasis; the maximum urine concentrations recorded are not, however, remarkable in relation to some other mammals adapted to desert conditions (Table 24.6).

Faecal water

The percentage of total free water intake excreted in the faeces varies from 14 to 25% (Anderson, 1983) and the partition of excreted water between urinary and non-urinary routes has been postulated as a factor in the aetiology of FUS (Jackson & Tovey, 1977).

PRESCRIPTION DIETS

The increased availability of a range of prescription diets is a welcome development as an aid to treatment of both acute and chronic disease. Many owners appreciate the opportunity to participate in the treatment and nursing of a sick animal and the availability of a range of diets which have particular nutritional characteristics provides clinicians with an opportunity to involve clients in the nursing and management of patients.

However, a great deal remains to be done to quantify dietary management in a wide range of canine and feline diseases. Much of the current knowledge is empirical or derivative from comparable, but not necessarily identical, conditions in man. As the use of prescription diets increases, however, the accumulated clinical experience should provide a basis for the more quantitative development of this field, both in the prevention and treatment of small animal disease.

Appendix 24.1 Minimum requirements for growing kittens (units per kg of diet, dry basis).[a]

Nutrient	Unit	Amount	Nutrient	Unit	Amount
Fat[b]			Phenylalanine	g	4
Linoleic acid	g	5	Taurine	mg	400
Arachidonic acid	mg	200	Threonine	g	7
			Tryptophan	g	1.5
Protein$_c$ (N × 6.25)	g	240	Valine	g	6
Arginine	g	10			
Histidine	g	3	Minerals		
Isoleucine	g	5	Calcium	g	8
Leucine	g	12	Phosphorus	g	6
Lysine	g	8	Magnesium	mg	400
Methionine plus cystine (total	g	7.5	Potassium$_d$	g	4
sulfur amino acids)			Sodium	mg	500
Methionine	g	4	Chloride	g	1.9
Phenylalanine plus tyrosine	g	8.5	Iron	mg	80

continued on p. 592

Appendix 24.1 *Continued*

Nutrient	Unit	Amount	Nutrient	Unit	Amount
Copper	mg	5	Riboflavin	mg	4
Iodine	μg	350	Vitamin B$_6$ (pyridoxine)	mg	4
Zinc	mg	50	Niacin	mg	40
Manganese	mg	5	Pantothenic acid	mg	5
Selenium	μg	100	Folacin (folic acid[f])	μg	800
			Biotin[f]	μg	70
Vitamins			Vitamin B$_{12}$	μg	20
Vitamin A (retinol)	mg	1 (3333 IU)	(cyanocobalamin)		
Vitamin D (cholecalciferol)	μg	12.5 (500 IU)			
Vitamin E$_e$ (α-tocopherol)	mg	30 (30 IU)	Choline[g]	g	2.4
Vitamin K$_f$ (phylloquinone)	μg	100	Myo-inositol[h]	–	–
Thiamin	mg	5			

[a] Based on a diet with an ME concentration of 5.0 kcal*/g dry matter fed to 10- to 20-week-old kittens. If dietary energy density is greater or lesser, it is assumed that these requirements should be increased or decreased proportionately. Nutrient requirement levels have been selected based on the most appropriate optimal response (i.e., growth, nitrogen retention, metabolite concentration or excretion, lack of abnormal clinical signs, etc.) of kittens fed a purified diet. Some of these requirements are known adequate amounts rather than minimum requirements. Since diet processing (such as extruding or retorting) may destroy or impair the availability of some nutrients, and since some nutrients, especially the trace minerals, are less available from some natural feedstuffs than from purified diets, increased amounts of these nutrients should be included to ensure that the minimum requirements are met. The minimum requirements presented in this table assume availabilities similar to those present in purified diets.

[b] No requirement for fat is known apart from the need for essential fatty acids and as a carrier of fat-soluble vitamins. Some fat normally enhances the palatability of the diet.

[c] Assuming that all the minimum essential amino acid requirements are met.

[d] The minimum potassium requirement increases with protein intake.

[e] This minimum should be adequate for a moderate to low-fat diet. It may be expected to increase three- to four-fold with a high PUFA diet, especially when fish oil is present.

[f] These vitamins may not be required in the diet unless antimicrobial agents or antivitamin compounds are present in the diet.

[g] Choline is not essential in the diet but if this quantity of choline is not present the methionine requirement should be increased to provide the same quantity of methyl groups.

[h] A dietary requirement for myo-inositol has not been demonstrated for the cat. However, almost all published studies in which purified diets have been used have included myo-inositol at 150 to 200 mg/kg diet and no studies have tested a myo-inositol-free diet.

Note: The minimum requirements of all the nutrients are not known for the adult cat at maintenance. It is known that these levels of nutrients are adequate and that protein and methionine can be reduced to 140 and 3 g/kg diet, respectively. It is likely that the minimum requirements of all the other nutrients are also lower for maintenance than for the growing kitten.

The minimum requirements of all the nutrients are not known for reproduction for the adult male or female cat. It is known that with the following modifications the Nutrient Allowances as recommended in the 1978 NRC report are adequate for gestation and lactation (in units/kg purified diet, note these recommendations are based on 4.0 kcal*/g dry diet): arachidonate, 200 mg; zinc, 40 mg; vitamin A, 5500 IU; and taurine, 500 mg. It is probable that the minimum requirements for growing kittens in this table would satisfy all requirements for reproduction if the following were modified as shown: vitamin A, 6000 IU/kg diet, and taurine, 500 mg/kg diet.

* 1 kcal = 4.184 kJ.

Reproduced from NRC (1986) with permission.

REFERENCES

Adolph E.S. (1947) Tolerance to heat and dehydration in several species of mammals. *Am. J. Physiol.* **151**, 564–75.

Aguirre G.D. (1978) Retinal degeneration associated with the feeding of dog food to cats. *J. Am. Vet. Med. Assoc.* **172**, 791.

Anderson R.S. (1973) Obesity in the dog and cat. In Grunsell C.S.G. & Hill F.W.G. (eds) *The Veterinary Annual*, 13th issue, pp. 182–6.

Anderson R.S. (1982) Water balance in the dog and cat. *J. Small Anim. Pract.* **23**, 588–98.

Anderson R.S. (1983) Fluid balance and diet. In Van Marthens (ed) *Proceedings of the 7th Kalkan Symposium for the Treatment of Small Animal Diseases*, pp. 19–26.

Baines F.M. (1981) Milk substitutes and the hand rearing of orphaned puppies and kittens. *J. Small Anim. Pract.* **22**, 555–78.

Ballard F.J. (1965) Glucose utilization in mammalian liver. *Comp. Biochem. Physiol.* **14**, 437–43.

Bartoshuk L.M., Hamed M.A. & Parks L.H. (1971) Taste of water in the cat: Effects on sucrose preference. *Science* **171**, 699–701.

Bennett D. (1976) Nutrition and bone disease in the dog and cat. *Vet. Rec.* **98**, 313–21.

Blaxter A., Lievesley P., Gruffydd-Jones T. & Wotton P. (1986) Periodic muscle weakness in Burmese kittens. *Vet. Rec.* **118**, 619–20.

Buffington C.A., Cook N.E., Rogers Q.R. & Morris J.G. (1989) The role of diet in feline struvite urolithiasis syndrome. In Burger I.H. & Rivers J.P.W. (eds) *Nutrition of the Dog and Cat*. Pergamon, Oxford, pp. 357–80.

Campbell J.R. & Douglas T.A. (1965) The effect of low calcium intake and vitamin D supplements on bone structure in young growing dogs. *Brit. J. Nutr.* **19**, 339.

Carpenter J.A. (1956) Species differences in taste preferences. *J. Comp. Physiol. Psychol.* **49**, 139–44.

Castonguay T.W. (1981) Dietary dilution and intake in the cat. *Physiol. Behav.* **27**, 547–9.

Chew R.M. (1965) Water metabolism in mammals. In Mayer M.V. & Van Gelder R.G. (eds) *Physiological Mammalogy*, vol. 2. Academic Press, New York, pp. 44–178.

Coman B.J. & Brunner H. (1972) Food habits of the feral house cat in Victoria. *Journal of Wildlife Management* **38**, 848.

Cordy D.R. & Stillinger C.J. (1953) Steatitis 'yellow fat disease' in kittens. *N. Amer. Vet.* **34**, 714–6.

Davidson M.G. (1992) Thiamin deficiency in a colony of cats. *Vet. Rec.* **130**, 94–7.

Davis S.M.J. (1987) *The Archeology of Animals*. Batsford, London, p. 133.

Dow S.W., Le Couteur R.A., Fettman M.V. & Spurgeon T. (1987) Potassium depletion in cats: Hypokalemic polymyopathy. *J. Am. Vet. Med. Ass.* **191**, 1563–8.

Eberhard T. (1954) Food habits of Pennsylvania house cats. *Journal of Wildlife Management* **19**, 284.

Edney A.T.B. (1973) Feeding behaviour and preferences in cats. *Feline Advisory Bureau Bulletin* **12**, 2–4.

English P.B. & Seawright A.A. (1964) Deforming cervical spondylosis of the cat. *Austral. Vet. J.* **40**, 376–81.

Frings H. (1951) Sweet taste in the cat and the taste spectrum. *Experientia* **7**, 424–6.

Fry P.D. (1989) Hypovitaminosis A in the cat. *Veterinary International* **1**, 16–23.

Gaskell C.J., Leedale A.H. & Douglas S.W. (1975) Pansteatitis in the cat: a report of four cases. *J. Small Anim. Pract.* **16**, 117–21.

Gershoff S.N., Legg M.A., O'Connor F.J. & Hegsted D.M. (1957) The effect of vitamin D deficient diets containing various Ca:P ratios on cats. *J. Nutr.* **63**, 79.

Holme D.W. (1982) Practical use of prepared foods for dogs and cats. In Edney A.T.B. (ed) *Dog and Cat Nutrition*, 1st edn. Pergamon, Oxford, pp. 47–59.

Hopkins A.L. (1989) Sporadic feline polymyopathy. *Vet. Rec.* **125**, 17.

Jackson O.F. & Tovey J.D. (1977) Water balance studies in domestic cats. *Feline Practice* **6**, 10–7.

Kane E. (1989) Feeding behaviour of the cat. In Burger I.H. & Rivers J.P.W. (eds) *Nutrition of the Dog and Cat. Waltham Symposium No. 7*. Cambridge University Press, pp. 147–58.

Kane E., Morris J.G. & Rogers Q.R. (1981a) Acceptability and digestibility by adult cats of diets made with various sources and levels of fat. *J. Anim. Sci.* **53**, 1516–23.

Kane E., Morris J.G., Rogers J.G., Ihirke P.J. & Cupps P.T. (1981b) Zinc deficiency in the cat. *J. Nutr.* **111**, 488–95.

Kane E., Rogers Q.R., Morris J.G. & Leung P.M.B. (1981c) Feeding behaviour of the cat fed laboratory and commercial diets. *Nutrition Research* **1**, 499–507.

Keen C.L., Lonnerdal B., Clegg M.S., Hurley L.S., Morris J.G., Rogers Q.R. & Rucker R.B. (1982) Developmental changes in the composition of cats' milk: Trace elements, minerals, protein, carbohydrate and fat. *J. Nutr.* **112**, 1763–9.

Kendall P.T., Holme D.W. & Smith P.M. (1982) Comparative evaluation of net digestive and absorptive efficiency in dogs and cats fed a variety of contrasting diet types. *J. Small Anim. Pract.* **23**, 577–87.

Kendall P.T., Blaza S.E. & Smith P.M. (1983) Comparative digestible energy requirements of adult Beagles and domestic cats for body weight maintenance. *J. Nutr.* **113**, 1946–55.

Kendall P.T., Burger I. & Smith P.M. (1985) Methods of estimation of the metabolizable energy content of cat foods. *Feline Practice* **15**, 38–44.

Krook L., Barrett R.B., Usui K. & Wolke R.E. (1963) Nutritional secondary hyperparathyroidism in the cat. *Cornell Vet.* **53**, 225–40.

Loveridge G.G. (1986) Body weight changes and energy intakes of cats during gestation and lactation. *Animal Technology* **37**, 7–15.

Loveridge G.G. (1987) Some factors affecting kitten growth. *Animal Technology* **88**, 9–18.

Loveridge G.G. & Rivers J.P.W. (1989) Body weight changes and energy intakes of cats during pregnancy and lactation. In Burger I.H. & Rivers J.P.W. (eds) *Nutrition of the Dog and Cat.* Cambridge University Press, pp. 113–32.

MacDonald M.L., Rogers Q.R. & Morris J.G. (1984) Nutrition of the cat, a mammalian carnivore. *Ann. Rev. Nutr.* **4**, 521–62.

McLean J.G. & Monger E.A. (1989) Factors determining the essential fatty acid requirements of the cat. In Burger I.H. & Rivers J.P.W. (eds) *Nutrition of the Dog and Cat.* Cambridge University Press, pp. 329–42.

Michell A.R. (1989) Salt intake, animal health and hypertension: should sleeping dogs lie? In Burger I.H. & Rivers J.P.W. (eds) *Nutrition of the Dog and Cat.* Pergamon, Oxford, pp. 275–92.

Miller S.A. & Allison J.B. (1958) The dietary nitrogen requirements of the cat. *J. Nutr.* **64**, 493.

Morris J.G. & Rogers Q.R. (1989) Comparative aspects of nutrition and metabolism of dogs and cats. In Burger I.H. & Rivers J.P.W. (eds) *Nutrition of the Dog and Cat.* Pergamon, Oxford, pp. 35–66.

Morris J.G., Trudell J. & Pencovic T. (1977) Carbohydrate digestion by the domestic cat Felis catus. *Br. J. Nutr.* **37**, 365–73.

Morris J.G., Rogers Q.R. & Pacioretty L.M. (1989) Taurine: an essential nutrient for cats. *J. Small Anim. Pract.* **31**, 502–9.

Mugford R.A. (1977) External influences in the feeding of carnivores. In Kare M.R. & Miller O. (eds) *The Chemical Senses and Nutrition.* Academic Press, New York, pp. 25–50.

Mugford R.A. & Thorne C.J. (1980) Comparative studies of meal patterns in pet and laboratory housed dogs and cats. In Anderson R.S. (ed) *Nutrition of the Dog and Cat.* Pergamon, Oxford, pp. 3–14.

Munday H.S. & Earle K.E. (1991) Energy requirements of the queen during lactation and kittens from birth to 12 weeks. *J. Nutr.* **121**, 543–4.

NRC (1986) *Nutrient Requirements of Cats.* National Academy Press, Washington DC.

Paul A.A. & Southgate D.A.T. (1978) *The Composition of Foods*, 4th edn. HMSO, London.

Peterson M.E., Kintzer P.P., Cavanagh P.G., Fox P.R., Ferguson D.C., Johnson G.F. & Becker D.V. (1983) Feline hyperthyroidism: Pretreatment, clinical and laboratory evaluation of 131 cases. *J. Am. Vet. Med. Assoc.* **183**, 103–10.

Pion P.D., Kittelson M.D., Rogers Q.R. & Morris J.G. (1987) Myocardial failure in cats associated with low plasma taurine: a reversible cardiomyopathy. *Science* **237**, 764–8.

Pfaffman C. (1955) Gustatory nerve impulses in rat, cat and rabbit. *J. Neurophysiol.* **18**, 429–40.

Rainbird A.L. (1988) Feeding throughout life. In Edney A.T.B. (ed) *Dog and Cat Nutrition*, 2nd edn. Pergamon, Oxford, pp. 75–96.

Rivers J.P.W., Frankel T.L., Juttla S. & Hay A.W.M. (1979) Vitamin D in the nutrition of the cat. *Proc. Nutr. Soc.* **38**, 36A (Abstr.).

Robinson K.W. & Lee D.H.K. (1941) Reactions of the cat to hot atmospheres. *Proc. R. Soc. Queensland* **53**, 159–70.

Rogers Q.R. & Morris J.G. (1979) Essentiality of amino acids for the growing kitten. *J. Nutr.* **109**, 718–23.

Rogers Q.R., Morris J.G. & Freedland R.A. (1977) Lack of hepatic enzymatic adaptation to low and high levels of dietary protein in the adult cat. *Enzyme* **22**, 348–56.

Schaeffer M.C., Rogers Q.R. & Morris J.G. (1989) Protein in the nutrition of dogs and cats. pp. 159–205. In Burger I.H. & Rivers J.P.W. (eds) *Nutrition of the Dog and Cat.* Cambridge University Press, pp. 329–42.

Schneck G.W. & Cumberland V. (1968) The effect of 10 percent dietary fat addition on the growth rate of cats. *Vet. Rec.* **83**, 486–8.

Seawright A.A., English P.B. & Gartner R.J.W. (1967) Hypervitaminosis A and deforming cervical spondylosis of the cat. *J. Comp. Pathol.* **77**, 29–39.

Thrall B.E. & Miller L.G. (1976) Water turnover in cats fed dry rations. *Feline Practice* **6**, 10–17.

Walker A.D., Weaver A.D., Anderson R.S., Crighton G.W., Fennell C., Gaskell C.J. & Wilkinson G.T. (1977) An epidemiological survey of the feline urological syndrome. *J. Small Anim. Pract.* **18**, 283–301.

Willeburg P. (1984) Epidemiology of naturally occurring feline urological syndrome. *Veterinary Clinics of North America* **14**, 455–69.

Chapter 25 / Endoparasites

A. I. WRIGHT

INTRODUCTION

The endoparasites of the cat comprise a variety of species which are found in each of the major taxonomic groups. With a few exceptions, they are seldom a cause of more than mild clinical disease and their incidence depends entirely on the lifestyle of the individual cat. Unlike the dog whose diet is usually strictly controlled by the owner, a cat allowed to roam freely may supplement its food from the wild and as a consequence acquires more parasites from this source than directly from other cats. Most cat parasites have an indirect life cycle involving infection of intermediate hosts which enable the parasites to be concentrated, protected and dispersed in the environment to a degree that virtually guarantees successful transmission. The intermediate hosts include arthropods, molluscs, amphibians, reptiles, birds and mammals, and more than one may be involved in transmission. They can act as true intermediate hosts, which are essential for successful development of larval stages of the parasite, or as transport hosts, which simply carry the parasite passively, as when an earthworm ingests parasite eggs or larvae, disseminating them by passage through the gut. The term 'paratenic host' is used in those instances where the immature stage of a parasite is trapped permanently in the tissues, depending on predation by cats for completion of development. Cats which are housed throughout their lives and fed entirely on cooked or tinned meat can be protected from parasites which utilize intermediate hosts. However, other ingenious modes of trans-

mission evolved by parasites still defy effective control; for example, the common roundworm *Toxocara cati* passes from dam to offspring via the milk, thus ensuring establishment of a worm burden in very young kittens.

Without doubt, the most important aspects of cat parasites, both external as well as internal, are the problems they pose as zoonoses. Toxocaral infection of man resulting in the disease visceral larva migrans is believed to be caused almost entirely by the dog ascarid *Toxocara canis*, but *T. cati* and *Toxascaris leonina*, both found in cats, are potentially able to infest man and should not be entirely dismissed as a possible cause of the disease. A more serious threat from the cat is toxoplasmosis, an infestation by a protozoan parasite which depends on the cat for development of its sexual stages. Asexually reproducing forms are able to develop in the tissues of all warm-blooded animals and such infestations are widespread, but fortunately only an occasional cause of disease. Human toxoplasmosis may be a congenital infestation or acquired later in life, either directly from cat faeces or from meat contaminated with the parasite. In man, the disease can cause severe damage to central nervous tissues with involvement of the eye and the lymphatic system. Toxoplasmosis can be of considerable economic importance in some farm livestock; in Britain, for example, it is one of the commonest causes of ovine abortion. Cryptosporidiosis and giardiasis, both occurring in cats, are now frequently diagnosed human infestations. The former is without doubt a zoonosis, but there is still uncertainty about the transmissibility of

Giardia from animals to man. There will be an increasing demand for the small animal practitioner to prove or disprove the presence of these infestations in family pets.

The remarkable extent to which some cat parasites succeed in contaminating the environment is due to their ability to survive outside the primary feline host. The eggs of *Toxocara* and the oocysts of *Toxoplasma* remain viable for months or even years under suitable conditions, and the tissue forms of these parasites remain dormant in many cases for the lifetime of their respective intermediate hosts. The prevention of infestation of cats by parasites necessitates restriction of freedom to a degree which most owners would be unable to impose and indeed would regard as undesirable. It must be assumed that the average household pet cat allowed to roam and forage at random will acquire some of the parasites described here, and it is important therefore that their nature and potential pathogenicity for all their hosts be fully appreciated.

COMMON HELMINTH PARASITES

Tapeworms

Dipylidium caninum

Despite its name, this tapeworm is common in cats. Fleas are the usual intermediate hosts, but the biting louse *Felicola subrostratus* is another source of infection. Adult worms live in the small intestine attached by the scolex, which bears four suckers and a retractable rostellum armed with five or six rows of rose-thorn-shaped hooks. The scolex is pinhead-sized and the slender strobila has a narrow 'neck' region and numerous segments, which assume a characteristic cucumber-seed-shape as they mature. These tapeworms may grow up to 40–50 cm in length, but most specimens rarely exceed 25 cm in the cat. The greater the number present, the shorter in length individual worms tend to be. They are often found in considerable numbers, several hundred having been recorded on occasions.

Each mature segment has a double set of male and female reproductive organs and a genital opening on either side, visible in the gravid segment as opaque indentations. The gravid segments contain egg capsules, each encompassing a cluster of from 10 to 20 eggs. For completion of the life cycle, the eggs must be ingested by larval fleas, which have chewing mouthparts and feed on organic debris in the host's bedding. The onchosphere released from the egg migrates into the body cavity of the larval flea and forms a cysticercoid, which persists through the pupal to the adult stage of the flea. Infestation of the cat occurs when fleas are accidentally swallowed while grooming. All stages of biting lice can ingest the egg, and cysticercoids develop as in fleas.

Gravid segments are shed in the faeces and also pass from the rectum independently of bowel movement to contaminate the perineal hair and the bedding. Most cats remove perineal contamination, but desiccated segments may be found on the long-haired breeds. Fresh segments are 1 cm in length and cream-coloured with a reddish-brown centre formed by the mass of dark egg capsules. Egg capsules are about 200 μm in length and just visible to the naked eye as dark granules when the segment is teased open in water. Segments move sluggishly for a time but soon rupture to release the egg capsules. Absence of egg capsules in segments may be a cause of confusion in identification. When completely desiccated, the segments are brittle, amber-coloured flakes no more than 3–4 mm in length. Soaking for several minutes in normal saline will restore their shape, but egg capsules are unlikely to be present.

Surveys of the incidence of intestinal parasites of cats based on observations at autopsy show *D. caninum* to be common in Britain. For example, an infection rate of over 50% was recorded at Aberystwyth and Glasgow, 44.5% in London, 12.7% in Liverpool, and 13.0% in Swansea. From these surveys and others recently reviewed by Nichol *et al.* (1981), it is apparent that faecal examination for the detection of tapeworms is unreliable where this method alone is employed – the incidence of tapeworms is always much lower than that recorded by autopsy examination. Tapeworm segments, egg capsules and free eggs appear intermittently in the faeces and can easily be missed.

Of the intermediate hosts of *D. caninum*, cat and dog fleas are more likely to transmit infestation than lice, as the latter have become scarce following the introduction of modern insecticides to which they are so vulnerable.

Taenia taeniaeformis

The above-mentioned review of the incidence of endoparasites of cats (Nichol *et al.*, 1981) indicates that *T. taeniaeformis* is recorded much less frequently than *Dipylidium caninum* in all the surveys. The highest incidence of 15% was recorded in Glasgow and Swansea. All the other surveys based on autopsy findings give a figure below 10%. This tapeworm is always present in low numbers in the small intestine; it is unusual to find more than three or four in an individual. Morphologically, they are easily distinguished from *D. caninum* by being much larger and stouter worms. Individuals grow to 50 cm in length and have a relatively large head with four suckers and a double row of hooks on the rostellum. There is no narrow 'neck' region behind the scolex and the mature segments have a posterior margin wider than the anterior end giving the strobila a distinctive serrated appearance and the gravid segments a flattened bell-shape. Each segment has a single set of male and female reproductive organs and the genital openings are irregularly unilateral.

The intermediate stage of *T. taeniaeformis* is called *Cysticercus fasciolaris* and develops in the liver of rats, mice, voles and squirrels. This larval stage differs from that of other taeniid tapeworms in having, in addition to the scolex, a short strobila of segments terminating with a small bladder. It is tightly packed into a pea-sized cyst formed by a host tissue reaction. The cystic stage is infective for cats in about 60 days and after ingestion the adult tapeworm is mature in 16–18 days. Gravid segments are shed in the faeces and, like *Dipylidium*, may migrate from the rectum independently of bowel movement. They can be distinguished easily from those of *Dipylidium* by their different shape and unilateral genital pore.

When broken open in water, large numbers of dark-brown eggs are released, measuring 40 μm in diameter and not enclosed in egg capsules. It is important to distinguish between the two tapeworms because treatment must be accompanied by measures to prevent reinfestation, the epidemiology of each being entirely different. Both species of tapeworm may occur together, and tend to infest cats over 1 year of age.

Species of *Taenia* tapeworms other than *T. taeniaeformis* are extremely uncommon in cats and there are only two records in recent years.

Echinococcus

Echinococcus granulosus does not reach sexual maturity in the cat and experimental infections are short-lived, so that cats can be disregarded as a source of hydatid disease. *Echinococcus multilocularis*, which does reach sexual maturity in the cat, does not occur in Britain.

Clinical signs

The majority of tapeworm infestations are symptomless and often remain undetected in cats, which bury their faeces outdoors. However, occasionally, and more especially in the finer breeds of cat such as Siamese and Burmese, obvious abdominal discomfort is sometimes seen. The shedding of segments may cause anal irritation and excessive attention to the perineal region. Diarrhoea and weight loss, despite popular belief, are not features of tapeworm infestations. The most unpleasant aspect of tapeworms is the aesthetic objection by the owner to the constant shedding of gravid segments about the house.

Treatment and control

Cestocides suitable for cats include bunamidine hydrochloride, niclosamide and praxiquantel. Individual idiosyncracy to these drugs may be seen and care should be taken when using them for the first time. Bunamidine and praxiquantel cause disintegration of the tapeworms before they are voided. None of these anthelminthics has any effect on roundworms. Of the more recently introduced anthelminthics, mebendazole and fenbendazole have some action against *Taenia* but not *Dipylidium*, and nitroscanate is unsuitable for cats. Apparent failure to treat successfully is nearly always due to reinfestation; this is certain to occur if no measures are taken to break the tapeworm's life cycle. When *Dipylidium* infestation is diagnosed, the cat in question and all other cats and dogs in contact must be treated for ectoparasites, and likely flea habitats in the environment destroyed. In most cases, it is not possible to prevent free-roaming cats from hunting rodents, and owners must be warned that reinfestation with *T. taeniaeformis* after treatment should be expected. Periodic treatment every 2 months or so may be necessary to keep cats free from tapeworms, but it should be stressed that they are relatively harmless, and with the exception of a few records of human infection with *Dipylidium* (acquired by inadvertently swallowing an infected flea or louse), the tapeworms of the cat are of no public health significance.

Roundworms

Ascarids

Two ascarids are found in the small intestine of the cat, *Toxocara cati* (= *T. mystax*) and *Toxascaris leonina*, the former being much the commoner species. The majority of surveys (e.g. Nichol *et al.*, 1981) show *T. cati* to be the most prevalent of all endoparasites, the incidence decreasing with age from a 30% infection rate in kittens under 3 months of age, to below 10% in adult and aged cats. The much less common *T. leonina* is usually recorded in surveys in less than 5% of the cat population. The difference in life cycles and epidemiology of the two worms explains this disparity in incidence.

T. cati is a large white worm, with the male measuring about 10 cm and the female up to 15 cm, but they are often much shorter in length. At the anterior end there is a pair of cervical alae which give the worms an arrow-headed appearance, and the male caudal region ends in a short finger-like process barely perceptible to the naked eye. *T. leonina* is similar in appearance but usually smaller and has lanceolate cervical alae and no finger-like appendage in the male. The egg of *T. cati* is subspherical, measuring about 75 μm with a thick pitted shell stained a light-brown colour. The egg of *T. leonina* is about the same size, but the shell is smooth and colourless. In both species the egg contains an ensegmented ovum when passed in the faeces.

LIFE CYCLE OF *T. CATI*

The life cycle of *T. cati* is less complicated than that of *T. canis* in the dog. There are three modes of infestation: by ingestion of embryonated eggs; from larvae in the milk of suckling queens; and from larvae in paratenic hosts. Embryonation of the eggs to the infective L_2 stage takes at least 4 weeks and considerably longer out-of-doors during the winter. When embryonated eggs are ingested, the larvae undergo a liver-to-lung migration and eventually return to the small intestine, where they grow to maturity and commence laying eggs about 6–7 weeks after infestation. However, this route is probably of little importance in kittens where the most potent source of infestation is via the milk; larvae are present in the milk throughout lactation. These larvae are derived from the tissues of the queen, especially mammary tissues, where they have been stored as L_2 larvae acquired both before and during pregnancy and throughout lactation. It should be noted that intrauterine infection, which invariably occurs in dogs infected with *T. canis*, does not occur in *T. cati* infections. When the embryonated eggs of T. cati are ingested by earthworms, beetles, rodents or birds, the L_2 migrates into the tissues of these paratenic hosts and remains there until eaten by a cat. An interesting feature of *T. cati* is that when larvae are acquired from the milk or in paratenic hosts, there is no liver-to-lung migration, development to maturity occurring entirely in the gut. Virtually all kittens become infected when they suckle and later in life ingestion of embryonated eggs and predation of paratenic hosts maintain a low level of infestation in adult cats.

LIFE CYCLE OF *T. LEONINA*

This ascarid is acquired by ingestion of the embryonated egg containing the L_2 larvae or by the predation of the same species of hosts which harbour the L_2 of *T. cati*. However, there is a slight diffcrence in that *T. leonina* develops from L_2 to L_3 in these hosts, which must be regarded therefore as true intermediate rather than paratenic hosts. Whichever is the source of infestation, there is no liver-to-lung migration and the prepatent period is at least 8 weeks. Because there is neither intrauterine nor transmammary infection, *T. leonina* is seldom seen in cats under 6 months of age and it always tends to be present in smaller numbers than *T. cati*.

CLINICAL SIGNS

Clinical disease due to ascarids is less frequent in cats than in dogs and is confined mainly to kittens during the first 8 weeks of life that acquire a heavy infestation of *T. cati* while suckling. As there is no liver-to-lung migration following infestation via this route, the pathogenic effects are confined to the gut. A burden comprising several dozen worms can cause unthriftiness, diarrhoea, a poor coat and an accumulation of gas in the intestines, which gives kittens a characteristic wormy pot-bellied appearance.

DIAGNOSIS, TREATMENT AND CONTROL

Often the most conspicuous evidence of infestation is the presence of worms in vomit or faeces. The distinctive eggs of the two species of ascarids can be detected in faeces by the standard McMaster slide technique, but they are unlikely to be present in kittens before 8 weeks of age.

Several anthelminthics are suitable for cats and their use has been reviewed by Connan (1979). Piperazine salts given in tablet form are both safe and easy to administer. Their efficacy against immature worms in the intestines is less than for adults and repeat treatments are advisable. It is important to give the correct dose of piperazine according to bodyweight as neurotoxic and other signs have been recorded in a kitten overdosed with this drug (Goddard & Johnston, 1986).

Of the benzimidazoles, both mebendazole and fenbendazole given orally are highly efficient against ascarids but have the disadvantage of having to be given daily for a number of days. The organophosphorus anthelminthic dichlorvos may be given in tablet form, but should be used with care as it is relatively toxic for cats.

A suitable regime of treatment for kittens would be a routine dose at 4–6 weeks of age, followed by treatment every 3 weeks up to 4 months of age. Subsequent treatments depend on the degree of access to infestation from a contaminated environment, or the availability of paratenic hosts. Free-roaming cats and cats kept in catteries with outside soil and grass runs are likely to carry a low burden of ascarids all their lives and therefore should be routinely treated at least twice a year. There is at present no way to destroy larvae in the body tissues and so prevent transmammary infection, but pregnant queens should be treated and prevented from acquiring infestation throughout pregnancy and lactation.

Soil in gardens contaminated by faeces containing ascarid eggs is likely to become a permanent source of infection. The eggs are extremely resistant and can remain viable for 2 or 3 years if protected from sunlight and desiccation. The feline habit of burying faeces, although to some extent reducing the amount of contamination, is likely to favour longevity of ascarid eggs. The destruction of eggs contaminating cages, pens and concrete runs is best achieved by heat treatment using boiling water containing a detergent, or by steam sterilization.

HUMAN VISCERAL LARVA MIGRANS

This disease is acquired by the accidental ingestion by humans of the embryonated eggs of the ascarids of the dog and cat. The larvae of all three species migrate in the tissues of a wide variety of mammals and birds, including man, who acts as yet another paratenic host. By far the most important for man is the dog ascarid *T. canis*, which is believed to be responsible for the majority of human visceral larva migrans. There is serological, histopathological and epidemiological evidence to suggest that *T. cati* is unlikely to be implicated, although it should not be completely disregarded as a possible cause. The opportunity for human infection to occur from cats is less than for dogs, because cats out-of-doors bury their faeces and tend to avoid contaminating recreation areas used by the public such as parks, playing fields and sand pits.

A survey by Woodruff and de Savigny (1982) highlights the difference between dogs and cats as a source of larva migrans. Using the immunosorbent assay technique (ELISA) they showed that 15.7% of dog breeders exhibiting at shows had significant toxocaral serum antibodies indicating present or past infestation, compared with only 1.5% positive in a similar group of cat breeders, and 2.6% positive in healthy adults in the general population. Moreover, in Iceland, where dogs have long been prohibited in order to control hydatidosis, the human population showed no serological evidence of toxocaral infestation despite a large population of cats. There can be no doubt that cats are capable of contaminating the environment with faecal-borne infections because the incidence of toxoplasmal antibodies in Iceland is similar to that of humans in Britain.

The authors conclude that cats clearly constitute a much lower risk to the general population than do dogs in respect of toxocaral infestation, but not in respect of toxoplasmal infestation. As larva migrans appears to be a canine zoonosis, it is not proposed to give a detailed description of the disease and readers should refer to the excellent accounts given by Woodruff (1970), and Beresford-Jones and Jacobs (1979).

Aelurostrongylus abstrusus

The lungworm of the cat is recognized as a common infestation in most parts of the world. It is a typical metastrongyloid nematode living in the lungs as an adult and utilizing a range of molluscan intermediate hosts, and an even greater variety of paratenic hosts which preserve, concentrate and confectionate the parasite and aid its dispersal. The majority of infestations are benign, and there is evidence that in the absence

of superinfestation, the burden is spontaneously shed after 3–4 months, after which the cat is strongly resistant to reinfestation. However, occasionally the worms may cause quite severe respiratory signs, although it is not certain whether this is due to heavy infestation or decreased resistance.

The adult worms live in the terminal bronchioles, alveolar ducts, and the smaller branches of the pulmonary artery. They are very small, slender worms, the males measuring about 5 mm and the females 9 mm in length, but they are difficult to recover intact as they lie embedded in lung tissues. Eggs are laid embryonated into the alveoli where the L_1 hatches and ascends the air passages to be coughed up and swallowed, appearing in the faeces as a small 0.36 mm long sluggish larva possessing a characteristic S-shaped kink in the tail. The L_1 can survive several months and further development only takes place in the intermediate host. Most of the common species of slugs and snails are suitable, and the larvae actively penetrate the integument and undergo two ecdyses in the muscle of the foot. They are now L_3 and as such are infective for cats. The molluscan intermediate host may be eaten by various paratenic hosts, in which the larvae are found unchanged in many tissues such as the gastrointestinal tract, submucosa and subserosa, lungs, diaphragm and adipose tissue. After ingestion of the infected intermediate or paratenic host by a cat, the L_3 penetrates the intestinal tract and travels to the lungs via the lymphatics and bloodstream. The prepatent period is from 34 to 42 days.

The only aspect of the life cycle which is imperfectly understood is whether infestation of cats occurs by ingestion of the molluscan intermediate host or one of the paratenic hosts. Cats are not known to eat slugs and snails and when molluscs are experimentally fed they tend to provoke vomiting. The paratenic hosts include amphibians, reptiles, rodents and birds. In Britain birds are probably the principal source of infection for cats; small rodents such as mice and voles are vegetarian, and the insectivorous shrews appear to be unpalatable to cats. The slow-worm is another possible paratenic host. As many as 600 infective larvae have been found in an individual snail and they can survive in this host for at least 2 years and for an indefinite period in the paratenic host.

The course of experimental infestation of cats and the histopathology of lungworms has been studied in detail by Hamilton (1966a, 1967). He found that as few as 50 infective larvae caused lung lesions, but in the region of 800 were necessary to produce respiratory signs. When an infecting dose of 1600–3200 was given, severe signs developed which were potentially lethal. Dyspnoea and coughing, even at rest but especially on exertion, were the commonest signs. In severe infestations, a chronic cough developed with increasing dyspnoea, inanition, anorexia and fever. Harsh lung sounds or moist rales may be heard on auscultation, and occasionally sneezing and oculonasal discharge occurs. Severity of infestation reaches a peak at 6–12 weeks, after which the signs subside and the disease spontaneously resolves. Larvae first appear in the faeces at about 5 weeks after infestation and increase to a peak at 10–14 weeks; they then gradually decline and eventually disappear altogether by week 24. Small numbers of adults may persist in the lungs for many months, although they do not produce larvae unless the cat is stressed.

PATHOLOGY

Lesions are confined to the thoracic cavity. In the mildest cases, which can result from as few as 50 infective larvae, pinpoint-sized greyish nodules occur throughout the lungs. In more severe infestations nodules up to 10 mm in diameter are seen, especially beneath the pleura, giving it an irregular surface. They are firm greyish-yellow lesions which tend to coalesce when numerous. The pleural cavity may contain thick milky fluid, rich in eggs and larvae. In most cases, the bronchial lymph nodes are enlarged. These lesions form 2–4 weeks after infestation, reach maximum size at 6–14 weeks, and almost completely regress by week 24.

Histopathological changes have been followed chronologically by Hamilton (1966a). The earliest lesions are formed by aggregates of eosinophils, lymphocytes and macrophages in bronchioles and alveoli, with hypertrophy of the smooth muscle of the walls of bronchioles, alveolar ducts, and the media layer of branches of the pulmonary artery. Adult worms and eggs in various stages of development are seen in section and in time these provoke a marked cellular reaction, often with central necrosis and calcification of the nodular mass. Epithelialization of the surrounding lung tissue is a feature and as the parasitic colonies decline 4–6 months after infestation, the outstanding feature of the lungs is numerous masses of hypertrophied bronchiolar and ductal smooth muscle, and marked medial hypertrophy and hyperplasia of the pulmonary artery branches. Residual lesions may persist for several years and even a lifetime. Studying the lungs of 256 randomly selected cats, Hamilton (1966b) found in 34.7% lesions of hypertrophy and hyperplasia of pulmonary arteries indistinguishable from those produced by experimental lungworm infestation. He concludes that lungworms are the probable cause of this apparently widespread lesion of cat lungs. Hamilton (1968a) also showed that a good acquired immunity developed to infestation, reinfestation causing respiratory signs but no shedding of larvae in the faeces. Immunity seems to be related to the presence of a small residual population of adults.

DIAGNOSIS, TREATMENT AND CONTROL

The only reliable method of diagnosing infestation is the demonstration of the characteristic larvae in faeces, best recovered from fresh samples by Baermann apparatus. However, larvae may appear intermittently, and are completely absent in the early and later stages of infestation. Hamilton (1968b) reported using the indirect fluorescent antibody test on cat serum and found it to be highly specific for *A. abstrusus*, but the test did not differentiate between active and past infestation. Lesions are visible radiologically but they are probably not specific enough to be diagnostic.

Of the anthelminthics available for treatment, only tetramisole hydrochloride has been recommended, at a dosage rate of 30–45 mg/kg. Five doses are recommended diluted with water and given orally every other day. Profuse salivation after administration can be controlled by atropine premedication. It is probable that some of the later benzimidazoles and ivermectin would be effective, but as yet no controlled trials on cats with lungworm infestation have been carried out.

In the hunting cat which has free access to the intermediate and paratenic hosts, there is no way of preventing infestation. However, it must be stressed that infestations are self-limiting and most are symptomless.

Ollulanus tricuspis

This minute nematode is found coiled on the stomach wall under a layer of mucus; the males measure 0.7 mm and the females 1.0 mm in length. The life cycle is direct, infestation passing from cat to cat by infective L_3 in the vomit, but larvae may also develop to adults endogenously without leaving the stomach. A review of this worm in the cat is given by Hasslinger (1984). Although generally regarded as non-pathogenic, there are a number of reports from the USA of chronic fibrosing gastritis associated with *Ollulanus* infestation (e.g. Hargis *et al.*, 1983). Its presence can be detected by examination of vomit or stomach washings for L_3, which are generally absent from the faeces. When suspected of causing gastritis, treatment with mebendazole or fenbendazole is recommended.

UNUSUAL HELMINTH PARASITES

Uncinaria stenocephala

The common hookworm of dogs does not seem capable of establishing itself in cats and there is no record of this worm from cats in Britain.

Capillaria aerophila

These nematodes live in the trachea and bronchi of the dog, cat and fox. They are fine slender worms measuring 25–30 mm in length, lying closely adherent to the mucous membrane of the air passages. The life cycle is direct and the characteristic bipolar eggs containing an unsegmented ovum are coughed up and swallowed, to pass in the faeces. The parasite is rare and most likely to be found in cats sharing the same habitat as foxes.

It is important to remember that when examining the faeces of hunting cats, the presence of strongyle-type or bipolar eggs may constitute spurious parasitism, the eggs having been derived from nematodes of wild animals. There is only one record of hookworm eggs in cat faeces in the UK (Else *et al.*, 1977) but it cannot be assumed that the eggs came from a hookworm infestation in the cat in question.

TOXOPLASMOSIS AND OTHER COCCIDIAL INFECTIONS

Toxoplasma gondii

The protozoan parasite *Toxoplasma gondii* was discovered in 1908 in gondis, a species of North African rodent. During the next 50 years, observations all over the world showed that infection was widespread in warm-blooded animals, including man, and that it was an occasional cause of clinical disease. The development of serological diagnostic tests for the parasite revealed symptomless infections to be commonplace and it is now accepted that probably all mammals and birds are susceptible. Remarkably, it was not until 1970 that the coccidian nature of *T. gondii* was confirmed, with felids playing a key role as the hosts which support the sexual stages of the life cycle (Hutchison *et al.*, 1970).

The coccidia belong to the class Sporozoa, a group characterizied by an alternation of asexual with sexual phases of reproduction. There have been several revisions of the classification of this group and the matter is still unresolved. The important genera of veterinary importance are *Toxoplasma*, *Eimeria*, *Isospora*, *Sarcocystis*, *Cryptosporidium* and *Besnoitia*. The life cycles and specific details of these protozoa are given by Levine (1985).

The life cycle of *T. gondii* is as follows.

Unsporulated oocysts are shed in the faeces of felids and ultimately sporulate to form two sporocysts, each containing four sporozoites. These can infect all felids and all the intermediate hosts. In felids the sporozoites undergo a typical coccidian life cycle, with a series of asexual schizogony generations succeeded by the sexual gametogony generation, all in the intestinal epithelial cells. After fertilization of macrogametes by microgametes, oocysts form and are shed unsporulated in the faeces. On ingestion of the sporulated oocysts by one of the vast range of intermediate hosts, which includes felids, the sporozoites released in the intestines penetrate the wall to enter any type of nucleated cell in the body where rapid asexual division occurs. The product of this multiplication, the tachyzoites, form aggregates within the lining of the parasitized cell known as pseudocysts. The multiplication of tachyzoites is associated with the acute stage of toxoplasmosis; zoites from the pseudocysts invade other host cells, travelling via the blood or lymphatics, or spreading locally to adjacent tissue and across serous cavities. Cells of the reticuloendothelial system are most likely to be invaded. The majority of intermediate hosts survive this phase and tachyzoites are then influenced by developing host immunity and adopt a slower rate of multiplication. These zoites are known as bradyzoites and colonies become surrounded by a true cyst wall, the infection now entering a chronic phase. Tissue cysts may contain a few or many thousands of bradyzoites; they are long-lived, surviving months or years and probably persist for the lifetime of most hosts, even surviving the death of the host for a while. In addition to acquiring infection by ingestion of sporulated oocysts, both the final (felid) and intermediate hosts can become infected by ingesting animal tissues containing the cystic forms. In the cat, either source can produce a tissue infection, but it is not known what initiates extraintestinal invasion.

Ingestion is not the only means of acquiring *Toxoplasma*: the organism can enter via the conjunctival, nasal, pharyngeal or respiratory membranes, or percutaneously. Milk and eggs may be a source of infection and also blood transfusions and organ transplants in man. Transplacental infection from mother to fetus occurs and venereal transmission via the semen has been demonstrated in sheep. Vertical transmission through several generations of laboratory rodents is recognized.

This extraordinarily pervasive parasite is helped in its spread and persistence in the environment by the remarkable degree of resistance of the oocyst and tissue cyst stages, which live at a reduced metabolic rate insulated from harmful elements by a protective wall. The role of wildlife in the epidemiology of toxoplasmosis is important where the territories of wild and domestic animals overlap, and the picture is further complicated by the presence of vectors and transport hosts, such as arthropods and earthworms, which may carry infection for a limited period. Thus the cycle cat–earthworm or arthropod–bird or rodent–cat could be an important route of transmission. The coccidial cycle in cats occurs in the epithelial cells of the small intestine, but the time of onset of oocyst production and its duration is variable and seems to depend on the type of infecting organism and the interval between infecting doses. Thus, Wallace (1973) found that when tissue cysts were fed to cats the prepatent period was only 3 or 4 days and persisted for about 2 weeks, whereas infection with sporulated oocysts gave rise to oocysts 3–7 weeks later and then for only a few days. Other observations tend to confirm that infection from intermediate hosts is a more potent and certain mode of infection for cats than oocysts direct from another cat. Not all infections result in the establishment of the parasite, but it should be assumed that whenever a cat eats infected meat or intermediate hosts, the intestinal cycle may be initiated and infectious oocysts result. Most healthy exposed cats having once shed oocysts following infection will not shed them again; if they do so the numbers voided are greatly reduced compared with the initial infection. Young cats first encountering infection soon after weaning are most susceptible and may excrete millions of oocysts during the patent period.

Clinical toxoplasmosis in cats

Because any body tissue is susceptible to invasion the signs of toxoplasmosis are extremely variable, often ill-defined and easily confused with other diseases. Following infection the majority of healthy cats show no signs because any pathological effect is quickly terminated by an immune response. Signs are likely to be seen in young cats or in cats which are immunosuppressed as a result of concomitant disease or therapy with immunosuppressive drugs. The most frequently observed early signs are lethargy, malaise, loss of appetite and pyrexia. Pneumonia with respiratory distress is a feature of toxoplasmosis in cats, and hepatitis and jaundice, diarrhoea, prostration, pancreatitis and lymphadenopathy may occur at a later stage. The central nervous system can be affected producing signs of ataxia, incoordination, hyperaesthesia, personality changes, circling, head pressing, and faecal and urinary incontinence. When the eye is involved the primary focus of damage is the retina followed by anterior uveitis. There may be abnormal pupil size and responsiveness to light, and eventual blindness. Vainisi and Campbell (1969) describe active ocular lesions in ten cats with toxoplasmosis. Toxoplasmosis in the cat can be confused with panleucopenia, lymphosarcoma and feline infectious peritonitis. It may also be a complication of infection with the feline immunodeficiency virus (Witt *et al.*, 1989). Detailed descriptions of clinical toxoplasmosis in cats are given by Frenkel (1978), Frenkel and Holzworth (1987), and Barlough and Jacobson (1988).

Diagnosis

The presence of *Toxoplasma* in both clinical and non-clinical infections may be difficult to establish. Faecal examination for the presence of oocysts is usually of little use as few cases of clinical disease occur at the time oocysts are shed. The oocysts measure $10 \times 12 \mu m$ but accurate identification requires considerable skill in differentiating them from similar parasitic cysts. Diagnosis therefore relies on the demonstration of antibodies to *Toxoplasma* in serum samples. Ideally two samples taken at an interval of 2–3 weeks should be tested simultaneously by the same technique in order to avoid day-to-day variations of the given test. A four-fold or greater increase in antibody titre in a cat with clinical signs is indicative of toxoplasmosis. The four standard serological tests are the Sabin–Feldman dye test (SFD), modified agglutination (MA), indirect haemagglutination (IHA) and latex agglutination (LA).

Dubey and Thulliez (1989) studied these techniques on the serum of seven cats fed tissue cysts. The subsequent symptomless infections were followed for 950 days. The MA test was the most sensitive but IHA and LA were easier to perform using kits suitable for the practice laboratory. The LA test kit is available in the UK*. The dye test has the disadvantage of requiring the handling of live virulent *T. gondii* and is therefore unsuitable for the practice laboratory. Whichever technique is chosen it is important to interpret the results correctly according to the test, and the laboratory which carries out the work should provide data for significant titres. A significant titre in a healthy cat suggests that the cat is immune and an unlikely source of oocysts. The absence of antibodies in a healthy cat suggests susceptibility and the likelihood of shedding oocysts following infection. In acute clinical toxoplasmosis, the antibody level will probably be low and tends to rise very slowly; death may occur before antibody is detectable. In chronic disease the level of antibody resembles that found in the normal cat population, which tends to show an increasing infection rate with increasing age.

When death occurs following acute disease, tissues or impression smears stained with H&E may show the presence of *Toxoplasma* in lesions of focal necrosis affecting many organs of the body. The sites most frequently affected are lungs, liver, CNS, heart, lymph nodes, digestive tract, pancreas and spleen. Parker *et al.* (1981) studied experimental infections in specific-pathogen-free cats. They found pneumonitis to be a constant feature with multifocal lesions rapidly compromising pulmonary function. Necrosis of

---

* Toxoreagent; Eiken Chemical Co. Ltd., Tokyo.

pneumocytes and other cells was the primary pathogenic event with *Toxoplasma* bodies present in almost all types of cell in the lung including macrophages and neutrophil leucocytes.

Affected organs such as liver, heart, pancreas and spleen are usually visibly swollen with red or yellow foci depending on the age of the lesion. Active lesions contain free tachyzoites in a variety of cells, whereas resolving or old lesions contain encysted bradyzoites. Care must be taken in the interpretation of histopathological changes. Only tachyzoites present in characteristic necrotic lesions indicate active disease; encysted bradyzoites may not be the cause of the signs elicited before death.

When extracts of tissues are injected intraperitoneally in mice there is usually a symptomless infection which must be confirmed histologically by finding tissue cysts, or demonstrating serum antibodies to *Toxoplasma*. Such a finding does not of course confirm that toxoplasmosis was the cause of death.

Treatment and control
Treatment should be reserved for cats showing clinical signs regardless of titre. In young cats especially, toxoplasmosis can be rapidly fatal and it is essential to treat as soon as possible. The most satisfactory treatment is a combination of sulphadimidine and pyrimethamine, which act synergistically by inhibiting the biosynthesis of folinic acid essential to *Toxoplasma*. The sulphonamide is given orally at a dosage rate of 60–100 mg/kg bodyweight daily, preferably divided into four doses, and pyrimethamine at 0.5–1.0 mg/kg as a single oral daily dose. The parasites are only inhibited by these drugs and treatment should continue for 1–2 weeks until the immune response of the cat confers adequate protection. Mammals can utilize folinic acid directly so in order to avoid side-effects following treatment, folinic acid in the form of brewer's or baker's yeast should be fed simultaneously.

Control of toxoplasmosis is difficult because measures to prevent infection of cats are usually impracticable. Cats which hunt or are fed on raw meat are sure to become infected, in all probability developing the symptomless form of the intestinal phase during which millions of oocysts may be shed in the faeces over a period of about 4–14 days after infection. Subsequent infections may or may not result in the shedding of oocysts, depending on the degree of acquired resistance. Cats shedding oocysts are a potential danger to other animals and to man, although most authorities believe that the tissue forms of *Toxoplasma* in flesh are a more potent source of infection for all animals including cats and humans (Frenkel & Dubey, 1972). Clinical illness in cats is the result of the tissue phase, which is unable to pass infection in the form of oocysts in the faeces. However, such cats must be regarded as a hazard for human contacts, especially young children and pregnant women. The organism may be present in secretions and exudates from acutely ill cats and, as already explained, may enter another host by a variety of routes. When acute toxoplasmosis is recognized, euthanasia rather than treatment of the affected cat should be considered if there is a risk to human contacts.

The extent and duration of contamination of the environment with cat faeces has been studied by Frenkel *et al.* (1975) who showed that oocysts can remain viable in moist soil for over a year. Their recommendations for control may be possible in some circumstances, but for the average household cat they are difficult to apply. Cats should be confined to prevent hunting and fed dry, canned or cooked food. The faeces of hunting cats using litter trays should be disposed of by burning, and contaminated equipment disinfected by dry heat or boiling water. Transmission of *Toxoplasma* to man can be reduced by washing hands after contact with soil and raw meat, and cooking meat by heating it to at least 66°C in order to kill tissue cysts. Human toxoplasmosis, its clinical aspects, histopathology and epidemiology, are described by Beverley (1974). In farm animals, toxoplasmosis is a common cause of abortion, still-birth and embryonic death in sheep in Britain. An account of ovine toxoplasmosis is given by Beverley *et al.* (1975), and the method of spread from cats to sheep is discussed by Plant *et al.* (1974). For further information on all aspects of *Toxoplasma* infection in animals and man readers should consult Dubey and Beattie (1988).

Isospora infection
(*I. felis* and *I. rivolta*)

Until recently, species in the genus *Isospora* have been regarded as similar to the genus *Eimeria*, the main difference being based on oocyst morphology. *Isospora* oocysts sporulate to form two sporocysts each with four sporozoites, whereas the oocysts of *Eimeria* contain four sporocysts each with two sporozoites. However, the *Isospora* spp. of cats and dogs are now known to have evolved a more elaborate life cycle than *Eimeria*; in addition to the normal intestinal coccidian life cycle, they utilize rodent paratenic hosts in which sporozoites derived from oocysts are found encysted in extra-intestinal tissues. Cats therefore become infected from two sources: oocysts shed by cats, and tissue forms in rodents; the parasite resembles *Toxoplasma* but differs in having a strictly limited range of paratenic hosts (Dubey & Frenkel, 1972).

Although a common and widespread infection, coccidiosis is seldom a cause of clinical disease in cats, probably because their fastidious nature precludes the possibility of ingestion of food grossly contaminated by faeces containing oocysts. Most infections are symptomless and probably derive from paratenic hosts, but heavy infections have been reported as a cause of diarrhoea with the passage of blood and mucus, tenesmus, and scalding of the perineum and tail. Such severe signs are only likely to be seen in kittens kept in very unhygienic conditions.

Oocysts may be found during routine faecal examination and require differentiation from those of *Toxoplasma*, *Sarcocystis* and *Cryptosporidium*. The surveys of endoparasites of cats mentioned in the sections on tapeworms and roundworms show a variable incidence of cats shedding *Isospora* oocysts, with *I. felis* apparently more prevalent than *I. rivolta* and both confined to cats below the ages of 3 and 5 years respectively (Nichol *et al.*, 1981), suggesting that a strong immunity to infection develops with age.

Diagnosis, treatment and control
Oocysts can be demonstrated by direct microscopic examination of faecal smear or by the standard flotation technique used for nematode eggs. *I. felis* measures $30 \times 40\,\mu m$ and *I. rivolta* $20 \times 25\,\mu m$ (*T. gondii* = $10 \times 12\,\mu m$). In the absence of reinfection, coccidiosis is a self-limiting disease, but treatment with sulphadimidine at a dosage rate of 0.25 g daily for 4 days would effect a cure.

Strict attention to hygiene will prevent clinical disease, but light infections are to be expected, especially in young cats allowed to hunt rodents.

Sarcocystis infection
Sarcocystis infects the mucosal cells of the intestine of the definitive carnivore host (dog, cat, man, etc.), undergoing a coccidian-type life cycle with the production of oocysts which may infect a range of intermediate host species. Infection of the definitive host is usually symptomless, but multiplication by schizogamy in the intermediate host and subsequent invasion of skeletal and cardiac muscle and also viscera may produce a systemic reaction. The life cycle is completed when the definitive host consumes the tissues of the intermediate host in which the parasite has entered a resting cystic stage.

Several species of *Sarocystis* are now recognized in the cat, the specific names combining the intermediate and definitive hosts, e.g. *S. bovifelis*, *S. ovifelis* and *S. porcifelis*. *S. cuniculi* is another species found in cat and rabbit.

The oocysts of *Sarcocystis* are sporulated when passed in the faeces of the predator host, having formed two sporocysts each containing four sporozoites. However, the sporocysts are usually free in the faeces, and having an average measurement of $12 \times 9\,\mu m$, resemble in size the oocysts of *Toxoplasma*. Levine (1985) gives a comprehensive account of the genus *Sarcocystis* and related coccidia.

Cryptosporidiosis

Cryptosporidium is a genus containing species of coccida that tend to infect young animals with a poorly developed immune system, or individuals whose immunity has been compromised, as in FeLV infection. The organisms are not host-specific and cross-infections occur between domesticated animals and also man. The life cycle is similar to that of other coccidia, with a pre-patent period of 3–7 days. However, there are some important aspects of development which are not seen in other enteric coccidial infections. No invasion of intestinal mucosal cells occurs and the pathogenesis of the disease is imperfectly understood. Two types of oocyst are produced; a resistant oocyst which is found in the faeces and becomes immediately infective, and oocysts which release infective stages (sporozoites) in the intestine to cause auto-infection.

Poochna and Pippin (1982) describe clinical cryptosporidiosis in a cat in which persistent diarrhoea and anorexia were prominent features. Bennett *et al.* (1985) report three cases of feline cryptosporidiosis; two of these were clinically ill with persistent diarrhoea, but the other one, a kitten, was clinically normal but excreting oocysts in the faeces and living in a household where a child was infected. Diagnosis depends on the demonstration of oocysts by a modified Ziehl–Nielsen stain of faecal smears (Henriksen & Pohlenz, 1981). Sporozoites appear as bright-red granules in the oocysts.

Unlike coccidiosis, the presence of *Cryptosporidium* oocysts is strongly suggestive of causal involvement in cases of persistent diarrhoea. There is as yet no specific treatment for cryptosporidiosis other than symptomatic. Oocysts are very resistant but can be destroyed by 5% ammonium hydroxide, 4% sodium hypochlorite, 10% formalin, freezing, and by heating to 60°C for 30 minutes. With increasing awareness of human cryptosporidiosis, the zoonotic nature of this parasite will focus attention on infections in cats, whether symptomless or associated with diarrhoea.

Giardiasis

The zoonotic nature of *Giardia* sp. is still in doubt but until the question is resolved it would be wise to assume that animals may be a reservoir of human infection. These protozoans live in the small intestine as motile, pear-shaped flagellate trophozoites about $13 \times 7\,\mu m$ in size. Each trophozoite has two nuclei, and one surface is a concave adhesive disc enabling it to attach to intestinal microvilli. There is no evidence of sexual reproduction and multiplication is by binary fission. The *Giardia* parasite is excreted in the faeces as a cyst containing two fused trophozoites. Trophozoites also appear unencysted in faeces but soon die in this form.

Attempts have been made to create species of *Giardia* for each host, e.g. *G. cati*, *G. canis*, *G. bovis*, etc., but until the taxonomy is finally established the term *Giardia duodenalis* (syn. *G. lamblia*) group is to be preferred (Levine, 1985). Morphologically these 'species' are all identical and differentiation, if it exists, will probably be decided by cross-infection experiments or by iso-enzyme or DNA typing techniques.

Clinical signs
Giardia infection may be symptomless in cats but when signs do occur, diarrhoea, either intermittent or continuous with weight loss, is the principal feature. Faeces are mucoid and have a strong odour, and there is evidence of steatorrhoea as a consequence of malabsorption. Pyrexia and vomiting may or may not be evident. Detailed descriptions of feline giardiasis are given by Brightman and Slonka (1976), Kirkpatrick and Farrell (1984), and Kirkpatrick and Laczak (1985). The signs are probably largely due to malabsorption following physical and biochemical changes in the gut mucosa. Immunological responses of the host appear to play a part, together with host–parasite competition for nutrients and gross alterations in gut flora.

The demonstration of trophozoites or cysts in the faeces is the standard method of diagnosis. A centrifugal flotation technique for cysts using zinc sulphate yields the best results (Kirkpatrick & Farrell, 1982).

In fresh watery faeces, trophozoites may be seen in a direct smear but they must not be confused with commensal protozoa; staining with iodine will reveal structural details. Examination every other day on three occasions is recommended because excretion of the parasites is intermittent. The use of a fibre-optic endoscope or gelatin capsule to retrieve material directly from the duodenum may be a more reliable method of recovering *Giardia*.

Treatment

Oral metronidazole at a dosage rate of 22 mg/kg bodyweight twice daily for 5 days is an effective treatment for cats (Zimmer, 1987). The trophozoites found in faeces soon perish but the more persistent cysts are destroyed by freezing, boiling or desiccation. Sodium hypochlorite 1% is an effective surface disinfectant.

EXOTIC PARASITES

Cats entering Britain are required to be quarantined for 6 months under the Rabies Order and although there is no obligation to diagnose and treat endoparasitic infections during this period, it is desirable to do so. The following parasites may be detected on routine examination of faeces, urine, blood, etc.

Ancylostoma tubaeforme

This feline hookworm lives in the small intestine and lays a strongyloid egg containing an ovum in an early stage of segmentation measuring 75 μm in length. *A. braziliense*, the canine hookworm, has been recorded in cats.

Strongyloides stercoralis **and** *S. cati*

These minute nematodes live in the small intestine and lay eggs measuring 40 μm and containing an L_1 larva. *S. stercoralis* is important because the L_3 can infect man by skin penetration.

Trichuris serrata

The whipworm of the cat lives in the caecum and lays distinctive eggs with bipolar plugs similar to those of *Capillaria*.

Spirocerca lupi

Spirocercosis is much more likely to be encountered in the dog than the cat. The adult worms live in the oesophagus and stomach, where they provoke the development of fibrous nodules. The eggs passed in the faeces are elongate and thick-walled, measuring 40 μm in length. Beetles act as intermediate hosts and paratenic hosts play an important part in transmission.

Capillaria feliscati

This small hair-like nematode lives in the bladder of cats and bipolar eggs are passed in the urine.

Dirofilaria immitis

Infestation with heartworm is less common in cats than in dogs, and cats appear to be more resistant to infestation. The number of worms establishing are fewer than in the dog and microfilariae are absent from the blood of most infected cats. Coughing, dyspnoea, vomiting, weight loss and lethargy are the usual presenting signs and sudden death without warning as a result of heart failure or respiratory failure is not uncommon. Adult worms may die following a short-lived infestation and cause severe pulmonary thromboembolism. Haematological examination of infected cats reveals anaemia, eosinophilia, basophilia and hyperglobulinaemia. With microfilariae frequently absent from the blood, diagnosis is based on clinical, haematological and radiological examination coupled with IFA and ELISA tests which unfortunately are not very reliable. Treatment with thiacetarsamide to kill the adult worms is usually successful and well tolerated, but sudden deaths have occurred from thromboembolism 1–2 weeks after administration. For fuller details of this disease readers should refer to Rawlings (1986).

Joyeuxiella pasqualei

This tapeworm resembles *Dipylidium* and is especially common in Africa and the Middle East. The life cycle involves both beetles and lizards acting as intermediate hosts. Unlike *Dipylidium*, the egg capsules contain only a single egg.

Diphyllobothrium latum

This and species of the related genus *Spirometra* may be encountered in cats. The eggs are operculate and yellow in colour, measuring about 75 μm in length.

Other operculate eggs in cat faeces could be those of flukes belonging to one of several genera and readers are referred to standard textbooks of veterinary parasitology for their identification.

The cysts of *Entamoeba histolytica* have been recorded in cat faeces.

REFERENCES

General

Dunn A.M. (1978) *Veterinary Helminthology*, 2nd edn. William Heinemann, London.

Soulsby E.J.L. (1982) *Helminths, Arthropods and Protozoa of Domesticated Animals*, 3rd edn. Baillière Tindall & Cassell, London.

Urquhart G.M., Armour J., Duncan J.L., Dunn A.M. & Jennings F.W. (1987) *Veterinary Parasitology*. Longman Scientific and Technical, London.

Specific topics

Barlough J.E. & Jacobson M.S. (1988) *Toxoplasmosis*. Cornell Feline Health Centre, No. 9, pp. 1–5.

Bennett M., Baxby D., Blundell N., Gaskell C.J., Hare C.A. & Kelly D.F. (1985) Cryptosporidiosis in the domestic cat. *Vet. Rec.* **116**, 73–4.

Beresford-Jones W.P. & Jacobs D.E. (1979) Endoparasites. In Chandler E.A. (ed) *Canine Medicine and Therapeutics*, 2nd edn. Blackwell Scientific Publications, Oxford.

Beverley J.K.A. (1974) Some aspects of toxoplasmosis, a worldwide zoonosis. In Soulsby E.J.L. (ed) *Parasitic Zoonoses*. Academic Press, New York.

Beverley J.K.A., Hutchinson W.M., Allsup T.N., Spence J.B. & Watson W.A. (1975) Studies on the spread of *Toxoplasma gondii* to sheep. *Br. Vet. J.* **131**, 130.

Brightman A.H. & Slonka G.F. (1976) A review of five clinical cases of giardiasis in cats. *J. Am. Anim. Hosp. Ass.* **12**, 492–7.

Connan R.M. (1979) Use of anthelminthics in dogs and cats. In Yoxall A.T. & Hird J.F.R. (eds) *Pharmacological Basis of Small Animal Medicine*. Blackwell Scientific Publications, Oxford.

Dubey J.P. & Beattie C.P. (1988) *Toxoplasmosis of Animals and Man*. CRC Press, Boca, Raton, Florida.

Dubey J.P. & Frenkel J.K. (1972) Extra-intestinal stages of *Isospora felis* and *I. rivolta* (Protozoa: Eimeriidae) in cats. *J. Protozool.* **19**, 89.

Dubey J.P. & Thulliez Ph. (1989) Serological diagnosis of toxoplasmosis in cats fed *Toxoplasma gondii* tissue cysts. *J. Am. Vet. Med. Ass.* **94**(9), 1297–9.

Else R.W., Bagnall B.G., Phaff J.J.G. & Potter C. (1977) Endo- and ecto-parasites of dogs and cats: a survey from practices in the East Anglian Region, B.S.A.V.A. *J. Small Anim. Pract.* **18**, 731–7.

Frenkel J.K. (1978) Toxoplasmosis in cats: diagnosis, treatment and prevention. *Comp. Immunol. Microbiol. Infect. Dis.* **1**, 15.

Frenkel J.K. & Dubey J.P. (1972) Toxoplasmosis and its prevention in cats and man. *J. Infect. Dis.* **126**, 664.

Frenkel J.K. & Holzworth J. (1987) Toxoplasmosis. In Holzworth J. (ed) *Diseases of the Cat*, vol. 1. W.B. Saunders, Philadelphia, pp. 369–90.

Frenkel J.K., Ruiz A. & Chinchilla M. (1975) Soil survival of *Toxoplasma* oocysts in Kansas and Costa Rica. *Am. J. Trop. Med. Hyg.* **24**, 439.

Goddard P.C. & Johnston A.M. (1986) Piperazine toxicity in a kitten. *Vet. Rec.* **119**, 635.

Hamilton J.M. (1966a) Experimental lungworm disease of the cat. *J. Comp. Path.* **76**, 147.

Hamilton J.M. (1966b) Pulmonary arterial disease of the cat. *J. Comp. Path.* **76**, 133.

Hamilton J.M. (1967) The number of *Aelurostrongylus abstrusus* larvae required to produce pulmonary disease in the cat. *J. Comp. Path.* **77**, 343.

Hamilton J.M. (1968a) Passive immunization in lungworm infection of the cat. *J. Comp. Path.* **78**, 331.

Hamilton J.M. (1968b) Immunofluorescence as a diagnostic procedure in lungworm disease of the cat. *Vet. Rec.* **83**, 401.

Hargis A.M., Prieur D.J. & Blanchard J.L. (1983) Prevalence, lesions and differential diagnosis of *Ollulanus tricuspis* infection in cats. *Vet. Pathol.* **20**, 71–9.

Hasslinger M.A. (1984) *Ollulanus tricuspis*, the stomach worm of the cat. *Feline Pract.* **14**(5), 32–5.

Henriksen S.Aa. & Pohlenz J.F.C. (1981) Staining of *Cryptosporidium* by a modified Ziehl–Nielsen technique. *Acta. Vet. Scand.* **22**, 594–6.

Hutchison W.M., Dunachie J.F., Siim J.C. & Work K. (1970) Coccidian-like nature of *Toxoplasma gondii*. *Br. Med. J.* **i**, 142.

Kirkpatrick C.E. & Farrell J.P. (1982) Giardiasis. *Compend. Cont. Educ. Pract. Vet.* **4**, 367–78.

Kirkpatrick C.E. & Farrell J.P. (1984) Feline giardiasis. Observations on natural and induced infections. *Am. J. Vet. Res.* **45**, 2182–8.

Kirkpatrick C.E. & Laczak J.P. (1985) Giardiasis in a cattery. *J. Am. Vet. Med. Assoc.* **187**, 161–2.

Levine N.D. (1985) *Veterinary Protozoology*. Iowa State University Press, Ames.

Nichol S., Ball S.J. & Snow K.R. (1981) Prevalence of intestinal parasites in domestic cats from the London area. *Vet. Rec.* **109**, 252.

Parker G.A., Langloss J.M., Dubey J.P. & Hoover E.A.

(1981) Pathogenesis of acute toxoplasmosis in specific pathogen-free cats. *Vet. Pathol.* **18**, 786–803.

Plant J.W., Richardson N. & Moyle G.G. (1974) *Toxoplasma* infection and abortion in sheep associated with feeding of grain contaminated with cat faeces. *Aust. Vet. J.* **50**, 19.

Poochna K.B. & Pippin C. (1982) Intestinal cryptosporidiosis in the cat. *Vet. Path.* **19**, 708–10.

Rawlings C.A. (1986) Heartworm disease in dogs and cats. W.B. Saunders, Philadelphia.

Vainisi S.J. & Campbell L.H. (1969) Ocular toxoplasmosis in cats. *J. Am. Vet. Med. Ass.* **154**(2), 141–52.

Wallace G.D. (1973) The role of the cat in the natural history of *Toxoplasma gondii. Am. J. Trop. Med. Hyg.* **22**, 313.

Witt C.J., Moench T.R., Gittelsohn A.M., Bishop B.D. & Childs J.E. (1989) Epidemiologic aberrations on feline immunodeficiency virus and *Toxoplasma gondii* co-infection in cats in Baltimore, Md. *J. Am. Vet. Med. Ass.* **194**(2), 229–33.

Woodruff A.W. (1970) Toxocariasis. *Br. Med. J.* **iii**, 663.

Woodruff A.W. & de Savigny D.H. (1982) Toxocaral and toxoplasmal antibodies in cat breeders and in Icelanders exposed to cats but not to dogs. *Br. Med. J.* **i**, 309.

Zimmer J.F. (1987) Treatment of feline giardiasis with metronidazole. *Cornell Vet.* **77**, 383–8.

Chapter 26 / Behavioural Problems

R. A. MUGFORD

INTRODUCTION

The distinction between amusing eccentricity and irritating, expensive or dangerous behavioural problems in companion animals is a fine one which usually depends upon the circumstances and expectations of the owner. The majority of behavioural patterns in cats which owners complain about are expressions of normal activity in unacceptable contexts; for instance, territorial aggression, marking with urine or predation upon birds. Predation upon rodents is usually tolerated. Only a minority of cats exhibit deviant behaviour which has no parallel in the repertoire of wild or feral forms. The more extensive our knowledge of the biology and social behaviour of wild cats (see Turner & Bateson, 1988), the more rarely will the behaviour of an individual pet cat justify the term abnormal.

Abnormal behaviours such as textile eating in Siamese may have a genetic basis, whereas certain forms of aggression can be related to distinctive neurological or other medical conditions. Some acquired behaviours may reasonably be categorized as abnormal because they are disabling for the individual concerned: for example, phobias, which are learned but excessive reactions to commonplace stimuli.

Incidence

It is difficult to estimate the type and frequency of behavioural problems in a population of pet cats, and those reported to veterinary surgeons probably represent only a minority of the total. How-

ever, some idea was given by Stead (1982), who found that 8% of requests for euthanazing cats concerned healthy animals with behavioural problems.

The author's referral practice is concerned with behaviour modification of companion animals, and fewer than 10% are cats, the rest being mainly dogs. This small proportion of cat cases could have two explanations: either feline behavioural problems make a relatively minor legal, medical and economic impact upon the owner and the community in general, or cats are less problem-prone than dogs.

Some guide to the relative frequencies of feline behavioural problems liable to be encountered in veterinary practice is given in Table 26.1, which is derived from a sample of 100 cases referred to the author.

More than half of all cases are concerned with some aspect of cats' eliminative behaviour: urination, defecation or spraying. Social behaviours such as aggression are much less frequent sources of problems in cats than in dogs.

Diagnosis

There is a widespread notion amongst pet owners and some veterinary surgeons that it is difficult to modify the behaviour of cats: they have independent natures and are liable to opt out of training sessions. However, there is a considerable fund of knowledge about cat behaviour to be drawn from selected research in comparative psychology, ethology, endocrinology and psychopharmacology, some of which has potential for

Table 26.1 Type and frequency of behavioural problems in 520 cats referred to the author.

Problem	%
Inappropriate urination and defecation	29
Spraying	22
Fighting	20
Aggression towards people	8
Self-mutilation	6
Fearfulness	4
Disturbed feeding	3
Others	8

resolving behavioural problems in cats and dogs. The first priority in any programme of behaviour modification is to define the problem from the animal's history, ideally supplemented by direct observation and testing in the home environment. Questioning of the owner should establish the following.

1 What exactly does the cat do?
2 Where does it do it?
3 When did it start?
4 When does it do it?
5 People, other cats and dogs in the home.
6 Access to the outdoors, e.g. by a cat-flap.
7 What treatment has already been tried?

The clinical history of the animal may have a direct or an indirect bearing upon its behaviour. For instance, metabolic disturbances such as renal failure, diabetes mellitus, or the presence of cystitis or bladder calculi can all increase the frequency of urinations and modify the choice of locations on which to urinate. Despite successful treatment of the original clinical cause of the disturbed excretory behaviour, the cat may continue to urinate in the wrong places.

A differential diagnosis to establish why the cat does what it does is rarely so simple as in the example given above. Information provided by the owner may not be sufficient to establish causation and thus effective treatment. A home visit with an open-ended time commitment for inspecting the environment and observing the cat may be necessary to understand the context within which a problem behaviour occurs. It is often useful to construct a protocol during this visit, which the owner can continue to use for recording the time, place and context of relevant behaviours.

Owner psychology

There are few absolute or standard causes of feline behavioural problems, and appropriate solutions for one case may be inappropriate for another superficially identical case. The selection of techniques and the vigour with which a strategy for treatment is pursued depend upon many factors, but must include the habits, commitment, needs and expectations of the whole family towards the pet. If there is significant variation in attitudes between various family members, a typed report is an invaluable device to prevent family conflict and misunderstanding of instructions. There may not be a solution to the cat's behavioural problem which will satisfy all members of the family. For example, very occasional lapses in toilet habits may be best dealt with by leading a discussion about the relatively minor risks of zoonotic disease from cats, rather than engaging in complicated regimes of house training.

INAPPROPRIATE URINATION AND DEFAECATION

It is widely assumed that cats are naturally secretive in their toilet habits, covering their urine and faeces in order to avoid detection by predators. Ethological studies of feral cats do not confirm this view and it is quite common for both urine and faeces to be deposited as territory markers (Macdonald, 1980). Uncovered, communal middens are sometimes utilized by feral and domestic cats. Accordingly, complaints from cat owners that their pet prefers the carpet, bed or Chippendale to the prescribed garden or litter tray must be viewed in a broad biological context. Terms such as 'dirty', 'lazy', or 'wilful' are often used to describe cats that urinate or defecate in inappropriate locations and various unpleasant punishments may be employed by owners faced with such problems. Actions such as rubbing cats' noses in excreta are still remarkably common and of course are ineffectual and to be deplored.

The acts of urination and defaecation are not necessarily performed close together in time or space. It is quite common for a cat to use the appropriate litter tray or soil for one, but an inappropriate location for the other. Activity and feeding increase the likelihood of defaecation occurring, but they have little influence upon the timing of urination.

Many of the author's cases involve cats that have suddenly changed their pattern of eliminative behaviour, but in a minority of cases clients were never able to train their kitten to use a litter tray. Sudden breakdown in toilet habits is sometimes traceable to a distinct event, such as an episode of diarrhoea, laying a new carpet, disrupted lifestyle or punishment whilst eliminating in a neighbouring garden. Such events may have initiated the problem, but other factors can maintain it and be a complicating variable in designing effective treatment. Eight general factors need consideration when dealing with toileting problems.

Clinical causes

Gastrointestinal upsets and any condition that provokes distress can induce both short- and long-term changes to accustomed toileting habits of cats. Aside from a comprehensive medical work-up on such cases, dietary management which reduces the volume of stools and improves their consistency may help the cat to re-establish desirable eliminative behaviours. Urinary incontinence may arise from many medical conditions of which feline urological syndrome (FUS) is probably the most significant.

Social adjustment

Chronic social stress arising from antagonism with another cat in the household, cats in the vicinity, other animals or people, can both initiate and maintain an excretory problem. The practitioner should look for scars as evidence of fighting and question the owner about recent introductions of animals or people. Are there other changes in emotional responses which support this view? Is the absence of the owner a source of distress to an overly-attached or loving cat?

Litter preference

A common initiating cause of changed toilet habits in cats referred to the author is climatic: many cats do not like to dig wet or frozen soil. The criteria for selection of one material over another for defaecation or urination purposes seem to be marginal and owners should not expect their cat to pay a great penalty for selecting the desired litter over the undesired. Simple provision of a covering over dry, friable soil is all that may be necessary.

Cats often exhibit distinctive preferences or aversions to alternative litters, and some commercial preparations may be avoided because of their physical composition or odour. Preference tests between dry soil, sand and clay-based proprietary litters usually show the former of these as most attractive to cats presenting excretion problems. The odour of disturbed soil fungi (such as occurs in newly dug gardens) attracts investigation and elimination by cats, and this response can be exploited whilst re-training cats to use a litter tray.

Substrate preference

Borchelt and Voith (1981) suggested that the substrate underlying the litter in a tray is a critical factor governing scratching or covering behaviour in cats. Idiosyncratic scratch preferences for smooth surfaces such as plastic or linoleum, granular material such as soil, or carpets can develop independently of litter or location preference. The author has encountered one such case in a long-haired cat that consistently scratched then defaecated on the carpet beside its litter tray. Lining the litter tray with off-cuts of carpet immediately re-established the desired response.

Location preference

The location and design of litter trays may be unsatisfactory for individual cats. Size and stability are obviously important, but a common mistake committed by owners of confined cats is to juxtapose litter tray and food bowl, usually in the kitchen. For many (but not all) cats, the presence of food discourages urination, defaecation and spraying. The location allocated by the owner for the cat's toilet may be avoided because something unpleasant occurred there in the past; alternative locations should be offered in such cases.

Olfactory preference

The odour of urine and faeces attracts some cats but repels others. Reasons for these contrasting reactions have not been found. Scrupulous cleaning of the tray and surrounding area and clean litter may be aversive if it has removed or modified all odours of prior eliminations. Such individuals are conservative in their eliminative habits, and tend to revisit the same location.

Cats which avoid contaminated sites and will only use a litter tray once tend to urinate or defaecate at many inappropriate locations within the house. For such individuals, the owner should offer many clean litter trays: perhaps as many as one per room.

Learned preference

As was mentioned earlier, some cats use personal or communal middens, which are often in hidden locations such as behind or inside furniture. Their presence may not be immediately apparent to the owner. In such cases, it may be necessary to retrain the cat to the use of a litter tray by confining it to a cage or pen in a new environment, such as a cattery. Having established use of the litter tray in a novel environment, the cat can be reintroduced to the home with a litter tray near the former midden.

Genetic influences

Reference has already been made to the substantial individual differences in cats' eliminative behaviour. Both Borchelt in the USA (personal communication) and the author see disproportionate numbers of Persian cats that are reluctant to use litter trays. Cats of this breed tend to be rather inactive, even indolent, and access to litter trays may have to be made especially easy.

Treatment of house-soiling cats

1 Examine social relationships: reduce stress and ban punishment from the owner.
2 Change the diet to a highly digestible, low-fibre recipe which produces firm stools.
3 Examine and improve the design, location and availability of indoor litter trays.
4 Establish litter and substrate preferences by experiment.
5 Thoroughly clean previously used and undesired toilet locations, using a biological washing powder in warm water or a proprietary, enzyme-based cleaning solution.
6 Feed the cat at *undesired* toilet locations, well away from litter trays.
7 Deny access to the undesired locations, e.g. close door or cover with furniture.
8 In difficult or chronic cases, re-establish use of a litter tray in a confined environment (e.g. hospitalize cat). After one week, return to one room with the same litter tray. Gradually, allow greater access to the home.

SPRAYING

Urine spraying is a quite normal part of feline social behaviour that should not necessarily be mistaken for a lapse in toilet manners (Turner & Bateson, 1988). The majority of cats spray urine outdoors at some time, but less commonly indoors when living in a stable, single-cat household. The frequency of spraying is reliably increased where the cat is in competition with others for social rank or physical resources, and the greater the number of cats, the greater the likelihood of one or more of them spraying. Apart from social disorganization as an initiating factor in spraying, there are a number of transient factors which may turn a non-sprayer into a sprayer. The most obvious is reproduction, and females often spray during oestrus to attract males; similarly, intact males spray to attract receptive females. Medical and behavioural factors should be considered when treating spraying cases.

Clinical causes

There are considerable individual variations in the posture adopted by cats that are urinating, defecating or spraying. The usual posture for spraying is from an upright position, tail held high and quivering as a stream of urine is projected horizontally. Scratching or burying movements rarely follow spraying as they usually do after eliminative urination. However, intermediate postures between the stand of spraying and crouch of urination sometimes occur, making it difficult to establish whether one is dealing with marking or eliminative behaviour. The best distinction is probably on the basis of volume of urine expressed: typically less than 1 ml/spray but greater than 20 ml/urination.

Disease of the lower urinary tract, such as in feline urological syndrome (FUS), can increase the frequency of attempted urination, decrease the volume and modify the posture. Urine analysis and the animal's history should distinguish between FUS and spraying for behavioural reasons.

Social interactions

Mention has already been made of the relationship between the number of cats in a household and spraying. It may only be possible to resolve a chronic spraying problem in a crowded household by removing or separating incompatible individuals. This should be done on a trial and error basis with periods of 1 week per manipulation. Rarely, cats spray in response to the presence of a particular person, because of a family crisis or stress from an antagonistic dog. Cats should be allowed to get away from social or environmental stressors by providing escape routes, cubby-holes and safe-havens.

The source of social stress that initiates a spraying problem can often be outside the household, notably fighting with neighbouring cats. Local feral cats may be invading the client's house in order to take food.

Endocrine factors

Males are more likely to spray than females, and intact males more likely than castrates. It is not certain whether spraying behaviour is directly influenced by hormones or whether spraying frequency varies as an indirect consequence of social dominance. Castration of intact male cats immediately stops spraying in about 50% of cases (Hart & Barrett, 1973) and a further third stop eventually. Spaying is indicated when queens only spray during oestrus, though overall, spayed females are as likely to spray as intact cats.

Hart (1938) and co-workers have explored the use of progestagens in treating a variety of feline and canine behavioural problems, including spraying in cats. Two compounds are particularly useful for controlling spraying: megestrol acetate* (MA) for oral dosing or medroxy progesterone acetate† (MPA) by injection. Their mode of action is not understood, but it seems likely to be due to their non-specific calming effects rather than any anti-gonadotrophic qualities.

Relatively high doses of both compounds are required to exert a therapeutic effect over spraying, at which levels serious side-effects can be anticipated in vulnerable individuals or with long-term administration (Borchelt & Voith, 1981). Pathologies of the reproductive tract are likely in intact females, and progestagens have been implicated in provoking hyperplasia of mammary tissues, reliably increasing food and water intake, incidence of diabetes in older individuals and behavioural depression in some cats. In the author's experience, more such negative side-effects are associated with MA than with MPA. At least oral administration of MA can be stopped immediately in response to such problems whereas the depot MPA will take several weeks to dissipate.

Learning

Some cats spray for no apparent social reason: it becomes a routine signalling behaviour that is time- and place-specific. There is a small possibility that spraying can be suppressed or at least redirected by well-tried and appropriate

* Ovarid; Glaxovet, Uxbridge, Middlesex, UK.
† Perlutex (Leo) or Promone-E (Upjohn).

punishment. Direct hitting or similar physical punishment is usually useless and is often counter-productive, alienating the cat from its owner and inducing more of the social stress that may have initiated the problem. A thrown light object or sprayed water is an ideal punishment, so long as they seem to occur independently of the owner. A long-lasting place-avoidance can be simply induced by placing an electrically charged mat near where the cat habitually sprays. In the author's practice, this has proved to be a reliable and stress-free procedure.

Proprietary chemical repellants, usually based upon powerful aromas in spray form, are not usually effective in deterring chemical marking in cats. Indeed, some are as malodorous as stale urine itself and invite further 'cover' marking by the cat.

Genetics

Some purebred cats are seen with much higher frequency of indoor spraying than other breeds or cross-breeds. The Burmese is most over-represented for spraying in the author's practice, as it is also most likely to present various unwanted aggressive behaviours.

Treatment

1 Castration and spaying should be a first line of treatment in entire cats. In neutered individuals, progestagen therapy may also be warranted. The regime favoured by the author is as follows:

MA: 2.5 mg/day for 10 days. Stop for 5 days and review. If problem continues/recommences dose @ 5 mg/day for 5 days. Stop for 5 days and review, then decrease dose to minimum for behavioural effect.

MPA is usually administered as a single s.c. or i.m. dose of 50–100 mg. If the cat does respond to MPA the therapeutic effect may last from days to months. Long-term learning or social readjustments may occur which permanently remove the motive to spray.

2 Social isolation of the spraying cat from other cats should be attempted if there is evidence of fighting or conflict. For instance, close off the cat flap or use a selective magnetic model which denies outside neighbourhood cats access to the patient's home.

3 Cleaning of sprayed surfaces is vital, but in practice this may not be easy. A warm solution of a concentrated biological washing powder will remove the components of dried urine more efficiently than regular household cleaners. This may be followed by wiping with an organic solvent such as absolute alcohol.

4 Punishment by the owner should not be attempted, but an electrically charged mat* may be useful in denying the cat access to particular locations where it habitually sprays indoors.

5 In the minority of cats where stress is the primary cause of spraying, petting and kindness from the owner should be prescribed. Safe havens and bolt-holes from other pets, children, etc. are essential. Mild tranquilizers such as diazepam, 1–2 mg/kg/day, may be warranted in the short term.

6 Neurosurgery in the form of olfactory trachotomy has been evaluated by Hart (1981) as a last option for treating spraying cats. Animals apparently made a good recovery and stopped spraying, but serious side-effects from experimentally induced anosmia in other species may also be expected in cats: changes in social behaviour, feeding and biological rhythms.

7 Rehoming of the recidivist sprayer to a single-cat, indoor home is, in the author's experience, often a worthwhile alternative to euthanasia.

AGGRESSION

The understanding and treatment of unwanted aggression in companion animals is a vital aspect of veterinary practice because one is attempting to protect animals and people from potentially serious physical assault and mental distress. An aggressive cat can deliver multiple bites and scratches to another cat, a dog or human being with dramatic speed and bloody effect; so one

---

* Invisible Gate; Contech Electronics, British Columbia, Canada.

must be confident that the advice is right. Aggression is not a unitary concept, but rather a general term encompassing several distinctive behaviours governed by a variety of physiological mechanisms.

The cat has been a favourite subject for neurophysiological research and including neural and biochemical control of aggression (Boudreau & Tsuchitani, 1973). Experimental stimulation and lesions to the temporal lobe, limbic system and hypothalamus have demonstrated diffuse control of aggression. There has been relatively little clinical or histopathological work to correlate naturally occurring disturbances in behaviour with the presence of tumour- or trauma-induced lesions to these brain areas. Disturbances to other behavioural systems besides aggression tend to occur with hypothalamic tumours; for example, to feeding, drinking and activity rhythms. Practical treatment of feline aggression cases mainly concerns endocrine therapy (including gonadectomy) and less commonly involves changes in husbandry, environment or specific training. In respect of damage-limitation from cat scratches, it is now possible to temporarily 'disarm' cat claws by fitting soft latex covers (see 'Furniture scratching' below). Prospects for treating aggressive cats vary from excellent to poor, depending upon the context and motivation within which the behaviour occurs.

Territorial aggression

Both entire and neutered cats will defend territory, regardless of their hormonal state (Turner & Bateson, 1988). Repeated and serious injury may be sustained by cats attempting to defend or extend their territory, but short of confinement there is not much the owner or practitioner can do to manipulate relationships between the pet and its neighbours.

Most antagonistic cats develop a regime of avoidance, where they allocate their use of time and space so as not to make contact. Owners can assist this process by liaising with other cat owners in the neighbourhood on the times that their pets are allowed outdoors. Defendable space should also be offered to a cat resident in its owner's garden: a simple box or platform 1 m off the ground, with a 0.2–0.3 m circular opening from which invading cats can be viewed.

In-household fighting

Two or more cats may live in harmony for many years but suddenly start ferocious fights. Fighting may occur as competition over some critical resource (usually the owner), or may occur in response to some change of routine. The most common provocative factor is separation of the cats, especially if a strange body odour is acquired by one of the cats.

The period of separation may be for less than 24 hours, such as when one of a pair of cats is anaesthetized for a minor veterinary procedure, hospitalized or boarded apart from its feline companion.

Such problems are best avoided by keeping cats together on a continuous basis. If one cat has to be separated, say for surgery, it should be reintroduced to its companions whilst confined in a mesh crate from which visual and olfactory contact can be re-established. If fighting is severe, short-term oral progestagen therapy is justified for all of the individuals concerned. In extreme cases of sudden-onset fighting between cats of the same household, sedation may also be warranted to manage the effects of stress.

Burmese cats are over-represented for fighting in the author's practice, usually between like-sex cohorts but rarely also when a male is separated from a female. If there is any history of conflict between Burmese cats it is best they are not separated, even for veterinary treatment.

Maternal aggression

Rarely does a queen with kittens attack human beings, but maternal aggression towards dogs is quite common. Clients should be warned to protect the family dog because these attacks can be unexpected and inflict serious injury. Occasionally, post-parturient personality changes occur in cats as in other animals, and these may be related to hormonal changes or to mineral imbalance, especially hypocalcaemia. The clinician should also consider this variable when treating cases of maternal cannibalism.

Fear-induced aggression

This behaviour is the typical reaction of a domestic cat to restraint under strange or stressful circumstances, such as in a veterinary surgery. For practical purposes one avoids such situations unless appropriately dressed and trained to handle cats.

Pain-induced aggression

Pain is a powerful factor in eliciting aggression in cats, as in other animals. It is probably the most common reason that children are hurt by cats. The levels or pain tolerated by individuals varies greatly and can only be briefly modified by drugs (see Chapter 27).

Aggression to owners

The biological determinants of aggression are supplemented by experience of the outcome of previous incidents. If an aggressive attack upon another cat, a dog or owner brings some advantage to the cat, it is more likely to be repeated. Learning processes of this sort are undoubtedly the basis for many reported incidents of cats suddenly beginning to attack their owners. A playful pat to the ankles of the owner, inadvertently reinforced by feeding or opening a door, can be quickly consolidated into more determined ambush and injuries. The speed with which the behaviour develops and the subtlety of the pay-offs for attacks may lead the owner to suspect, mistakenly, pathological process. For example, the author was presented with a Siamese female that had begun to bite judges and handlers in cat shows. The first incident concerned an inexperienced handler who dropped the cat whilst it was still behaving well. Subsequent aggression was consistently rewarded by the cat being quickly returned to its show cage. The case was success-fully treated by setting new, calm handling criteria before the cat was released.

The herb catmint, *Nepeta faassenii* and other species, along with its derivatives can provoke dramatic emotional changes in cats, and rarely, unprovoked attacks upon the owner. The behaviour of cats under the influence of catnip is highly idiosyncratic and many show no reaction at all. In the author's practice, four cases have been encountered where the timing of attacks upon the owner coincided with provision of new catnip toys. This factor should be routinely explored at time of history taking.

Predation

Hunting in cats is a hybrid behaviour which incorporates elements of play, aggression and feeding. There are marked familial tendencies, which may be caused by both inherited factors and by schooling of kittens to hunt by the dam. Once a cat has learned to become a proficient hunter, the behaviour is self-reinforcing and is not motivated by the need for food.

A number of punishing and ambush techniques are described in the popular literature to discourage predation of birds or other animals, but none can be recommended to clients. The fitting of a collar and bell is usually only a brief handicap to a hunting cat. Surgically declawed cats are unable to make the first grasp-hold of birds, and the same handicap to hunting can also be imposed by fitting latex nail-covers to cats' fore-paws (see 'Furniture scratching' below). Finally, unwanted hunting by cats can be responsibly avoided by constructing an outdoor run or an 'aviary' in reverse, which is probably preferable to keeping cats permanently indoors.

FEEDING

When allowed the opportunity to self-regulate from an ad lib food supply, cats take large numbers of meals, evenly spaced across 24 hours (6–18 meals/day: Mugford & Thorne, 1980). The majority of cats are very proficient at relating intake to need and it is unusual to encounter major feeding problems that are solely of behavioural origin. Disturbed feeding behaviour is more likely to be due to disease processes, but exceptions will be dealt with here.

The selection habits or preferences of cats for various food items have been exhaustively researched by the pet food companies and are the subject of endless anecdotes amongst owners. The general findings are: cooked meats are preferred to raw meat; liver is the most preferred offal; food at blood heat is always preferred to food above or below 38°C; and moisture content of cat foods is not an important factor in palatability, but variety or regular changes of brands and flavours augment intake. However, substantial individual differences and eccentricities in feeding habits and preferences are found amongst pet cats.

Inappetence

Loss of appetite can be an indication of many clinical illnesses, but it can also be a response to stress. Separation from the owner is a common initiating factor in inappetence cases, either because of excessive social attachment or dependence, or because owner and cat have shared common mealtimes (social facilitation). If the owner has to be away from home or the cat boarded, the cat should be accustomed to feeding out of the presence of the owner and outside his or her mealtimes.

Social attachments of cats to humans and animal members of households is often underestimated as a factor in general health and liveliness. A case seen by the author confirmed this attachment between cats within a household: one of a 4-year-old pair died and the survivor would not eat for 2 weeks. Feeding recommenced when the cat was temporarily re-homed: a changed environment reduced the importance of previous long-standing social relationships.

Pharmacological intervention may (rarely) be justified in dealing with apparently unhappy, inappetent cats, the drug of choice being diazepam, 2.5–5 mg IV; B-complex vitamins given by injec-

tion are sometimes a useful stimulus to the appetite of an anorexic cat.

Obesity

There are many cause of obesity and in domestic cats it may be because owners indulge their animals in excessive quantities of palatable food. However, endogenous factors arising from faulty hypothalamic control, early feeding habits (particularly infrequent, gorged meals) and endocrine status are probably more important causes of obesity in cats than the composition of the diet. Forced dietary restriction of obese cats should be carefully managed as individuals fed substantially below normal maintenance levels can become irritable, emotionally upset and relatively inactive.

Depraved appetite

The Siamese breed of cat is notable because it sometimes develops irrational appetites for textiles, plastics and other non-nutritive items. Large quantities of wool, string, aluminium and textiles have been consumed in cases presented to the author, and life-threatening intestinal obstruction may result. Treatment takes three forms: prevention (by keeping the cat away from favoured items); retraining (by some form of punishment); and dietary changes. Of the latter, free access to high-fibre dry food can be helpful where bouts of pica coincide with hunger. In extreme cases, we recommend the patient be indulged with chopped woollen fibres from discarded clothes. No nutritional basis for this behaviour has been demonstrated, but there is a genetic aspect because particular lines of Siamese and littermates can be affected with identical compulsions to eat fabrics.

Obsessive compulsive disorders

The term 'stereotypy' has traditionally been used to describe the repetitive performance of behaviours that serve no obvious purpose. Cats are liable to display a number of such signs when confronted with stressful situations, for instance extreme confinement, overcrowding, unpredictable punishment or the threat of punishment (for review, see Leuscher *et al.*, in press). The variety of obsessive compulsive disorders (OCDs) displayed by cats seems to be endless, from the most common complaint of excessive grooming, tail-chasing, star-gazing, panic-running and many more bizarre signs of visual hallucinations.

Self-mutilation can be rapid in onset and life-threatening in scale. In the author's practice, biting of the tail and scratching of the head and ears are the most common focus for referred cases of self-mutilating cats. Treatment of feline OCDs should naturally be determined by underlying causation; the first priority is to eliminate possible sources of stress and conflict. In practice, this may not always be attainable, and pharmacological approaches will be needed. Diazepam at 1–2 mg/kg/day is probably the drug of first choice, but other sedatives and anticonvulsants may assist in particular cases.

Tail-chasing is also seen in cats as a variant of normal play: most seem to occasionally dissociate their tail from the rest of their body. Differential diagnosis should focus upon referred pain from spinal nerves, peripheral neuritis from traumatic injury to the tail and ectoparasites. An Elizabethan collar may give temporary respite to the problem if the tail is chewed; vinyl claw covers may be used to prevent damage if the tail or body is scratched (see 'Furniture scratching' below). In extreme cases, the tail may have to be amputated close to the sacro-coccygeal junction, and in the author's experience this need not have adverse sequelae.

The neuropharmacology of OCDs in animals is linked with dopamine turnover and endogenous opiates, and performance of stereotypies has been experimentally controlled by administering morphine antagonists such as naloxone, nalmefine and diprenorphine (Dodman *et al.*, 1988). Unfortunately, this approach only usually offers short-term relief, but longer-acting compounds and delivery systems are under development.

Boredom and lack of play opportunities may be a factor in some cases of OCD, and more time should be spent by owners playing with their cats, investing in play-chase toys and generally enriching the environment.

FURNITURE/FABRIC SCRATCHING

This normal behaviour is connected with removal of loose, keratinous scales from the claws, and scent and visual marking. Once a tradition of scratching a particular item or substrate develops, it can be difficult for owners to redirect their cat towards something less valuable than furniture or draperies. The problem is best dealt with early by training kittens to use specially provided scratch posts, indoors and out. A number of commercial repellents are available, but in the author's experience, strongly scented furniture polish is the most practical.

Surgical declawing is commonly requested by American cat owners. In theory at least, such cats should have impaired climbing ability. However, most apparently compensate well, particularly indoor-living cats. No substantial scientific study into the behavioural effects of declawing cats has been performed and ethical reservations of non-American veterinarians will doubtless continue until such work is done. Official policy of the UK's Royal College of Veterinary Surgeons is that surgical declawing is not an acceptable procedure where it is conducted for the convenience of its owner.

An interesting humane alternative to surgical declawing has recently been devised by an American veterinarian (Wexler, 1990). Soft vinyl pads* are fitted over the cat's claws and glued in position. The claw covers remain in position for 6–10 weeks during which time retraining can be attempted, or they may be refitted on a regular basis. Studies by the author show that such cats continue to perform the actions of 'scratching' at the usual sites but without penetration. The same procedure is highly effective at reducing any other damage from scratching, both to the cat itself in self-mutilating cases, or to other cats in aggressive cats; it can also be used to handicap hunting cats.

---

* Feline Soft Paws Inc.; Lafayette, Louisiana, USA.

PROBLEMS OF
SOCIAL ATTACHMENT

The process of social attachment to conspecifics, humans and other species occurs in kittens between the ages of 2 and 16 weeks or thereabouts (Karsh, 1983). Much as in puppies (Beaver, 1980), adoption of kittens not previously exposed to humans can be problematic when they are more than 10 weeks of age, though feral kittens taken as pets at less than this age are likely to form affectionate relationships with humans. Nevertheless, many exceptions to these predictions of critical eras of socialization are encountered in feline practice; tender loving care of ex-feral and semi-dependent cats is in many cases sufficient to build a tolerant relationship with one or even several humans.

The small animal practitioner may occasionally encounter cats reported to avoid particular individuals within a family. One should not assume that such personal antipathies arise from intentional mistreatment, but they sometimes occur as one of several superstitious behaviours in under-socialized cats. Treatment should concentrate upon reducing the cat's social access to other members of the family, thereby re-directing its attention and affection towards the rejected person. The latter should also feed the cat.

Excessive dependence or attachment to people in general, or to the owner in particular, is much less common in cats than in dogs. Mention has already been made of separation anxiety symptoms in cats: anorexia, emotional changes, even self-mutilation. Therapy to reduce social attachment should take the form of frequent (initially brief) periods of leaving the cat alone. All affection should be re-scheduled to follow a period of separation: periods in between should see less affection exhanged between owner and cat.

MISCELLANEOUS PROBLEMS
OF LEARNED ORIGIN

Cats are very competent at mastering complex tasks and have been widely used to study the process of learning. Acquisition of new behav-iours, desirable or problematic, can occur very quickly under rather subtle reinforcement contingencies. Access to food, warmth, liberty, conspecifics and of course the owner continuously affect the flow of behaviour in cats, and it is very easy for owners inadvertently to reinforce expression of undesired behaviours.

Owners are usually best advised to avoid direct punishment of their cat, except by loud noises or water spray. Extinction of the undesired behaviour can often quickly be accomplished by ensuring that it is no longer rewarded, but in some cases a counter-conditioning programme which introduces new behaviour to disrupt the old may be attempted. This technique is usually referred to by psychologists as response-substitution and can be used to treat a variety of behavioural problems in companion animals. For example, there are two options for dealing with a cat that attacks its owner's ankles before feeding. One is to punish the cat, but that will probably induce undesired secondary effects, such as fear of the owner and conflict about food. Response-substitution does not require any punishment: the cat is trained to jump onto a distinctive spot (e.g. a chair) every time a hand-held buzzer sounds. Compliance brings a dry catfood pellet during training trials. Once the response is established, mealtimes may be preceded by requiring the cat to jump onto the chair and out of range of the owner's ankles.

REFERENCES

General

- Beaver B. (1980) *Veterinary aspects of Feline Behavior.* C.V. Mosby, St Louis.
- Hart B.L. (1978) *Feline Behavior.* Veterinary Practice Publishing Company, Santa Barbara.
- Turner D.C. & Bateson P. (1988) *The Domestic Cat. The Biology of its Behaviour.* Cambridge University Press.

Specific topics

Borchelt P.L. & Voith V.L. (1981) Elimination behavior problems in cats. *Compend. Cont. Educ. Pract. Vet.* **3**, 730–7.

Boudreau J.C. & Tsuchitani C. (1973) *Sensory Neurophysiology*. Van Nostrand Reinhold, New York.

Dodman N.H., Shuster L., White S.D., Court M.H., Parker D., & Dixon R. (1988) Use of narcotic antagonists to modify stereotypic self-licking, self-chewing, and scratching behaviour in dogs. *J. Am. Vet. Med. Ass.* **193**, 815–9.

Hart B.L. (1981) Handling behavioural problems in a busy practice. *Proceedings of the Congress of the Royal Netherlands Veterinary Association*, pp. 125–27.

Hart B.L. & Barrett R.E. (1973) Effects of castration on fighting, roaming, and urine spraying in adult male cats. *J. Am. Vet. Med. Ass.* **63**, 290–2.

Karsh E.B. (1983) The effects of early handling on the development of social bonds between cats and people. In Katcher A.H. & Beck A.M. (eds) *New Perspectives on our Lives with Companion Animals*. University of Pennsylvania Press, Philadelphia.

Luescher V.A., McKeown D.B. & Halip J. *Veterinary Clinics of North America*. W.B. Saunders, Philadelphia (in press).

MacDonald D.W. (1980) Patterns of scent marking with urine and faeces amongst carnivore communities. In Stoddart M. (ed) *Olfaction in Mammals*. Academic Press, London.

Mugford R.A. & Thorne R. (1980) Comparative studies of meal patterns in pet and laboratory-housed dogs and cats. In Anderson R.S. (ed) *Nutrition of the Dog and Cat*. Pergamon Press, Oxford.

Stead A.C. (1982) Euthanasia in the dog and cat. *J. Small Anim. Pract.* **23**, 37–43.

Chapter 27 / Clinical Pharmacology and Therapeutics

R. J. EVANS

INTRODUCTION

The cat is a species in which the practice of drug therapy is particularly difficult. References to iatrogenic intoxications and to unusual drug sensitivities abound in the literature (Yeary, 1965; Wilkinson, 1968, 1980; Atkins & Johnson, 1975) and the folklore of feline therapeutics. Some of these responses have been well studied and their pharmacological or pharmacokinetic basis has been demonstrated. This chapter discusses the pharmacological and pharmacokinetic principles which underlie practical therapeutics and its particular pitfalls in the cat.

PHARMACOLOGICAL AND PHARMACOKINETIC PRINCIPLES

The fate of any chemical agent administered to or acquired by an animal is complex. Its absorption will be influenced by the route of acquisition, by the physiological state of the recipient and by the chemical nature and formulation of the material itself.

Once absorbed, the compound will be distributed in one or more body compartments. It may be confined to the circulation, may permeate the extracellular compartment or the total body water, or it may be selectively concentrated in particular organs. Its distribution may change with time if equilibrium between compartments is slow.

Wherever it has access to its specific site of action or receptor, the agent will exert its primary pharmacological or toxicological action in a concentration-dependent fashion, provided that its concentration exceeds any necessary threshold level. Side-effects may arise from subsidiary actions at other sites or from undesirable consequences of the primary action. Drug receptor interactions and receptor-response coupling are discussed by Baggott (1988) and Rang and Dale (1987).

The drug circulating in the vascular compartment is also continually exposed to the processes of metabolism and elimination, which generally inactivate the compound and clear it from the blood and then from the body (Gibson & Skett, 1986; Hladky, 1990). In some cases metabolism may result in the formation of an active principle from an inactive precursor (prodrug) or the conversion of one active compound to another. The major site of drug metabolism is the liver. Many of the therapeutic difficulties encountered in the cat are the consequence of an unusual pattern of hepatic drug metabolism in this species. This may represent an adaptation to extreme carnivorism: in free-living animals the major source of chemically unusual foreign compounds will be ingested plant material. Drug excretion occurs mainly via the urine and bile. Many drugs partition into milk and it is wise to recognize this when dealing with nursing queens.

Hepatic drug metabolism

Drug metabolism within the liver occurs in two phases. Phase I is also known as the non-synthetic or degradative phase. The reactions in this phase involve oxidation, reduction or hydrolysis. In consequence, the drug may be changed in activity, may be inactivated, or in some cases an inactive precursor may be changed to an active metabolite. The products of phase I reactions also tend to be more water-soluble and less lipid-soluble than the parent compound and to bear reactive groups which act as substrates for phase II activity.

Phase II reactions are known as synthetic or conjugation reactions. They involve the coupling of the drug, or a product of phase I, to an endogenous compound. The endogenous substrates commonly employed as conjugating agents in mammals are carbohydrates, amino acids, acetic acid or inorganic sulphate. In the majority of mammals glucuronide formation is the major phase II reaction.

Species variation is encountered in phase I reactions and, in general, activity is inversely related to body size (Walker, 1978). The cat is in good accord with this generalization for many phase I reactions, although a few phase I reactions do occur relatively slowly in the cat. Much more species variation occurs in phase II reactions and the cat has unusual features in this respect. The cat has a metabolic deficit of glucuronic acid conjugation, which is the major phase II reaction in mammals. As an example, we may consider the formation of glucuronide from phenol, which proceeds 65–100 times as fast in many species (e.g. pig and goat) as it does in the cat (Smith, 1978; Gibson & Skett, 1986). Glucuronide formation is also limited, although less severely so, in other carnivores, including the dog and ferret. Interestingly, the cat's conjugation deficit is not absolute: while only 1–3% of doses of phenol, 1-naphthol or paracetamol undergo glucuronide conjugation, 60% of a similar dose of phenolphthalein is glucuronidated. Progesterone and testosterone also undergo substantial glucuronic acid conjugation. The major part of the poorly glucuronidated compounds is converted to the sulphate conjugate, which is a much slower reaction. Possibly as a further compensation for its glucuronidation deficiency, the cat also makes some unusual conjugates, notably phosphate and glycyltaurine derivatives.

The phase II reactions have been discussed in some detail because the cat's glucuronidation defect is of major significance. Its consequences will emerge further in the following sections.

Excretion of drugs

The kidney is the major organ for elimination of drugs and their metabolites. Because of the importance of water-solubility for renal excretion, the latter is relatively slow in the cat, being limited by the rate at which water-soluble conjugates are formed in the liver. Thus, the overall rate of elimination of many drugs in the cat is slower than in other species.

The pH dependence of renal drug elimination is important in treating intoxications. Many drugs, toxic agents or metabolites are weak acids or bases, While the un-ionized forms of these weak electrolytes are subject to passive resorption in the renal tubules, the ionized forms are not. Thus, their rate of elimination may be enhanced by increasing the ionized proportion of the whole in the renal tubules. This may be achieved for weak acids by alkalinizing the urine and for weak alkalis by acidifying the urine. Elimination may be further increased by enhancing urine flow. The technique of forced alkaline diuresis, and to a lesser extent that of forced acid diuresis, is of substantial clinical value in speeding elimination of intoxicant in overdose and poisoning cases.

Time course of drug-effect and plasma drug concentrations

Pharmacokinetic principles predict the variation with time of drug concentration in the plasma. This is correlated closely with the pharmacological or toxicological effect of the agent since these are usually concentration-dependent. Pharmacokinetics is therefore a potent tool for predicting the drug doses and dosage intervals required to maintain therapeutically effective plasma concentrations and for adjustment of these in the light of species or individual variations.

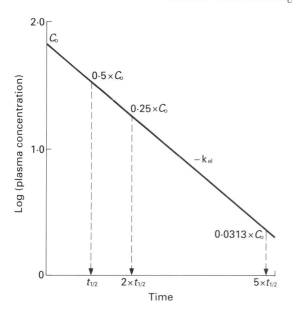

Fig. 27.1 The change in plasma concentration following an intravenous injection of a drug. After an initial phase of distribution and mixing, the concentration falls exponentially with the concentration halving at a fixed interval (the elimination half-life $t_{1/2}$.) C_0 = notional zero-time concentration. $-k_{el}$ = eliminate rate constant.

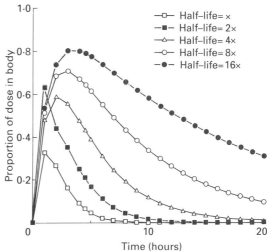

Fig. 27.2 The time course of drug plasma concentration after administration by a non-intravenous route. After administration the concentration rises to a peak as absorption occurs and then falls exponentially by elimination once absorption is complete. The curves show the effect of variation in elimination half-life. With increasing elimination half-life the peak is higher and slightly later but drug persists for substantially longer.

Single doses

If a single dose of a drug is given intravenously, an instantaneous peak concentration is reached in the plasma. The plasma concentration falls initially by mixing and distribution and then exponentially, with a fixed half-life, by elimination (Fig. 27.1). A constant fraction is eliminated in unit time. If the drug is given by any other route, the peak concentration is delayed and lessened by an amount dependent upon the rate of absorption by that route. The peak concentration is also affected by dose, although the time course is little altered. Alteration of elimination rates has only a slight effect on peak concentration, but has a major effect on plasma concentration at times beyond the first half-life after dosing (Fig. 27.2)

The plateau principle: repeated dosing

With multiple dosing, since more than four half-lives are required for complete elimination, administration of the drug at intervals shorter than this leads inevitably to drug accumulation. With exponential elimination, the absolute rate of elimination will increase as drug accumulates (Fig. 27.3). Eventually a plateau state will be reached at which the amount administered in any one dose will be eliminated in the interval before the next dose is given. The plasma concentration then fluctuates about a mean value. Repeated dosing gives a pattern of drug concentration characterized by the time course of accumulation, the extent of accumulation and the size of the fluctuations between adjacent doses. Ninety-seven percent of the plateau level is reached after five half-lives and this time is independent of dosage and dose interval. The full therapeutic effect is thus not achieved for five half-lives. Faster accumulation can be achieved by giving large loading doses before dropping to the maintenance doses; this procedure is not recommended in the cat since high peak levels may be reached and give acute intoxication (Fig. 27.4).

The average plasma concentration maintained

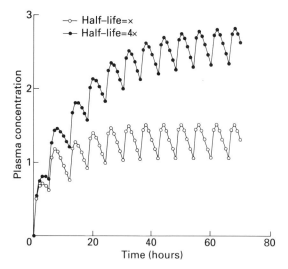

Fig. 27.3 The accumulation of drug to a plateau level with repeat dosing. It takes 4–5 half-lives to reach the plateau level regardless of the half-life. Thus if the half-life is lengthened, approach to plateau is delayed in absolute terms. At a fixed dose rate a higher plateau level is also achieved if the elimination half-life is longer.

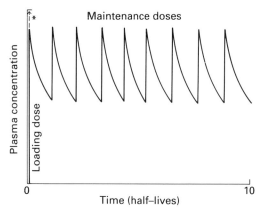

Fig. 27.4 The principle of using a loading dose to achieve the plateau concentration with rapidity. Thereafter the plasma concentration may be maintained by maintenance doses of the usual size. *Note that only a small over estimate (dotted line) of the loading dose may be needed to overshoot the safe peak maximum and induce toxicity and that because of the general tendency to low elimination rate constants the cat is particularly prone to this hazard.

at plateau is dependent only on the total amount of drug given per unit time (i.e. dosage rate = dose/dose interval) and the elimination rate constant. It can be seen from this that with a given regimen of administration per unit time, any drug which has slow elimination in the cat will reach a higher plateau level than species in which elimination is faster. This has led to many problems. Doses extrapolated from other species without regard to elimination rate, have led to accumulated high plasma concentrations and development of toxicity; aspirin administration is a case in point (see below). If the elimination rate constant for aspirin in the cat is determined, a dosage regime can be calculated which will achieve therapeutic rather than toxic plasma concentrations. The agent can thus be used safely, but the dose required is much smaller than might be anticipated from extrapolation.

The fluctuations about the plateau are determined by the size of the dose and dosage interval. The dosage interval is selected primarily by considering the fluctuations that can be tolerated without excessive toxicity at the one extreme or loss of therapeutic efficacy at the other. In view of the cat's susceptibility to intoxication, small doses at a dosage interval equal to or less than an elimination half-life are probably desirable rather than splitting the whole into larger less-frequent doses. Dosage levels need to be reduced in hepatic or renal disease because of slowed elimination.

The pharmacokinetic factors affecting dosage regimens matters are discussed in greater detail in Baggott (1977), Evans (1991a) and Hladky (1990).

ANTIMICROBIAL USAGE IN THE CAT

Antimicrobial drugs are commonly considered to be both effective and safe therapeutic agents. There is a considerable element of truth in this since many of these compounds have a wide therapeutic ratio with a large margin of safety. The penicillins are perhaps the best example of this relative safety. The combined efficacy and safety of the penicillins arises from a low toxicity and their bactericidal nature.

Not all antimicrobial agents share the advantageous therapeutic ratio of penicillin and its derivatives, and thus side-effects may arise at or near the therapeutic plasma level of such agents (Adams, 1975; English, 1985). These include cardiovascular depression, respiratory difficulties, neuromuscular blockade, hypersensitivity and immune-mediated disorders, altered metabolism of other drugs and target organ toxicity; their occurrence is influenced by the need to maintain an effective plasma concentration. Errors in dose or dosage interval, or failure to take account of the specific pharmacokinetic properties of the drug in the cat may lead to low plasma concentrations with failure to achieve any therapeutic effect, or alternatively may result in high drug concentrations and intoxication. Apart from the manifestation of idiosyncrasy and hypersensitivity by individual animals, two classes of undesirable effects commonly arise with the use of antibacterials: gastrointestinal disturbance and specific organ toxicity. Both of these effects are dose-related.

Gastrointestinal disturbance and associated effects

Practically all individuals receiving therapeutic doses of an antimicrobial undergo alterations in the normal microbial flora of the gastrointestinal tract. Alterations also occur in the microflora of the respiratory and genitourinary tracts. The changes in flora vary according to the drug used. Often these changes cause no ill-effects, but sometimes they may be deleterious. Nutritional disturbances may arise and diarrhoea is a common consequence of antimicrobial therapy. Occasionally more serious sequelae arise: sometimes a drug-resistant organism, which has been freed from competition by suppression of other organisms, proliferates and causes enterocolitis and even Gram-negative septicaemia, which may be fatal. The organisms giving rise to superinfection are often extremely difficult to treat with available anti-infective agents.

The broader the spectrum of an antimicrobial, the greater is the probability of such emergence of a single component of the normal flora and the production of superinfection. Superinfection is most commonly seen with tetracyclines, chloramphenicol and with mixed broad-spectrum therapy. Unfortunately, there is little specific information about the incidence of superinfection in cats receiving antibacterial therapy.

Specific organ toxicity

This is much better documented in the cat than is superinfection. The specific toxicities induced by individual drugs are discussed below. They are a significant determinant of drug use in the cat.

Implementation of therapy

Effective use of antibiotics in the cat depends upon the application of the usual microbiological laboratory aids to identify the organism and the drugs to which it is sensitive. It is not the object of this chapter to discuss the principles of choice of antibiotics in relation to specific infections; this is well documented elsewhere (Greene, 1984; Knifton, 1984; Prescott & Baggott, 1988).

The possibility that harmful consequences may arise from the therapeutic or prophylactic use of antimicrobial agents should never discourage their use when they are definitely indicated. They should, however, be used with great circumspection when required. The potential consequences are such that they should be used hesitantly or not at all in the absence of a clear specific indication.

β-lactam antibiotics

Penicillins

The penicillins are the most commonly used of the β-lactam antibiotics (which also include the cephalosporins, cephamycins and monobactams). They are bactericidal by virtue of inhibiting the transpeptidase enzymes which are involved in the cross-linking of the peptidoglycan of the bacterial cell wall. This is the final stage of cell wall synthesis and when it is inhibited the bacterial cell is no longer protected against osmotic lysis. The naturally occurring and semi-synthetic penicillins are valuable therapeutic agents in the cat. They have high therapeutic indices and very high dose levels can be employed safely. Their usefulness is enhanced by the variety of activity spectra now available amongst the semi-synthetic derivatives.

The penicillins most commonly employed in the cat are penicillin G (benzylpenicillin) in a variety of formulations, and the broad-spectrum semi-synthetic drugs, notably ampicillin and amoxycillin, the latter either alone or in combination with clavulanic acid (Bogan, 1977; Bywater, 1978; Bywater *et al.*, 1985). The soluble sodium, potassium or calcium salts will produce high blood levels rapidly with rapid excretion thereafter. These are probably the most useful formulations since evidence is emerging that with bactericidal antibiotics there is considerable elimination of organisms by host defences for some hours after peak levels of antibiotic have been achieved.

Procaine benzylpenicillin and benzathine benzylpenicillin are of low solubility and give slow release and low plasma levels. All these properties are more marked with the benzathine complex. These formulations are very inefficient ways to use benzylpenicillin in view of the long time taken to achieve therapeutic levels and the low peak levels attained. These formulations ought to have little place in the treatment of infection.

It is claimed that the incidence of penicillin-induced anaphylaxis in the cat is low and this is probably correct. Adverse reactions are seen, however, particularly following use of the longer-acting formulations, and it has been suggested that procaine intoxications may be the real cause of many of these reactions (Yeary, 1965). One case of a pemphigus foliaceous-like skin eruption associated with the use of ampicillin has been recorded (Mason & Day, 1987).

Penicillin G is predominantly active against Gram-positive organisms, including anaerobes, which are more susceptible to this agent than to other penicillins, together with a few Gram-negative organisms, for example *Haemophilus* spp. It has the disadvantages of being susceptible to hydrolysis by gastric acid, so that it cannot be administered orally, and of being destroyed by bacterial β-lactamase (penicillinase) enzymes.

The isolation of the 6-aminopenicillanic acid nucleus allowed the production of many modified semi-synthetic penicillins thus permitting manipulation of the antibacterial spectrum and production of acid-stable of β-lactamase-resistant penicillins. Ampicillin and amoxycillin have less marked activity against Gram-positive organisms than does penicillin G but have significant activity against Gram-negative bacteria including some enterobacteria. Activity against *Proteus* spp., *Pseudomonas aeruginosa* and *Klebsiella* spp. is poor. Both are resistant to acid hydrolysis and so can be administered orally but are susceptible to β-lactamase. Their use in the cat is increasing rapidly, although there are strong arguments for reserving them for use in situations where their broad-spectrum activity is indicated. Both are destroyed by β-lactamase. The two agents are pharmacologically equivalent, but amoxycillin is pharmacokinetically superior, being better absorbed than ampicillin after oral administration and giving higher peak plasma concentrations (Bywater, 1978). There is less disturbance of the gastrointestinal flora. Amoxycillin also has a more rapid bactericidal action.

The bioavailability and pharmacokinetics of ampicillin in the cat have been studied in some detail. The half-life of ampicillin is 73 minutes and excretion is primarily renal (Mercer *et al.*, 1977). The percentage of the administered dose absorbed varies with the formulation and the route of administration. With administration of ampicillin trihydrate subcutaneously (SC), 56% of the dose was absorbed. When anhydrous ampicillin was administered, 28% was absorbed from intramuscular (IM) injection, 18% from oral suspension and 42% from capsules *per os* (PO). Even with intramuscular administration, twice daily dosing is adequate, Bogan (1977) has, however, suggested that dosing should be three or four times daily. As pointed out above, there is no need to maintain the plasma concentration when using penicillins, and twice daily dosing is therapeutically effective (Bywater, 1978).

Amoxycillin plus clavulanate (co-amoxiclav)
As noted above amoxycillin has the disadvantage of being susceptible to β-lactamases. Clavulanic acid is a compound produced by *Streptomyces clavigerus* which structurally resembles the penicillins. It has no significant antibacterial activity but is a potent inhibitor of many β-lactamases. The inhibition of β-lactamases is irreversible. Clavulanic acid can be administered orally. If clavulanic acid is given in combination with a penicillin it protects the penicillin from inactivation by β-lactamase and potentiates bactericidal activity against the penicillinase-producing organisms. It is useful in situations where amoxycillin would normally be employed and sensitivity testing shows the organism to be resistant to amoxycillin alone but sensitive to the combination (Bywater *et al.*, 1985). Both components are excreted by the renal tubule, reaching high concentrations in urine, and the combination is effective in bacterial cystitis due to β-lactamase-producing *E. coli* (Senior *et al.*, 1985).

Cephalosporins
The cephalosporins are also bactericidal β-lactam antibiotics with a similar mechanism of action to the penicillins. They are active against Gram-positive organisms but many cephaloporins also have marked activity against Gram-negative bacteria. Their pharmacokinetics are similar to those of the penicillins since they are generally cleared by renal tubular excretion. They often have little susceptibility to the action of β-lactamase. A number of semi-synthetic derivatives are available, often classified by division into three 'generations'. These agents are well tolerated in the cat and they may have some use in the treatment of penicillin-resistant infections and in some individuals with penicillin hypersensitivity. It is worthy of note that in man there is cross-allergenicity between penicillins and cephalosporins, but this is only partial. Thus, patients allergic to penicillin can often, but not always, be safely treated with cephalosporins. In man high

doses produce renal damage, but this does not appear to be a problem in cats.

First-generation cephalosporins include cephalothin, cephaloridine and cephalexin. They are active against a wide range of Gram-positive organisms, and some Gram-negative bacteria including *Haemophilus* spp., *Pasteurella* spp., *E. coli*, *Salmonella* spp. and *Klebsiella*.

Second-generation cephalosporins include cefoxitin, cefuroxime and cefachlor. They are more active against Gram-negative bacteria partly by virtue of lesser susceptibility to β-lactamases.

Cefotaxime has a half-life of 0.5–1.5 hours in the cat (McElroy *et al.*, 1986), but the therapeutic concentrations are not yet clearly defined.

The veterinary use of cephalosporins is often limited by their high cost. First- and second-generation cephalosporins have utility in the treatment of penicillinase-resistant staphylococcal infections, streptococcal infections, and urinary tract infections with susceptible organisms. Cephalexin (Crosse & Burt, 1984; Silley *et al.*, 1988) and cefachlor can be administered orally. Cephalexin has an oral bioavailability of approximately 66% and plasma concentrations peak around 2.5 hours after oral administration (Silley *et al.*, 1988). Its half-life is approximately 1.5 hours.

Third-generation cephalosporins have much-enhanced activity against the Enterobacteriaceae at the expense of reduced activity against Gram-positive organisms. They presently have little application in cats.

Aminoglycosides and aminocyclitols
The aminoglycosides and aminocyclitols are a group of antibiotics characterized by the presence of amino-sugar glycoside groups. The aminoglycosides and aminocyclitols are bactericidal agents with a rather broad spectrum of activity. They are mainly active against Gram-negative anaerobes but have some efficacy against a few Gram-positive organisms, mycobacteria and mycoplasmas. Their mechanism of action is by binding to the 30S subunit of bacterial ribosomes causing faulty codon-anticodon pairing with consequent misreading of the genetic code and thus the syn-

thesis of non-functional proteins. None of these drugs is adequately absorbed from the gut. They penetrate the CSF poorly and are relatively rapidly excreted by the normal kidney. The aminoglycosides are mainly used to treat infections by Gram-negative bacteria. Resistance to aminoglycosides may develop and bacteria that acquire resisitance to one aminoglycoside may exhibit resistance to others. Serious toxicity is a severe limitation to the usefulness of these agents. The aminoglycosides all have a similar spectrum of toxicity. Ototoxicity, affecting both the auditory and vestibular components of VIII cranial nerve function, is marked. Neurotoxicity also occurs as an acute effect and may give rise to respiratory failure. Nephrotoxicity is also an important adverse effect. The cat is particularly sensitive to the ototoxic action.

Streptomycin and dihydrostreptomycin are the most commonly used aminoglycosides. Others of lesser importance are gentamicin, neomycin, kanamycin, framomycin and spectinomycin.

Streptomycin and dihydrostreptomycin

There is some disagreement as to whether significant toxicity occurs at clinical dose levels. A suitable dosage regime is 10 mg/kg 12-hourly. Wilkinson (1968) suggests that normal therapeutic doses may give rise to nausea, salivation, vomiting and ataxia, and that large doses cause restlessness, dyspnoea and loss of concentration. Certainly, prolonged therapy gives VIII nerve damage with the appearance of nystagmus and imbalance which are usually reversible. The histopathological findings in the cat are consistent and unusual in that severe damage involves the cristae rather than the maculae.

The author's view is that streptomycin is not contraindicated in the cat, but it is wise to use it only when essential and then with great care, particularly in kittens, in aged animals or in the presence of renal disease. Courses should be as short as possible: they should not exceed 7 days and preferably should be shorter. In urinary tract infection, the genitourinary antibacterial activity of these drugs can be increased by alkalinizing the urine.

Gentamicin

Gentamicin resembles streptomycin in many ways. It is particularly active against *Pseudomonas aeruginosa* and *Proteus* spp. and its main use is in the treatment of localized, respiratory tract or urinary tract infections by these agents and by *E. coli* and in life-threatening Gram-negative septicaemia. Endotoxinaemia has relatively little effect on the pharmacokinetics of the drug: slight but statistically significant alterations are noted (Jernigan *et al.*, 1988a,b). In the latter situation, it may usefully be combined with ampicillin. Gentamicin may also be used for the treatment of infections by staphylococci sensitive only to this drug. It has a half-life of 10–15 hours (Jacobson *et al.*, 1985).

There is relatively little experience with this drug in cats, but doses of 4 mg/kg twice on the first day and then once every 24 hours, or of 2 mg/kg 12-hourly or 3 mg/kg 8-hourly appear not to give rise to intoxication (Jernigan *et al.*, 1988a). Such a regimen is satisfactory provided that renal function is normal and treatment is not continued beyond 10 days. The dosing interval should be increased if renal function is impaired (Evans, 1991b). At dose levels above those recommended, moderate to severe ataxia, nephrotoxicity and death may occur. Unfortunately, there are no data available on the plasma concentrations associated with toxicity in the cat.

Neomycin

Given systemically, neomycin may cause respiratory failure acutely, or chronic toxicity with renal and VIII nerve damage may develop. The major use for neomycin is, however, for topical application, notably for otitis externa in which situation absorption is minimal and toxicity should not arise. Topical neomycin may be a potent sensitizing agent. Treatment of diarrhoea with oral neomycin is best avoided since iatrogenic disturbance may be substituted for self-limiting illness.

Kanamycin

At a dose level of 6 mg/kg IM or SC 12-hourly, kanamycin may be used for the treatment of systemic infections by *Proteus* spp. or *E. coli*.

Again, courses should be short and the same precautions should be exercised as for gentamicin use.

Framomycin and spectinomycin
There is little information about the use of these drugs in the cat. For this reason they are probably best avoided.

Tetracyclines

The tetracyclines, as their name implies, are a group of antibiotics based on a complex four-ringed nucleus. Tetracycline, oxytetracycline and chlortetracycline are commonly employed and are relatively water-soluble. Minocycline and doxycycline are newer, relatively more lipid-soluble agents which are gaining in importance. The tetracyclines have a very wide spectrum of antibacterial activity and are also effective against chlamydiae, rickettsiae and mycoplasmas. Their usefulness has decreased as a result of increasing bacterial resistance, but they remain the agents of choice for treatment of feline infectious anaemia and of chlamydial infections. They are bacteriostatic rather than bactericidal.

The tetracyclines are adequately absorbed after oral administration. Absorption of the older tetracyclines is impaired by the presence of food, particularly milk and dairy products which are high in calcium, since they chelate calcium ions. Absorption of minocycline and doxycycline is not affected by food. The tetracyclines are widely distributed in most tissues but do not readily enter transcellular fluids, particularly the CSF. Minocycline and doxycycline reach such sites much more readily and attain adequate concentrations in CSF, tears and prostatic fluid. The older tetracyclines are excreted in the bile and urine without metabolism. Minocycline undergoes some metabolism and doxycycline is excreted primarily via the bile. These agents are therefore preferable to the older tetracyclines if there is renal failure.

The tetracyclines have been widely used and have a reputation for safety which is perhaps not altogether deserved. Because of the breadth of their spectrum, the opportunity for one species of the gut flora to overgrow and produce superinfection is great: anorexia, vomiting and diarrhoea are not uncommon. Stomatitis may also develop and Wilkinson (1968) suggests that hepatic damage may occur. These problems are such that it is wise to reserve the tetracyclines for use in infections not responding to narrow-spectrum agents, and for the specific conditions mentioned above rather than using them indiscriminately in inadequately diagnosed infections. Normal therapeutic doses may result in deposition in the teeth and bones of growing animals with obvious staining of the teeth. Inflammation and pain may be produced at injection sites.

Chloramphenicol

Chloramphenicol is a potent, potentially toxic, bacteriostatic antibiotic. Chloramphenicol's mechanism of action is inhibition of the petidyl transferase associated with the 50S subunit of bacterial ribosomes thus inhibiting bacterial protein synthesis. Its spectrum of antibacterial activity is very wide, including marked effectiveness against several Gram-negative organisms and against rickettsiae. It is also effective against chlamydiae and mycoplasmas. Mammalian mitochondria possess 70S ribosomes which are inhibited by chloramphenicol and this accounts in part for its mammalian toxicity. The compound contains a nitrobenzene moiety which may be responsible for other aspects of its mammalian toxicity. The dealkylation of chloramphenicol proceeds very slowly in the cat. It inhibits drug-metabolizing enzymes and may thus prolong the action of pentobarbitone (Adams & Dixit, 1970). Chloramphenicol is generally rapidly absorbed with a high bioavailability (Watson, 1979a,b) following oral or IM administration, widely and rapidly distributed, about 33% being protein-bound, and eliminated with a half-life of approximately 5 hours (Davis *et al.*, 1972). Oral bioavailability from the palmitate salt is, however, poor (Watson, 1979a). There is no difference in absorption between doses administered orally as capsules or tablets (Watson, 1980a,b). 50 mg/

adult cat twice daily may be a suitable dosage regimen.

There are good reasons why the use of chloramphenicol should be limited. Its toxicity in the cat is well documented (Penny *et al.*, 1968, 1970; Watson, 1980c). When cats were given 50 mg/kg i.m. daily in divided doses, a severe, frequently fatal syndrome developed over 1–3 weeks. The signs were severe inappetence, marked depression and terminal diarrhoea. The animals showed severe bone marrow aplasia with leucopenia. Agranulocytosis was severe, the white cell count falling to around 2.0×10^9/l. There was no significant decrease in packed cell volume (PCV). Bone marrow taps were dry after 21 days. At 14 days bone marrow biopsy revealed marked hypocellularity with a marked decrease in the proportion of erythroid cells. There was vacuolation of the cytoplasm and occasionally the nucleus of many early cells of both the myeloid and erythroid series. These effects may be exaggerated in cats with prior bone-marrow depression. Thus, at doses only four times those employed therapeutically, severe toxicity develops. It is not clear whether this occurs with normal therapeutic doses, but it is wise to employ chloramphenicol systemically only in life-threatening infections in which the organism is sensitive to no less toxic antibiotic. In Britain the recommendations of the Royal College of Veterinary Surgeons and the British Veterinary Association must be borne in mind. The responsible use of chloramphenicol in small animal practice has been discussed by Knifton (1987) and Harper (1987). Its major applications are for ocular infections and brain abscesses. Although chloramphenicol is indicated for ophthalmic use, there is evidence that significant amounts of chloramphenicol can be absorbed from topical ocular applications. Although chloramphenicol has been advocated for the prophylaxis and treatment of secondary invasion by *E. coli* in panleucopenia, ampicillin, amoxycillin or gentamicin are clearly to be preferred in this situation, in view of the severe bone marrow depression already present.

Sulphonamides and sulphonamide combinations with trimethoprim

The sulphonamides are safe and useful antimicrobial agents with a wide spectrum of activity including both Gram-positive and Gram-negative organisms and also chlamydiae. They are bacteriostatic, acting by inhibiting synthesis of folic acid by competition with *p*-aminobenzoic acid. Folate is essential for one-carbon transfer in the synthesis of certain amino acids and of thymine and purines. Bacterial protein and nucleic acid synthesis are thus inhibited through lack of these precursors. The usefulness of the sulphonamides has been declining because of increasing bacterial resistance. Sulphonamide-trimethoprim combinations, which produce a bactericidal effect by the synergistic action of two bacteriostatic drugs, have largely replaced simple sulphonamides. Trimethoprim also acts upon folate metabolism, in this case by inhibiting the enzyme dihydrofolate reductase and thus the conversion of dihydrofolate to the active form tetrahydrofolic acid. The combinations have a similar spectrum of activity to simple sulphonamide preparations, but are much more effective against Gram-negative bacteria (except *Pseudomonas*) and resistance develops less readily.

Potentiated sulphonamides have a narrower margin of safety in the cat than in the dog (Craig & White, 1976). Acute toxicity can arise from oral overdosage but is transient. Ataxia, sedation and anorexia are noted.

Chronic intoxication may develop during prolonged dosing. Anorexia, depression and unthriftiness are encountered. Crystalluria is fortunately uncommon in cats, but occurs occasionally and gives rise to haematuria, albuminuria and oliguria. Crystalluria may be prevented by encouraging fluid intake while therapy is in progress. If crystalluria occurs, administration of sodium bicarbonate to produce urinary alkalinization and increase sulphonamide solubility is of value.

Blood dyscrasias with bone marrow depression, agranulocytosis and anaemia may occur, as may hypersensitivity reactions. In both cases the drug should be withdrawn.

Macrolides

Erythromycin

Erythromycin is a complex antibiotic based upon a cyclic lactone linked with amino sugars through glycosidic bonds. It is bacteriostatic but may be bactericidal at high concentrations. It acts to inhibit bacterial protein synthesis, binding to the 50S subunit of bacterial ribosomes and interfering with the translocation step. It has a moderately broad spectrum of activity, being effective against the majority of Gram-positive organisms but few Gram-negative organisms. It is a relatively safe agent in cats although it may disturb the gastro-intestinal flora and induce gastroenteritis when given orally. It is irritant on injection and therefore oral administration is the most commonly used route. Its major use is in the treatment of staphylococcal and streptococcal infections, particularly when the organism involved is resistant to penicillins.

Fluoroquinolones

The fluoroquinolones, such as ciprofloxacin and norfloxacin, are inhibitors of DNA-gyrase (Neer, 1988). They are broad-spectrum bactericidal antimicrobials. As yet few data exist about their use in the cat but enrofloxacin has recently been licensed for use in cats.

Metronidazole

Metronidazole is a heterocyclic antibacterial which is active against protozoa and fastidious anaerobes and protozoa. It can be used in combination with other antimicrobials without interference with activity. It is extremely valuable in the treatment of anaerobe infections.

Griseofulvin

Griseofulvin is an antifungal antibiotic which binds to β-tubulin and interferes with mitosis by disruption of the mitotic spindle. The drug is active only against dermatophytes. The drug acts within the keratinized squames and arrives there by incorporation into immature skin cells followed by transfer within the cells as they mature. This incorporation takes many weeks and therapy for 6 weeks or more is required. In cases where there is nail-bed infection much more prolonged administration is needed.

Griseofulvin has significant toxicity in the cat (Helton *et al.*, 1986). Gastric irritation can result in vomiting following dosing when there is no food in the stomach. High-dose therapy with griseofulvin can result in anaemia in some individuals (Kunkle & Meyer, 1987). Griseofulvin has been widely used for the treatment of ringworm in cats, including pregnant queens. However, two reports suggest griseofulvin is teratogenic, especially when administered in the first third of pregnancy. Cleft palates in kittens (Gillick & Bulmer, 1972) and decreased kitten survival rates are reported to occur, as are limb abnormalities, cranium bifidum, spina bifida and exencephaly (Scott *et al.*, 1975). Griseofulvin should, therefore, not be used in pregnant cats.

ANALGESIA

The cat is frequently denied the benefit of analgesia. This is perhaps in part due to the stoical nature of the species. None the less it is most unfortunate since any circumstance likely to induce pain in man may also be presumed to be painful in the cat. Certainly the choice of an analgesic which is both safe and effective is difficult. Adequate analgesia can, however, be achieved in the cat without undesirable side-effects provided sufficient circumspection is exercised in the choice of treatment and this should be the objective whenever a patient is likely to be suffering pain.

The drugs with analgesic activity may be divided pharmacologically into two classes: the opioid (or narcotic) analgesics and the non-steroidal anti-inflammatory drugs which are analgesics. Both groups present problems when used in cats, but of differing kinds.

The opioid analgesics

The narcotic analgesics are potent agents derived from opium or resembling morphine in their action. The term 'opiates' refers to agents which are closely related chemical analogues of morphine. The term 'opioid' embraces all substances having morphine-like actions which are antagonized by naloxone. The latter term thus includes opiates and endogenous neuropeptides as well as synthetic narcotic analgesics with little or no chemical resemblance to morphine. Opioids act within the central nervous system both to reduce transmission of nociceptive impulses and to modify the cortical response to perceived pain. They are effective against both acute and chronic pain of visceral or somatic origin and regardless of severity. Their use is primarily in the control of severe pain, or pain of visceral origin or postoperative pain (Heavner, 1970). The affective cortical component (euphoria) in morphine's action is an important part of its analgesic action. In addition to these pain-alleviating and dissociative effects, opioids are also depressant and cause sleepiness. They depress the cough reflex and reduce the sensitivity of the respiratory centre to carbon dioxide tension, thus decreasing respiratory drive. They induce nausea and vomiting by an action on the chemoreceptor trigger zone. They also have marked gastrointestinal effects to increase the tone of smooth muscle and to decrease motility leading to severe constipation.

Morphine and the synthetic opioids are now known to be potent mimetics of endogenous neuropeptide modulators which are involved in the gating of pain pathways, and also in the control of emotional responses (Jaffe & Martin, 1990). There are three classes of these neuropeptides: the enkephalins, the endorphins and dynorphin. Opioid receptors have been characterized on the basis both of actions *in vivo* (μ, κ and σ receptors) and by *in vitro* ligand-binding studies (μ, κ and δ receptors). These studies have ascribed the following actions to the various receptor types:

μ – supraspinal analgesia, respiratory depression, euphoria
κ – spinal analgesia, sedation
σ – dysphoria/mania, hallucinations

The binding of ligands to the various receptors has been studied in considerable detail and only a brief outline is possible here. There is no clear-cut evidence from binding studies for receptor sites corresponding to physiologically defined σ receptors nor is there any known function of δ receptors.

The agents binding to opioid receptors can be divided roughly into three categories, although the picture is complicated by differing actions at the different receptor types:

1 Pure agonists: these include most of the more typical morphine-like drugs such as morphine, codeine, fentanyl, pethidine and etorphine. Their action is predominantly at μ receptors, but they have variable activity at δ and κ receptors.
2 Mixed agonist-antagonists: these agents have partial morphine-like activity but also an ability to antagonize some actions of morphine. They include nalorphine, pentazocine, butorphanol and buprenorphine. These agents are partial agonists or competitive antagonists at μ receptors but are κ and σ agonists.
3 Antagonists: these agents produce very little or no effect when administered in the absence of other opioids. They bind to all opioid receptors and block the action of other opioids. The most important is naloxone, which preferentially antagonizes μ receptors although it also blocks κ, δ and σ receptors.

Morphine

It is commonly believed that morphine and narcotic analgesics have a violent excitatory action in the cat and that this is a powerful contraindication to the use in that species. This belief has also led to the view that the action of morphine in the cat is fundamentally different to that in other species. Both of these beliefs are misguided; morphine certainly does have a role as an analgesic in the cat.

Early studies on the effect of morphine in the cat describe dose-dependent behavioural changes. At doses of 0.1–0.2 mg/kg there was definite depression and marked narcosis which lasted several hours. With doses of 2–5 mg/kg cats became apprehensive and shy, but not aggressive. Cats given 10–15 mg/kg showed motor unrest and severe startle responses. At 20 mg/kg there was profound motor excitation, ataxia and seizures. While some reports mention mania, rage and aggressive behaviour at the higher dose levels, others do not. High doses of any opioid may induce hyperthermia.

It clearly emerges from this that the action of morphine in the cat is biphasic. Low doses of the drug produce narcosis and adcquatc analgesia; higher doses produce release phenomena and excitement. Thus, stimulation is a consequence of overdosage of cats with morphine. The dose requirement for narcosis and analgesia in the cat is low. These conclusions have been amply confirmed in a re-evaluation of morphine in cats by Davis and Donnelly (1968).

Morphine at low doses (0.1 mg/kg SC) induced analgesia and narcosis without excitement. The same dose level given postoperatively by slow intravenous injection produced tranquil patients with a useful level of analgesia, but slightly delayed recovery. No change in respiratory pattern was detectable. Morphine given subcutaneously is rapidly absorbed with a peak plasma concentration at 1 hour and a half-life of 3 hours. There is extensive tissue localization of the drug (V_D = 1.35 l/kg) and effective analgesia is maintained up to 4 hours after injection. Thus, used with care and precision, morphine is a valuable analgesic in the cat. Morphine overdosage or respiratory depression may be reversed by nalorphine or naloxone intravenously, intramuscularly, or subcutaneously.

Pethidine (meperidine)

Many practices will prefer to have available pethidine rather than morphine. It has been thought that pethidine should be avoided in the cat because of dose-related excitation similar to that seen with morphine. The therapeutic dose is in the range 2.5–10 mg/kg given subcutaneously; at this dose there is little depression and there is no excitement. At a dose of 22 mg/kg (IV) moderate excitement of short duration is induced; thus, again, excitation is a consequence of overdosage. Pethidine is rapidly converted to norpethidine. Davis and Donnelly (1968) report a plasma half-life of 0.7 h for the drug; on this basis one might expect analgesia to be short-lived and they report that analgesia was present at 2 hours but not at 4 h after injection. They suggest that the half-life

is too short for its practical use in pain relief. Thus, there is still some doubt about the value of the drug in the cat. However, administered 3-hourly rather than 4-hourly, it would appear to have some practical value in short-term pain relief.

Codeine

Codeine is methylmorphine and is metabolized to morphine. Its pharmacological properties closely resemble those of morphine: it has approximately 15% of the analgesic potency of morphine. Its potency in most other actions is only about one-tenth of that of morphine, but it produces marked constipation. There is little specific information about codeine in the cat, but clinical experience shows it to be a useful analgesic for the treatment of moderate pain in the cat at a dose of 0.25–1.0 mg/kg PO. The constipating effect may sometimes limit its long-term use. Care should be exercised in prescribing codeine preparations also containing aspirin or paracetamol. In view of the toxicity of these drugs in the cat (see below), such preparations should be avoided and single ingredient codeine phosphate preparations prescribed.

Dextropropoxyphene

Dextropropoxyphene produces CNS effects qualitatively similar to those produced by codeine. In equi-analgesic doses, side-effects are similar to those of codeine except that dextropropoxyphene has the advantage that it does not produce constipation.

Davis and Donnelly (1968) found that an oral dose of 32 mg/kg was safe and effective in the cat; 2.2 mg/kg IM was also effective with analgesia detectable 2 and 4 hours after injection. No indications as to an appropriate dosing interval can be given since the pharmacokinetics of this agent have not been determined in the cat. Higher doses or intravenous injection produced some incoordination and mydriasis.

It seems that dextropropoxyphene should be a useful analgesic for moderate pain in the cat, but there is little practical clinical experience with the drug in cats. Many preparations of dextropropoxyphene also contain aspirin or paracetamol, and these compound preparations should be avoided.

Buprenorphine

Buprenorphine is a mixed agonist-antagonist. It is a potent analgesic, particularly at the spinal level, and acts for 4–8 hours. Unlike most other narcotic analgesics its effects are only partially reversed by naloxone but doxapram may be used to reverse respiratory depression. It has little effect on cardiovascular function and does not induce vomiting. It is probably now the opiate analgesic of choice in the cat.

Butorphanol

Butorphanol also has useful analgesic activity at doses which do not induce behavioural abnormalities or sedation (Swayer & Rech, 1987). A dose of 0.1–0.2 mg/kg IV produces visceral analgesia for 5–6 hours, whilst subcutaneous administration of 0.8 mg/kg results in somatic analgesia for around 2 hours.

Lomotil

Lomotil is a symptomatic antidiarrhoeal agent containing diphenoxylate hydrochloride and atropine. Diphenoxylate is a congener of pethidine. Excitement, restlessness, mydriasis and in more severe cases blindness, ataxia and goose-stepping have been encountered in cats treated with lomotil but these reactions may be idiosyncratic (Ormerod et al., 1978; Bogan & Lauder, 1981). Lomotil should be used with care and the dose of diphenoxylate should not exceed 0.5–1 mg/kg; however, given these precautions it is useful for the symptomatic control of diarrhoea (Maarsboom et al., 1962; Bogan & Lauder, 1981).

Antipyretic, anti-inflammatory analgesics: non-steroidal anti-inflammatory drugs (NSAIDs)

The NSAIDs are a diverse group of small organic molecules with an analgesic action which is predominantly mediated in the periphery. They do, however, have some central nervous system actions. They are much less potent than the opioids and are employed in mild pain or pain of somatic

Table 27.1 Antipyretic analgesics and non-steroidal anti-inflammatory agents.

Salicylates (T)	Fenemates (I)
Acetoxy-5-acetyl salicylic acid	Flufenamic acid
Acetylsalicylic acid (aspirin)	Meclofenamic acid
Diflusinal	Mefenamic acid
Salicylamide	Toflkenamic acid
Sodium salicylate	Flunixin
	Clonixin
Anilides (N)	
Acetanilide	Propionoic acids (I)
Aminopyrine	Ibuprofen
Antipyrine	Flurbiprofen
Paracetamol	Fenoprofen
Phenacetin	Benoxaprofen
	Indoprofen
Pyrazolones (T)	Pirprofen
Oxyphenbutazone	Carprofen
Phenylbutazone	Ketoprofen
Sulphinpyrazone	Naproxen
Acetic acids (I)	Oxicams
Indomethacin	Piroxicam
Indoxole	Miloxicam
Sulindac	Isoxicam
Tolmetin	Tenoxicam
Zomepirac	
Diclofenac	
Fenclofenac	
Isoxepac	

T: Significant toxicity in the cat: usable with care.
N: Not usable in the cat: extremely toxic.
I: Insufficient information available: likely to be significantly or extremely toxic in the cat.

origin. Aspirin may be considered as the archetype of this group. Aspirin has three major pharmacological activities: it is analgesic; it is anti-inflammatory; and it is antipyretic. It also has well-documented side-effects (see below). There are six major subgroups of antipyretic analgesics (Table 27.1).

Pharmacological mediators of pain and acute inflammation

It would be inappropriate to give a detailed account of this subject here; the reader is referred to Dale and Foreman (1989) and to Lees *et al.* (1991). It is, however, necessary to discuss the matter briefly in order to clarify the interactions of pain, inflammation and pyrogenesis, and to elucidate the actions and side-effects of the aspirin-like analgesics.

Acute inflammation and pain generation are closely integrated responses to noxious insults involving cellular, vascular and nervous responses to soluble mediators released from damaged cells. The haemostatic response is also activated via effects on the vascular wall and upon blood platelets. Exogenous pyrogens induce the release of endogenous pyrogen, a term used to describe the pyrogenic activity of a number of peptides released from leucocytes, including interleukin-1, tumour necrosis factor and γ-interferon. Endogenous pyrogen in turn acts upon the hypothalamic thermoregulatory centres to induce prostaglandin synthesis and increase the set point, which results in fever. Unfortunately the mechanisms of chronic inflammation are presently obscure and it is unlikely that the mediators discussed above have a major role in its pathophysiology (Lees *et al.*, 1991).

The role of histamine, 5-hydroxytryptamine and bradykinin in these responses has long been appreciated. More recently, it has become apparent that a family of closely related derivatives of the essential fatty acids play a major role in the response to noxious stimuli. These mediators are the prostaglandins, the thromboxanes and the leukotrienes, known collectively as eicosanoids. The eicosanoids are synthesized from arachidonic acid, which is mobilized from membrane lipids by phospholipase A_2 when cells are injured. Arachidonic acid is converted by an enzyme, cyclo-oxygenase, to an endoperoxide PGG_2, which is the precursor of both other prostaglandins and the thromboxanes. A second enzyme, lipoxygenase, converts arachidonic acid to 5-hydroperoxyeicosatetraenoic acid (5-HPETE), the precursor of the leukotrienes. These agents have direct inflammatory and haemostatic effects on local cells, blood vessels and blood platelets and sensitize pain-mediating nerve fibres to the stimulatory action of bradykinin. Bradykinin itself releases

prostaglandins from peripheral tissues. Platelet-activating factor is another lipid mediator which is derived from membrane phospholipids and has potent effects on vascular permeability and tone as well as on platelets and leucocytes.

Mechanism of action
The major NSAIDs are all inhibitors of cyclo-oxygenase and thus of prostaglandin synthesis, although the drugs vary in their effectiveness in inhibiting prostaglandin synthesis in different organs. The drugs display their three important activities with differentially varying potency. All three actions can largely be attributed to inhibition of prostaglandin synthesis, the variations in potency correlating with the degree of synthesis inhibition in particular organs. In particular, paracetamol is analgesic but not anti-inflammatory and unusually its analgesic action is centrally mediated: this correlates with failure to inhibit prostaglandin synthesis in the periphery, while doing so effectively in the brain. There may, however, be significant contributions to the clinical response to these drugs due to other actions which are independent of their inhibition of eicosanoid synthesis. A number of the NSAIDs associate directly with cell membranes modifying membrane fluidity and signal transduction mechanisms. These effects may modify the chemotactic, bactericidal and adhesion properties of leucocytes and contribute to the anti-inflammatory action. The NSAIDs are analgesic in chronic inflammation but it is uncertain whether they exert an anti-inflammatory effect in this phase of disease.

Adverse effects
Aspirin and other members of this group of drugs have well-known side-effects including the induction of a bleeding diathesis, bone marrow suppression with agranulocytosis, gastrointestinal ulceration, haemorrhage, vomiting and diarrhoea. Many of these toxic effects are related to inhibition of prostaglandin synthesis. Gastrointestinal effects are most commonly encountered. Some also produce severe anaemia in the cat (see below).

The toxicity of these drugs in cats is poorly

documented and this, coupled with lack of knowledge of bioavailability on oral administration, is a factor which seriously limits their application in feline medicine. The properties of the individual agents are discussed below.

Salicylates

Aspirin (acetylsalicylic acid) is the archetype of this group; others include salicylamide and acetoxy-5-acetylsalicylic acid. Only aspirin is in common use. The major properties of the drug have been outlined above.

Aspirin has a poor reputation in the cat. All too often, cases of aspirin poisoning are encountered, commonly after uninformed administration of the drug by owners. This prominence of aspirin toxicity has led many to suggest that aspirin should not be used in the treatment of cats. However, as Yeary and Swanson (1973) point out, the adoption of such attitudes could lead to the cat becoming a therapeutic orphan. The sensitivity of the cat to salicylates is due to slow drug metabolism (Davis & Westfall, 1972). With knowledge of its pharmacokinetics, aspirin can be used safely in the cat and is probably the first choice NSAID as an anti-inflammatory agent and an antipyretic in this species. It can be useful also to inhibit thrombus formation in cats with cardiomyopathy, thus reducing the risk of aortic embolism.

The pharmacokinetics of aspirin in the cat has been investigated by a number of authors. Aspirin is converted to salicylate by de-acetylation, a process which has a half-life of 8 minutes. The half-life of salicylate, which also has analgesic, antipyretic and anti-inflammatory actions, is much more prolonged and varies with dose; at a dose level of 5 mg/kg it is 22 hours, at 25 mg/kg, 45 hours. This dose-dependence may reflect saturation of elimination mechanisms at higher doses. If aspirin is given regularly, plasma levels form a plateau very close to the predicted value. By contrast with its effect in the dog, chloramphenicol administration does not modify the half-life of salicylate in the cat. The therapeutic plasma concentration for salicylate is in the range 10–20 mg/dl; the lethal plasma concentration is 60 mg/dl. Because of the long half-life, small or

infrequent doses are required to maintain the plateau in the therapeutic range. A suitable dosage regime is to give 5–25 mg/kg daily PO. The author gives no more than 350 mg/adult cat in any one week. Paediatric aspirin tablet may be helpful in prescribing these small doses. If such a protocol is followed, prolonged treatment is possible without toxic effects. Owners should be firmly instructed about the hazards of exceeding the dosage regime.

Doses of aspirin higher than 33 mg/kg can produce toxic signs in 1–2 days, and doses above 80 mg/kg daily are lethal in 7–20 days. The hazard is increased in kittens.

The clinical signs of poisoning are depression, poor appetite and incoordination followed by vomiting, diarrhoea, weight loss, icterus, coma and death. In some recipients there may be nystagmus, aggressive behaviour and convulsions. Electrolyte imbalance and aciduria develop and there is a non-responsive anaemia with increased numbers of Heinz bodies. The white cell count is increased and there is a left shift. Stimulation and then depression of the respiratory centre occurs giving hyperpnoea followed by apnoea, and hyperpyrexia also occurs (Herrgesell *et al.*, 1967). There is a severe haemorrhagic gastroenteritis and toxic hepatitis, and inhibition of platelet function and hypoprothrombinaemia lead to ecchymotic haemorrhage. These features are prominent post-mortem findings (Larson, 1963).

The treatment of aspirin poisoning aims to correct the acid–base balance and to induce alkaline diuresis (Zontine & Uno, 1969). Alkaline diuresis will increase aspirin excretion. Lactated Ringer's solution or glucose saline and bicarbonate should be administered intravenously and frusemide given by injection. Urine pH should be maintained at 8.0 or above for 36–48 hours. Glucose, B-complex vitamins and glucocorticoids may be of assistance in limiting liver damage.

Aniline derivatives

Paracetamol is the only agent in this group in common use; phenacetin and acetanilide are obsolete, aminopyrine and antipyrine are not used in small animals. All of these agents are extremely toxic in the cat, and should not be employed therapeutically. Unfortunately, misguided owners may give paracetamol to their animal, and cases of paracetamol poisoning may therefore be encountered from time to time. The condition is frequently fatal.

Fatal intoxication may arise following a total dose as low as 125 mg (Davis, 1985), and the cat is considerably more susceptible to the toxic effects of paracetamol than is the dog (Hjelle & Grauer, 1986). This is a consequence of the poor capacity of feline liver to both glucuronidate or sulphate paracetamol (Cullison, 1984). Cats, however, rarely show liver failure, which is a late feature in intoxication of other species, but suffer from acute hypoxia due to oxidative damage to erythrocytes. It is suggested that this is a consequence of the marked susceptibility of feline haemoglobin to oxidation to methaemoglobin. The mechanism is uncertain although reduced red cell glutathione concentrations are noted (Hjelle & Grauer, 1986). Haemoglobin may catalyse the conversion of paracetamol to reactive metabolites within the red cell, which may in turn deplete glutathione with methaemoglobinaemia resulting secondarily (Cullison, 1984; Hjelle & Grauer, 1986). Nephrotoxicity is also rarely seen in cats.

Clinical signs may appear within 2 hours. Early signs are pale mucous membranes, facial oedema, salivation, anorexia and lethargy. Conjunctival oedema, vomiting and dilated unreactive pupils may also be noted. Body temperature is often decreased, although it may be normal or even elevated in some patients, and pulse rate is increased. The methaemoglobinaemia gives rise to chocolate-brown discoloration of the blood, intravascular haemolysis and anoxia. The impaired oxygen transport results in dyspnoea, with moist rales and tachycardia. After about 4 hours muddy cyanosis of the mucous membranes and perioral skin may be apparent, as may haemoglobinuria; the urine may also be intensely brown and haematuria may also be present. Later, icterus develops as a consequence of both haemolysis and hepatic necrosis. There is a vigorous regenerative anaemia with Heinz bodies present. Serum alanine aminotransferase and unconjugated bilirubin concen-

trations are elevated. Hyperaesthesia and fits may occur terminally.

On post-mortem examination the carcass is cyanosed and chocolate-brown coloration of the blood is usually noted. The liver and kidneys are swollen and may be petechiated. Pulmonary oedema may also be present.

Treatment of paracetamol poisoning hinges on the use of agents which are precursors of glutathione; the most effective of these is *N*-acetyl-L-cysteine (St Omer & McKnight, 1980; Gaunt *et al.*, 1981; Lorenzana, 1985). Ascorbate may also be of value for its ability to reduce methaemoglobin to haemoglobin (Lorenzana, 1985; Hjelle & Grauer, 1986). It has been claimed that 1.6% sodium sulphate solution intravenously may be as effective as acetylcysteine (Savides *et al.*, 1985). Gastric lavage and blood transfusion are helpful; other supportive therapy is also of importance. A detailed treatment regimen is documented by Lorenzana (1985).

Aminonicotinic acids

None of these agents is presently licensed for use in the cat, although flunixin is licensed for use in dogs. The pharmacokinetics of flunixin has been examined in cats. After oral dosing in the cat flunixin has a bioavailability close to 100% and the elimination half-life is 1–3 hours (Lees & Taylor, 1991; McKellar, May & Lees, 1991). Because of this short half life cumulation is very unlikely to occur with daily or twice daily administration. Its efficacy as an inhibitor of feline cyclo-oxygenase has also been demonstrated and thus it may be expected to be efficacious in cats. As yet, however, there is no information concerning its toxicity in the cat and its use can not therefore presently be recommended.

Pyrazolone derivatives

These are phenylbutazone, oxyphenbutazone and sulphinpyrazone. Phenylbutazone is a potent anti-inflammatory agent with poor analgesic activity. In a clinical paper on cervical spondylosis it is recorded that the use of 12–16 mg/kg administered twice daily on alternate weeks for courses of treatment as long as 1 year produced no signs of toxicity (English & Seawright, 1964). In a toxicological study, administration of 44 mg/kg daily caused death in 4 out of 5 cats after 13 to 20 doses. The fifth cat was destroyed *in extremis*. The clinical signs observed were decreased appetite, weight loss, loss of hair, vomiting, progressive dehydration and decreased faecal output, although the faeces remained soft and unformed. Three cats became anaemic with no evidence of haemolysis or regeneration. There was a variable neutrophilia. Bone marrow biopsy revealed decreased cellularity, an increased myeloid/erythroid ratio, maturation arrest of myeloid cells with foamy cytoplasmic vacuolaton and increased mitosis (Penny *et al.*, 1968). At post-mortem examination ulceration and inflammation were noted in the stomach and inflammation in the small intestine. No purpura or haemorrhage was present despite thrombocytopenia. Hepatocellular and renal tubular changes were also noted. The exact cause of death was uncertain.

At least one preparation containing phenylbutazone is licensed for use in cats. At a dose rate of 5–7 mg/kg daily PO, and certainly not in excess of 15 mg/kg daily as two divided doses, is recommended for the cat. If a dose rate of 12–15 mg/kg is used, the maximum duration of treatment should be 5 days. It seems wise even with lower dose rates to ensure that courses are kept as short as possible and the drug should be withheld if inappetance or depression develops.

Indoline derivatives, anthranilic acid derivatives, propionic acids and oxicams

These three groups of drugs are predominantly anti-inflammatory. There is a dearth of information concerning their administration to cats. The exceptions are ketoprofen and flufenamic acid.

Ketoprofen is licensed for use in the cat both in oral and injectable formulations. It has good bioavailability (approximately 94%). Its half life is short (1–2.25 hours) so that, with once daily dosing, there is little risk of cumulative increase in plasma concentration. Ketoprofen is highly bound to plasma proteins and passes into inflammatory exudates and synovial fluid, in which circumstances levels are higher and the persistence prolonged compared with those for plasma. Dose

rates in the range 1–2 mg/kg once daily are recommended.

Flufenamic acid has been reported to be toxic in the cat (Carlisle, 1983). With low dose levels (5 mg/kg for 36 days) depression and inappetance were seen. With intermediate doses (15 mg/kg for 3 days followed by 7.5 mg/kg for 28 days) ataxia, vomiting, diarrhoea, hyperaesthesia and hyperexcitability and paralysis were also noted. When the drug was administered at a dose level of 80 mg/kg for 4 days two out of three cats became comatose. A dose-related elevation in blood urea was seen in all cats receiving the drug. It would seem wise to await pharmacological and pharmacokinetic evaluation in the cat before employing members of the group other than ketoprofen clinically in this species.

Anti-inflammatory steroids

Glucocorticoids

As discussed, the non-steroidal anti-inflammatory agents have limited use in the cat in our present state of knowledge. The anti-inflammatory glucocorticoids and their synthetic congeners have considerable use. In particular, they are indicated in a number of inflammatory conditions in which hypersensitivity is a pathophysiological mechanism. Notably, these are labial granuloma, miliary dermatitis and flea allergy (after elimination of fleas) and the components of the eosinophilic granuloma complex. The general clinical pharmacology of these agents has been discussed by Keen (1986). No special considerations apply to the choice of glucocorticoids in the cat and, indeed, the cat is less susceptible to many of the side-effects of glucocorticoids than is the dog, but they should none the less be employed with circumspection. It should be noted that there are a few reports of localized hair loss, skin-thinning and subcutaneous calcification after the subcutaneous injection of glucocorticoid preparations in the nape.

In the treatment of immune-mediated conditions, prednisolone is the agent of choice. It is essential to initiate therapy with high dosage rates; 2–4 mg/kg may be used daily (in two divided doses) for 5–7 days or until a satisfactory clinical response is achieved. A rather longer period of high-dose treatment may be required in some circumstances, particularly with skin conditions, whereas others, for example haematological conditions, usually respond rapidly. The dose is then reduced gradually over 6–16 weeks to 0.125 mg/kg on alternate days before ceasing. This is to allow recovery from the adrenocortical suppression which follows high doses. In some animals signs may reappear after the cessation of this course or may fail to disappear completely. In these animals low-dose maintenance therapy may be required throughout life. It is important to minimize adrenocortical suppression in these circumstances. Alternate day therapy maintains a useful therapeutic response while limiting the degree of adrenocortical depression. It is suggested that dosing at the time when endogenous glucocorticoid levels are highest also limits suppression. Since the cat is a nocturnal animal, it is thus wise to administer prednisolone in the evening.

Megestrol acetate and medroxyprogesterone acetate

Megestrol acetate is a 17,a-acetoxy-6-methyl synthetic analogue of progesterone with progestogenic activity. It has a diverse range of physiological actions and is widely used in feline practice. Its use in breeding control and in behaviour modification is beyond the scope of this chapter and is discussed in Chapters 7 and 26.

In addition to its reproductive and behavioural effects, megestrol acetate appears clinically to have a valuable anti-inflammatory action in the cat, although it is difficult to demonstrate anti-inflammatory activity in experimental systems. The mechanism of the anti-inflammatory action of megestrol acetate in the cat is not known. Medroxyprogesterone acetate, which also has the 6-methyl substitution, has similar effects. There is evidence that medroxyprogesterone has glucocorticoid activity and mimics glucocorticoid-induced adrenocortical suppression and growth hormone release. It is not clear whether the glucocorticoid activity is due to the administered compounds or to metabolites.

Regardless of its mechanism of action, megestrol acetate appears to have some value in the treat-

ment of labial granuloma, miliary dermatitis and eosinophilic granuloma, although it is difficult to predict the response in individual patients. A dose of 2.5–5.0 mg should be given two or three times weekly until lesions start to regress and then once weekly until a satisfactory clinical response has been obtained. Some patients may show exacerbation when therapy is withdrawn and these cases may require weekly or fortnightly maintenance administration of 1.2–2.5 mg.

It must be noted that megestrol acetate administration is not without adverse effects. Long-term use in entire queens is to be avoided since endometritis and pyometra may result; stump pyometra has been recorded in neutered females. Obesity may be a problem (Chen & Bellenger, 1987). Prolonged courses occasionally induce benign mammary hyperplasia (Hinton & Gaskell, 1977). The condition is painless although physically inconvenient and is usually localized to one or two glands; biopsy is important in differentiating it from neoplasia. Very rarely mixed mammary tumours or adenocarcinomata may follow megestrol acetate therapy, although it is not clear that it is a direct consequence. Perhaps the most serious adverse effect of megestrol acetate is to induce marked adrenocortical suppression (Chastain *et al.*, 1981; Middleton *et al.*, 1987). Both prednisolone and megestrol acetate may induce glucose intolerance (Middleton & Watson, 1985; Peterson, 1987) and diabetes mellitus may ensue (Herrtage *et al.*, 1985).

Anticonvulsants

In the cat generalized tonic-clonic seizures (grand-mal) epilepsy and focal seizures with secondary general spread are commonly seen. In animals which show recurrent seizures occurring with significant frequency prevention of further seizures is a major therapeutic aim. In status epilepticus termination of the fit is the immediate objective. Anticonvulsants should, ideally, suppress motor cortex firing activity whilst having negligible effects on other neural responses. Particularly, they should not produce excessive sedation, which is a common side-effect of the agents employed as anticonvulsants. Since drugs employed in the prophylaxis of seizures are usually given for several years and because high doses may be necessary, the pharmacokinetic properties of the drugs are important. Their tendency to cumulate, as well as chronic or acute side-effects, are all of practical importance in the selection, institution and maintenance of therapy. Because there is a risk of rebound seizures if plasma levels fall below the therapeutic range, owner compliance to ensure that doses are not omitted is of great importance and the pharmacokinetic properties of the drug are relevant since they determine the significance of missed doses. Unfortunately there have been relatively few investigations of the pharmacokinetics of anticonvulsants in the cat. Tolerance may develop to both the anticonvulsant and the sedative effects of anti-epileptic drugs and, although development of tolerance to their seizure-inhibiting effect is rarely if ever clinically significant, tolerance to sedation is important in allowing safe and effective therapy. During repetitive dosing approximately five elimination half-lives are required to achieve a steady-state plasma concentration of drug. Because of this time required for steady-state conditions to become established, the time course of development of tolerance to sedation, and the natural interseizure interval, several weeks of observation with a given agent or dose rate should be allowed to elapse before a judgment is made as to whether the therapeutic regimen is appropriate. Diazepam and phenobarbitone are the anticonvulsants of choice in feline epilepsy and will be discussed in detail, but pertinent features of the pharmacology of some other drugs will also be presented.

Phenobarbitone
Phenobarbitone is the most appropriate barbiturate for the treatment of seizures since it has a much wider therapeutic index than other barbiturates between doses which induce sedation or hypnosis and those required for the anticonvulsant action.

The mechanism of the anticonvulsant action of phenobarbitone is uncertain. Barbiturates interact with receptors for the inhibitory central neurotransmitter γ-aminobutyric acid (GABA). The

GABA$_A$ receptor consists of four subunits which in addition to bearing the GABA binding site form a chloride channel through the neuronal membrane. Opening of the channel, which is induced by GABA-binding, results in increased chloride conductance of the membrane and stabilizes the neuron against firing by making its membrane potential more polarized. Barbiturate binding sites may exist in association with GABA$_A$ receptors and result in increased chloride channel opening thus stabilizing the neuron against firing. However, although barbiturates can be shown to potentiate GABA-mediated neurotransmission the effect is rather feeble, requires concentrations at the upper limit of the anticonvulsant range, and is also better correlated with the sedative and hypnotic potency of the barbiturates than with their anticonvulsant potency.

The major side-effects of phenobarbitone are sedation and hypnosis. Tolerance to these develops relatively rapidly but they are none the less commonly the factor which limits the efficacy of prophylaxis at high dose levels. On withdrawal rebound seizures may arise and therapy should therefore be terminated by gradually reducing the dose over a period of many weeks. Phenobarbitone induces hepatic mixed function oxidase and may accelerate the elimination of other drugs. The terminal phase half-life of phenobarbitone in the cat is 34–43 hours (Frey, 1989). The plasma concentration yielding effective control varies widely.

Frey (1989) recommends that phenobarbitone therapy be initiated with a daily dose rate of 3–6 mg/kg bodyweight divided into two or three portions, continuing with two doses per day once sedation has faded. At least 2 weeks will be required before the efficacy of prophylaxis can be assessed. If necessary the dose should then be increased and a further 2 weeks allowed to elapse before control and adverse effects are again evaluated. The maximum recommended daily dose is 15 mg/kg.

Primidone
Primidone will not be considered in detail. It has been generally thought that primidone is toxic for

cats. Frey (1989) claims, however, that primidone in doses up to 40 mg/kg is well tolerated with minimal side-effects, and Sawchuck *et al.* (1985) report that no hepatotoxicity occurs at this dose level. It is possible therefore that the drug might be of some value in cats. However, its metabolism and mechanism of action are such that phenobarbitone is still preferable, particularly in view of the paucity of clinical experience with the drug in the treatment of cats. Primidone is metabolized by the liver to phenobarbitone and phenylethyl-malonamide (PEMA), both of which are active (Bogan & Smith, 1968). Primidone has anticonvulsant activity but much of its effect is thought to be due to phenobarbitone since during long-term therapy this reaches steady-state concentrations substantially higher than those of the parent drug. Although less conversion of primidone to phenobarbitone occurs in cats (Sawchuck *et al.*, 1985) and primidone also has a longer half-life than in dogs or man and the parent drug must thus contribute relatively more to the action, phenobarbitone still exerts the major effect. At high doses conversion to phenobarbitone is less and also hepatocellular damage may result. Thus both to obtain certainty of action and avoid adverse effects, phenobarbitone is preferable.

Diazepam

Diazepam is one of a number of benzodiazepines which are employed as anti-epileptic agents in man. There is no information concerning the pharmacokinetics or use of other benzodiazepines in cats and detailed discussion will therefore be limited to diazepam. The benzodiazepines are ineffective in the absence of normal GABA levels in the CNS and associate with a binding site associated with the $GABA_A$ receptor. The binding results in increased affinity of GABA for its binding site and an increased frequency of opening of the chloride channel. Benzodiazepines thus potentiate the inhibitory action of GABA and stabilize the cell reducing neuronal firing rate.

In man diazepam is metabolized by the liver to *N*-desmethyldiazepam, temazepam and to oxazepam, all of which have anticonvulsant activity. In cats *N*-desmethyldiazepam accumulates slowly and does not reach particularly high concentrations. Oxazepam achieves very low concentrations and does so only 8 hours after administration of a single dose (Frey, 1989). Thus the parent compound must make a greater contribution to the anticonvulsant action than in man. In the cat the elimination half-life is probably around 15–20 hours.

Diazepam is useful for seizure prophylaxis and also for the treatment of status epilepticus (see Chapter 2). Frey (1989) suggests that diazepam is the drug of choice for the treatment of feline epilepsy and suggests a dose rate of 0.5–2.0 mg/kg daily divided in three doses. Tolerance to the anticonvulsant action does not develop and effective long-term control of seizures is possible (Frey & Schwartz-Porsche, 1985).

Phenytoin

Phenytoin (diphenylhydantoin) is a membrane-stabilizing drug which blocks voltage-gated sodium channels in a use-dependent fashion and thus stabilizes excitable membranes. It also has effects on neurotransmission mediated by GABA and by 5-hydroxytryptamine. The relationship of these effects to its anticonvulsant action remains obscure. In cats the half-life is extremely long, being in the range 24–108 hours (Roye *et al.*, 1973). The extreme variability in half-life may be due to saturation of metabolism or elimination at high doses leading to zero-order elimination. There is always therefore considerable risk of accumulation of the drug to toxic plasma concentrations. Adverse effects in cats include dermal atrophy (Barthold *et al.*, 1980), gingival hyperplasia, marked sedation, incoordination and anorexia. These factors, coupled with the absence of clinical experience with the drug in cats, mean that the drug is best avoided in this species. If it is employed therapeutic monitoring of plasma concentrations is essential (Frey, 1989).

Valproic acid

Valproic acid is active against all forms of epilepsy. Its anticonvulsant mechanism is uncertain. Potentiation of GABA-mediated neurotransmission has been reported and a number of explanations have been offered for this. The drug activates glutamic acid decarboxylase, which is the synthetic enzyme for GABA, and also inhibits GABA-transaminase, which degrades it. Brain GABA levels become elevated and there is increased release of GABA from neurons in the presence of valproate. Other possible mechanisms also exist, however, and valproate has recently been shown to block voltage-gated sodium channels in a use-dependent fashion and also to potentiate release of γ-hydroxybutyrate, a putative inhibitory neurotransmitter. In cats its half-life is approximately 8 hours (van Djuin & Beckmann, 1975). The drug may have possible clinical utility in the cat but presently there is no experience with it in this species.

Anticonvulsant of choice

In summary, therefore, diazepam and phenobarbitone are the only drugs which can presently be recommended for the prophylaxis of feline seizures (Frey, 1986). The author has until recently thought phenobarbitone to be the drug of choice in feline epilepsy and has more experience of the use of that drug than of diazepam. There is, however, no doubt that diazepam is effective and the arguments put forward by Frey (1989) in favour of diazepam as the drug of choice are persuasive.

APPETITE STIMULATION

Diazepam has an additional use in the cat – the stimulation of appetite in cats which are anorexic, when it is used at a dose rate of 0.1–0.5 mg/kg intravenously (Macy & Gasper, 1985). Benzodiazepines have this effect in a number of species but it is particularly marked in cats. The pharmacology of appetite control is extremely complex and the mechanism of action of diazepam in this respect remains uncertain. There is evidence that GABA receptors are involved in regulation of eating and that benzodiazepine inverse agonists, stimulatory agents that reduce the effectiveness of GABA-mediated transmission by binding to benzodiazepine receptors thereby decreasing chloride channel opening, reduce appetite. Conversely stimulation of GABA receptors, probably involved in hunger/satiety mechanisms, stimulates appetite. This may involve altering the balance between GABA-mediated and serotoninergic, noradrenergic or dopaminergic transmission since central serotoninergic and dopaminergic mechanisms are important for normal eating and benzodiazepines reduce the effectiveness of amphetamine as an appetite suppressant.

TRANQUILLIZERS AND SEDATIVES

From time to time it may be necessary to sedate animals for travel, for reduction of locomotor activity or for minor procedures not requiring general anaesthesia. Two major groups of drugs have been used for this purpose: these are the phenothiazines and the benzodiazepines. Phenobarbitone is also useful for this purpose.

Phenothiazines

The phenothiazines are profound depressants of a large number of physiological functions. They interact with central nervous system dopamine, muscarinic, 5-HT and H_1 receptors inducing blockade, central α-receptors to give facilitation, and block peripheral α-adrenergic transmission. Ideally, tranquillizers would decrease locomotor activity and responses to external stimuli without impairing consciousness. Unfortunately, those in use in veterinary medicine produce marked sedation, although arousal is easily accomplished. In addition, in a proportion of animals paradoxical excitement may occur yielding an unmanageable patient; in the author's view this is sufficient to contraindicate widespread use in cats. Phenothiazines are hypotensive and suppress cardiovascular reflexes even at quite low dose levels, and in large doses they also depress respiratory rate. These agents are contraindicated in shock and should be used with great caution in weak, debilitated or aged individuals or in patients with cardiovascular disease. Depression of the thermoregulatory centres may give rise to hypothermia. High doses may induce tremors of the extremities and head, loss of righting reflexes, shivering, marked lethargy, diarrhoea and anal sphincter relaxation. These effects are reversible on withdrawal of the drug, but may take several days to subside.

Phenothiazines are antiemetic. This effect is neither marked nor particularly consistent in the cat, but they can produce useful protection against travel sickness and this is the main indication for their use.

These agents lower rather than raise the seizure threshold and their use in animals with convulsions is strictly contraindicated.

Other phenothiazines, and also organophosphorus compounds, have synergistic effects and these combinations should be avoided. Phenothiazines potentiate the activity of procaine and should not be used with it.

For details of their use as premedicating agents, standard textbooks of anaesthesia should be consulted (e.g. Hall & Clarke, 1991).

Chlorpromazine, promazine and acepromazine are in common use, acepromazine being most widely employed. Their properties are very similar but acepromazine is the most potent. They may be used orally, intramuscularly, subcutaneously or intravenously, and doses may be repeated 1–4 times daily. The manufacturers' data sheets should be consulted for details of doses.

Benzodiazepines

The benzodiazepines have a hypnotic action in high doses and are perhaps best described as anxiolytic in low doses. They also produce muscle relaxation. There is no autonomic blockade and minimal disturbance of cardiovascular or respiratory function. Paradoxical excitement is not seen. They have no antiemetic activity. High doses may produce temporary incoordination.

Diazepam (see above) has properties which make it very useful as a sedative for cats. Despite its lack of antiemetic activity, it is particularly useful as a sedative for car travel. The dose rate is generally 0.25–0.5 mg/kg PO and this may be repeated at 8-hour intervals. Occasional animals may require 1 mg/kg.

Phenobarbitone

In low doses phenobarbitone also has anxiolytic and sedative properties and reduces locomotor activity. It is useful for these purposes in the cat

and also for breaking undesirable behavioural habits. The dose should be titrated in the individual, but will usually lie in the range 3–15 mg once or twice daily. With repeated use, tolerance develops over a period of days and the dose may then need to be increased.

DRUGS ACTING UPON THE CARDIOVASCULAR SYSTEM

The range of drugs acting on the cardiovascular system that has been employed in cats is extremely limited. There is a need to use positive inotropes – drugs that enhance contractile force – in heart failure associated with cardiomyopathies. Digoxin has been the positive inotrope generally used in the cat, but the bipyridine inhibitors of phosphodiesterase III may prove to have utility, and for the treatment of cardiogenic shock dopamine and dobutamine are indicated. In other species there is increasing emphasis on the use of vasodilator drugs to decrease preload and afterload but there is as yet little experience with these agents in the cat. In circumstances when antidysrhythmic therapy is required in the cat, blockade of sympathetic drive to the heart is often also desirable and propranolol is the agent commonly employed. Loop diuretics are commonly used to reduce circulating volume and relieve oedema and effusions associated with heart failure. In many cases there is no specific pharmacokinetic information for these agents in the cat and use has been based on empirical trial, there being few reports of thorough clinical trials.

Positive inotropic agents

Digoxin
The cardiac glycosides are steroidal glycosides isolated from a variety of plants which have a positive inotropic effect. They include digoxin, digitoxin and ouabain. Only digoxin is commonly used in the cat. These drugs are inhibitors of the sodium-potassium ATPase (the sodium pump) which expels sodium ions from cells in exchange for potassium ions. This raises intracellular sodium levels which in turn affects carrier-mediated sodium–calcium exchange across the membrane

of the myocardial cells raising intracellular calcium levels. Calcium mobilization is the key step
in excitation-contraction coupling in cardiac
muscle, and increased calcium levels thus enhance the force of cardiac contraction. This improved contractility shifts the failing heart onto a
higher Starling curve, allowing cardiac output to
be maintained at a lower left ventricular end
diastolic pressure. Cardiac glycosides also decrease sinus rate, slow atrioventricular conduction and increase vagal tone. These effects make
digitalis useful for controlling supraventricular
tachyarrhythmias.

Congestive heart failure associated with the
various forms of cardiomyopathy is being increasingly recognized in the cat. In advanced dilative
cardiomyopathy positive inotropes are the cor-
nerstone of therapy and digoxin is generally employed. Toxic effects, however, limit its utility.
Inappetence, salivation, persistent vomiting and
depression are encountered. The lethal effect is
due to cardiac toxicity and has features similar to
those in other species. The LD_{50} for oral digoxin
in the cat is 0.8 mg/kg. There is an important
interaction between potassium ions and cardiac
glycosides. At low potassium concentrations inhibition of the sodium pump by cardiac glycosides
is increased and at high potassium concentrations
it is decreased. At low potassium concentrations
the dysrhythmogenic potential of the glycosides is
increased. Thus hypokalaemia may precipitate
digoxin toxicity as may acid–base disturbances as
a consequence of their effect on potassium levels.

Digitalization of cats is a hazardous procedure
and mild or early cases of cardiomyopathy are
best managed without this, but severe cases
may benefit from it. Digoxin is the cardiac glycoside of choice. Cats should never be digitalized
rapidly.

Digoxin is about 15–20% bound to plasma
proteins in the cat (Baggot & Davis, 1973) and has
a half-life of approximately 33 hours (Bolton &
Powell, 1982). Erichsen *et al.* (1978, 1980) have
evaluated the use of digoxin in the cat with particular attention to dosage regimes and plasma
levels. Cats were given equal doses of digoxin as
elixir, tablets or crushed tablets on food. The

highest peak plasma concentration followed administration of elixir; the lowest, only one-third
of that following elixir, resulted from administering the crushed tablet on food. Cats given elixir at
a dose rate of 0.011 mg/kg for 4 days showed a
60% increase in peak concentration and a 230%
increase in trough concentration over 4 days.
Males had plasma levels 50–100% higher than
those in females, but showed no significant
ECG changes. Secondary concentration peaks
occurring 1–24 hours after dosing may be due to
enterohepatic cycling of drug and in man this is
associated with eating. These peaks introduce
variability into the cumulation of drug. Toxic
plasma levels are above 2.4 ng/ml and there is
no evidence that the cat is particularly sensitive
(Bolton & Powell, 1982).

Cats absorb digoxin slowly from tablets and the
bioavailability of the drug varies. Solid digoxin is
variably solubilized in the upper gut where it
is best absorbed and this results in lower and
variable concentrations. The administration of
crushed tablets with food delays gastric emptying
and digoxin is lost due to hydrolysis by gastric
acid. By contrast, digoxin as elixir is absorbed
more uniformly and completely in a shorter time.
Elixir also has the advantage of greater flexibility
and accuracy in matching dose to body weight.
Although the higher peak values with elixir may
present some risk of toxicity, the advantages of
using it seem to outweigh this.

Cats given a single toxic dose (0.11 mg/kg)
of elixir showed depression, vomiting, salivation
and anorexia followed by minimal ECG changes,
and were clinically ill for 48–96 hours.

It is wise to digitalize cats using the maintenance dose rather than attempting the use of
loading doses. The dosage is in the range 0.002–
0.008 mg/kg daily in two equal doses and requires
individual adjustment. Signs of toxicity develop
before ECG changes, so that there is time to
adjust the dose before serious dysrhythmias develop. If vomiting or other toxic signs develop,
the drug should be withheld for two or three
doses before resuming at a reduced dose level. In
the interim electrolyte levels should be evaluated.
If there is hypokalaemia and no heart block

0.1 g of potassium chloride should be given p.o. divided into several small doses.

It is vital that clients understand the dosage regime, the cumulative properties of the drug and the significance of signs of toxicity.

Bipyridines

Increases in intracellular cyclic AMP have a positive inotropic effect in cardiac muscle and induce vasodilation in peripheral vascular smooth muscle. Phosphodiesterase III (PDE III) is a phosphodiesterase isoenzyme which selectively degrades cyclic AMP. Inhibitors of PDE III thus increase cyclic AMP levels and are useful agents in the treatment of cardiac failure since they are both positive inotropes and peripheral vasodilators. A number of bipyridine compounds are selective PDE II inhibitors. None is licensed for use in veterinary medicine but amrinone (now withdrawn) and milrinone have been used in dogs; as improved compounds are introduced they may have application as positive inotropes in feline cardiomyopathies.

Sympathomimetic amines

Animals with cardiomyopathy, particularly advanced dilative cardiomyopathy, may present in cardiogenic shock due to low-output failure. Two amines which are agonists at adrenergic β_1-receptors exert a direct positive inotropic effect and are useful in the emergency reversal of cardiogenic shock. They do, however, have significant adverse effects.

Dopamine is a natural catecholamine and the precursor of noradrenaline. It is an agonist at β_1-receptors and at high concentrations also stimulates noradrenaline release. It has a specific vasodilator action on renal, cerebral, mesenteric and coronary vessels due to activation of dopaminergic receptors present in these vascular beds. It induces an increase in cardiac output, increased renal blood flow and, at low doses, a slight fall in blood pressure. At high doses there is a small rise in blood pressure. The pressor response is due to activation of α-receptors in other vascular beds. It may also cause tachydysrhythmias.

Dobutamine is a synthetic sympathomimetic amine which is relatively selective for cardiac β_1-receptors, mediating the inotropic effect. Its relative lack of effect on a, β_2-, dopaminergic, or chronotropic β_1-receptors results in selective increase in cardiac contractility, with little effect on heart rate or rhythmicity and with only a slight increase in peripheral resistance. It does not, however, have the beneficial effects on renal and coronary perfusion seen with dopamine.

Both agents must be given by intravenous infusion. Dopamine has been employed in cats at an infusion rate of 5–10 µg/kg/min and dobutamine at 5–20 µg/kg/min.

Antidysrhythmic drugs

Propranolol

Propranolol is a non-selective blocker of catecholaminergic β-receptors. It thus protects against catecholamine-induced tachycardia, inotropy and dysrhythmias. It also has a quinidine-like action to block voltage-gated sodium channels although this probably contributes little to its anti-arrhythmic action. It decreases the firing rate of sino-atrial and ectopic pacemaker tissue and slows orthodromic and antidromic conduction reducing re-entry excitation. Because it increases the AV nodal refractory period it is useful for slowing ventricular rate in supraventricular tachydysrhythmias. The drug is well absorbed from the gut but is efficiently cleared from the portal blood by the liver. Oral doses must therefore be considerably higher than intravenous doses for the same therapeutic effect. Propranolol is useful in hypertrophic cardiomyopathy at a dose of 0.3–1.0 mg/kg once heart failure is responding to therapy. In hyperthyroidism there is an upregulation of myocardial β-receptors and increased catecholaminergic actions contribute to the pathophysiology of the tachycardia, dysrhythmias, increased blood pressure and cardiac hypertrophy seen in this condition. Propranolol is useful in reducing heart rate and force as an adjunct to specific antithyroid therapy.

Side-effects commonly encountered include depression, anorexia and, less frequently, vomiting and diarrhoea. Propranolol potentiates airway constriction by blocking β_2-receptors and should not be used in the presence of feline asthma. In heart failure, care must be exercised, however, since propranolol can potentiate the failure by reducing myocardial contractility. It may also induce hypotension. Since it blocks sympathetic drive to the heart and slows cardiac conduction it is also contraindicated in heart block. Indeed it may itself induce heart block. Rapid cessation of long-term therapy may result in rebound arrhythmias and the drug should therefore be tailed off gradually over several weeks.

Vasodilators

Vasodilator drugs can be of value in the treatment of cardiac failure by reducing preload and afterload, and in consequence myocardial workload and oxygen demand. They may particularly be of value in advanced dilated cardiomyopathy.

Nitroglycerine

Nitroglycerine ointment has been used in dilated cardiomyopathy. Nitroglycerine is a potent venodilator, the predominant effect of which is to reduce preload. Its mechanism is probably direct activation of particulate guanylate cyclase of vascular smooth muscle leading to increased intracellular cyclic GMP concentrations, reduced intracellular free calcium concentrations and vasodilation. It may, however, lead to pooling in the venous circulation and marked hypotension, thus it is not ideal. The oral and parenteral formulations have short half-lives and duration of action. They are thus unsuitable for veterinary use. Ointment containing 2% nitroglycerine is, however, much more practicable since the duration of action can be as long as 3 hours due to slow percutaneous absorption of the drug. For cats, a segment of ointment about 1/8 to 1/4 inch long is extruded from the tube nozzle and is rubbed into a hairless or shaved area of skin. The site of application should be one which the animal cannot reach to lick: the inner surface of the ear pinna is often used. There is significant risk of absorption of drug through the fingers and gloves should be worn for applying the ointment.

Hydralazine

Hydralazine is a direct-acting arteriolar vasodilator whose mechanism of action is unknown. It has a marked dilator effect in the coronary, mesenteric, renal and cerebral vascular beds but relatively little effect on those of skin or skeletal muscle. It thus reduces afterload, and consequently stroke volume and cardiac output are increased. The increased renal blood flow and consequent increase in glomerular filtration rate (GFR) is clinically valuable. There is some favourable experience with the drug in the cat for the treatment of dilated cardiomyopathy at a dose rate of 0.5–0.8 mg/kg b.i.d. orally. It is suggested that the initial oral dose in the cat should be 2.5 mg, which may be increased by titration to a maximum of 10 mg. The effects are seen within 1 h, peak after 3–5 hours and last approximately 12 hours (Kittleson, 1983).

Diuretics

Loop diuretics have an extremely potent diuretic effect by inhibiting resorption of sodium and chloride in the thick portion of the ascending limb of the loop of Henle. The use of loop diuretics to reduce circulating volume, ventricular filling and thus cardiac distension and heart work is an important element in the control of cardiac failure. In many cases loop diuretics may be sufficient as the sole form of drug therapy. Oedema and effusions are also relieved. Care must be taken that circulating volume is not reduced to the level at which reduced venous return compromises cardiac output and induces low-output failure. Loop diuretics increase excretion of sodium, chloride, potassium and hydrogen ions and water. The potassium loss may cause hypokalaemia and thus may potentiate the action of cardiac glycosides and precipitate toxicity. Excessive use may result in metabolic acidosis. Cats are particularly responsive to loop diuretics and care must be exercised to avoid overdosing.

Furosemide (frusemide)

Furosemide is the loop diuretic of choice in the cat because of its marked efficacy coupled with extensive clinical experience in its use. The drug is highly protein bound and not significantly metabolized. Oral absorption is rapid and efficient. Renal excretion occurs by glomerular filtration and tubular secretion and the half-life is around 15–20 minutes. It is valuable in the management of cardiac failure associated with hypertrophic or dilated cardiomyopathy. The dose requires individual adjustment in the light of the response, but is usually in the range 2.25–5 mg/kg IV once or twice daily for the first 24–48 hours for emergency diuresis when initiating therapy in hypertrophic cardiomyopathy with severe cardiac failure. The response is rapid, diuresis ensuing within minutes, being maximal after about half an hour and persisting for 2–3 hours. Subsequently oral dosing with 1–2 mg/kg once or twice daily is appropriate for long-term maintenance therapy and also for cases of dilated cardiomyopathy. With oral dosing diuresis begins after an hour, the maximal effect occurs after about 2 hours and persists for 4–6 hours. The lowest practical maintenance dose should be used and in some cases of hypertrophic cardiomyopathy less frequent administration may be sufficient, for example dosing every second or even third day.

The therapy of feline acquired heart disease is discussed in detail in Chapter 11.

CHEMOTHERAPY OF NEOPLASMS

The drug therapy of neoplasms is an area requiring considerable skill and experience. Such therapy is becoming more commonly practised in the cat than formerly and whilst specialist opinion may be sought for the initiation of therapy the duration of therapy is such that its continuation and surveillance will often be continued outside specialist centres and in some cases may be initiated by veterinarians in general practice.

Chemotherapy is rarely the sole element in the treatment of neoplasia and surgery and radiotherapy may also have major roles. Control of pain and the management of paraneoplastic syndromes is also of considerable importance. The therapeutic ratio for cytotoxic drugs is low and the effects of toxicity may seriously compromise the patient and can result in death. Careful judgment based on detailed clinical evaluation (MacEwen *et al.*, 1987) and cytological or histopathological diagnosis is therefore required in each individual case to decide whether chemotherapy is appropriate and to select the appropriate regimen. This is particularly so in the case of cats where cytotoxic treatment generally results in temporary remission rather than radical cure. Chemotherapy can, however, be of value (i) in the management of neoplasms which are not amenable to surgical excision or to radiotherapy, (ii) in the prolongation of the disease-free period following irradiation or excision, and (iii) in the prevention and control of metastatic disease.

The cell cycle

Proliferating cells, whether normal or neoplastic, progress through a well-defined sequence of phases involving synthesis of RNA and protein, DNA replication and cell division by mitosis. This sequence is known as the cell cycle and the phases are as follows:

1 *G_1 (prereplicative) and G_0 (resting) phases.* Immediately following mitosis there is a resting phase with respect to DNA synthesis. During this period proliferating cells synthesize substantial amounts of RNA and protein. RNA synthesis increases towards the end of the phase. This is G_1 phase. Alternatively cells may enter a much more prolonged phase of 'rest' during which they perform vegetative functions but may subsequently return to active cell division. This phase, in which cells are out of the cell cycle, is called G_0. Cells in G_0 are generally not susceptible to the effects of cytotoxic drugs. Because of this the proportion of the cell population in G_0 relative to those in other phases of the cell cycle is important in determining the fractional kill of tumour cells and the effectiveness of chemotherapy.

2 *S (DNA synthesis) phase.* S phase follows G_1 and during this phase the DNA content of the cell nucleus is duplicated.

3 *G_2 (premitotic interval) phase.* In the G_2 phase, which follows the S phase, DNA synthesis is again halted but RNA and protein synthesis continue.

Chapter 27

Table 27.2 The major anti-tumour drugs used in feline therapeutics.

Plant alkaloid spindle poisons	*Antimetabolites*
Vincristine	Cytosine arabinoside
Alkylating agents	*Enzymes*
Cyclophosphamide	L-asparaginase
Chlorambucil	
Melphalan	*Enzyme inhibitors*
	Methotrexate
Hormones	Hydroxyurea
Prednisolone	
Cytotoxic antibiotics	
Bleomycin	
Doxorubicin	

4 M (mitotic) phase. The M phase (mitosis) is associated with a decrease in the synthetic rates of protein and RNA and there is assembly of the microtubules which comprise the mitotic spindle.

Some cytotoxic drugs have their action on specific phases of the cell cycle, because of their modes of action, whereas others are phase non-specific.

Mechanisms of action and properties

The major drugs employed in tumour chemotherapy in cats are listed in Table 27.2. These agents act at many different sites to inhibit cell growth and division or to cause cell death. The various sites at which these agents may act are discussed further below.

Alkylating agents

The alkylating agents commonly used in chemotherapy are all nitrogen mustards which form covalent bonds with DNA, generally cross-linking the two DNA strands and inhibiting DNA replication and its function as a template for RNA synthesis. The alkylating agents are non-phase-specific in their action.

Cyclophosphamide is the alkylating agent which is most widely used in feline practice. It is inactive and is converted by the mono-oxygenase system in the liver to 4-hydroxycyclophosphamide, which in turn reversibly forms aldophosphamide. Aldophosphamide is transported to

other tissues where it is converted to phosphoramide mustard (the active agent) and to acrolein, which is toxic. Acrolein may result in chemical cystitis with haematuria, increased urinary frequency and dysuria but fortunately this is uncommon in cats. The agent may be administered by the oral or the intravenous routes.

Alkylating agent-like cross-linking agents

Cisplatin (*cis*-diaminedichloroplatinum) is a coordination complex containing a central platinum atom surrounded by two chloride ions and two ammonia groups. Its precise mechanism of action is uncertain but it seems probable that it acts analogously to the alkylating agents and thus cross-links DNA. It should not be used in cats since in this species it induces damage to the pulmonary microvasculature with consequent pulmonary oedema (Knapp *et al.*, 1987).

Antimetabolites and enzyme inhibitors

The antimetabolites and enzyme inhibitors inhibit the biosynthesis of precursors of DNA and are S phase-specific. Methotrexate inhibits the enzyme dihydrofolate reductase, which is required for the formation of tetrahydrofolate, the active form of the methyl group donor. It thus inhibits nucleotide formation and nucleic acid synthesis. Methotrexate can be administered by the oral or the intravenous route.

Cytosine arabinoside (cytarabine) is an analogue of the natural nucleoside 2'-deoxycytidine. It differs in having the inverted hydroxyl configuration on the 2' carbon of the pentose so that the sugar is arabinose rather than ribose. Cytarabine enters cells and is phosphorylated to its triphosphate. The drug is incorporated into both DNA and RNA to a limited extent but its cytotoxic action is predominantly due to inhibition of DNA polymerase by the triphosphate.

Hydroxyurea is an analogue of urea which inhibits ribonucleotide reductase thus interfering with the conversion of ribonucleotides to deoxyribonucleotides and inhibiting DNA synthesis. Its use is in the control of polycythaemia rubra vera.

5-Fluorouracil may induce severe CNS disturbances and shock in cats, which can be fatal. Its use in cats is therefore contraindicated.

Cytotoxic antibiotics

Many cytotoxic antibiotics are intercalating agents, i.e. compounds whose molecules insinuate between adjacent base pairs in the DNA helix. They thus inhibit both DNA and RNA synthesis. Doxorubicin is the most widely used of these agents. It is cell cycle phase non-specific. It requires slow intravenous administration via an indwelling catheter into a continuously flowing infusion of saline. Care must be taken to avoid extravascular spillage since severe sloughing may arise and result in indolent ulceration. The drug has significant nephrotoxicity in cats and this may be the major limiting factor in clinical use (Cotter *et al.*, 1985). It may be useful in combination with cyclophosphamide for the treatment of non-haemopoietic neoplasms (Maudlin *et al.*, 1988).

Bleomycin is a metal-chelating glycopeptide antibiotic. It is thought to act by chelating ferrous iron and interaction of the chelate with oxygen to generate superoxide and hydroxyl radicals. Free radical-induced damage then degrades DNA with chain fragmentation and release of free bases. Bleomycin is effectively G_2 phase-specific although it also has lesser effects in the S phase and M phase.

Enzymes

L-Asparaginase is a preparation of a bacterial enzyme which hydrolyses L-asparagine in the extracellular fluid. Non-neoplastic cells synthesize L-asparagine and are not dependent on extracellular sources. Neoplastic lymphocytes are unable to do so and require extracellular arginine for protein synthesis. Thus the enzyme is effective in lymphomas since it inhibits the cells by removing this extracellular source of arginine. It is usually administered by intraperitoneal injection. Being a foreign protein L-asparaginase may induce anaphylaxis.

Hormones

Glucocorticoids are used in two contexts in the chemotherapy of neoplasms. Because of its cytolytic effect on lymphocytes prednisolone is of value in combination protocols for the treatment of lymphoid neoplasms, whether solid or leukaemic. By virtue of its anti-inflammatory properties it is also used in a number of protocols for the treatment of other neoplasms as a means of reducing the side-effects induced by chemotherapeutic agents such as the cystitis induced by cyclophosphamide.

Plant alkaloid mitotic spindle poisons

Vincristine and vinblastine bind to the protein β-tubulin, which constitutes the spindle elements in mitosis, with consequent arrest of cell division in metaphase. Vincristine is widely used in treatment protocols for feline neoplasms (Golden & Langston, 1988). It should be administered intravenously with great care to avoid perivascular spillage.

Use of anti-neoplastic agents

The differing biochemical sites of action and phase specificities of the cytotoxic drugs underlie the use of these agents in combination. Combinations of agents result in cumulative functional lesions of cells with much greater therapeutic effect than can be achieved with single agents whilst minimizing adverse effects. The development of resistance of tumour cells to the drugs may also be slowed by the use of combination therapy. The differing phase specificity of the agents used coupled with any differential timespan for recovery from drug-induced inhibition of normal and neoplastic cells determines strategies of dose pulsing which allow a selective effect on the cells of the neoplasm while sparing sensitive normal tissues such as bone marrow and gastrointestinal mucosal cells.

Adverse effects

The occurrence of adverse effects is the major limitation in the use of chemotherapeutic agents in the treatment of neoplasia. Adverse effects to cytotoxic drugs are not as commonly a problem in cats as they are in the dog. None the less it is extremely important to monitor the patient for the possible development of toxic effects and to modify or stop therapy as appropriate should they arise.

Anorexia and vomiting

Anorexia is commonly encountered during chemotherapy. Vomiting may occur during therapy with many of the agents discussed although less commonly in the cat than in the dog. Cyclophosphamide and the other alkylating agents, methotrexate and doxorubicin, are particularly likely to produce anorexia or induce vomiting. Vomiting may be controlled by the use of antiemetics such as metoclopramide, domperidone or prochlorperazine. Dexamethasone may also be of value in reducing the frequency of occurrence of vomiting and may be used in combination with the antiemetics noted above.

Bone marrow suppression

With the exception of prednisolone, which is not myelosuppressive and indeed is mildly stimulatory to bone marrow, all the cytotoxic agents discussed above can induce decreased production of the formed elements of the blood. Because of the short lifespans of granulocytes and of blood platelets, myelosuppression usually presents as leucopenia, usually as a consequence of neutropenia, together with thrombocytopenia. Associated with these cytopenias there is increased susceptibility to infections and occasionally haemorrhagic complications may result. Anaemia may be present as part of the effects of the primary disease and is exacerbated by myelosuppression. Should the neutrophil count fall below $3 \times 10^9 l^{-1}$ the dose of cytotoxic drugs should be reduced and prophylaxis instituted with a broad-spectrum antimicrobial (see above). If pyrexia and depression are associated with leucopenia, septicaemia may be present and antimicrobial therapy may be required (see above).

Therapy of haemopoietic neoplasms

Lymphoproliferative disease

A number of combination therapy regimens have been employed in the treatment of lymphoma and acute lymphocytic leukaemia (ALL).

MacEwen *et al.* (1979, 1981) have reported protocols which combine vincristine as an inhibitor of mitosis, cyclophosphamide as an alkylating agent, methotrexate or cytosine arabinoside as antimetabolites and prednisolone as a lymphocytolytic. The protocol is initiated with two cycles

of therapy delivered over 8 weeks with subsequent cycles of treatment over periods of up to 3 years. Complete remission resulted in 69% of treated cats with a mean survival time of 210 days (MacEwen *et al.*, 1987). Twenty-three percent of treated cats showed a partial response with mean survivals of 80 days. A similar protocol based upon L-asparaginase, vincristine, cyclophosphamide (or chlorambucil if chemical cystitis is problematical) and prednisolone has been described by Squires and Gorman (1990). In a study of 75 cats with lymphoma, Jeglum *et al.* (1987) employed a combination of vincristine, cyclophosphamide and methotrexate. The median survival time was 8 weeks with extremes of 2 days and 4 years. They found that addition of prednisolone or L-aparaginase to the regimen was without benefit. There was marked variability in the median survival time depending upon the form of the disease. The shortest survival time was in mediastinal lymphoma ($1\frac{1}{2}$ months); renal lymphoma had a median survival time of 5 months, alimentary lymphoma 11 months and multicentric lymphoma 21 months.

Feline cases of chronic lymphocytic leukaemia (CLL) or multiple myeloma have been treated successfully using melphalan and prednisolone (Couto, 1989).

Myeloproliferative disease

Myeloproliferative disease is a clinically and cytologically diverse collection of conditions. In the cat myeloid dysplasia is relatively common (see Chapter 4) and often progresses to frank leukaemia rather rapidly. Chemotherapy of myeloid dysplasia is not indicated and once transition to leukaemia occurs such treatment is generally unsuccessful.

Malignant mastocytosis

Prednisolone may be used in the treatment of splenic or disseminated mast cell malignancy following splenectomy. The H_2-receptor antagonists cimetidine or ranitidine have value in reducing gastric acid secretion and gastric and duodenal ulceration secondary to mast cell tumours. Combination chemotherapy with vincristine, cyclophosphamide and doxorubicin has been attempted for subcutaneous mast cell tumours but with poor success and wide surgical excision followed by prednisolone is the preferred approach.

For information about the treatment of other neoplasms and further discussion the reader is referred to MacEwen *et al.* (1987) and Squires and Gorman (1990).

REFERENCES

Adams H.R. (1975) Acute adverse effects of antibiotics. *J. Amer. Vet. Med. Assoc.* **166**, 983–7.

Adams H.R. & Dixit B.N. (1970) Prolongation of pentobarbital anesthesia by chloramphenicol in dogs and cats. *J. Amer. Vet. Med. Assoc.* **156**, 902–5.

Atkins C.E. & Johnson R.K. (1975) Clinical toxicities of cats. *Vet. Clin. North Am.* **5**, 623–52.

Baggot J.D. (1977) *Principles of Drug Disposition in Domestic Animals: The Basis of Veterinary Clinical Pharmacology.* W.B. Saunders, Philadelphia.

Baggot J.D. (1988) Pharmacodynamics. In Booth N.H. & McDonald L.E. (eds) *Veterinary Pharmacology and Therapeutics*, 6th edn. Iowa State University Press, Ames, pp. 25–72.

Baggot J.D. & Davis L.E. (1973a) Plasma protein binding of digitoxin and digoxin in several mammalian species. *Res. Vet. Sci.* **15**, 81–7.

Baggot J.D. & Davis L.E. (1973b) Comparative study on plasma protein binding of diphenylhydantoin. *Comp. Gen. Pharmacol.* **4**, 399–405.

Barthold S.W., Kaplan B.J. & Schwartz A. (1980) Reversible dermal atrophy in a cat treated with phenytoin. *Vet. Pathol.* **17**, 469–76.

Bogan J.A. (1977) Treatment of small animals with ampicillin and amoxycillin. *Vet. Rec.* **101**, 473.

Bogan J.A. & Lauder I. (1981) Lomotil in cats. *Vet. Rec.* **108**, 523.

Bogan J. & Smith M. (1968) The relation between primidone and phenobarbitone blood levels. *J. Pharm. Pharmacol.* **20**, 64–8.

Bogan J.A. & Snow D.H. (1976) Mixed blessing. *Vet. Rec.* **99**, 56.

Bolton G.R. & Powell A.A. (1982) Plasma kinetics of digoxin in the cat. *Amer. J. Vet. Res.* **43**, 1994–9.

Bywater R.J. (1978) Treatment of animals with ampicillin and amoxycillin. *Vet. Rec.* **102**, 44.

Bywater R.J., Hewett G.R. & Marshall A.B. (1985) Efficacy of clavulanate-potentiated amoxycillin in experimental and clinical skin infections. *Vet. Rec.* **116**, 177–9.

Carlisle C.H. (1983) Toxicity of flufenamic acid in the cat. *J. Small Anim. Pract.* **24**, 653–8.

Chastain C.B., Graham C.L. & Nichols C.E. (1981) Adrenocortical suppression in cats given megestrol acetate. *Amer. J. Vet. Res.* **42**, 2029–35.

Chen J.C. & Bellenger C.R. (1987) Obese appearance, mammary development and retardation of hair growth following megestrol acetate administration to cats. *J. Small Anim. Pract.* **28**, 1161–7.

Cotter S.M., Kanki P.J. & Simon M. (1985) Renal disease in five cats treated with adriamycin. *J. Amer. Anim. Hosp. Assoc.* **21**, 405–9.

Craig G.R. & White G. (1976) Studies in dogs and cats dosed with trimethoprim and sulphadiazine. *Vet. Rec.* **98**, 82–6.

Crosse R. & Burt D.G. (1984) Antibiotic concentrations in the serum of dogs and cats following a single oral dose of cephalexin. *Vet. Rec.* **115**, 106–7.

Dale M.M. & Foreman J.C. (eds) (1989) *Textbook of Immunopharmacology*, 2nd edn. Blackwell Scientific Publications, Oxford.

Davis L.E. (1980) Clinical pharmacology of salicylates. *J. Amer. Vet. Med. Assoc.* **176**, 65–6.

Davis L.E. & Donnelly E.J. (1968) Analgesic drugs in the cat. *J. Amer. Vet. Med. Assoc.* **153**, 1161–7.

Davis L.E. & Westfall B.A. (1972) Species differences in biotransformation and excretion of salicylate. *Amer. J. Vet. Res.* **33**, 1253–62.

Davis L.E., Neff C.A., Baggott J.D. & Powers T.E. (1972) The pharmacokinetics of chloramphenicol in domesticated animals. *Amer. J. Vet. Res.* **33**, 2259–66.

English P.B. (1985) Adverse reactions to antimicrobial agents in the dog and cat. *Vet. Ann.* **25**, 292–301.

English P.B. & Seawright A.A. (1964) Deforming cervical spondylosis of the cat. *Austral. Vet. J.* **40**, 376–81.

Erichsen D.F., Harris S.G. & Upson D.W. (1978) Plasma levels of digoxin in the cat: some clinical applications. *J. Amer. Anim. Hosp. Assoc.* **14**, 734–7.

Erichsen D.F., Harris S.G. & Upson D.W. (1980) Therapeutic and toxic plasma concentrations of digoxin in the cat. *Amer. J. Vet. Res.* **41**, 2049–58.

Evans R.J. (1991a) Clinical pharmacology: the rational basis of therapeutics: In Chandler E.A., Price C.J., Sutton J.B. & Thompson D.J. (eds) *Canine Medicine and Therapeutics*, 3rd edn. Blackwell Scientific Publications, Oxford, pp. 829–56.

Evans R.J. (1992) Effects of renal dysfunction on plasma drug concentrations and their consequences for dosage regimens. *Proc. Assoc. Vet. Pharm. Therap.* **14**, 26–40.

Frey H.H. (1986) Use of anticonvulsants in small animals. *Vet. Rec.* **118**, 484–6.

Frey H.H. (1989) Anticonvulsant drugs used in the treatment of epilepsy. *Problems in Veterinary Medicine* **4**, 558–77.

Frey H.H. & Schwartz-Porsche D. (1986) Pharmakologische Grundlagen der Behandlung der Epilepsie bei Hund and Katze. *Tierartz. Praxis* **13**, 541–9.

Gaunt S.D., Baker D.C. & Green R.A. (1981) Clinicopathological evaluation of *N*-acetylcysteine therapy in acetaminophen toxicosis in the cat. *Amer. J. Vet. Res.* **42**, 1982–4.

Gibson G.G. & Skett P. (1986) *Introduction to Drug Metabolism*. Chapman & Hall, London.

Gillick A. & Bulmer W.S. (1972) Griseofulvin – a possible teratogen. *Canad. Vet. J.* **13**, 244.

Golden D.L. & Langston V.C. (1988) Uses of vincristine and vinblastine in dogs and cats. *J. Amer. Vet. Med. Assoc.* **193**, 1114–7.

Greene C.E. (1984) *Clinical Microbiology and Infectious Diseases of the Dog and Cat*. W.B. Saunders, Philadelphia.

Hall L.W. & Clarke K.W. (1991) *Veterinary Anaesthesia*, 9th edn. Baillière Tindall, London.

Harper R.C. (1987) The responsible use of chloramphenicol in small animal practice: 2. Clinical considerations. *J. Small. Anim. Pract.* **28**, 543–7.

Heavner J.E. (1970) Morphine for postsurgical use in cats. *J. Amer. Vet. Med. Assoc.* **156**, 1018–9.

Helton K.A., Nesbitt G.H. & Caciolo P.L. (1986) Griseofulvin toxicity in cats: literature review and report of seven cases. *J. Amer. Anim. Hosp. Assoc.* **22**, 453–8.

Herrgesell J.D. (1967) Aspirin poisoning in the cat. *J. Amer. Vet. Med. Assoc.* **151**, 452–5.

Herrtage M.E., Barnett K.C. & MacDougall D.F. (1985) Diabetic retinopathy in a cat with megestrol acetate-induced diabetes. *J. Small Anim. Pract.* **26**, 595–601.

Hinton M. & Gaskell C.J. (1977) Non-neoplastic mammary hypertrophy in the cat associated either with pregnancy or oral progestagen therapy. *Vet. Rec.* **100**, 277–80.

Hjelle J.J. & Grauer G.F. (1986) Acetaminophen-induced toxicosis in dogs and cats. *J. Amer. Vet. Med. Assoc.* **188**, 742–6.

Hladky S.B. (1990) *Pharmacokinetics*. Manchester University Press, Manchester.

Jacobson E.R., Groff J.M., Gronwall R.R., Moreland A.F. & Chung M. (1985) Serum concentrations of gentamicin in cats. *Amer. J. Vet. Res.* **46**, 1356–8.

Jaffe J.H. & Martin W.R. (1990) Opioid analgesics and antagonists. In Goodman G.G., Rall T.W., Nies A.S. & Taylor P. (eds) *The Pharmacological Basis of Therapeutics*, 8th edn. Pergamon Press, New York, pp. 485–521.

Jernigan A.D., Hatch R.C., Wilson R.C., Brown J. & Tuler S.M. (1988a) Pharmacokinetics of gentamicin in cats given *Escherichia coli* endotoxin. *Amer. J. Vet. Res.* **49**, 603–7.

Jernigan A.D., Hatch R.C., Wilson R.C., Brown J. & Crowell W.A. (1988b) Pathologic changes and tissue gentamicin concentrations after intravenous gentamicin administration in clinically normal and endotoxemic cats. *Amer. J. Vet. Res.* **49**, 613–7.

Jernigan A.D., Wilson R.C., Hatch R.C. & Kemp D.T. (1988c) Pharmacokinetics of gentamicin after intravenous, intramuscular and subcutaneous administration in cats. *Amer. J. Vet. Res.* **49**, 32–5.

Keen P.M. (1986) Uses and abuses of corticosteroids. *Vet. Ann.* **27**, 45–62.

Knapp D.W., Richardson R.C. & DeNicola D.B. (1987) Cisplatin toxicity in cats. *J. Vet. Intern. Med.* **1**, 29–32.

Knifton A. (1984) Selection of antibiotics in small animal practice. *Vet. Rec.* **115**, 38–40.

Knifton A. (1987) The responsible use of chloramphenicol in small animal practice: 1. Pharmacological considerations. *J. Small Anim. Pract.* **28**, 537–42.

Kunkle G.A. & Meyer D.J. (1987) Toxicity of high doses of griseofulvin in cats. *J. Amer. Vet. Med. Assoc.* **191**, 322–3.

Larson E.J. (1963) Toxicity of low doses of aspirin in the cat. *J. Amer. Vet. Med. Assoc.* **143**, 837–40.

Lees P., May S.A. & McKellar Q.A. (1991) Pharmacology and therapeutics of non-steroidal anti-inflammatory drugs in the dog and cat: 1. General pharmacology. *J. Small Anim. Pract.* **32**, 183–93.

Lorenzana R.M. (1985) Paracetamol poisoning in cats. *Vet. Rec.* **117**, 135.

McElroy D., Ravis W.R. & Clark C.H. (1986) Pharmacokinetics of cefotaxime in the domestic cat. *Amer. J. Vet. Res.* **47**, 86–8.

MacEwen E.G., Mooney S., Brown N.O. & Hayes A.A. (1987) Management of feline neoplasms; surgery, immunotherapy and chemotherapy. In Holzworth J. (ed) *Diseases of the Cat: Medicine and Surgery*, vol. 1. pp. 597–617.

McGee T.M. & Olszewski J. (1962) Streptomycin sulphate and dihydrostreptomycin toxicity. *Arch. Otolaryngol.* **75**, 295–303.

McKellar Q.A., May S.A. & Lees P. (1991) Pharmacology and therapeutics of non-steroidal anti-inflammatory drugs in the dog and cat: 2. Individual agents. *J. Small Anim. Pract.* **32**, 225–35.

Macy D.W. & Gasper P.W. (1985) Diazepam-induced eating in anorexic cats. *J. Amer. Anim. Hosp. Assoc.* **21**, 17–20.

Marsboom R., Hofkens C., Martelmans J. & Vercruysse J. (1962) Diphenoxylate, a useful drug in the symptomatic treatment of acute and chronic diarrhoea in domestic and wild animals. *Vet. Rec.* **74**, 1043–6.

Mason K.V. & Day M.J. (1987) A pemphigus foliaceus-like eruption associated with the use of ampicillin in a cat. *Austr. Vet. J.* **64**, 223–4.

Maudlin G.N., Matus R.E., Patnaik A.K., Bond B.R. & Mooney S.C. (1988) Efficacy and toxicity of doxorubicin and cyclophosphamide used in the treatment of selected malignant tumours in 23 cats. *J. Vet. Intern. Med.* **2**, 60–5.

Mercer H.P., Garg R.C., Powers J.D. & Powers T.E. (1977) Bioavailability and pharmacokinetics of several dosage forms of ampicillin in the cat. *Amer. J. Vet. Res.* **38**, 1353–9.

Middleton D.J. & Watson A.D.J. (1985) Glucose intolerance in cats given short term therapies of prednisolone and megestrol acetate. *Amer. J. Vet. Res.* **46**, 2623–5.

Middleton D.J., Watson A.D.J., Howe C.J. & Caterson I.D. (1987) Suppression of cortisol responses to exogenous adrenocorticotrophic hormone and the occurrence of side effects attributable to glucocorticoid excess in cats during therapy with megestrol acetate and prednisolone. *Canad. J. Vet. Res.* **51**, 60–5.

Neer M.T. (1988) Clinical pharmacologic features of fluoroquinolone antimicrobial drugs. *J. Amer. Vet. Med. Assoc* **193**, 577–80.

Ormerod E., Bogan J.A. & Lauder I.M. (1978) Toxic effects of Lomotil in cats. *Vet. Rec.* **102**, 110.

Penney B.E. & White R.J. (1978) Narcotic analgesics in the domestic cat. *Vet. Clin. N. Amer.* **8**, 317–33.

Penny R.H.C., Carlisle C.H., Prescott C.W. & Davidson H.A. (1968) Toxic effects of phenylbutazone on the cat. *Brit. Vet. J.* **124**, 562–8.

Penny R.H.C., Carlisle C.H., Prescott C.W. & Davidson H.A. (1970) Further observations on the effect of chloramphenicol on the haemopoietic system of the cat. *Brit. Vet. J.* **126**, 453–8.

Petersen M.E. (1987) Effects of megestrol acetate on glucose tolerance and growth hormone secretion in the cat. *Res. Vet. Sci.* **42**, 354–7.

Prescott J.F. & Baggott J.D. (1988) *Antimicrobial Therapy in Veterinary Medicine.* Blackwell Scientific Publications, Boston.

Rang H.P. & Dale M.M. (1987) *Pharmacology.* Churchill Livingstone, Edinburgh, pp. 3–33.

Roye D.B., Serrano E.E., Hammer R.M. & Wilder B.J. (1973) Plasma kinetics of diphenylhydantoin in dogs and cats. *Amer. J. Vet. Res.* **34**, 947–54.

Savides M.C., Oehme F.W. & Leipold H.W. (1985) Effects of various treatments on acetaminophen toxicosis and biotransformation in cats. *Amer. J. Vet. Res.* **46**, 1485–9.

Sawchuk S.A., Parker A.J., Neff-Davis C. & Davis L.E. (1985) Primidone in cats. *J. Amer. Anim. Hosp. Assoc.* **21**, 647–50.

Scheer M. (1987) Concentrations of active ingredients in the serum and in tissues after oral and parenteral adminstration of Baytril. *Vet. Med. Rev. GFR* **2**, 104–18.

Scott F.W., DeLa Schultz R.D., Bistner S.I. & Riis R.C. (1975) Teratogenesis in cats associated with griseofulvin therapy. *Teratol.* **11**, 79.

Senior D.F., Gaskin J.M., Buergelt C.D., Franks P.P. & Keefe T.J. (1985) Amoxycillin and clavulanic acid combination in the treatment of experimentally induced bacterial cystitis in cats. *Res. Vet. Sci.* **39**, 42–6.

Short C.R., Hardy M.L., Clarke C.R., Taylor W. & Baggot J.D. (1986) The nephrotoxic potential of gentamicin in the cat: a pharmacokinetic and histopathologic investigation. *J. Vet. Pharmacol. Therap.* **9**, 325–9.

Silley P., Rudd A.P., Symington W.M. & Tait A.J. (1988) Pharmacokinetics of cephalexin in dogs and cats after oral, subcutaneous and intramuscular administration. *Vet. Rec.* **122**, 15–7.

Smith R.L. (1978) Extrapolation of animal results to man. In Gorrod J.W. & Beckett A.H. (eds) *Drug Metabolism in Man.* Taylor & Francis, London.

Squires R.A. & Gorman N.T. (1990) Antineoplastic chemotherapy in cats. *In Practice* **12**, 101–11.

Stanton M.E. & Legendre A.M. (1986) Effects of cyclophosphamide in dogs and cats. *J. Amer. Vet. Med. Assoc.* **188**, 1319–22.

St. Omer V.V. & McKnight E.D. (1980) Acetylcysteine for the treatment of acetaminophen toxicosis in the cat. *J. Amer. Vet. Med. Assoc.* **176**, 911–3.

Swayer D.C. & Rech R.H. (1987) Analgesic and behavioral effects of butorphanol, nalbuphine and pentazocine in the cat. *J. Amer. Anim. Hosp. Assoc.* **23**, 438–46.

Walker C.H. (1978) Species differences in microsomal monooxygenase activity and their relationship to biological half-lives. *Drug Metabolism Reviews* **7**(2), 295–323.

Watson A.D.J. (1979a) Effect of ingesta on the systemic availatility of chloramphenicol from two oral preparations in cats. *J. Vet. Pharmacol. Therap.* **2**, 117–21.

Watson A.D.J. (1979b) Plasma chloramphenicol concentrations in cats after parenteral administration of chloramphenicol sodium succinate. *J. Vet. Pharmacol. Therap.* **2**, 123–7.

Watson A.J.D. (1980a) Systemic availability of chloramphenicol from tablets and capsules in cats. *J. Vet. Pharmacol. Therap.* **3**, 45–51.

Watson A.J.D. (1980b) Oral chloramphenicol dosage regimens in cats. *J. Vet. Pharmacol. Therap.* **3**, 145–9.

Watson A.J.D. (1980c) Further observations on chloramphenicol toxicosis in cats. *Amer. J. Vet. Res.* **41**, 293–4.

Wilkinson G.T. (1968) A review of drug toxicity in the cat. *J. Small Anim. Pract.* **9**, 21–32.

Wilkinson G.T. (1980) Cat. In *The Therapeutic Jungle. University of Sydney Postgraduate Symposium.*

Yeary R.A. (1965) Systemic toxic effects of chemotherapeutic agents in domestic animals. *Vet. Clin. North Am.* **5**, 51–69.

Yeary R.A. & Swanson W. (1973) Aspirin dosages for the cat. *J. Amer. Vet. Med. Assoc.* **163**, 1177–8.

Zontine W.J. & Uno T. (1969) Acute aspirin toxicity in a cat. *Vet. Med. Small. Anim. Clinic.* **64**, 680–2.

Chapter 28 / Poisoning

I. H. BURGER AND P. A. FLECKNELL

INTRODUCTION

Clinical cases of poisoning apparently occur less commonly in the cat than in other domestic animals. It is possible that the true incidence is higher, however, and that many cases are mis-diagnosed, since unless a clear history of contact with toxic material is provided, a firm diagnosis is often impossible, even at autopsy. There are so many substances which are potentially poisonous to the cat that it is impossible to include details of all of them in this text. For this reason and the fact that there is relatively little specific information on the effects of many substances on the cat, we have restricted our discussion to those materials with which the cat is most likely to come into contact and those for which there is at least some documentation of toxic effects on the cat itself. Even so, many of these reports are the descriptions of single cases and generalization from these may be misleading. Given these problems, however, a general approach to a suspected case of poisoning can be adopted, which will provide rational treatment and a reasonable degree of success.

Before considering clinical treatment, however, it is useful to review briefly the behaviour of the cat in relation to the toxic hazards that it may encounter. Cats are less likely to ingest poisons that have a noticeable taste or smell, since their close inspection of potential food will often deter them from eating it. However, although it is often stated that cats chew their food more thoroughly than dogs, and so are more likely to detect unusual-tasting material, this is by no

means a universal characteristic – many cats will eat their food very rapidly, with minimal mastication. A cat's hunting instincts may increase the risk from certain poisons, since it may catch and eat rodents or birds which have been poisoned and so ingest the material itself. The most significant behavioural pattern that increases the incidence of ingestion of poisons is grooming of the coat. Cats have an inquisitive nature and whilst this often stops short of eating poisonous material, their close inspection of the substances will often result in contamination of their fur and subsequent grooming will result in ingestion of the poison. Aside from its behavioural characteristics, the cat has an increased or altered susceptibility to some materials compared with the dog, owing to differences in some of its metabolic pathways.

DIAGNOSIS

As mentioned previously, unless a definite history of contact with a poison is available, a general diagnosis of poisoning is usually made with difficulty and diagnosis of a specific toxicosis is often impossible. There are, however, certain clinical signs that may be of use and these are summarized in Table 28.1. Sudden onset of clinical illness involving neurological disturbances or vomiting and diarrhoea, or respiratory distress, may all lead to a suspicion of poisoning. All of these, however, may be the acute manifestation of a long-standing illness. On the other hand, poisoning is unlikely to be suspected in cats with a history of chronic illness, and hence some cases

Table 28.1 Clinical signs.

Clinical sign	Poison
Abdominal pain	Sodium chlorate, fluoroacetate, thallium, arsenic, acids, alkalis, phenols
Ataxia	Chlorphenoxy acids, hexachlorobenzene, organochlorines, organophosphates, metaldehyde, alphachloralose, arsenic, mercury, ethylene glycol, bromethalin
Convulsions	Glyphosate, organochlorines, organophosphates, metaldehyde, alphachloralose, fluoroacetate, strychnine, zinc phosphate, crimidine, aniline dyes, phenols, benzoic acid
Coma	Alphachloralose, zinc phosphide, arsenic, ethylene glycol, phenols, carbon monoxide
Cyanosis	Organophosphates, metaldehyde
Depression/weakness	Chlorphenoxy acids, triazines, alphachloralose, calciferol, zinc phosphide, arsenic, lead, mercury, aniline dyes, carbon monoxide, ethylene glycol, petroleum spirit
Diarrhoea	Warfarin, calciferol, sodium chlorate, fluoroacetate, arsenic, bleach, phenols, acids, alkalis
Dyspnoea/respiratory distress	Paraquat/diquat, glyphosate, triazines, thallium, aniline dyes, warfarin
Muscle twitching	Triazines, organochlorines, organophosphates, metaldehyde, strychnine, carbon monoxide
Polydipsia	Arsenic, calciferol
Salivation	Organophosphates, acids, alkalis, metaldehyde
Vomiting	Chlorphenoxy acids, organochlorines, phenols, bleach, aniline dyes, acids, alkalis, lead, arsenic, crimidine, fluoroacetate, ethylene glycol

will remain undiagnosed. Diagnosis of poisoning must therefore be made only after all of the possible aetiological agents of the illness have been considered.

Post-mortem examination may enable a conclusive diagnosis to be reached, but unless the potential causes can be narrowed to one or two possibilities, chemical analysis of tissues is likely to be unproductive and expensive. If a definite poison is suspected, a specialist analytical laboratory should be contacted for advice on which tissues should be stored for analysis, but this should not preclude a full post-mortem examination being undertaken.

TREATMENT

In cases where a definite history of poisoning exists, treatment can be tailored to suit the individual poison, and, if available, a specific antidote administered (Table 28.2 and see in text

Table 28.2 Specific antidotes.

Poison	Antidote
Sodium chlorate	1% sodium thiosulphate: orally
Organophosphates	Atropine sulphate: 0.2–0.25 mg/kg bodyweight (BW) intravenously
Warfarin	Vitamin K_1: 5–7 mg/kg BW intravenously then 2–5 mg/kg BW intramuscularly
Crimidine	Pyridoxine: 20 mg/kg BW intravenously
Arsenic	Dimercaprol: 3 mg/kg BW intramuscularly 4-hourly for 1–2 days (see text)
Lead	CaEDTA: 75–100 mg/kg BW intravenously or subcutaneously in divided doses (see text)
Mercury	Dimercaprol: as for arsenic poisoning and/or *N*-acetyl-*d*-l-penicillamine: 3–4 mg/kg BW orally 6-hourly
Ethylene glycol	20% ethanol: 5 mg/kg BW intraperitoneally

under individual poisons). In many cases this will not be possible, either because the specific poison is not known, or no specific antidote is available. In these cases, symptomatic treatment and supportive therapy are all that can be given.

Initially, when an owner telephones to report the cat's contact with a poison, the following advice should be given. If the animal has material on its skin, then prevent it from licking its skin by physically restraining it. If it is showing signs of central nervous system excitement, warn the owner to take care in handling – preferably wrap it in a blanket or large towel with only the head exposed to prevent it from injuring itself or its handler. In all cases, get the animal to the surgery as soon as possible.

It is often suggested that the owner should be instructed to administer an emetic, for example table salt, a washing soda crystal, or hydrogen peroxide, to induce vomiting if ingestion of poisonous material is suspected. These agents are very variable in their effects in the cat, and a distraught owner may spend an undue amount of time attempting to administer the emetic to the animal. The delay in receiving expert attention can have serious consequences. If possible, the suspected poison should be brought to the surgery, along with the patient. Proprietary products usually have a clear analysis of their contents, but old containers may have been used to store other materials, and this may result in inappropriate treatment.

On initial presentation of a case of suspected poisoning, it is important to carry out a thorough clinical examination, even if a clear history of ingestion of the poison is available. This will help ensure the detection of any pre-existing disease that could complicate therapy. If the animal is known to have ingested poisonous material and is still asymptomatic, then further absorption should be prevented by removal of the material from the stomach. Most standard emetics, even when administered correctly, are not particularly useful in the cat and adequate removal can usually only be achieved by gastric lavage. The cat should be anaesthetized and intubated using a cuffed endotracheal tube (2.5–3.5 mm outside diameter). A soft rubber tube, about 8 mm external diameter and about 30 cm in length, should be used for stomach tubing.

Mark on the tube the distance from the animal's nose to the xiphoid cartilage, then pass the tube and gradually introduce about 50–100 ml of tap water into the stomach. Gently massage the stomach through the body wall and lower the end of the tube to allow the gastric contents to escape. If very little material is removed in this way, then the contents should be gently aspirated with a 50 ml syringe whilst massaging the stomach. The procedure should be repeated until clear water is aspirated from the stomach tube. The stomach should then be filled with a mixture of activated charcoal and water (20 ml in 100 ml of water), drained 10 minutes later and refilled with the same mixture to attempt to absorb any remaining poison. If clinical signs of poisoning have developed, then the risk of anaesthesia must be balanced against the need for effective gastric lavage. If it is decided that anaesthesia is undesirable, then activated charcoal and water may be administered by mouth. Great care should be taken in administering this charcoal mixture in animals with central nervous system (CNS) depression, since accidental inhalation of material can easily occur.

If the cat's coat has been contaminated with poisonous material, then the affected areas should be thoroughly cleaned as soon as practicable. This is best achieved by clipping or shaving the fur and then washing the skin with warm soapy water. If the material is tar or oil, then warm vegetable oil can be used as a solvent to assist in its removal. If complete removal is impossible, or the cat's condition precludes such manipulations, then further licking must be prevented either by bandaging the area, or by use of an Elizabethan collar, until complete removal can be achieved. Following cleaning of the coat, the cat should be thoroughly dried to help prevent the development of hypothermia.

Supportive treatment

Many cases of poisoning will require intensive nursing and the use of a wide range of supportive measures to aid recovery. Of primary importance in most instances is to ensure that respiratory function is adequate. If possible, the animal's respiratory rate should be monitored using a suitable apnoea alarm* to provide adequate warning of respiratory failure.

Respiratory depression should be treated by the use of respiratory stimulants such as doxapram† at 5 mg/kg bodyweight. Repeated dosage every 20–30 minutes may be necessary. If a suitable infusion pump is available (e.g. MS18 syringe driver‡) then doxapram can be given by continuous infusion. If cyanosis of the visible mucous membranes is detected, oxygen should be administered and ventilation assisted by manual compression of the thorax. Supplementation of inspired air with oxygen is also often beneficial in cases with less severe respiratory depression. A simple 'oxygen tent' can be produced by placing a wire cat basket in a large clear plastic bag. Oxygen is introduced at one side and an outlet made at the other end. If prolonged severe respiratory depression occurs, or if there is blockage of the pharynx with mucus or vomit, then the animal should be intubated, or, exceptionally, a tracheostomy performed. As an emergency measure respiration can then be maintained using a Rees-modified T-piece with periodic ventilation using the reservoir bag.

When using a T-piece in this way, it is important to increase the gas flow rate to three or four times that normally used to try to minimize any rebreathing. Prolonged artificial ventilation requires use of a mechanical ventilator and careful monitoring of the patient.

A second major complication in treating poisoning is disturbance of body temperature. Careful monitoring is important; in a sedated or unconscious patient this is best achieved by using an electronic thermometer and rectal probe to provide a continually up-dated read-out. Hyperthermia can be controlled by use of ice packs, but this should be undertaken carefully, as it is easy to cool the animal excessively. Hypothermia should be treated by providing supplemental heating and insulating the animal. Insulation alone is relatively ineffective in reversing the fall in body temperature. Care should be taken in rewarming an animal that shows signs of shock, since the rapid cutaneous capillary dilation which results can cause a precipitous fall in blood pressure, which may be fatal. In these cases, procedures to maintain fluid balance and support circulatory function must first be instituted.

If the animal has a history of fluid or blood loss, then appropriate replacement therapy will be necessary. Even in cases where no noticeable loss has occurred, adequate fluid intake should be ensured by the intravenous administration of lactated Ringer's solution (40 ml/kg bodyweight per 24 hours), at rates not exceeding 15 ml/kg bodyweight per hour. If the ingested poison is excreted by the kidneys then diuretics (furosemide (frusemide), 2–4 mg/kg bodyweight intramuscularly) should be administered together with intravenous fluids. It is essential to monitor urine production, however, ideally by catheterizing the bladder, to ensure that renal function is adequate to cope with the additional fluid load.

If the animal appears to be in pain, then an analgesic should be administered (buprenorphine*, 0.005 mg/kg bodyweight i.m. repeated 8-hourly; pethidine, 2.5 mg/kg i.m. repeated 4-hourly). Pethidine should be used with caution if respiratory depression is present.

Convulsions, hyperactivity or excitement can be controlled by the administration of diazepam† or midazolam‡. Intravenous injection (2 mg/kg) is the preferred method of administration, but both agents are rapidly absorbed following intraperitoneal injection (in about 10–15 minutes). Repeated dosage may be required every 3–4 hours, depending upon effect. If the animal survives the acute phase of poisoning, supportive therapy must be continued until normal body functions are restored. Recumbent animals should be turned every 4 hours, to help prevent hypostatic congestion of the lungs, and any pressure points (e.g. elbows and hocks) massaged to prevent the development of pressure sores.

* Veterinary Drug Company; Veterinary Instrumentation, Donnington, UK.
† Dopram V; Willows Francis, Crawley, W. Sussex, UK.
‡ Graseby Dynamics.

* Temgesic; Reckitt & Coleman, Hull, UK.
† Valium: Roche Products Ltd, Welwyn Garden City, UK.
‡ Hypnovel; Roche Products Ltd.

If severe diarrhoea has developed, this can be controlled by a mixture of activated charcoal (to continue to absorb toxin), kaolin and water. If damage to the gastrointestinal tract is suspected, then antibiotics should be administered to help prevent systemic infection with gut organisms. Fluid therapy should be continued. If irritant or caustic material has been ingested, the damage to the oral membranes may cause prolonged inappetence and in these cases use of a pharyngostomy tube to supply the animal's nutritional fluid requirements should be considered (Böhning *et al.*, 1970). Even when the animal appears to have recovered from the harmful effects of the poison, a regular, thorough clinical examination should be undertaken over the following few weeks to enable early detection of any chronic toxic effects.

SPECIFIC HAZARDS

Herbicides

Sodium chlorate

This is the traditional 'total' plant killer which is still widely used, although more sophisticated selective herbicides are now extensively available. There is little specific information on cats but symptoms in other species include methaemoglobinaemia, abdominal pain, diarrhoea and haematuria. Treatment in other species is with methylene blue, intravenously at a dose of 10 mg/kg bodyweight, to counteract the methaemoglobinaemia, but it has been suggested that this is effective only in early stages of the poisoning. Furthermore, the cat is very sensitive to methylene blue and therefore we consider that this is an unsuitable antidote for use in cats. An alternative is 1% sodium thiosulphate orally and other suggested treatment includes gastric lavage and blood transfusion. The fairly high LD_{50} values reported for sodium chlorate (several g/kg bodyweight for rodents) should not disguise the fact that this substance is a strong oxidant and a very dangerous chemical.

The typical post-mortem change is the dark-brown colour of blood, liver and lungs resulting from methaemoglobin formation.

Paraquat and diquat

These are the bipyridyl herbicides which work on contact with the plant and are rapidly inactivated on reaching the soil. Nevertheless, they are very poisonous substances if ingested with a reported oral LD_{50} in the cat of around 50 mg/kg bodyweight for paraquat. There appears to be no specific information on diquat in the cat but data for other species suggest it is less toxic with an LD_{50} of about 200 mg/kg bodyweight. Paraquat poisoning has been described in cats which show symptoms similar to those seen in other animals: respiratory distress with radiographic evidence of pulmonary consolidation. Treatment is very difficult because there is still no effective antidote to these substances. Johnson and Huxtable (1976) reported that the use of a corticosteroid resulted in improvement in the condition of a cat poisoned with paraquat, but they were uncertain whether this was due to the treatment itself. Very variable effects are seen with these chemicals and in man apparently lethal doses have been ingested with the patient making a full, sometimes uneventful recovery. It has been suggested that supportive therapy in cats should follow the same measures recommended for man: these include the use of bentonite, cathartics, gastric lavage and haemodialysis. Superoxide dismutase enzyme is currently being studied in rats as a possible therapeutic aid in breaking down the superoxide anion produced in the lungs by paraquat. Cruickshank (1982) recommends the use of cyanocobalamin (vitamin B_{12}) as an effective antidote in mild paraquat poisoning in dogs, although this may be another case where recovery is not due solely to the treatment given.

Post-mortem changes are most noticeable in the lungs which are a purple-red colour and congested. Enlargement of the liver may also occur.

Chlorphenoxy acids

This group includes substances such as 2,4-dichlorophenoxyacetic acid (2,4-D), 2,4,5-trichlorophenoxyacetic acid (2,4,5-T) and silvex.

They are selective weedkillers which act as plant growth regulators (analogues of hormones) rather than as contact poisons and are used extensively for removing weeds from lawns. They act preferentially on dicotyledonous plants. Their acute toxicity is not quoted for the cat, but in dogs oral LD_{50} values of approximately 100 mg/kg bodyweight have been reported for 2,4-D and 2,4,5-T. Clinical signs include loss of appetite, depression, incoordination, muscle weakness and weight loss. Large doses may also cause vomiting. Some recent evidence suggests that some of these chemicals (notably 2,4,5-T) may not be as safe as was previously thought because they contain the potent carcinogen dioxin as a contaminant or they are carcinogenic *per se* (Anon, 1982a). However, this remains a controversial area and these particular compounds are currently the subject of much research including epidemiological studies in man.

No specific antidote has been reported for this group. Treatment is by emesis and gastric lavage, followed by general supportive therapy. Post-mortem changes include haemorrhagic gastritis.

Glyphosate

This substance (*N*-phosphonomethylglycine) is a herbicide which acts systemically by leaf absorption. Very little information is available on the effects of glyphosate in domestic animals, but its acute toxicity seems to be very low with oral LD_{50} values of up to 4 g/kg bodyweight and 1.6 g/kg bodyweight reported for rats and mice respectively. Administration of lethal doses of this chemical to rats has been accompanied by severe stress, enhanced breathing, hyperthermia and asphyxial convulsions. It has been suggested that uncoupling of mitochondrial oxidative phosphorylation may be a primary lesion in acute glyphosate poisoning (Bababunmi *et al.*, 1978) and in this case the treatment should be mainly symptomatic: correction of hyperthermia with ice packs, maintenance of fluid balance, and the use of sedatives such as diazepam.

Triazines

The triazines include substances such as amino-triazol, atrazine and simazine. They are used mostly to clear weeds from paths and drives. Acute toxicity values do not seem to be available for cats but oral LD_{50} values for rodents are reported to be in the range of 1–5 g/kg bodyweight, which means they are of low toxicity (similar to glyphosate) and the likelihood of them causing poisoning is correspondingly low. Suschetet *et al.* (1974) fed 0.01 and 0.05% atrazine in the diet of rats for 6 months and observed only mild effects such as a reduction in the growth rate (caused partly by a decrease in food intake), a slight leucopenia, some disturbances to thiamin and riboflavin metabolism and some changes in the weights of various organs. No histological lesions attributable to the treatment were observed. Where acute effects occur they consist of anorexia, depression, dyspnoea and muscle spasms. The suggested treatment is emetics followed by general supportive therapy similar to that described for the chlorphenoxy acids.

Fungicides

Hexachlorobenzene (HCB)

HCB is employed as a fungicidal agent in the treatment of seeds where it has been used to replace mercury compounds. It should not be confused with benzene hexachloride (lindane) which is discussed later in the section on insecticides. The cat was reported to be the most sensitive of four laboratory species investigated (the others were mice, rats and rabbits) with an oral LD_{50} of 1.7 g/kg bodyweight. Although of fairly low acute toxicity, HCB causes a variety of ill-effects during and after prolonged exposure. These include porphyria, blood cell disorders, neurological disorders, hepatomegaly and decreased weight gain.

No antidotes have been reported to be successful (Booth & McDowell, 1975). Intakes as low as 10 mg/kg bodyweight per day in cats can cause adverse effects over 35 days; the no-effect dose (over 24 days) was around 0.5–0.6 mg/kg bodyweight per day (Hansen *et al.*, 1977).

Pentachlorophenol (PCP)

This substance has been used extensively as a fungicide, usually for preserving timber, although it is being increasingly replaced by less toxic alternatives. The oral LD_{50} for most species is about 50 mg/kg bodyweight and although no value is reported for the cat, PCP poisoning has been described in this species. In one outbreak, Munro *et al.* (1977) reported the deaths of 11 cats in 1 year at a cattery. PCP was suspected as the toxic agent and was found to be present in samples of sawdust and shavings used for bedding. With one exception, all cats died suddenly and the most consistent post-mortem signs were kidney enlargement, liver degeneration and profuse haemorrhages into the abdominal or thoracic cavities. A similar outbreak of suspected PCP poisoning in cats was reported by Peet *et al.* (1977). Phenol compounds present a significant hazard for cats as a result both of their inefficient, easily saturated detoxifying mechanism for these substances and their habit of grooming themselves by extensive licking, a factor which has been discussed earlier. Like glyphosate, PCP is an uncoupler of oxidative phosphorylation and produces similar signs of poisoning, although it is much more toxic than the herbicide. There is no specific antidote and treatment is similar to that suggested for glyphosate.

Insecticides and molluscicides

Insecticides of vegetable origin

Under this heading we can include pyrethrum, rotenone and nicotine. Pyrethrum and rotenone (the active constituent of the derris plant or powders) are considered to be relatively non-toxic to the cat. Pyrethrum has been used successfully in flea collars for cats (see below). Rotenone has been reported to cause liver damage in cats ingesting it from their fur when applied as a dust. Nicotine is more toxic than the other two compounds with a minimum oral lethal dose as low as 20–100 mg reported for the cat and it is also easily absorbed through the intact skin. However, when used as an insecticide, it is unlikely to cause poisoning in cats. It is more of a hazard to dogs;

puppies have suffered nicotine poisoning after eating cigar or cigarette ends, but this is unlikely to occur in the much more fastidious cat.

Organochlorines

These insecticides, also called the chlorinated hydrocarbons, were first used about 40 years ago as highly effective controllers of the malarial mosquito. Perhaps the best known of the group is DDT, but there are many others including lindane (benzene hexachloride, BHC), endrin, dieldrin, aldrin, methoxyclor and toxaphene. To avoid any confusion in nomenclature it should be pointed out that lindane is the gamma isomer of hexachlorocyclohexane (HCH). This is the more recent (and chemically correct) name for benzene hexachloride (BHC), but the latter is still used.

Cats are generally considered to be more susceptible than other animals to this group of chemicals, but this may be related more to their grooming habits than to increased sensitivity *per se* (see previous section on PCP). For example, the lowest oral lethal dose of DDT for the cat (250 mg/kg bodyweight) is little different to that for the dog (300 mg/kg bodyweight). Also, the long-term no-adverse-effect level reported for lindane in the cat is about 1 mg/kg bodyweight per day, which is similar to that quoted for the dog (Herbst & Bodenstein, 1972). Nevertheless, these chemicals vary greatly in their toxicity and it is unwise to make too many generalizations about their degree of potency. Endrin is far more dangerous than DDT with a lowest oral lethal dose for the cat as low as 5 mg/kg bodyweight; this compound seems to be more toxic to other species as well. In addition to ingestion, cats can be exposed via dusting powders or by lying or walking on surfaces treated with the chemical and then licking their feet and fur. Sawdust contaminated with dieldrin has also been implicated in cat deaths (Anon, 1977).

The principal reaction of these chemicals is on the CNS. The first signs appear 1–4 hours after ingestion or 12–24 hours after skin application. Restlessness, hypersensitivity, vomiting and lack of coordination are usually the first signs, which are followed typically by convulsions which may become almost continuous. Cats also show greater extensor rigidity and opisthotonos than other animals. These effects may alternate with quieter phases and the dominance of one over the other may indicate the identity of the poison. For lindane and DDT the excited state is dominant, whereas for toxaphene it is the depressed phase. Gruffydd-Jones *et al.* (1981) described a case of chronic dieldrin poisoning in cats exposed to floors treated with a preparation of the chemical to control woodworm. No muscle tremors were noted but there was depression with gross emaciation in the queens and marked hair loss around the face of the tom cats. This case was of particular interest as the cats were not allowed access to the treated floors until 6 weeks after application of dieldrin, by which time all noticeable odour had dispersed and the wood appeared dry. There have been further similar reports of dieldrin toxicity on cats, and it is now recommended that cats are kept out of treated rooms for at least 7–8 weeks, possibly several months (Anon, 1984; Grisedale, 1984).

Phenobarbitone (10–20 mg/kg bodyweight) is the compound of choice to control the convulsions and may be administered intravenously, intraperitoneally or orally. Calcium or sodium gluconate (2–4 ml of a 10% solution, intravenously) has been reported to reduce mortality in organochlorine poisoning. General supportive treatment should be given with particular attention to maintaining adequate renal output since these compounds are excreted in the urine. There are no characteristic post-mortem signs, but widespread small haemorrhages and lung congestion have been observed.

Accidents involving the organochlorine insecticides are now fairly uncommon as the use of these chemicals has greatly declined in recent years. Although they are very effective at controlling insects, especially those carrying disease, the organochlorines persist in the environment (e.g. in the fatty tissues of the body) and are particularly toxic to birds and fish. For this reason, other insecticides with greater biodegradability have been developed, the most common examples of these are the organophosphorus and carbamate compounds which are discussed in the following section.

Organophosphorus and carbamate compounds
Among the compounds included under this heading are parathion, malathion, dichlorvos and diazinon (organophosphates) and pirimicarb, carbaryl and methiocarb (carbamates). The two groups are different as regards their general chemical structure, but will be considered together as they have the same mode of action. These substances are now widely used (for the reasons outlined above) and have been responsible for many cases of poisoning. Although their toxicity varies considerably, for example from less than 1 mg/kg bodyweight (oral LD_{50}) for parathion to over 100 mg/kg bodyweight for malathion, they all act via inhibition of the enzyme acetylcholinesterase. This enzyme breaks down acetylcholine (ACh), which is the transmitter substance at neuromuscular junctions and parasympathetic nerve endings. Inhibition of the cholinesterase enzyme allows ACh to accumulate and the signs of poisoning are mainly secondary to this effect. The accumulation of transmitter is categorized under three broad groups of clinical signs: muscarinic (parasympathetic), nicotinic (neuromuscular) and CNS effects. The muscarinic effects include profuse salivation, gastrointestinal hypermotility with abdominal pain, vomiting, diarrhoea, excessive lacrimation and cyanosis. The nicotinic and CNS effects start with excessive and uncontrollable muscle stimulation which can lead to paralysis, and convulsions which can lead to coma. Death is usually attributed to respiratory failure.

The preferred treatment is atropine sulphate and its efficacy in cats has been demonstrated. Atropine temporarily blocks the action of ACh at muscarinic and CNS sites, although it has little effect at nicotinic sites. Since overdosage with atropine can be harmful, it must be administered with caution. It is difficult to quote a precise dose rate as this will vary depending upon the build-up of ACh at the receptor sites. Initially, approximately 0.2–0.25 mg/kg bodyweight of atropine sulphate should be administered by *slow* intravenous injection. If the cat is cyanosed, this should be treated by assisting ventilation and administering oxygen. The dose of atropine may need to be doubled in seriously affected animals, and in most cases repeated administration of atropine will be required. Dose rates should be adjusted according to clinical response, but the possibility of over-atropinization must be carefully monitored. Oximes such as pralidoxime (2-PAM) are specific antidotes for organophosphate poisoning as they correct the biochemical abnormality by breaking down the phosphorylated enzyme complex (thereby releasing the native enzyme) and combining with the organophosphate making it more readily excretable. Thus, pralidoxime can also restore the action of cholinesterase at nicotinic sites. The recommended dosage is 20–40 mg/kg bodyweight. Zenger (1988) describes the successful treatment of organophosphate (fenthion) poisoning in two cats using pralidoxime chloride. A dose of 20 mg/kg bodyweight was given, intravenously or subcutaneously, at 12-hourly intervals without concurrent atropine administration. Response to treatment was dramatic with complete remission after only four injections. Most authorities warn that pralidoxime therapy is contraindicated in carbamate poisoning because it may actually assist in the inactivation of cholinesterase. However, it has been suggested that these warnings were based upon work with carbaryl and do not apply to most other carbamate insecticides (Buck, 1979). In any event, it is important that the oxime is administered as soon as possible after poisoning because the inactivated cholinesterase becomes more resistant to reactivation as the complex ages.

There are no characteristic post-mortem changes but inflammation of the alimentary tract has been reported. Pancreatitis can occur after organophosphate poisoning in dogs but was not observed in cats (Frick *et al.*, 1987).

Cordoba *et al.* (1983) reported that dogs given a high dose (30 mg/kg bodyweight) of an organophosphate (dichlorvos) showed blood acidosis. By restoring acid–base balance with repeated intravenous injections of sodium bicarbonate, they achieved a marked improvement in the

animals with a survival rate of 11 out of 13. Although this work has been reported only in dogs, it could offer another important method of treatment for this type of poisoning.

Flea collars

Flea collars are essentially continuous contact insecticides – usually organophosphates or carbamates – and represent a potential hazard that can easily be overlooked. Reports of adverse reactions include ataxia and depression due to the anticholinesterase effects of the organophosphates contained in some collars, and contact dermatitis. Both conditions resolve rapidly on removal of the collar. Such reactions appear to be rare, but are much more likely to be seen when several organophosphate preparations are used simultaneously. For example, use of an insecticide spray on a cat already wearing a flea collar can rapidly produce signs of poisoning. Insecticide strips used in some households may contain the same material as flea collars, and this can lead to overdosage with organophosphorus compounds. Some anthelminthic preparations also contain organophosphates. Waltner-Toews (1981) discusses a case in which the use of a flea medallion containing dichlorvos (and related chemicals) and a spray containing carbaryl caused poisoning in a cat, which then succumbed to haemobartonellosis as a complication associated with the stress of the chemical poisoning. Whetstone (1986) warns that some individual cats may be particularly sensitive to flea collars. Their use may also render cats more sensitive to drugs such as phenothiazine and the barbiturates because their potency can be increased by organophosphates. However, two developments may help to increase the efficacy of these aids while decreasing their possible hazard (Bledsoe *et al.*, 1982). They are the use of insect growth hormones or regulators and the microencapsulation of pesticides, which allows long-term control of insect pests but dramatically reduces the risk of toxicity to the pet.

Diethanolamine

In the USA, Sundlof and Mayhew (1983) reported a debilitating and often lethal syndrome in cats and dogs following use of a proprietary flea repellant containing diethanolamine as the active ingredient. The substance was given mainly in the food (at about 44 mg/kg bodyweight per day) and was associated with ataxia, paresis and ascending paralysis. The product was voluntarily withdrawn from the market.

Metaldehyde
Metaldehyde, a polymer of acetaldehyde, is widely used as a slug killer, sometimes mixed with bran and usually sold in the form of pellets containing 4–6% of the active substance. Some slug baits contain other chemicals, the most common being methiocarb, which is one of the carbamate pesticides (see above). Slug pellets seem to be very attractive to pets and many instances of poisoning have been described. In a survey of 34 veterinary practices in Australia, Studdert (1985) reported that snail and slug baits were the most common cause of poisoning in dogs and cats. Fatality rates were fairly high: in cats 16.7% for metaldehyde and 50% for methiocarb. To combat this problem some modern preparations now contain substances which are repellent to pets. The LD_{50} for metaldehyde is not quoted for the cat but seems to be around 500 mg/kg bodyweight for most species. Clinical signs of poisoning in the cat are similar to those in the dog. They include lack of coordination, muscle tremors, hypersalivation and hyperaesthesia, which may be followed by collapse and coma. The muscle tremors are continuous and cannot be initiated by external stimuli, unlike those seen in strychnine poisoning (see below). Nystagmus is reported to be a characteristic sign in cats poisoned with metaldehyde. Hyperthermia and temporary blindness have also been observed as a feature of this syndrome.

Treatment aims to control the muscle tremors, prevent further absorption of the poison and provide supportive therapy. Diazepam (2–3 mg/kg bodyweight) should be administered intraperitoneally or intravenously to control tremors, followed by gastric lavage to remove the poison. Fluid balance should be maintained and general supportive treatment given as described previ-

ously. The hypersalivation and severe muscle spasms may interfere with respiration and produce cyanosis, requiring assisted ventilation and administration of oxygen. Vitamin B_{12} has also been reported to be a useful antidote in dogs poisoned with metaldehyde (but see comments in section on paraquat). The characteristic post-mortem sign of metaldehyde poisoning is the smell of acetaldehyde in the stomach.

Rodenticides

Warfarin and related compounds
These are perhaps the most common and best known of the rodenticides. All are structurally related to coumarin and belong to one of two chemical groups: hydroxycoumarins and indandiones. They are now also divided into so-called first and second generation compounds. Substances such as warfarin (hydroxycoumarin), and diphacinone and pindone (indandiones) are first-generation chemicals which generally require repeated doses to produce an effect. Newer second-generation compounds like the hydroxycoumarins brodifacoum and bromadiolone are usually effective after a single exposure (Mount, 1988). All act in the same way by reducing the clotting ability of the blood through interference with vitamin K activity, thereby inhibiting the formation of prothrombin. The normal activity of the animal is then enough to produce fatal internal haemorrhage.

The toxicity of these compounds varies for individuals in a given species. For the first-generation compounds small repeated doses are more toxic than single large ones. In cats a single dose of between 5 and 50 mg/kg bodyweight is lethal whereas 1 mg/kg over 5 days will produce the same effect. Commercial preparations usually contain at least 0.005% of active ingredient and ingestion of baits is reported to be the most common source of toxicity in cats. Poisoning may also arise from the ingestion of rodents which have died from the effects of the chemical, but this is more likely with the second-generation anticoagulants.

The clinical signs are variable but usually consist of pale mucous membranes, bloody diarrhoea, lameness and irregular heart beat. If haemorrhage involves the brain, CNS signs will occur including rapid death, which is one of the possibilities that can result from a massive dose of the poison. Treatment should involve minimal or very gentle handling of the animal to avoid further bruising. The specific antidote is vitamin K_1. Traditionally it has been advised that this should be given intravenously but Mount (1988) warns that this may run the risk of anaphylaxis, and suggests subcutaneous, intramuscular or oral routes of administration as viable alternatives. An initial dose of 5–7 mg/kg bodyweight followed by 2–5 mg/kg for 2–4 days is the suggested treatment for warfarin. However, the dosage depends on the type of poison. The indandiones and second-generation hydroxycoumarins require a longer course of treatment as they have much longer half-lives than warfarin. For these compounds a vitamin K_1 intake of 5 mg/kg per day for 2–3 weeks is recommended with an assessment of blood coagulation status after 2 weeks, if possible. It should also be noted that the water-soluble vitamin K analogues such as menadione (vitamin K_3) are not as effective as antidotes in this type of poisoning as they are inferior to vitamin K_1 in restoring blood-clotting time to normal. In severe cases, whole blood transfusion and oxygen therapy may be necessary. Intrathoracic haemorrhage may cause severe dyspnoea and thoracocentesis may be required. As expected, post-mortem changes include multiple haemorrhages in most organs and muscles.

It is worth noting that coumarin-derived anticoagulants are widely used as therapeutic agents for the treatment of thrombosis in man, and a large number of drugs have been found to interact with these substances. Compounds found to potentiate the effects include some antibiotics (penicillin, tetracycline, ampicillin and sulphonamides) which may be used in cats. A review by the Royal College of Pathologists (1982) discusses these effects. It has also been reported that large doses of vitamin E increase the effects of anticoagulant drugs by increasing vitamin K requirements (Anon, 1982b).

Alphachloralose

Alphachloralose is used as a mouse poison, and acts by both stimulating and depressing the CNS. The minimum lethal dose for cats is quoted as 100 mg/kg bodyweight with LD_{50} values around 500 mg/kg bodyweight. Commercial preparations usually contain about 2–4% of the active compound. Cats have occasionally shown mild signs of poisoning after consuming mice still containing the chemical in the gut. The clinical signs are very variable and include ataxia and hyperactivity or sedation and coma. Cats which have eaten large doses can later show extreme aggression, convulsions and unconsciousness. Hypothermia ultimately follows the ingestion of large quantities and it is for this reason that alphachloralose is particularly effective against very small animals, which have a large surface area relative to weight and therefore lose body heat more rapidly than larger species.

Treatment is with emetics if poisoning is noted soon after ingestion (say 30 minutes). In most cases, it is advisable that medication (including the use of sedatives or stimulants) is avoided, but 2–3 mg/kg bodyweight of diazepam intraperitoneally has been suggested as one possible treatment to counteract the convulsions. General supportive therapy, in particular maintenance of body temperature and keeping the animal roused to stimulate body metabolism, is usually sufficient to ensure recovery.

Calciferol

This substance (vitamin D_2) is used alone or in combination with anticoagulants and acts by causing hypercalcaemia and calcification of various parts of the body, notably the arteries and kidneys. The minimal lethal dose in the dog is reported to be 4 mg/kg bodyweight (approximately 160 000 IU/kg bodyweight) and cats are said to be more susceptible. This may be explained by the fact that, even during growth, cats seem to be almost totally independent of a supply of this vitamin, either from the diet or from the action of sunlight (ultraviolet light) on lipid compounds in the skin (Rivers *et al.*, 1979). Their dietary requirement of vitamin D_2 is therefore very low and toxic effects may occur with lower intakes than those reported for other animals. Nevertheless, as commercial preparations of this rodenticide usually contain only 0.1% of the active compound, a cat would have to eat a fairly large quantity of bait to induce acute toxicity. The clinical signs include anorexia, hypercalcaemia, constipation or diarrhoea, lethargy, spinal arching, polydipsia and polyuria. Treatment is symptomatic and consists of a diet with low calcium, high salt and a high fluid intake (Moore *et al.*, 1988). Sunlight should be avoided and, for the reasons given earlier, this part of the treatment may be particularly important for cats.

Fluoroacetate and fluoroacetamide

Fluoroacetate and fluoroacetamide are often referred to as compounds 1080 and 1081 respectively. Fluoroacetate acts via a 'lethal synthesis' in the body, so-called because it is metabolized to fluorocitrate, which blocks the action of the citric acid cycle and causes inhibition of cellular respiration. However, the fact that characteristic signs of poisoning occur before citrate concentrations increase has led researchers to propose other mechanisms as responsible for the toxic effects. One suggestion is that the primary action in fluoroacetate poisoning is a reduction in the levels of ionizable calcium by the chelating effect of the citrate accumulating as a result of the enzyme block (Roy Shapira *et al.*, 1980). Increased ammonia concentration in the brain has been associated with the onset of convulsions in fluoroacetate poisoning in the dog, but in the cat it has been reported that ammonia in the CNS has only a secondary role in initiating CNS dysfunction (Raabe, 1981). Fluoroacetate is very toxic to domestic animals, with LD_{50} values as low as 0.3–0.5 mg/kg bodyweight quoted for the cat. Fluoroacetamide is less toxic than the acetate, presumably because it is metabolized *in vivo* to fluoroacetate, which prevents a substantial build-up of the final toxic agent. The cat may be intoxicated both directly and through ingestion of poisoned rodents.

Clinical signs may not appear until a latent period of 30 minutes to 2½ hours. These signs are primarily cardiac and nervous in cats consisting of abdominal pain, restlessness, vomiting, diarrhoea, hyperaesthesia to light and touch reflexes, convulsions, tachycardia, cardiac arrhythmia and ventricular fibrillation. Unlike convulsions in strychnine poisoning (see next section), those caused by fluoroacetate are not induced by external stimuli.

There is no specific antidote. Glycerol monoacetin (0.1–0.5 mg/kg bodyweight i.m.) may be given hourly for several hours, up to a total of 2–4 mg/kg bodyweight, to inhibit the conversion of fluoroacetate to fluorocitrate, but its efficacy is disputed. Supportive therapy and the control of convulsions with diazepam (2 mg/kg bodyweight) are generally considered to be the first two priorities. Gammie (1980) describes the successful treatment of fluoroacetate poisoning in a cat through the use of 5 ml 10% calcium gluconate (subcutaneous), 8 mg diazepam (5 mg intramuscular and 3 mg subcutaneous), 5 mg furosemide (intramuscular) and supplementary oxygen. Postmortem changes are not specific, but include cyanosis and congested liver and kidneys.

Despite their toxicity, these substances do not pose a serious environmental hazard in Britain because their use is strictly controlled.

Strychnine

Strychnine is an indole alkaloid, derived from seeds of the plants *Strychnos nux-vomica* and *S. ignatti*, which has been used as an animal poison for many centuries. Although it is now permitted in Britain only for controlling moles, it is used widely abroad and is sometimes used illegally in Britain, for example in poisoned bait for foxes. Strychnine is an extremely toxic substance with a reported oral minimal lethal dose for cats of 0.75 mg/kg bodyweight. As commercial preparations usually contain around 0.3% of the active compound, a 4 kg cat would need to consume only 1 g of bait to receive a lethal dose. Strychnine appears to affect the CNS by interfering with postsynaptic inhibition so that the controlling effects are eliminated. It is believed that this action is via selective competitive antagonism of the amino acid glycine, which is known to be an inhibitory neurotransmitter in the spinal cord.

Clinical signs can appear within a few minutes to several hours after ingestion. The presence of food in the stomach can delay the onset of poisoning because strychnine is absorbed poorly from the stomach but much more readily from the small intestine. Early signs are general nervousness and apprehension, an increase in muscle tone and twitching of skeletal muscles. Violent convulsions may happen spontaneously or be precipitated by stimuli such as noise, a sudden draught of air, movement of the surface on which the animal is lying, or a sudden bright light. There is extreme extensor rigidity and breathing may cease momentarily by contraction of the diaphragm and the thoracic and abdominal muscles.

The convulsions are interspersed with periods of relaxation and, if untreated, death can rapidly occur due to brain anoxia during one of the seizures. There is no specific antidote: the first objective of treatment is to control the convulsions with diazepam (2 mg/kg bodyweight IV or 2–3 mg/kg bodyweight IP). In the early stages of poisoning, before convulsions have occurred, emesis with apomorphine is recommended by some, but it may exacerbate the convulsions when they develop. Following control of convulsions with diazepam, general anaesthesia should be induced (e.g. with intravenous thiopentone), the cat intubated, and gastric lavage carried out with tannic acid (1–2%) to precipitate any remaining strychnine, or with potassium permanganate (1:1000 to 1:2000) to oxidize it. Following recovery from anaesthesia, sedation should be continued by repeated administration of diazepam, and the cat protected from external stimuli. General supportive treatment should also be given. Strychnine is eliminated from the body within 10–12 hours and hence survival beyond this period is encouraging. There are no characteristic post-mortem signs. Rigor mortis occurs rapidly after death from strychnine poisoning and the remains of the poisoned bait (or prey) may often be found in the cat's stomach.

Zinc phosphide

This is one of the older rodenticides, but is still used occasionally. Its toxic effect relies on the liberation of phosphine gas in the alimentary tract. The lethal dose in most animals seems to lie between 20 and 40 mg/kg bodyweight. Commercial preparations usually contain between 2.5 and 5% of the chemical. Clinical signs are rather variable and include marked anorexia, lethargy and coma, but hyperkinesis, convulsions and rigor may also occur and it is possible to confuse the symptoms with strychnine or fluoroacetate poisoning. There is no recommended treatment, but gastric lavage or emesis may be effective. Postmortem signs include gastroenteritis, pulmonary oedema and venous congestion. The characteristic garlic-like smell of phosphine is often detected on the breath or after the alimentary tract is opened.

Thallium

This was once a popular rodenticide but its high toxicity and frequency of poisoning in pets and children have led to restrictions in its use. Nevertheless, many instances of thallium poisoning in the cat have been documented (Zook *et al.*, 1968). The usual preparation is in the form of its acetate and sulphate salts and the minimum oral lethal dose for the cat is about 10 mg/kg bodyweight. The clinical signs of poisoning can be conveniently divided into acute and subacute/chronic. In the acute form symptoms appear 12 hours to a few days after ingestion and consist of anorexia, vomiting and abdominal pain; there may also be respiratory distress. Death can occur any time between 5 or 14 days later. The subacute/chronic form is characterized primarily by cutaneous lesions and within a few days the skin around the mouth and eyes becomes dry, crusted and erythematous. Hair loss occurs around the face and the skin lesions can progress over the remainder of the face and eventually over the whole body. Other subacute signs include incoordination, ataxia and loss of the landing and righting reflexes.

The treatment of thallium poisoning is generally disappointing. Emesis and gastric lavage can be carried out if the poisoning is fairly recent. Specific antidotes such as diphenyl thiocarbazone have been used, but some authorities say they are inadvisable because of redistribution of thallium, particularly in the CNS. The treatment of choice now seems to be Prussian blue (ferric ferrocyanide) given orally at an intake of about 250 mg/kg bodyweight per day subdivided into 2 to 4 fractions. Prussian blue acts by absorbing thallium in the gut and preventing its redistribution throughout the body. As Prussian blue is not absorbed from the gastrointestinal tract, the thallium will eventually be excreted in the faeces. General supportive therapy is very important and should include parenteral fluids and electrolytes, B-complex vitamins and antibiotics. The severe skin lesions should be treated with appropriate soothing ointments or lotions.

Post-mortem signs include ulcerative lesions along the gastrointestinal tract, necrosis of cardiac and skeletal muscle, pulmonary oedema and the characteristic skin lesions described earlier.

Crimidine

This chemical (also called Castrix) is used widely in Europe (though not in Britain) and several cases of accidental poisoning in cats have been reported. Crimidine is a structural analogue of pyridoxine (vitamin B_6) and acts by antagonizing the normal function of this vitamin. The reported oral LD_{50} values for rodents are in the region of 2.5–5 mg/kg bodyweight. Commercial preparations contain between 0.1 and 0.15% of the active compound. Clinical signs include violent convulsions which, like those occurring in strychnine poisoning, alternate with periods of calm. Vomiting is also reported to occur. The specific antidote is pyridoxine, intravenously at 20 mg/kg bodyweight; diazepam can be used to control the convulsions. Lung oedema is found on post-mortem examination in some cases.

Bromethalin

Bromethalin is a relatively new rodenticide which acts by uncoupling oxidative phosphorylation, but the toxic effects are different from those seen with pentachlorophenol and glyphosate. Bromethalin causes an accumulation of fluid in the CNS which results in pressure on the axons and subsequent neurological effects. This is thought to arise from a lack of ATP which weakens the sodium/potassium gradient in the nerve cells (van Lier & Cherry, 1988). Cats are reported to be the most susceptible species (more so than the rat!), with a minimal lethal dose of around 0.5 mg/kg bodyweight (Dorman *et al.*, 1990). As the concentration in bait is usually 0.01%, a lethal intake could occur from the ingestion of as little as 20 g. Typical signs of poisoning in the cat are pelvic limb ataxia, loss of the pelvic limb deep pain response, vocalization and decerebrate posture. Death occurs due to paralysis. Post-mortem changes in the CNS appear as a diffuse spongy degeneration of the white matter and intramyelinic oedema (Dorman *et al.*, 1990). At present there seems to be no effective therapy. The use of superactivated charcoal, osmotic diuretics and corticosteroids is recommended but these measures were reported to be ineffective in cats (Dorman *et al.*, 1990).

DOMESTIC HAZARDS

Acids and alkalis

Strong acids and alkalis are very unlikely to be ingested, but spillage on the coat, followed by attempts to clean the area, may result in poisoning. Clinical signs in other species consist of abdominal pain, vomiting and damage to mucous membranes or skin. A systemic acidosis (acids) or alkalosis (alkalis) may develop. Treatment consists of neutralizing the material with magnesium hydroxide or vinegar respectively. The skin should be washed with copious amounts of water and if significant quantities of material are believed to have been ingested, olive oil should be given by mouth. The most effective treatment is gastric lavage with the appropriate neutralizing agent. Lavage should be performed carefully, as ingestion of large quantities of caustic material can produce oesophageal or gastric burns, and predispose to oesophageal rupture. If severe oesophageal or gastric damage is suspected, radiographic examination should be carried out. Pain should be controlled by the administration of pethidine or buprenorphine.

Aniline dyes

These are present in crayons, pencils and shoe polish, and are toxic to cats. Clinical signs of poisoning include depression, dyspnoea, vomiting and convulsions, and the development of methaemoglobinaemia. Treatment to minimize absorption of material should be carried out as described above. If severe methaemoglobinaemia develops, blood transfusions may be required.

Aspirin

Aspirin is toxic to cats at dose rates that would be considered therapeutically appropriate for other species. Clinical signs of poisoning include a severe haemorrhagic gastroenteritis, panting, which is sometimes followed by respiratory depression, seizures, vomiting' and collapse. Repeated exposure to low dosages of aspirin produces chronic toxic effects including bone marrow depression, anaemia, thrombocytopenia and liver damage (Penny *et al.*, 1967).

Treatment consists of gastric lavage and general supportive therapy. If respiratory depression develops, analeptics may be useful. Acidosis is a feature of aspirin poisoning and hence fluid therapy with the addition of sodium bicarbonate may be of value in correcting the acidosis and promoting renal excretion of salicylates.

Studies of pharmacokinetics of aspirin in the cat (Davis & Donnelly, 1968) have demonstrated that in this species it is an extremely stable drug, with a plasma half-life of 37.6 hours. Based on these findings, various suggestions of dosage regimes have been stated, for example 25 mg every other day (see Chapter 27).

Bleach

Domestic bleach has a caustic action if in concentrated solution; if diluted bleach is ingested it causes gastrointestinal disturbances with vomiting and diarrhoea. As with many other materials, poisoning is most likely to follow soiling of the coat with the material. Treatment consists of gastric lavage and administration of olive oil as a demulcent.

Carbon monoxide

With the phasing out of coal gas for domestic supplies, the main source of carbon monoxide is now petrol engine exhaust fumes and incomplete combustion in domestic fires as a result of poor ventilation. Clinical signs include depression, twitching of the skeletal muscles, pyrexia and a cherry-red colour to the mucous membranes. Treatment consists of artificial ventilation, with oxygen if necessary. Prolonged administration of supplemental oxygen may be required.

Ethylene glycol

The commonest source of this material is as the major constituent of antifreeze: it has a sweet taste that is apparently quite palatable to cats. The compound is metabolized to glycolic acid, glyoxylate and oxalate, all of which are toxic to the cat. Clinical signs of poisoning occur within 12 hours and include ataxia, progressive incoordination, depression, loss of reflex responses, coma and death. Occasionally animals may develop convulsions (Penumarthy & Oehme, 1975). In less severe cases, onset of illness may be delayed until 12–24 hours following ingestion, and tachycardia, tachypnoea and pulmonary oedema are the predominant clinical signs (Grauer & Thrall, 1982). The most commonly seen manifestation of poisoning occurs 24–72 hours after ingestion of material and results from renal failure. Oliguria, uraemia, vomiting and severe depression are noted, followed by coma and death. This stage of poisoning is associated with formation of calcium oxalate crystals in the renal tubules, resulting in renal damage.

Treatment must be commenced as rapidly as possible. Ethanol (20% solution, 5 ml/kg bodyweight) should be administered intraperitoneally. This reduces the rate of metabolism of ethylene glycol and hence the production of toxic metabolites. Since metabolic acidosis is a consistent feature of ethylene glycol poisoning, sodium bicarbonate should also be administered (6 ml of 5% bicarbonate/kg bodyweight, IP). Treatment should be repeated every 6 hours. General supportive therapy, particularly to maintain fluid balance, is also important. Fluid output must be monitored carefully, however, to avoid overhydration in cases with renal failure.

Petroleum spirit

Spillage on the skin of large quantities of petrol can result in the development of ataxia, depression and in severe cases muscular twitching, mydriasis and convulsions. Treatment is symptomatic, coupled with thorough cleaning of the skin.

Phenols, cresols and related compounds

The cat has a greater susceptibility to the toxic effects of these substances compared with other species of domestic animal (see earlier section on pentachlorophenol). They are contained in a variety of products, in disinfectants and wood preservatives, for example. Poisoning results in hyperptyalism, abdominal pain, occasionally diarrhoea or vomiting, weakness, convulsions and eventual circulatory collapse and death. There is no specific antidote and general supportive treatment should be given. Sufficient soiling of the skin to cause clinical illness can occur following contact with floors or utensils which have been cleaned with undiluted household disinfectants.

Quaternary ammonium disinfectants

Disinfectants containing quaternary ammonium compounds are widely used, and have been considered to be relatively non-toxic to cats. Exposure to undiluted disinfectant has been shown to result in anorexia, hyperptyalism, depression, dehydration, stomatitis with mucosal ulceration, ulceration of the skin, and development of a nasal and ocular discharge (Trapani *et al.*, 1982).

These findings emphasize the care that is needed to use disinfectants only at their recommended dilutions.

TOXIC METALS

Arsenic

Arsenic and its derivatives are now used less frequently than they were and the incidence of poisoning with these substances has decreased. However, they still find some use as rodenticides and herbicides. The soluble inorganic arsenic compounds such as sodium arsenite are the most dangerous; organic compounds such as arsanilic and cacodylic acids are less toxic. The lowest oral lethal dose recorded for the cat (for sodium arsenate) is 20 mg/kg bodyweight, and the lowest dose that produced toxicity is reported to be 5 mg/kg (Furr & Buck, 1974). One of the most common sources of arsenic poisoning in cats in the USA is an ant poison containing sodium arsenate as the active principle (Hornfeldt & Borys, 1986). The effects of arsenic can be acute (1–2 days) or subacute (up to 7 days) and the clinical signs are characterized by vomiting, diarrhoea and intense abdominal pain followed by extreme weakness, thirst, anorexia, dehydration and ataxia. These can lead to subnormal temperature, collapse, coma and death. Arsenic exerts its action by combining with and blocking the thiol groups at the active sites of a number of enzymes. The specific antidote is dimercaprol (British Anti-Lewisite, BAL) which itself contains two thiol groups and chelates arsenic, thereby hastening its release from the body and restoring the enzyme thiol groups to normal activity. The recommended dosage of dimercaprol is 3 mg/kg bodyweight IM every 4 hours for the first 1–2 days, reducing to every 6–8 hours on the next day and then twice a day for a further 10 days (maximum) or until recovery is complete. Sodium thiosulphate (20% solution) is sometimes recommended as an effective alternative, injected intravenously at 20–40 mg/kg bodyweight (double this if the dose is oral) two or three times daily for 3 days. Supportive therapy is strongly recommended and this includes the use of electrolyte solutions, B-complex vitamins and perhaps anti-biotics to control secondary infections.

The characteristic post-mortem lesion is severe gastrointestinal inflammation, but degeneration of liver and kidneys is often seen.

Lead

Although lead poisoning is relatively common in dogs (particularly puppies), it seems to be comparatively rare in cats. This may be due to the more fastidious eating habits of cats, but some cases can go undetected because of the lack of obvious specific signs. It is difficult to give precise figures for a toxic dose and it is probably more useful to concentrate on the characteristic signs of lead poisoning. Nevertheless, chronic intakes of 2 mg/kg bodyweight per day and above have been reported to cause toxic signs in the dog. More than 10 mg/kg bodyweight per day is rapidly toxic.

The most common source of lead is paint (particularly old paint which contains a high proportion of lead) but linoleum, putty and metallic lead objects can also be hazardous.

Lead inhibits haemoglobin synthesis and thus causes anaemia, but it is the presence of lead in the liver, kidneys and the CNS that causes the major signs of lead poisoning. The signs associated with acute toxicity can be divided into two main categories: gastrointestinal and nervous. Some reports describe only pronounced neurological signs in cats including hyperactivity, frantic behaviour and, in some affected animals, dilation of the pupils. However, reports by Jacobs (1981) and Watson (1981) – both in Persian cats – describe symptoms of lethargy, poor appetite and intermittent vomiting. In both cases, the probable source of the lead was old paint being sanded or scraped off preparatory to redecoration. In one cat blood lead concentration was increased to 0.7 parts/10^6 (mg/l). However, blood lead is not always the best indicator of lead toxicity and there is some disagreement as to the normal blood lead levels in cats, with reported values ranging from 0.05 to 0.2 parts/10^6. Blood levels in some affected cats have been reported to be as low as 0.2–0.3 parts/10^6 (Prescott, 1983). The urinary concentration of delta-amino levulinic acid (DALA) can be a useful indicator of lead poisoning, particularly to monitor the effectiveness of chelation therapy. DALA is a metabolite that accumulates as a result of impairment or blocking of haemoglobin synthesis. Normal values are reported to be less than 38 µM, which can rise to several hundred during lead poisoning. Basophilic stippling of erythrocytes is also a frequent, though not invariable, feature of lead poisoning.

The standard treatment is calcium disodium ethylenediamine tetra-acetate (CaEDTA), which chelates the lead and removes it from the body. The recommended total daily dose is 75–100 mg/kg bodyweight given in two to four divided doses by slow intravenous injection or subcutaneously for 5 days. The CaEDTA should be diluted in a 1–4% solution for subcutaneous injection as it is painful when given by this route. D-penicillamine at 12.5 mg/kg bodyweight orally four times a day was reported to be superior to CaEDTA in dogs given lead in a laboratory investigation (Green *et al.*, 1978). This drug may also be useful if anti-lead therapy is to be given in the client's home, but it does have some undesirable side-effects such as vomiting and anorexia. In severe lead poisoning, supportive therapy with diazepam to control convulsions and fluid therapy to combat dehydration is also indicated. Severe convulsions are usually indicative of cerebral oedema, which will require treatment with mannitol and dexamethasone. There are no characteristic post-mortem signs.

Mercury

Mercury poisoning has been well documented in man and many other animal species and has usually resulted from the use of mercury salts as fungicides for seed grains or from the build-up of mercury in foodstuffs. The latter can arise when metallic mercury (which is of relatively low oral toxicity) is converted to more toxic compounds, particularly organic derivatives such as ethyl- or methylmercury, by the action of microorganisms. The compounds can then accumulate in animals (particularly fish) which are ultimately used as food sources.

The cat has been found to display symptoms of excessive mercury intake similar to those shown by man and has therefore been used as an animal model to investigate the effects of mercury ingestion. Consequently, unlike the normal situation where little or no information is available for the cat, there are many reports on methylmercury intoxication in cats. The effects of acute mercury exposure with relatively large doses of methylmercury (>1 mg/kg bodyweight) are different to those resulting from chronic doses. Acute effects seem to be confined mainly to the lung vascular structure while chronic effects are neurological in nature and include impairment of motor co-ordination (loss of balance and the righting reflex, abnormal gait), muscle weakness (especially of the hindlimbs) and changes in temperament and behaviour. It is these chronic signs which are more likely to be encountered and which have been extensively investigated in the cat. In regions where methylmercury concentrations in fish are very high, poisoning may occur in domestic cats if fish constitutes an appreciable part of their diet (Gruber *et al.*, 1978).

By surveying the reports of chronic poisoning by methylmercury, it is possible to compile a fairly close correlation between intake, length of feeding and appearance of symptoms, with the apparent no-effect level decreasing as the time of exposure is increased. An intake of 0.75 mg/kg bodyweight per day was reported to cause symptoms in 2 days and death in 30 days (Khera, 1973a). With a level of 0.6 mg/kg bodyweight per day, clinical signs appeared in 10 weeks (Gruber *et al.*, 1978). Charbonneau *et al.* (1976), in an extensive study, observed clinical signs with a range of intakes as follows: 0.176 mg/kg bodyweight per day, 14 weeks; 0.074 mg/kg bodyweight per day, 40 weeks; 0.046 mg/kg bodyweight per day, slight neurological impairment after 60 weeks which did not progress in subsequent weeks. Interestingly, an intake of 0.25 mg/kg bodyweight per day administered to 4-day-old kittens for 16–17 weeks (i.e. during their rapid growth phase) produced no ill-effects (Khera, 1973b), which suggests that

kittens are less susceptible than adult cats to methylmercury intoxication.

The standard treatment for mercury poisoning is dimercaprol (see section on arsenic) and/or *N*-acetyl-*d*-l-penicillamine (3–4 mg/kg bodyweight orally, every 6 hours), but related and more effective substitutes such as 2,3-dimercaptosuccinic acid are under investigation. The post-mortem signs of mercury poisoning are confined to microscopic changes in the brain and dorsal root ganglia and consist primarily of neuronal degeneration. The highest levels of mercury are found in liver and kidney with elevated levels also found in the brain and blood.

Other toxic metals

There are many other metals which are known to be toxic when ingested at high intakes and these include substances that are essential nutrients (at lower concentrations) such as copper, zinc and iron. Nevertheless, these are unlikely to be encountered as acute poisons in cats. The other important toxic metal not mentioned so far is cadmium, which is used in areas such as electroplating, plastics, paints and batteries. Information on cadmium has been accumulating in recent years and it is now known to be a highly toxic substance. As far as we are aware, acute poisoning has not been described in cats; however, a recent long-term study in beagles suggests that intakes up to 1 mg/kg bodyweight/day over a period of 8 years can be tolerated with no overt adverse effects or changes in clinical chemistry (Kodama *et al.*, 1990). In man symptoms of cadmium poisoning include skeletal deformities, muscular pain and kidney malfunction. Diethyldithiocarbamate has been reported to be an effective treatment of acute cadmium poisoning in mice under laboratory conditions (Gale *et al.*, 1981).

TOXIC SUBSTANCES IN FOOD

Food components

There are very few foods which when fed to cats are poisonous *per se*. It is usually the accidental

Chapter 28

contamination of wholesome food with a poisonous substance that gives rise to food being implicated as toxic and the most likely substances
involved will be those that have been discussed in
the preceding sections. Nevertheless, there are a
few reports of poisoning in which food itself has
been implicated and perhaps the best-known case
in cats is vitamin A toxicity, which has been
associated with the feeding of large quantities of
raw liver. This results in a crippling bone disease
with tenderness of the extremities accompanied
by tooth loss and gingivitis. Seawright *et al.*
(1967) showed that feeding 15 mg vitamin A/kg
bodyweight per day for 41 weeks produced no
adverse effects, but doses of 17 mg/kg bodyweight
per day and above induced skeletal lesions (15 mg
vitamin A is equivalent to 50 000 IU). The vitamin
appeared to be more toxic when fed as raw liver
than as a pure preparation.

Onion poisoning has been described in many
species including farm animals and dogs.
Kobayashi (1981) reported a haemolytic anaemia
and an increase in Heinz bodies in erythrocytes of
cats that had consumed onion soup. The author
also observed haemoglobinuria when large
amounts of soup were given. Nevertheless, it
must be remembered that cats normally have
a small percentage of erythrocytes with Heinz
bodies and, unlike the dog, observation of Heinz
body formation in cats is not useful as a diagnostic
aid in this condition, unless the proportion of
affected cells is very high. The onion poisoning
was not considered to pose a clinical problem
unless ingestion was continuous.

Poisoning from cocoa and related products
has been described on a number of occasions in
dogs: the toxic principle is the methylxanthine
derivative, theobromine. The symptoms are
vomiting, diarrhoea, sudden collapse and death.
The oral LD_{50} for cats is quoted as 200 mg/kg
bodyweight and, as cocoa contains around 1.5–
2% theobromine (Sutton, 1981), it would theoretically need only 40–50 g of cocoa to provide
a potentially lethal dose. Although we are not
aware of any reported cases of cocoa poisoning
in cats, it must present a possible source of
intoxication.

Additives and contaminants

The best known incident of food additive toxicity
in the cat is benzoic acid, which is used as a
human food preservative but is not permitted in
any animal feeds within the EC. Bedford and
Clarke (1972) found that the highest intake that
could be fed safely was 200 mg/kg bodyweight.
An intake of 300 mg/kg bodyweight caused mild
hyperaesthesia from which the cat recovered, and
higher doses caused aggression, hyperaesthesia
and death. The susceptibility of cats to benzoic
acid arises from their inability to detoxify this
substance sufficiently quickly – a deficiency which
is also responsible for their hypersensitivity to
aspirin, paracetamol and phenol compounds (see
Chapter 27). Benzyl alcohol poisoning has been
reported in cats that received lactated Ringer's
solution containing benzyl alcohol as a preservative (Cullison *et al.*, 1983). On entering the
body, benzyl alcohol is rapidly oxidized to benzoic
acid, and hence is toxic in the cat. At the time of
writing, none of the commercial preparations of
lactated Ringer's solution which are available in
Britain contain benzyl alcohol.

Propylene glycol (PG) has been used as a
humectant in semi-moist cat foods, where it exerts
a preservative action by binding water thereby
making it unavailable for food spoilage organisms.
In 1986 the US National Research Council stated
that high levels of PG caused Heinz body formation in cats (see above) and might result in
haemolytic anaemia (NRC, 1986). Some recent
research now indicates that the main action
of PG is on erythrocyte survival time, whereas
haemolytic anaemia was not observed (Christopher *et al.*, 1989; Hickman *et al.*, 1990). These
effects were seen with dietary concentrations of
PG similar to those used in semi-moist products
(typically 5–15%). Whether this effect is actually
detrimental to the health of the cat is open to
question but it was recently reported that the
erythrocytes of cats fed a commercial diet containing 8.3% PG were more susceptible to oxidant
stress. It must remain a possibility, therefore,
that PG can decrease the cat's ability to respond
to challenges posed by certain diseases or chemi-

cals (Weiss *et al.*, 1990). As a result of the uncertainties surrounding its safety-in-use, PG was delisted as a permitted additive for cat foods in the European Community in 1991.

Of the various food contaminants that may affect cats, bacterial and fungal toxins are the ones most likely to be involved in outbreaks of poisoning. Staphylococcal food poisoning has been shown to affect cats – in fact kittens have been used as the test animal for investigations into this toxin. Botulinum toxin is also toxic to cats, but the occurrence of botulism in Britain is very rare. Cats (and particularly dogs) are much more resistant to botulism than are other animals, including man (Prévot *et al.*, 1953). Feline salmonellosis has been documented (Timoney *et al.*, 1978), with symptoms of gastroenteritis and septicaemia. Antibiotics and supportive therapy were used in the treatment of the disease.

The adverse effects of fungal toxins (mycotoxins) have been well documented in many species of animals, particularly farm livestock. These toxins include substances such as ergot, ochratoxin and aflatoxin. The adverse effects can be one of three general forms: acute, chronic and secondary. Acute poisoning usually affects the liver and can result in hepatitis, jaundice and related disturbances. The chronic and secondary effects are not usually manifested as overt disease, but in farm animals result in a general loss of performance, such as reduction in feed and reproductive efficiency, and an increased susceptibility to infection (Pier *et al.*, 1980). Aflatoxin is probably the most toxic of this group of compounds with an oral LD_{50} of 0.55 mg/kg bodyweight reported for the cat, which classifies it as one of the most susceptible species along with the dog, pig, rabbit and duck. In dogs, 5 µg/kg bodyweight per day fed for 10 weeks (5 days per week) did not cause morphological changes (Armbrecht *et al.*, 1971), but the authors estimated, using regression analysis data from higher intakes, that even this low intake would induce adverse effects in about 3 years. For a dose of 1 µg/kg bodyweight per day the induction time was estimated to be beyond the dog's normal lifespan. There

does not seem to be a specific antidote to aflatoxin, but the area is the subject of current research. Activated charcoal, anabolic steroids and oxytetracycline are among the substances reported to be beneficial in aflatoxin poisoning.

Food allergy

There are many reports of allergic reactions of cats to food; however, the overall scale of the problem is difficult to ascertain. Values between 1 and 30% have been suggested for the incidence of food allergy in causing skin problems and dermatitis in small animals, but the true figure is generally thought to be fairly low. The usual sites affected in allergic responses to food in the cat are the skin and/or alimentary tract and incriminated substances include beef, fish and cow's milk. The use of an elimination diet for 3–5 days is the recommended cause of action and usually results in a successful outcome. The subject has been reviewed by Wills (1991).

POISONOUS PLANTS AND ANIMALS

There seem to be relatively few references to plant or animal poisoning in the cat. Hanna (1986) suggests that the Araceae family contains the houseplants most commonly recognized as toxic. This includes species such as *Philodendron*. Laurel, ivy, laburnum and the pine needles of Christmas trees have also been reported in poisoning incidents. It is most unlikely that there is a specific antidote. Treatment involves removal of as much material as possible from the gastrointestinal tract, the use of an absorbent such as activated charcoal and general supportive therapy (Hanna, 1986; Hoskins, 1989). Leroux (1986) and Hoskins (1989) both give comprehensive lists of houseplants which can be implicated in poisoning incidents in cats. It should also be noted that many cats (particularly those housed mainly or solely indoors) habitually chew the leaves of house plants, some of which contain irritant or poisonous substances. Owners should be advised to provide an alternative source of foliage, such as grass, to minimize this problem. Mushroom (*Amanita* spp.) poisoning has also been reported in cats and can be of two main types. With *A. muscaria* (fly agaric) the toxic principle is muscarine, which produces excessive cholinergic activity manifested as profuse salivation, vomiting and diarrhoea. Treatment is with atropine (see section on organophosphates and carbamates). In the other type of poisoning, for example with *A. pantherina* (false blusher), the toxic agents resemble atropine in their mode of action and the use of atropine is therefore contraindicated (Ridgway, 1978). In this case, gastric lavage, activated charcoal and general supportive measures are recommended together with carefully controlled doses of physostigmine (0.25–0.5 mg total subcutaneously). The latter is a cholinesterase inhibitor which overcomes the action of atropine, in effect the muscarine treatment in reverse.

The only poisonous snake in Britain is the common adder. Its venom is of low potency but it is still capable of inflicting lethal bites on small animals. Cats are much less likely to be attacked than dogs as they tend to avoid snakes; they are also said to have greater resistance to the venom. The symptoms of poisoning are not particularly characteristic and usually consist of an initial excited phase followed by depression and collapse. Perhaps the most useful aid to diagnosis is the presence of fang marks. In a Swedish study Kangstrom (1989) reported on 170 dogs and 54 cats which had been bitten by *Vipera berus*. The most common sites were the face and feet; oedema, sometimes with haemorrhage, was the most obvious clinical sign. The mortality rate was low: two cats and six dogs, around 3.5% for both species. Post-mortem findings included extensive haemorrhage and damage to the heart, liver and kidneys. Suggested treatment is prednisolone (3 mg/kg), antibiotics and intravenous infusion of electrolytes or blood. If possible the specific antivenin should also be used, injected intramuscularly, or intravenously in serious cases. Other 'remedies' such as potassium permanganate, suction or incision of the bite, and the use of antihistamines should be avoided.

Bee and wasp stings are unlikely to represent a serious hazard unless the cat is attacked by a swarm or has been previously exposed to the venom and become hypersensitized, after which anaphylactic shock can result from only one sting. In serious cases 1–5 ml of a 1:10 000 adrenaline solution should be injected subcutaneously. For single stings, neutralization with an alkali such as dilute ammonia (for bee stings) or a dilute acid such as vinegar (for wasps) is usually recommended. The use of a domestic meat tenderizer such as papain is said to provide rapid relief of pain. Antihistamines or corticosteroids should be used to control any inflammation or oedema and may be particularly indicated for serious cases.

Probably the only other hazard in this category likely to be encountered by the cat in Britain is the common toad, which secretes various noxious substances from glands in the head. Cats which have bitten or mouthed toads show symptoms of poisoning such as excessive salivation and general distress. However, the animal usually recovers fairly rapidly and, in general, no specific treatment is necessary.

REFERENCES

Anon (1977) Contaminated sawdust kills animals. *New Scientist* **74**, 233.

Anon (1982a) Phenoxy herbicides, trichlorophenols and soft tissue sarcomas. *Lancet* i, 1051–2.

Anon (1982b) Vitamin K, vitamin E and the coumarin drugs. *Nutr. Rev.* **40**, 180–2.

Anon (1984) Dieldrin poisoning. *Vet. Rec.* **114**, 282.

Armbrecht B.H., Geleta J.N., Shalkop W.T. & Durbin C.G. (1971) A subacute exposure of Beagle dogs to aflatoxin. *Toxicol. Appl. Pharmacol.* **18**, 579–85.

Bababunmi E.A., Olorunsogo O.O. & Bassir O. (1978) Toxicology of glyphosate in rats and mice. *Toxical. Appl. Pharmacol.* **45**, 319–20.

Bedford P.G.C. & Clarke E.G.C. (1972) Experimental benzoic acid poisoning in the cat. *Vet. Rec.* **90**, 53–8.

Bledsoe B., Fadok B.A. & Bledsoe M.E. (1982) Current therapy and new developments in indoor flea control. *J. Am. Anim. Hosp. Assoc.* **18**, 415–22.

Böhning R.H., DeHoff W.D., McElhinney A. & Hofstra P.C. (1970) Pharyngostomy for maintenance of the anoretic animal *J. Am. Vet. Med. Assoc.* **156**, 611–5.

Booth N.H. & McDowell J.R. (1975) Toxicity of hexachlorobenzene and associated residues in edible animal tissues. *J. Am. Vet. Med. Assoc.* **165**, 591–5.

Buck W.B. (1979) Clinical toxicosis induced by insecticides in dogs and cats. *Vet Med. Small Anim. Clin.* **74**, 1119–24.

Charbonneau S.M., Munro I.C., Nera E.A., Armstrong F.A.J., Willes R.F., Bryce F. & Nelson R.F. (1976) Chronic toxicity of methylmercury in the adult cat. Interim report. *Toxicology* **5**, 337–49.

Christopher M.M., Perman V. & Eaton J.W. (1989) Contribution of propylene glycol-induced Heinz body formation to anemia in cats. *J. Am. Vet. Med. Assoc.* **194**, 1045–56.

Cordoba D., Cadavid S., Angulo D. & Ramos I. (1983) Organo-phosphate poisoning: modifications in acid-base equilibrium and use of sodium bicarbonate as an aid in the treatment of toxicity in dogs. *Vet. Hum. Toxicol.* **25**, 1–3.

Cruickshank A.K. (1982) Metaldehyde and paraquat poisoning. *Vet. Rec.* **111**, 149–50.

Cullison R.F., Menard P.D. & Buck W.B. (1983) Toxicosis in cats from use of benzyl alcohol in lactated Ringer's solution. *J. Am. Vet. Med. Assoc.* **182**, 61.

Davis L.E. & Donnelly E.J. (1968) Analgesic drugs in the cat. *J. Am. Vet. Med. Assoc.* **153**, 1161–7.

Dorman D.C., Parker A.J., Dye J.A. & Buck W.B. (1990) Bromethalin neurotoxicosis in the cat. *Prog. Vet. Neurol.* **1**, 189–96.

Frick T.W., Dalo S., O'Leary J.F., Runge W., Borner J.W., Baraniewski H., Dressel T., Shearen J.G. & Goodale R.L. (1987) Effects of insecticide, diazinon, on pancreas of dog, cat and guinea pig. *J. Environ. Toxicol. Oncol.* **7**, 1–11.

Furr A.A. & Buck W.B. (1974) Sodium arsenate toxicity in the domestic cat induced by a commercial ant bait. *Vet. Hum. Toxicol.* **16**, 41–2.

Gale G.R., Smith A.B. & Walker Jr E.M. (1981) Diethyldithiocarbamate in treatment of acute cadmium poisoning. *Ann. Clin. Lab. Sci.* **11**, 476–83.

Gammie J. (1980) Sodium fluoroacetate poisoning in a cat. *Canad. Vet. J.* **21**, 64.

Grauer G.F. & Thrall M.A. (1982) Ethylene glycol (antifreeze) poisoning in the dog and cat. *J. Am. Anim. Hosp. Assoc.* **18**, 492–7.

Green R.A., Selby L.A. & Zumwalt R.W. (1978) Experimental lead intoxication in dogs: a comparison of blood lead and urinary delta-amino levulinic acid following intoxication and chelation therapy. *Canad. J. Comp. Med.* **42**, 205–13.

Grisedale I.M. (1984) Dieldrin poisoning in cats. *Vet. Rec.* **114**, 363.

Gruber T.A., Costigan P., Wilkinson G.T. & Seawright A.A. (1978) Chronic methylmercurialism in the cat. *Aust. Vet. J.* **54**, 155–60.

Gruffydd-Jones T.J., Evans R.J. & Sullivan K. (1981) Dieldrin poisoning of cats after woodworm treatment. *Vet. Rec.* **108**, 540.

Hanna G. (1986) Plant poisoning in canines and felines. *Vet. Hum. Toxicol.* **28**, 38–40.

Hansen L.G., Schafer R.F., White V.A. & Hoffman W.E. (1977) Toxicity of pure hexachlorobenzene and HCB-contaminated pork to cats. *J. Food Safety* **1**, 137–45.

Herbst M. & Bodenstein G. (1972) Toxicology of lindane. In Ullman E. (ed) *Lindane-monograph of an insecticide*. Verlag K. Schillinger, Freiburg.

Hickman M.A., Rogers Q.R. & Morris J.G. (1990) Effect of diet on Heinz body formation in kittens. *Am. J. Vet. Res.* **50**, 475–8.

Hornfeldt C.S. & Borys D.J. (1986) Inorganic arsenic poisoning in cats. *Fel. Pract.* **16**(5), 20–4.

Hoskins J.D. (1989) Plants and their clinical importance. *Vet. Technician* **10**, 93–102.

Jacobs G. (1981) Lead poisoning in a cat. *J. Am. Vet. Med. Assoc.* **179**, 1396–7.

Johnson R.P. & Huxtable C.R. (1976) Paraquat poisoning in a dog and cat. *Vet. Rec.* **98**, 189–91.

Kangstrom L.E. (1989) Snake bite (*Vipera berus*) in dogs and cats (Swedish). *Svensk Vet.* **41**, 38–46.

Khera K.S. (1973a) Teratogenic effects of methylmercury in the cat: note on the use of this species as a model for teratogenicity studies. *Teratology* **8**, 293–304.

Khera K.S. (1973b) Effects of methylmercury in cats after pre- or post-natal treatment. *Teratology* **7**, 20A.

Kobayashi K. (1981) Onion poisoning in the cat. *Fel. Pract.* **11**(1), 22–27.

Kodama Y., Matsuno K. & Tsuchiya, K. (1990) Cadmium distribution in blood and urine of dogs after long-term oral administration of cadmium. *Toxicol. Environ. Chem.* **27**, 73–80.

Leroux V. (1986) Poisoning of pets by house plants (French). *Point Vet.* **18**, 45–55.

Moore F.M., Kudisch M., Richter K. & Faggella A. (1988) Hypercalcemia associated with rodenticide poisoning in three cats. *J. Am. Vet. Med. Assoc.* **193**, 1099–100.

Mount M.E. (1988) Diagnosis and therapy of anticoagulant rodenticide intoxications. *Vet. Clin. N. Am. Small Anim. Pract.* **18**, 115–30.

Munro I.B., Ostler D.C., Machin A.F. & Quick M.P. (1977) Suspected poisoning by pentachlorophenol in sawdust. *Vet. Rec.* **101**, 525–526.

NRC (1986) *Nutrient Requirements of Cats*. National Academy Press, Washington DC, p. 35.

Peet R.L., MacDonald G. & Keefe A. (1977) Possible pentachlorophenol poisoning in cats. *Aust. Vet. J.* **53**, 602.

Penny R.H.C., Carlise C.H., Prescott C.W. & Davidson H.A. (1967) Effects of aspirin (acetylsalicylic acid) on the haemopoietic system of the cat. *Brit. Vet. J.* **123**, 154–60.

Penumarthy L. & Oehme F.W. (1975) Ethylene glycol toxicosis in cats. *Am. J. Vet. Res.* **36**, 209–12.

Pier A.C., Richard J.L. & Cysewski S.J. (1980) Implications of mycotoxins in animal disease. *J. Am. Vet. Med. Assoc.* **176**, 719–24.

Prescott C.W. (1983) Clinical findings in dogs and cats with lead poisoning. *Aust. Vet. J.* **60**, 270–1.

Prévot A.R., Brygoo E.R. & Sillioc R. (1953) Botulism and its five toxins (French). *Ann. Inst. Pasteur* **85**, 559–61.

Raabe W.A. (1981) Ammonia and disinhibition in the cat motor cortex by ammonium acetate, monofluoroacetate and insulin-induced hypoglycaemia. *Brain Res.* **210**, 311–22.

Ridgway R.L. (1978) Mushroom (Amanita pantherina) poisoning. *J. Am. Vet. Med. Assoc.* **172**, 681–2.

Rivers J.P.W., Frankel T.L., Juttla S. & Hay A.W.M. (1979) Vitamin D in the nutrition of the cat. *Proc. Nutr. Soc.* **38**, 36A.

Roy Shapira A., Taitelman U. & Bursztein S. (1980) Evaluation of the role of ionised calcium in sodium fluoroacetate (1080) poisoning. *Toxicol. Appl. Pharmacol.* **56**, 216–20.

Royal College of Pathologists – Standing Advisory Committee for Haematology (1982) Drug interaction with coumarin-derivative anticoagulants. *Brit. Med. J.* **285**, 274–5.

Seawright A.A., English P.B. & Gartner R.J.W. (1967) Hypervitaminosis A and deforming cervical spondylosis of the cat. *J. Comp. Path.* **77**, 29–39.

Studdert V.P. (1985) Epidemiological features of snail and slug bait poisoning in dogs and cats. *Aust. Vet. J.* **62**, 269–71.

Sundlof S.F. & Mayhew I.G. (1983) A neuroparalytic syndrome associated with an oral flea repellant containing diethanolamine. *Vet. Hum. Toxicol.* **25**, 247–9.

Suschetet M., Leclerc J., Lhussier M & Loisel W. (1974) Toxicity and nutritional effects in the rat of two herbicides: picloram and atrazine (French). *Ann. Nutr. Alim.* **28**, 29–47.

Sutton R.H. (1981) Cocoa poisoning in a dog. *Vet. Rec.* **109**, 563–5.

Timoney J.F., Neibert H.C. & Scott F.W. (1978) Feline salmonellosis: a nosocomial outbreak and experimental studies. *Cornell Vet.* **68**, 211–9.

Trapani M., Brooks D.L. & Tillman P.C. (1982) Quaternary ammonium toxicosis in cats. *Lab. Anim. Sci.* **32**, 520–2.

van Lier R.B.L. & Cherry L.D. (1988) The toxicity and mechanism of action of bromethalin: a new single-feeding rodenticide. *Fundam. Appl. Toxicol.* **11**, 664–72.

Waltner-Toews D. (1981) Organo-phosphate poisoning and haemobartonellosis in a cat. *Mod. Vet. Pract.* **62**, 48.

Watson A.D.J. (1981) Lead poisoning in a cat. *J. Small Anim. Pract.* **22**, 85–9.

Weiss D.J., McClay C.B., Christopher M.M., Murphy M. & Perman V. (1990) Effects of propylene glycol-containing diets on acetaminophen-induced methemoglobinemia in cats. *J. Am. Vet. Med. Assoc.* **196**, 1816–9.

Whetstone J.S. (1986) Toxicity from commercial flea collars. *Fel. Pract.* **16**(5), 5.

Wills, J. (1991) Dietary hypersensitivity in cats. *In Practice* **13**, 87–91.

Zenger E. (1988) Treatment of fenthion toxicity in two cats. *Calif. Vet.* **42**(6), 5–6.

Zook B.C., Holzworth J & Thornton G.W. (1986) Thallium poisoning in cats. *J. Am. Vet. Med. Assoc.* **153**, 285–99.

GENERAL READING

Coppock R.W., Mostrom M.S. & Lillie L.E. (1988) The toxicology of detergents, bleaches, antiseptics and disinfectants in small animals. *Vet. Hum. Toxicol.* **30**, 463–73.

Evans R.J. (1988) Toxic hazards to cats. *Vet. Ann.* **28**, 251–60.

Fikes J.D. (1990) Organophosphorus and carbamate insecticides. *Vet. Clin. N. Am. Small Anim. Pract.* **20**, 353–67.

Harvey D.G. (1981) Has it been poisoned? *Brit. Vet. J.* **137**, 317–36.

Humphreys D.J. (1988) *Veterinary Toxicology*, 3rd edn. Baillière Tindall, London.

Meehan A.P. (1984) *Rats and mice. Their biology and control.* Rentokil, East Grinstead, UK.

Moraillon R. & Pinault L. (1978) Diagnosis and treatment of common intoxicants in carnivores (French). *Rec. Med. Vet.* **154**, 137–50.

Surber E.E. (1983) Common household toxicities in cats. *Vet Med./Small Anim. Clin.* **78**, 535–46.

Valentine W.M. (1990) Pyrethrin and pyrethroid insecticides. *Vet. Clin. N. Am. Small Anim. Pract.* **20**, 375–82.

Index

dermatitis (flea-allergy
  dermatitis) 8–9, 39, 47,
  Plate 1.21
papulocrustous dermatitis 72–3
Flea collars 39, 41–2, 664
Flea infestation 35, 39, 364, **Plate
  1.16**
  diagnosis 8, 10, 11
  feline symmetric alopecia 68, 69
  lesions on owners 39, **Plate 1.17**
Fleas, *Dipylidium* transmission
  596, 597
Flucytosine (5-fluorocytosine)
  127, 255
Fludrocortisone 425, 426
Flufenamic acid 640
Fluid intake *see* Water intake
Fluid therapy
  Addisonian crisis 426
  feline panleucopenia 448
  feline urological syndrome 243,
    244
  in poisoning 659
  uraemic crisis 236–7
Flunixin 151, 639
Fluorescein angiography, retina
  352
Fluorescein dye-impregnated strips
  337
Fluorescent antibody tests
  conjunctivitis 333
  rabies 525, 526
Fluoroacetamide poisoning 667
Fluoroacetate poisoning 667
Fluoroquinolone antibiotics 633
5-Fluorouracil 650
Fly-strike (myiasis) 35, 40
Folic acid 592
Follicle-stimulating hormone (FSH)
  273, 418
Follicular cysts (milia) 63
Folliculitis 24
Food hypersensitivity (allergy) 47,
  48, 675, **Plate 1.22**
  diagnosis 9, 14–15
  diarrhoea 307
Food intolerance 307
Food poisoning 675
Foods 587–90
  additives and contaminants
    674–5
  daily allowances 580
  energy content 575, 576
  nutrient content 588–9
  taste and palatability 574, 582
  taurine content 580
  toxins in 673–5
  see also Canned foods; Diet; Dry
    cat foods; Nutrition
Foreign bodies
  abscess formation 557, 558
  external auditory meatus 365–6

gastric 299
  intestinal 307, *308*
  laryngeal 257
  nasal cavity 256
  oesophageal 295, **Plate 8.6**
  oral 291
  orbit 325
  pharyngeal 292
  skin lesions 41
Forelimbs, arrested development
  174
Fostering 279
Fourth cranial nerve (trochlear)
  101
  palsies 103–4
Foxes
  rabies in Europe 526–8
  rabies vaccination 530–1
Fractures 132
  compound 138
  pathological 139, 141, 173
  teeth 291
Framomycin 631
Free-range cats
  FeLV infection 475–6
  roundworm infestations 599
Frontal sinuses 257
  chronic rhinitis 253–4, *255*
Frostbite 43–4, 364
Frusemide (furosemide)
  brain oedema 92
  cardiac disease 410, 411–12,
    648–9
  promoting excretion of poisons
    659
  renal disease 236, 238–9
Fundus, ocular 351, 352, **Plates
  9.17–18**
Fungal culture 12–13
Fungal infections 564–5
  bone 138–9
  central nervous system 127
  diagnosis 12–13
  hypersensitivity dermatosis
    49–51
  kittens 282
  lower urinary tract 245
  otitis externa 74, 366
  pneumonia 258–9
  skin 29–34
  see also Mycoses; *specific
    infections*
Fungal toxins 675
Fungicide poisoning 661–2
Furniture scratching 620
Furosemide *see* Frusemide
Furunculosis 24, 71

GABA (γ-aminobutyric acid) 642,
  643–4
Gait, incoordination *see* Ataxia

Gastric diseases 298–301
Gastric emptying, delayed 300–1
Gastric lavage 658
Gastric neoplasia 299, 300
Gastric ulceration 299–300
Gastrinoma, pancreatic 299, 306,
  433
Gastritis 298–9, **Plate 8.8**
  Ollulanus tricuspis 298, 299,
    602
Gastro-oesophageal reflux 294,
  295
Gastrocnemius muscle/tendon
  contracture 182
Gastrointestinal disease 287–318
  antibiotics inducing 627
  chlamydial infection 299, 546
  FIV infection 497
  inappropriate defecation 613
  polyarthritis with 158, 159
Gastrostomy, tube 301
Genital system 269–78
  chlamydial infection 545
Gentamicin 630
Gentian violet 32
Gestation, duration of 270
Giant cell sarcoma 168, *169*
Giant cell tumour (osteoclastoma)
  167–8
  extraskeletal 61
Giardia infections (giardiasis)
  304, 607–8, **Plate 8.10**
  clinical signs 607–8
  transmission to man 595–6, 607
  treatment 608
Gingivitis 288–90
  anaemia 198
  idiopathic chronic 289–90, 458
  lymphocytic-plasmacytic 290,
    Plate 8.3
Glaucoma 342, 348–50
  diagnostic techniques 348–9
  primary 349
  secondary 344, 348, 349
  treatment 349–50
Globoid cell leucodystrophy 112
Glomerular filtration rate (GFR)
  233
Glomerulonephritis 229–30,
  237–8
Glossopharyngeal nerve (IX) 106
Glucocorticoids 640
  adrenal cortical 454
  adverse skin reactions 50, 73,
    Plate 1.33
  arthritis 151, 153–4
  brain oedema 91–2
  chemotherapy of neoplasms 651
  diarrhoea 302
  eosinophilic granuloma complex
    66, 288
  feline infectious peritonitis 511